Appetite and Satiety Control-Gut Mechanisms

Appetite and Satiety Control-Gut Mechanisms

Editors

Christine Feinle-Bisset
Michael Horowitz

MDPI • Basel • Beijing • Wuhan • Barcelona • Belgrade • Manchester • Tokyo • Cluj • Tianjin

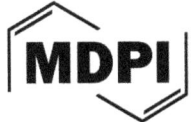

Editors

Christine Feinle-Bisset
Adelaide Medical School
The University of Adelaide
Adelaide
Australia

Michael Horowitz
Adelaide Medical School
The University of Adelaide
Adelaide
Australia

Editorial Office
MDPI
St. Alban-Anlage 66
4052 Basel, Switzerland

This is a reprint of articles from the Special Issue published online in the open access journal *Nutrients* (ISSN 2072-6643) (available at: www.mdpi.com/journal/nutrients/special_issues/Satiety_and_Appetite_Control).

For citation purposes, cite each article independently as indicated on the article page online and as indicated below:

LastName, A.A.; LastName, B.B.; LastName, C.C. Article Title. *Journal Name* **Year**, *Volume Number*, Page Range.

ISBN 978-3-0365-2348-4 (Hbk)
ISBN 978-3-0365-2347-7 (PDF)

© 2021 by the authors. Articles in this book are Open Access and distributed under the Creative Commons Attribution (CC BY) license, which allows users to download, copy and build upon published articles, as long as the author and publisher are properly credited, which ensures maximum dissemination and a wider impact of our publications.

The book as a whole is distributed by MDPI under the terms and conditions of the Creative Commons license CC BY-NC-ND.

Contents

About the Editors ix

Christine Feinle-Bisset and Michael Horowitz
Appetite and Satiety Control—Contribution of Gut Mechanisms
Reprinted from: *Nutrients* **2021**, *13*, 3635, doi:10.3390/nu13103635 1

Van B. Lu, Fiona M. Gribble and Frank Reimann
Nutrient-Induced Cellular Mechanisms of Gut Hormone Secretion
Reprinted from: *Nutrients* **2021**, *13*, 883, doi:10.3390/nu13030883 7

Amanda J. Page
Gastrointestinal Vagal Afferents and Food Intake: Relevance of Circadian Rhythms
Reprinted from: *Nutrients* **2021**, *13*, 844, doi:10.3390/nu13030844 43

Charles-Henri Malbert
Vagally Mediated Gut-Brain Relationships in Appetite Control-Insights from Porcine Studies
Reprinted from: *Nutrients* **2021**, *13*, 467, doi:10.3390/nu13020467 61

Nicholas V. DiPatrizio
Endocannabinoids and the Gut-Brain Control of Food Intake and Obesity
Reprinted from: *Nutrients* **2021**, *13*, 1214, doi:10.3390/nu13041214 79

Allison W. Rautmann and Claire B. de La Serre
Microbiota's Role in Diet-Driven Alterations in Food Intake: Satiety, Energy Balance, and Reward
Reprinted from: *Nutrients* **2021**, *13*, 3067, doi:10.3390/nu13093067 95

Lea Decarie-Spain and Scott E. Kanoski
Ghrelin and Glucagon-Like Peptide-1: A Gut-Brain Axis Battle for Food Reward
Reprinted from: *Nutrients* **2021**, *13*, 977, doi:10.3390/nu13030977 109

Kirsteen N. Browning and Kaitlin E. Carson
Central Neurocircuits Regulating Food Intake in Response to Gut Inputs—Preclinical Evidence
Reprinted from: *Nutrients* **2021**, *13*, 908, doi:10.3390/nu13030908 131

Marlou P. Lasschuijt, Kees de Graaf and Monica Mars
Effects of Oro-Sensory Exposure on Satiation and Underlying Neurophysiological Mechanisms—What Do We Know So Far?
Reprinted from: *Nutrients* **2021**, *13*, 1391, doi:10.3390/nu13051391 149

Dan M. Livovsky and Fernando Azpiroz
Gastrointestinal Contributions to the Postprandial Experience
Reprinted from: *Nutrients* **2021**, *13*, 893, doi:10.3390/nu13030893 165

Russell Keast, Andrew Costanzo and Isabella Hartley
Macronutrient Sensing in the Oral Cavity and Gastrointestinal Tract: Alimentary Tastes
Reprinted from: *Nutrients* **2021**, *13*, 667, doi:10.3390/nu13020667 181

Lizeth Cifuentes, Michael Camilleri and Andres Acosta
Gastric Sensory and Motor Functions and Energy Intake in Health and Obesity—Therapeutic Implications
Reprinted from: *Nutrients* **2021**, *13*, 1158, doi:10.3390/nu13041158 203

Jennifer Wilbrink, Gwen Masclee, Tim Klaassen, Mark van Avesaat, Daniel Keszthelyi and Adrian Masclee
Review on the Regional Effects of Gastrointestinal Luminal Stimulation on Appetite and Energy Intake: (Pre)clinical Observations
Reprinted from: *Nutrients* **2021**, *13*, 1601, doi:10.3390/nu13051601 233

Peyman Rezaie, Vida Bitarafan, Michael Horowitz and Christine Feinle-Bisset
Effects of Bitter Substances on GI Function, Energy Intake and Glycaemia-Do Preclinical Findings Translate to Outcomes in Humans?
Reprinted from: *Nutrients* **2021**, *13*, 1317, doi:10.3390/nu13041317 253

Cong Xie, Weikun Huang, Richard L. Young, Karen L. Jones, Michael Horowitz, Christopher K. Rayner and Tongzhi Wu
Role of Bile Acids in the Regulation of Food Intake, and Their Dysregulation in Metabolic Disease
Reprinted from: *Nutrients* **2021**, *13*, 1104, doi:10.3390/nu13041104 275

Mona Farhadipour and Inge Depoortere
The Function of Gastrointestinal Hormones in Obesity—Implications for the Regulation of Energy Intake
Reprinted from: *Nutrients* **2021**, *13*, 1839, doi:10.3390/nu13061839 291

Dimitris Papamargaritis and Carel W. le Roux
Do Gut Hormones Contribute to Weight Loss and Glycaemic Outcomes after Bariatric Surgery?
Reprinted from: *Nutrients* **2021**, *13*, 762, doi:10.3390/nu13030762 309

Ian Chapman, Avneet Oberoi, Caroline Giezenaar and Stijn Soenen
Rational Use of Protein Supplements in the Elderly—Relevance of Gastrointestinal Mechanisms
Reprinted from: *Nutrients* **2021**, *13*, 1227, doi:10.3390/nu13041227 335

Rebecca O'Rielly, Hui Li, See Meng Lim, Roger Yazbeck, Stamatiki Kritas, Sina S. Ullrich, Christine Feinle-Bisset, Leonie Heilbronn and Amanda J. Page
The Effect of Isoleucine Supplementation on Body Weight Gain and Blood Glucose Response in Lean and Obese Mice
Reprinted from: *Nutrients* **2020**, *12*, 2446, doi:10.3390/nu12082446 351

Lucas Baumard, Zsa Zsa R. M. Weerts, Ad A. M. Masclee, Daniel Keszthelyi, Adina T. Michael-Titus and Madusha Peiris
Effect of Obesity on the Expression of Nutrient Receptors and Satiety Hormones in the Human Colon
Reprinted from: *Nutrients* **2021**, *13*, 1271, doi:10.3390/nu13041271 363

Bryant Avalos, Donovan A. Argueta, Pedro A. Perez, Mark Wiley, Courtney Wood and Nicholas V. DiPatrizio
Cannabinoid CB_1 Receptors in the Intestinal Epithelium Are Required for Acute Western-Diet Preferences in Mice
Reprinted from: *Nutrients* **2020**, *12*, 2874, doi:10.3390/nu12092874 377

Carme Grau-Bové, Alba Miguéns-Gómez, Carlos González-Quilen, José-Antonio Fernández-López, Xavier Remesar, Cristina Torres-Fuentes, Javier Ávila-Román, Esther Rodríguez-Gallego, Raúl Beltrán-Debón, M Teresa Blay, Ximena Terra, Anna Ardévol and Montserrat Pinent
Modulation of Food Intake by Differential TAS2R Stimulation in Rat
Reprinted from: *Nutrients* **2020**, *12*, 3784, doi:10.3390/nu12123784 393

Ryan Jalleh, Hung Pham, Chinmay S. Marathe, Tongzhi Wu, Madeline D. Buttfield, Seva Hatzinikolas, Charles H. Malbert, Rachael S. Rigda, Kylie Lange, Laurence G. Trahair, Christine Feinle-Bisset, Christopher K. Rayner, Michael Horowitz and Karen L. Jones
Acute Effects of Lixisenatide on Energy Intake in Healthy Subjects and Patients with Type 2 Diabetes: Relationship to Gastric Emptying and Intragastric Distribution
Reprinted from: *Nutrients* **2020**, *12*, 1962, doi:10.3390/nu12071962 . . . . **407**

Dan M. Livovsky, Claudia Barber, Elizabeth Barba, Anna Accarino and Fernando Azpiroz
Abdominothoracic Postural Tone Influences the Sensations Induced by Meal Ingestion
Reprinted from: *Nutrients* **2021**, *13*, 658, doi:10.3390/nu13020658 . . . . **415**

Daniel R. Crabtree, William Buosi, Claire L. Fyfe, Graham W. Horgan, Yannis Manios, Odysseas Androutsos, Angeliki Giannopoulou, Graham Finlayson, Kristine Beaulieu, Claire L. Meek, Jens J. Holst, Klaske Van Norren, Julian G. Mercer, Alexandra M. Johnstone and on behalf of the Full4Health-Study Group
Appetite Control across the Lifecourse: The Acute Impact of Breakfast Drink Quantity and Protein Content. The Full4Health Project
Reprinted from: *Nutrients* **2020**, *12*, 3710, doi:10.3390/nu12123710 . . . . **425**

Avneet Oberoi, Caroline Giezenaar, Alina Clames, Kristine Bøhler, Kylie Lange, Michael Horowitz, Karen L. Jones, Ian Chapman and Stijn Soenen
Whey Protein Drink Ingestion before Breakfast Suppressed Energy Intake at Breakfast and Lunch, but Not during Dinner, and Was Less Suppressed in Healthy Older than Younger Men
Reprinted from: *Nutrients* **2020**, *12*, 3318, doi:10.3390/nu12113318 . . . . **451**

About the Editors

Christine Feinle-Bisset

Prof Christine Feinle-Bisset is a nutritional scientist with an undergraduate degree from the University of Stuttgart-Hohenheim (Germany). Following a PhD in gastrointestinal physiology at the University of Sheffield, UK, and a postdoctoral position at the University of Zurich, Switzerland, she joined the University of Adelaide in 2000, and was appointed to Professor in 2010. Her research is clinical and relates to the impact of nutrients on appetite, GI motor and hormone function and perception, in health, obesity and functional dyspepsia. Her work has contributed significantly to current concepts of the role of gastrointestinal mechanisms in the regulation of energy intake in health and obesity, and symptom generation in functional dyspepsia. Prof Feinle-Bisset has authored over 200 scientific papers with >12800 citations.

Michael Horowitz

Prof Michael Horowitz is Professor of Medicine, University of Adelaide, and Director of the Endocrine and Metabolic Unit, Royal Adelaide Hospital. He is a clinician scientist with a career in translational clinical research focussing on the relevance of gastrointestinal function to diabetes, appetite regulation, critical illness and ageing. These research interests are complementary to his clinical activities as an endocrinologist. The outcomes of his work, particularly relating to the impact of gastric emptying in blood glucose control of type 1 and, particularly, type 2 diabetes have led to major improvements in management. Prof Horowitz is the author of 732 scientific papers which have been cited 54,330 times.

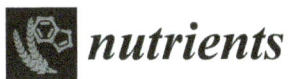

Editorial

Appetite and Satiety Control—Contribution of Gut Mechanisms

Christine Feinle-Bisset [1,2,*] and Michael Horowitz [1,2,3]

1. Adelaide Medical School, Faculty of Health and Medical Sciences, University of Adelaide, Adelaide, SA 5000, Australia; michael.horowitz@adelaide.edu.au
2. Centre of Research Excellence in Translating Nutritional Science to Good Health, University of Adelaide, Adelaide, SA 5000, Australia
3. Endocrine & Metabolic Unit, Royal Adelaide Hospital, Adelaide, SA 5000, Australia
* Correspondence: christine.feinle@adelaide.edu.au

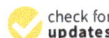

Citation: Feinle-Bisset, C.; Horowitz, M. Appetite and Satiety Control—Contribution of Gut Mechanisms. *Nutrients* 2021, *13*, 3635. https://doi.org/10.3390/nu13103635

Received: 6 October 2021
Accepted: 15 October 2021
Published: 17 October 2021

Publisher's Note: MDPI stays neutral with regard to jurisdictional claims in published maps and institutional affiliations.

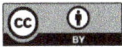

Copyright: © 2021 by the authors. Licensee MDPI, Basel, Switzerland. This article is an open access article distributed under the terms and conditions of the Creative Commons Attribution (CC BY) license (https://creativecommons.org/licenses/by/4.0/).

The prevalence of obesity, and its comorbidities, particularly type 2 diabetes, cardiovascular and hepatic disease and certain cancers, continues to rise at an alarming rate worldwide [1,2]. This reflects, in part, the suboptimal therapeutic options available for both the prevention and management of obesity. Paradoxically, despite an increasingly obesogenic environment, particularly in Western societies, undernutrition is also extremely common and associated with major adverse consequences for quality of life and healthcare utilisation [3,4]. Older individuals, in particular, may be predisposed to malnutrition as a result of the 'physiological' anorexia of ageing. Accordingly, an improved understanding of the mechanisms which regulate appetite and energy intake is of pivotal importance.

Appetite and energy intake are modulated by a diverse range of factors—the latter are both 'central' and 'peripheral' [5,6]. The regulation of energy intake has been, and continues to be, investigated in both animal and human studies. The focus of animal studies has often been to define mechanisms, with the implicit caveat that findings may not be directly applicable to humans. Moreover, subjective perceptions of appetite cannot be evaluated in animals. In contrast, studies in humans have traditionally addressed phenomenology, as invasive mechanistic studies are not feasible. The application of novel, sophisticated techniques, particularly related to imaging as well as molecular biology, has substantially advanced our understanding of the peripheral and central components of the mechanisms controlling appetite and energy intake in humans. This has led to a redefinition of many concepts, including the relative importance of central versus peripheral mechanisms, recognising that the gastrointestinal tract, particularly gut hormones, plays a critical role [7].

During meal ingestion, the oral cavity is exposed to the texture, taste and smell of the food [8]. As food enters the stomach, it is mixed with gastric secretions to produce chyme and progressively distends the stomach to induce a feeling of fullness. As gastric emptying progresses, specialised receptors, located on enteroendocrine cells, are activated by intestinal contents, including nutrients, nutrient digestion products and metabolites, bile acids and other food components, such as bitter substances, triggering the release of gut hormones [9,10]. The latter, in turn, modulate the motor functions of the stomach to further regulate gastric emptying and also activate specialised receptors on vagal afferents to transmit meal-related signals to the brain, leading to meal termination and modulation of reward perception [7]. In recent years, there has been substantial interest in characterising the contribution of the microbiota to the regulation of ingestive behaviour. It is now clear that a number of eating-related disorders, including obesity, are associated with dysregulations of gastrointestinal signalling involved in the regulation of eating [7].

Given the major advance in knowledge in the field, this Special Issue is timely, providing a comprehensive overview of the gastrointestinal mechanisms underlying the regulation of appetite and energy intake, as a series of definitive reviews by international authorities. These reviews address gut-related mechanisms, including nutrient sensing, gut hormones, gastrointestinal motility, gut-brain communication and the roles of the vagus, diet and the microbiota, as well as the abnormalities associated with eating disorders, specifically obesity and the anorexia of ageing. The reviews are divided into two sections; the first focuses on preclinical research, and the second on knowledge derived from stu-dies in humans, including the implications for the management of metabolic diseases and eating-related disorders. The reviews are complemented by a number of important original papers.

Lu and colleagues [11] discuss the cellular mechanisms that underlie the secretion of gut hormones released in response to dietary macronutrients and their digestion products, with a focus on the 'incretin' hormones, glucagon-like peptide-1 (GLP-1) and glucose-dependent insulinotropic polypeptide (GIP). It is now appreciated that the nutrient-induced release of gut hormones involves a range of mechanisms. An improved understanding of these mechanisms is likely to lead to the identification of novel targets for the management of disordered eating. Page summarises current knowledge about the transmission of gastrointestinal luminal, meal-related signals to the brain via the vagus nerve, the modulatory role of circadian rhythms on vagal responsiveness to luminal signals and the influences of obesity and light cycle disruptions—the latter simulating shift-work [12]. Malbert addresses vagally mediated gut–brain relationships, focusing on important insights derived from studies in pigs [13], particularly in relation to the sensing of information from the stomach, intestines and portal vein by vagal afferents and the central processing of this information, as evaluated by sophisticated imaging techniques. DiPatrizio summarises the evidence that supports an important modulatory role for endocannabinoids in transmitting signals along the gut-brain axis via direct and indirect interactions with vagal afferents [14]. Endocannabinoids activate cannabinoid receptors on vagal afferents directly and also indirectly by mediating nutrient-induced gut hormone secretion from enteroendocrine cells. It is increasingly appreciated that disturbances in the composition of the gut microbiota are associated with a number of dysfunctions, including autoimmune, psychiatric, neurological and metabolic disorders—the latter includes obesity and type 2 diabetes. While knowledge relating to the importance of the microbiota in the regulation of energy intake is still in its infancy, there is increasing evidence that diet-induced changes in the composition of the microbiota impact both eating behaviour and body weight. The review by Rautmann and de la Serre summarises the current understanding of the pathways by which the microbiota may modulate eating behaviour, including gut hormone release and signalling along the vagus nerve [15]. The reinforcing properties of food have the capacity to drive decisions based on reward incentives rather than metabolic needs and are, thus, of potential importance to the regulation of food intake. The review by Decarie-Spain and Kanoski [16] addresses the roles of the gut hormones, ghrelin and GLP-1, in modulating food reward-motivated behaviours, with a particular focus on the opposing effects of the two hormones on a number of behavioural constructs related to food reward and reinforcement. The sensory information from the GI tract enters the central nervous system via the nucleus of the solitary tract, where it is integrated with inputs from other brainstem, midbrain and forebrain nuclei. This information is then transmitted to the dorsal motor nucleus of the vagus, from where feedback signals to the periphery are coordinated. Browning and Carson [17] provide an insightful overview of these circuits and the key centres involved in the regulation of gastric functions, with relevance to the regulation of food intake.

The subjective sensory experience of food, including its appearance, smell, taste and texture, is recognised to play an important role in the regulation of energy intake. Lasschuijt and colleagues [18] discuss the contributions of orosensory factors during food ingestion and mastication, including the palatability and texture of foods, on appetite and energy intake, as well as the central neurophysiological mechanisms that mediate the responses to orosensory exposure. Food ingestion is also associated with and driven by a hedonic experience, including a sense of satisfaction and changes in mood, which are fundamental to a positive postprandial experience. Livovski and Azpiroz review the relationship of this experience with the sensory inputs provided by physiological stimuli that are elicited in the process of meal consumption [19].

The composition of a meal is detected in the oral cavity and throughout the lumen of the gastrointestinal tract. In addition to the four basic taste qualities, sweet, sour, salty and bitter, there is now evidence for the existence of additional tastes, including fat, umami, kokumi and carbohydrate. Keast and colleagues provide an overview of these tastes, their sensing in the oral cavity and gastrointestinal lumen, and their implications for food consumption [20]. As a receptacle and storage organ for food, often for many hours post-consumption, the stomach plays a critical role in the acute regulation of food intake. Distension of the stomach by a meal induces fullness, providing a satiation signal, and gastric emptying regulates the delivery of nutrients to the small intestine triggering gut hormone secretion and nutrient absorption. Cifuentes and colleagues discuss the motor and sensory functions of the stomach, including their assessment using state of the art techniques, the relationship between gastric functions and the regulation of energy intake and the dysfunctions in obesity and consequent implications for effective management [21]. Once dietary nutrients are present in the small intestinal lumen, their effects appear to be region-dependent, with early studies demonstrating that the administration of nutrients directly into the distal small intestine (ileum) potently slows gastric emptying, a phenomenon termed the 'ileal brake'. It is now recognised that similar 'intestinal brakes' exist for the effects of nutrients to reduce appetite and energy intake. Wilbrink and colleagues summarise current knowledge relating to the effects of nutrients administered into the proximal and distal small intestine on appetite and energy intake [22]. In particular, their review highlights the region-dependency of intestinal nutrient-induced modulation of appetite. Bitter substances have recently attracted substantial interest, subsequent to the recognition of their capacity to stimulate gastrointestinal functions (particularly the release of gut hormones and slowing of gastric emptying) that are integral to the regulation of energy intake. Rezaie and colleagues discuss the mechanisms underlying intestinal bitter sensing, the gastrointestinal effects of bitter substances in both preclinical and clinical settings, whether current evidence is indicative of potent energy intake-suppressant effects of bitter substances and the potential clinical implications for the management of obesity [23]. The important contribution of bile acids to a number of gastrointestinal and metabolic functions, including the secretion of gut hormones, is increasingly appreciated. Xie and colleagues summarise the role of bile acids, previously regarded as 'detergents', in the regulation of energy intake and body weight, with a focus on the secretion of gut hormones and the changes in obesity and type 2 diabetes [24]. It is clear that bile acids are important signalling molecules, although their precise contribution to the regulation of appetite and energy intake remains to be determined.

Obesity is characterised by dysregulations in the mechanisms controlling energy balance, including energy intake. Farhadipour and Depoortere review the evidence that gut hormone secretion is altered in obesity, reflecting changes in the functionality of gastrointestinal nutrient receptors and the effects of different weight loss strategies [25]. That bariatric surgery is the most effective strategy to achieve long-term weight loss in obesity is likely to be attributable to the markedly enhanced secretion of some gut hormones. Papamargaritis and le Roux discuss current knowledge derived from clinical studies relating to the effects of bariatric surgery on gut hormones and its associated effects to reduce food intake and suppress appetite [26]. In contrast to obesity, which is characterised by relative overconsumption of food, 'healthy' ageing is associated with a decline in hunger and the desire to eat, making individuals more susceptible (e.g., as a result of intercurrent illness) to malnutrition and a loss of bodily function, particularly of muscle. Chapman and colleagues summarise the age-related changes in gastrointestinal functions that regulate appetite and energy intake and the implications for the use of dietary supplements, particularly those rich in protein, to cover nutritional requirements and minimise age-related muscle loss [27].

The review articles are accompanied by eight important original articles—the latter attest to the diversity of the work in this field. Preclinical studies investigated the effect of dietary supplementation with the amino acid isoleucine on body weight and blood glucose in lean and obese mice [28]; the effects of obesity on the expression of nutrient receptors and gut hormones in tissue samples of the human colon [29]; the impact of cannabinoid CB1 receptors in the intestinal epithelium on acute dietary preferences for a Western diet in mice [30]; the involvement of specific bitter receptor subtypes, hTAS2R5, hTAS2R14 and hTAS2R39, in the enteroendocrine secretion of CCK, GLP-1 and PYY from intestinal segments in response to a number of bitter agonists; and the relationship with food intake in rats [31]. Clinical studies related to the acute effects of the short-acting GLP-1 receptor agonist lixisenatide (used widely in the management of type 2 diabetes) on energy intake, and the relationship with gastric emptying and intragastric meal distribution, in both health and type 2 diabetes [32]. Other studies investigated the effects of manipulating abdominothoracic postural tone on sensations of digestive 'well-being' and bloating induced by meal ingestion [33], and the effects of protein-containing drinks on appetite, food consumption and gut hormones across the life span [34,35].

We believe that this Special Issue provides a comprehensive overview of the gastrointestinal mechanisms contributing to appetite and energy intake regulation. Over the last decade, there have been substantial advances in our understanding of a number of areas—from the sensing of meal content, texture and palatability, signal transmission to the brain, signal processing and the translation into behavioural responses, through to the characterisation of dysfunctions in eating-related disorders, specifically obesity and the anorexia of ageing. Hence, while classically, the brain was viewed as the centre of appetite control mechanisms, it is now clear that many of the signals that activate the pathways involved in appetite control originate in the gastrointestinal tract. The powerful effects of bariatric surgery on gut hormone release, appetite suppression and sustained weight loss attest to this. The challenge for the next decade is to translate this knowledge, particularly that relating to the cellular mechanisms underlying nutrient sensing and gut hormone release, into effective dietary and pharmaceutical approaches for both the prevention and management of eating-related disorders.

Funding: Christine Feinle-Bisset acknowledges support by a Senior Research Fellow (grant number 1103020, 2016–2021) from the National Health and Medical Research Council of Australia.

Conflicts of Interest: The authors declare no conflict of interest.

References

1. Jackson, S.E.; Llewellyn, C.H.; Smith, L. The obesity epidemic—Nature via nurture: A narrative review of high-income countries. *SAGE Open Med.* **2020**, *8*, 2050312120918265. [CrossRef]
2. Ng, M.; Fleming, T.; Robinson, M.; Thomson, B.; Graetz, N.; Margono, C.; Mullany, E.C.; Biryukov, S.; Abbafati, C.; Abera, S.F.; et al. Global, regional, and national prevalence of overweight and obesity in children and adults during 1980–2013: A systematic analysis for the Global Burden of Disease Study. *Lancet* **2014**, *384*, 766–781. [CrossRef]
3. Soenen, S.; Chapman, I.M. Body Weight, Anorexia, and Undernutrition in Older People. *J. Am. Med. Dir. Assoc.* **2013**, *14*, 642–648. [CrossRef] [PubMed]
4. Newman, A.B.; Yanez, D.; Harris, T.; Duxbury, A.; Enright, P.L.; Fried, L.P.; Cardiovascular Study Research Group. Weight Change in Old Age and its Association with Mortality. *J. Am. Geriatr. Soc.* **2001**, *49*, 1309–1318. [CrossRef]
5. Camilleri, M. Peripheral Mechanisms in Appetite Regulation. *Gastroenterology* **2015**, *148*, 1219–1233. [CrossRef] [PubMed]
6. Woods, S.C.; D'Alessio, D.A. Central Control of Body Weight and Appetite. *J. Clin. Endocrinol. Metab.* **2008**, *93*, s37–s50. [CrossRef] [PubMed]
7. Steinert, R.E.; Feinle-Bisset, C.; Asarian, L.; Horowitz, M.; Beglinger, C.; Geary, N. Ghrelin, CCK, GLP-1, and PYY(3–36): Secretory Controls and Physiological Roles in Eating and Glycemia in Health, Obesity, and after RYGB. *Physiol. Rev.* **2017**, *97*, 411–463. [CrossRef] [PubMed]
8. McCrickerd, K.; Forde, C. Sensory influences on food intake control: Moving beyond palatability. *Obes. Rev.* **2016**, *17*, 18–29. [CrossRef] [PubMed]
9. Rasoamanana, R.; Darcel, N.; Fromentin, G.; Tomé, D. Nutrient sensing and signalling by the gut. *Proc. Nutr. Soc.* **2012**, *71*, 446–455. [CrossRef]

10. Raka, F.; Farr, S.; Kelly, J.; Stoianov, A.; Adeli, K. Metabolic control via nutrient-sensing mechanisms: Role of taste receptors and the gut-brain neuroendocrine axis. *Am. J. Physiol. Endocrinol. Metab.* **2019**, *317*, E559–E572. [CrossRef] [PubMed]
11. Lu, V.; Gribble, F.; Reimann, F. Nutrient-Induced Cellular Mechanisms of Gut Hormone Secretion. *Nutrients* **2021**, *13*, 883. [CrossRef] [PubMed]
12. Page, A. Gastrointestinal Vagal Afferents and Food Intake: Relevance of Circadian Rhythms. *Nutrients* **2021**, *13*, 844. [CrossRef]
13. Malbert, C.-H. Vagally Mediated Gut-Brain Relationships in Appetite Control-Insights from Porcine Studies. *Nutrients* **2021**, *13*, 467. [CrossRef] [PubMed]
14. DiPatrizio, N. Endocannabinoids and the Gut-Brain Control of Food Intake and Obesity. *Nutrients* **2021**, *13*, 1214. [CrossRef] [PubMed]
15. Rautmann, A.W.; de La Serre, C.B. Influence of the Gut Microbiota on Food Intake: Satiety, Energy Balance, and Reward. *Nutrients* **2021**, *13*, 3067. [CrossRef] [PubMed]
16. Decarie-Spain, L.; Kanoski, S. Ghrelin and Glucagon-Like Peptide-1: A Gut-Brain Axis Battle for Food Reward. *Nutrients* **2021**, *13*, 977. [CrossRef] [PubMed]
17. Browning, K.; Carson, K. Central Neurocircuits Regulating Food Intake in Response to Gut Inputs—Preclinical Evidence. *Nutrients* **2021**, *13*, 908. [CrossRef]
18. Lasschuijt, M.; de Graaf, K.; Mars, M. Effects of Oro-Sensory Exposure on Satiation and Underlying Neurophysiological Mechanisms—What Do We Know So Far? *Nutrients* **2021**, *13*, 1391. [CrossRef] [PubMed]
19. Livovsky, D.; Azpiroz, F. Gastrointestinal Contributions to the Postprandial Experience. *Nutrients* **2021**, *13*, 893. [CrossRef] [PubMed]
20. Keast, R.; Costanzo, A.; Hartley, I. Macronutrient Sensing in the Oral Cavity and Gastrointestinal Tract: Alimentary Tastes. *Nutrients* **2021**, *13*, 667. [CrossRef]
21. Cifuentes, L.; Camilleri, M.; Acosta, A. Gastric Sensory and Motor Functions and Energy Intake in Health and Obesity—Therapeutic Implications. *Nutrients* **2021**, *13*, 1158. [CrossRef] [PubMed]
22. Wilbrink, J.; Masclee, G.; Klaassen, T.; van Avesaat, M.; Keszthelyi, D.; Masclee, A. Review on the Regional Effects of Gastrointestinal Luminal Stimulation on Appetite and Energy Intake: (Pre)clinical Observations. *Nutrients* **2021**, *13*, 1601. [CrossRef] [PubMed]
23. Rezaie, P.; Bitarafan, V.; Horowitz, M.; Feinle-Bisset, C. Effects of Bitter Substances on GI Function, Energy Intake and Glycaemia-Do Preclinical Findings Translate to Outcomes in Humans? *Nutrients* **2021**, *13*, 1317. [CrossRef] [PubMed]
24. Xie, C.; Huang, W.; Young, R.; Jones, K.; Horowitz, M.; Rayner, C.; Wu, T. Role of Bile Acids in the Regulation of Food Intake, and Their Dysregulation in Metabolic Disease. *Nutrients* **2021**, *13*, 1104. [CrossRef]
25. Farhadipour, M.; Depoortere, I. The Function of Gastrointestinal Hormones in Obesity—Implications for the Regulation of Energy Intake. *Nutrients* **2021**, *13*, 1839. [CrossRef]
26. Papamargaritis, D.; le Roux, C. Do Gut Hormones Contribute to Weight Loss and Glycaemic Outcomes after Bariatric Surgery? *Nutrients* **2021**, *13*, 762. [CrossRef]
27. Chapman, I.; Oberoi, A.; Giezenaar, C.; Soenen, S. Rational Use of Protein Supplements in the Elderly—Relevance of Gastrointestinal Mechanisms. *Nutrients* **2021**, *13*, 1227. [CrossRef] [PubMed]
28. O'Rielly, R.; Li, H.; Lim, S.M.; Yazbeck, R.; Kritas, S.; Ullrich, S.S.; Feinle-Bisset, C.; Heilbronn, L.; Page, A.J. The Effect of Isoleucine Supplementation on Body Weight Gain and Blood Glucose Response in Lean and Obese Mice. *Nutrients* **2020**, *12*, 2446. [CrossRef] [PubMed]
29. Baumard, L.; Weerts, Z.; Masclee, A.; Keszthelyi, D.; Michael-Titus, A.; Peiris, M. Effect of Obesity on the Expression of Nutrient Receptors and Satiety Hormones in the Human Colon. *Nutrients* **2021**, *13*, 1271. [CrossRef]
30. Avalos, B.; Argueta, D.; Perez, P.A.; Wiley, M.; Wood, C.; DiPatrizio, N.V. Cannabinoid CB_1 Receptors in the Intestinal Epithelium Are Required for Acute Western-Diet Preferences in Mice. *Nutrients* **2020**, *12*, 2874. [CrossRef] [PubMed]
31. Grau-Bové, C.; Miguéns-Gómez, A.; González-Quilen, C.; Fernández-López, J.-A.; Remesar, X.; Torres-Fuentes, C.; Ávila-Román, J.; Rodríguez-Gallego, E.; Beltrán-Debón, R.; Blay, M.T.; et al. Modulation of Food Intake by Differential TAS2R Stimulation in Rat. *Nutrients* **2020**, *12*, 3784. [CrossRef] [PubMed]
32. Jalleh, R.; Pham, H.; Marathe, C.S.; Wu, T.; Buttfield, M.D.; Hatzinikolas, S.; Malbert, C.H.; Rigda, R.S.; Lange, K.; Trahair, L.G.; et al. Acute Effects of Lixisenatide on Energy Intake in Healthy Subjects and Patients with Type 2 Diabetes: Relationship to Gastric Emptying and Intragastric Distribution. *Nutrients* **2020**, *12*, 1962. [CrossRef]
33. Livovsky, D.; Barber, C.; Barba, E.; Accarino, A.; Azpiroz, F. Abdominothoracic Postural Tone Influences the Sensations Induced by Meal Ingestion. *Nutrients* **2021**, *13*, 658. [CrossRef]
34. Crabtree, D.; Buosi, W.; Fyfe, C.; Horgan, G.; Manios, Y.; Androutsos, O.; Giannopoulou, A.; Finlayson, G.; Beaulieu, K.; Meek, C.; et al. Appetite Control across the Lifecourse: The Acute Impact of Breakfast Drink Quantity and Protein Content. The Full4Health Project. *Nutrients* **2020**, *12*, 3710. [CrossRef]
35. Oberoi, A.; Giezenaar, C.; Clames, A.; Bøhler, K.; Lange, K.; Horowitz, M.; Jones, K.; Chapman, I.; Soenen, S. Whey Protein Drink Ingestion before Breakfast Suppressed Energy Intake at Breakfast and Lunch, but Not during Dinner, and Was Less Suppressed in Healthy Older than Younger Men. *Nutrients* **2020**, *12*, 3318. [CrossRef] [PubMed]

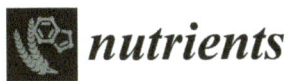

Review

Nutrient-Induced Cellular Mechanisms of Gut Hormone Secretion

Van B. Lu, Fiona M. Gribble * and Frank Reimann *

Wellcome Trust-MRC Institute of Metabolic Science Metabolic Research Laboratories, Cambridge University, Addenbrookes Hospital, Cambridge CB2 0QQ, UK; vl285@medschl.cam.ac.uk
* Correspondence: fmg23@cam.ac.uk (F.M.G.); fr222@cam.ac.uk (F.R.)

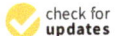

Abstract: The gastrointestinal tract can assess the nutrient composition of ingested food. The nutrient-sensing mechanisms in specialised epithelial cells lining the gastrointestinal tract, the enteroendocrine cells, trigger the release of gut hormones that provide important local and central feedback signals to regulate nutrient utilisation and feeding behaviour. The evidence for nutrient-stimulated secretion of two of the most studied gut hormones, glucagon-like peptide 1 (GLP-1) and glucose-dependent insulinotropic polypeptide (GIP), along with the known cellular mechanisms in enteroendocrine cells recruited by nutrients, will be the focus of this review. The mechanisms involved range from electrogenic transporters, ion channel modulation and nutrient-activated G-protein coupled receptors that converge on the release machinery controlling hormone secretion. Elucidation of these mechanisms will provide much needed insight into postprandial physiology and identify tractable dietary approaches to potentially manage nutrition and satiety by altering the secreted gut hormone profile.

Keywords: enteroendocrine cells; chemosensory; GIP; GLP-1; nutrients; hormones

Citation: Lu, V.B.; Gribble, F.M.; Reimann, F. Nutrient-Induced Cellular Mechanisms of Gut Hormone Secretion. *Nutrients* **2021**, *13*, 883. https://doi.org/10.3390/nu13030883

Academic Editor: Christine Feinle-Bisset

Received: 18 January 2021
Accepted: 5 March 2021
Published: 9 March 2021

Publisher's Note: MDPI stays neutral with regard to jurisdictional claims in published maps and institutional affiliations.

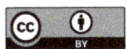

Copyright: © 2021 by the authors. Licensee MDPI, Basel, Switzerland. This article is an open access article distributed under the terms and conditions of the Creative Commons Attribution (CC BY) license (https://creativecommons.org/licenses/by/4.0/).

1. Introduction

The food we eat is composed of water and macronutrients including carbohydrates, fats, and proteins. These nutrients trigger physiological responses to initiate digestion, absorption, and metabolism of nutrients to allow for their biochemical utilisation in the body. Furthermore, nutrients activate neuronal and hormonal signalling to the brain to regulate food intake and appetite. The gastrointestinal tract plays a key role in mediating the physiological effects induced by ingested nutrients. It has long been long known that specialised cells lining the gut epithelium can sense changes in luminal content and respond by releasing chemicals. Bayliss and Starling [1] described the first gut hormone secretin, and demonstrated its release following delivery of acidic solutions into the small intestine. Similarly, nutrients ingested or liberated following digestion can stimulate hormone secretion from enteroendocrine cells (EECs), which are specialised gut epithelial cells that reside within the polarized absorptive epithelial layer. The anatomy of "open" type EECs, with a slender apical process that extends to the intestinal lumen and a basolateral surface facing the interstitial space and circulatory system, link luminal composition to a variety of secreted chemical signals thus making EECs prime candidates to serve as intestinal nutrient sensors. EECs may also form additional extensions that interact with local neuronal and glial cells [2,3] to further expand the range of physiological responses to detected nutrients.

Gut responses triggered by nutrients extend beyond detection of the physical presence of substances within the intestinal lumen. Although classical studies demonstrated osmotic pressure within the stomach as an important factor in determining the rate of gastric emptying into the duodenum [4], the addition of physiological or hyperosmotic solutions of sodium chloride into the intestine were not sufficient to trigger gut hormone secretion [5], supporting the notion that nutrient-stimulated hormone release involves specific mechanisms. Moreover, nutrient-stimulated release can be disrupted using pharmacological and genetic approaches targeting transporter and carrier proteins as well as luminal and epithelial enzymes involved in digestion and absorption. This chapter will review the cellular mechanisms recruited by various nutrients to stimulate hormone secretion from the gastrointestinal tract, with a focus on mechanisms within EECs that release two important gut hormones implicated in glucose homeostasis and appetite regulation: glucagon-like peptide 1 (GLP-1) and glucose-dependent insulinotropic polypeptide (formerly known as gastric inhibitory peptide, GIP).

2. Enteroendocrine Cells That Release GLP-1 and GIP

EECs are a collection of endocrine cells of the gastrointestinal tract, releasing over 30 different hormones into the bloodstream [6] that act locally, peripherally or centrally to initiate physiological responses. Although EECs are sparse and account for only 1% of the total epithelial cell number, they are scattered along the entire gastrointestinal tract from the stomach to the rectum covering a substantial area and thus together comprise the largest endocrine organ in the body. EECs arise from local intestinal stem cells and are in a continuous state of cell turnover, being replaced every 3–5 days in the small intestine [7].

Collectively, EECs secrete a range of hormones that regulate glucose homeostasis, gut motility, appetite, adiposity, and epithelial cell proliferation. Notably, GLP-1 and GIP act as incretin hormones, amplifying insulin secretion following oral glucose administration [8,9], and account for 50–70% of total postprandial insulin secretion. Exaggerated incretin hormone release following bariatric surgery contributes to the beneficial outcomes of weight loss [10] and glycaemic control [11] and mimetics of GLP-1 are effective treatments for Type 2 diabetes [12], with some agents additionally licenced to treat obesity.

EECs are traditionally categorised into distinct cell types based on their hormonal signature. For instance, EECs that release GIP or GLP-1 are traditionally classified as K- and L-cells, respectively. However, immunohistochemical studies [13,14] and transcriptomic profiling of different EEC populations [15–17] have revealed an unexpected degree of overlap between EECs within the proximal small intestine, including those expressing GLP-1 and GIP. Indeed, the data suggest that individual EECs can express a much broader range of gut hormones than originally believed, which may be exploited in future therapeutic strategies. Although individual gut hormones are produced by overlapping populations of EECs, they each have a distinct longitudinal distribution along the gut [18–20] with the highest number of GIP-producing K-cells being found in the proximal small intestine, predominantly the duodenum [21,22], and GLP-1-producing L-cells more broadly located along the gut but increasing in numbers more distally with the highest density of L-cells in the distal small intestine and colon [23] (Figure 1).

EECs in the proximal gut are well placed to respond acutely to incoming nutrient loads and are postulated to contribute more than distally located EECs to nutrient-driven satiety [24]. Most ingested nutrients are absorbed within the proximal small intestine and compared with the distal gut, the upper small intestine receives more vagal afferent innervation, which forms part of a neural circuit that mediates satiety [25,26]. The physiological roles of nutrient-sensing mechanisms in EECs of the distal gut remain elusive, although colonic EECs may respond to locally produced microbial products [27] and lipid metabolites [28] and provide signals reflective of long-term dietary history. However, the beneficial metabolic effects of increased nutrient exposure and recruitment of distal EECs following bariatric surgery suggest these mechanisms may be exploited for effective weight and blood glucose control.

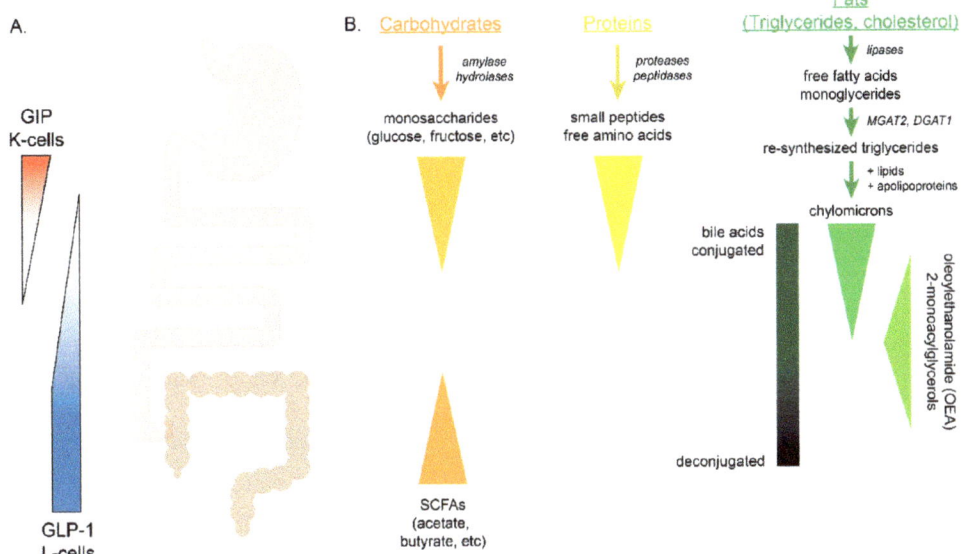

Figure 1. Overview of macronutrient digestion. (**A**) Schematic representation of the distribution of glucose-dependent insulinotropic polypeptide (GIP) expressing K-cells and glucagon-like peptide 1 (GLP-1) expressing L-cells along the longitudinal intestinal axis. (**B**) Schematic representation of major sites of macronutrient digestion and absorption for carbohydrates, proteins and fats along the longitudinal intestinal axis. The breakdown of macronutrients denoted above primary location of nutrient absorption. Whereas absorbed monosaccharides and amino acids are exported from the intestinal epithelium as such, the majority of free fatty acids and monoglycerides are stepwise re-synthesised within the epithelium by MGAT2 and DGAT1 into triglycerides, which together with other lipophilic substances are secreted as chylomicrons. The production of lipid metabolites, such as OEA and 2-monoacylglycerides, which are synthesized following absorption of dietary fats, is represented in light green. Conjugated bile acids released following fat detection in the proximal small intestine is deconjugated in the distal intestine by colonic gut bacteria, as indicated by a dark green bar. Few macronutrients escape absorption in the small intestine, but bacterial fermentation of "indigestible fibres" provides SCFA as another nutritional source in the large intestine. Abbreviations: DGAT1, diacylglyceride-acyltransferase-1; GIP, glucose-dependent insulinotropic polypeptide; GLP-1, glucagon-like peptide 1; MGAT2, monoacylglyceride-acyltransferase-2; OEA, oleoylethanolamide; SCFAs, short-chain fatty acids.

This review will focus on mechanisms of GLP-1 and GIP secretion and suppression of appetite and food intake, but it is worth mentioning other co-released gut hormones from EECs that also mediate physiological effects on food intake and may act in concert with GIP and GLP-1.

Cholecystokinin (CCK) is a peptide hormone secreted by a subset of EECs, classically designated as I-cells [29]; though significant protein levels of CCK are also produced in the brain and peripheral nervous system [30,31]. CCK plays an important role facilitating digestion in the small intestine by stimulating bile release from the gallbladder and enzyme secretion from the pancreas [32], and CCK also reduces food intake when administered peripherally [33,34] or centrally [35] via a number of mechanisms [36]. CCK is produced along the entire small intestine, with the highest density of CCK hormone-expressing cells in the duodenum [19,20,37]. Several transcriptomic [16,17,37] and immunohistochemical [37,38] studies demonstrated co-expression of CCK with other gut hormones including GIP, GLP-1, secretin and neurotensin. A recent transcriptomic analysis of all EEC populations in the small intestine revealed overlap of CCK expression in the majority of EEC cell types defined by hormonal expression profile [15]. The co-expression of CCK and incretin hormones within the same individual EECs suggests similar nutrient-sensing mechanisms can trigger multiple hormone release. However, carbohydrates were a modest secretagogue of CCK release despite being a potent stimulus for GIP and GLP-1 secretion [39–41]. Within EECs expressing multiple gut hormones, storage vesicles containing only CCK have been reported [42]; however, possible mechanisms to selectively mobilise specific vesicular pools remain to be elucidated.

Secretin is another peptide hormone transcriptionally co-expressed with a variety of gut peptides [15], including GLP-1 and GIP [16,17,37,43], which switches on during EEC maturation [44]. Levels of secretin are elevated postprandially and play roles in gastric acid secretion, pancreatic bicarbonate release [45] and promoting satiety. Peripheral administration of secretin decreased food intake in rats [46,47] which was mediated by vagal afferent signalling [48]. Secretin producing EECs (S-cells) are found throughout the small intestine, with the highest immunoreactivity in the duodenum [19,20,37] and are also found in the colon of adult and developing mice [49].

Xenin [50] is a 25 amino acid length neurotensin-like peptide released from GIP-expressing K-cells [51], although of questionable physiological significance as it is produced from a cytoplasmic coat protein [52] with no clear evidence of how it might reach the lumen of secretory vesicles. Secretion of xenin is elevated after a meal and possibly triggered by the anticipation of food [53]. Xenin has been reported to enhance GIP-mediated insulin secretion [54] via activation of cholinergic neurons innervating β cells. Intravenous (IV) injection of synthetic xenin stimulated jejunal motility in dogs [55] and increased contraction frequency in humans [56]. Intracerebroventricular (ICV) injection of xenin reduced food intake and weight gain in mice and this effect was abolished in neurotensin receptor 1 (Ntsr1)-deficient mice [57,58]. Neurotensin (NTS) is a peptide hormone widely distributed in the central and peripheral nervous system and expressed in a subpopulation of EECs (N-cells). Both glucose and fat triggered NTS release [59–61] and centrally administered NTS reduces appetite [57,62,63], with peripheral satiety effects mediated primarily by Ntsr1 receptors located on vagal afferent neurons [58,64]. The greatest expression of NTS protein is found in the ileum [19,37,65] and co-localises with a number of gut hormones including the incretin hormones GLP-1 and GIP [16,17,37,66]. Interestingly, NTS was localised to a population of vesicles distinct from those staining for GLP-1 in the distal ileum [66], which may result from EECs expressing *Gcg* and *Nts* at different times during development and maturation. Although the independent release of NTS from this distinct pool of vesicles may be possible, GLP-1 and NTS were found to be co-secreted across a range of different stimuli [66].

Oxyntomodulin (OXM) is a circulating gut hormone produced from the same proglucagon precursor peptide as GLP-1, and can activate both GLP-1 and glucagon receptors (GLP1R, GCGR, respectively) [67]. ICV and intraperitoneal (IP) injections of oxyntomodulin in rats inhibit food intake and promote weight loss [68,69] and in mouse models, both GCGR and GLP1R activity were shown to contribute to the weight loss phenotype [70]. In a randomised double-blind placebo controlled cross-over study, IV oxyntomodulin administration reduced energy intake and significantly reduced hunger scores [71]. Long acting peptides combining GCGR and GLP1R activity are in clinical trials for the treatment of type 2 diabetes and obesity [72].

Peptide YY (PYY) hormone is co-located with GLP-1 in L-cells, and is found at highest levels in the ileum and colon [18–20] where it is co-released with GLP-1 [73–75]. IP or IV administration of PYY3-36 suppressed food intake in rodents and humans [76,77], analogous to the effects of GLP-1. Interestingly, direct stimulation of gut hormone release from distal L-cells, which increased both GLP-1 and PYY levels, reduced food intake as a result of PYY signalling through Y2 receptors [78]. However, not all studies have been able to reproduce the anorexigenic actions of exogenously administered PYY [79–81]. In studies describing a PYY-induced reduction in feeding, mechanisms proposed to mediate this effect include the vagal-brainstem-hypothalamic circuit [25,82,83], inhibition of gastric acid secretion [84,85] and delayed gastrointestinal motility/small intestinal transit [86–88].

Another hormonal product co-expressed in GLP-1 expressing L-cells of the distal colon and rectum is insulin-like peptide 5 (INSL5). INSL5 protein is co-stored in the same vesicles and co-released with GLP-1 and PYY following stimulation [74]. Unlike GLP-1 and PYY, however, INSL5 appears to exert orexigenic actions, as peripheral injection of INSL5 increased food intake in mice, an effect lost in mice deficient in its cognate receptor, relaxin family peptide receptor 4, Rxfp4 [89]. The overall importance of INSL5 in regulating feeding behaviour is unclear as ablation of *Insl5* expression in mice resulted in no obvious feeding deficit [90] and a subtle orexigenic effect of selective distal L-cell stimulation became apparent only when the opposing and overriding anorexigenic PYY effect was blocked with a Y2R-inhibitor [78]. The physiological rationale for distal EECs co-releasing hormones with opposing actions on food intake has yet to be reconciled.

3. Models to Study Nutrient-Sensing Mechanisms in the Gut

A variety of in vitro and ex vivo experimental models have been developed to study the mechanisms regulating EECs function. In combination with in vivo models and clinical studies that measure food intake following ingestion of nutrients, a comprehensive understanding of nutrient-stimulated responses in the gastrointestinal tract has been revealed.

Studies utilising intestinal cell line models of EECs provided initial insights into nutrient-sensing mechanisms in EECs. The most commonly used murine and human models for GLP-1 secretion are GLUTag [91] and NCI-H716 cells [92,93], respectively. GLUTag cells, derived from oncogenic tumours from the large bowel, respond to a range of nutrient and hormonal stimuli [94], whereas NCI-H716 cells, derived from a poorly differentiated adenocarcinoma of the human caecum, also respond to a range of nutrient stimuli [95] but possess altered regulation of proglucagon gene expression [96]. The secretin tumour cell line, STC-1 [97], derived from a mouse small intestinal neuroendocrine carcinoma, secretes a variety of small intestinal gut hormones including GIP, GLP-1, secretin and CCK. Subclones of STC-1 cells have been generated to produce lines with increased GIP expression or secretion [98–100]. Conflicting reports on the sensitivity of STC-1 cells to glucose emphasized the need for studies using primary intestinal cell models. Initial attempts to culture primary EECs involved elutriation to purify and enrich the K- or L-cell population from canine intestinal epithelia [101,102] or the use of fetal rat intestinal tissue [103]. Optimised culturing techniques, including enrichment of intestinal crypts or the deep folds of the intestinal epithelium have permitted studies from primary cultures of adult mouse [104] and human [105] intestinal tissue. The development of transgenic mouse models labelling K- and L-cell populations [104,106] has allowed transcriptomic and single-cell recording approaches to be applied to specific EEC populations and advanced our understanding of the signalling pathways recruited following specific nutrient exposure. Renewable cell culture technologies such as intestinal organoids [107] have been used to study EECs and have confirmed many nutrient-stimulated signalling mechanisms described in primary intestinal preparations [108] but more importantly provide a means to interrogate nutrient-sensing mechanisms in human EEC populations by labelling specific populations of EECs with fluorescent proteins under the control of hormonal promoters [109,110].

Two-dimensional cultures of these in vitro cell models permit access to EECs for membrane recordings and intracellular measurements. They also allow nutrients to bind targets on EECs that may be inaccessible from the luminal side of the intestine, by-passing nutrient absorptive and transport mechanisms. Three-dimensional organoid models maintain a polarized epithelium in culture, and as the luminal epithelial surface is directed towards the central organoid domain, exogenously applied nutrients may still by-pass transport and absorptive pathways. To investigate nutrient-sensing mechanisms under more physiological settings, ex vivo preparations such as Ussing chambers [111–113] and vascular perfused intestinal models have been used by several laboratories [114,115]. Properly prepared, both models retain tight junctions between epithelial cells and maintain the polarity of the epithelial layer. The location of receptors and sites of action of nutrients can be determined in these models by application of nutrients to the isolated apical or basolateral surface. Hormone secretion from L-cells has been monitored in these models either by collection of perfusate or media from the basolateral side combined with immunoassays [112], or by measurement of trans-epithelial short circuit currents [113].

Finally, in vivo models allow assessment of nutrient ingestion or infusion and effects on food intake and feeding behaviour. In rodents and humans, diets may be altered to control for macronutrient composition, but the palatability and other sensory attributes of food (e.g., odour) should be considered, as inputs from lingual sensors and olfactory centres can also impact feeding behaviour. Nutrients may also be delivered directly into the intestine by oral gavage or by insertion of a nasoenteral feeding tube into the stomach, duodenum, or jejunum. Alternatively, catheters may be surgically inserted to directly infuse nutrients into the lumen of a specified intestinal region, which however, if infused distal to the sphincter of Oddi, may not mix physiologically with pancreatic exocrine secretions and bile, thus altering the digestion of macronutrients. Studies involving human participants are relevant in translating our understanding of the cellular mechanisms underlying nutrient-sensing but can be particularly challenging. Measurements of hunger are subjective and dependent on previous eating habits. Moreover, multiple factors such as alterations in gut motility may unexpectedly modify gastrointestinal responses to nutrients. For instance, the effect of nutrients on hunger scores was attenuated in older participants [116].

4. Cellular Mechanisms of Nutrient-Induced Gut Hormone Secretion

The suppression of food intake following oral ingestion or direct infusion of nutrients into the intestine is associated with a rise in the release of GLP-1 and GIP [117–119]. Nutrient-induced gut hormone secretion entails recruitment of specific cellular mechanisms that are influenced by rates of digestion and absorption as well as expression of nutrient-specific transporters and receptors.

4.1. Carbohydrates

Complex carbohydrates cannot be absorbed across the intestinal wall and therefore must be broken down to monosaccharides before they are transported across cell membranes. Amylases from saliva and pancreatic secretions initiate enzymatic digestion and a combination of hydrolases expressed on enterocytes complete the breakdown of ingested carbohydrates to monosaccharides.

Mechanisms of glucose-stimulated GLP-1 and GIP secretion have been intensively investigated as glucose is a potent secretagogue and there is interest in understanding the role of both incretin hormones in the pathology and therapeutics of Type 2 diabetes (T2D). In humans, glucose can be detected in the proximal duodenum within 5 min of ingestion of liquid glucose load, correlating with the time for first rapid elevation of GLP-1 and GIP concentrations in the bloodstream [120]. The early rise in GIP levels is readily attributed to arrival of nutrients in the duodenum with its high local density of GIP-expressing K-cells. However, the rapid rise in GLP-1 occurs well before glucose can reach the distal portion of the gut, and most of the glucose ingested is absorbed in the proximal small intestine with very little passing more distally to where the majority of GLP-1 expressing L-cells reside [120]. Measurements of glucose concentrations in the distal gut of several species after a meal confirm low levels of glucose [121]; however, levels at the ileo-caecal junction can rise as high as 10 mM after a meal [122]. The most likely mechanism to account for the rapid phase of GLP-1 secretion is the activation of proximal GLP-1 expressing cells [123], rather than recruitment of neuronal or humoral signals from the proximal to distal intestine, as patients with ileal resections maintained the rapid phase of GLP-1 secretion [124].

Glucose-stimulated release of GLP-1 and GIP from EECs requires absorption of carbohydrates. Monosaccharides are transported into cells by active and facilitative glucose transporters. Active glucose transporters, including the sodium-glucose linked transporter 1 (SGLT1), are located on the apical surface of the intestinal epithelial layer [125–127] and *Sglt1* is expressed in GIP- and GLP-1-releasing EECs [104,106,110] (Figure 2). Sodium-coupled active transporters carry glucose into cells, against its concentration gradient, along with sodium ions (Na^+) down the Na^+ concentration gradient established by basolateral Na/K-ATPase activity. The movement of 2 Na$^+$ ions per glucose molecule by SGLT1 produces a small electrogenic current which is sufficient to depolarise the cell membrane potential and trigger action potential firing in GLUTag cells [128]. The sensitivity of L-cells to release GLP-1 in response to glucose closely mirrors the binding potency of SGLT1 for glucose [129] supporting the role of SGLT1 as the primary glucose-sensing mechanism for GLP-1 expressing cells. Non-metabolisable sugars such as alpha-methyl-glucopyranoside and 3-O-methylglucose [130,131] are also substrates for SGLT1 and stimulate GIP and GLP-1 secretion in vivo [115,132] and activating SGLT1 using various substrates reduced food intake [24]. Further supporting the essential role of SGLT1 in glucose-stimulated incretin hormone release, the SGLT1 inhibitor phloridzin or knock-out of *Sglt1* reduced glucose-triggered GLP-1 and GIP release [115,132,133]. However, whilst glucose triggered GIP-secretion is essentially absent in *Sglt1*-knock-out mice, the profile of GLP-1 release after an oral glucose challenge in *Sglt1*-deficient mice is complex as there is significantly reduced GLP-1 release at early time points (<15 min), but elevated GLP-1 release at later times (1–2 h) [134]. The amplified delayed phase of GLP-1 release in this model is thought to be due to reduced glucose absorption in the proximal gut and delivery of more glucose to the distal intestine that seems to activate SGLT1-independent glucose-sensing mechanisms, possibly involving fermentation to short chain fatty acids. Another sodium-glucose co-transporter, SGLT3, has been described in GLUTag cells [128] and enteric neurons of the submucosal and myenteric plexus [135], but whether SGLT3 contributes to glucose-sensing in EECs is not clear. Interestingly, the human variant of SGLT3 has been reported to have lost its capacity to transport glucose and operates as a glucose-sensitive sodium channel [135]. Facilitative glucose transporters are differentially expressed along the gastrointestinal tract [125] and generally localised to the basolateral surface to facilitate glucose efflux into the bloodstream. Transient apical translocation of glucose transporters has also been implicated in the absorption of glucose into intestinal cells [136,137]. Transient GLUT2 insertion into the brush border shortly after high glucose exposure would allow rapid glucose uptake when SGLT1 capacity is saturated and maintain the Na$^+$ concentration gradient for other cellular processes, but this hypothesis remains controversial [138,139].

Glucose-sensitive tissues, including enteroendocrine K- and L-cells, express glucokinase (GCK), usually the rate-limiting enzyme in the breakdown of glucose [14,17,104,106,140,141]. The relatively low affinity of GCK for glucose links glycolytic fluxes to physiologically relevant extracellular glucose concentrations. However, patients with inactivating mutations in GCK did not exhibit impaired GLP-1 or GIP secretion following an oral glucose challenge [142], suggesting GCK is not the primary glucose sensor for the gut. Potassium channels sensitive to ATP (K_{ATP} channels) are described in a number of glucose-responsive tissues as a mechanism to link the nutrient status of a cell to membrane electrical excitability. The generation of ATP following catabolism of glucose increases the intracellular ATP to ADP ratio, leading to the closure of K_{ATP} channels and depolarisation of the membrane potential that may trigger action potential firing or activation of voltage-gated calcium channels to facilitate Ca^{2+} entry into the cell [143]. K_{ATP} channels are composed of a pore forming subunit (Kir6.1/2) and a sulphonylurea receptor (SUR1/2), and both Kir6.2 and SUR1 are highly expressed in GIP- and GLP-1-expressing EECs [104,106,144]. In electrophysiological recordings from GLP-1 expressing cells, glucose depolarises the cell membrane potential, triggers an increase in electrical activity and stimulates GLP-1 secretion [104,110,145]. Closure of K_{ATP} channels by tolbutamide stimulated a similar increase in action potential firing frequency and diazoxide, a K_{ATP} channel opener, blocked the effects of high glucose on cell excitability and GLP-1 release [104,145,146]. Much less is known about the electrical activity of GIP-expressing K-cells, but tolbutamide stimulated an increase in GIP secretion in primary small intestinal cultures [106] and in STC-1 cells high glucose triggered membrane depolarisation and extracellular Ca^{2+} entry to stimulate CCK release [147]. However, the finding of functional K_{ATP} channels in EECs does not imply that they are involved in glucose-triggered hormone release, and evidence that K_{ATP} channels regulate glucose-stimulated incretin hormone secretion in vivo is lacking. Mice deficient in Kir6.2 expression maintained elevated GIP release after an oral glucose load [148] and sulfonylureas had no effect on peak GLP-1 and GIP responses to an oral glucose tolerance test in human participants [149,150]. This discrepancy around the impact of K_{ATP} channels on regulating gut hormone secretion could be a result of low resting K_{ATP} channel activity in vivo compared to in vitro culturing conditions.

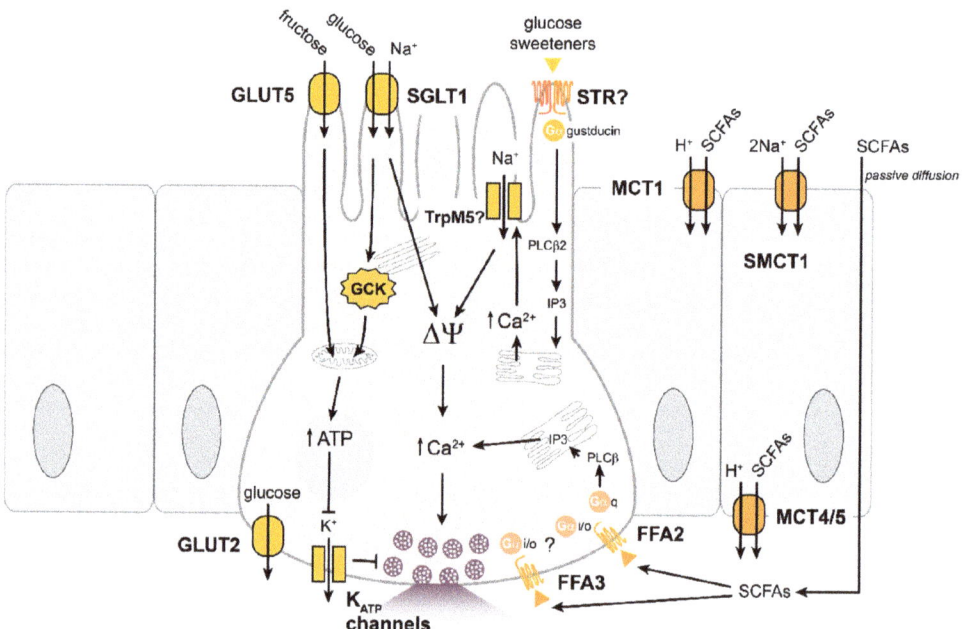

Figure 2. Carbohydrate-sensing mechanisms in incretin hormone secreting EECs. Schematic of EEC with apical process (top) and basolateral surface (bottom) populated with secretory vesicles containing incretin hormones. Enterocytes shown in grey beside EEC. Glucose sensing by incretin-secreting EECs is critically dependent on sodium coupled uptake via SGLT1. Other sensors have been described, but are controversial (labelled with a question mark) or appear to be of limited physiological relevance. When SGLT1 is inhibited, GLP-1 secretion is elevated at later time points, possibly downstream of fermentation to short-chain fatty acids, which target G-protein coupled fatty acid receptors FFA2 and FFA3. These have been depicted on the basolateral membrane in analogy to the location of FFA1 (see text for details). Transport mechanisms of SCFAs across the intestinal epithelium illustrated in enterocytes on the right. Abbreviations: ATP, adenosine triphosphate; FFA2 or 3, Free fatty acid receptors; GCK, glucokinase; GLUT2, glucose transporter 2; GLUT5, glucose transporter 5; IP3, inositol triphosphate; K_{ATP}, ATP sensitive potassium channel; MCT1 or 4/5, monocarboxylate transporters; PLCβ, phospholipase C beta; SCFAs, short-chain fatty acids; SGLT1, sodium-glucose linked transporter 1; SMCT1, sodium-coupled monocarboxylate transporter 1; STR, sweet taste receptor; TrpM5, transient receptor potential cation channel subfamily M member 5; ΔΨ, membrane depolarization.

Other carbohydrates, such as galactose, are handled by the intestine in a similar way to glucose. However, some other dietary carbohydrates, such as fructose, can recruit different mechanisms in EECs. Fructose is not as satiating as glucose in rats [24,26] and monkeys [151] but was found to have similar or greater satiating potential in humans [152,153]. Fructose can stimulate GLP-1 and GIP secretion [60,106,115,128]; though some studies found fructose did not stimulate GIP [60,132] or GLP-1 [154] release. Fructose is not a substrate for SGLT1 but is transported into cells by the apical transporter GLUT5 [155] and possibly GLUT2. GLUT5 is abundant in the gut epithelium, with higher expression in the proximal small intestine [156]. GIP- and GLP-1 expressing cells of the intestine expressed *Slc2a5*, the gene encoding GLUT5 [104,106]. Fructose is fully metabolised, like glucose, and can recruit metabolic pathways such as K_{ATP} channel closure to induce gut hormone secretion. In GLUTag cells, fructose triggered membrane depolarisation and action potential firing, and a decrease in conductance consistent with closure of K_{ATP} channels [128]. Furthermore, fructose stimulated GLP-1 secretion was abolished by treatment with the K_{ATP} channel opener diazoxide [60], but other studies have found that mice lacking the pore-forming subunit Kir6.2 maintained fructose-stimulated GIP and GLP-1 release [157].

Sweet taste receptors (STRs) expressed in the gut can also detect glucose and other natural or synthetic sweeteners; however, a number of conflicting reports in the field have prevented a consensus view on their glucose-sensing role in EECs. Sweet taste receptors were first described in oral lingual taste cells [158] and comprise heterodimeric GPCRs from the type 1 taste receptor family, T1R2 and T1R3 [159]. STRs in the tongue couple to α-gustducin and activate the calcium-sensitive transient receptor potential cation channel subfamily M member 5 (TrpM5) to allow Na^+ entry into cells and trigger membrane depolarisation. Components of the STR signalling pathway have been identified in isolated cells of the intestinal epithelium and co-localised with GLP-1 and GIP [160–163]; however, it is unclear if all elements are expressed in the same EEC to reconstitute functional STR signalling [164]. Furthermore, expression of the genes encoding the STR subunits *Tas1R2* and *Tas1R3* were not readily detectable in GIP or GLP-1-expressing cells [104,106,110]. Agonists of STRs, such as sucralose, stimulated GLP-1 release from GLUTag [165] and NCI-H716 cells [162], but did not enhance GIP or GLP-1 secretion from murine primary intestinal epithelial cultures [104,106]. Artificial sweeteners were also unable to replicate glucose-stimulated GIP [163] or GLP-1 levels [166] in rats and humans, and although mice lacking α-gustducin or T1R3 exhibited reduced GIP and GLP-1 responses [161,162], inhibiting STRs with gurmarin or blocking TrpM5 channels did not inhibit luminal glucose stimulated GIP and GLP-1 secretion [167]. Further work is needed to clarify the role, if any, of STRs, and the accompanying transduction pathway in gut endocrine cells.

4.2. Proteins

Dietary proteins are broken down to small peptides by enzymes in the stomach and pancreas, then further digested by peptidases on the brush border to smaller di- and tripeptides and free amino acids. Amino acids are primarily recycled to produce proteins in the body but can also be used to generate energy when carbohydrate or lipid stores are depleted. In comparison to carbohydrates, the number of different products that arise from the breakdown of ingested proteins is vast; however, specific amino acids or small peptides can elicit specific responses from EECs. In classical studies, intraduodenal infusion of specific amino acids was more potent at stimulating GIP over CCK secretion [168]. The specificity of responses could permit targeting of peptide/amino acid-sensing pathways in incretin hormone releasing cells to manage food intake and satiety.

Several combinations of peptides or protein hydrolysates have been shown to stimulate hormone secretion from EECs through a variety of mechanisms. Peptones, consisting of a soluble mix of amino acids and peptides derived from partial protein hydrolysis, potently stimulated GLP-1 and GIP secretion from GLUTag and STC-1 cells [100,169], which involved upregulation of proglucagon gene expression but not alteration in K_{ATP} channel activity; arguing against metabolic production of ATP from dietary protein as the primary mechanism for peptide-stimulated gut hormone secretion. In NCI-H716 cells, meat hydrolysates triggered GLP-1 release by recruiting the MAPK signalling pathway but did not alter proglucagon gene expression [170], perhaps highlighting species variation in protein/peptide-sensing in the gut.

In murine primary colonic L-cells, the non-metabolisable dipeptide glycine-sarcosine (Gly-Sar) stimulated GLP-1 secretion [171], likely involving the H$^+$/peptide co-transporter, PEPT1, as higher pH, an inhibitor of PEPT1 (4-aminomethylbenzoic acid) and knock-out of *Pept1* abolished dipeptide stimulated GLP-1 release and intracellular Ca^{2+} responses in vitro (Figure 3). Transport by PEPT1 is electrogenic and activation of PEPT1 has been shown to depolarise the cell membrane potential and activate voltage-gated calcium channels, which can contribute to hormone secretion from EECs [172]. Further work is required, however, to ascertain the role of PEPT1 as a dipeptide sensor in EECs in vivo. Similarly, the role of another electrogenic amino-acid transporter located at the apical site of the intestinal epithelium, B(0)AT-1 (*Slc6a19*), needs to be further explored. B(0)AT-1 knock-out mice showed elevated GIP and GLP-1 responses upon refeeding compared to their wild type littermates, which at least for GLP-1 might reflect increased delivery of nutrients to the more distal intestine [173].

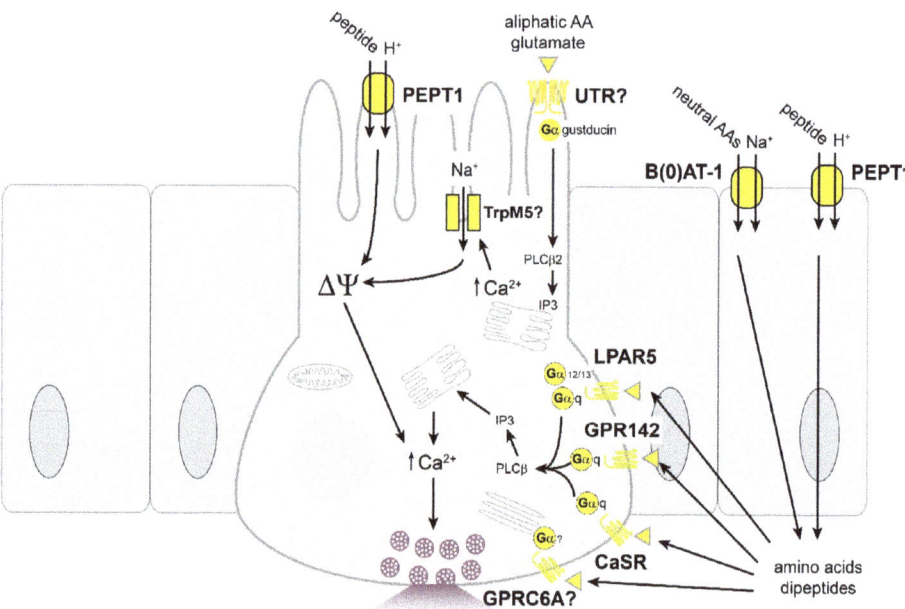

Figure 3. Protein-sensing mechanisms in incretin hormone secreting EECs. Schematic as in Fig2. Good evidence exists for a role of PEPT1, CaSR and GPR142 in incretin secretion, however, the exact locations of receptors and transporters are incompletely defined. Controversial contributors are marked with a question mark (see text for details). Abbreviations: AA, amino acid; B(0)AT-1, sodium-dependent neutral amino acid transporter; CaSR, calcium-sensing receptor; GPR142, G-protein coupled-receptor 142; GPRC6A, G protein-coupled receptor family C group 6 member A; IP3, inositol triphosphate; LPAR5, lysophosphatidic acid receptor 5; PEPT1, H$^+$/peptide co-transporter; PLCβ, phospholipase C beta; TrpM5, transient receptor potential cation channel subfamily M member 5; UTR, umami taste receptor; ΔΨ, membrane depolarization.

The calcium sensing receptor, CaSR, is expressed in L-cells of the small intestine and colon and also contributes to the stimulatory responses to amino acids, dipeptides and peptones in L-cells [171,174]. Agonists of CaSR triggered GLP-1 release and selective CaSR antagonists reduced peptone-triggered GLP-1 release from rodent primary intestinal cultures [171,175]. This role of CaSR in amino acid-sensing in L-cells is comparable to its involvement in peptone triggered release of CCK from STC-1 and primary CCK-releasing EECs [176] supporting a common mechanism of amino acid sensing across EEC populations. CaSR responds to a broad range of amino acids and in other intestinal epithelial cell models the receptor couples to the phosphatidylinositol pathway resulting in elevation of intracellular Ca^{2+} [177]. In murine primary L-cells, however, peptone triggered GLP-1 release was inhibited by nifedipine and lanthanum, suggesting roles for L-type Ca^{2+} channels and TRP channels, respectively, as alternative signalling pathways downstream of CaSR recruitment [174]. In the perfused rat small intestinal model, CaSR agonists were shown to access basolaterally located receptors to trigger GLP-1 release [178].

There are several other GPCRs that have been implicated in amino acid responses in EECs. The lysophosphatidic acid receptor 5 (LPAR5, also known as GPR92/93), is highly expressed in the intestinal mucosal layer particularly in the duodenum [179]. This promiscuous receptor couples to various G-proteins, including Gαq and Gα12/13 [180]. LPAR5 is proposed to mediate peptone-sensing in CCK-expressing EECs [179]; however, expression of *Lpar5* transcript was not detected in colonic L-cells and GLP-1 secretion was not impaired in primary cultures from *Lpar5*-deficient mice [171] suggesting LPAR5 is not a major contributor to amino acid-sensing in L-cells.

GPR142 is a Gαq-coupled receptor activated by aromatic amino acids such as tryptophan and phenylalanine. In vivo, oral dosing of aromatic amino acids increased plasma GIP levels which were abolished in *Gpr142* knock-out animals [181,182]. Interestingly, aromatic amino acids also evoked a rapid rise in plasma GLP-1 levels after oral gavage but this was maintained in *Gpr142*-deficient mice [182]. GPR142 seems also not to be required for gut hormone responses to dietary protein, as mixed protein delivered orally to mice triggered a robust increase in GIP and GLP-1 secretion that was maintained in *Gpr142*-deficient mice [181].

Taste receptors composed of T1R1/T1R3 subunits, which form the umami taste receptor, respond to a broad spectrum of aliphatic amino acids including L-glutamate [159,183]. This receptor is allosterically modulated by purine nucleotides, such as inosine-5-monophosphate (IMP), to potentiate amino acid responses. However, even though genes encoding the components of the umami taste receptor, *Tas1R1* and *Tas1R3*, were not enriched in GLP-1 or GIP-expressing cells [104,106,110], umami receptor dependent GLP-2 secretion has been reported [184]. In lingual taste cells, residual sensitivity to oral glutamate and IMP was observed in double *Tas1R1/Tas1R3* knock-outs [185] suggesting other receptors may be involved in mediating glutamate-triggered taste responses. Alternative candidate receptors including ionotropic and metabotropic glutamate receptors (mGluR1/4) have been identified in taste cells [186,187]; even though expression and a defensive role of mGluR4 activation in the duodenal mucosa has been demonstrated [188], the question of whether similar mechanisms are utilised in EECs remains to be studied.

GPRC6A is another receptor that responds to a broad spectrum of amino acids, particularly basic ones [189]. GPRC6A is activated by multiple ligands besides amino acids, including the hormones osteocalcin and testosterone, and is allosterically modulated by Ca^{2+} [190]. GPRC6A colocalised with GLP-1 expressing cells in the small intestine [191], though the majority of GPRC6A-positive cells were not immunoreactive for GLP-1. However, in another study, *Gprc6a* expression was low in primary L-cells [171] and of all the GPCRs associated with amino acid detection, *Gprc6a* was found at lowest abundance in STC-1 cells [192]. Although GPRC6A contributed to ornithine triggered GLP-1 release from GLUTag cells, ornithine did not stimulate GLP-1 secretion from primary L-cells [193].

More work is needed in the area of amino acid sensing mechanisms in the gut as several amino acids exert potent effects on gastrointestinal function and feeding behaviour, but the exact mechanisms remain to be fully elucidated. Tryptophan, for instance, can potently suppress energy intake and inhibit gastric emptying [194]. Although GLP-1 release from EECs can reduce food intake and slow gastric emptying rates, only modest changes in GLP-1 levels were reported by several groups following tryptophan administration [195,196] and studies that reported an increase in GLP-1 levels following tryptophan administration found GPR142 not to be involved [182]. GIP secretion was markedly increased after an oral tryptophan ingestion [181], but GIP is proposed to have the opposite effect and increase the gastric emptying rate [197]. Another amino acid with an incompletely characterised mechanism of action is glutamine, which triggers incretin hormone secretion from GLUTag, primary L- and K-cells and in human participants [104,106,198–200]. A sodium-dependent electrogenic transporter may be involved in glutamine sensing as both glutamine and asparagine triggered depolarising currents when applied to GLUTag cells [198] and transcripts for several electrogenic amino acid transporters are expressed in GLUTag cells. However, under non-electrogenic conditions where the cell membrane potential is pre-emptively depolarised to negate the effect of small currents generated by electrogenic transporters, glutamine could still enhance GLP-1 release [198]. Intracellular calcium and cAMP levels are elevated in GLP-1 expressing cells following glutamine application [201] suggesting the activation of additional pathways. The rise in intracellular calcium was dependent on extracellular Na^+ and Ca^{2+}, so recruitment of voltage-gated calcium channels following activation of a sodium-dependent electrogenic transporter is possible. CaSR may also be involved as the CaSR inhibitor Calhex 231 reduced glutamine stimulated GIP and GLP-1 release [174,175]. Studies in other endocrine cell models have demonstrated that CaSR can also couple to Gαs to stimulate adenylyl cyclase activity and cAMP production [202].

4.3. Fats

Fats are highly effective at suppressing energy intake and appetite [203,204], stimulating GIP secretion [118], and eliciting sustained GLP-1 release [118,205]. The stimulatory effects of dietary lipids on incretin hormone secretion were found to be dependent on fatty acid chain length and saturation [206–209]; however, other studies demonstrated the importance of metabolism and absorption for fat-stimulated GLP-1 and GIP secretion [210].

The processing of lipids after ingestion is more involved than carbohydrates or proteins. Dietary lipids in the form of triglycerides, cholesterol, phospholipids and fat-soluble vitamins are first emulsified by bile salts to promote efficient hydrolysis and absorption. Triglycerides are broken down to monoglycerides and fatty acids by pancreatic lipases released into the intestinal lumen. Hydrolysis of triglycerides is essential for EEC lipid-sensing as orlistat, a lipase inhibitor, attenuated postprandial GIP and GLP-1 secretion [211–214]. The breakdown products generated by lipases aggregate with bile acids to form micelles, facilitating uptake by enterocytes. Within enterocytes, triglycerides are re-synthesised from fatty acids and monoglycerides, and packaged with lipoproteins and other lipids to form chylomicrons. Chylomicrons are released from enterocytes from the basolateral surface and enter the lymphatic system through the central lacteal of the villus. Physiological concentrations of chylomicrons [215] significantly stimulated GLP-1 and GIP secretion in murine and human duodenal cultures [216]. The formation of chylomicrons seems to be required for lipid-stimulated release of incretin hormones as pluronic L-81, a surfactant that inhibits chylomicron synthesis [217], impaired lipid-stimulated release of GLP-1 and GIP [218,219]. Furthermore, murine knock-outs of genes responsible for re-esterification of absorbed free-fatty acids and monoglycerides prior to their incorporation into chylomicrons, monocaylglyceride-acyltransferase-2 (MGAT2) and diacylglyceride-acyltransferase-1 (DGAT1), reduced secretion of GIP from the upper GI tract following an oral triglyceride load [220]. However, MGAT2 and DGAT1 knock-out animals exhibited delayed GLP-1 responses to an oral triglyceride load, likely because impairment of fat absorption increased delivery of lipids more distally to regions of the intestine with a higher density of GLP-1-producing L-cells, leading to activation of other non-chylomicron-mediated mechanisms of GLP-1 release [221]. A neuronally mediated circuit has also been implicated in regulating feeding responses following lipid ingestion, as vagal deafferentation blocked the ability of oleate and corn oil infusions to reduce food intake [222] and silencing neuronal activity with tetracaine or capsaicin prevented duodenal lipid suppression of feeding in sham-fed rats [223,224].

The cellular mechanisms underlying lipid-stimulated GLP-1 and GIP secretion involve G-protein coupled receptors of the free-fatty acid (FFA) receptor family (Figure 4). The free-fatty acid receptor 1 (FFA1), known previously as the orphan receptor GPR40 [225,226], is highly expressed in K- and L-cells [104,106,110] and FFA1 colocalised with gut hormones GIP and GLP-1 [227]. FFA1 binds medium to long chain fatty acids and mediates lipid-induced incretin hormone release, as mice lacking *Ffar1* expression exhibited impaired release of GIP and GLP-1 following consumption of a high fat diet [227]. FFA1 couples primarily to Gαq proteins, which recruit phosphatidylinositol signalling pathways, but with some ligands has also been suggested to couple to Gαs proteins to elevate cAMP levels [228]. Heterologous expression studies suggested that Gαi/o proteins may also contribute to the downstream signalling associated with FFA1 activation [229]. In pancreatic β cells, activation of FFA1 was associated with activation of transient receptor potential cation channel subfamily C member 3, TrpC3 [230] and in mouse GLP-1 expressing cells TrpC3 activation downstream of FFA1 generated depolarising currents to increase electrical excitability and GLP-1 secretion [108]. A similar increase in electrical excitability following FFA1 activation was observed in human GLP-1 expressing L-cells, but the mechanism did not appear to involve TrpC3 channels [110]. The other known GPCR of the free-fatty acid receptor family responsive to long-chain fatty acids is FFA4, formerly known as GPR120 [231]. FFA4 has been identified in the intestine, particularly in GIP-expressing K-cells [106,232,233] and GLP-1-expressing L-cells [104,110]. FFA4 is activated by unsaturated long-chain fatty acids such as α-linoleate, docosahexaenoic acid (DHA), palmitoleate and oleate. Activation of FFA4 by long-chain fatty acids promotes secretion of GLP-1 [231] and knock-down of *Ffar4* in STC-1 cells reduced GLP-1 secretion induced by α-linolenic acid [231]. Mice deficient in *Ffar4* or treated with a pharmacological inhibitor of FFA4 exhibited reduced GIP responses to an oral lard oil challenge [233]. However, the relative contributions of FFA1 and FFA4 in mediating lipid-stimulated GIP secretion remain incompletely resolved. One study found that knock-out of *Ffar1* but not *Ffar4* reduced GIP release following an oral olive oil challenge, although double knock-out of both receptors was more effective at reducing lipid-stimulated GIP secretion than either single knock-out [234]. By contrast, another study reported that mice deficient in *Ffar1* or *Ffar4* exhibited reduced GIP secretion following oral corn oil ingestion, with a greater reduction in *Ffar1* knock-out animals [235]. In this study, it was noted that the simultaneous reduction in CCK secretion further impaired GIP secretion, likely downstream of reduced gallbladder contraction, as GIP levels were partially restored following exogenous CCK replacement, particularly in the *Ffar4* knock-out group. Like FFA1, FFA4 couples to Gαq-dependent pathways to mediate GLP-1 secretion, but Gαi/o pathways have been implicated in other FFA4 expressing cells including gastric ghrelin-secreting cells [236] and pancreatic δ cells [237]. Recruitment of protein kinase C ζ, which is not a target of diacylglycerol downstream of FFA1/4 activation, was implicated in oleic acid-induced GLP-1 release from GLUTag cells [238], although details of the pathway remain uncertain. Recruitment of the transient receptor potential channel TrpM5 has been linked to FFA4 activation by linoleic acid to stimulate CCK release from STC-1 cells [239], mirroring the involvement of TrpC3 in L-cells downstream of FFA1 activation [108]. Although the reported recruitment of different Trp channels downstream of FFA1 and FFA4 might reflect functional differences between these receptors, the possibility of cell line or species-specific responses cannot be ruled out.

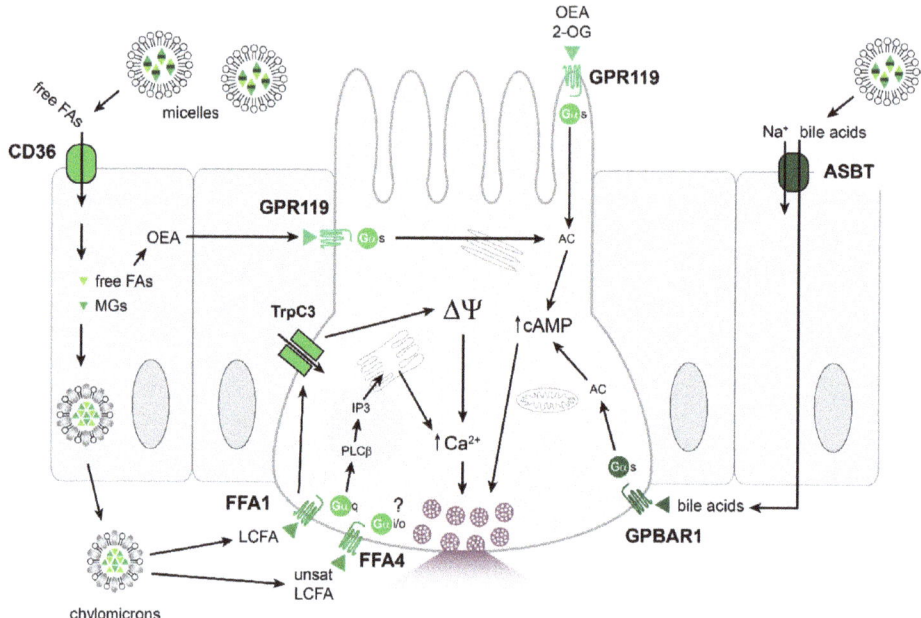

Figure 4. Fat-sensing mechanisms in incretin hormone secreting EECs. Lipid sensing appears dominated by activation of G-protein coupled receptors. Contrary to what had been thought originally, these do not directly sample the luminal contents, but are shielded behind lipid absorption by enterocytes, with the possible exception of the mono-acyl-glyceride sensor GPR119. Absorption of micelles and formation of chylomicrons through enterocytes is illustrated on the left. Bile acids, which assist in the emulsification and breakdown of fatty acids, also stimulate incretin hormone secretion and the mechanism of bile acid-sensing in EECs is illustrated in dark green on right side of EEC. Transport route for conjugated bile acids in the small intestine via ASBT, illustrated in enterocyte on the right. See text for details. Abbreviations: 2-OG, 2-oleoylglycerol; AC, adenylyl cyclase; ASBT, sodium-dependent bile acid transporter; cAMP, cyclic adenosine monophosphate; CD36, cluster of differentiation also known as fatty acid translocase; FA; fatty acid; FFA1, free fatty acid receptor 1; FFA4, free fatty acid receptor 4; GPBAR1, G-protein coupled bile acid receptor 1; GPR119, G-protein coupled receptor 119; IP3, inositol triphosphate; LCFA, long-chain fatty acid; MG; monoglycerides; OEA, oleoylethanolamide; PLCβ, phospholipase C beta; TrpC3, transient receptor potential cation channel subfamily C member 3; ΔΨ, membrane depolarization.

Another GPCR involved in lipid sensing in the gastrointestinal tract is GPR119, which is also enriched in K- and L-cells [104,106,110,234,240]. A number of endogenous lipid substrates bind GPR119 receptors including: oleoylethanolamide (OEA), a lipid amide synthesized in the small intestine during absorption of dietary fats [241]; 2-oleoylglycerol (2-OG) and other 2-monoacylglycerols, natural digestion products of intestinal triacylglycerol digestion [242]; N-oleoyldopamine [243] and lysophosphatidylcholine [244]. The selectivity of the above-mentioned lipid-derivatives for GPR119 still needs to be addressed as OEA was able to suppress food intake in *Gpr119*-deficient mice suggesting other targets of OEA [245]. It has been reported, for example, that OEA is an endogenous substrate for the nuclear receptor PPAR-α which can also influence satiety and lipid uptake [241,246,247]. Application of OEA to various in vitro L-cell models, however, triggered GPR119-dependent GLP-1 secretion [240]. Oral administration of OEA to humans increased plasma GLP-1 and GIP levels [242], and small synthetic agonists of GPR119 elevated GIP and GLP-1 levels in mice [248] and decreased food intake in rats [249]. Whilst it is possible that local production of OEA in the small intestine modulates GPR119 activity [250], it is unclear if sufficient OEA is generated to activate the receptor [251]. Nevertheless, GPR119 seems to be an important sensor of ingested fat, as there was reduced GIP secretion following an oral triglyceride challenge in *Gpr119* knock-out animals, [234], and impaired oil-triggered GLP-1 release in mice lacking *Gpr119* in L-cells [252]. The GLP-1 response to GPR119 agonism is more prominent in the distal gut, as it was impaired in mice lacking L-cells in the terminal ileum and large intestine [28]. Mirroring this finding, GPR119 agonists were more effective at triggering GLP-1 release in vitro from murine colonic than small intestinal cultures, and elevated cAMP in ~70% of colonic L-cells but only 50% of small intestinal L-cells [252]. By contrast, GPR119 agonism was a relatively poor stimulus of GLP-1 secretion from human colonic cultures [105], although this might reflect species-specific differences in the receptor or in vitro preparation. In a clinical study, multiple dosing of a GPR119 agonist JNJ-38431055 in subjects with T2D increased plasma GLP-1 and GIP levels, but this did not translate into improvements in 24 h blood glucose control [253]. GPR119 couples to Gαs proteins to increase cAMP levels [234,252]. Thus, in conjunction with Gαq-signalling pathways downstream of FFA1/4, the magnitude of gut hormone secretion following fat ingestion is amplified beyond activation of a single GPCR. This feature may underlie the effectiveness of fats in stimulating robust incretin hormone responses.

As mentioned above, lipid absorption is critical for lipid-induced GIP secretion, and impairment of luminal fat digestion or epithelial absorption reduced GIP release. Receptors for free fatty acids (FFA1) are located on the basolateral face of EECs [254] so free-fatty acids can only access receptors to trigger hormone release following their absorption across the epithelium. GPR119, by contrast, is reported to be located apically as well as basolaterally [255].

Free fatty acids can enter enterocytes by the fatty acid transporter CD36. Expression of CD36 is described in oral taste bud cells [256,257] and intestine, though levels are higher in the proximal than distal intestine [258]. CD36 is an integral membrane protein which mediates the cellular uptake of long-chain fatty acids and has been linked to lingual and small intestinal fat detection and transport [241,259,260]. Mice lacking CD36 exhibit reduced chylomicron formation [261] and reduced fatty acid and cholesterol uptake in the proximal, but not distal intestine [262]. CD36 knock-out mice are also insensitive to the suppression of food intake mediated by duodenal lipid infusion [241]. Such participation of CD36 in lipid signalling mechanisms is likely indirect. As discussed above, transepithelial transport of fatty acids is necessary to target basolaterally located free-fatty acid receptors, and CD36 was also postulated to assist in FFA4 signalling by accumulating long-chain fatty acids in the vicinity of low affinity FFA4 receptors [263]. In addition, uptake of fatty acids is required for the synthesis of OEA and its precursor N-oleoyl-phosphatidylethanolamine (NOPE), and mice lacking CD36 had reduced OEA production and OEA-induced satiety [241].

4.4. Other: Bile Acids

Bile acids are released into the gut lumen following fat detection in the duodenum and release of CCK from EECs which stimulates gall bladder contraction. Bile acids contribute to the emulsification of dietary lipids, aiding digestion, and can also activate selective G-protein coupled bile acid receptors (GPBAR1) also known as Takeda G-protein coupled receptor 5 (TGR5) [264,265], as well as the nuclear farnesoid X receptor, FXR [266].

Early studies in anesthetised dogs found that intra-ileal infusion of bile increased secretion of proglucagon gene products [267,268]. EEC cell line models and mouse primary intestinal epithelial cultures confirmed that bile acids stimulated GLP-1 release [269–271] alongside clinical studies showing that luminal bile acids increased GLP-1 and PYY release [272,273]. Intraluminal infusion of bile into human participants and rodents also triggered a strong GIP secretory response [274,275].

Bile acid triggered gut hormone release is dependent on GPBAR1 as selective agonists of the receptor, designed with preferential activity for GPBAR1 over the nuclear bile acid receptor FXR, triggered GLP-1 release and mice lacking the receptor exhibited abrogated GLP-1 secretory responses to bile acids [112,269,276]. Ex vivo intestinal models demonstrated that only basolaterally accessible selective GPBAR1 agonists were able to elicit GLP-1 release [112,277], indicating that absorption of bile acids is critical for their effectiveness in triggering gut hormone secretion. Conjugated bile acids require transport into cells by the apical sodium-dependent bile acid transporter, ASBT [278], which is predominantly expressed in the terminal ileum. Consequently, blocking the absorption of bile acids with an inhibitor of ASBT blocked the effectiveness of bile acids to trigger GLP-1 release [112,277]. In the colon where expression of ASTB is lower, bile acids gain access to basolaterally located GPBAR1 following deconjugation and dehydroxylation by gut bacteria, which improves bile acid permeability and potency at GPBAR1 [265] and negates the dependence of bile acid-triggered GLP-1 release on ASBT [277]. Binding to GPBAR1 activates adenylyl cyclase cAMP production [112,270,271] downstream of Gαs proteins, and elevations in intracellular Ca^{2+} have also been reported in cell models of GLP-1 releasing cells following application of bile acids [112,269]. The activation of GPBAR1 in GLP-1 expressing cells increased evoked action potential activity and increased calcium currents through L-type voltage-gated calcium channels [108]. Bile acids may also increase the size of the L-cell population in the intestinal epithelium [276]. By contrast, FXR receptor activity inhibited GLP-1 production in L-cells [279], and the consequences of simultaneous activation of intestinal GPBAR1 and FXR receptors by bile acids still need to be reconciled. Bile acids may also contribute to reducing food intake by GLP-1 independent mechanisms: for example, GPBAR1 expression was found on inhibitory motor neurons in the myenteric plexus, corresponding with reduced spontaneous intestinal contractile activity following bile acid application [280].

4.5. Other: Short-Chain Fatty Acids (SCFAs)

Colonic fermentation of undigested dietary fibre by gut bacteria produces high concentrations of SCFAs in the intestinal lumen. In humans, SCFAs were most abundant in the caecum and ascending colon, whereas levels of circulating SCFA were substantially lower [27].

SCFA signalling is mediated by G-protein coupled receptors of the free-fatty acid receptor family. Free-fatty acid receptor 2 (FFA2), formerly known as GPR43 [281,282], is activated by SCFAs of 2–4 carbon lengths but acetate (C2) and propionate (C3) are the most potent. *Ffar2* expression is highest in the distal gut and using an antibody raised against rat FFA2, the receptor co-localised with PYY, and presumably GLP-1, in rats [283] and humans [284]. FFA2 was also described in serotonin-containing mast cells but not enterochromaffin cells, clarifying a mechanism for SCFA stimulation of colonic motility [285]. An *Ffar2*-reporter mouse line confirmed *Ffar2* expression in intestinal mast cells; however, there was weak association with EECs [286]. FFA2 is postulated to couple to G-proteins of the Gαq/11 and Gαi/o family, though the pathways recruited in EECs are incompletely elucidated. Activation of FFA2 produces a rise in intracellular calcium in murine L-cells [286,287], presumably by canonical Gαq-coupled pathways involving phospholipase C-dependent production of inositol-3-phosphate and Ca^{2+} release from intracellular stores. The free-fatty acid receptor 3 (FFA3), formerly known as GPR41 [288], is the other member of the FFA receptor family responsive to SCFAs. It preferentially binds SCFAs of three to five carbon lengths and couples to G-proteins of the Gαi/o family. FFA3 is localised to the colonic mucosa and co-localises with PYY [289]. In an *Ffar3*-reporter mouse model, a widespread pattern of *Ffar3* expression was described in EECs, including GLP-1 and GIP-expressing cells, as well as peripheral neuronal ganglia associated with enteric, sensory and autonomic signalling [286,290]. The cellular mechanism of FFA3 signalling in EECs has not been elucidated, though in neurons has been shown to involve inhibition of voltage-gated calcium channels by a G$\beta\gamma$-mediated mechanism [291]. Other receptors responsive to SCFAs include the olfactory receptor subfamily 51E (OR51E1 in human, Olfr558 in mouse; OR51E2 in human, Olfr78 in mouse), and GPR109A, also known as the niacin receptor.

In murine primary colonic cultures, SCFAs stimulated GLP-1 release through FFA2-dependent [292] or both FFA2 and FFA3-dependent mechanisms [287]. A selective FFA2 agonist, Compound 1, also stimulated GLP-1 secretion [293]. SCFA-stimulated GLP-1 release did not involve pertussis toxin-sensitive pathways and SCFAs triggered a rise in intracellular calcium in GLP-1-producing EECs, suggesting Gαq-coupled pathways are responsible for mediating the stimulatory effects of SCFAs on EECs. Furthermore, a selective inhibitor of Gαq signalling FR900359 abolished SCFA-triggered GLP-1 release and an FFA2 agonist with biased activity for Gαi-signalling, AZ1729, did not trigger GLP-1 secretion [294]. The molecular details of FFA3 involvement in stimulating GLP-1 release are still unclear, given that FFA3 seems to signal exclusively through inhibitory Gαi/o-coupled pathways. In an isolated perfused colon model, basolaterally applied SCFAs triggered release of GLP-1 which was more pronounced following enhancement of cAMP levels [295]. Given the high production of SCFA luminally, localisation of receptors on the basolateral surface may be a mechanism preventing continuous activation or saturation of SCFA receptors. However, the receptors involved in enhancing GLP-1 release following SCFA administration in this ex vivo model were not clear as selective FFA2 or FFA3 agonists and antagonists had no effect. Perhaps another SCFA receptor is involved or synergistic activation of both FFA2 and FFA3 is required for mediating the effects of SCFAs on GLP-1 expressing cells. Basolateral, rather than apical sensing of SCFA on GLP-1 secreting cells is, however, further supported by the correlation of circulating rather than faecal SCFA concentrations with GLP-1 in fasting humans [296].

As mentioned previously, FFA3 co-localised with GIP in the proximal small intestine [286]. SCFAs can arise in the proximal small intestine from fermentation by oral microbiota [297] but at much lower concentrations compared with the distal intestine, or from pathological bacterial overgrowth. Generation of SCFAs in the proximal small intestine is associated with suppression of GIP release by an FFA3-dependent mechanism [298].

Prolonged SCFA exposure can also alter gene expression, including genes encoding gut hormones. Proglucagon expression increased in STC-1 cells after 24 h incubation with SCFAs and in the colon of rats fed chow diets enriched with fermentable fibre [299]. In human cell line models of EECs, there was little increase in proglucagon expression following SCFA treatment, but a pronounced increase in PYY expression following butyrate treatment which was mediated by histone deacetylase (HDAC) inhibition and FFA2 [300]. SCFA have also been reported to alter the number of GLP-1 producing L-cells, but whereas an increase in L-cell number was observed following chronic SCFA exposure in mouse and human intestinal organoids in vitro [301], SCFA appeared to suppress L-cell number and function in germ free mice recolonised with SCFA producing bacteria [302,303].

5. Effect of GLP-1 and GIP on Food Intake and Weight Loss

The consensus view is that exogenous administration of GLP-1 reduces energy intake and appetite in rodents [304] and humans [305–307]. The anorexigenic actions of GLP-1 extend to long-acting mimetics such as exenatide, liraglutide and semaglutide [308–311] and persist in Type 2 diabetic and obese individuals, thus supporting the use of GLP-1 receptor agonists in weight management therapies.

The effect of GIP on food intake is more controversial. Administration of GIP or a long-acting analogue acyl-GIP, at doses sufficient to produce positive metabolic effects, had no effect on body weight in mice [312] or hunger scores and food ingestion in humans [197], and in a recent double-blind crossover study, there was no significant change in food intake in overweight/obese individuals given GIP along with an IV glucose infusion that mimicked the blood glucose rise after an oral glucose challenge [313]. Animal models with diminished GIP activity including *Gipr* knockout mice [314], enteroendocrine K-cell ablation [315], and GIPR antagonism [316,317] show reduced body weight gain associated with diet-induced obesity. By contrast, overexpression of GIP in mice also led to decreased energy intake and reduced weight gain associated with diet-induced obesity [318]. Interpretation of these studies may be complicated by confounding factors such as GIP stimulation of pancreatic insulin and glucagon secretion, which can themselves modulate appetite [319,320], and compensatory changes in the absence of functional GIP signalling [321]. Furthermore, GIP has a complicated pharmacology as certain peptides declared to be antagonists of GIPR in fact display partial agonist activity [322,323] and interspecies differences in GIPR pharmacology exist [322]. Recent studies have favoured a reduction of food intake as a consequence of pharmacological GIPR agonism [324], but further studies will be required to fully elucidate the molecular mechanisms governing GIP action on food intake.

Despite the controversy surrounding GIP action on food intake, there is growing interest in developing agonists that target two or more receptors involved in metabolic control, including receptors for the incretin hormones GLP-1 and GIP. Studies in mice demonstrated that co-administration of GIP and GLP-1 analogues enhanced body weight loss and improved glycaemic control in obese mice [312,325,326]. Dual GIP/GLP-1 agonists are in development as potential new anti-diabetic and anti-obesity treatments. The pharmacological reasoning for this approach is to amplify the beneficial metabolic effects whilst lowering doses and adverse side effect profiles of the individual components. Promising improvements in blood glucose control were obtained with the acylated unimolecular dual GIP/GLP-1 agonist RG7697/NNC0090-2746 in healthy [327] and T2D patients [328] and significant reductions in body weight were achieved but the magnitude was possibly similar to liraglutide treatment alone [329]. However, another dual GIP/GLP-1 agonist tirzepatide (LY3298176) displayed improved efficacy over the selective GLP-1 receptor agonist dulaglutide [330,331].

6. Gut Hormone-Mediated Mechanisms of Satiety

Infusion of various nutrients into the small intestine is associated with greater suppression of food intake than nutrients that are delivered intravenously [332,333], strongly supporting a gut-derived mechanism for satiety. GLP-1 and GIP released from the gastrointestinal tract can initiate satiety signals through a variety of mechanisms ranging from direct modulation of gastrointestinal function to recruitment of central circuits involved in feeding behaviours.

The actions of GLP-1 and GIP on gastric emptying and gastric acid secretion are well studied. Briefly, postprandial GLP-1 is associated with delayed gastric emptying [334] whereas GIP was found to have the opposite effect of increasing the gastric emptying rate [197]. Vagal afferent fibres were necessary for mediating GLP-1 effects on gastric emptying [335] along with cholinergic signalling and GLP1R activation [336], which is consistent with GLP1R expression described in the gastric antrum and pylorus [337]. Other gut hormones such as CCK and PYY also control gastric emptying rates [338]. Vagal innervation was also necessary in mediating the inhibitory effects of GLP-1 on gastric acid secretion [339] as vagotomised patients did not exhibit an inhibitory response to GLP-1 [340]. Peripheral infusion of GIP also inhibited gastric acid secretion, albeit at supraphysiological concentrations [341] and involved a reduction in postprandial gastrin release.

Gut hormones also internally regulate intestinal motility and luminal transit in response to a high nutrient load. Infusion of physiological levels of GLP-1 slowed intestinal motility in the fed and fasted state in rats [342] and humans [342,343], and was reversed by the GLP1R antagonist Exendin(9–39) [342]. Exogenous GIP also reduced intestinal transit in mice, which was blocked by a somatostatin receptor antagonist [344], but by comparison GLP-1 was more potent than GIP in abolishing myoelectric activity in the small bowel of rats [345].

Overall, by modulating various aspects of gastrointestinal function (gastric emptying, gastric acid secretion and intestinal motility), GLP-1 and GIP can slow the digestion of nutrients allowing more efficient nutrient breakdown and absorption. This serves to increase exposure of proximal EECs to nutrients. The slowing of gastrointestinal activity can also increase distension of the stomach and intestinal wall, and consequent activation of stretch-activated mechanoreceptors directly signals to the brain to control feeding and enhances the perception of fullness [346].

Neuronal mechanisms play an integral role in mediating the satiating effects of GLP-1 and possibly GIP. The effect of peripherally administered GLP-1 on food intake was ablated after bilateral subdiaphragmatic total vagotomy [25] in rats, and the suppression of short-term food intake following intraduodenal nutrient infusion was eliminated by selective vagal rhizotomy of the celiac branch, which abolishes afferent vagal inputs to the intestine [26]. Both findings highlight the significance of vagal signalling in appetite control. Vagal afferent neurons project peripherally to visceral organs, including much of the small intestine and the proximal third of the large intestine. A subpopulation of vagal afferent neurons express receptors for GLP-1 [337,347,348] but single-cell transcriptomics studies were unable to resolve expression of receptors for GIP in nodose neurons. GLP-1 directly stimulated activity in vagal afferent neurons [349] and augmented Ca^{2+} responses in GLP1R-expressing nodose neurons in vitro [337]. Vagal afferent neurons project to two brainstem regions: the area postrema and the nucleus of the solitary tract (NTS). GLP1R expression, staining and ligand binding have been detected in a number of brain regions, including the area postrema, ventromedial hypothalamus, arcuate and paraventricular nuclei [350–353]. Sensory afferent inputs into the hindbrain are essential for mediating the suppression of feeding by nutrients as chemical destruction of these neurons by capsaicin abolished this inhibition [354,355]. Some neurons in the NTS also produce and release GLP-1 [356] but these neurons do not express GLP1R or respond to exogenous GLP-1 [357,358]. Although vagal afferent signalling is important in mediating some effects of GLP-1 on feeding control, the route of intestinal GLP-1 to activate vagal afferent neurons is unclear. Vagal afferents, particularly neurons that express gut hormone receptors, do not appear to innervate the basolateral surface of L-cells [348,359], although *Glp1r*-expressing enteric neurons have been identified [337], which may be involved in relaying signals. Diffusion of GLP-1 in the vicinity of its site of release from L-cells may contribute to non-synaptic activation of local nerve endings, and could act in tandem with other mediators released from EECs such as glutamate [360] or ATP [361] to exert its effects on food intake.

Central injection of GLP-1 into the cerebral ventricles [304,362–364] or hypothalamus [365] reduces food intake. These centrally mediated effects of GLP-1 were dependent on GLP1R signalling as they were not observed in *Glp1r* KO animals [366] or in the presence of the GLP1R antagonist exendin(9–39) [362,367]. Whilst some of the central GLP1R sites are involved in the satiating effects of peripherally supplied GLP1R agonists, it is becoming clear that activation of GLP-1 expressing neurons in the NTS recruits additional anorexic circuits [358].

There is increasing support for a central mechanism mediating food intake reduction by GIP. Central administration of GIP decreased food intake and body weight and combined with GLP-1 produced a synergistic reduction of food consumption [367]. Furthermore, *Gipr* expression has been described in the arcuate, dorsomedial, and paraventricular nuclei in the hypothalamus and activation of *Gipr* expressing cells in this region suppressed food intake [368]. Many questions remain, including whether circulating GIP released from K-cells in the proximal small intestine activates centrally expressed GIPR, which are also found in the area postrema [368], as well as the identity and relative importance of the circuitry mediating GIP-mediated suppression of food intake.

Besides its role in mediating homeostatic feeding, GLP-1 is also implicated in circuits driving food reward and motivation. Activation of GLP-1 producing preproglucagon neurons in the NTS seems to be of minor importance for homeostatic feeding control, but becomes relevant under stress, one of which is overeating, presumably involving stomach stretching [369]. In this context it is important to note that *Glp1r* is expressed by neurons in the ventral tegmental area (VTA) and nucleus accumbens, brain regions associated with reward and desire. Exendin-4, a GLP-1 mimetic, or GLP-1 injected peripherally reduced palatable food intake and reward-motivated behaviour and a similar effect was observed when exendin-4 was injected directly into the VTA [370,371]. In agreement with these findings, injection of the GLP1R antagonist, Exendin(9–39), into the nucleus accumbens increased meal size and palatability of sucrose solutions [372].

7. Future Directions

There are still many unresolved issues in our understanding of nutrient-induced gut hormone secretory mechanisms, including the role of GLP-1 produced in the distal GI tract. GLP-1 is produced in large quantities in the distal small intestine and colon, regions of the intestine not typically reached by ingested nutrients, where its release may follow different regulatory mechanisms including control by metabolites of gut microbiota and neurohormonal pathways. Recent studies identified the possible importance of distal L-cells in mediating responses to lipid-derivatives, melanocortin receptor 4 agonists and lipopolysaccharides [28]. Another question is whether therapeutic activation of GPCRs in EECs could trigger sufficient gut hormone release to produce significant metabolic benefits or satiation. Injectable GLP1 receptor agonists and the levels of GLP-1 achieved following bariatric surgery are far in excess of levels expected in a normal healthy postprandial state. The feasibility of targeting nutrient-sensing receptors in EECs also needs to be properly assessed. Many of these receptors respond to a range of ligands but the potential importance of biased downstream signalling is not known. Finally, desensitisation of nutrient-sensing receptors in EECs has not been investigated in-depth, but could arise from the prolonged exposure of EECs to saturating concentrations of nutrients in the postprandial state or with altered dietary status such as in models of diet-induced obesity, which have been shown to alter expression levels of peptide hormone receptors expressed on vagal afferent neurons [373]. Further complications or, alternatively considered, treatment options arise from cross talk between different EECs, notably the apparent chronic paracrine inhibition of L-cells by somatostatin [374] released from nearby D-cells, which themselves express a number of nutrient sensing receptors, as shown by RNAseq for D-cells in the stomach [375].

8. Conclusions

Nutrient absorption and stimulation of gut hormone secretion occur predominantly in the proximal small intestine. However, as demonstrated by the effectiveness of bariatric surgery to deliver nutrients more distally along the gut, distal GLP-1 producing L-cells represent a vast source of endogenous GLP-1 that can potentially be exploited to suppress appetite and increase insulin secretion. Future work is needed to reveal the physiological importance of distal GLP-1 producing L-cells and identify strategies to recruit these cell populations for improved glucose homeostasis and appetite regulation.

Author Contributions: V.B.L., F.M.G., F.R. wrote, revised, and approved the submitted version of this review. All authors have read and agreed to the published version of the manuscript.

Funding: V.B.L., F.M.G. and F.R. were funded by a Wellcome Joint Investigator Award to FR and FMG (106262/Z/14/Z and 106263/Z/14/Z) and the Metabolic Diseases Unit (MRC_MC_UU_12012/3).

Institutional Review Board Statement: Not applicable.

Informed Consent Statement: Not applicable.

Data Availability Statement: Data sharing not applicable.

Conflicts of Interest: The FR/FMG lab receives additional grant support from AstraZeneca and Eli Lilly for unrelated work. FMG is a consultant for Kallyope (New York, NY, USA).

References

1. Bayliss, W.M.; Starling, E.H. The mechanism of pancreatic secretion. *J. Physiol.* **1902**, *28*, 325–353. [CrossRef]
2. Bohórquez, D.V.; Chandra, R.; Samsa, L.A.; Vigna, S.R.; Liddle, R.A. Characterization of basal pseudopod-like processes in ileal and colonic PYY cells. *J. Mol. Histol.* **2010**, *42*, 3–13. [CrossRef]
3. Bohórquez, D.V.; Samsa, L.A.; Roholt, A.; Medicetty, S.; Chandra, R.; Liddle, R.A. An Enteroendocrine cell—enteric glia connection revealed by 3D electron microscopy. *PLoS ONE* **2014**, *9*, e89881. [CrossRef]
4. McSwiney, B.A.; Spurrell, W.R. Influence of osmotic pressure upon the emptying time of the stomach. *J. Physiol.* **1933**, *79*, 437–442. [CrossRef]
5. Knapper, J.; Heath, A.; Fletcher, J.; Morgan, L.; Marks, V. GIP and GLP-1(7–36) amide secretion in response to intraduodenal infusions of nutrients in pigs. *Comp. Biochem. Physiol. Part C Pharm. Toxicol. Endocrinol.* **1995**, *111*, 445–450. [CrossRef]
6. Rehfeld, J.F. The new biology of gastrointestinal hormones. *Physiol. Rev.* **1998**, *78*, 1087–1108. [CrossRef]
7. Umar, S. Intestinal stem cells. *Curr. Gastroenterol. Rep.* **2010**, *12*, 340–348. [CrossRef] [PubMed]
8. Creutzfeldt, M.W. The incretin concept today. *Diabetologia* **1979**, *16*, 75–85. [CrossRef] [PubMed]
9. Elrick, H.; Stimmler, L.; Hlad, C.J.; Arai, Y. Plasma insulin response to oral and intravenous glucose administration. *Clin. Endocrinol. Metab.* **1964**, *24*, 1076–1082. [CrossRef]
10. Le Roux, C.W.; Welbourn, R.; Werling, M.; Osborne, A.; Kokkinos, A.; Laurenius, A.; Lönroth, H.; Fändriks, L.; Ghatei, M.A.; Bloom, S.R.; et al. Gut hormones as mediators of appetite and weight loss after Roux-en-Y gastric bypass. *Ann. Surg.* **2007**, *246*, 780–785. [CrossRef] [PubMed]
11. Jørgensen, N.B.; Dirksen, C.; Bojsen-Møller, K.N.; Jacobsen, S.H.; Worm, D.; Hansen, D.L.; Kristiansen, V.B.; Naver, L.; Madsbad, S.; Holst, J.J. Exaggerated glucagon-like peptide 1 response is important for improved β-cell function and glucose tolerance after Roux-en-Y gastric bypass in patients with Type 2 diabetes. *Diabetes* **2013**, *62*, 3044–3052. [CrossRef]
12. Hansen, K.B.; Vilsbøll, T.; Knop, F.K. Incretin mimetics: A novel therapeutic option for patients with type 2 diabetes—A review. *Diabetes Metab. Syndr. Obes. Targets* **2010**, *3*, 155–163.
13. Mortensen, K.; Christensen, L.L.; Holst, J.J.; Orskov, C. GLP-1 and GIP are colocalized in a subset of endocrine cells in the small intestine. *Regul. Pept.* **2003**, *114*, 189–196. [CrossRef]
14. Theodorakis, M.J.; Carlson, O.; Michopoulos, S.; Doyle, M.E.; Juhaszova, M.; Petraki, K.; Egan, J.M. Human duodenal enteroendocrine cells: Source of both incretin peptides, GLP-1 and GIP. *Am. J. Physiol. Metab.* **2006**, *290*, E550–E559. [CrossRef] [PubMed]
15. Haber, A.L.; Biton, M.; Rogel, N.; Herbst, R.H.; Shekhar, K.; Smillie, C.; Burgin, G.; DeLorey, T.M.; Howitt, M.R.; Katz, Y.; et al. A single-cell survey of the small intestinal epithelium. *Nat. Cell Biol.* **2017**, *551*, 333–339. [CrossRef]
16. Egerod, K.L.; Engelstoft, M.S.; Grunddal, K.V.; Nøhr, M.K.; Secher, A.; Sakata, I.; Pedersen, J.; Windeløv, J.A.; Füchtbauer, E.-M.; Olsen, J.; et al. A major lineage of enteroendocrine cells coexpress CCK, secretin, GIP, GLP-1, PYY, and neurotensin but not somatostatin. *Endocrinology* **2012**, *153*, 5782–5795. [CrossRef] [PubMed]
17. Habib, A.M.; Richards, P.; Cairns, L.S.; Rogers, G.J.; Bannon, C.A.M.; Parker, H.E.; Morley, T.C.E.; Yeo, G.S.H.; Reimann, F.; Gribble, F.M.; et al. Overlap of endocrine hormone expression in the mouse intestine revealed by transcriptional profiling and flow cytometry. *Endocrinology* **2012**, *153*, 3054–3065. [CrossRef] [PubMed]
18. Jorsal, T.; Rhee, N.A.; Pedersen, J.; Wahlgren, C.D.; Mortensen, B.; Jepsen, S.L.; Jelsing, J.; Dalbøge, L.S.; Vilmann, P.; Hassan, H.; et al. Enteroendocrine K and L cells in healthy and Type 2 diabetic individuals. *Diabetologia* **2018**, *61*, 284–294. [CrossRef] [PubMed]
19. Roberts, G.P.; Larraufie, P.; Richards, P.; Kay, R.G.; Galvin, S.G.; Miedzybrodzka, E.L.; Leiter, A.; Li, H.J.; Glass, L.L.; Ma, M.K.; et al. Comparison of human and murine enteroendocrine cells by transcriptomic and peptidomic profiling. *Diabetes* **2019**, *68*, 1062–1072. [CrossRef] [PubMed]
20. Sjölund, K.; Sandén, G.; Håkanson, R.; Sundler, F. Endocrine cells in human intestine: An immunocytochemical study. *Gastroenterology* **1983**, *85*, 1120–1130. [CrossRef]
21. Bryant, M.G.; Bloom, S.R.; Polak, J.M.; Hobbs, S.; Domschke, W.; Mitznegg, P.; Ruppin, H.; Demling, L. Measurement of gut hormonal peptides in biopsies from human stomach and proximal small intestine. *Gut* **1983**, *24*, 114–119. [CrossRef]
22. Buchan, A.M.J.; Polak, J.M.; Capella, C.; Solcia, E.; Pearse, A.G.E. Electronimmunocytochemical evidence for the K cell localization of gastric inhibitory polypeptide (GIP) im man. *Histochem. Cell Biol.* **1978**, *56*, 37–44. [CrossRef] [PubMed]
23. Eissele, R.; Göke, R.; Willemer, S.; Harthus, H.-P.; Vermeer, H.; Arnold, R.; Göke, B. Glucagon-like peptide-1 cells in the gastrointestinal tract and pancreas of rat, pig and man. *Eur. J. Clin. Investig.* **1992**, *22*, 283–291. [CrossRef] [PubMed]
24. Meyer, J.H.; Hlinka, M.; Tabrizi, Y.; Dimaso, N.; Raybould, H.E. Chemical specificities and intestinal distributions of nutrient-driven satiety. *Am. J. Physiol. Integr. Comp. Physiol.* **1998**, *275*, R1293–R1307. [CrossRef] [PubMed]
25. Abbott, C.R.; Monteiro, M.; Small, C.J.; Sajedi, A.; Smith, K.L.; Parkinson, J.R.; Ghatei, M.A.; Bloom, S.R. The inhibitory effects of peripheral administration of peptide YY3–36 and glucagon-like peptide-1 on food intake are attenuated by ablation of the vagal–brainstem–hypothalamic pathway. *Brain Res.* **2005**, *1044*, 127–131. [CrossRef] [PubMed]

26. Walls, E.K.; Phillips, R.J.; Wang, F.B.; Holst, M.C.; Powley, T.L. Suppression of meal size by intestinal nutrients is eliminated by celiac vagal deafferentation. *Am. J. Physiol. Integr. Comp. Physiol.* **1995**, *269*, R1410–R1419. [CrossRef] [PubMed]
27. Cummings, J.H.; Pomare, E.W.; Branch, W.J.; Naylor, C.P.; Macfarlane, G.T. Short chain fatty acids in human large intestine, portal, hepatic and venous blood. *Gut* **1987**, *28*, 1221–1227. [CrossRef]
28. Panaro, B.L.; Yusta, B.; Matthews, D.; Koehler, J.A.; Song, Y.; Sandoval, D.A.; Drucker, D.J. Intestine-selective reduction of Gcg expression reveals the importance of the distal gut for GLP-1 secretion. *Mol. Metab.* **2020**, *37*, 100990. [CrossRef]
29. Buffa, R.; Solcia, E.; Go, V.L.W. Immunohistochemical identification of the cholecystokinin cell in the intestinal mucosa. *Gastroenterology* **1976**, *70*, 528–532. [CrossRef]
30. Hökfelt, T.; Herrera-Marschitz, M.; Seroogy, K.; Ju, G.; A Staines, W.; Holets, V.; Schalling, M.; Ungerstedt, U.; Post, C.; Rehfeld, J.F.; et al. Immunohistochemical studies on cholecystokinin (CCK)-immunoreactive neurons in the rat using sequence specific antisera and with special reference to the caudate nucleus and primary sensory neurons. *J. Chem. Neuroanat.* **1988**, *1*, 11–51.
31. Rehfeld, J. Immunochemical studies on cholecystokinin. II: Distribution and molecular heterogeneity in the central nervous system and small intestine of man and hog. *J. Biol. Chem.* **1978**, *253*, 4022–4030. [CrossRef]
32. Kerstens, P.; Lamers, C.; Jansen, J.; De Jong, A.; Hessels, M.; Hafkenscheid, J. Physiological plasma concentrations of cholecystokinin stimulate pancreatic enzyme secretion and gallbladder contraction in man. *Life Sci.* **1985**, *36*, 565–569. [CrossRef]
33. Gibbs, J.; Smith, G.P. Cholecystokinin and satiety in rats and rhesus monkeys. *Am. J. Clin. Nutr.* **1977**, *30*, 758–761. [CrossRef] [PubMed]
34. Gibbs, J.; Young, R.C.; Smith, G.P. Cholecystokinin decreases food intake in rats. *J. Comp. Physiol. Psychol.* **1973**, *84*, 488–495. [CrossRef]
35. Saito, A.; Williams, J.A.; Goldfine, I.D. Alterations in brain cholecystokinin receptors after fasting. *Nat. Cell Biol.* **1981**, *289*, 599–600. [CrossRef]
36. Little, T.J.; Horowitz, M.; Feinle-Bisset, C. Role of cholecystokinin in appetite control and body weight regulation. *Obes. Rev.* **2005**, *6*, 297–306. [CrossRef] [PubMed]
37. Sykaras, A.G.; Demenis, C.; Cheng, L.; Pisitkun, T.; McLaughlin, J.T.; Fenton, R.A.; Smith, C.P. Duodenal CCK cells from male mice express multiple hormones including ghrelin. *Endocrinology* **2014**, *155*, 3339–3351. [CrossRef] [PubMed]
38. Roth, K.A.; Kim, S.; Gordon, J.I. Immunocytochemical studies suggest two pathways for enteroendocrine cell differentiation in the colon. *Am. J. Physiol. Liver Physiol.* **1992**, *263*, G174–G180. [CrossRef]
39. Gerspach, A.C.; Steinert, R.E.; Schönenberger, L.; Graber-Maier, A.; Beglinger, C. The role of the gut sweet taste receptor in regulating GLP-1, PYY, and CCK release in humans. *Am. J. Physiol. Metab.* **2011**, *301*, E317–E325. [CrossRef]
40. Hopman, W.P.M.; Jansen, J.B.M.J.; Lamers, C.B.H.W. Comparative Study of the effects of equal amounts of fat, protein, and starch on plasma cholecystokinin in man. *Scand. J. Gastroenterol.* **1985**, *20*, 843–847. [CrossRef]
41. Liddle, R.A.; Goldfine, I.D.; Rosen, M.S.; Taplitz, R.A.; Williams, J.A. Cholecystokinin bioactivity in human plasma. Molecular forms, responses to feeding, and relationship to gallbladder contraction. *J. Clin. Investig.* **1985**, *75*, 1144–1152. [CrossRef]
42. Fothergill, L.J.; Callaghan, B.; Hunne, B.; Bravo, D.M.; Furness, J.B. Costorage of enteroendocrine hormones evaluated at the cell and subcellular levels in male mice. *Endocrinology* **2017**, *158*, 2113–2123. [CrossRef]
43. Rindi, G.; Ratineau, C.; Ronco, A.; E Candusso, M.; Tsai, M.; Leiter, A.B. Targeted ablation of secretin-producing cells in transgenic mice reveals a common differentiation pathway with multiple enteroendocrine cell lineages in the small intestine. *Development* **1999**, *126*, 4149–4156.
44. Beumer, J.; Artegiani, B.; Post, Y.; Reimann, F.; Gribble, F.; Nguyen, T.N.; Zeng, H.; Born, M.V.D.; Van Es, J.H.; Clevers, H.; et al. Enteroendocrine cells switch hormone expression along the crypt-to-villus BMP signalling gradient. *Nat. Cell Biol.* **2018**, *20*, 909–916. [CrossRef]
45. Afroze, S.; Meng, F.; Jensen, K.; McDaniel, K.; Rahal, K.; Onori, P.; Gaudio, E.; Alpini, G.; Glaser, S.S. The physiological roles of secretin and its receptor. *Ann. Transl. Med.* **2013**, *1*, 29. [PubMed]
46. Cheng, C.Y.Y.; Chu, J.Y.S.; Chow, B.K.C. Central and peripheral administration of secretin inhibits food intake in mice through the activation of the melanocortin system. *Neuropsychopharmacology* **2010**, *36*, 459–471. [CrossRef] [PubMed]
47. Motojima, Y.; Kawasaki, M.; Matsuura, T.; Saito, R.; Yoshimura, M.; Hashimoto, H.; Ueno, H.; Maruyama, T.; Suzuki, H.; Ohnishi, H.; et al. Effects of peripherally administered cholecystokinin-8 and secretin on feeding/drinking and oxytocin-mRFP1 fluorescence in transgenic rats. *Neurosci. Res.* **2016**, *109*, 63–69. [CrossRef] [PubMed]
48. Chu, J.Y.S.; Cheng, C.Y.Y.; Sekar, R.; Chow, B.K.C. Vagal afferent mediates the anorectic effect of peripheral secretin. *PLoS ONE* **2013**, *8*, e64859. [CrossRef]
49. Lopez, M.J.; Upchurch, B.H.; Rindi, G.; Leiter, A.B. Studies in Transgenic mice reveal potential relationships between secretin-producing cells and other endocrine cell types. *J. Biol. Chem.* **1995**, *270*, 885–891. [CrossRef] [PubMed]
50. Feurle, G.; Hamscher, G.; Kusiek, R.; Meyer, H.; Metzger, J. Identification of xenin, a xenopsin-related peptide, in the human gastric mucosa and its effect on exocrine pancreatic secretion. *J. Biol. Chem.* **1992**, *267*, 22305–22309. [CrossRef]
51. Anlauf, M.; Weihe, E.; Hartschuh, W.; Hamscher, G.; Feurle, G.E. Localization of xenin-immunoreactive cells in the duodenal mucosa of humans and various mammals. *J. Histochem. Cytochem.* **2000**, *48*, 1617–1626. [CrossRef] [PubMed]
52. Feurle, G. Xenin—A review. *Peptides* **1998**, *19*, 609–615. [CrossRef]

53. Feurle, G.E.; Ikonomu, S.; Partoulas, G.; Stoschus, B.; Hamscher, G. Xenin plasma concentrations during modified sham feeding and during meals of different composition demonstrated by radioimmunoassay and chromatography. *Regul. Pept.* **2003**, *111*, 153–159. [CrossRef]
54. Wice, B.M.; Wang, S.; Crimmins, D.L.; Diggs-Andrews, K.A.; Althage, M.C.; Ford, E.L.; Tran, H.; Ohlendorf, M.; Griest, T.A.; Wang, Q.; et al. Xenin-25 potentiates glucose-dependent insulinotropic polypeptide action via a novel cholinergic relay mechanism. *J. Biol. Chem.* **2010**, *285*, 19842–19853. [CrossRef]
55. Feurle, G.E.; Heger, M.; Niebergall-Roth, E.; Teyssen, S.; Fried, M.; Eberle, C.; Singer, M.V.; Hamscher, G. Gastroenteropancreatic effects of xenin in the dog. *J. Pept. Res.* **2009**, *49*, 324–330. [CrossRef] [PubMed]
56. Feurle, G.E.; Pfeiffer, A.; Schmidt, T.; Dominguez-Munoz, E.; Malfertheiner, P.; Hamscher, G. Phase III of the migrating motor complex: Associated with endogenous xenin plasma peaks and induced by exogenous xenin. *Neurogastroenterol. Motil.* **2001**, *13*, 237–246. [CrossRef]
57. Cooke, J.H.; Patterson, M.; Patel, S.R.; Smith, K.L.; Ghatei, M.A.; Bloom, S.R.; Murphy, K.G. Peripheral and central administration of xenin and neurotensin suppress food intake in rodents. *Obesity* **2009**, *17*, 1135–1143. [CrossRef]
58. Kim, E.R.; Mizuno, T.M. Role of neurotensin receptor 1 in the regulation of food intake by neuromedins and neuromedin-related peptides. *Neurosci. Lett.* **2010**, *468*, 64–67. [CrossRef]
59. Dakka, T.; Cuber, J.C.; Chayvialle, J.A. Functional coupling between the active transport of glucose and the secretion of intestinal neurotensin in rats. *J. Physiol.* **1993**, *469*, 753–765. [CrossRef]
60. Kuhre, R.E.; Gribble, F.M.; Hartmann, B.; Reimann, F.; Windeløv, J.A.; Rehfeld, J.F.; Holst, J.J. Fructose stimulates GLP-1 but not GIP secretion in mice, rats, and humans. *Am. J. Physiol. Liver Physiol.* **2014**, *306*, G622–G630. [CrossRef] [PubMed]
61. Walker, J.P.; Fujimura, M.; Sakamoto, Y.; Greeley, G.H.; Townsend, C.M.; Thompson, J.C. Importance of the ileum in neurotensin released by fat. *Surgery* **1985**, *98*, 224–229.
62. Hawkins, M.F. Central nervous system neurotensin and feeding. *Physiol. Behav.* **1986**, *36*, 1–8. [CrossRef]
63. Luttinger, D.; King, R.A.; Sheppard, D.; Strupp, J.; Nemeroff, C.B.; Prange, A.J. The effect of neurotensin on food consumption in the rat. *Eur. J. Pharm.* **1982**, *81*, 499–503. [CrossRef]
64. Remaury, A.; Vita, N.; Gendreau, S.; Jung, M.; Arnone, M.; Poncelet, M.; Culouscou, J.-M.; Le Fur, G.; Soubrié, P.; Caput, D.; et al. Targeted inactivation of the neurotensin type 1 receptor reveals its role in body temperature control and feeding behavior but not in analgesia. *Brain Res.* **2002**, *953*, 63–72. [CrossRef]
65. Polak, J.M.; Sullivan, S.N.; Bloom, S.R.; Buchan, A.M.J.; Facer, P.; Brown, M.R.; Pearse, A.G.E. Specific localisation of neurotensin to the N cell in human intestine by radioimmunoassay and immunocytochemistry. *Nat. Cell Biol.* **1977**, *270*, 183–184. [CrossRef] [PubMed]
66. Grunddal, K.V.; Ratner, C.F.; Svendsen, B.; Sommer, F.; Engelstoft, M.S.; Madsen, A.N.; Pedersen, J.; Nøhr, M.K.; Egerod, K.L.; Nawrocki, A.R.; et al. Neurotensin is coexpressed, coreleased, and acts together with GLP-1 and PYY in enteroendocrine control of metabolism. *Endocrinology* **2016**, *157*, 176–194. [CrossRef] [PubMed]
67. Pocai, A.; Carrington, P.E.; Adams, J.R.; Wright, M.; Eiermann, G.; Zhu, L.; Du, X.; Petrov, A.; Lassman, M.E.; Jiang, G.; et al. Glucagon-like peptide 1/glucagon receptor dual agonism reverses obesity in mice. *Diabetes* **2009**, *58*, 2258–2266. [CrossRef] [PubMed]
68. Dakin, C.L.; Gunn, I.; Small, C.J.; Edwards, C.M.B.; Hay, D.L.; Smith, D.M.; Ghatei, M.A.; Bloom, S.R. Oxyntomodulin inhibits food intake in the rat. *Endocrinology* **2001**, *142*, 4244–4250. [CrossRef]
69. Dakin, C.L.; Small, C.J.; Batterham, R.L.; Neary, N.M.; Cohen, M.A.; Patterson, M.; Ghatei, M.A.; Bloom, S.R. Peripheral oxyntomodulin reduces food intake and body weight gain in rats. *Endocrinology* **2004**, *145*, 2687–2695. [CrossRef]
70. Kosinski, J.R.; Hubert, J.; Carrington, P.E.; Chicchi, G.G.; Mu, J.; Miller, C.; Cao, J.; Bianchi, E.; Pessi, A.; Sinharoy, R.; et al. The glucagon receptor is involved in mediating the body weight-lowering effects of oxyntomodulin. *Obesity* **2012**, *20*, 1566–1571. [CrossRef]
71. Cohen, M.A.; Ellis, S.M.; Le Roux, C.W.; Batterham, R.L.; Park, A.; Patterson, M.M.; Frost, G.S.; Ghatei, M.A.; Bloom, S.R. Oxyntomodulin suppresses appetite and reduces food intake in humans. *J. Clin. Endocrinol. Metab.* **2003**, *88*, 4696–4701. [CrossRef]
72. Parker, V.E.R.; Robertson, D.; Wang, T.; Hornigold, D.C.; Petrone, M.; Cooper, A.T.; Posch, M.G.; Heise, T.; Plum-Moerschel, L.; Schlichthaar, H.; et al. Efficacy, safety, and mechanistic insights of cotadutide, a dual receptor glucagon-like peptide-1 and glucagon agonist. *J. Clin. Endocrinol. Metab.* **2019**, *105*, 803–820. [CrossRef] [PubMed]
73. Adrian, T.; Ferri, G.-L.; Bacarese-Hamilton, A.; Fuessl, H.; Polak, J.; Bloom, S. Human distribution and release of a putative new gut hormone, peptide YY. *Gastroenterology* **1985**, *89*, 1070–1077. [CrossRef]
74. Billing, L.J.; Smith, C.A.; Larraufie, P.; Goldspink, D.A.; Galvin, S.; Kay, R.G.; Howe, J.D.; Walker, R.; Pruna, M.; Glass, L.; et al. Co-storage and release of insulin-like peptide-5, glucagon-like peptide-1 and peptide YY from murine and human colonic enteroendocrine cells. *Mol. Metab.* **2018**, *16*, 65–75. [CrossRef] [PubMed]
75. Pedersen-Bjergaard, U.; Høt, U.; Kelbæk, H.; Schifter, S.; Rehfeld, J.F.; Faber, J.; Christensen, N.J. Influence of meal composition on postprandial peripheral plasma concentrations of vasoactive peptides in man. *Scand. J. Clin. Lab. Investig.* **1996**, *56*, 497–503. [CrossRef]
76. Batterham, R.L.; Cowley, M.A.; Small, C.J.; Herzog, H.; Cohen, M.A.; Dakin, C.L.; Wren, A.M.; Brynes, A.E.; Low, M.J.; Ghatei, M.A.; et al. Gut hormone PYY3–36 physiologically inhibits food intake. *Nat. Cell Biol.* **2002**, *418*, 650–654. [CrossRef]

77. Halatchev, I.G.; Ellacott, K.L.J.; Fan, W.; Cone, R.D. Peptide YY3–36Inhibits food intake in mice through a melanocortin-4 Receptor-independent mechanism. *Endocrinology* **2004**, *145*, 2585–2590. [CrossRef]
78. Lewis, J.E.; Miedzybrodzka, E.L.; Foreman, R.E.; Woodward, O.R.M.; Kay, R.G.; Goldspink, D.A.; Gribble, F.M.; Reimann, F. Selective stimulation of colonic L cells improves metabolic outcomes in mice. *Diabetologia* **2020**, *63*, 1396–1407. [CrossRef]
79. Babu, M.; Purhonen, A.; Bansiewicz, T.; Mäkelä, K.; Walkowiak, J.; Miettinen, P.; Herzig, K. Effect of total colectomy and PYY infusion on food intake and body weight in rats. *Regul. Pept.* **2005**, *131*, 29–33. [CrossRef] [PubMed]
80. Boggiano, M.M.; Chandler, P.C.; Oswald, K.D.; Rodgers, R.J.; Blundell, J.E.; Ishii, Y.; Beattie, A.H.; Holch, P.; Allison, D.B.; Schindler, M.; et al. PYY3–36 as an anti-obesity drug target. *Obes. Rev.* **2005**, *6*, 307–322. [CrossRef]
81. Tschöp, M.; Castañeda, T.R.; Joost, H.G.; Thöne-Reineke, C.; Ortmann, S.; Klaus, S.; Hagan, M.M.; Chandler, P.C.; Oswald, K.D.; Benoit, S.C.; et al. Does gut hormone PYY3–36 decrease food intake in rodents? *Nat. Cell Biol.* **2004**, *430*, 1–3. [CrossRef]
82. Fu-Cheng, X.; Anini, Y.; Chariot, J.; Castex, N.; Galmiche, J.-P.; Rozé, C. Mechanisms of peptide YY release induced by an intraduodenal meal in rats: Neural regulation by proximal gut. *Pflügers Arch.* **1997**, *433*, 571–579. [CrossRef]
83. Koda, S.; Date, Y.; Murakami, N.; Shimbara, T.; Hanada, T.; Toshinai, K.; Niijima, A.; Furuya, M.; Inomata, N.; Osuye, K.; et al. The role of the vagal nerve in peripheral PYY3–36-induced feeding reduction in rats. *Endocrinology* **2005**, *146*, 2369–2375. [CrossRef]
84. Yang, H.; Tache, Y. PYY in brain stem nuclei induces vagal stimulation of gastric acid secretion in rats. *Am. J. Physiol. Liver Physiol.* **1995**, *268*, G943–G948. [CrossRef]
85. Zeng, N.; Walsh, J.; Kang, T.; Wu, S.; Sachs, G. Peptide YY inhibition of rat gastric enterochromaffin-like cell function. *Gastroenterology* **1997**, *112*, 127–135. [CrossRef]
86. Lin, H.C.; Zhao, X.T.; Wang, L.; Wong, H. Fat-induced ileal brake in the dog depends on peptide YY. *Gastroenterology* **1996**, *110*, 1491–1495. [CrossRef] [PubMed]
87. Savage, A.P.; E Adrian, T.; Carolan, G.; Chatterjee, V.K.; Bloom, S.R. Effects of peptide YY (PYY) on mouth to caecum intestinal transit time and on the rate of gastric emptying in healthy volunteers. *Gut* **1987**, *28*, 166–170. [CrossRef]
88. Wiley, J.W.; Lu, Y.; Owyang, C. Mechanism of action of peptide YY to inhibit gastric motility. *Gastroenterology* **1991**, *100*, 865–872. [CrossRef]
89. Grosse, J.; Heffron, H.; Burling, K.; Hossain, M.A.; Habib, A.M.; Rogers, G.J.; Richards, P.; Larder, R.; Rimmington, D.; Adriaenssens, A.A.; et al. Insulin-like peptide 5 is an orexigenic gastrointestinal hormone. *Proc. Natl. Acad. Sci. USA* **2014**, *111*, 11133–11138. [CrossRef]
90. Lee, Y.S.; De Vadder, F.; Tremaroli, V.; Wichmann, A.; Mithieux, G.; Bäckhed, F. Insulin-like peptide 5 is a microbially regulated peptide that promotes hepatic glucose production. *Mol. Metab.* **2016**, *5*, 263–270. [CrossRef]
91. Drucker, D.J.; Jin, T.; Asa, S.L.; Young, T.A.; Brubaker, P.L. Activation of proglucagon gene transcription by protein kinase—A in a novel mouse enteroendocrine cell line. *Mol. Endocrinol.* **1994**, *8*, 1646–1655. [CrossRef] [PubMed]
92. De Bruïne, A.P.; Dinjens, W.N.M.; Pijls, M.M.J.; Linden, E.P.M.V.D.; Rousch, M.J.M.; Moerkerk, P.T.; De Goeij, A.F.P.M.; Bosnian, F.T. NCI-H716 cells as a model for endocrine differentiation in colorectal cancer. *Virchows Arch. B* **1992**, *62*, 311–320. [CrossRef]
93. Park, J.G.; Oie, H.K.; Sugarbaker, P.H.; Henslee, J.G.; Chen, T.R.; Johnson, B.E.; Gazdar, A. Characteristics of cell lines estab-lished from human colorectal carcinoma. *Cancer Res.* **1987**, *47*, 6710–6718. [PubMed]
94. Brubaker, P.L.; Schloos, J.; Drucker, D.J. Regulation of glucagon-like peptide-1 synthesis and secretion in the GLUTag Enteroendocrine cell line. *Endocrinology* **1998**, *139*, 4108–4114. [CrossRef] [PubMed]
95. Reimer, R.A.; Darimont, C.; Gremlich, S.; Nicolas-Métral, V.; Rüegg, U.T.; Macé, K. A human cellular model for studying the regulation of glucagon-like peptide-1 secretion. *Endocrinology* **2001**, *142*, 4522–4528. [CrossRef]
96. Cao, X.; Flock, G.; Choi, C.; Irwin, D.M.; Drucker, D.J. Aberrant regulation of human intestinal proglucagon gene expression in the NCI-H716 cell line. *Endocrinology* **2003**, *144*, 2025–2033. [CrossRef] [PubMed]
97. Rindi, G.; Grant, S.G.; Yiangou, Y.; Ghatei, M.A.; Bloom, S.R.; Bautch, V.L.; Solcia, E.; Polak, J.M. Development of neuroen-docrine tumors in the gastrointestinal tract of transgenic mice. Heterogeneity of hormone expression. *Am. J. Pathol.* **1990**, *136*, 1349–1363.
98. Cheung, A.T.; Dayanandan, B.; Lewis, J.T.; Korbutt, G.S.; Rajotte, R.V.; Bryer-Ash, M.; Boylan, M.O.; Wolfe, M.M.; Kieffer, T.J. Glucose-dependent insulin release from genetically engineered K cells. *Science* **2000**, *290*, 1959–1962. [CrossRef] [PubMed]
99. Kieffer, T.J.; Huang, Z.; McIntosh, C.H.; Buchan, A.M.; Brown, J.C.; Pederson, R.A. Gastric inhibitory polypeptide release from a tumor-derived cell line. *Am. J. Physiol. Metab.* **1995**, *269*, E316–E322. [CrossRef]
100. Ramshur, E.B.; Rull, T.R.; Wice, B.M. Novel insulin/GIP co-producing cell lines provide unexpected insights into Gut K-cell function In Vivo. *J. Cell. Physiol.* **2002**, *192*, 339–350. [CrossRef]
101. Aponte, G.W.; Taylor, I.L.; Soll, A.H. Primary culture of PYY cells from canine colon. *Am. J. Physiol. Liver Physiol.* **1988**, *254*, G829–G836. [CrossRef]
102. Kieffer, T.J.; Buchan, A.M.; Barker, H.; Brown, J.C.; Pederson, R.A. Release of gastric inhibitory polypeptide from cultured canine endocrine cells. *Am. J. Physiol. Metab.* **1994**, *267*, E489–E496. [CrossRef] [PubMed]
103. Brubaker, P.L.; Vranic, M. Fetal rat intestinal cells in monolayer culture: A new In Vitro System to study the glucagon-like immunoreactive peptides. *Endocrinology* **1987**, *120*, 1976–1985. [CrossRef] [PubMed]
104. Reimann, F.; Habib, A.M.; Tolhurst, G.; Parker, H.E.; Rogers, G.J.; Gribble, F.M. Glucose sensing in L cells: A primary cell study. *Cell Metab.* **2008**, *8*, 532–539. [CrossRef] [PubMed]
105. Habib, A.M.; Richards, P.; Rogers, G.J.; Reimann, F.; Gribble, F.M. Co-localisation and secretion of glucagon-like peptide 1 and peptide YY from primary cultured human L cells. *Diabetologia* **2013**, *56*, 1413–1416. [CrossRef] [PubMed]

106. Parker, H.E.; Habib, A.M.; Rogers, G.J.; Gribble, F.M.; Reimann, F. Nutrient-dependent secretion of glucose-dependent insulinotropic polypeptide from primary murine K cells. *Diabetologia* **2009**, *52*, 289–298. [CrossRef] [PubMed]
107. Sato, T.; Vries, R.G.; Snippert, H.J.; Van De Wetering, M.; Barker, N.; Stange, D.E.; Van Es, J.H.; Abo, A.; Kujala, P.; Peters, P.J.; et al. Single Lgr5 stem cells build crypt-villus structures In Vitro without a mesenchymal niche. *Nature* **2009**, *459*, 262–265. [CrossRef] [PubMed]
108. Goldspink, D.A.; Lu, V.B.; Billing, L.J.; Larraufie, P.; Tolhurst, G.; Gribble, F.M.; Reimann, F. Mechanistic insights into the detection of free fatty and bile acids by ileal glucagon-like peptide-1 secreting cells. *Mol. Metab.* **2018**, *7*, 90–101. [CrossRef]
109. Beumer, J.; Puschhof, J.; -Martinez, J.B.; Martínez-Silgado, A.; Elmentaite, R.; James, K.R.; Ross, A.; Hendriks, D.; Artegiani, B.; Busslinger, G.A.; et al. High-resolution mRNA and secretome atlas of human enteroendocrine cells. *Cell* **2020**, *182*, 1062–1064. [CrossRef]
110. Goldspink, D.A.; Lu, V.B.; Miedzybrodzka, E.L.; Smith, C.A.; Foreman, R.E.; Billing, L.J.; Kay, R.G.; Reimann, F.; Gribble, F.M. Labeling and characterization of human GLP-1-secreting L-cells in primary ileal organoid culture. *Cell Rep.* **2020**, *31*, 107833. [CrossRef]
111. Ussing, H.H.; Zerahn, K. Active transport of sodium as the source of electric current in the short-circuited isolated frog skin. *Acta Physiol. Scand.* **1951**, *23*, 110–127. [CrossRef]
112. Brighton, C.A.; Rievaj, J.; Kuhre, R.E.; Glass, L.L.; Schoonjans, K.; Holst, J.J.; Gribble, F.M.; Reimann, F. Bile acids trigger GLP-1 release predominantly by accessing basolaterally located G protein—coupled bile acid receptors. *Endocrinology* **2015**, *156*, 3961–3970. [CrossRef]
113. Joshi, S.; Tough, I.R.; Cox, H.M. Endogenous PYY and GLP-1 mediatel-glutamine responses in intestinal mucosa. *Br. J. Pharm.* **2013**, *170*, 1092–1101. [CrossRef] [PubMed]
114. Wen, J.; Phillips, S.F.; Sarr, M.G.; Kost, L.J.; Holst, J.J. PYY and GLP-1 contribute to feedback inhibition from the canine ileum and colon. *Am. J. Physiol. Liver Physiol.* **1995**, *269*, G945–G952. [CrossRef]
115. Ritzel, U.; Fromme, A.; Ottleben, M.; Leonhardt, U.; Ramadori, G. Release of glucagon-like peptide-1 (GLP-1) by carbohydrates in the perfused rat ileum. *Acta Diabetol.* **1997**, *34*, 18–21. [CrossRef]
116. Cook, C.G.; Andrews, J.M.; Jones, K.L.; Wittert, G.A.; Chapman, I.M.; Morley, J.E.; Horowitz, M. Effects of small intestinal nutrient infusion on appetite and pyloric motility are modified by age. *Am. J. Physiol. Content* **1997**, *273*, R755–R761. [CrossRef]
117. Lavin, J.H.; Wittert, G.A.; Andrews, J.; Yeap, B.; Wishart, J.M.; Morris, H.A.; Morley, J.E.; Horowitz, M.; Read, N.W. Interaction of insulin, glucagon-like peptide 1, gastric inhibitory polypeptide, and appetite in response to intraduodenal carbohydrate. *Am. J. Clin. Nutr.* **1998**, *68*, 591–598. [CrossRef]
118. Elliott, R.M.; Morgan, L.M.; Tredger, J.A.; Deacon, S.; Wright, J.; Marks, V. Glucagon-like peptide-1(7–36) amide and glucose-dependent insulinotropic polypeptide secretion in response to nutrient ingestion in man: Acute post-prandial and 24-h secretion patterns. *J. Endocrinol.* **1993**, *138*, 159–166. [CrossRef]
119. Herman, G.A.; Bergman, A.; Stevens, C.; Kotey, P.; Yi, B.; Zhao, P.; Dietrich, B.; Golor, G.; Schrodter, A.; Keymeulen, B.; et al. Effect of single oral doses of sitagliptin, a dipeptidyl peptidase-4 inhibitor, on incretin and plasma glucose levels after an oral glucose tolerance test in patients with Type 2 diabetes. *J. Clin. Endocrinol. Metab.* **2006**, *91*, 4612–4619. [CrossRef]
120. Schirra, J.; Katschinski, M.; Weidmann, C.; Schäfer, T.; Wank, U.; Arnold, R.; Göke, B. Gastric emptying and release of incretin hormones after glucose ingestion in humans. *J. Clin. Investig.* **1996**, *97*, 92–103. [CrossRef] [PubMed]
121. Ferraris, R.P.; Yasharpour, S.; Lloyd, K.C.; Mirzayan, R.; Diamond, J.M. Luminal glucose concentrations in the gut under normal conditions. *Am. J. Physiol. Liver Physiol.* **1990**, *259*, G822–G837. [CrossRef]
122. Stephen, A.M.; Haddad, A.C.; Phillips, S.F. Passage of carbohydrate into the colon. Direct measurements in humans. *Gastroenterology* **1983**, *85*, 589–595. [CrossRef]
123. Sun, E.W.; De Fontgalland, D.; Rabbitt, P.; Hollington, P.; Sposato, L.; Due, S.L.; Wattchow, D.A.; Rayner, C.K.; Deane, A.M.; Young, R.L.; et al. Mechanisms controlling glucose-induced GLP-1 secretion in human small intestine. *Diabetes* **2017**, *66*, 2144–2149. [CrossRef]
124. Nauck, M.A.; Siemsgluss, J.; Orskov, C.; Holst, J.J. Release of glucagon-like peptide 1 (GLP-1 [7–36 amide]), gastric inhibi-tory polypeptide (GIP) and insulin in response to oral glucose after upper and lower intestinal resections. *Zeitschrift Gastroenterologie* **1996**, *34*, 159–166.
125. Yoshikawa, T.; Inoue, R.; Matsumoto, M.; Yajima, T.; Ushida, K.; Iwanaga, T. Comparative expression of hexose transporters (SGLT1, GLUT1, GLUT2 and GLUT5) throughout the mouse gastrointestinal tract. *Histochem. Cell Biol.* **2011**, *135*, 183–194. [CrossRef]
126. Yoshida, A.; Takata, K.; Kasahara, T.; Aoyagi, T.; Saito, S.; Hirano, H. Immunohistochemical localization of Na(+)-dependent glucose transporter in the rat digestive tract. *Histochem. J.* **1995**, *27*, 420–426. [CrossRef]
127. Hwang, E.-S.; Hirayama, B.A.; Wright, E.M. Distribution of the SGLT1 Na+glucose cotransporter and mRNA along the crypt-villus axis of rabbit small intestine. *Biochem. Biophys. Res. Commun.* **1991**, *181*, 1208–1217. [CrossRef]
128. Gribble, F.M.; Williams, L.; Simpson, A.K.; Reimann, F. A novel glucose-sensing mechanism contributing to glucagon-like peptide-1 secretion from the GLUTag cell line. *Diabetes* **2003**, *52*, 1147–1154. [CrossRef] [PubMed]
129. Díez-Sampedro, A.; Lostao, M.; Wright, E.; Hirayama, B. Glycoside binding and translocation in Na+-dependent glucose cotransporters: Comparison of SGLT1 and SGLT3. *J. Membr. Biol.* **2000**, *176*, 111–117. [CrossRef]

130. Landau, B.R.; Bernstein, L.; Wilson, T.H. Hexose transport by hamster intestine in vitro. *Am. J. Physiol. Content* **1962**, *203*, 237–240. [CrossRef] [PubMed]
131. Csáky, T.Z.; Glenn, J.E. Urinary recovery of 3-methylglucose administered to rats. *Am. J. Physiol. Content* **1956**, *188*, 159–162. [CrossRef]
132. Sykes, S.; Morgan, L.M.; English, J.; Marks, V. Evidence for preferential stimulation of gastric inhibitory polypeptide secretion in the rat by actively transported carbohydrates and their analogues. *J. Endocrinol.* **1980**, *85*, 201–207. [CrossRef]
133. Gorboulev, V.; Schürmann, A.; Vallon, V.; Kipp, H.; Jaschke, A.; Klessen, D.; Friedrich, A.; Scherneck, S.; Rieg, T.; Cunard, R.; et al. Na+-D-glucose cotransporter SGLT1 is pivotal for intestinal glucose absorption and glucose-dependent incretin secretion. *Diabetes* **2011**, *61*, 187–196. [CrossRef]
134. Powell, D.R.; Smith, M.; Greer, J.; Harris, A.; Zhao, S.; Dacosta, C.; Mseeh, F.; Shadoan, M.K.; Sands, A.; Zambrowicz, B.; et al. LX4211 increases serum glucagon-like peptide 1 and peptide YY levels by reducing sodium/glucose cotransporter 1 (SGLT1)–mediated absorption of intestinal glucose. *J. Pharm. Exp.* **2013**, *345*, 250–259. [CrossRef]
135. Díez-Sampedro, A.; Hirayama, B.A.; Osswald, C.; Gorboulev, V.; Baumgarten, K.; Volk, C.; Wright, E.M.; Koepsell, H. A glucose sensor hiding in a family of transporters. *Proc. Natl. Acad. Sci. USA* **2003**, *100*, 11753–11758. [CrossRef]
136. Kellett, G.L.; Helliwell, P.A. The diffusive component of intestinal glucose absorption is mediated by the glucose-induced recruitment of GLUT2 to the brush-border membrane. *Biochem. J.* **2000**, *350*, 155–162. [CrossRef]
137. Affleck, J.A.; Helliwell, P.A.; Kellett, G.L. Immunocytochemical detection of GLUT2 at the rat intestinal brush-border membrane. *J. Histochem. Cytochem.* **2003**, *51*, 1567–1574. [CrossRef]
138. Scow, J.S.; Iqbal, C.W.; Jones, T.W.; Qandeel, H.G.; Zheng, Y.; Duenes, J.A.; Nagao, M.; Madhavan, S.; Sarr, M.G.; Madhaven, S.; et al. Absence of evidence of translocation of GLUT2 to the apical membrane of enterocytes in everted intestinal sleeves. *J. Surg. Res.* **2011**, *167*, 56–61. [CrossRef] [PubMed]
139. Röder, P.V.; Geillinger, K.E.; Zietek, T.S.; Thorens, B.; Koepsell, H.; Daniel, H. The role of SGLT1 and GLUT2 in intestinal glucose transport and sensing. *PLoS ONE* **2014**, *9*, e89977. [CrossRef]
140. Parker, H.E.; Adriaenssens, A.; Rogers, G.; Richards, P.; Koepsell, H.; Reimann, F.; Gribble, F.M. Predominant role of active versus facilitative glucose transport for glucagon-like peptide-1 secretion. *Diabetologia* **2012**, *55*, 2445–2455. [CrossRef]
141. Jetton, T.L.; Liang, Y.; Pettepher, C.C.; Zimmerman, E.C.; Cox, F.G.; Horvath, K.; Matschinsky, F.M.; Magnuson, M.A. Analysis of upstream glucokinase promoter activity in transgenic mice and identification of glucokinase in rare neuroen-docrine cells in the brain and gut. *J. Biol. Chem.* **1994**, *269*, 3641–3654. [CrossRef]
142. Murphy, R.; Tura, A.; Clark, P.M.; Holst, J.J.; Mari, A.; Hattersley, A.T. Glucokinase, the pancreatic glucose sensor, is not the gut glucose sensor. *Diabetologia* **2008**, *52*, 154–159. [CrossRef]
143. Rorsman, P. The pancreatic beta-cell as a fuel sensor: An electrophysiologist's viewpoint. *Diabetologia* **1997**, *40*, 487–495. [CrossRef] [PubMed]
144. Nielsen, L.B.; Ploug, K.B.; Swift, P.; Ørskov, C.; Jansen-Olesen, I.; Chiarelli, F.; Holst, J.J.; Hougaard, P.; Pörksen, S.; Holl, R.; et al. Co-localisation of the Kir6.2/SUR1 channel complex with glucagon-like peptide-1 and glucose-dependent insulinotrophic polypeptide expression in human ileal cells and implications for glycaemic control in new onset type 1 diabetes. *Eur. J. Endocrinol.* **2007**, *156*, 663–671. [CrossRef]
145. Reimann, F.; Gribble, F.M. Glucose-sensing in glucagon-like peptide-1-secreting cells. *Diabetes* **2002**, *51*, 2757–2763. [CrossRef] [PubMed]
146. Kuhre, R.E.; Frost, C.R.; Svendsen, B.; Holst, J.J. Molecular mechanisms of glucose-stimulated GLP-1 secretion from perfused rat small intestine. *Diabetes* **2014**, *64*, 370–382. [CrossRef] [PubMed]
147. Mangel, A.W.; Prpic, V.; Snow, N.D.; Basavappa, S.; Hurst, L.J.; Sharara, A.I.; Liddle, R.A. Regulation of cholecystokinin secretion by ATP-sensitive potassium channels. *Am. J. Physiol. Liver Physiol.* **1994**, *267*, G595–G600. [CrossRef] [PubMed]
148. Tsukiyama, K.; Yamada, Y.; Miyawaki, K.; Hamasaki, A.; Nagashima, K.; Hosokawa, M.; Fujimoto, S.; Takahashi, A.; Toyoda, K.; Toyokuni, S.; et al. Gastric inhibitory polypeptide is the major insulinotropic factor in K(ATP) null mice. *Eur. J. Endocrinol.* **2004**, *151*, 407–412. [CrossRef] [PubMed]
149. Stephens, J.; Bodvarsdottir, T.; Wareham, K.; Prior, S.; Bracken, R.; Lowe, G.; Rumley, A.; Dunseath, G.; Luzio, S.; Deacon, C.; et al. Effects of short-term therapy with glibenclamide and repaglinide on incretin hormones and oxidative damage associated with postprandial hyperglycaemia in people with type 2 diabetes mellitus. *Diabetes Res. Clin. Pract.* **2011**, *94*, 199–206. [CrossRef] [PubMed]
150. El-Ouaghlidi, A.; Rehring, E.; Holst, J.J.; Schweizer, A.; Foley, J.; Holmes, D.; Nauck, M.A. The dipeptidyl peptidase 4 inhibitor vildagliptin does not accentuate glibenclamide-induced hypoglycemia but reduces glucose-induced glucagon-like peptide 1 and gastric inhibitory polypeptide secretion. *J. Clin. Endocrinol. Metab.* **2007**, *92*, 4165–4171. [CrossRef]
151. Moran, T.H.; McHugh, P.R. Distinctions among three sugars in their effects on gastric emptying and satiety. *Am. J. Physiol. Integr. Comp. Physiol.* **1981**, *241*, R25–R30. [CrossRef] [PubMed]
152. Rayner, C.K.; Park, H.S.; Wishart, J.M.; Kong, M.-F.; Doran, S.M.; Horowitz, M. Effects of intraduodenal glucose and fructose on antropyloric motility and appetite in healthy humans. *Am. J. Physiol. Integr. Comp. Physiol.* **2000**, *278*, R360–R366. [CrossRef] [PubMed]
153. Kong, M.-F.; Chapman, I.; Goble, E.; Wishart, J.; Wittert, G.; Morris, H.; Horowitz, M. Effects of oral fructose and glucose on plasma GLP-1 and appetite in normal subjects. *Peptides* **1999**, *20*, 545–551. [CrossRef]

154. Shima, K.; Suda, T.; Nishimoto, K.; Yoshimoto, S. Relationship between molecular structures of sugars and their ability to stimulate the release of glucagon-like peptide-1 from canine ileal loops. *Eur. J. Endocrinol.* **1990**, *123*, 464–470. [CrossRef]
155. Burant, C.; Takeda, J.; Brot-Laroche, E.; Bell, G.; Davidson, N. Fructose transporter in human spermatozoa and small intestine is GLUT5. *J. Biol. Chem.* **1992**, *267*, 14523–14526. [CrossRef]
156. Rand, E.B.; De Paoli, A.M.; Davidson, N.O.; Bell, G.I.; Burant, C.F. Sequence, tissue distribution, and functional characterization of the rat fructose transporter Glutam. *J. Physiol. Liver Physiol.* **1993**, *264*, G1169–G1176. [CrossRef]
157. Seino, Y.; Ogata, H.; Maekawa, R.; Izumoto, T.; Iida, A.; Harada, N.; Miki, T.; Seino, S.; Inagaki, N.; Tsunekawa, S.; et al. Fructose induces glucose-dependent insulinotropic polypeptide, glucagon-like peptide-1 and insulin secretion: Role of adenosine triphosphate-sensitive K+channels. *J. Diabetes Investig.* **2015**, *6*, 522–526. [CrossRef]
158. Wong, G.T.; Gannon, K.S.; Margolskee, R.F. Transduction of bitter and sweet taste by gustducin. *Nat. Cell Biol.* **1996**, *381*, 796–800. [CrossRef] [PubMed]
159. Nelson, G.; Chandrashekar, J.; Hoon, M.A.; Feng, L.; Zhao, G.; Ryba, N.J.P.; Zuker, C.S. An amino-acid taste receptor. *Nat. Cell Biol.* **2002**, *416*, 199–202. [CrossRef]
160. Rozengurt, N.; Wu, S.V.; Chen, M.C.; Huang, C.; Sternini, C.; Rozengurt, E. Colocalization of the α-subunit of gustducin with PYY and GLP-1 in L cells of human colon. *Am. J. Physiol. Liver Physiol.* **2006**, *291*, G792–G802. [CrossRef]
161. Kokrashvili, Z.; Mosinger, B.; Margolskee, R.F. Taste signaling elements expressed in gut enteroendocrine cells regulate nutrient-responsive secretion of gut hormones. *Am. J. Clin. Nutr.* **2009**, *90*, 822S–825S. [CrossRef]
162. Jang, H.-J.; Kokrashvili, Z.; Theodorakis, M.J.; Carlson, O.D.; Kim, B.-J.; Zhou, J.; Kim, H.H.; Xu, X.; Chan, S.L.; Juhaszova, M.; et al. Gut-expressed gustducin and taste receptors regulate secretion of glucagon-like peptide-1. *Proc. Natl. Acad. Sci. USA* **2007**, *104*, 15069–15074. [CrossRef]
163. Fujita, Y.; Wideman, R.D.; Speck, M.; Asadi, A.; King, D.S.; Webber, T.D.; Haneda, M.; Kieffer, T.J. Incretin release from gut is acutely enhanced by sugar but not by sweeteners In Vivo. *Am. J. Physiol. Metab.* **2009**, *296*, E473–E479. [CrossRef] [PubMed]
164. Bezençon, C.; Le Coutre, J.; Damak, S. Taste-signaling proteins are coexpressed in solitary intestinal epithelial cells. *Chem. Senses* **2007**, *32*, 41–49. [CrossRef]
165. Margolskee, R.F.; Dyer, J.; Kokrashvili, Z.; Salmon, K.S.H.; Ilegems, E.; Daly, K.; Maillet, E.L.; Ninomiya, Y.; Mosinger, B.; Shirazi-Beechey, S.P. T1R3 and gustducin in gut sense sugars to regulate expression of Na+-glucose cotransporter. *Proc. Natl. Acad. Sci. USA* **2007**, *104*, 15075–15080. [CrossRef] [PubMed]
166. Ma, J.; Chang, J.; Checklin, H.L.; Young, R.L.; Jones, K.L.; Horowitz, M.; Rayner, C.K. Effect of the artificial sweetener, sucralose, on small intestinal glucose absorption in healthy human subjects. *Br. J. Nutr.* **2010**, *104*, 803–806. [CrossRef]
167. Saltiel, M.Y.; Kuhre, R.E.; Christiansen, C.B.; Eliasen, R.; Conde-Frieboes, K.W.; Rosenkilde, M.M.; Holst, J.J. Sweet taste receptor activation in the gut is of limited importance for glucose-stimulated GLP-1 and GIP secretion. *Nutrients* **2017**, *9*, 418. [CrossRef]
168. Thomas, F.; Sinar, D.; Mazzaferri, E.; Cataland, S.; Mekhjian, H.; Caldwell, J.; Fromkes, J. Selective release of gastric inhibitory polypeptide by intraduodenal amino acid perfusion in man. *Gastroenterology* **1978**, *74*, 1261–1265. [CrossRef]
169. Cordier-Bussat, M.; Bernard, C.; Levenez, F.; Klages, N.; Laser-Ritz, B.; Philippe, J.; Chayvialle, J.A.; Cuber, J.C. Peptones stimulate both the secretion of the incretin hormone glucagon-like peptide 1 and the transcription of the proglucagon gene. *Diabetes* **1998**, *47*, 1038–1045. [CrossRef]
170. Reimer, R.A. Meat hydrolysate and essential amino acid-induced glucagon-like peptide-1 secretion, in the human NCI-H716 enteroendocrine cell line, is regulated by extracellular signal-regulated kinase1/2 and p38 mitogen-activated protein kinases. *J. Endocrinol.* **2006**, *191*, 159–170. [CrossRef] [PubMed]
171. Diakogiannaki, E.; Pais, R.; Tolhurst, G.; Parker, H.E.; Horscroft, J.; Rauscher, B.; Zietek, T.; Daniel, H.; Gribble, F.M.; Reimann, F.; et al. Oligopeptides stimulate glucagon-like peptide-1 secretion in mice through proton-coupled uptake and the calcium-sensing receptor. *Diabetologia* **2013**, *56*, 2688–2696. [CrossRef]
172. Matsumura, K.; Miki, T.; Jhomori, T.; Gonoi, T.; Seino, S. Possible role of PEPT1 in gastrointestinal hormone secretion. *Biochem. Biophys. Res. Commun.* **2005**, *336*, 1028–1032. [CrossRef] [PubMed]
173. Jiang, Y.; Rose, A.J.; Sijmonsma, T.P.; Bröer, A.; Pfenninger, A.; Herzig, S.; Schmoll, D.; Bröer, S. Mice lacking neutral amino acid transporter B0AT1 (Slc6a19) have elevated levels of FGF21 and GLP-1 and improved glycaemic control. *Mol. Metab.* **2015**, *4*, 406–417. [CrossRef]
174. Pais, R.; Gribble, F.M.; Reimann, F. Signalling pathways involved in the detection of peptones by murine small intestinal enteroendocrine L-cells. *Peptides* **2016**, *77*, 9–15. [CrossRef] [PubMed]
175. Mace, O.J.; Schindler, M.; Patel, S. The regulation of K- and L-cell activity by GLUT2 and the calcium-sensing receptor CasR in rat small intestine. *J. Physiol.* **2012**, *590*, 2917–2936. [CrossRef]
176. Liou, A.P.; Sei, Y.; Zhao, X.; Feng, J.; Lu, X.; Thomas, C.; Pechhold, S.; Raybould, H.E.; Wank, S.A. The extracellular calcium-sensing receptor is required for cholecystokinin secretion in response to l-phenylalanine in acutely isolated intestinal I cells. *Am. J. Physiol. Liver Physiol.* **2011**, *300*, G538–G546. [CrossRef] [PubMed]
177. Rey, O.; Young, S.H.; Jacamo, R.; Moyer, M.P.; Rozengurt, E. Extracellular calcium sensing receptor stimulation in human colonic epithelial cells induces intracellular calcium oscillations and proliferation inhibition. *J. Cell. Physiol.* **2010**, *225*, 73–83. [CrossRef]
178. Modvig, I.M.; Kuhre, R.E.; Holst, J.J. Peptone-mediated glucagon-like peptide-1 secretion depends on intestinal absorption and activation of basolaterally located Calcium-sensing receptors. *Physiol. Rep.* **2019**, *7*, e14058. [CrossRef]

179. Choi, S.; Lee, M.; Shiu, A.L.; Yo, S.J.; Halldén, G.; Aponte, G.W. GPR93 activation by protein hydrolysate induces CCK transcription and secretion in STC-1 cells. *Am. J. Physiol. Liver Physiol.* **2007**, *292*, G1366–G1375. [CrossRef] [PubMed]
180. Lee, C.-W.; Rivera, R.; Gardell, S.; Dubin, A.E.; Chun, J. GPR92 as a New G12/13- and Gq-coupled lysophosphatidic acid receptor that increases cAMP, LPA5. *J. Biol. Chem.* **2006**, *281*, 23589–23597. [CrossRef]
181. Rudenko, O.; Shang, J.; Munk, A.; Ekberg, J.P.; Petersen, N.; Engelstoft, M.S.; Egerod, K.L.; Hjorth, S.A.; Wu, M.; Feng, Y.; et al. The aromatic amino acid sensor GPR142 controls metabolism through balanced regulation of pancreatic and gut hormones. *Mol. Metab.* **2019**, *19*, 49–64. [CrossRef]
182. Lin, H.V.; Efanov, A.M.; Fang, X.; Beavers, L.S.; Wang, X.; Wang, J.; Valcarcel, I.C.G.; Ma, T. GPR142 controls tryptophan-induced insulin and incretin hormone secretion to improve glucose metabolism. *PLoS ONE* **2016**, *11*, e0157298. [CrossRef]
183. Li, X.; Staszewski, L.; Xu, H.; Durick, K.; Zoller, M.; Adler, E. Human receptors for sweet and umami taste. *Proc. Natl. Acad. Sci. USA* **2002**, *99*, 4692–4696. [CrossRef] [PubMed]
184. Wang, J.-H.; Inoue, T.; Higashiyama, M.; Guth, P.H.; Engel, E.; Kaunitz, J.D.; Akiba, Y. Umami receptor activation increases duodenal bicarbonate secretion via glucagon-like peptide-2 release in rats. *J. Pharm. Exp.* **2011**, *339*, 464–473. [CrossRef] [PubMed]
185. Blonde, G.D.; Travers, S.P.; Spector, A.C. Taste sensitivity to a mixture of monosodium glutamate and inosine 5′-monophosphate by mice lacking both subunits of the T1R1 + T1R3 amino acid receptor. *Am. J. Physiol. Integr. Comp. Physiol.* **2018**, *314*, R802–R810. [CrossRef]
186. Lin, W.; Kinnamon, S.C. Physiological evidence for ionotropic and metabotropic glutamate receptors in rat taste cells. *J. Neurophysiol.* **1999**, *82*, 2061–2069. [CrossRef] [PubMed]
187. Bigiani, A.; De Lay, R.J.; Chaudhari, N.; Kinnamon, S.C.; Roper, S.D. Responses to glutamate in rat taste cells. *J. Neurophysiol.* **1997**, *77*, 3048–3059. [CrossRef]
188. Akiba, Y.; Watanabe, C.; Mizumori, M.; Kaunitz, J.D. Luminal l-glutamate enhances duodenal mucosal defense mechanisms via multiple glutamate receptors in rats. *Am. J. Physiol. Liver Physiol.* **2009**, *297*, G781–G791. [CrossRef]
189. Wellendorph, P.; Hansen, K.B.; Balsgaard, A.; Greenwood, J.R.; Egebjerg, J.; Bräuner-Osborne, H. Deorphanization of GPRC6A: A promiscuous l-α-Amino acid receptor with preference for basic amino acids. *Mol. Pharm.* **2004**, *67*, 589–597. [CrossRef]
190. Pi, M.; Quarles, L.D. Multiligand specificity and wide tissue expression of GPRC6A reveals new endocrine networks. *Endocrinology* **2012**, *153*, 2062–2069. [CrossRef]
191. Mizokami, A.; Yasutake, Y.; Higashi, S.; Kawakubo-Yasukochi, T.; Chishaki, S.; Takahashi, I.; Takeuchi, H.; Hirata, M. Oral administration of osteocalcin improves glucose utilization by stimulating glucagon-like peptide-1 secretion. *Bone* **2014**, *69*, 68–79. [CrossRef]
192. Wang, H.; Murthy, K.S.; Grider, J.R. Expression patterns of l-amino acid receptors in the murine STC-1 enteroendocrine cell line. *Cell Tissue Res.* **2019**, *378*, 471–483. [CrossRef]
193. Oya, M.; Kitaguchi, T.; Pais, R.; Reimann, F.; Gribble, F.; Tsuboi, T. The G protein-coupled receptor family C group 6 subtype A (GPRC6A) receptor is involved in amino acid-induced glucagon-like peptide-1 secretion from GLUTag cells. *J. Biol. Chem.* **2013**, *288*, 4513–4521. [CrossRef] [PubMed]
194. Carney, B.I.; Jones, K.L.; Horowitz, M.; Sun, W.M.; Hebbard, G.; Edelbroek, M.A.L. Stereospecific effects of tryptophan on gastric emptying and hunger in humans. *J. Gastroenterol. Hepatol.* **1994**, *9*, 557–563. [CrossRef] [PubMed]
195. Steinert, R.E.; Luscombe-Marsh, N.D.; Little, T.J.; Standfield, S.; Otto, B.; Horowitz, M.; Feinle-Bisset, C. Effects of intraduodenal infusion of L-tryptophan on ad libitum eating, antropyloroduodenal motility, glycemia, insulinemia, and gut peptide secretion in healthy men. *J. Clin. Endocrinol. Metab.* **2014**, *99*, 3275–3284. [CrossRef] [PubMed]
196. McVeay, C.; Fitzgerald, P.C.E.; Ullrich, S.S.; Steinert, R.E.; Horowitz, M.; Feinle-Bisset, C. Effects of intraduodenal administration of lauric acid and L-tryptophan, alone and combined, on gut hormones, pyloric pressures, and energy intake in healthy men. *Am. J. Clin. Nutr.* **2019**, *109*, 1335–1343. [CrossRef] [PubMed]
197. Edholm, T.; Degerblad, M.; Grybäck, P.; Hilsted, L.; Holst, J.J.; Jacobsson, H.; Efendic, S.; Schmidt, P.T.; Hellström, P.M. Differential incretin effects of GIP and GLP-1 on gastric emptying, appetite, and insulin-glucose homeostasis. *Neurogastroenterol. Motil.* **2010**, *22*, 1191. [CrossRef] [PubMed]
198. Reimann, F.; Williams, L.; Xavier, G.D.S.; Rutter, G.A.; Gribble, F.M. Glutamine potently stimulates glucagon-like peptide-1 secretion from GLUTag cells. *Diabetologia* **2004**, *47*, 1592–1601. [CrossRef]
199. Greenfield, J.R.; Farooqi, I.S.; Keogh, J.M.; Henning, E.; Habib, A.M.; Blackwood, A.; Reimann, F.; Holst, J.J.; Gribble, F.M. Oral glutamine increases circulating glucagon-like peptide 1, glucagon, and insulin concentrations in lean, obese, and Type 2 diabetic subjects. *Am. J. Clin. Nutr.* **2008**, *89*, 106–113. [CrossRef]
200. Chang, J.; Wu, T.; Greenfield, J.R.; Samocha-Bonet, D.; Horowitz, M.; Rayner, C.K. Effects of intraduodenal glutamine on incretin hormone and insulin release, the glycemic response to an intraduodenal glucose infusion, and antropyloroduodenal motility in health and Type 2 diabetes. *Diabetes Care* **2013**, *36*, 2262–2265. [CrossRef]
201. Tolhurst, G.; Zheng, Y.; Parker, H.E.; Habib, A.M.; Reimann, F.; Gribble, F.M. Glutamine triggers and potentiates glucagon-like peptide-1 secretion by raising cytosolic Ca2+ and cAMP. *Endocrinology* **2011**, *152*, 405–413. [CrossRef]
202. Mamillapalli, R.; Wysolmerski, J. The calcium-sensing receptor couples to Gαs and regulates PTHrP and ACTH secretion in pituitary cells. *J. Endocrinol.* **2009**, *204*, 287–297. [CrossRef] [PubMed]
203. Geoghegan, J.G.; A Cheng, C.; Lawson, C.; Pappas, T.N. The effect of caloric load and nutrient composition on induction of small intestinal satiety in dogs. *Physiol. Behav.* **1997**, *62*, 39–42. [CrossRef]

204. Chapman, I.M.; A Goble, E.; A Wittert, G.; Horowitz, M. Effects of small-intestinal fat and carbohydrate infusions on appetite and food intake in obese and nonobese men. *Am. J. Clin. Nutr.* **1999**, *69*, 6–12. [CrossRef]
205. Herrmann, C.; Göke, R.; Richter, G.; Fehmann, H.-C.; Arnold, R.; Göke, B. Glucagon-like peptide-1 and glucose-dependent insulin-releasing polypeptide plasma levels in response to nutrients. *Digestion* **1995**, *56*, 117–126. [CrossRef] [PubMed]
206. Thomsen, C.; Rasmussen, O.; Lousen, T.; Holst, J.J.; Fenselau, S.; Schrezenmeir, J.; Hermansen, K. Differential effects of saturated and monounsaturated fatty acids on postprandial lipemia and incretin responses in healthy subjects. *Am. J. Clin. Nutr.* **1999**, *69*, 1135–1143. [CrossRef] [PubMed]
207. Rocca, A.S.; Brubaker, P.L. Stereospecific effects of fatty acids on proglucagon-derived peptide secretion in fetal rat intestinal cultures. *Endocrinology* **1995**, *136*, 5593–5599. [CrossRef]
208. Kwasowski, P.; Flatt, P.R.; Bailey, C.J.; Marks, V. Effects of fatty acid chain length and saturation on gastric inhibitory polypeptide release in obese hyperglycaemic (ob/ob) mice. *Biosci. Rep.* **1985**, *5*, 701–705. [CrossRef]
209. Feltrin, K.L.; Little, T.J.; Meyer, J.H.; Horowitz, M.; Smout, A.J.P.M.; Wishart, J.; Pilichiewicz, A.N.; Rades, T.; Chapman, I.M.; Feinle-Bisset, C. Effects of intraduodenal fatty acids on appetite, antropyloroduodenal motility, and plasma CCK and GLP-1 in humans vary with their chain length. *Am. J. Physiol. Integr. Comp. Physiol.* **2004**, *287*, R524–R533. [CrossRef]
210. Maggio, C.A.; Koopmans, H.S. Food intake after intragastric meals of short-, medium-, or long-chain triglyceride. *Physiol. Behav.* **1982**, *28*, 921–926. [CrossRef]
211. Pilichiewicz, A.; O'Donovan, D.; Feinle, C.; Lei, Y.; Wishart, J.M.; Bryant, L.; Meyer, J.H.; Horowitz, M.; Jones, K.L. Effect of lipase inhibition on gastric emptying of, and the glycemic and incretin responses to, an oil/aqueous drink in Type 2 diabetes mellitus. *J. Clin. Endocrinol. Metab.* **2003**, *88*, 3829–3834. [CrossRef] [PubMed]
212. Enç, F.Y.; Öneş, T.; Akın, H.L.; DeDe, F.; Turoğlu, H.T.; Ülfer, G.; Bekiroğlu, N.; Haklar, G.; Rehfeld, J.F.; Holst, J.J.; et al. Orlistat accelerates gastric emptying and attenuates GIP release in healthy subjects. *Am. J. Physiol. Liver Physiol.* **2009**, *296*, G482–G489. [CrossRef]
213. Ellrichmann, M.; Kapelle, M.; Ritter, P.R.; Holst, J.J.; Herzig, K.-H.; Schmidt, W.E.; Schmitz, F.; Meier, J.J. Orlistat inhibition of intestinal lipase acutely increases appetite and attenuates postprandial glucagon-like peptide-1-(7-36)-Amide-1, cholecystokinin, and peptide YY concentrations. *J. Clin. Endocrinol. Metab.* **2008**, *93*, 3995–3998. [CrossRef] [PubMed]
214. Beglinger, S.; Drewe, J.; Schirra, J.; Göke, B.; D'Amato, M.; Beglinger, C. Role of fat hydrolysis in regulating glucagon-like peptide-1 secretion. *J. Clin. Endocrinol. Metab.* **2010**, *95*, 879–886. [CrossRef]
215. Rajalahti, T.; Lin, C.; Mjøs, S.A.; Kvalheim, O.M. Serum fatty acid and lipoprotein subclass concentrations and their associations in prepubertal healthy Norwegian children. *Metabolomics* **2016**, *12*, 1–10. [CrossRef] [PubMed]
216. Psichas, A.; Larraufie, P.F.; Goldspink, D.A.; Gribble, F.M.; Reimann, F. Chylomicrons stimulate incretin secretion in mouse and human cells. *Diabetologia* **2017**, *60*, 2475–2485. [CrossRef] [PubMed]
217. Fatma, S.; Yakubov, R.; Anwar, K.; Hussain, M.M. Pluronic L81 enhances triacylglycerol accumulation in the cytosol and inhibits chylomicron secretion. *J. Lipid Res.* **2006**, *47*, 2422–2432. [CrossRef]
218. Shimotoyodome, A.; Fukuoka, D.; Suzuki, J.; Fujii, Y.; Mizuno, T.; Meguro, S.; Tokimitsu, I.; Hase, T. Coingestion of acylglycerols differentially affects glucose-induced insulin secretion via glucose-dependent insulinotropic polypeptide in C57BL/6J mice. *Endocrinology* **2009**, *150*, 2118–2126. [CrossRef]
219. Lu, W.J.; Yang, Q.; Yang, L.; Lee, D.; D'Alessio, D.; Tso, P. Chylomicron formation and secretion is required for lipid-stimulated release of incretins GLP-1 and GIP. *Lipids* **2012**, *47*, 571–580. [CrossRef]
220. Okawa, M.; Fujii, K.; Ohbuchi, K.; Okumoto, M.; Aragane, K.; Sato, H.; Tamai, Y.; Seo, T.; Itoh, Y.; Yoshimoto, R. Role of MGAT2 and DGAT1 in the release of gut peptides after triglyceride ingestion. *Biochem. Biophys. Res. Commun.* **2009**, *390*, 377–381. [CrossRef]
221. Liu, J.; McLaren, D.G.; Chen, D.; Kan, Y.; Stout, S.J.; Shen, X.; Murphy, B.A.; Forrest, G.; Karanam, B.; Sonatore, L.; et al. Potential mechanism of enhanced postprandial glucagon-like peptide-1 release following treatment with a diacylglycerol acyltransferase 1 inhibitor. *Pharm. Res. Perspect.* **2015**, *3*, e00193. [CrossRef]
222. Sclafani, A.; Ackroff, K.; Schwartz, G.J. Selective effects of vagal deafferentation and celiac-superior mesenteric ganglionectomy on the reinforcing and satiating action of intestinal nutrients. *Physiol. Behav.* **2003**, *78*, 285–294. [CrossRef]
223. Tamura, C.S.; Ritter, R.C. Intestinal capsaicin transiently attenuates suppression of sham feeding by oleate. *Am. J. Physiol. Integr. Comp. Physiol.* **1994**, *267*, R561–R568. [CrossRef]
224. Greenberg, D.; Smith, G.P.; Gibbs, J. Intraduodenal infusions of fats elicit satiety in sham-feeding rats. *Am. J. Physiol. Integr. Comp. Physiol.* **1990**, *259*, R110–R118. [CrossRef] [PubMed]
225. Kotarsky, K.; Nilsson, N.E.; Flodgren, E.; Owman, C.; Olde, B. A human cell surface receptor activated by free fatty acids and thiazolidinedione drugs. *Biochem. Biophys. Res. Commun.* **2003**, *301*, 406–410. [CrossRef]
226. Briscoe, C.P.; Tadayyon, M.; Andrews, J.L.; Benson, W.G.; Chambers, J.K.; Eilert, M.M.; Ellis, C.; Elshourbagy, N.A.; Goetz, A.S.; Minnick, D.T.; et al. The orphan G protein-coupled receptor GPR40 is activated by medium and long chain fatty acids. *J. Biol. Chem.* **2003**, *278*, 11303–11311. [CrossRef] [PubMed]
227. Edfalk, S.; Steneberg, P.; Edlund, H. Gpr40 is expressed in enteroendocrine cells and mediates free fatty acid stimulation of incretin secretion. *Diabetes* **2008**, *57*, 2280–2287. [CrossRef] [PubMed]

228. Hauge, M.; Vestmar, M.A.; Husted, A.S.; Ekberg, J.P.; Wright, M.J.; Di Salvo, J.; Weinglass, A.B.; Engelstoft, M.S.; Madsen, A.N.; Lückmann, M.; et al. GPR40 (FFAR1)—Combined Gs and Gq signaling In Vitro is associated with robust incretin secretagogue action Ex Vivo and In Vivo. *Mol. Metab.* **2015**, *4*, 3–14. [CrossRef] [PubMed]
229. Qian, J.; Gu, Y.; Wu, C.; Yu, F.; Chen, Y.; Zhu, J.; Yao, X.; Bei, C.; Zhu, Q. Agonist-induced activation of human FFA1 receptor signals to extracellular signal-regulated kinase 1 and 2 through Gq- and Gi-coupled signaling cascades. *Cell. Mol. Biol. Lett.* **2017**, *22*, 1–12. [CrossRef]
230. Yamada, H.; Yoshida, M.; Ito, K.; Dezaki, K.; Yada, T.; Ishikawa, S.-E.; Kakei, M. Potentiation of glucose-stimulated insulin secretion by the GPR40–PLC–TRPC pathway in pancreatic β-Cells. *Sci. Rep.* **2016**, *6*, 25912. [CrossRef]
231. Hirasawa, A.; Tsumaya, K.; Awaji, T.; Katsuma, S.; Adachi, T.; Yamada, M.; Sugimoto, Y.; Miyazaki, S.; Tsujimoto, G. Free fatty acids regulate gut incretin glucagon-like peptide-1 secretion through GPR120. *Nat. Med.* **2005**, *11*, 90–94. [CrossRef]
232. Tanaka, T.; Yano, T.; Adachi, T.; Koshimizu, T.-A.; Hirasawa, A.; Tsujimoto, G. Cloning and characterization of the rat free fatty acid receptor GPR120: In Vivo effect of the natural ligand on GLP-1 secretion and proliferation of pancreatic β cells. *Naunyn-Schmiedeberg's Arch. Pharmacol.* **2008**, *377*, 515–522. [CrossRef] [PubMed]
233. Iwasaki, K.; Harada, N.; Sasaki, K.; Yamane, S.; Iida, K.; Suzuki, K.; Hamasaki, A.; Nasteska, D.; Shibue, K.; Joo, E.; et al. Free fatty acid receptor GPR120 is highly expressed in enteroendocrine K cells of the upper small intestine and has a critical role in GIP secretion after fat ingestion. *Endocrinology* **2015**, *156*, 837–846. [CrossRef] [PubMed]
234. Ekberg, J.H.; Hauge, M.; Kristensen, L.V.; Madsen, A.N.; Engelstoft, M.S.; Husted, A.-S.; Sichlau, R.; Egerod, K.L.; Timshel, P.; Kowalski, T.J.; et al. GPR119, a major enteroendocrine sensor of dietary triglyceride metabolites coacting in synergy with FFA1 (GPR40). *Endocrinology* **2016**, *157*, 4561–4569. [CrossRef] [PubMed]
235. Sankoda, A.; Harada, N.; Iwasaki, K.; Yamane, S.; Murata, Y.; Shibue, K.; Thewjitcharoen, Y.; Suzuki, K.; Harada, T.; Kanemaru, Y.; et al. Long-chain free fatty acid receptor GPR120 mediates oil-induced GIP secretion through CCK in male mice. *Endocrinology* **2017**, *158*, 1172–1180. [CrossRef] [PubMed]
236. Engelstoft, M.S.; Park, W.-M.; Sakata, I.; Kristensen, L.V.; Husted, A.S.; Osborne-Lawrence, S.; Piper, P.K.; Walker, A.K.; Pedersen, M.H.; Nøhr, M.K.; et al. Seven transmembrane G protein-coupled receptor repertoire of gastric ghrelin cells. *Mol. Metab.* **2013**, *2*, 376–392. [CrossRef]
237. Stone, V.M.; Dhayal, S.; Brocklehurst, K.J.; Lenaghan, C.; Winzell, M.S.; Hammar, M.; Xu, X.; Smith, D.M.; Morgan, N.G. GPR120 (FFAR4) is preferentially expressed in pancreatic delta cells and regulates somatostatin secretion from murine islets of Langerhans. *Diabetologia* **2014**, *57*, 1182–1191. [CrossRef]
238. Iakoubov, R.; Izzo, A.; Yeung, C.; Whiteside, C.I.; Brubaker, P.L. Protein kinase Cζ is required for oleic acid-induced secretion of glucagon-like peptide-1 by intestinal endocrine L cells. *Endocrinology* **2007**, *148*, 1089–1098. [CrossRef]
239. Shah, B.P.; Liu, P.; Yu, T.; Hansen, D.R.; Gilbertson, T.A. TRPM5 is critical for linoleic acid-induced CCK secretion from the enteroendocrine cell line, STC-1. *Am. J. Physiol. Physiol.* **2012**, *302*, C210–C219. [CrossRef] [PubMed]
240. Lauffer, L.M.; Iakoubov, R.; Brubaker, P.L. GPR119 is essential for oleoylethanolamide-induced glucagon-like peptide-1 secretion from the intestinal enteroendocrine L-cell. *Diabetes* **2009**, *58*, 1058–1066. [CrossRef]
241. Schwartz, G.J.; Fu, J.; Astarita, G.; Li, X.; Gaetani, S.; Campolongo, P.; Cuomo, V.; Piomelli, D. The lipid messenger OEA links dietary fat intake to satiety. *Cell Metab.* **2008**, *8*, 281–288. [CrossRef]
242. Hansen, K.B.; Rosenkilde, M.M.; Knop, F.K.; Wellner, N.; Diep, T.A.; Rehfeld, J.F.; Andersen, U.B.; Holst, J.J.; Hansen, H.S. 2-oleoyl glycerol is a GPR119 agonist and signals GLP-1 release in humans. *J. Clin. Endocrinol. Metab.* **2011**, *96*, E1409–E1417. [CrossRef]
243. Chu, Z.-L.; Carroll, C.; Chen, R.; Alfonso, J.; Gutierrez, V.; He, H.; Lucman, A.; Xing, C.; Sebring, K.; Zhou, J.; et al. N-oleoyldopamine enhances glucose homeostasis through the activation of GPR119. *Mol. Endocrinology* **2010**, *24*, 161–170. [CrossRef]
244. Soga, T.; Ohishi, T.; Matsui, T.; Saito, T.; Matsumoto, M.; Takasaki, J.; Matsumoto, S.-I.; Kamohara, M.; Hiyama, H.; Yoshida, S.; et al. Lysophosphatidylcholine enhances glucose-dependent insulin secretion via an orphan G-protein-coupled receptor. *Biochem. Biophys. Res. Commun.* **2005**, *326*, 744–751. [CrossRef]
245. Lan, H.; Vassileva, G.; Corona, A.; Liu, L.; Baker, H.; Golovko, A.; Abbondanzo, S.J.; Hu, W.; Yang, S.; Ning, Y.; et al. GPR119 is required for physiological regulation of glucagon-like peptide-1 secretion but not for metabolic homeostasis. *J. Endocrinol.* **2009**, *201*, 219–230. [CrossRef] [PubMed]
246. Fu, J.; Oveisi, F.; Gaetani, S.; Lin, E.; Piomelli, D. Oleoylethanolamide, an endogenous PPAR-α agonist, lowers body weight and hyperlipidemia in obese rats. *Neuropharmacology* **2005**, *48*, 1147–1153. [CrossRef]
247. Fu, J.; Gaetani, S.; Oveisi, F.; Verme, J.L.; Serrano, A.; De Fonseca, F.R.; Rosengarth, A.; Luecke, H.; Di Giacomo, B.; Tarzia, G.; et al. Oleylethanolamide regulates feeding and body weight through activation of the nuclear receptor PPAR-α. *Nat. Cell Biol.* **2003**, *425*, 90–93. [CrossRef] [PubMed]
248. Chu, Z.-L.; Carroll, C.; Alfonso, J.; Gutierrez, V.; He, H.; Lucman, A.; Pedraza, M.; Mondala, H.; Gao, H.; Bagnol, D.; et al. A role for intestinal endocrine cell-expressed G protein-coupled receptor 119 in glycemic control by enhancing glucagon-like peptide-1 and glucose-dependent insulinotropic peptide release. *Endocrinology* **2008**, *149*, 2038–2047. [CrossRef] [PubMed]
249. De Fonseca, F.R.; Navarro, M.; Gómez, R.; Escuredo, L.; Nava, F.; Fu, J.; Murillo-Rodríguez, E.; Giuffrida, A.; LoVerme, J.; Gaetani, S.; et al. An anorexic lipid mediator regulated by feeding. *Nature* **2001**, *414*, 209–212. [CrossRef]
250. Fu, J.; Astarita, G.; Gaetani, S.; Kim, J.; Cravatt, B.F.; Mackie, K.; Piomelli, D. Food intake regulates oleoylethanolamide formation and degradation in the proximal small intestine. *J. Biol. Chem.* **2007**, *282*, 1518–1528. [CrossRef] [PubMed]

251. Overton, H.A.; Babbs, A.J.; Doel, S.M.; Fyfe, M.C.; Gardner, L.S.; Griffin, G.; Jackson, H.C.; Procter, M.J.; Rasamison, C.M.; Tang-Christensen, M.; et al. Deorphanization of a G protein-coupled receptor for oleoylethanolamide and its use in the discovery of small-molecule hypophagic agents. *Cell Metab.* **2006**, *3*, 167–175. [CrossRef]
252. Moss, C.E.; Glass, L.L.; Diakogiannaki, E.; Pais, R.; Lenaghan, C.; Smith, D.M.; Wedin, M.; Bohlooly, M.-Y.; Gribble, F.M.; Reimann, F. Lipid derivatives activate GPR119 and trigger GLP-1 secretion in primary murine L-cells. *Peptides* **2016**, *77*, 16–20. [CrossRef]
253. Katz, L.B.; Gambale, J.J.; Rothenberg, P.L.; Vanapalli, S.R.; Vaccaro, N.; Xi, L.; Sarich, T.C.; Stein, P.P. Effects of JNJ-38431055, a novel GPR119 receptor agonist, in randomized, double-blind, placebo-controlled studies in subjects with Type 2 diabetes. *Diabetes Obes. Metab.* **2012**, *14*, 709–716. [CrossRef] [PubMed]
254. Christensen, L.W.; Kuhre, R.E.; Janus, C.; Svendsen, B.; Holst, J.J. Vascular, but not luminal, activation of FFAR1 (GPR40) stimulates GLP-1 secretion from isolated perfused rat small intestine. *Physiol. Rep.* **2015**, *3*, e12551. [CrossRef] [PubMed]
255. Tough, I.R.; Forbes, S.; Herzog, H.; Jones, R.M.; Schwartz, T.W.; Cox, H.M. Bidirectional GPR119 agonism requires peptide YY and glucose for activity in mouse and human colon mucosa. *Endocrinology* **2018**, *159*, 1704–1717. [CrossRef]
256. Simons, P.J.; Kummer, J.A.; Luiken, J.J.; Boon, L. Apical CD36 immunolocalization in human and porcine taste buds from circumvallate and foliate papillae. *Acta Histochem.* **2011**, *113*, 839–843. [CrossRef] [PubMed]
257. Fukuwatari, T.; Kawada, T.; Tsuruta, M.; Hiraoka, T.; Iwanaga, T.; Sugimoto, E.; Fushiki, T. Expression of the putative membrane fatty acid transporter (FAT) in taste buds of the circumvallate papillae in rats. *FEBS Lett.* **1997**, *414*, 461–464. [CrossRef] [PubMed]
258. Chen, M.; Yang, Y.; Braunstein, E.; Georgeson, K.E.; Harmon, C.M. Gut expression and regulation of FAT/CD36: Possible role in fatty acid transport in rat enterocytes. *Am. J. Physiol. Metab.* **2001**, *281*, E916–E923. [CrossRef]
259. Laugerette, F.; Passilly-Degrace, P.; Patris, B.; Niot, I.; Febbraio, M.; Montmayeur, J.-P.; Besnard, P. CD36 involvement in orosensory detection of dietary lipids, spontaneous fat preference, and digestive secretions. *J. Clin. Investig.* **2005**, *115*, 3177–3184. [CrossRef]
260. Drover, V.A.; Nguyen, D.V.; Bastie, C.C.; Darlington, Y.F.; Abumrad, N.A.; Pessin, J.E.; London, E.; Sahoo, D.; Phillips, M.C. CD36 mediates both cellular uptake of very long chain fatty acids and their intestinal absorption in mice. *J. Biol. Chem.* **2008**, *283*, 13108–13115. [CrossRef]
261. Nauli, A.M.; Nassir, F.; Zheng, S.; Yang, Q.; Lo, C.; Von Lehmden, S.B.; Lee, D.; Jandacek, R.J.; Abumrad, N.A.; Tso, P.; et al. CD36 is important for chylomicron formation and secretion and may mediate cholesterol uptake in the proximal intestine. *Gastroenterology* **2006**, *131*, 1197–1207. [CrossRef]
262. Nassir, F.; Wilson, B.; Han, X.; Gross, R.W.; Abumrad, N.A. CD36 is important for fatty acid and cholesterol uptake by the proximal but not distal intestine. *J. Biol. Chem.* **2007**, *282*, 19493–19501. [CrossRef]
263. Martin, C.; Passilly-Degrace, P.; Gaillard, D.; Merlin, J.-F.; Chevrot, M.; Besnard, P. The lipid-sensor candidates CD36 and GPR120 are differentially regulated by dietary lipids in mouse taste buds: Impact on spontaneous fat preference. *PLoS ONE* **2011**, *6*, e24014. [CrossRef]
264. Maruyama, T.; Miyamoto, Y.; Nakamura, T.; Tamai, Y.; Okada, H.; Sugiyama, E.; Nakamura, T.; Itadani, H.; Tanaka, K. Identification of membrane-type receptor for bile acids (M-BAR). *Biochem. Biophys. Res. Commun.* **2002**, *298*, 714–719. [CrossRef]
265. Kawamata, Y.; Fujii, R.; Hosoya, M.; Harada, M.; Yoshida, H.; Miwa, M.; Fukusumi, S.; Habata, Y.; Itoh, T.; Shintani, Y.; et al. A G protein-coupled receptor responsive to bile acids. *J. Biol. Chem.* **2003**, *278*, 9435–9440. [CrossRef]
266. Makishima, M.; Okamoto, A.Y.; Repa, J.J.; Tu, H.; Learned, R.M.; Luk, A.; Hull, M.V.; Lustig, K.D.; Mangelsdorf, D.J.; Shan, B.; et al. Identification of a nuclear receptor for bile acids. *Science* **1999**, *284*, 1362–1365. [CrossRef]
267. Namba, M.; Matsuyama, T.; Nonaka, K.; Tarui, S. Effect of intraluminal bile or bile acids on release of gut glucagon-like immunoreactive materials in the dog. *Horm. Metab. Res.* **1983**, *15*, 82–84. [CrossRef]
268. Namba, M.; Matsuyama, T.; Itoh, H.; Imai, Y.; Horie, H.; Tarui, S. Inhibition of pentagastrin-stimulated gastric acid secretion by intraileal administration of bile and elevation of plasma concentrations of gut glucagon-like immunoreactivity in anesthetized dogs. *Regul. Pept.* **1986**, *15*, 121–128. [CrossRef]
269. Thomas, C.; Gioiello, A.; Noriega, L.; Strehle, A.; Oury, J.; Rizzo, G.; Macchiarulo, A.; Yamamoto, H.; Mataki, C.; Pruzanski, M.; et al. TGR5-mediated bile acid sensing controls glucose homeostasis. *Cell Metab.* **2009**, *10*, 167–177. [CrossRef]
270. Parker, H.E.; Wallis, K.; Le Roux, C.W.; Wong, K.Y.; Reimann, F.; Gribble, F.M. Molecular mechanisms underlying bile acid-stimulated glucagon-like peptide-1 secretion. *Br. J. Pharm.* **2011**, *165*, 414–423. [CrossRef]
271. Katsuma, S.; Hirasawa, A.; Tsujimoto, G. Bile acids promote glucagon-like peptide-1 secretion through TGR5 in a murine enteroendocrine cell line STC-1. *Biochem. Biophys. Res. Commun.* **2005**, *329*, 386–390. [CrossRef]
272. Wu, T.; Bound, M.J.; Standfield, S.D.; Gedulin, B.; Jones, K.L.; Horowitz, M.; Rayner, C.K. Effects of rectal administration of taurocholic acid on glucagon-like peptide-1 and peptide YY secretion in healthy humans. *Diabetes Obes. Metab.* **2012**, *15*, 474–477. [CrossRef]
273. Adrian, T.E.; Ballantyne, G.H.; Longo, W.E.; Bilchik, A.J.; Graham, S.; Basson, M.D.; Tierney, R.P.; Modlin, I.M. Deoxycholate is an important releaser of peptide YY and enteroglucagon from the human colon. *Gut* **1993**, *34*, 1219–1224. [CrossRef]
274. Kuhre, R.E.; Albrechtsen, N.J.W.; Larsen, O.; Jepsen, S.L.; Balk-Møller, E.; Andersen, D.B.; Deacon, C.F.; Schoonjans, K.; Reimann, F.; Gribble, F.M.; et al. Bile acids are important direct and indirect regulators of the secretion of appetite- and metabolism-regulating hormones from the gut and pancreas. *Mol. Metab.* **2018**, *11*, 84–95. [CrossRef]
275. Burhol, P.G.; Lygren, I.; Waldum, H.; Jorde, R. The effect of duodenal infusion of bile on plasma VIP, GIP, and secretin and on duodenal bicarbonate secretion. *Scand. J. Gastroenterol.* **1980**, *15*, 1007–1011. [CrossRef] [PubMed]

276. Lund, M.L.; Sorrentino, G.; Egerod, K.L.; Kroone, C.; Mortensen, B.; Knop, F.K.; Reimann, F.; Gribble, F.M.; Drucker, D.J.; De Koning, E.J.; et al. L-cell differentiation is induced by bile acids through GPBAR1 and paracrine GLP-1 and serotonin signaling. *Diabetes* **2020**, *69*, 614–623. [CrossRef]
277. Christiansen, C.B.; Trammell, S.A.J.; Albrechtsen, N.J.W.; Schoonjans, K.; Albrechtsen, R.; Gillum, M.P.; Kuhre, R.E.; Holst, J.J. Bile acids drive colonic secretion of glucagon-like-peptide 1 and peptide-YY in rodents. *Am. J. Physiol. Liver Physiol.* **2019**, *316*, G574–G584. [CrossRef]
278. Balakrishnan, A.; Wring, S.A.; Polli, J.E. Interaction of native bile acids with human apical sodium-dependent bile acid transporter (hASBT): Influence of steroidal hydroxylation pattern and C-24 conjugation. *Pharm. Res.* **2006**, *23*, 1451–1459. [CrossRef]
279. Trabelsi, M.-S.; Daoudi, M.; Prawitt, J.; Ducastel, S.; Touche, V.; Sayin, S.I.; Perino, A.; Brighton, C.A.; Sebti, Y.; Kluza, J.; et al. Farnesoid X receptor inhibits glucagon-like peptide-1 production by enteroendocrine L cells. *Nat. Commun.* **2015**, *6*, 7629. [CrossRef]
280. Poole, D.P.; Godfrey, C.; Cattaruzza, F.; Cottrell, G.S.; Kirkland, J.G.; Pelayo, J.C.; Bunnett, N.W.; Corvera, C.U. Expression and function of the bile acid receptor GpBAR1 (TGR5) in the murine enteric nervous system. *Neurogastroenterol. Motil.* **2010**, *22*, 814–e228. [CrossRef] [PubMed]
281. Le Poul, E.; Loison, C.; Struyf, S.; Springael, J.-Y.; Lannoy, V.; Decobecq, M.-E.; Brezillon, S.; Dupriez, V.; Vassart, G.; Van Damme, J.; et al. Functional characterization of human receptors for short chain fatty acids and their role in polymorphonuclear cell activation. *J. Biol. Chem.* **2003**, *278*, 25481–25489. [CrossRef]
282. Brown, A.J.; Goldsworthy, S.M.; Barnes, A.A.; Eilert, M.M.; Tcheang, L.; Daniels, D.; Muir, A.I.; Wigglesworth, M.J.; Kinghorn, I.; Fraser, N.J.; et al. The orphan G protein-coupled receptors GPR41 and GPR43 are activated by propionate and other short chain carboxylic acids. *J. Biol. Chem.* **2003**, *278*, 11312–11319. [CrossRef]
283. Karaki, S.-I.; Mitsui, R.; Hayashi, H.; Kato, I.; Sugiya, H.; Iwanaga, T.; Furness, J.B.; Kuwahara, A. Short-chain fatty acid receptor, GPR43, is expressed by enteroendocrine cells and mucosal mast cells in rat intestine. *Cell Tissue Res.* **2006**, *324*, 353–360. [CrossRef] [PubMed]
284. Karaki, S.-I.; Tazoe, H.; Hayashi, H.; Kashiwabara, H.; Tooyama, K.; Suzuki, Y.; Kuwahara, A. Expression of the short-chain fatty acid receptor, GPR43, in the human colon. *J. Mol. Histol.* **2008**, *39*, 135–142. [CrossRef] [PubMed]
285. Fukumoto, S.; Tatewaki, M.; Yamada, T.; Fujimiya, M.; Mantyh, C.; Voss, M.; Eubanks, S.; Harris, M.; Pappas, T.N.; Takahashi, T.; et al. Short-chain fatty acids stimulate colonic transit via intraluminal 5-HT release in rats. *Am. J. Physiol. Integr. Comp. Physiol.* **2003**, *284*, R1269–R1276. [CrossRef]
286. Nøhr, M.K.; Pedersen, M.H.; Gille, A.; Egerod, K.L.; Engelstoft, M.S.; Husted, A.S.; Sichlau, R.M.; Grunddal, K.V.; Poulsen, S.S.; Han, S.; et al. GPR41/FFAR3 and GPR43/FFAR2 as cosensors for short-chain fatty acids in enteroendocrine cells vs FFAR3 in enteric neurons and FFAR2 in enteric leukocytes. *Endocrinology* **2013**, *154*, 3552–3564. [CrossRef] [PubMed]
287. Tolhurst, G.; Heffron, H.; Lam, Y.S.; Parker, H.E.; Habib, A.M.; Diakogiannaki, E.; Cameron, J.; Grosse, J.; Reimann, F.; Gribble, F.M.; et al. Short-chain fatty acids stimulate glucagon-like peptide-1 secretion via the g-protein-coupled receptor FFAR2. *Diabetes* **2011**, *61*, 364–371. [CrossRef]
288. Nilsson, N.E.; Kotarsky, K.; Owman, C.; Olde, B. Identification of a free fatty acid receptor, FFA2R, expressed on leukocytes and activated by short-chain fatty acids. *Biochem. Biophys. Res. Commun.* **2003**, *303*, 1047–1052. [CrossRef]
289. Tazoe, H.; Otomo, Y.; Karaki, S.-I.; Kato, I.; Fukami, Y.; Terasaki, M.; Kuwahara, A. Expression of short-chain fatty acid receptor GPR41 in the human colon. *Biomed. Res.* **2009**, *30*, 149–156. [CrossRef]
290. Nøhr, M.; Egerod, K.; Christiansen, S.; Gille, A.; Offermanns, S.; Schwartz, T.; Møller, M. Expression of the short chain fatty acid receptor GPR41/FFAR3 in autonomic and somatic sensory ganglia. *Neuroscience* **2015**, *290*, 126–137. [CrossRef]
291. Won, Y.-J.; Lu, V.B.; Puhl, H.L.; Ikeda, S.R. β-Hydroxybutyrate modulates N-type calcium channels in rat sympathetic neurons by acting as an agonist for the G-protein-coupled receptor FFA3. *J. Neurosci.* **2013**, *33*, 19314–19325. [CrossRef]
292. Psichas, A.; Sleeth, M.L.; Murphy, K.G.; Brooks, L.J.; A Bewick, G.; Hanyaloglu, A.C.; A Ghatei, M.; Bloom, S.R.; Frost, G. The short chain fatty acid propionate stimulates GLP-1 and PYY secretion via free fatty acid receptor 2 in rodents. *Int. J. Obes.* **2015**, *39*, 424–429. [CrossRef]
293. Forbes, S.; Stafford, S.; Coope, G.; Heffron, H.; Real, K.; Newman, R.; Davenport, R.; Barnes, M.; Grosse, J.; Cox, H.; et al. Selective FFA2 agonism appears to act via intestinal PYY to reduce transit and food intake but does not improve glucose tolerance in mouse models. *Diabetes* **2015**, *64*, 3763–3771. [CrossRef]
294. Bolognini, D.; Moss, C.E.; Nilsson, K.; Petersson, A.U.; Donnelly, I.; Sergeev, E.; König, G.M.; Kostenis, E.; Kurowska-Stolarska, M.; Miller, A.; et al. A novel allosteric activator of free fatty acid 2 receptor displays unique gi-functional bias. *J. Biol. Chem.* **2016**, *291*, 18915–18931. [CrossRef]
295. Christiansen, C.B.; Gabe, M.B.N.; Svendsen, B.; Dragsted, L.O.; Rosenkilde, M.M.; Holst, J.J. The impact of short-chain fatty acids on GLP-1 and PYY secretion from the isolated perfused rat colon. *Am. J. Physiol. Liver Physiol.* **2018**, *315*, G53–G65. [CrossRef]
296. Müller, M.; Hernández, M.A.G.; Goossens, G.H.; Reijnders, D.; Holst, J.J.; Jocken, J.W.E.; Van Eijk, H.; Canfora, E.E.; Blaak, E.E. Circulating but not faecal short-chain fatty acids are related to insulin sensitivity, lipolysis and GLP-1 concentrations in humans. *Sci. Rep.* **2019**, *9*, 1–9. [CrossRef] [PubMed]

297. Høverstad, T.; Bjørneklett, A.; Midtvedt, T.; Fausa, O.; Bøhmer, T. Short-chain fatty acids in the proximal gastrointestinal tract of healthy subjects. *Scand J. Gastroenterol.* **1984**, *19*, 1053–1058.
298. Lee, E.-Y.; Zhang, X.; Miyamoto, J.; Kimura, I.; Taknaka, T.; Furusawa, K.; Jomori, T.; Fujimoto, K.; Uematsu, S.; Miki, T.; et al. Gut carbohydrate inhibits GIP secretion via a microbiota/SCFA/FFAR3 pathway. *J. Endocrinol.* **2018**, *239*, 267–276. [CrossRef] [PubMed]
299. Zhou, J.; Martin, R.J.; Tulley, R.T.; Raggio, A.M.; McCutcheon, K.L.; Shen, L.; Danna, S.C.; Tripathy, S.; Hegsted, M.; Keenan, M.J.; et al. Dietary resistant starch upregulates total GLP-1 and PYY in a sustained day-long manner through fermentation in rodents. *Am. J. Physiol. Metab.* **2008**, *295*, E1160–E1166. [CrossRef] [PubMed]
300. Larraufie, P.; Martin-Gallausiaux, C.; Lapaque, N.; Dore, J.; Gribble, F.M.; Reimann, F.; Blottiere, H.M. SCFAs strongly stimulate PYY production in human enteroendocrine cells. *Sci. Rep.* **2018**, *8*, 1–9. [CrossRef] [PubMed]
301. Petersen, N.; Reimann, F.; Bartfeld, S.; Farin, H.F.; Ringnalda, F.C.; Vries, R.G.J.; Brink, S.V.D.; Clevers, H.; Gribble, F.M.; De Koning, E.J.P.; et al. Generation of L cells in mouse and human small intestine organoids. *Diabetes* **2014**, *63*, 410–420. [CrossRef]
302. Arora, T.; Akrami, R.; Pais, R.; Bergqvist, L.; Johansson, B.R.; Schwartz, T.W.; Reimann, F.; Gribble, F.M.; Bäckhed, F. Microbial regulation of the L cell transcriptome. *Sci. Rep.* **2018**, *8*, 1207. [CrossRef]
303. Wichmann, A.; Allahyar, A.; Greiner, T.U.; Plovier, H.; Östergren, G.L.; Larsson, T.; Drucker, D.J.; Delzenne, N.M.; Cani, P.; Bäckhed, F.; et al. Microbial modulation of energy availability in the colon regulates intestinal transit. *Cell Host Microbe* **2013**, *14*, 582–590. [CrossRef]
304. De Fonseca, F.R.; Navarro, M.; Alvarez, E.; Roncero, I.; Chowen, J.A.; Maestre, O.; Gómez, R.; Muñoz, R.M.; Eng, J.; Blázquez, E.; et al. Peripheral versus central effects of glucagon-like peptide-1 receptor agonists on satiety and body weight loss in Zucker obese rats. *Metabolism* **2000**, *49*, 709–717. [CrossRef] [PubMed]
305. Näslund, E.; Barkeling, B.; King, N.; Gutniak, M.; Blundell, J.; Holst, J.; Rössner, S.; Hellström, P. Energy intake and appetite are suppressed by glucagon-like peptide-1 (GLP-1) in obese men. *Int. J. Obes.* **1999**, *23*, 304–311. [CrossRef] [PubMed]
306. Gutzwiller, J.-P.; Göke, B.; Drewe, J.; Hildebrand, P.; Ketterer, S.; Handschin, D.; Winterhalder, R.; Conen, D.; Beglinger, C. Glucagon-like peptide-1: A potent regulator of food intake in humans. *Gut* **1999**, *44*, 81–86. [CrossRef]
307. Flint, A.; Raben, A.; Astrup, A.; Holst, J.J. Glucagon-like peptide 1 promotes satiety and suppresses energy intake in humans. *J. Clin. Investig.* **1998**, *101*, 515–520. [CrossRef] [PubMed]
308. Kim, D.; MacConell, L.; Zhuang, N.; Kothare, P.A.; Trautmann, M.; Fineman, M.; Taylor, K. Effects of once-weekly dosing of a long-acting release formulation of exenatide on glucose control and body weight in subjects with Type 2 diabetes. *Diabetes Care* **2007**, *30*, 1487–1493. [CrossRef]
309. Holst, J.J. Incretin hormones and the satiation signal. *Int. J. Obes.* **2013**, *37*, 1161–1168. [CrossRef]
310. Astrup, A.; Rössner, S.; Van Gaal, L.; Rissanen, A.; Niskanen, L.; Al Hakim, M.; Madsen, J.; Rasmussen, M.F.; Lean, M.E. Effects of liraglutide in the treatment of obesity: A randomised, double-blind, placebo-controlled study. *Lancet* **2009**, *374*, 1606–1616. [CrossRef]
311. Knudsen, L.B.; Lau, J. The discovery and development of liraglutide and semaglutide. *Front. Endocrinol.* **2019**, *10*, 155. [CrossRef]
312. Finan, B.; Ma, T.; Ottaway, N.; Müller, T.D.; Habegger, K.M.; Heppner, K.M.; Kirchner, H.; Holland, J.; Hembree, J.; Raver, C.; et al. Unimolecular dual incretins maximize metabolic benefits in rodents, monkeys, and humans. *Sci. Transl. Med.* **2013**, *5*, 209. [CrossRef]
313. Bergmann, N.C.; Lund, A.; Gasbjerg, L.S.; Meessen, E.C.E.; Andersen, M.M.; Bergmann, S.; Hartmann, B.; Holst, J.J.; Jessen, L.; Christensen, M.B.; et al. Effects of combined GIP and GLP-1 infusion on energy intake, appetite and energy expenditure in overweight/obese individuals: A randomised, crossover study. *Diabetologia* **2019**, *62*, 665–675. [CrossRef]
314. Miyawaki, K.; Yamada, Y.; Ban, N.; Ihara, Y.; Tsukiyama, K.; Zhou, H.; Fujimoto, S.; Oku, A.; Tsuda, K.; Toyokuni, S.; et al. Inhibition of gastric inhibitory polypeptide signaling prevents obesity. *Nat. Med.* **2002**, *8*, 738–742. [CrossRef]
315. Althage, M.C.; Ford, E.L.; Wang, S.; Tso, P.; Polonsky, K.S.; Wice, B.M. Targeted ablation of glucose-dependent insulinotropic polypeptide-producing cells in transgenic mice reduces obesity and insulin resistance induced by a high fat diet. *J. Biol. Chem.* **2008**, *283*, 18365–18376. [CrossRef]
316. Pathak, V.; Gault, V.A.; Flatt, P.R.; Irwin, N. Antagonism of gastric inhibitory polypeptide (GIP) by palmitoylation of GIP analogues with N- and C-terminal modifications improves obesity and metabolic control in high fat fed mice. *Mol. Cell. Endocrinol.* **2015**, *401*, 120–129. [CrossRef] [PubMed]
317. Nakamura, T.; Tanimoto, H.; Mizuno, Y.; Okamoto, M.; Takeuchi, M.; Tsubamoto, Y.; Noda, H. Gastric inhibitory polypeptide receptor antagonist, SKL-14959, suppressed body weight gain on diet-induced obesity mice. *Obes. Sci. Pr.* **2018**, *4*, 194–203. [CrossRef] [PubMed]
318. Kim, S.-J.; Nian, C.; Karunakaran, S.; Clee, S.M.; Isales, C.M.; McIntosh, C.H.S. GIP-overexpressing mice demonstrate reduced diet-induced obesity and steatosis, and improved glucose homeostasis. *PLoS ONE* **2012**, *7*, e40156. [CrossRef]
319. Geary, N.; Smith, G.P. Pancreatic glucagon and postprandial satiety in the rat. *Physiol. Behav.* **1982**, *28*, 313–322. [CrossRef]
320. Schwartz, M.W.; Figlewicz, D.P.; Woods, S.C.; Porte, D.; Baskin, D.G. Insulin, neuropeptide Y, and food intake. *Ann. N. Y. Acad. Sci.* **1993**, *692*, 60–71. [CrossRef]
321. Pamir, N.; Lynn, F.C.; Buchan, A.M.J.; Ehses, J.; Hinke, S.A.; Pospisilik, J.A.; Miyawaki, K.; Yamada, Y.; Seino, Y.; McIntosh, C.H.S.; et al. Glucose-dependent insulinotropic polypeptide receptor null mice exhibit compensatory changes in the enteroinsular axis. *Am. J. Physiol. Metab.* **2003**, *284*, E931–E939. [CrossRef]

322. Sparre-Ulrich, A.H.; Hansen, L.S.; Svendsen, B.; Christensen, M.S.; Knop, F.K.; Hartmann, B.; Holst, J.J.; Rosenkilde, M.M. Species-specific action of (Pro3)GIP—A full agonist at human GIP receptors, but a partial agonist and competitive antagonist at rat and mouse GIP receptors. *Br. J. Pharm.* **2015**, *173*, 27–38. [CrossRef]
323. Gault, V.A.; O'Harte, F.P.; Harriott, P.; Flatt, P.R. Characterization of the cellular and metabolic effects of a novel enzyme-resistant antagonist of glucose-dependent insulinotropic polypeptide. *Biochem. Biophys. Res. Commun.* **2002**, *290*, 1420–1426. [CrossRef] [PubMed]
324. Mroz, P.A.; Finan, B.; Gelfanov, V.; Yang, B.; Tschöp, M.H.; DiMarchi, R.D.; Perez-Tilve, D. Optimized GIP analogs promote body weight lowering in mice through GIPR agonism not antagonism. *Mol. Metab.* **2019**, *20*, 51–62. [CrossRef] [PubMed]
325. Nørregaard, P.K.; Deryabina, M.A.; Shelton, P.T.; Fog, J.U.; Daugaard, J.R.; Eriksson, P.; Larsen, L.F.; Jessen, L. A novel GIP analogue, ZP 4165, enhances glucagon-like peptide-1-induced body weight loss and improves glycaemic control in rodents. *Diabetes Obes. Metab.* **2018**, *20*, 60–68. [CrossRef]
326. Gault, V.A.; Kerr, B.D.; Harriott, P.; Flatt, P.R. Administration of an acylated GLP-1 and GIP preparation provides added beneficial glucose-lowering and insulinotropic actions over single incretins in mice with Type 2 diabetes and obesity. *Clin. Sci.* **2011**, *121*, 107–117. [CrossRef] [PubMed]
327. Portron, A.; Jadidi, S.; Sarkar, N.; Di Marchi, R.; Schmitt, C. Pharmacodynamics, pharmacokinetics, safety and tolerability of the novel dual glucose-dependent insulinotropic polypeptide/glucagon-like peptide-1 agonist RG7697 after single subcutaneous administration in healthy subjects. *Diabetes Obes. Metab.* **2017**, *19*, 1446–1453. [CrossRef]
328. Schmitt, C.; Portron, A.; Jadidi, S.; Sarkar, N.; Di Marchi, R. Pharmacodynamics, pharmacokinetics and safety of multiple ascending doses of the novel dual glucose-dependent insulinotropic polypeptide/glucagon-like peptide-1 agonist RG7697 in people with Type 2 diabetes mellitus. *Diabetes Obes. Metab.* **2017**, *19*, 1436–1445. [CrossRef]
329. Frias, J.P.; Bastyr, E.J.; Vignati, L.; Tschöp, M.H.; Schmitt, C.; Owen, K.; Christensen, R.H.; DiMarchi, R.D. The sustained effects of a dual GIP/GLP-1 receptor agonist, NNC0090–2746, in patients with Type 2 diabetes. *Cell Metab.* **2017**, *26*, 343–352.e2. [CrossRef]
330. Frias, J.P.; Nauck, M.A.; Van, J.; Kutner, M.E.; Cui, X.; Benson, C.; Urva, S.; Gimeno, R.E.; Milicevic, Z.; Robins, D.; et al. Efficacy and safety of LY3298176, a novel dual GIP and GLP-1 receptor agonist, in patients with Type 2 diabetes: A randomised, placebo-controlled and active comparator-controlled phase 2 trial. *Lancet* **2018**, *392*, 2180–2193. [CrossRef]
331. Coskun, T.; Sloop, K.W.; Loghin, C.; Alsina-Fernandez, J.; Urva, S.; Bokvist, K.B.; Cui, X.; Briere, D.A.; Cabrera, O.; Roell, W.C.; et al. LY3298176, a novel dual GIP and GLP-1 receptor agonist for the treatment of Type 2 diabetes mellitus: From discovery to clinical proof of concept. *Mol. Metab.* **2018**, *18*, 3–14. [CrossRef]
332. Welch, I.; Saunders, K.; Read, N. Effect of ileal and intravenous infusions of fat emulsions on feeding and satiety in human volunteers. *Gastroenterology* **1985**, *89*, 1293–1297. [CrossRef]
333. Lavin, J.H.; Wittert, G.; Sun, W.M.; Horowitz, M.; Morley, J.E.; Read, N.W. Appetite regulation by carbohydrate: Role of blood glucose and gastrointestinal hormones. *Am. J. Physiol. Metab.* **1996**, *271*, E209–E214. [CrossRef]
334. Naslund, E.; Grybäck, P.; Bäckman, L.; Jacobsson, H.; Holst, J.J.; Theodorsson, H.E.; Hellstrom, P.M.; Juul, J. Distal small bowel hormones (Correlation with fasting antroduodenal motility and gastric emptying). *Dig. Dis. Sci.* **1998**, *43*, 945–952. [CrossRef]
335. Imeryüz, N.; Yeğen, B.Ç.; Bozkurt, A.; Coşkun, T.; Villanueva-Peñacarrillo, M.L.; Ulusoy, N.B. Glucagon-like peptide-1 inhibits gastric emptying via vagal afferent-mediated central mechanisms. *Am. J. Physiol. Liver Physiol.* **1997**, *273*, G920–G927. [CrossRef]
336. Schirra, J.; Nicolaus, M.; Woerle, H.J.; Struckmeier, C.; Katschinski, M.; Göke, B. GLP-1 regulates gastroduodenal motility involving cholinergic pathways. *Neurogastroenterol. Motil.* **2009**, *21*, 609–e22. [CrossRef]
337. Richards, P.; Parker, H.E.; Adriaenssens, A.E.; Hodgson, J.M.; Cork, S.C.; Trapp, S.; Gribble, F.M.; Reimann, F. Identification and characterization of GLP-1 receptor-expressing cells using a new transgenic mouse model. *Diabetes* **2014**, *63*, 1224–1233. [CrossRef]
338. Fitzgerald, P.C.E.; Manoliu, B.; Herbillon, B.; Steinert, R.E.; Horowitz, M.; Feinle-Bisset, C. Effects of L-phenylalanine on energy intake and glycaemia—impacts on appetite perceptions, gastrointestinal hormones and gastric emptying in healthy males. *Nutrients* **2020**, *12*, 1788. [CrossRef]
339. Layer, P.; Holst, J.J.; Grandt, D.; Goebell, H. Ileal release of glucagon-like peptide-1 (GLP-1). *Dig. Dis. Sci.* **1995**, *40*, 1074–1082. [CrossRef]
340. Wettergren, A.; Wojdemann, M.; Meisner, S.; Stadil, F.; Holst, J.J. The inhibitory effect of glucagon-like peptide-1 (GLP-1) 7–36 amide on gastric acid secretion in humans depends on an intact vagal innervation. *Gut* **1997**, *40*, 597–601. [CrossRef] [PubMed]
341. Villar, H.V.; Fender, H.R.; Rayford, P.L.; Bloom, S.R.; Ramus, N.I.; Thompson, J.C. Suppression of gastrin release and gastric secretion by gastric inhibitory polypeptide (GIP) and vasoactive intestinal polypeptide (VIP). *Ann. Surg.* **1976**, *184*, 97–102. [CrossRef]
342. Tolessa, T.; Gutniak, M.; Holst, J.J.; Efendic, S.; Hellström, P.M. Inhibitory effect of glucagon-like peptide-1 on small bowel motility. Fasting but not fed motility inhibited via nitric oxide independently of insulin and somatostatin. *J. Clin. Investig.* **1998**, *102*, 764–774. [CrossRef]
343. Halim, A.; Degerblad, M.; Sundbom, M.; Karlbom, U.; Holst, J.J.; Webb, D.-L.; Hellström, P.M. Glucagon-like peptide-1 inhibits prandial gastrointestinal motility through myenteric neuronal mechanisms in humans. *J. Clin. Endocrinol. Metab.* **2017**, *103*, 575–585. [CrossRef]
344. Ogawa, E.; Hosokawa, M.; Harada, N.; Yamane, S.; Hamasaki, A.; Toyoda, K.; Fujimoto, S.; Fujita, Y.; Fukuda, K.; Tsukiyama, K.; et al. The effect of gastric inhibitory polypeptide on intestinal glucose absorption and intestinal motility in mice. *Biochem. Biophys. Res. Commun.* **2011**, *404*, 115–120. [CrossRef]

345. Edholm, T.; Cejvan, K.; Efendic, S.; Schmidt, P.T.; Hellström, P.M.; Abdel-Halim, S.M. The incretin hormones GIP and GLP-1 in diabetic rats: Effects on insulin secretion and small bowel motility. *Neurogastroenterol. Motil.* **2009**, *21*, 313–321. [CrossRef]
346. Powley, T.L.; Phillips, R.J. Gastric satiation is volumetric, intestinal satiation is nutritive. *Physiol. Behav.* **2004**, *82*, 69–74. [CrossRef] [PubMed]
347. Kupari, J.; Häring, M.; Agirre, E.; Castelo-Branco, G.; Ernfors, P. An atlas of vagal sensory neurons and their molecular specialization. *Cell Rep.* **2019**, *27*, 2508–2523.e4. [CrossRef]
348. Egerod, K.L.; Petersen, N.; Timshel, P.N.; Rekling, J.C.; Wang, Y.; Liu, Q.; Schwartz, T.W.; Gautron, L. Profiling of G protein-coupled receptors in vagal afferents reveals novel gut-to-brain sensing mechanisms. *Mol. Metab.* **2018**, *12*, 62–75. [CrossRef] [PubMed]
349. Bucinskaite, V.; Tolessa, T.; Pedersen, J.; Rydqvist, B.; Zerihun, L.; Holst, J.J.; Hellström, P.M. Receptor-mediated activation of gastric vagal afferents by glucagon-like peptide-1 in the rat. *Neurogastroenterol. Motil.* **2009**, *21*, e78. [CrossRef] [PubMed]
350. Cork, S.C.; Richards, J.E.; Holt, M.K.; Gribble, F.M.; Reimann, F.; Trapp, S. Distribution and characterisation of Glucagon-like peptide-1 receptor expressing cells in the mouse brain. *Mol. Metab.* **2015**, *4*, 718–731. [CrossRef]
351. Jensen, C.B.; Pyke, C.; Rasch, M.G.; Dahl, A.B.; Knudsen, L.B.; Secher, A. Characterization of the glucagonlike peptide-1 receptor in male mouse brain using a novel antibody and In Situ hybridization. *Endocrinology* **2017**, *159*, 665–675. [CrossRef]
352. Ast, J.; Arvaniti, A.; Fine, N.H.F.; Nasteska, D.; Ashford, F.B.; Stamataki, Z.; Koszegi, Z.; Bacon, A.; Jones, B.J.; Lucey, M.A.; et al. Super-resolution microscopy compatible fluorescent probes reveal endogenous glucagon-like peptide-1 receptor distribution and dynamics. *Nat. Commun.* **2020**, *11*, 1–18. [CrossRef]
353. Gabery, S.; Salinas, C.G.; Paulsen, S.J.; Ahnfelt-Rønne, J.; Alanentalo, T.; Baquero, A.F.; Buckley, S.T.; Farkas, E.; Fekete, C.; Frederiksen, K.S.; et al. Semaglutide lowers body weight in rodents via distributed neural pathways. *JCI Insight* **2020**, *5*. [CrossRef]
354. Yox, D.P.; Stokesberry, H.; Ritter, R.C. Fourth ventricular capsaicin attenuates suppression of sham feeding induced by intestinal nutrients. *Am. J. Physiol. Integr. Comp. Physiol.* **1991**, *260*, R681–R687. [CrossRef]
355. Yox, D.P.; Ritter, R.C. Capsaicin attenuates suppression of sham feeding induced by intestinal nutrients. *Am. J. Physiol. Integr. Comp. Physiol.* **1988**, *255*, R569–R574. [CrossRef] [PubMed]
356. Larsen, P.; Tang-Christensen, M.; Holst, J.J.; Ørskov, C. Distribution of glucagon-like peptide-1 and other preproglucagon-derived peptides in the rat hypothalamus and brainstem. *Neuroscience* **1997**, *77*, 257–270. [CrossRef]
357. Hisadome, K.; Reimann, F.; Gribble, F.M.; Trapp, S. Leptin directly depolarizes preproglucagon neurons in the nucleus tractus solitarius. *Diabetes* **2010**, *59*, 1890–1898. [CrossRef] [PubMed]
358. Brierley, D.I.; Holt, M.K.; Singh, A.; de Araujo, A.; Vergara, M.; Afaghani, M.H.; Lee, S.J.; Scott, K.; Langhans, W.; Krause, E.; et al. Central and peripheral GLP-1 systems independently and additively suppress eating. *bioRxiv* **2020**. [CrossRef]
359. Powley, T.L.; Spaulding, R.A.; Haglof, S.A. Vagal afferent innervation of the proximal gastrointestinal tract mucosa: Chemoreceptor and mechanoreceptor architecture. *J. Comp. Neurol.* **2010**, *519*, 644–660. [CrossRef] [PubMed]
360. Kaelberer, M.M.; Buchanan, K.L.; Klein, M.E.; Barth, B.B.; Montoya, M.M.; Shen, X.; Bohórquez, D.V. A gut-brain neural circuit for nutrient sensory transduction. *Science* **2018**, *361*, 5236. [CrossRef]
361. Lu, V.B.; Rievaj, J.; O'Flaherty, E.A.; Smith, C.A.; Pais, R.; Pattison, L.A.; Tolhurst, G.; Leiter, A.B.; Bulmer, D.C.; Gribble, F.M.; et al. Adenosine triphosphate is co-secreted with glucagon-like peptide-1 to modulate intestinal enterocytes and afferent neurons. *Nat. Commun.* **2019**, *10*, 1029. [CrossRef]
362. Williams, D.L.; Baskin, D.G.; Schwartz, M.W. Evidence that intestinal glucagon-like peptide-1 plays a physiological role in satiety. *Endocrinology* **2008**, *150*, 1680–1687. [CrossRef] [PubMed]
363. Turton, M.D.; O'Shea, D.; Gunn, I.; Beak, S.A.; Edwards, C.M.B.; Meeran, K.; Choi, S.J.; Taylor, G.M.; Heath, M.M.; Lambert, P.D.; et al. A role for glucagon-like peptide-1 in the central regulation of feeding. *Nat. Cell Biol.* **1996**, *379*, 69–72. [CrossRef]
364. Tang-Christensen, M.; Larsen, P.J.; Göke, R.; Fink-Jensen, A.; Jessop, D.S.; Möller, M.; Sheikh, S.P. Central administration of GLP-1-(7–36) amide inhibits food and water intake in rats. *Am. J. Physiol. Integr. Comp. Physiol.* **1996**, *271*, R848–R856. [CrossRef]
365. Schick, R.R.; Zimmermann, J.P.; Walde, T.V.; Schusdziarra, V. Glucagon-like peptide 1-(7–36) amide acts at lateral and medial hypothalamic sites to suppress feeding in rats. *Am. J. Physiol. Integr. Comp. Physiol.* **2003**, *284*, R1427–R1435. [CrossRef] [PubMed]
366. Baggio, L.L.; Huang, Q.; Brown, T.J.; Drucker, D.J. Oxyntomodulin and glucagon-like peptide-1 differentially regulate murine food intake and energy expenditure. *Gastroenterology* **2004**, *127*, 546–558. [CrossRef] [PubMed]
367. Namkoong, C.; Kim, M.S.; Jang, B.-T.; Lee, Y.H.; Cho, Y.-M.; Choi, H.J. Central administration of GLP-1 and GIP decreases feeding in mice. *Biochem. Biophys. Res. Commun.* **2017**, *490*, 247–252. [CrossRef] [PubMed]
368. Adriaenssens, A.E.; Biggs, E.K.; Darwish, T.; Tadross, J.; Sukthankar, T.; Girish, M.; Polex-Wolf, J.; Lam, B.Y.; Zvetkova, I.; Pan, W.; et al. Glucose-dependent insulinotropic polypeptide receptor-expressing cells in the hypothalamus regulate food intake. *Cell Metab.* **2019**, *30*, 987–996.e6. [CrossRef]
369. Holt, M.K.; Richards, J.E.; Cook, D.R.; Brierley, D.I.; Williams, D.L.; Reimann, F.; Gribble, F.M.; Trapp, S. Preproglucagon neurons in the nucleus of the solitary tract are the main source of brain GLP-1, mediate stress-induced hypophagia, and limit unusually large intakes of food. *Diabetes* **2019**, *68*, 21–33. [CrossRef]
370. Mietlicki-Baase, E.G.; Ortinski, P.I.; Rupprecht, L.E.; Olivos, D.R.; Alhadeff, A.L.; Pierce, R.C.; Hayes, M.R. The food intake-suppressive effects of glucagon-like peptide-1 receptor signaling in the ventral tegmental area are mediated by AMPA/kainate receptors. *Am. J. Physiol. Metab.* **2013**, *305*, E1367–E1374. [CrossRef]

371. Dickson, S.L.; Shirazi, R.H.; Hansson, C.; Bergquist, F.; Nissbrandt, H.; Skibicka, K.P. The Glucagon-like peptide 1 (GLP-1) analogue, exendin-4, decreases the rewarding value of food: A new role for mesolimbic GLP-1 receptors. *J. Neurosci.* **2012**, *32*, 4812–4820. [CrossRef]
372. Dossat, A.M.; Diaz, R.; Gallo, L.; Panagos, A.; Kay, K.; Williams, D.L. Nucleus accumbens GLP-1 receptors influence meal size and palatability. *Am. J. Physiol. Metab.* **2013**, *304*, E1314. [CrossRef]
373. Kentish, S.; Li, H.; Philp, L.K.; O'Donnell, T.A.; Isaacs, N.J.; Young, R.L.; Wittert, G.A.; Blackshaw, L.A.; Page, A.J. Diet-induced adaptation of vagal afferent function. *J. Physiol.* **2011**, *590*, 209–221. [CrossRef]
374. Jepsen, S.L.; Grunddal, K.V.; Albrechtsen, N.J.W.; Engelstoft, M.S.; Gabe, M.B.N.; Jensen, E.P.; Ørskov, C.; Poulsen, S.S.; Rosenkilde, M.M.; Pedersen, J.; et al. Paracrine crosstalk between intestinal L- and D-cells controls secretion of glucagon-like peptide-1 in mice. *Am. J. Physiol. Metab.* **2019**, *317*, E1081–E1093. [CrossRef]
375. Adriaenssens, A.; Lam, B.Y.H.; Billing, L.; Skeffington, K.; Sewing, S.; Reimann, F.; Gribble, F. A transcriptome-led exploration of molecular mechanisms regulating somatostatin-producing D-Cells in the gastric epithelium. *Endocrinology* **2015**, *156*, 3924–3936. [CrossRef]

Review
Gastrointestinal Vagal Afferents and Food Intake: Relevance of Circadian Rhythms

Amanda J. Page [1,2]

1. Adelaide Medical School, University of Adelaide, Adelaide, SA 5000, Australia; amanda.page@adelaide.edu.au; Tel.: +61-8-8128-4840
2. Nutrition, Diabetes and Gut Health, Lifelong Health Theme, South Australian Health and Medical Research Institution (SAHMRI), Adelaide, SA 5000, Australia

Abstract: Gastrointestinal vagal afferents (VAs) play an important role in food intake regulation, providing the brain with information on the amount and nutrient composition of a meal. This is processed, eventually leading to meal termination. The response of gastric VAs, to food-related stimuli, is under circadian control and fluctuates depending on the time of day. These rhythms are highly correlated with meal size, with a nadir in VA sensitivity and increase in meal size during the dark phase and a peak in sensitivity and decrease in meal size during the light phase in mice. These rhythms are disrupted in diet-induced obesity and simulated shift work conditions and associated with disrupted food intake patterns. In diet-induced obesity the dampened responses during the light phase are not simply reversed by reverting back to a normal diet. However, time restricted feeding prevents loss of diurnal rhythms in VA signalling in high fat diet-fed mice and, therefore, provides a potential strategy to reset diurnal rhythms in VA signalling to a pre-obese phenotype. This review discusses the role of the circadian system in the regulation of gastrointestinal VA signals and the impact of factors, such as diet-induced obesity and shift work, on these rhythms.

Keywords: vagal afferents; circadian; food intake; gastrointestinal tract

1. Introduction

In response to a meal, the gastrointestinal tract sends humoral and neural signals to the central nervous system where it is combined with other signals ultimately leading to the termination of a meal. These satiety signals are not static, displaying a high degree of plasticity [1]. For example, gastric vagal afferents (VAs) display diurnal rhythms in their response to food related stimuli [2]. These rhythms are inversely associated with meal size and meal frequency and thus stomach content [2,3], such that in mice the nadir in gastric VA sensitivity during the dark phase is associated with an increase meal size and meal frequency, whereas the peak in sensitivity during the light phase is associated with reduced meal size and meal frequency [3]. This is important for the fine regulation of food intake to meet the daily fluctuations in energy demand and forms a component of the circadian systems role in energy homeostasis, namely temporal regulation of appetite and food intake as well as metabolic processes, such as anabolism and catabolism [4].

Circadian rhythms occur over ~24 h and are driven by endogenous clocks that form a sequence of interlocking molecular loops. The master clock is located in the suprachiasmatic nucleus (SCN) and receives input from the retina to allow entrainment to the light-dark cycle [5]. However, there are other clocks located both centrally and peripherally. For example, VA neurons express clock gene molecules which oscillate over a 24 h period [2]. Disruption of these VA rhythms, such as occurs in diet-induced obesity or shift work conditions, could lead to disruption in the timing of food intake contributing to the misalignment of metabolic processes and perpetuating the issue.

This review focusses on current knowledge on gastrointestinal VA satiety signalling, with particular emphasis on the diurnal regulation of these signals and the potential significance of these rhythms in the fine control of food intake. In addition, the impact of disrupted satiety signalling on food intake patterns and the development/maintenance of obesity will be discussed as well as the potential benefits of time restricted feeding.

2. Gastrointestinal Vagal Afferents

2.1. Subtypes of Gastrointestinal Vagal Afferents

Gastrointestinal VAs play an important role in food intake regulation [6], signalling to the hindbrain the arrival, amount and chemical composition of a meal. This information is then processed leading to reflex control of gut motility and secretions, required for the digestion and absorption of a meal, and sensations of satiety and fullness, that ultimately terminate a meal. Therefore, gastrointestinal VAs play an important role in limiting food intake and the size of a meal. Gastrointestinal VAs can be classified, based on their response to various stimuli, into three main groups, namely mechano-, chemo- and thermoreceptors, all with specific roles in gastrointestinal physiology, however, this review will focus on mechano- and chemoreceptors due to their known or suspected role in food intake regulation [7].

2.1.1. Mechanoreceptors

Mechanosensitive gastrointestinal VAs are important for sensing the amount and movement of food as it passes through the gastrointestinal tract. The receptive fields for mechanosensitive VAs are located within the mucosal and muscular layers of the gut wall [8] (Figure 1), and are categorised into tension, stretch, mucosal and tension-mucosal receptors depending on their response to specific mechanical stimuli [9,10]. These different types of afferent are discussed below:

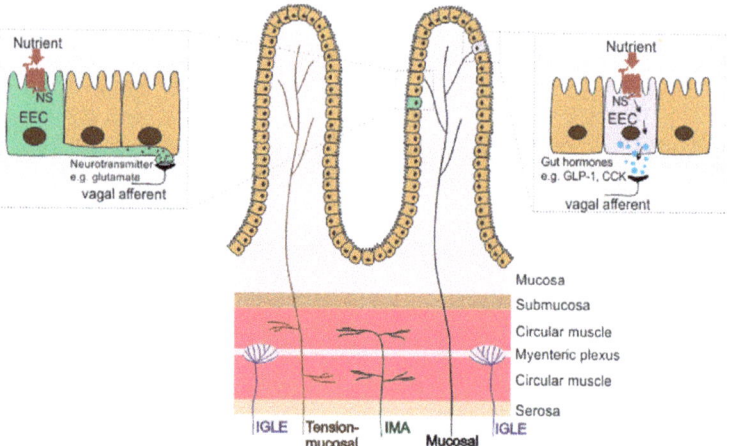

Figure 1. Schematic of the wall of the gastrointestinal tract with the location of the receptive fields of subclasses of gastrointestinal vagal afferents (VAs), including mechanosensitive (mucosal stroking) and/or chemosensitive mucosal afferents (Black), intraganglionic laminar endings (IGLEs, tension receptors; Purple), stretch sensitive intramuscular arrays (IMAs, stretch receptors; Green) and tension-mucosal afferents (Brown; sensitive to mucosal stroking and stretch). Chemosensing occurs via specialized enteroendocrine cells (EECs) that express nutrient receptors (NS) which when activated initiate an intracellular process culminating in: (1) the release of gut hormones, such as cholecystokinin (CCK) and glucagon-like peptide 1 (GLP-1) which subsequently act on peripheral VA terminals; or (2) the release of a neurotransmitter, such as glutamate, directly onto VA endings via neuropods that protrude from the basolateral surface of EECs.

Tension or Stretch Receptors

Tension receptors are generally slowly adapting, low threshold mechanoreceptors that respond to circular tension [11,12]. Tension receptors are thought to have specialized endings with a flattened leaf-like structure surrounding the myenteric ganglia termed intraganglionic laminar endings (IGLEs) [13,14]. Recently, a subpopulation of gastric IGLEs, which express glucagon-like peptide 1 receptor (GLP-1R), was activated by mechanical distension in vivo in mice [15,16]. In addition, there is a population of IGLEs in the small intestine, which express the oxytocin receptor gene (*Oxtr*) [15], which when activated by optogenetic and chemogenetic stimulation dramatically reduced food intake [15]. This suggests there are small intestinal mechanosensitive afferents which contribute to the regulation of food intake.

Gastrointestinal VA tension receptors were generally thought to be a homogenous population of afferents that detect both muscular tension and stretch [9,17]. However, stretch and tension are two completely different forces with tension the force required to maintain muscle length and stretch reflecting the need for muscle extension or contraction [9]. The identification of two morphologically distinct VA ending in the muscle layer of the gut raised the possibility of two distinct populations of stretch and tension receptors [18], with intramuscular arrays proposed as stretch receptors [9]. Intramuscular arrays are VA endings that run in parallel to muscle bundles in the muscularis externa [18–20].

Mucosal Receptors

Mucosal mechanoreceptors innervate the mucosal layer of the gastrointestinal tract and are fast adapting, low threshold mechanoreceptors activated by mucosal stroking, such as occurs when food particles pass over the receptive field. Mucosal receptors are relatively uninvestigated but, in the stomach, these receptors are thought to be involved in the control of gastric emptying, through the detection of food particle size, as well as the vomiting reflex [7,9,21,22], however, there is no direct in vivo evidence that this is the case.

Tension-Mucosal Receptors

Tension-mucosal receptors have been observed in the ferret oesophagus and respond to both circular tension and mucosal stroking [12]. However, using a similar approach a distinct population of tension-mucosal receptors could not be identified in the mouse [11]. This is possibly a consequence of the thinness of the oesophageal tissue in the mice, where low intensity mucosal stroking with von Frey hairs (e.g., 10 mg) can also stretch the underlying muscular layer making it impossible to distinguish between tension and tension-mucosal receptors [11]. Nonetheless, soon after their identification a similar subpopulation of colonic splanchnic and pelvic afferents, termed mucosal-muscular receptors, were identified in mice [23]. It has been suggested that these afferents have multiple endings that terminate in the muscular and mucosal layers of the gut wall [12,24]. However, although there is evidence that a single dorsal root ganglia neuron can receive input from a number of endings within the gut wall [25,26], including the mucosa, myenteric ganglia and circular muscle, the location of vagal tension-mucosal afferents remains to be determined and it is possible that a single ending in the subepithelial plexus is responsive to both stretch and mucosal stroking [10].

2.1.2. Chemoreceptors

Gastrointestinal VA chemoreceptors, located in the mucosal lamina propria of the gut wall, detect a wide range of stimuli, including changes in pH, osmolarity, gut hormones and nutrients [27] (Figure 1). While some chemosensitive afferents respond directly to nutrients, such as glucose [28], mucosal VAs do not make direct contact with the luminal content and instead chemosensing mechanisms are mediated by specialized epithelial cells in the gut wall, known as enteroendocrine cells (EECs), which express gut hormones. Different EECs express different specialized nutrient receptors with meal consumption and digestion resulting in a complex pattern of gut hormone release [29]. These hormones then act on their receptors on VA endings which signal to the brain and initiate the termination of food intake [30]. For example, glucose in the lumen of the small intestine induces release of the gut hormones glucagon-like peptide 1 (GLP-1) and 5-hydroxytryptamine (5-HT), which subsequently activate VA endings in the intestinal mucosa ultimately contributing to the regulation of gut motility (e.g., gastric emptying) and intestinal fluid secretion [30]. In addition, fatty acids and amino acids have been shown to induce cholecystokinin (CCK) release which subsequently activates VAs to induce satiety [31]. Further, VAs, in the distal intestine, have been shown to make synaptic connections with EECs via axon-like projections, known as neuropods, that protrude from the basolateral surface of EECs [32–36]. It has been demonstrated that infusion of sucrose evoked VA firing, through the release of glutamate from the neuropod onto the VA ending [37].

2.2. Gastrointestinal Vagal Afferents and Food Intake Regulation

Gastrointestinal VAs are important for the short term regulation of food intake and meal size. To date most of our knowledge relates to the role of VA mechanosensitive tension/stretch receptors and chemoreceptors and, therefore, these receptors will be the focus of this review. As food moves through the gastrointestinal tract the VA mechano- and chemoreceptor signalling occurs in a coordinated manner as outlined below:

2.2.1. Gastric Signals

As food enters and gradually fills the stomach it causes distension of the stomach wall which activates tension or stretch receptors innervating the stomach wall. These are one of the first signals to induce feelings of fullness and satiety [38–41]. The distension component of a meal can be reproduced in humans and separated from the nutrient component using a bag. Inflating a bag with air in the proximal stomach reduced hunger and induced a sensation of pressure-like fullness [38,40]. Distension of the proximal stomach by filling the bag with water induced feelings of fullness [42] and filling the bag with 400–800 mL of water reduced food intake in a volume-dependent manner [43]. Further, gastric distension, before or during a meal, reduced food intake in humans [41]. The antrum has also been shown to play a role in the perception of fullness and termination of a meal and it has been shown that fullness is directly related to the volume of a 350 mL glucose test drink in the distal stomach [44]. Further, after a mixed-nutrient drink subsequent energy intake was inversely associated with antral volume prior to the meal [45].

In a recent mouse study, Bai et al. showed that a subset of GLP-1R positive neurons are gastric IGLE mechanosensitive tension receptors [15]. Further, optogenetic and chemogenetic activation of these GLP-1R positive neurons inhibited food intake, albeit not to the same degree as activation of oxytocin receptor positive neurons which are predominantly small intestinal IGLE mechanosensitive tension receptors [15]. Nonetheless, it is clear that activation of tension receptors in the stomach initiates the satiety signalling.

2.2.2. Small Intestinal Signals

As gastric emptying occurs chyme enters the small intestine and the gastric distension signals diminish to be replaced by small intestinal signals. The intestine is the major site of macronutrient breakdown and nutrient absorption. However, the small intestine is not just the site of nutrient absorption but also nutrient detection with extensive sensory VA innervation of the small intestine, with peak density in the duodenum [10,46]. Recent evidence indicates mechanosensitive tension receptors in the duodenum play a more important role in satiety signalling than VA chemoreceptors [15]. However, there is a multitude of evidence to suggest that small intestinal VAs act as nutrient sensors, responding to gut hormones released from EECs upon exposure to nutrients to induce satiety.

Within the small intestine gut-hormone release is region and nutrient specific. For example, the gastrointestinal hormone CCK is released from I-cells, primarily in the duodenum and proximal jejunum, in response to luminal fatty acids and proteins [47–49]. In contrast, peptide YY (PYY) and GLP-1 are predominantly released from L-cells in the ileum and in humans distal (190 cm from the pylorus) glucose infusion substantially increased plasma GLP-1 levels, whereas proximal infusion (13 cm beyond the pylorus) had minimal effect on GLP-1 levels in healthy individuals and type 2 diabetic patients [50]. However, despite this PYY and GLP-1 have been observed in the porcine duodenum and jejunum suggesting a more global role for these hormones throughout the small intestine [51] and a study utilizing equicaloric intra-duodenal infusion of glucose and intralipid showed that fat is more potent at stimulating GLP-1 secretion compared to glucose in healthy males [52]. Co-expression of gut hormones, originally considered to be synthesized in distinct populations of EECs such as I-cells or L-cells, has been observed suggesting EECs are a single cell type which can produce an array of peptides depending on the location and environment [53]. PYY and GLP-1 are released in response to carbohydrates, fatty acids and amino acids. All these hormones have established anorexigenic effects and given their short plasma half-life, particularly for GLP-1, a local paracrine action is more probable than an endocrine action [54]. CCK has pronounced effects on food intake, reducing meal size and cumulative food intake [55]. The majority of the effects of CCK on food intake are due to action at CCKA receptors expressed on VAs [56,57]. PYY knockout mice are hyperphagic and exhibit a delayed satiety response to luminal nutrients, implying a role in the regulation of energy balance [58], whereas analogues of PYY, such as PYY (3–36), inhibit food intake [59]. Further, PYY receptors (Y2R) are expressed in VA neurons [60] and exogenous administration of PYY (3–36) increases VA firing [61]. In addition, bilateral subdiaphragmatic vagotomy led to the loss of PYYs anorexigenic effects [62]. However, treatment with capsaicin, to destroy VA fibres, had no effect on the inhibitory effect of PYY on food intake [63]. This could be due to non-specific effects on other fibre types [64] or the incomplete lesion induced using capsaicin [63]. The gut hormone GLP-1 has also been shown to increase satiation and reduce food intake. These effects are likely mediated via VAs as capsaicin treatment [63], bilateral sub-diaphragmatic vagotomy [62], and vagal deafferentation [65] resulted in loss of the anorexigenic effects of GLP-1 and its analogues. Further, GLP-1 receptors are expressed in rat VA neurons [66] and selective knockout of these receptors was associated with increased meal size, however, there was no long-term effects on energy balance [67]. Overall, it is likely that nutrients acting at specific sites on EECs initiate an intracellular process resulting in the release of a peptide/hormone, such as GLP-1, CCK, or PYY. Subsequently these hormones activate VA endings which send signals to the brain where it is processed leading to feelings of satiety and fullness, ultimately terminating a meal.

2.3. Plasticity of Gastrointestinal Afferents

Gastrointestinal VAs demonstrate a high degree of plasticity in order to precision match food intake to energy requirements. For example, after a fasting period energy demand is high and the first meal is increased, specifically the size and duration of the meal [68,69]. In fact, the size of this first meal has been shown to be directly associated with the length of the fasting period [69]. Further, it is known that gastric VA tension receptor responses to stretch are dampened after a fast [70]. Thus, more food would need to enter the stomach to signal the same response elicited in the fed state. This may, at least in part, explain why the first meal after a fast is increased compared to control. Whether the reduced mechanosensitivity depends on the length of the fasting period remains to be determined. A more chronic physiological adaptation occurs during pregnancy. During pregnancy gastric VA responses to stretch, assessed during the light phase, were attenuated in mice [71]. This is accompanied by an increase in food intake, predominantly due to an increase in meal size, during the light but not the dark phase and thus appears to be circadian in nature [71]. It is known that gastric VAs display diurnal rhythms in their response to food related stimuli [2], to regulate food intake over a 24 h period. The pregnancy data suggest that adjustments in the diurnal sensitivity of gastric VAs might play an important role in the fine tuning of food intake over longer periods of time, such as during pregnancy. However, this is speculative and requires further investigation.

Nonetheless, diurnal rhythms in gastric VA sensitivity to food related stimuli is another example of the plasticity of VAs and this will be discussed in the next section.

3. Circadian Regulation of Food Intake

3.1. Circadian System and Food Intake Patterns

The natural feeding behaviour in most living organisms is to spend one phase of the light-dark cycle in an active and feeding state and the other in a resting and fasting state [72]. For instance, humans and other diurnal mammals naturally spend the light phase in the active and feeding state, whereas, nocturnal mammals, such as rodents, are generally active and feeding during the dark phase. For example, ad libitum standard chow fed mice consume between 65 and 80% of food during the dark phase [3,73–75].

These rhythms are controlled by the circadian clock system which has a central clock located in the hypothalamic suprachiasmatic nucleus (SCN). The SCN influences other clocks located both centrally and peripherally [76] to temporally regulate metabolic processes over a 24 h period, giving rise to circadian rhythms in energy expenditure [77,78] and appetite/hunger [79–82]. In turn, the SCN is regulated by the light-dark cycle, through information received from the retina via the retinohypothalamic tract [5]. The molecular mechanisms driving circadian oscillations in the SCN consist of a series of interlocking transcriptional-translational molecular feedback loops. Briefly, clock genes consist of positive and negative elements. Positive elements include Circadian Locomotor Output Cycles Kaput (Clock), Brain and Muscle ARNT-Like 1 (BMAL1) and neuronal PAS domain protein 2 (NPAS2). Heterodimers of these positive elements, including BMAL1/Clock or BMAL1/NPAS2, enter the nucleus and stimulate the transcription of negative elements, such as period 1, 2 and 3 (Per1–3) and cryptochrome 1 and 2 (Cry1–2) [83–85]. In turn, the protein products of these transcriptional factors translocate to the nucleus and inhibit the activity of the BMAL1/Clock complex, ultimately inhibiting their own transcription and allowing the build up of the BMAL1/Clock complex to initiate a new cycle. In addition, there are also numerous nuclear receptors, including REV-ERB and ROR, which are considered to be core components of the clock system [86]. The heterodimer BMAL1/Clock has been shown to activate the transcription of REV-ERBα, which subsequently represses the transcription of BMAL1 [87,88]. These nuclear receptors enable bi-directional communication between the circadian system and other physiological systems and allows clock rhythms to be influenced by, for example, hormonal signals and cellular redox status [89–91].

Data using genetically modified mice with knockout or mutated clock genes provide compelling evidence for the role of clock molecules in the regulation of diurnal rhythms in food intake. For example, diurnal feeding rhythms in homozygous Clock mutant mice are greatly attenuated and the mice are also hyperphagic [92,93]. Similarly, loss or attenuation of feeding rhythms and/or hyperphagia has been observed in other clock gene mutant mice, such as BMAL1 [94], Cry1–2 [95,96] and Per2 mutant mice.

There are connections between the SCN and other regions in the hypothalamus and beyond involved in energy homeostasis, including but not limited to the arcuate nucleus (ARC), dorsal medial hypothalamus (DMH) and paraventricular nucleus [97–100]. These connections are essential for the day-to-day organization of physiological rhythms, such as food intake and energy expenditure. In addition to receiving projections and information from the SCN, many sites within the hypothalamus, including the ARC and DMH, possess their own circadian oscillators [101]. This has been demonstrated in cultured brain slices from PER2::Luciferase reporter mice and in long-term electrophysiological recordings [102]. The ARC and DMH have established roles in food intake regulation [103] and both regions are critical in driving diurnal rhythms in feeding behaviour. For instance, there are diurnal rhythms in the expression of ARC neuropeptides involved in food intake regulation, such as neuropeptide Y (NPY) [104], pro-opiomelanocortin (POMC) [105], and cocaine and amphetamine regulated transcript (CART) [105,106]. In rats, targeted destruction of ARC leptin- or NPY-responsive neurons, using saponin conjugated ligands, resulted in a disruption of the diurnal feeding rhythms [107,108]. In addition, deletion of the NPY receptors Y2 and Y4 altered daily feeding patterns [109]. In contrast, selective deletion of POMC neurons had no effect on diurnal rhythms in feeding behaviour in mice [110], although altered feeding rhythms were observed in Per2 knockout mice and linked to disruption in the diurnal rhythms of α-melanocyte-stimulating hormone, a POMC cleavage product [111]. Other central sites are involved in the control of feeding behaviour, however, there are numerous reviews on this area [100,112] and the focus of this review is gastrointestinal VAs.

Similar clock oscillators are located in peripheral tissue, including the gastrointestinal tract, adipose tissue and muscle, and the SCN sends neural or hormonal signals to these clocks to align and prevent the dampening of these rhythms [113]. For example, the neural links, e.g., VAs, between the gut and the central nervous system have also been shown to contain clock oscillators [2].

3.2. Circadian Vagal Afferent Signalling

The diurnal sensitivity of gastric VAs to food related stimuli is a good example of the high degree of plasticity these afferents exhibit (Figure 2). Gastric VA mucosal and tension receptors display diurnal rhythms in their response to mucosal stroking, using calibrated von Frey hairs, and stretch, respectively, with peak responses during the light phase and a nadir during the dark phase in mice [2]. In addition, these oscillations in gastric VA mechanosensitivity are inversely associated with the amount of food present in the stomach [2]. Meal size varies considerably between the light and dark phase in rodents, with larger and more frequent meals in the active dark phase when energy requirements are high [114]. Activation of VA tension receptors, by gastric distension has been shown to induce satiety [39] and, therefore, reduced sensitivity of gastric tension receptors, during the active dark phase, would permit more food to be consumed before satiation is reached. Whilst this is the only report of gastrointestinal VA circadian rhythmicity it has been shown that colonic afferents also exhibit circadian variation in their response to mechanical stimulation [115]. In this study it was observed that the spinal afferent mediated pain response to colonic distension was greater during the dark than the light phase in rats [115].

Although gastric VAs are predominantly mechanosensitive, the response of gastric VAs to food related stimuli can be modulated by peptides and hormones, including gastric hormones such as the 'hunger hormone' ghrelin. Ghrelin receptors are expressed in VA cell bodies and ghrelin attenuates gastric VA responses to mechanical stimuli. Of particular significance are the nutritional status dependent inhibitory effects of ghrelin on mucosal receptor mechanosensitivity; with inhibition observed in fasted mice but not *ad libitum* fed mice [70]. However, over a 24 h period, despite the distinct feed-fast episodes, the inhibitory effect of ghrelin on mouse gastric VAs did not display diurnal rhythms [3], suggesting a prolonged fast is required to elicit these effects. In addition, ghrelin plasma levels display circadian rhythms with a peak and trough during the inactive and active phases, respectively, in rodents and humans [116,117], therefore, it is unlikely to be mediating diurnal rhythms in gastric VA mechanosensitivity, as peak gastric VA sensitivity (Figure 2) occurs at about the same time as peak ghrelin levels in mice.

As stated earlier, gastrointestinal VA signals impact on the reflex control of gut motility. Although the focus of this review is food intake, it is important to recognize that changes in gut motility may be a consequence of changes in VA sensitivity. For example, it has been shown that gastric emptying half-time, of a solid not liquid meal, in humans is significantly longer in the evening (8 p.m.) compared to a morning (8 a.m.) meal [118]. This could be due to the diurnal sensitivity of gastric VAs responses to the meal which would presumably lead to diurnal reflex control of gastric emptying, however, this requires further investigation.

3.2.1. Nutrient and Gut Hormone Signals

In the gastrointestinal tract other mechanisms involved in gut to brain signalling via VAs may be responsible for circadian regulation of satiety signals, such as the nutrient sensing mechanisms within the intestine. For example, T1R2, a component of the sweet taste receptor, displayed circadian rhythmicity with peak expression in the mouse proximal jejunum, just prior to the commencement of the dark phase [119]. In theory, as these sweet taste receptors are co-localised with gut hormones, such as GLP-1, in EECs within the small intestine [120,121] and carbohydrates (e.g., glucose and sucrose) stimulate secretion of GLP-1 from EEC lines [121], diurnal rhythms in sweet taste receptors should lead to diurnal rhythms in GLP-1 secretion in response to the same nutrient load. However, there was no apparent difference in GLP-1 or PYY secretion, in response to a standard liquid Ensure meal given in the middle of the dark or light phase in rats [122], which is consistent with the lack of diurnal rhythms in T1R2 in the rat jejunum [123]. Further, research is required to clarify the role if any of the circadian system in gastrointestinal nutrient sensing and possible species variations.

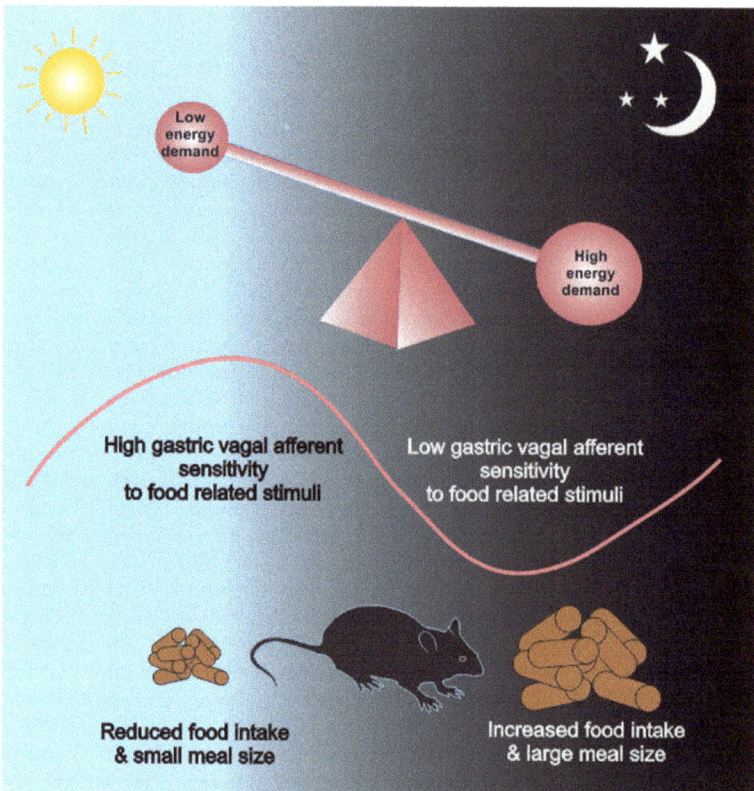

Figure 2. Schematic of the relationship between energy demand (e.g., during the active dark phase (dark grey region) verses inactive light phase (light blue region)), gastric vagal afferent (VA) sensitivity to food related stimuli (pink line) and food intake and meal size in mice. During the light phase the mice are resting and energy demand is low. Further, gastric VA sensitivity is high and associated with reduced food intake and meal size. Conversely, during the dark phase mice are active and consequently energy demand is high. In addition, gastric VA sensitivity is low and associated with increased food intake and meal size.

3.2.2. Gut Microbiota

The gut microbiota may also play a role in regulating diurnal rhythms in gastrointestinal VA function. Bacterial-derived molecules can influence VA function either directly or indirectly via activation of receptors on EECs (see review [124]). For example, receptors for short-chain fatty acids (SCFAs), produced by the gut microbiota, are present on EECs and the SCFA propionate has been shown to stimulate the release of PYY and GLP-1, both in vitro and in vivo in humans [125–127], which can subsequently activate intestinal VAs. Up to 60% of total microbial composition oscillates over a 24 h period, translating to 20% of commensal species in the mouse and 10% in humans [128]. In addition, there are daily rhythms in SCFA production [129], which is dependent on the timing of food intake and the supply of substrate (dietary fibre) for microbiota production of SCFAs. Therefore, it is possible a disruption in food intake patterns, such as occurs in shift workers, would lead to disruption in SCFA production which could conceivably lead to disruption in gastrointestinal VA satiety signalling that would further disrupt food intake patterns, perpetuating the situation. However, this is highly speculative and requires more detailed investigation. The host circadian clock has also been shown to regulate microbiota production of SCFAs, with disruption of SCFA production observed in Bmal knockout mice [130]. However, this is restored by dark-phase time restricted feeding, suggesting that disruption of SCFA production in Bmal knockout mice is secondary to changes in the timing of food intake.

3.2.3. Disrupted Circadian Signalling

High Fat Diet-Induced Obesity

Disruption of the diurnal rhythms in gastric VA satiety signalling may impact on food intake and contribute to metabolic disorders. In high fat diet-induced obese mice the diurnal rhythm in gastric VA satiety signalling was lost and associated with a loss or attenuation in the diurnal patterns of food intake [3] (Figure 3). For example, in high fat diet-induced obese mice there was an increase in meal size during the light phase, to levels equivalent to meal size in the dark phase [3]. This loss of diurnal rhythms in gastric VA mechanosensitivity is probably due to the obese state rather than the high fat diet as circadian rhythms in gastric VA mechanosensitivity were still observed two and four weeks after commencement of the high fat diet, at stages when there is no significant difference or the point of transition to increased weight gain, respectively, compared to standard chow fed mice [3,131]. The loss of diurnal rhythms in high fat diet-induced obese mice is predominantly due to a loss of the peak gastric VA mechanosensitivity observed during the light phase [2], allowing more food to be consumed when mice are inactive and energy demand is low. Jejunal VA responses to distension and chemical (e.g., CCK) stimuli are also attenuated during the light phase in high fat diet-induced obese mice [132] and, therefore, it is possible that jejunal VAs have a similar circadian profile as gastric VAs, although to date this remains to be determined. Further, the attenuated response, observed during the light phase, does not return to normal upon return to a standard chow diet for an equivalent time on the high fat diet [133]. This reduction in gastric VA tension receptor mechanosensitivity is consistent with the observed reduction in neural activation, in response to gastric distension, within the hypothalamus of obese individuals [134]. In addition, the failure of gastric VAs to revert back to the lean phenotype has also been observed in the neuronal responses to food intake in the brain of post-obese individuals [135]. It is acknowledged that chronic feeding of an energy dense and palatable diet leads to obesity [136], which once established is defended against weight loss [137] or weight perturbations [138]. It is possible the reduction in gastric VA responses to distension may contribute to the difficulty in maintaining weight loss.

Disrupted Light Cycle

Long-term misalignment of the circadian system, such as occurs in shift work, is a risk factor for metabolic disorders, including obesity [139–142]. This is a huge problem as ~15–20% of the working population are shift workers, including those on permanent night shifts or on rotating or irregular schedules [143–145]. As stated previously, animals and humans normally exhibit diurnal rhythms in food intake with the majority of food consumed during the natural active/wake period. These daily rhythms in food intake are aligned with other zeitgebers, such as the light cycle and activity, where they can act synergistically to promote synchronization of daily rhythms, including appetite, anabolism and catabolism. Misalignment of these zeitgebers can occur for a number of reasons, including shift work, exposure to long hours of artificial light and even dim light during the dark phase, and result in disruption of the syncrony of daily physiological and behavioural rhythms. For example, shift workers who are active during the rest period and exposed to long hours of artificial light also eat meals around their working hours [146–149] resulting in increased food intake during a period when they normally rest. Interestingly, although total energy intake is similar between night and day shift workers [150], the pattern of food intake is altered with night shift workers spreading food intake across a 24 h period with no extended fasting periods [151]. In addition, shift workers usually revert back to a more social daytime schedule on their days off, imposing a jet-lag model as physiological processes attempt to adjust to the new schedule. Similarly, the ready availability of artificial light has extended the length of the day period which has, subsequently, led to an extension of the feeding period. For example, a smart-phone application designed to monitor food intake has been used to demonstrate that feeding episodes span over 15 h/day in >50% of participants [152].

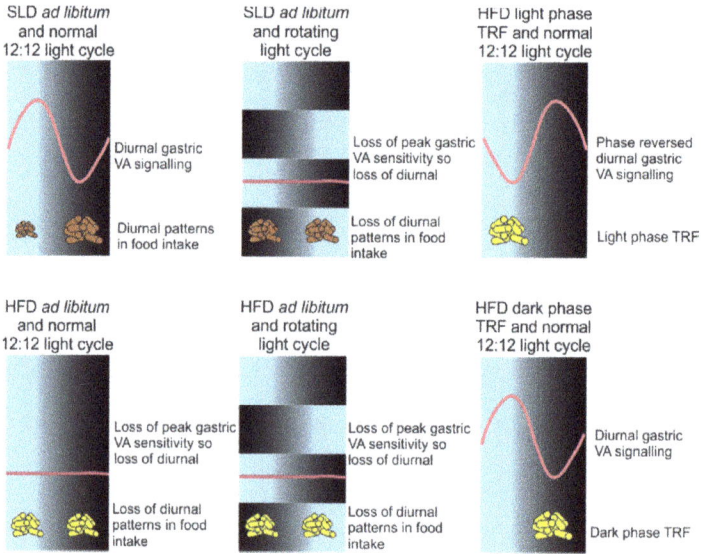

Figure 3. Schematic of the effect of circadian desynchrony on diurnal gastric vagal afferent (VA) responses to food related stimuli (e.g., stretch or mucosal stroking) in mice. On a normal standard laboratory diet (SLD) gastric VAs display diurnal rhythms in sensitivity to food related stimuli, with associated diurnal rhythms in food intake. In high fat diet-induced obese mice and/or mice exposed to a rotating light cycle diurnal rhythms in gastric VA responses to food related stimuli are lost and associated with a disruption in diurnal food intake patterns. High fat diet-fed mice exposed to a time restricted feeding (TRF) protocol, where food is restricted to the 12 h light phase or 12 h dark phase, retain diurnal rhythms in gastric VA responses to food related stimuli.

There are a number of animal models of shift work, including alterations in activity and/or sleep or light exposure [153], which have shown that circadian misalignment promotes metabolic disturbances, such as obesity [153–155]. For example, weight gain was higher in mice exposed to dim light at night compared to mice exposed to a normal light-dark cycle and, despite no change in overall 24 h food intake, there was disrupted feeding patterns due to increased light phase food intake [156–158]. Further, in a mouse rotating light cycle model of shift work, diurnal rhythms in gastric VA sensitivity to food related stimuli was ablated and accompanied by disruptions in diurnal food intake patterns [159].

In this study the lean standard laboratory and obese high fat diet-fed mice exposed to the rotating light cycle gained more weight than their counterparts on a normal 12 h light-12 h dark cycle, despite the fact there was no overall change in 24 h energy intake [159]. Therefore, diurnal gastric VA mechanosensitivity is susceptible to disturbances in the light-dark cycle and the obese state. These disturbances are associated with changes in food intake patterns and likely contribute to the difficulty in losing and maintaining weight loss. It is unclear whether the disruption in diurnal rhythms in VA sensitivity is causing the disruption in food intake or vice versa but, in spite of this, time restricted protocols to re-establish fed-fasting regimes is an attractive option to reinforce circadian rhythms.

3.2.4. Time Restricted Feeding

The timing of food intake episodes is another important regulator for central and peripheral clocks [160]. Time restricted feeding, where food intake is limited to a specific number of hours per day (6–12 h), provides a mechanism to re-establish diurnal rhythms in fed/fasting states, realigning and reinforcing circadian rhythms. Time restricted feeding has been shown to protect against metabolic disease in high fat diet-fed mice without reducing energy intake [161]. Further, time restricted feeding prevented obesity in mouse models of jetlag or shift work [162]. The metabolic benefits of time restricted feeding have been reviewed extensively [163] and, therefore, this review will focus on gastrointestinal VA satiety signalling and the impact of time restricted feeding on these signals. Early light phase time restricted feeding (800–1400 h), in humans, reduced appetite and, perhaps more important in terms of gastrointestinal VA function, increased feelings of fullness [164]. Twelve-hour time-restricted feeding in the light or dark phase prevented the loss of diurnal rhythms in gastric VA satiety signalling in high fat diet-induced obese mice, albeit the rhythms were phase reversed when the feeding was restricted to the light phase [131]. It remains to be determined whether time restricted feeding will reverse the loss of rhythms in VA sensitivity in established high fat diet-induced obesity [3] or shift work conditions [159] and, therefore, whether time restricted feeding is a potential solution to the lack of reversal of these afferents, to the pre-obese diurnal phenotype, upon return to a normal diet in mice [133]. Further, it remains to be established whether a time restricted feeding protocol is only required for a short period to switch the VA phenotype back to the pre-obese state or whether there needs to be a maintenance protocol, such as time restricted feeding for 3–4 days per week.

4. Conclusions

Gastrointestinal VAs play an essential role in the short-term regulation of food intake. The sensitivity of these afferents is not static, displaying diurnal sensitivity to food related stimuli in order to finely control food intake, over a 24 h period, to match the daily fluctuations in energy demand. Disruption of these diurnal rhythms, such as occurs in diet-induced obesity and shift work, is associated with disrupted food intake patterns which, without increases in energy intake, can lead to weight gain due to misalignment of metabolic processes with food intake. In diet-induced obesity the loss of these rhythms can be prevented using a time restricted feeding protocol. It remains to be determined whether time restricted feeding will reverse the loss of diurnal signals in established diet-induced obesity.

Funding: The author was funded by an Australian National Health and Medical Research Council (NHMRC) project grant (APP1046289) for studies related to this review.

Conflicts of Interest: The author declares no conflict of interest. The NHMRC had no input in the content or the decision to write this review.

References

1. Kentish, S.J.; Page, A.J. Plasticity of gastro-intestinal vagal afferent endings. *Physiol. Behav.* **2014**, *136*, 170–178. [CrossRef]
2. Kentish, S.J.; Frisby, C.L.; Kennaway, D.J.; Wittert, G.A.; Page, A.J. Circadian variation in gastric vagal afferent mechanosensitivity. *J. Neurosci.* **2013**, *33*, 19238–19242. [CrossRef]
3. Kentish, S.J.; Vincent, A.D.; Kennaway, D.J.; Wittert, G.A.; Page, A.J. High-Fat Diet-Induced Obesity Ablates Gastric Vagal Afferent Circadian Rhythms. *J. Neurosci.* **2016**, *36*, 3199–3207. [CrossRef]
4. Armstrong, S. A chronometric approach to the study of feeding behavior. *Neurosci. Biobehav. Rev.* **1980**, *4*, 27–53. [CrossRef]
5. Ma, M.A.; Morrison, E.H. Neuroanatomy, Nucleus Suprachiasmatic. In *StatPearls*; StatPearls Publishing: Treasure Island, FL, USA, 2019.
6. Schwartz, M.W.; Woods, S.C.; Porte, D., Jr.; Seeley, R.J.; Baskin, D.G. Central nervous system control of food intake. *Nature* **2000**, *404*, 661–671. [CrossRef]
7. Kentish, S.J.; Page, A.J. The role of gastrointestinal vagal afferent fibres in obesity. *J. Physiol.* **2015**, *593*, 775–786. [CrossRef]
8. Wang, Y.B.; De Lartigue, G.; Page, A.J. Dissecting the Role of Subtypes of Gastrointestinal Vagal Afferents. *Front. Physiol.* **2020**, *11*, 643. [CrossRef] [PubMed]
9. Phillips, R.J.; Powley, T.L. Tension and stretch receptors in gastrointestinal smooth muscle: Re-evaluating vagal mechanoreceptor electrophysiology. *Brain Res. Rev.* **2000**, *34*, 1–26. [CrossRef]
10. Brookes, S.J.; Spencer, N.J.; Costa, M.; Zagorodnyuk, V.P. Extrinsic primary afferent signalling in the gut. *Nat. Rev. Gastroenterol. Hepatol.* **2013**, *10*, 286–296. [CrossRef] [PubMed]
11. Page, A.J.; Martin, C.M.; Blackshaw, L.A. Vagal mechanoreceptors and chemoreceptors in mouse stomach and esophagus. *J. Neurophysiol.* **2002**, *87*, 2095–2103. [CrossRef] [PubMed]
12. Page, A.J.; Blackshaw, L.A. An in vitro study of the properties of vagal afferent fibres innervating the ferret oesophagus and stomach. *J. Physiol.* **1998**, *512*, 907–916. [CrossRef] [PubMed]
13. Zagorodnyuk, V.P.; Chen, B.N.; Brookes, S.J.H. Intraganglionic laminar endings are mechano-transduction sites of vagal tension receptors in the guinea-pig stomach. *J. Physiol.* **2001**, *534*, 255–268. [CrossRef] [PubMed]
14. Zagorodnyuk, V.P.; Brookes, S.J. Transduction sites of vagal mechanoreceptors in the guinea pig esophagus. *J. Neurosci.* **2000**, *20*, 6249–6255. [CrossRef] [PubMed]
15. Bai, L.; Mesgarzadeh, S.; Ramesh, K.S. Genetic Identification of Vagal Sensory Neurons That Control Feeding. *Cell* **2019**, *179*, 1129–1143.e1123. [CrossRef]
16. Williams, E.K.; Chang, R.B.; Strochlic, D.E.; Umans, B.D.; Lowell, B.B.; Liberles, S.D. Sensory Neurons that Detect Stretch and Nutrients in the Digestive System. *Cell* **2016**, *166*, 209–221. [CrossRef] [PubMed]
17. Iggo, A. Tension receptors in the stomach and the urinary bladder. *J. Physiol.* **1955**, *128*, 593–607. [CrossRef]
18. Berthoud, H.R.; Powley, T.L. Vagal Afferent Innervation of the Rat Fundic Stomach: Morphological Characterization of the Gastric Tension Receptor. *J. Comp. Neurol.* **1992**, *319*, 261–276. [CrossRef]
19. Fox, E.A.; Phillips, R.J.; Martinson, F.A.; Baronowsky, E.A.; Powley, T.L. Vagal afferent innervation of smooth muscle in the stomach and duodenum of the mouse: Morphology and topography. *J. Comp. Neurol.* **2000**, *428*, 558–576. [CrossRef]
20. Powley, T.L.; Hudson, C.N.; McAdams, J.L.; Baronowsky, E.A.; Phillips, R.J. Vagal Intramuscular Arrays: The Specialized Mechanoreceptor Arbors That Innervate the Smooth Muscle Layers of the Stomach Examined in the Rat. *J. Comp. Neurol.* **2016**, *524*, 713–737. [CrossRef] [PubMed]
21. Becker, J.M.; Kelly, K.A. Antral control of canine gastric emptying of solids. *Am. J. Physiol. Gastrointest. Liver Physiol.* **1983**, *8*, 334–338. [CrossRef]
22. Andrews, P.L.; Wood, K.L. Vagally mediated gastric motor and emetic reflexes evoked by stimulation of the antral mucosa in anaesthetized ferrets. *J. Physiol.* **1988**, *395*, 1–16. [CrossRef]
23. Brierley, S.M.; Jones, R.C.; Gebhart, G.F.; Blackshaw, L.A. Splanchnic and pelvic mechanosensory afferents signal different qualities of colonic stimuli in mice. *Gastroenterology* **2004**, *127*, 166–178. [CrossRef] [PubMed]
24. Brierley, S.M.; Jones, R.C., 3rd; Xu, L.; Gebhart, G.F.; Blackshaw, L.A. Activation of splanchnic and pelvic colonic afferents by bradykinin in mice. *Neurogastroenterol. Motil.* **2005**, *17*, 854–862. [CrossRef]
25. Spencer, N.J.; Kyloh, M.; Beckett, E.A.; Brookes, S.; Hibberd, T. Different types of spinal afferent nerve endings in stomach and esophagus identified by anterograde tracing from dorsal root ganglia. *J. Comp. Neurol.* **2016**, *524*, 3064–3083. [CrossRef]
26. Spencer, N.J.; Hu, H. Enteric nervous system: Sensory transduction, neural circuits and gastrointestinal motility. *Nat. Rev. Gastroenterol. Hepatol.* **2020**, *17*, 338–351. [CrossRef] [PubMed]
27. Powley, T.L.; Phillips, R.J. Gastric satiation is volumetric, intestinal satiation is nutritive. *Physiol. Behav.* **2004**, *82*, 69–74. [CrossRef] [PubMed]
28. Grabauskas, G.; Song, I.; Zhou, S.; Owyang, C. Electrophysiological identification of glucose-sensing neurons in rat nodose ganglia. *J. Physiol.* **2010**, *588*, 617–632. [CrossRef] [PubMed]
29. Mace, O.J.; Tehan, B.; Marshall, F. Pharmacology and physiology of gastrointestinal enteroendocrine cells. *Pharmacol. Res. Perspect.* **2015**, *3*, e00155. [CrossRef]
30. Raybould, H.E. Gut chemosensing: Interactions between gut endocrine cells and visceral afferents. *Auton. Neurosci.* **2010**, *153*, 41–46. [CrossRef] [PubMed]
31. Dockray, G.J. Luminal sensing in the gut: An overview. *J. Physiol. Pharmacol.* **2003**, *54*, 9–17. [PubMed]

32. Kaelberer, M.M.; Bohorquez, D.V. The now and then of gut-brain signaling. *Brain Res.* **2018**, *1693*, 192–196. [CrossRef]
33. Bohorquez, D.V.; Chandra, R.; Samsa, L.A.; Vigna, S.R.; Liddle, R.A. Characterization of basal pseudopod-like processes in ileal and colonic PYY cells. *J. Mol. Histol.* **2011**, *42*, 3–13. [CrossRef] [PubMed]
34. Bohorquez, D.V.; Liddle, R.A. Axon-like basal processes in enteroendocrine cells: Characteristics and potential targets. *Clin. Transl. Sci.* **2011**, *4*, 387–391. [CrossRef]
35. Bohorquez, D.V.; Samsa, L.A.; Roholt, A.; Medicetty, S.; Chandra, R.; Liddle, R.A. An enteroendocrine cell-enteric glia connection revealed by 3D electron microscopy. *PLoS ONE* **2014**, *9*, e89881. [CrossRef]
36. Bohorquez, D.V.; Shahid, R.A.; Erdmann, A. Neuroepithelial circuit formed by innervation of sensory enteroendocrine cells. *J. Clin. Investig.* **2015**, *125*, 782–786. [CrossRef] [PubMed]
37. Kaelberer, M.M.; Buchanan, K.L.; Klein, M.E. A gut-brain neural circuit for nutrient sensory transduction. *Science* **2018**, *361*. [CrossRef] [PubMed]
38. Feinle, C.; Grundy, D.; Read, N.W. Effects of duodenal nutrients on sensory and motor responses of the human stomach to distension. *Am. J. Physiol. Gastrointest. Liver Physiol.* **1997**, *273*, G721–G726. [CrossRef]
39. Wang, G.; Tomasi, D.; Backus, W. Gastric distention activates satiety circuitry in the human brain. *Neuroimage* **2008**, *39*, 1824–1831. [CrossRef]
40. Distrutti, E.; Azpiroz, F.; Soldevilla, A.; Malagelada, J.R. Gastric wall tension determines perception of gastric distention. *Gastroenterology* **1999**, *116*, 1035–1042. [CrossRef]
41. Kissileff, H.R.; Carretta, J.C.; Geliebter, A.; Pi-Sunyer, F.X. Cholecystokinin and stomach distension combine to reduce food intake in humans. *Am. J. Physiol. Regul. Integr. Comp. Physiol.* **2003**, *285*, R992–R998. [CrossRef]
42. Melton, P.M.; Kissileff, H.R.; Pi-Sunyer, F.X. Cholecystokinin (CCK-8) affects gastric pressure and ratings of hunger and fullness in women. *Am. J. Physiol.* **1992**, *263*, R452–R456. [CrossRef]
43. Geliebter, A.; Westreich, S.; Gage, D. Gastric distention by balloon and test-meal intake in obese and lean subjects. *Am. J. Clin. Nutr.* **1988**, *48*, 592–594. [CrossRef]
44. Jones, K.L.; Doran, S.M.; Hveem, K. Relation between postprandial satiation and antral area in normal subjects. *Am. J. Clin. Nutr.* **1997**, *66*, 127–132. [CrossRef]
45. Sturm, K.; Parker, B.; Wishart, J. Energy intake and appetite are related to antral area in healthy young and older subjects. *Am. J. Clin. Nutr.* **2004**, *80*, 656–667. [CrossRef]
46. Jagger, A.; Grahn, J.; Ritter, R.C. Reduced vagal sensory innervation of the small intestinal myenteric plexus following capsaicin treatment of adult rats. *Neurosci. Lett.* **1997**, *236*, 103–106. [CrossRef]
47. Liou, A.P.; Sei, Y.; Zhao, X. The extracellular calcium-sensing receptor is required for cholecystokinin secretion in response to l-phenylalanine in acutely isolated intestinal I cells. *Am. J. Physiol. Gastrointest. Liver Physiol.* **2011**, *300*, G538–G546. [CrossRef] [PubMed]
48. Rehfeld, J.F. Immunochemical studies on cholecystokinin. II. Distribution and molecular heterogeneity in the central nervous system and small intestine of man and hog. *J. Biol. Chem.* **1978**, *253*, 4022–4030. [CrossRef]
49. Cummings, D.E.; Overduin, J. Gastrointestinal regulation of food intake. *J. Clin. Investig.* **2007**, *117*, 13–23. [CrossRef]
50. Zhang, X.; Young, R.L.; Bound, M. Comparative Effects of Proximal and Distal Small Intestinal Glucose Exposure on Glycemia, Incretin Hormone Secretion, and the Incretin Effect in Health and Type 2 Diabetes. *Diabetes Care* **2019**, *42*, 520–528. [CrossRef] [PubMed]
51. Mortensen, K.; Christensen, L.L.; Holst, J.J.; Orskov, C. GLP-1 and GIP are colocalized in a subset of endocrine cells in the small intestine. *Regul. Pept.* **2003**, *114*, 189–196. [CrossRef]
52. Wu, T.; Rayner, C.K.; Watson, L.E.; Jones, K.L.; Horowitz, M.; Little, T.J. Comparative effects of intraduodenal fat and glucose on the gut-incretin axis in healthy males. *Peptides* **2017**, *95*, 124–127. [CrossRef]
53. Habib, A.M.; Richards, P.; Cairns, L.S. Overlap of endocrine hormone expression in the mouse intestine revealed by transcriptional profiling and flow cytometry. *Endocrinology* **2012**, *153*, 3054–3065. [CrossRef]
54. Meier, J.J.; Nauck, M.A.; Kranz, D. Secretion, Degradation, and Elimination of Glucagon-Like Peptide 1 and Gastric Inhibitory Polypeptide in Patients with Chronic Renal Insufficiency and Healthy Control Subjects. *Diabetes* **2004**, *53*, 654–662. [CrossRef]
55. Ballinger, A.B.; Clark, M.L. L-phenylalanine releases cholecystokinin (CCK) and is associated with reduced food intake in humans: Evidence for a physiological role of CCK in control of eating. *Metabolism* **1994**, *43*, 735–738. [CrossRef]
56. Dockray, G.J. Cholecystokinin. *Curr. Opin. Endocrinol. Diabetes Obes.* **2012**, *19*, 8–12. [CrossRef] [PubMed]
57. Lin, L.; Thomas, S.R.; Kilroy, G.; Schwartz, G.J.; York, D.A. Enterostatin inhibition of dietary fat intake is dependent on CCK-A receptors. *Am. J. Physiol. Regul. Integr. Comp. Physiol.* **2003**, *285*, R321–R328. [CrossRef]
58. Batterham, R.L.; Heffron, H.; Kapoor, S. Critical role for peptide YY in protein-mediated satiation and body-weight regulation. *Cell Metab.* **2006**, *4*, 223–233. [CrossRef] [PubMed]
59. Batterham, R.L.; Cowley, M.A.; Small, C.J. Gut hormone PYY(3-36) physiologically inhibits food intake. *Nature* **2002**, *418*, 650–654. [CrossRef] [PubMed]
60. Burdyga, G.; De Lartigue, G.; Raybould, H.E. Cholecystokinin Regulates Expression of Y2 Receptors in Vagal Afferent Neurons Serving the Stomach. *J. Neurosci.* **2008**, *28*, 11583–11592. [CrossRef]
61. Koda, S.; Date, Y.; Murakami, N. The role of the vagal nerve in peripheral PYY3-36-induced feeding reduction in rats. *Endocrinology* **2005**, *146*, 2369–2375. [CrossRef]

62. Abbott, C.R.; Monteiro, M.; Small, C.J. The inhibitory effects of peripheral administration of peptide YY(3-36) and glucagon-like peptide-1 on food intake are attenuated by ablation of the vagal-brainstem-hypothalamic pathway. *Brain Res.* **2005**, *1044*, 127–131. [CrossRef]
63. Talsania, T.; Anini, Y.; Siu, S.; Drucker, D.J.; Brubaker, P.L. Peripheral exendin-4 and peptide YY(3-36) synergistically reduce food intake through different mechanisms in mice. *Endocrinology* **2005**, *146*, 3748–3756. [CrossRef] [PubMed]
64. Browning, K.N.; Babic, T.; Holmes, G.M.; Swartz, E.; Travagli, R.A. A critical re-evaluation of the specificity of action of perivagal capsaicin. *J. Physiol.* **2013**, *591*, 1563–1580. [CrossRef] [PubMed]
65. Labouesse, M.A.; Stadlbauer, U.; Weber, E.; Arnold, M.; Langhans, W.; Pacheco-López, G. Vagal Afferents Mediate Early Satiation and Prevent Flavour Avoidance Learning in Response to Intraperitoneally Infused Exendin-4. *J. Neuroendocrinol.* **2012**, *24*, 1505–1516. [CrossRef] [PubMed]
66. Nakagawa, A.; Satake, H.; Nakabayashi, H. Receptor gene expression of glucagon-like peptide-1, but not glucose-dependent insulinotropic polypeptide, in rat nodose ganglion cells. *Auton. Neurosci.* **2004**, *110*, 36–43. [CrossRef] [PubMed]
67. Krieger, J.P.; Arnold, M.; Pettersen, K.G.; Lossel, P.; Langhans, W.; Lee, S.J. Knockdown of GLP-1 Receptors in Vagal Afferents Affects Normal Food Intake and Glycemia. *Diabetes* **2016**, *65*, 34–43. [CrossRef] [PubMed]
68. Larue-Achagiotis, C.; Le Magnen, J. Changes of meal patterns induced by food deprivation: Metabolic correlates. *Neurosci. Biobehav. Rev.* **1980**, *4*, 25–27. [CrossRef]
69. Le Magnen, J.; Devos, M.; Larue-Achagiotis, C. Food deprivation induced parallel changes in blood glucose, plasma free fatty acids and feeding during two parts of the diurnal cycle in rats. *Neurosci. Biobehav. Rev.* **1980**, *4*, 17–23. [CrossRef]
70. Kentish, S.; Li, H.; Philp, L.K. Diet-induced adaptation of vagal afferent function. *J. Physiol.* **2012**, *590*, 209–221. [CrossRef]
71. Li, H.; Clarke, G.S.; Christie, S. Pregnancy-related plasticity of gastric vagal afferent signals in mice. *Am. J. Physiol. Gastrointest. Liver Physiol.* **2021**, *320*, G183–G192. [CrossRef]
72. Hastings, M.H.; Reddy, A.B.; Maywood, E.S. A clockwork web: Circadian timing in brain and periphery, in health and disease. *Nat. Rev. Neurosci.* **2003**, *4*, 649–661. [CrossRef]
73. Christie, S.; Vincent, A.D.; Li, H. A rotating light cycle promotes weight gain and hepatic lipid storage in mice. *Am. J. Physiol. Gastrointest. Liver Physiol.* **2018**, *315*, G932–G942. [CrossRef]
74. Honma, K.; Hikosaka, M.; Mochizuki, K.; Goda, T. Loss of circadian rhythm of circulating insulin concentration induced by high-fat diet intake is associated with disrupted rhythmic expression of circadian clock genes in the liver. *Metabolism* **2016**, *65*, 482–491. [CrossRef]
75. Kohsaka, A.; Laposky, A.D.; Ramsey, K.M. High-fat diet disrupts behavioral and molecular circadian rhythms in mice. *Cell Metab.* **2007**, *6*, 414–421. [CrossRef]
76. Patton, A.P.; Hastings, M.H. The suprachiasmatic nucleus. *Curr. Biol.* **2018**, *28*, R816–R822. [CrossRef] [PubMed]
77. Krauchi, K.; Wirz-Justice, A. Circadian rhythm of heat production, heart rate, and skin and core temperature under unmasking conditions in men. *Am. J. Physiol.* **1994**, *267*, R819–R829. [CrossRef] [PubMed]
78. Spengler, C.M.; Czeisler, C.A.; Shea, S.A. An endogenous circadian rhythm of respiratory control in humans. *J. Physiol.* **2000**, *526*, 683–694. [CrossRef] [PubMed]
79. Scheer, F.A.; Morris, C.J.; Shea, S.A. The internal circadian clock increases hunger and appetite in the evening independent of food intake and other behaviors. *Obesity* **2013**, *21*, 421–423. [CrossRef]
80. Owens, D.S.; Macdonald, I.; Benton, D.; Sytnik, N.; Tucker, P.; Folkard, S. A preliminary investigation into individual differences in the circadian variation of meal tolerance: Effects on mood and hunger. *Chronobiol. Int.* **1996**, *13*, 435–447. [CrossRef]
81. Sargent, C.; Zhou, X.; Matthews, R.W.; Darwent, D.; Roach, G.D. Daily Rhythms of Hunger and Satiety in Healthy Men during One Week of Sleep Restriction and Circadian Misalignment. *Int. J. Environ. Res. Public Health* **2016**, *13*, 170. [CrossRef] [PubMed]
82. Wehrens, S.M.T.; Christou, S.; Isherwood, C. Meal Timing Regulates the Human Circadian System. *Curr. Biol.* **2017**, *27*, 1768–1775.e1763. [CrossRef] [PubMed]
83. Bunger, M.K.; Wilsbacher, L.D.; Moran, S.M. Mop3 is an essential component of the master circadian pacemaker in mammals. *Cell* **2000**, *103*, 1009–1017. [CrossRef]
84. Gekakis, N.; Staknis, D.; Nguyen, H.B. Role of the CLOCK protein in the mammalian circadian mechanism. *Science* **1998**, *280*, 1564–1569. [CrossRef]
85. Reick, M.; Garcia, J.A.; Dudley, C.; McKnight, S.L. NPAS2: An analog of clock operative in the mammalian forebrain. *Science* **2001**, *293*, 506–509. [CrossRef] [PubMed]
86. Kojetin, D.J.; Burris, T.P. REV-ERB and ROR nuclear receptors as drug targets. *Nat. Rev. Drug Discov.* **2014**, *13*, 197–216. [CrossRef] [PubMed]
87. Preitner, N.; Damiola, F.; Lopez-Molina, L. The orphan nuclear receptor REV-ERBalpha controls circadian transcription within the positive limb of the mammalian circadian oscillator. *Cell* **2002**, *110*, 251–260. [CrossRef]
88. Sato, T.K.; Panda, S.; Miraglia, L.J. A functional genomics strategy reveals Rora as a component of the mammalian circadian clock. *Neuron* **2004**, *43*, 527–537. [CrossRef] [PubMed]
89. Balsalobre, A. Clock genes in mammalian peripheral tissues. *Cell Tissue Res.* **2002**, *309*, 193–199. [CrossRef] [PubMed]
90. Cermakian, N.; Boivin, D.B. The regulation of central and peripheral circadian clocks in humans. *Obes. Rev.* **2009**, *10*, 25–36. [CrossRef]

91. Zhang, E.E.; Kay, S.A. Clocks not winding down: Unravelling circadian networks. *Nat. Rev. Mol. Cell Biol.* **2010**, *11*, 764–776. [CrossRef]
92. Turek, F.W.; Joshu, C.; Kohsaka, A. Obesity and metabolic syndrome in circadian Clock mutant mice. *Science* **2005**, *308*, 1043–1045. [CrossRef] [PubMed]
93. Pitts, S.; Perone, E.; Silver, R. Food-entrained circadian rhythms are sustained in arrhythmic Clk/Clk mutant mice. *Am. J. Physiol. Regul. Integr. Comp. Physiol.* **2003**, *285*, R57–R67. [CrossRef] [PubMed]
94. Storch, K.F.; Weitz, C.J. Daily rhythms of food-anticipatory behavioral activity do not require the known circadian clock. *Proc. Natl. Acad. Sci. USA* **2009**, *106*, 6808–6813. [CrossRef]
95. Zhang, E.E.; Liu, Y.; Dentin, R. Cryptochrome mediates circadian regulation of cAMP signaling and hepatic gluconeogenesis. *Nat. Med.* **2010**, *16*, 1152–1156. [CrossRef]
96. Iijima, M.; Yamaguchi, S.; Van der Horst, G.T.; Bonnefont, X.; Okamura, H.; Shibata, S. Altered food-anticipatory activity rhythm in Cryptochrome-deficient mice. *Neurosci. Res.* **2005**, *52*, 166–173. [CrossRef] [PubMed]
97. Moore, R.Y. Organization of the mammalian circadian system. *Ciba Found. Symp.* **1995**, *183*, 88–99; discussion 100–106. [PubMed]
98. Stephan, F.K.; Berkley, K.J.; Moss, R.L. Efferent connections of the rat suprachiasmatic nucleus. *Neuroscience* **1981**, *6*, 2625–2641. [CrossRef]
99. Vrang, N.; Larsen, P.J.; Moller, M.; Mikkelsen, J.D. Topographical organization of the rat suprachiasmatic-paraventricular projection. *J. Comp. Neurol.* **1995**, *353*, 585–603. [CrossRef] [PubMed]
100. Challet, E. The circadian regulation of food intake. *Nat. Rev. Endocrinol.* **2019**, *15*, 393–405. [CrossRef] [PubMed]
101. Abe, M.; Herzog, E.D.; Yamazaki, S. Circadian rhythms in isolated brain regions. *J. Neurosci.* **2002**, *22*, 350–356. [CrossRef] [PubMed]
102. Guilding, C.; Hughes, A.T.; Brown, T.M.; Namvar, S.; Piggins, H.D. A riot of rhythms: Neuronal and glial circadian oscillators in the mediobasal hypothalamus. *Mol. Brain* **2009**, *2*, 28. [CrossRef] [PubMed]
103. Williams, K.W.; Elmquist, J.K. From neuroanatomy to behavior: Central integration of peripheral signals regulating feeding behavior. *Nat. Neurosci.* **2012**, *15*, 1350–1355. [CrossRef] [PubMed]
104. Akabayashi, A.; Levin, N.; Paez, X.; Alexander, J.T.; Leibowitz, S.F. Hypothalamic neuropeptide Y and its gene expression: Relation to light/dark cycle and circulating corticosterone. *Mol. Cell Neurosci.* **1994**, *5*, 210–218. [CrossRef]
105. Steiner, R.A.; Kabigting, E.; Lent, K.; Clifton, D.K. Diurnal rhythm in proopiomelanocortin mRNA in the arcuate nucleus of the male rat. *J. Neuroendocrinol.* **1994**, *6*, 603–608. [CrossRef]
106. Xu, B.; Kalra, P.S.; Farmerie, W.G.; Kalra, S.P. Daily changes in hypothalamic gene expression of neuropeptide Y, galanin, proopiomelanocortin, and adipocyte leptin gene expression and secretion: Effects of food restriction. *Endocrinology* **1999**, *140*, 2868–2875. [CrossRef]
107. Li, A.J.; Wiater, M.F.; Oostrom, M.T. Leptin-sensitive neurons in the arcuate nuclei contribute to endogenous feeding rhythms. *Am. J. Physiol. Regul. Integr. Comp. Physiol.* **2012**, *302*, R1313–R1326. [CrossRef]
108. Wiater, M.F.; Mukherjee, S.; Li, A.J. Circadian integration of sleep-wake and feeding requires NPY receptor-expressing neurons in the mediobasal hypothalamus. *Am. J. Physiol. Regul. Integr. Comp. Physiol.* **2011**, *301*, R1569–R1583. [CrossRef] [PubMed]
109. Edelsbrunner, M.E.; Painsipp, E.; Herzog, H.; Holzer, P. Evidence from knockout mice for distinct implications of neuropeptide-Y Y2 and Y4 receptors in the circadian control of locomotion, exploration, water and food intake. *Neuropeptides* **2009**, *43*, 491–497. [CrossRef]
110. Richard, C.D.; Tolle, V.; Low, M.J. Meal pattern analysis in neural-specific proopiomelanocortin-deficient mice. *Eur. J. Pharmacol.* **2011**, *660*, 131–138. [CrossRef]
111. Yang, S.; Liu, A.; Weidenhammer, A. The role of mPer2 clock gene in glucocorticoid and feeding rhythms. *Endocrinology* **2009**, *150*, 2153–2160. [CrossRef]
112. Bechtold, D.A.; Loudon, A.S. Hypothalamic clocks and rhythms in feeding behaviour. *Trends Neurosci.* **2013**, *36*, 74–82. [CrossRef] [PubMed]
113. Ohdo, S. Chronotherapeutic strategy: Rhythm monitoring, manipulation and disruption. *Adv. Drug Deliv. Rev.* **2010**, *62*, 859–875. [CrossRef] [PubMed]
114. Rosenwasser, A.M.; Boulos, Z.; Terman, M. Circadian organization of food intake and meal patterns in the rat. *Physiol. Behav.* **1981**, *27*, 33–39. [CrossRef]
115. Gschossmann, J.M.; Buenger, L.; Adam, B. Diurnal variation of abdominal motor responses to colorectal distension and plasma cortisol levels in rats. *Neurogastroenterol. Motil.* **2001**, *13*, 585–589. [CrossRef]
116. Bodosi, B.; Gardi, J.; Hajdu, I.; Szentirmai, E.; Obal, F., Jr.; Krueger, J.M. Rhythms of ghrelin, leptin, and sleep in rats: Effects of the normal diurnal cycle, restricted feeding, and sleep deprivation. *Am. J. Physiol. Regul. Integr. Comp. Physiol.* **2004**, *287*, R1071–R1079. [CrossRef]
117. Shiiya, T.; Nakazato, M.; Mizuta, M. Plasma Ghrelin Levels in Lean and Obese Humans and the Effect of Glucose on Ghrelin Secretion. *J. Clin. Endocrinol. Metab.* **2002**, *87*, 240–244. [CrossRef] [PubMed]
118. Goo, R.H.; Moore, J.G.; Greenberg, E.; Alazraki, N.P. Circadian variation in gastric emptying of meals in humans. *Gastroenterology* **1987**, *93*, 515–518. [CrossRef]
119. Page, A.J.; Christie, S.; Symonds, E.; Li, H. Circadian regulation of appetite and time restricted feeding. *Physiol. Behav.* **2020**, *220*, 112873. [CrossRef]

120. Steinert, R.E.; Gerspach, A.C.; Gutmann, H.; Asarian, L.; Drewe, J.; Beglinger, C. The functional involvement of gut-expressed sweet taste receptors in glucose-stimulated secretion of glucagon-like peptide-1 (GLP-1) and peptide YY (PYY). *Clin. Nutr.* **2011**, *30*, 524–532. [CrossRef]
121. Jang, H.-J.; Kokrashvili, Z.; Theodorakis, M.J. Gut-expressed gustducin and taste receptors regulate secretion of glucagon-like peptide-1. *Proc. Natl. Acad. Sci. USA* **2007**, *104*, 15069–15074. [CrossRef]
122. Moghadam, A.A.; Moran, T.H.; Dailey, M.J. Alterations in circadian and meal-induced gut peptide levels in lean and obese rats. *Exp. Biol. Med.* **2017**, *242*, 1786–1794. [CrossRef]
123. Bhutta, H.; Deelman, T.; Ashley, S.; Rhoads, D.; Tavakkoli, A. Disrupted Circadian Rhythmicity of the Intestinal Glucose Transporter SGLT1 in Zucker Diabetic Fatty Rats. *Dig. Dis. Sci.* **2013**, *58*, 1537–1545. [CrossRef]
124. Fetissov, S.O. Role of the gut microbiota in host appetite control: Bacterial growth to animal feeding behaviour. *Nat. Rev. Endocrinol.* **2017**, *13*, 11–25. [CrossRef]
125. Chambers, E.S.; Morrison, D.J.; Frost, G. Control of appetite and energy intake by SCFA: What are the potential underlying mechanisms? *Proc. Nutr. Soc.* **2015**, *74*, 328–336. [CrossRef] [PubMed]
126. Chambers, E.S.; Viardot, A.; Psichas, A. Effects of targeted delivery of propionate to the human colon on appetite regulation, body weight maintenance and adiposity in overweight adults. *Gut* **2015**, *64*, 1744–1754. [CrossRef]
127. Samuel, B.S.; Shaito, A.; Motoike, T. Effects of the gut microbiota on host adiposity are modulated by the short-chain fatty-acid binding G protein-coupled receptor, Gpr41. *Proc. Natl. Acad. Sci. USA* **2008**, *105*, 16767–16772. [CrossRef] [PubMed]
128. Thaiss, C.A.; Zeevi, D.; Levy, M. Transkingdom control of microbiota diurnal oscillations promotes metabolic homeostasis. *Cell* **2014**, *159*, 514–529. [CrossRef] [PubMed]
129. Tahara, Y.; Yamazaki, M.; Sukigara, H. Gut Microbiota-Derived Short Chain Fatty Acids Induce Circadian Clock Entrainment in Mouse Peripheral Tissue. *Sci. Rep.* **2018**, *8*, 1395. [CrossRef] [PubMed]
130. Segers, A.; Desmet, L.; Thijs, T.; Verbeke, K.; Tack, J.; Depoortere, I. The circadian clock regulates the diurnal levels of microbial short-chain fatty acids and their rhythmic effects on colon contractility in mice. *Acta Physiol.* **2018**, e13193. [CrossRef]
131. Kentish, S.J.; Hatzinikolas, G.; Li, H.; Frisby, C.L.; Wittert, G.A.; Page, A.J. Time-Restricted Feeding Prevents Ablation of Diurnal Rhythms in Gastric Vagal Afferent Mechanosensitivity Observed in High-Fat Diet-Induced Obese Mice. *J. Neurosci.* **2018**, *38*, 5088–5095. [CrossRef]
132. Daly, D.M.; Park, S.J.; Valinsky, W.C.; Beyak, M.J. Impaired intestinal afferent nerve satiety signalling and vagal afferent excitability in diet induced obesity in the mouse. *J. Physiol.* **2011**, *589*, 2857–2870. [CrossRef]
133. Kentish, S.J.; O'Donnell, T.A.; Frisby, C.L.; Li, H.; Wittert, G.A.; Page, A.J. Altered gastric vagal mechanosensitivity in diet-induced obesity persists on return to normal chow and is accompanied by increased food intake. *Int. J. Obes.* **2014**, *38*, 636–642. [CrossRef]
134. Tomasi, D.; Wang, G.-J.; Wang, R. Association of Body Mass and Brain Activation during Gastric Distention: Implications for Obesity. *PLoS ONE* **2009**, *4*, e6847. [CrossRef] [PubMed]
135. DelParigi, A.; Chen, K.; Salbe, A.D. Persistence of abnormal neural responses to a meal in postobese individuals. *Int. J. Obes. Relat. Metab. Disord.* **2004**, *28*, 370–377. [CrossRef] [PubMed]
136. Lemonnier, D.; Suquet, J.P.; Aubert, R.; De Gasquet, P.; Pequignot, E. Metabolism of the mouse made obese by a high-fat diet. *Diabete Metab.* **1975**, *1*, 77–85.
137. Levin, B.E.; Dunn-Meynell, A.A. Defense of body weight against chronic caloric restriction in obesity-prone and -resistant rats. *Am. J. Physiol. Regul. Integr. Comp. Physiol.* **2000**, *278*, R231–R237. [CrossRef]
138. Ravussin, Y.; Gutman, R.; Diano, S. Effects of chronic weight perturbation on energy homeostasis and brain structure in mice. *Am. J. Physiol. Regul. Integr. Comp. Physiol.* **2011**, *300*, R1352–R1362. [CrossRef]
139. Cappuccio, F.P.; Taggart, F.M.; Kandala, N.B. Meta-analysis of short sleep duration and obesity in children and adults. *Sleep* **2008**, *31*, 619–626. [CrossRef]
140. Di Lorenzo, L.; De Pergola, G.; Zocchetti, C. Effect of shift work on body mass index: Results of a study performed in 319 glucose-tolerant men working in a Southern Italian industry. *Int. J. Obes. Relat. Metab. Disord.* **2003**, *27*, 1353–1358. [CrossRef] [PubMed]
141. Shimba, S.; Ogawa, T.; Hitosugi, S. Deficient of a clock gene, brain and muscle Arnt-like protein-1 (BMAL1), induces dyslipidemia and ectopic fat formation. *PLoS ONE* **2011**, *6*, e25231. [CrossRef] [PubMed]
142. Suwazono, Y.; Dochi, M.; Sakata, K. A longitudinal study on the effect of shift work on weight gain in male Japanese workers. *Obesity* **2008**, *16*, 1887–1893. [CrossRef] [PubMed]
143. Agnes, P.T.; Isabella, B.; Jorge, C. *Sixth European Working Conditions Survey—Overview Report*; Eurofound: Brussels, Belgium, 2016.
144. Bureau of Labor Statistics. *Workers on Flexible and Shift Schedules in 2004 Summary*; US Bureau of Labor Statistics: Washington, DC, USA, 2005.
145. Australian Bureau of Statistics. *Working Time Arrangements, Australia, November 2012*; ABS: Canberra, Australia, 2012.
146. Knutsson, A. Health disorders of shift workers. *Occup. Med.* **2003**, *53*, 103–108. [CrossRef]
147. Vener, K.J.; Szabo, S.; Moore, J.G. The effect of shift work on gastrointestinal (GI) function: A review. *Chronobiologia* **1989**, *16*, 421–439.
148. Pasqua, I.C.; Moreno, C.R. The nutritional status and eating habits of shift workers: A chronobiological approach. *Chronobiol. Int.* **2004**, *21*, 949–960. [CrossRef]

149. Lennernas, M.; Hambraeus, L.; Akerstedt, T. Shift related dietary intake in day and shift workers. *Appetite* **1995**, *25*, 253–265. [CrossRef] [PubMed]
150. Cayanan, E.A.; Eyre, N.A.B.; Lao, V. Is 24-h energy intake greater during night shift compared to non-night shift patterns? A systematic review. *Chronobiol. Int.* **2019**, *36*, 1599–1612. [CrossRef]
151. Shaw, E.; Dorrian, J.; Coates, A.M. Temporal pattern of eating in night shift workers. *Chronobiol. Int.* **2019**, *36*, 1613–1625. [CrossRef]
152. Gill, S.; Panda, S. A Smartphone App Reveals Erratic Diurnal Eating Patterns in Humans that Can Be Modulated for Health Benefits. *Cell Metab.* **2015**, *22*, 789–798. [CrossRef]
153. Opperhuizen, A.L.; Van Kerkhof, L.W.; Proper, K.I.; Rodenburg, W.; Kalsbeek, A. Rodent models to study the metabolic effects of shiftwork in humans. *Front. Pharmacol.* **2015**, *6*, 50. [CrossRef] [PubMed]
154. Barclay, J.L.; Husse, J.; Bode, B. Circadian desynchrony promotes metabolic disruption in a mouse model of shiftwork. *PLoS ONE* **2012**, *7*, e37150. [CrossRef]
155. De Oliveira, E.M.; Visniauskas, B.; Sandri, S. Late effects of sleep restriction: Potentiating weight gain and insulin resistance arising from a high-fat diet in mice. *Obesity* **2015**, *23*, 391–398. [CrossRef]
156. Fonken, L.K.; Lieberman, R.A.; Weil, Z.M.; Nelson, R.J. Dim light at night exaggerates weight gain and inflammation associated with a high-fat diet in male mice. *Endocrinology* **2013**, *154*, 3817–3825. [CrossRef]
157. Fonken, L.K.; Workman, J.L.; Walton, J.C. Light at night increases body mass by shifting the time of food intake. *Proc. Natl. Acad. Sci. USA* **2010**, *107*, 18664–18669. [CrossRef]
158. Aubrecht, T.G.; Jenkins, R.; Nelson, R.J. Dim light at night increases body mass of female mice. *Chronobiol. Int.* **2015**, *32*, 557–560. [CrossRef]
159. Kentish, S.J.; Christie, S.; Vincent, A.; Li, H.; Wittert, G.A.; Page, A.J. Disruption of the light cycle ablates diurnal rhythms in gastric vagal afferent mechanosensitivity. *Neurogastroenterol. Motil.* **2019**, *31*, e13711. [CrossRef] [PubMed]
160. Froy, O. Metabolism and circadian rhythms—Implications for obesity. *Endocr. Rev.* **2010**, *31*, 1–24. [CrossRef]
161. Hatori, M.; Vollmers, C.; Zarrinpar, A. Time-restricted feeding without reducing caloric intake prevents metabolic diseases in mice fed a high-fat diet. *Cell Metab.* **2012**, *15*, 848–860. [CrossRef] [PubMed]
162. Oike, H.; Sakurai, M.; Ippoushi, K.; Kobori, M. Time-fixed feeding prevents obesity induced by chronic advances of light/dark cycles in mouse models of jet-lag/shift work. *Biochem. Biophys. Res. Commun.* **2015**, *465*, 556–561. [CrossRef]
163. Chaix, A.; Manoogian, E.N.C.; Melkani, G.C.; Panda, S. Time-Restricted Eating to Prevent and Manage Chronic Metabolic Diseases. *Annu. Rev. Nutr.* **2019**, *39*, 291–315. [CrossRef] [PubMed]
164. Ravussin, E.; Beyl, R.A.; Poggiogalle, E.; Hsia, D.S.; Peterson, C.M. Early Time-Restricted Feeding Reduces Appetite and Increases Fat Oxidation But Does Not Affect Energy Expenditure in Humans. *Obesity* **2019**, *27*, 1244–1254. [CrossRef]

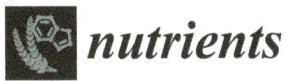

Review

Vagally Mediated Gut-Brain Relationships in Appetite Control-Insights from Porcine Studies

Charles-Henri Malbert [1,2,3]

[1] Aniscan Unit, INRAE, Saint-Gilles, 35590 Paris, France; charles-henri.malbert@inrae.fr
[2] National Academy of Medicine, 75000 Paris, France
[3] Adelaide Medical School, University of Adelaide, Adelaide, SA 5000, Australia

Abstract: Signals arising from the upper part of the gut are essential for the regulation of food intake, particularly satiation. This information is supplied to the brain partly by vagal nervous afferents. The porcine model, because of its sizeable gyrencephalic brain, omnivorous regimen, and comparative anatomy of the proximal part of the gut to that of humans, has provided several important insights relating to the relevance of vagally mediated gut-brain relationships to the regulation of food intake. Furthermore, its large size combined with the capacity to become obese while overeating a western diet makes it a pivotal addition to existing murine models, especially for translational studies relating to obesity. How gastric, proximal intestinal, and portal information relating to meal arrival and transit are encoded by vagal afferents and their further processing by primary and secondary brain projections are reviewed. Their peripheral and central plasticities in the context of obesity are emphasized. We also present recent insights derived from chronic stimulation of the abdominal vagi with specific reference to the modulation of mesolimbic structures and their role in the restoration of insulin sensitivity in the obese miniature pig model.

Keywords: miniature pig; pig model; functional brain imaging; molecular imaging; vagal afferents; single fiber recording; insulin resistance; GLP-1r; gastric barostat; gastric emptying; scintigraphy

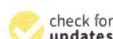

Citation: Malbert, C.-H. Vagally Mediated Gut-Brain Relationships in Appetite Control-Insights from Porcine Studies. *Nutrients* **2021**, *13*, 467. https://doi.org/10.3390/nu13020467

Academic Editor: Anders Sjodin
Received: 4 January 2021
Accepted: 28 January 2021
Published: 30 January 2021

Publisher's Note: MDPI stays neutral with regard to jurisdictional claims in published maps and institutional affiliations.

Copyright: © 2021 by the author. Licensee MDPI, Basel, Switzerland. This article is an open access article distributed under the terms and conditions of the Creative Commons Attribution (CC BY) license (https://creativecommons.org/licenses/by/4.0/).

1. Introduction

Large animal and murine models have contributed to the understanding of vagally mediated gut-brain relationships since the early recognition of the importance of this pathway for appetite control by Iggo in the UK and Mei [1] in France initially in cats [2] and subsequently in sheep [3]. Both pioneered the single fiber recording of mechanical and chemical vagal digestive afferents. Unfortunately, while the vagus is easy to dissect in these species, the carnivorous or the herbivorous regimens were only remotely close to dietary patterns in humans, raising uncertainties about translational relevance. Recently, genetic identification of the functional population of abdominal vagal afferent neurons in a murine model has been published [4]. The screening strategy is fundamentally based on the histological identification of the neuronal ending. However, the available electrophysiological evidence has been unable to associate one neuronal shape with a distinct functional outcome. For example, while intraganglionic laminar endings are certainly mechanosensitive [5], that does not preclude the possibility that other neuronal types are mechanosensitive. An alternative approach to evaluate the vagally driven appetite control is to investigate brain activity directly. Unfortunately, the primary integration site, the dorsal vagal complex (DVC), is challenging to reach with a microelectrode, necessitating irreversible, invasive surgery. Similarly, imaging the DVC is equally demanding in large animal models given the requirement for ultra-high field (7T) fMRI [6] or partial volume correction with nuclear imaging methods [7]. Unlike the primary integration area, secondary structures involved in cortical and sub-cortical projections of vagal neurons are more accessible to evaluation, when quantitative imaging methods are available in a gyrencephalic species, to facilitate translational interpretation. These methods include a

3D digital atlas of the pig [8] together with the co-registered templates [9] and adapted algorithms [10]. The strategies used to investigate appetite directly and indirectly in the pig model are initially reviewed. Meal-related modulation of gastric and intestinal vagal afferents relevant for appetite control are presented. Finally, the appetite-related effects of chronic stimulation of vagal abdominal trunks are described. A particular focus is on data derived from our laboratory.

2. Appetite, Satiety, and Their Measurements

Satiety and satiation are the critical players in the control of appetite. Satiety engulfs the many processes occurring between meals triggered by food consumption and it is usually measured in humans by subjective ratings of hunger and fullness, both of which are not feasible in any preclinical animal model [11]. Satiation occurs during a meal and brings the meal to its end while ultimately determining meal size. Perhaps surprisingly, in humans, the method for evaluating satiation is often limited to measurement of the size of a meal given that the approach is frequently more comprehensive in animal models [12]. For example, the refined analysis of the structure of the meal [13] aims to dissect the temporal evolution of satiation with a time resolution close that of the physiological processes.

The microstructure of a meal can be obtained readily in individually housed pigs with dedicated robotic feeders (Figure 1). In its most simple design, the device consists of a weight-sensitive sensor attached to the bottom of the trough [14]. Several issues were critical in acquiring and analyzing data recorded from these devices. While constant access to the trough was initially thought to be preferable, this proved not to be the case for several reasons. First, during the within-meal foraging, the pig secretes a large quantity of saliva that, after mixing with the pellets, renders the meal residues far less attractive. This reduction in palatability of the diet is almost impossible to quantify but is intuitively likely to compromise the assessment of satiation. Second, meaningful information from the time interval between two consecutive meals cannot be obtained, which is unfortunately not an index of satiety but rather a reflection of the boredom of the animal. These limitations were overcome by the incorporation of several modifications controlling the access to the trough using a vertical hatch and allowing the remains of the meal to be removed immediately before the initiation of a new meal by capsizing the trough. These improvements allowed the delivery of several meals per day with fresh pellets, accordingly, of stable palatability. Using dedicated algorithms, the rate and duration of meal ingestion, and the number of eating bouts per meal can be extracted from the continuous measurement of the weight of the trough after the detection and removal of foraging artifacts [15,16]. The incorporation of several devices side-by-side (Figure 1 B), and different diets, could be used to assess diet preferences [9,17].

The difficulty in assessing satiety in animal models leads us and others to investigate potential biological proxies. Probably the most promising of these arises from functional neuroimaging methods that are adaptable to the porcine model given that a suitable three-dimensional atlas of the brain is available [8] and integrated into the adequate neuroimaging tools [18]. In humans, fMRI and ^{15}O water PET rely on the hemodynamic response with a time resolution of several seconds. They are, accordingly, well suited to investigate satiation [19]. In animal models, these methods, particularly as anesthesia is mandatory for imaging, do not convey additional value. In contrast, SPECT (single photon emission tomography) after ^{99m}Tc-HMPAO administration can characterize brain activation, in the conscious pig, because (i) the penetration of the radioactive molecule is proportional to brain micro vascularization and (ii) it is possible to temporally disconnect the imaging and the stimulus. HMPAO, after its intravenous administration, crosses the brain-blood barrier freely as a lipophilic molecule and penetrates the neuron where bioconversion is achieved, rendering the molecule lipophobic thereby impairing its retro diffusion to the interstitial space [20]. Since this process occurs within 60 s, the distribution of the radioactivity represents a "snap-shoot" of the brain activity that persists for about two hours irrespective of the events occurring after HMPAO injection [21]. This period enables the performance of SPECT imaging in an anesthetized animal without altering the distribution of the radioactivity. The time resolution of the method has been proven to be useful in evaluating satiety during gastric distension [22] and chronic vagal stimulation [23].

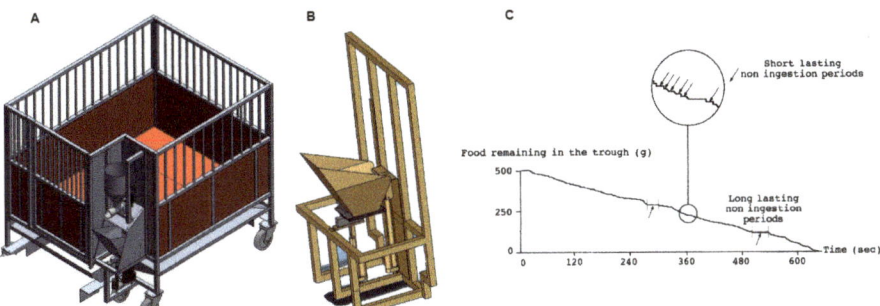

Figure 1. (**A**): Schematic of the individual cage, including the robotic feeder allowing multiple meals per day while analyzing the microstructure of each meal. Note the diet distributor affixed to the top of the feeder, consisting of a large reservoir connected to a worm driven by homemade software allowing precise delivery of the diet. (**B**). Close-up view of the bottom part of the robotic feeder, including the trough, capsize design, and the access door to ensure that the palatability of the diet is identical throughout the day. Three identical feeders can be positioned side by side for meal preference studies. (**C**). Recording of changes in the trough weight during a meal after removal of foraging artifacts. The close-up view illustrates periods of non-ingestion (arrows) during a single meal. Adapted from Ref. [15].

While the farm pig represents an easily accessible experimental animal, it is suboptimal since the animal weight is above 200 kg once adult. On the contrary, the miniature pig model allows experiments in adult obese animals with a body weight less than 100 kg. Several western diets with or without fructose have been used, in the miniature pig, to mimic the human metabolic syndrome. However, these dietary interventions were unable to reproduce the actual metabolic syndrome observed in humans—chronic hyperglycemia and hepatic steatosis [24,25]. Furthermore, in the miniature pig and more significantly in the Gottingen breed, the distribution of western diet ad libitum results in alternating periods of hyperphagia and voluntary starvation that extend over a couple of days, resulting in the impossibility to investigate experimentally induced changes in food intake [23]. The most common solution used to overcome this behavior is to supply a limited yet above the dietary requirement both in energy density (about 4000 instead of 2200 kcal per kg of diet) and volume (288 kcal per kg of body weight$^{0.75}$, i.e., 150% of the energy requirement). Nevertheless, the surprising resistance of the obese pig to type 2 diabetes is puzzling [26]. Indeed, the fasting plasma glucose is always less than 7 mmol/L, while the insulin sensitivity was less than 3 dL/kg.min/µU/mL* 1×10^{-3} for more than a month. Furthermore, since the obese pig does not present polydipsia or polyuria, the hallmark signs of diabetes, the threshold used to declare diabetes in humans is probably adequate for the pig [27]. On the contrary, the significant insulin resistance and moderate hyperglycemia suggest that the obese pig behaves as a permanent pre-diabetic. This concept is further supported by creating actual diabetes in the obese miniature pig after the additional administration of a small dose of streptozotocin that, alone, is unable to be effective in lean animals [12].

3. Gastric Emptying and Meal Distribution

In humans, the Adelaide team [28] and others [29] have demonstrated that the volume, and the physical characteristics of a meal are critical determinants of satiation. In the pig model, gastric emptying has been poorly investigated by noninvasive methods considered to be the "state of the art" in humans, particularly scintigraphic imaging [30]. Gastric cannulae with or without aspiration of gastric contents have been frequently used in the past and represent an inadequate approach for emptying estimation because of unavoidable numerous artifacts, low temporal resolution, and over-estimation of the emptying rate due to suppression of the gastroduodenal pressure gradient [31]. We pioneered a direct scintigraphic approach in conscious pigs (Figure 2 B), mimicking the method used and validated in humans and employed widely for both clinical and research purposes [32].

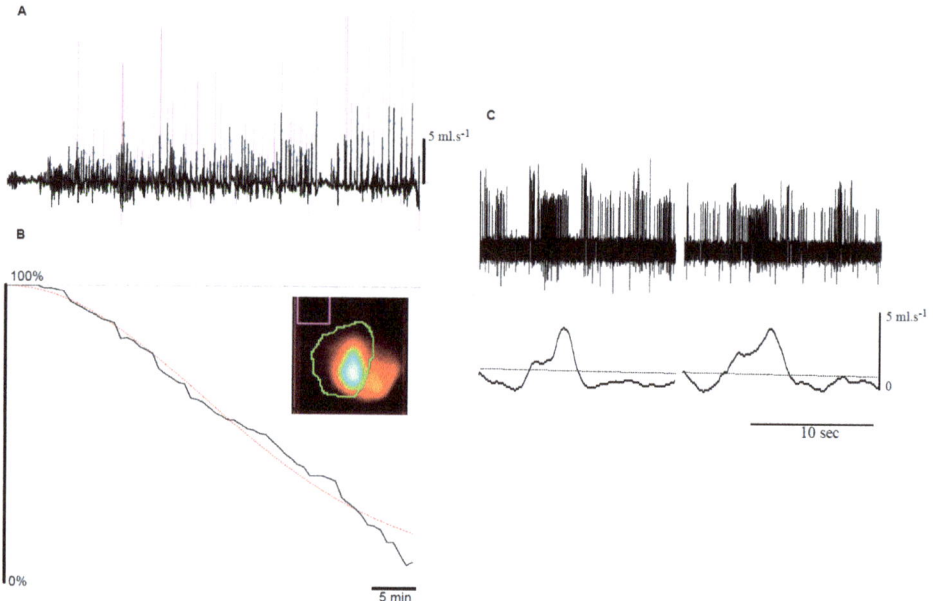

Figure 2. Pulsatile (i.e., "second-by-second") emptying and vagal information from duodenal vagal receptors sensitive to the stroke volume of individual pulses. (**A**). Transpyloric flow recording (black line) after a 500 mL glucose 10% meal, with detected pulses (dots) and associated stroke volume (proportional to the pink vertical lines). (**B**). Related "overall" emptying measured by scintigraphy of the same meal labeled with 30 MBq of ^{99m}Tc-DTPA. The red dotted line represents the power exponential fit of the residual counts per pixel present in the region of interest delineating the stomach (in green on the maximal intensity projection insert). (**C**). Concomitant recording of duodenal afferent neuronal activity with transpyloric passage of the fluid in anesthetized pig. Note the increased frequency of action potentials during the positive flow. Duodenal pressure at the level of the receptive field is constant (not shown).

Meal labeling has to be partially adapted to the porcine regimen that is at least comparable to humans due to its omnivorous status. As in humans, liquid test meals should be caloric, since water or isotonic saline empties very rapidly (half emptying time less than 15 min). A 500 mL-10% glucose meal [33] is readily ingested by, even poorly compliant, animals. The choices for solid and/or semi-solid meals are theoretically wider. Three test meals are associated with an almost equal quality of binding between the radioactive molecule and the meal constituents: scrambled eggs, grounded beef, and porridge. Of these, porridge is close to the typical cereal-based food for pigs [34]. Furthermore, once reduced into fine particles, it is possible to substitute oats with the animal's actual feed. Moreover, the half emptying time of this meal is around 2 h, which is compatible with the maximum duration for a pig to stay quietly in a sling frame. Grounded beef is arguably the optimal solid test meal for humans but, in pigs, large inter- and intraindividual variations in the emptying profile are observed with this meal [32], as it is with scrambled egg, which is usually widely used for clinical measurement of gastric emptying in humans.

A limiting factor, in pigs, for correct interpretation of scintigraphic gastric emptying data relates to the absence of readily available analysis software—those designed for use in humans are inadequate. This reflects several issues relating to animal behavior and its anatomical peculiarities. First, lateral imaging correction used to cancel the non-planar anatomy of the stomach is, not surprisingly, mandatory. Indeed, pigs do not tolerate being squeezed between a double head gamma camera, an approach to reduce the planar error. Second, motion generates major artifacts, which is a significant issue, as measurements of solid emptying requiring more prolonged data acquisition. These pitfalls can be addressed satisfactorily using dedicated software integrating depth correction and blur-detection image shifts and/or removal [35,36].

4. Gastric signals

4.1. Acute Gastric Distension

Several lines of evidence suggest that short-term control of food intake is related to the arrival and storage of the meal in the proximal part of the stomach [37]. Indeed, the experimental proxy of these events e.g., acute balloon distension suppresses food intake [38]. However, data in humans are inconclusive—a 400 mL balloon occupying 30% of the stomach failed to trigger a significant reduction in food intake [39–41]. Therefore, it remains unclear whether, if so, and to what extent the mechanical induced signals of gastric fundic and antral distension alter food intake within the meal time-frame. The gastric barostat overcomes the main limitation of a fixed volume distension because it maintains a constant gastric pressure despite the fundic relaxation induced by acute gastric distension [42]. Pressures equal or above 11 mmHg were found to increase meal duration, while volume distensions did not affect feeding behavior irrespective of the gastric bag volume [15]. The wall tension changes are likely to account for these differences, which also explains the discrepancies observed by others using only volume distension.

a. Vagal afferents during gastric distension

At the cervical level, the vagal trunk in the pig exhibits sufficient anatomical separation between its afferent and efferent branches [43] to allow recording of afferent vagal activity using extracellular electrodes during gastric distension. Furthermore, the distance between the recording site and the location of the stimulation is sufficient to avoid motion artifacts that could impair the quality of the single afferent recording [44]. These advantages overcome the difficulties of separating fiber bundles dispersed in a dense connective tissue unlike the scattered lose connective tissue in the cat or the rat. We capitalized on these assets to investigate the single neuron afferent response to gastric distension compared to isovolumetric and barostatic gastric distension in the pig [45]. Surprisingly, the observed increase in spiking activity was the opposite to that expected based on our previous experiment in conscious pigs [15]. Irrespective of distension pressure, volume distension was shown to be the most effective stimulus to increase spiking activity. For the largest volume distensions, there was no significant difference between volume and pressure distensions. Furthermore, some receptors sensitive to volume distension were quiescent during pressure distensions. The observed absence of response for some receptors, while a sustained elevation in pressure was maintained, suggests that, similar to "baro" receptors in the cardiovascular system, circumferential strain might be required to activate these receptors. This possibility has also been suggested based on in vitro recordings using rat explants [46,47]. Taken together, our observations and those obtained from in vitro experiments in rats argue strongly against the often-reported claim that gastric distension activates vagal afferent mechanoreceptors in a dose-dependent manner [48]. This implies that some sort of preconditioning of the distension-related information occurs at the periphery in turn alleviating the processing burden of the primary vagal integrating centers.

b. Central processing

Ultimately, following primary integration on the dorsal vagal nuclei, information encoding distention is processed by secondary brain networks. The engagement of these networks in humans has been studied by either PET ^{15}O or fMRI. In these studies, a balloon was orally placed in the stomach, and its volume quickly enlarged to elicit fullness or pain [49,50]. When inflation of the balloon is more gradual, the temporal limitation of the BOLD signal used for fMRI requires that the balloon is inflated and deflated every minute, a situation that mimics post-prandial distention only remotely [51]. Furthermore, the presence in the throat of a gastric tube connecting the distension device to the balloon potentially represents a substantial confounder exacerbating emotional salience [52]. Taking advantage of the precise determination of the maximal pressure achieved, and the temporal pressure changes, during a meal, we have recreated, in the conscious pig, the strains and stresses occurring at the gastric wall during a meal. Furthermore, the barostat bag was inserted through a permanent, surgically prepared access to the gastric lumen. Finally, brain tissue perfusion changes during the entire cycle associated with the virtual meal were detected using SPECT-HMPAO imaging—a time-independent representation of brain activation [22]. The major regions located along vagal-related ascending pathways were activated: brainstem, periaqueductal grey, thalamus, and olfactory bulb. Unrelated vagal regions were also engaged, such as the globus pallidus and the hippocampus/amygdala, suggesting that the reward network might also be involved during mild gastric (Figure 3) [53]. The importance of the reward network engagement through physical stimulation may be of particular relevance to the success of gastric bypass surgery in obese individuals [54,55].

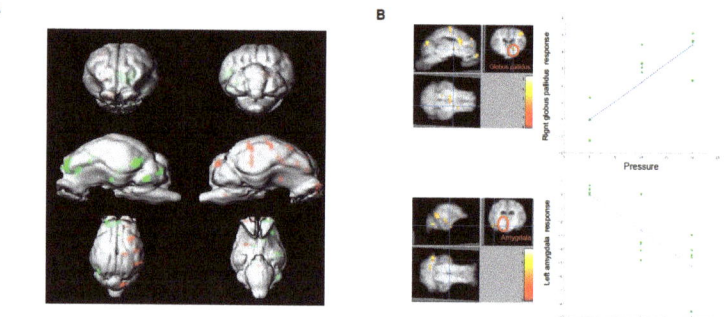

Figure 3. Brain activity during acute gastric distension measured by ^{99m}Tc HMPAO uptake in conscious growing pigs. (**A**). Statistical parameter mapping analysis of activated (green) and de-activated (red) brain areas during acute mild gastric distension versus no distension. (**B**). Relationship between gastric pressure and hemodynamic response in activated (Globus palidus) and de-activated areas (Amygdala).

The contribution of spinal afferents to the gastric afferent information is classically considered to be negligible, especially at low pressures, such as those occurring during a meal [56]. Unlike humans, the pig tolerates vagotomy without drainage [33] allowing the investigation of central processing of vagal vs. spinal gastric information. The brain areas engaged during distension changed following vagotomy [57]. As expected, brain structures related to vagal processing were modulated only before vagotomy, e.g., pons, thalamus, prefrontal, and amygdala-hippocampus cortices. However, after vagotomy, the activity of several brain areas still correlated with fundic pressure, e.g., colliculus superior, medulla, amygdala. These observations established both that the reward network is involved only by vagal afferent information occurring during gastric distension and that proximal gastric distension has the capacity to activate brain areas such as the amygdala when the vagal pathways have been severed, consistent with the concept of a significant spinal contribution even at a low distending pressure.

4.2. Chronic Gastric Distension

Permanent distension of the stomach with water or an air-filled balloon aimed to be an alternative therapy to bariatric surgery. These devices are in many cases well tolerated and relatively easy to insert and remove by endoscopy [58] but their efficacy in reducing weight and increasing satiety remains uncertain [59]. Using a miniature obese pig model, we have demonstrated that an air-filled balloon, after a couple of weeks, instead of reducing gastric volume, increased it by about one third [60]. This reflected an increase in fundic compliance measured by the pressure-volume slope during step-wise barostatic distension. Furthermore, we also observed a reduction in gastric emptying of a porridge meal, which is probably a consequence of the decreased gastric tone. These effects may well contribute to the limited efficacy of balloon therapy in obese patients.

The potential for a difference in brain processing related to the chronic presence of an intragastric balloon, especially in comparison with those occurring as a result of acute gastric distension, was also investigated. Unfortunately, it is impossible to standardize intragastric pressure in these circumstances since changes in pressure within the chronic balloon are not readily accessible. Nevertheless, the intragastric balloon (chronic distension) was associated with activation of the olfactory bulb, prefrontal cortex, nucleus accumbens, thalamus, posterior amygdala, and pons [61]. These brain structures were also engaged during acute distension, except the prefrontal cortex and the nucleus accumbens. The divergence between the minor behavioral consequence of chronic gastric distension on food intake, on the one hand, and the substantial reward network engagement, on the other, was unexpected. Furthermore, the activations of the prefrontal cortex and the nucleus accumbens by acute distension might only reflect the importance of these structures in hedonistic aspects. Indeed, the human prefrontal cortex and nucleus accumbens are specifically reactive to pleasant, rewarding stimuli and are not engaged by unpleasant stimuli [62].

5. Intestinal Signals

The importance of the pig model to current understanding of the role of intestinal nutrients to appetite control has been reviewed [63], particularly in relation to peripheral nutrient-sensing [64]. Recently, we showed that mimicking peripheral chemo-sensing with artificial sweeteners has a global impact on insulin sensitivity far beyond appetite control [65].

5.1. Transpyloric Flow

In several animal models, including the pig, gastric emptying is predominantly pulsatile rather than continuous, supplying nutrients as a series of gushes in the duodenum (Figure 2A) [66]. In these models, the flow pulses last about 4 s every 15 s, resulting in a stroke volume of 0.9 mL per pulse. The forward to backward flow ratio is about 4:1 and this has been confirmed in humans using Doppler ultrasonography [67]. The pulsatile arrival of nutrients in the intestine was not evident to gastric emptying measurements in humans using either scintigraphy or stable isotope breath test because of their much lower temporal resolution, but has potential consequences. The sudden passage of fluid results in irregular arrival of a significant volume of fluid within the narrow proximal duodenum, probably activating low threshold duodenal vagal mechanoreceptors (Figure 2C). Indeed, there is a linear relationship between the interspike distribution of duodenal vagal afferents and the stroke volume, but not the duration or the peak flow of flow pulses [68]. Furthermore, neither the circumferential strain recorded by a strain gauge affixed on the serosa nor the fluid velocity were related to the firing of receptors, suggesting that duodenal mechanoreceptors primary detect the stroke volume of the pulses. Despite evidence for vagal afferent coding, the contribution of pulsatile transpyloric flow to appetite control appears unimportant. Indeed, in humans, antropyloroduodenal pressures, plasma CCK concentration, and appetite are not modified by pulsatile versus constant infusion of lipid into the duodenum [69]. The situation might be different in obese after gastric bariatric surgery since it results in a much more rapid emptying [70] probably as a consequence of flow pulses of larger stroke volume. Unfortunately, experimental data is missing to support this hypothesis since Roux en Y surgery in the porcine model increases paradoxical glucose metabolism [71] and accordingly no attempt to record transpyloric flow, in these conditions, have been done in the porcine model.

5.2. Jejunal vs. Portal Signals

Vagally mediated appetite control is dependent on the integration of glucose-sensing mechanisms located in the brain, portal vein, and intestine [72]. The impact of obesity and insulin resistance on brain glucose sensing has been investigated extensively [73], but there is much less information about the hepato-portal sensor [74] probably, in part, because it is much less accessible.

There is indirect evidence for a neuronal circuit responsible for a regulatory response to portal hyperglycemia [75]. Unfortunately, there is a lack of direct confirmation of portal sensitive neurons, reflecting the sparsity of the portal innervation [4]. Nevertheless, it is clear that glucagon-like peptide-1 receptor (GLP-1r) is critical to portal vagally mediated glucose sensing [56,76]. We identified, in lean and obese mini-pigs, GLP-1-dependent portal glucose signaling, in vivo, using a novel ^{68}Ga labeled GLP-1r positron-emitting probe [77] that provided a quantitative in situ tridimensional representation of the portal sensor [78] (Figure 4). We also used this as a map for single-neuron electrophysiology driven by image-based abdominal navigation. In insulin-resistant animals, portal vagal afferents failed to inhibit their spiking activity during glucose infusion, a GLP-1r-dependent function. The importance of a reduction in portal GLP-1r binding potential, particularly between the splenic vein and the liver entrance, was further demonstrated by the suppression of the glucose effect on the afferent by pharmacological inhibition of the GLP-1r, in lean animals only. Accordingly, in the pig, obesity-induced insulin resistance leads to functional portal denervation with marked suppression of vagal sensitivity to portal glucose. The latter appears to be the consequence of a reduction in the density of GLP-1r, as indicated by diminished GLP-1r binding potential in obese insulin-resistant animals [79]. The concept of a functional denervation at the portal level suggests that it might be possible to restore pharmacologically the portal glucose sensor in obese insulin-resistant patient through the expression of GLP-1r.

Despite the importance of the portal sensor for glucose detection, in the pig, duodenal and portal glucose infusions were equally potent in reducing food intake [80]. Both duodenal and portal glucose infusions activated the dorsolateral prefrontal cortex and primary somatosensory cortex. Duodenal glucose infusion also induced activation of the prepyriform area, orbito-frontal cortex, caudate, and putamen [81]. This comparable effectiveness suggests that the intestinal vagal signal is poorly integrated centrally and/or is not essential to the central response to intestinal glucose, particularly as the glycemic response is also identical. Nevertheless, the substantial difference in brain matrix observed for portal vs. duodenal infusion with a comparable behavioral outcome is surprising and might reflect the limitation of SPECT-HMPAO imaging. Indeed, like fMRI, SPECT-HMPAO is at best semi-quantitative with a mandatory normalization using either the entire brain tissue or the cerebellum as a reference. This step, which is not required for PET when an arterial input function is simultaneously acquired, has the potential to generate artifactual activation, especially for low significance statistical threshold [82].

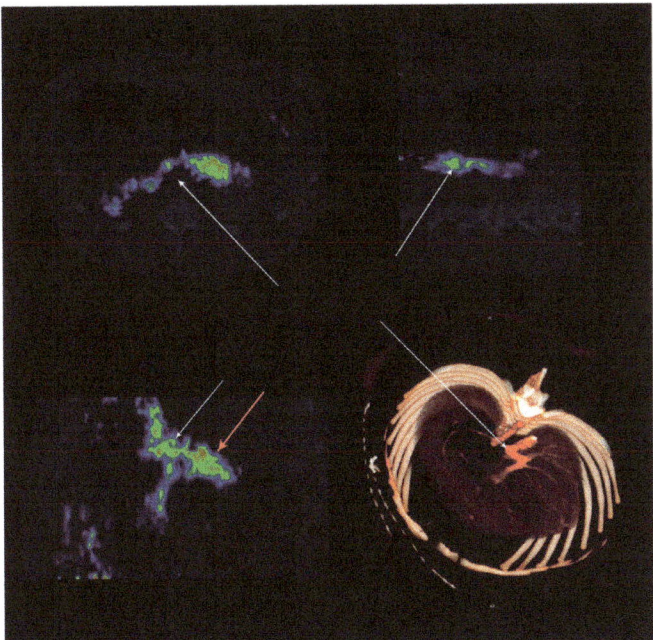

Figure 4. Hybrid PET-CT imaging of GLP-1r distribution along the portal vein using ^{68}Ga-DO3A-Exendin-4 (0.2MBq/Kg) was administered IV in adult miniature pigs. Each color pixel is coded to represent the binding potential of GLP-1r. Note the localization of the GLP-1r along the portal vein immediately before its entrance into the liver. The density of GLP-1r parallels that of the portal glucose sensor since the GLP-1r is critical for vagal signal transduction. Radioactive binding is not evident in obese adult miniature pigs due to the suppression of the glucose sensor. Adapted from Ref. [79].

6. Mimicking Abdominal Afferent Vagal Signaling

6.1. Importance of Vagal Afferents for Appetite

Despite the intricacies of the digestive vagal information, several attempts have been made to manipulate this information using electrical nerve stimulation. Vagotomy has historically been a therapy for peptic ulcers, where some obese patients experienced weight loss [83]. Based on these observations and trials of bilateral vagotomy as a treatment for obesity [84,85], even though the results were mitigated-a device aimed at inducing vagal blockade has been developed to generate weight loss. Not surprisingly, reflecting the extreme intricacy, even in vitro, of achieving effective nerve blockade, the therapy proved to be unsuccessful albeit safe in obese humans [86]. In contrast, our data in obese pigs [14,87] together with the important observations from murine models [88–90] demonstrated that vagal signals are attenuated in obese models suggesting that therapy must be based on stimulation rather than inhibition of the vagal signal. However, mimicking abdominal afferent vagal signaling using current pulses applied on the vagus represents only one option for the restoration of the vagal traffic between the gut and the brain. Alternatives solutions such as pharmacological modulation of the vagal sensors peripherally or modifications of the primary and secondary brain networks related to vagal inputs represent equally attractive, non-mutually exclusive, options for obesity treatment.

6.2. Vagal Afferents Plasticity

Vagal afferents are inherently plastic, and experimental evidence obtained in rats and mice shows that they can change the synaptic number, neuronal excitability, and neuropeptide expression in response to peripheral stimuli. These have been recently reviewed by de Lartigue and Xu [91]. Nevertheless, the possibility for vagal afferents to switch from expressing anorectic to orexigenic neuropeptides as a consequence of metabolic challenges is still a matter of debate [92]. On the contrary, the mitigation of vagal afferent mechanical sensing during obesity is firmly established [47,93]. However, the functional consequences of peripheral plasticity are still largely putative, mostly because equally important plasticity occurs in secondary projection areas of vagal afferents [94]. The final integration of the peripheral signals is intuitively more complex than the raw addition of central and peripheral plasticity, but the mathematical tools capable of handling these intermingled modulations quantitatively are scarce [95]. Furthermore, the demonstration of these in porcine model is still missing.

6.3. Early Outcomes of Abdominal Vagal Stimulation

Together with other groups [96], we initiated chronic vagal stimulation in pigs to investigate bilateral stimulation of the abdominal vagal nerves (VNS). The first attempt to identify the optimal location of the electrodes to suppress food intake was by Laskiewicz et al., in rats [97]. They reported that bilateral VNS is more effective than unilateral vagal stimulation [98]. Using the porcine model, we initially evaluated juxta-abdominal bilateral vagal stimulation in an attempt to minimize adverse cardiovascular effects. This location proved to decrease weight gain, food consumption, and sweet craving in both growing pigs [14] and adult obese minipigs [99]. However, in both normal-weight and obese animals, the reductions in food intake and body weight were modest. Indeed, in both situations, body weight and food intake continued to rise as the animals became older, although the rate at which this occurred was reduced by vagal stimulation. It is likely that the limited effects reflected the infra-optimal stimulation parameters since stimulation was achieved using two separate clinical VNS stimulators that were not working in synchronicity on both vagi. Furthermore, electrical compliance of these generators while sufficient for the small diameter of the human cervical vagal nerve may well have been inappropriate for the larger abdominal vagus of the pig [100]. Nevertheless, while recognizing that the methodology was suboptimal, an essential step was the demonstration that vagal stimulation did not modify gastric emptying in a large animal model [22] suggesting that epigastric fullness and other symptoms related to increased gastric retention are unlikely to occur and/or are not causative for the behavioral effects of vagal stimulation. The early trials in vagal stimulation, while being partly inconclusive, paved the way for more adequate technologies that we developed during the past years, including laparoscopically implantable electrode cuffs suitable for the abdominal vagus, double stage, high compliance, synchronous, current stimulator appropriate for chronic implantation, together with remote wireless monitoring of the changes in electrical impedance of the nerve-electrode complex representative of the interlocking between the cuff and the perineurium [23]. These technologies were applied incrementally in the experiments described in the next paragraphs.

6.4. Targeting the Appropriate Neuronal Type

The modest or negligible outcomes of VNS in obese humans may well reflect premature translation from animals to humans without sufficient information about the optimum stimulation profile, current intensity, and more generally therapy characteristics [96]. For example, the concept that the same stimulation current used at the cervical level to alleviate epilepsy would be effective at the abdominal level was naïve. Indeed, at the abdominal level, the majority of vagal neurons located either in the dorsal or ventral vagal trunks are small diameter myelinated and un-myelinated neurons, i.e., Adelta or C type [101]. Therefore, large current pulses are needed to depolarize the axon membrane and generate an action potential-more than 20 mA may be needed [102]. While they proved to be effective acutely, the use of these currents would be unrealistic in a chronic implant, since they generate damage to the electrode and the biological tissues [100]. In anesthetized animals, an innovative stimulation profile (named pulson) applied bilaterally on both abdominal vagal trunks can trigger action potentials in small-diameter neurons (C and Adelta types) [16]. The pulson profile is composed in a short series of very high frequency pulses (>100 Hz) that individually cannot depolarize the neuron. In conscious animals, this stimulation profile could increase the metabolism of the DVC and that of other brain areas that are primary or secondary projections from the DVC. Pulson stimulation was also able to halve the food intake within two weeks, unlike the classical millisecond stimulation pattern that takes several weeks to reduce the slope only [99]. Since this stimulation pattern required only about one-third of the charge needed for a long-lasting classical pulse to evoke an action potential, it has the potential to be used chronically without altering the integrity of the nerve [17,103,104]. Given its efficacy to reduce food intake, a feature never encounter before, this solution deserves further studies in animal model and in obese humans.

6.5. Central Effects of VNS

Regardless of the significant improvements in electrode placement, stimulation scheme, and hardware design in the last five years, early clues to refine stimulation parameters without waiting to observe changes in body weight are needed. It is probable that brain-imaging methods and the computational model of VNS [100,105] may be useful. Several studies have investigated the effect of left cervical VNS on brain function using PET and fMRI imaging both in animals and humans. In epileptic and depressive patients, cervical VNS induced a gradual brain response involving a change in dorsolateral prefrontal/cingulate cortical activities followed by dopaminergic activation of the limbic system [106] or limbic-connected structures [107]. A widespread engagement involving several functional brain networks [108] has also been identified.

We reported the only quantitative brain map of glucose metabolism induced by abdominal VNS in obese preclinical pig models (Figure 5). Using this unbiased analysis, statistical parameter mapping performed on quantitative glucose-uptake images showed that brain glucose uptake was increased in the stimulated animal but only in a limited number of brain areas [109] including the periaqueducal grey, the thalamic and hypothalamic areas, and part of the amygdala and the insular cortex (Figure 5C). More importantly, enhanced brain connectivity in several regions including the striatum, cingulate, insula, thalamus, amygdala, hippocampus, and mid-brain were identified. These changes were associated together with profound alterations in DAT and SERT binding potentials. DAT binding potential was decreased markedly in the striatum while SERT binding potential was doubled in the mid-brain [17], (Figure 5D). These changes may be fundamental to the reduced food intake induced by VNS since the mesolimbic dopamine reward system is central to the regulation of eating behavior [110], and dopamine receptors availability has been reported to be reduced in morbidly obese individuals [111].

6.6. VNS Improves Insulin Sensitivity

Animal studies provide persuasive evidence that acute vagal stimulation increases fasting insulin release from the pancreas [112]. In contrast, the effect of chronic vagal stimulation on insulin sensitivity has received much less attention. One study in Zucker rats suggested that chronic vagal stimulation may up-regulate insulin receptor expression in the brain, liver, and skeletal muscle [113]. In obese pigs, chronic bilateral vagal stimulation can restore fasting glucose metabolism. This effect is evident at the whole-body level and in the brain, the liver, and the skeletal muscle and is associated with reductions in fasting glucose and insulin. The observed changes in glucose metabolism in the brain were also area-specific, with particular involvement of an amygdala-cingulate network and, more generally, several parts of the limbic system. The importance of the cingulate in insulin secretion is of specific interest, since electrical stimulation of the dorsal cingulate cortex in the dog suppresses insulin secretion in response to an intravenous glucose load [114]. Similarly, there is evidence that the cingulate cortices are involved in the brain response to the GLP1 agonist, exenatide [115], which may also improve insulin sensitivity. While chronic bilateral vagal stimulation is exceptionally successful in the restoration of insulin sensitivity, long-term efficacy on primary outcomes remains to be established. A further challenge is to translate favorable trial outcomes to a real-world setting.

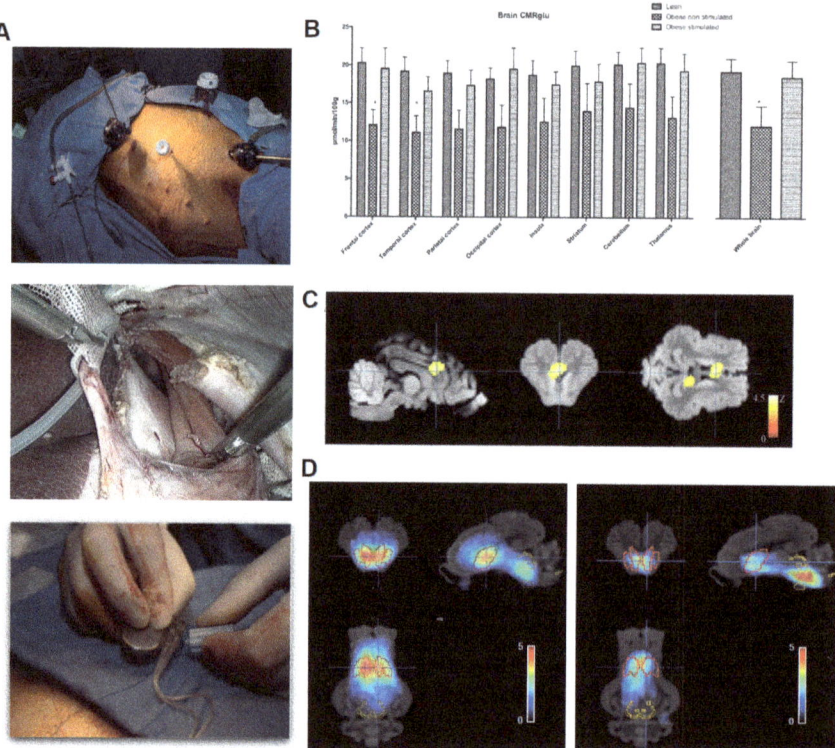

Figure 5. Brain metabolism and SERT/DAT expression in adult miniature pigs after chronic abdominal vagal stimulation. (**A**). Laparoscopic access to the abdominal vagus at the level of the lower esophageal sphincter in the obese miniature pig. Two cuffs with electrode pairs Pt-Ir are located around each vagal nerve after careful dissection and subsequent closure of the esophageal groove. The electrode leads were connected to purpose made, double current high compliance channels, neurostimulator that was implanted in a subcutaneous pocket [109]. (**B**). Quantitative changes in brain glucose uptake after several weeks of chronic vagal stimulation in lean and obese animals showing restoration of obesity-related impaired glucose metabolism by VNS. (**C**). Voxel-based statistical parametric mapping analysis showing the differences in glucose metabolism between the obese non-stimulated and obese-stimulated groups. The image was centered the dorsal anterior cingular cortex, which was the region most markedly affected by stimulation. (**D**). Pixel-wise modeled SPECT dynamic image after administration of ^{123}I ioflupane showing the binding potential of DAT/SERT overlaid on the MRI template. Red VOIs correspond to DAT-rich areas, whereas yellow VOIs represent SERT-rich areas. The left panel represents sham, whereas the right panel shows vagal stimulated obese miniature pigs. Adapted from Refs. [17,104].

7. Conclusions

In conclusion, the porcine model has provided unique data on the peripheral modulation of the vagal afferent information in lean and obese animals. Its size was adequate to translate recording tools from clinical to research setting while being possible to access invasively vagal activity—an ethical issue in human research. Furthermore, it has been demonstrated that the engagement of primary and secondary vagal projection brain areas was extremely sensitive to peripheral sensing of the vagal afferent and its modulation by diet and pathophysiological conditions such as obesity. This unpredicted behavior, uncorrelated with changes in satiation or satiety, militates for a stringent threshold during the analysis of brain activation maps within the scope of appetite control. It also points out the absolute requirement for quantitative analysis of these maps. Finally, the similarities of the abdominal vagus between the pig and the human, a condition fundamentally different from that observed in the murine models, constitute a driving force towards innovative therapy tools engulfing developments in material physics, electronics, and radiochemistry.

Author Contributions: C.-H.M. has made substantial contributions to the conception or design of the work; acquisition, analysis, interpretation of data; and the creation of new software used in the work. He has approved the submitted manuscript version and agrees to be personally accountable for the contribution presented in this paper and for ensuring that questions related to the accuracy or integrity of any part of the work, even that which the author was not personally involved, are appropriately investigated, resolved, and documented in the literature.

Funding: This research was funded by the Institute of Agronomic Research (Now INRAE), The Banque Publique d'investissement (BPI), The Agence Nationale de la Recherche (ANR) and the Britany Council.

Institutional Review Board Statement: The experiments were conducted in accordance with the current ethical standards of the European legislation after validation by an ethics Committee.

Informed Consent Statement: Not applicable.

Data Availability Statement: No new data were created or analyzed in this study. Data sharing is not applicable to this article.

Acknowledgments: The author acknowledges the involvement of INRA (now INRAE) in supporting the research topic presented in this manuscript through several public grants over the years. The author also acknowledges the financial support of ANR (Nutrisens and Savane programs) and of BPIFrance within the "Investments for the Future" program (Intense program). The author thanks the students that were involved, under his supervision, in the research topic in France and thanks the staff of the animal facilities of UEPR unit for ongoing animal care and surgery. The author also thanks E. Bobillier for the development of several research tools, including the robotic feed dispensers and part of the electrophysiology apparatus, L Leitner for his involvement in the early vagal recording in pigs, and the members of the Nuclear medicine department of Eugene Marquis hospital. The author also thanks the actual and past members of Aniscan imaging department for the administrative support. The author also thanks General Electric-Nuclear imaging department for their ongoing support.

Conflicts of Interest: The author declares no conflict of interest.

Abbreviations

BOLD	Blood-oxygen-level dependent
DAT	Dopamine active transporter
DVC	Dorsal vagal complex
fMRI	functional magnetic resonance imaging
GLP-1r	Glucagon like peptide-1 receptor
HMPAO	hexa-methyl-propyl-amineoxime
PET	Positron emission tomography
SPECT	Single photon emission computed tomography
SERT	sodium-dependent serotonin transporter
VNS	vagal nerve stimulation
VOI	volume of interest

References

1. Duclaux, R.; Mei, N.; Ranieri, F. Conduction velocity along the afferent vagal dendrites: A new type of fibre. *J. Physiol.* **1976**, *260*, 487–495. [CrossRef] [PubMed]
2. Iggo, A. Gastric mucosal chemoreceptors with vagal afferent fibres in the cat. *Q. J. Exp. Physiol. Cogn. Med. Sci.* **1957**, *42*, 398–409. [CrossRef] [PubMed]
3. Cottrell, D.F.; Iggo, A. Mucosal enteroceptors with vagal afferent fibres in the proximal duodenum of sheep. *J. Physiol.* **1984**, *354*, 497–522. [CrossRef] [PubMed]

4. Bai, L.; Mesgarzadeh, S.; Ramesh, K.S.; Huey, E.L.; Liu, Y.; Gray, L.A.; Aitken, T.J.; Chen, Y.; Beutler, L.R.; Ahn, J.S.; et al. Genetic identification of vagal sensory neurons that control feeding. *Cell* **2019**, *179*, 1129–1143. [CrossRef] [PubMed]
5. Zagorodnyuk, V.P.; Chen, B.N.; Costa, M.; Brookes, S.J. Mechanotransduction by intraganglionic laminar endings of vagal tension receptors in the guinea-pig oesophagus. *J. Physiol.* **2003**, *553*, 575–587. [CrossRef] [PubMed]
6. Sclocco, R.; Beissner, F.; Desbordes, G.; Polimeni, J.R.; Wald, L.L.; Kettner, N.W.; Kim, J.; Garcia, R.G.; Renvall, V.; Bianchi, A.M.; et al. Neuroimaging brainstem circuitry supporting cardiovagal response to pain: A combined heart rate variability/ultrahigh-field (7 T) functional magnetic resonance imaging study. *Philos. Trans. R. Soc. A Math. Phys. Eng. Sci.* **2016**, *374*, 20150189. [CrossRef] [PubMed]
7. Cai, P.Y.; Bodhit, A.; Derequito, R.; Ansari, S.; Abukhalil, F.; Thenkabail, S.; Ganji, S.; Saravanapavan, P.; Shekar, C.C.; Bidari, S.; et al. Vagus nerve stimulation in ischemic stroke: Old wine in a new bottle. *Front. Neurol.* **2014**, *5*, 107. [CrossRef]
8. Saikali, S.; Meurice, P.; Sauleau, P.; Eliat, P.-A.; Bellaud, P.; Randuineau, G.; Verin, M.; Malbert, C.-H. A three-dimensional digital segmented and deformable brain atlas of the domestic pig. *J. Neurosci. Methods* **2010**, *192*, 102–109. [CrossRef]
9. Sauleau, P.; Lapouble, E.; Val-Laillet, D.; Malbert, C.-H. The pig model in brain imaging and neurosurgery. *Animal* **2009**, *3*, 1138–1151. [CrossRef]
10. Malbert, C.H. AniMate. An open source software for absolute PET quantification. In Proceedings of the Annual Congress of the European Association of Nuclear Medicine 43, Barcelona, Spain, 15–19 October 2016.
11. Gibbons, C.; Hopkins, M.; Beaulieu, K.; Oustric, P.; Blundell, J.E. Issues in measuring and interpreting human appetite (satiety/satiation) and its contribution to obesity. *Curr. Obes. Rep.* **2019**, *8*, 77–87. [CrossRef]
12. Koopmans, S.J.; Schuurman, T. Considerations on pig models for appetite, metabolic syndrome and obese type 2 diabetes: From food intake to metabolic disease. *Eur. J. Pharmacol.* **2015**, *759*, 231–239. [CrossRef] [PubMed]
13. Doulah, A.; Farooq, M.; Yang, X.; Parton, J.; McCrory, M.A.; Higgins, J.A.; Sazonov, E. Meal microstructure characterization from sensor-based food intake detection. *Front. Nutr.* **2017**, *4*, 31. [CrossRef] [PubMed]
14. Biraben, A.; Guerin, S.; Bobillier, E.; Malbert, C.H. Central activation after chronic vagus nerve stimulation in pigs: Contribution of functional imaging. *Bull. Acad. Vet. Fr.* **2008**, *161*, 441–448.
15. Lepionka, L.; Malbert, C.-H.; LaPlace, J.P. Proximal gastric distension modifies ingestion rate in pigs. *Reprod. Nutr. Dev.* **1997**, *37*, 449–457. [CrossRef] [PubMed]
16. Malbert, C.-H.; Bobillier, E.; Picq, C.; Divoux, J.-L.; Guiraud, D.; Henry, C. Effects of chronic abdominal vagal stimulation of small-diameter neurons on brain metabolism and food intake. *Brain Stimul.* **2017**, *10*, 735–743. [CrossRef]
17. Malbert, C.-H.; Genissel, M.; Divoux, J.-L.; Henry, C. Chronic abdominal vagus stimulation increased brain metabolic connectivity, reduced striatal dopamine transporter and increased mid-brain serotonin transporter in obese miniature pigs. *J. Transl. Med.* **2019**, *17*, 78. [CrossRef]
18. Malbert, C.-H. *Brain Imaging during Feeding Behaviour*; Wiley Online Library: Angers, France, 2013.
19. De Graaf, C.; Blom, W.A.M.; Smeets, P.A.M.; Stafleu, A.; Hendriks, H.F.J. Biomarkers of satiation and satiety. *Am. J. Clin. Nutr.* **2004**, *79*, 946–961. [CrossRef]
20. Warwick, J.M. Imaging of brain function using SPECT. *Metab. Brain Dis.* **2004**, *19*, 113–123. [CrossRef]
21. Murase, K.; Tanada, S.; Fujita, H.; Sakaki, S.; Hamamoto, K. Kinetic behavior of technetium-99m-HMPAO in the human brain and quantification of cerebral blood flow using dynamic SPECT. *J. Nucl. Med.* **1992**, *33*, 135–143.
22. Lapouble, E.; Chauvin, A.; Guerin, S.; Malbert, C.-H. Regional Brain Activation during Proximal Gastric Distension in Pigs. In *Joint International Society Meeting in Neurogastroenterology and GI Motility*; Wiley-Blackwell: Boston, MA, USA, 2006.
23. Malbert, C.-H. Porc miniature modèle pour l'innovation thérapeutique—Stimulation vagale et syndrome métabolique. *Bull. Académie Vétérinaire Fr.* **2018**. [CrossRef]
24. Ochoa, M.; Malbert, C.-H.; Meurice, P.; Val-Laillet, D. Effects of chronic consumption of sugar-enriched diets on brain metabolism and insulin sensitivity in adult Yucatan minipigs. *PLoS ONE* **2016**, *11*, e0161228. [CrossRef]
25. Lee, S.S.; Alloosh, M.; Saxena, R.; Van Alstine, W.; Watkins, B.A.; Klaunig, J.E.; Sturek, M.; Chalasani, N. Nutritional model of steatohepatitis and metabolic syndrome in the Ossabaw miniature swine. *Hepatology* **2009**, *50*, 56–67. [CrossRef] [PubMed]
26. Bahri, S.; Horowitz, M.; Malbert, C.-H. Inward glucose transfer accounts for insulin-dependent increase in brain glucose metabolism associated with diet-induced obesity. *Obesity* **2018**, *26*, 1322–1331. [CrossRef] [PubMed]
27. Koopmans, S.J.; Mroz, Z.; Dekker, R.; Corbijn, H.; Ackermans, M.; Sauerwein, H. Association of insulin resistance with hyperglycemia in streptozotocin-diabetic pigs. *Metabolism* **2006**, *55*, 960–971. [CrossRef]
28. Horowitz, M.; Jones, K.; Edelbroek, M.A.L.; Smout, A.J.P.M.; Read, N.W. The effect of posture on gastric emptying and intra-gastric distribution of oil and aqueous meal components and appetite. *Gastroenterology* **1993**, *105*, 382–390. [CrossRef]
29. Janssen, P.; Berghe, P.V.; Verschueren, S.; Lehmann, A.; Depoortere, I.; Tack, J. Review article: The role of gastric motility in the control of food intake. *Aliment. Pharmacol. Ther.* **2011**, *33*, 880–894. [CrossRef]
30. Abell, T.L.; Camilleri, M.; Donohoe, K.; Hasler, W.L.; Lin, H.C.; Maurer, A.H.; McCallum, R.W.; Nowak, T.; Nusynowitz, M.L.; Parkman, H.P.; et al. Consensus recommendations for gastric emptying scintigraphy: A joint report of the American Neurogastroenterology and Motility Society and the Society of Nuclear Medicine. *Am. J. Gastroenterol.* **2008**, *103*, 753–763. [CrossRef]
31. Anderson, D.L.; Bartholomeusz, F.D.; Kirkwood, I.D.E.; Chatterton, B.; Summersides, G.; Penglis, S.; Kuchel, T.; Sansom, L. Liquid gastric emptying in the pig: Effect of concentration of inhaled isoflurane. *J. Nucl. Med.* **2002**, *43*, 968–971.

32. Malbert, C.-H.; Mathis, C.; Bobillier, E.; LaPlace, J.P.; Horowitz, M. Measurement of gastric emptying by intragastric gamma scintigraphy. *Neurogastroenterol. Motil.* **1997**, *9*, 157–165. [CrossRef]
33. Blat, S.; Guerin, S.; Chauvin, A.; Bobillier, E.; Le Cloirec, J.; Bourguet, P.; Malbert, C.-H. Role of vagal innervation on intragastric distribution and emptying of liquid and semisolid meals in conscious pigs. *Neurogastroenterol. Motil.* **2001**, *13*, 73–80. [CrossRef]
34. Blat, S.; Guerin, S.; Chauvin, A.; Bobillier-Chaumont, E.; Malbert, C.-H. Dorsal vagal trunk has a preponderant role to control gastric emptying in pigs. *Neurogastroenterol. Motil.* **1998**, *10*, 467.
35. Malbert, C.-H.; Biraben, A.; Guerin, S.; Chauvin, A. Gastric Emptying is Not Altered by Chronic Vagal Stimulation. In *Joint International Society Meeting in Neurogastroenterology and GI Motility*; Wiley-Blackwell: Boston, MA, USA, 2006.
36. Ménard, O.; Famelart, M.-H.; Deglaire, A.; Le Gouar, Y.; Guérin, S.; Malbert, C.-H.; Dupont, D. Gastric emptying and dynamic in vitro digestion of drinkable yogurts: Effect of viscosity and composition. *Nutrients* **2018**, *10*, 1308. [CrossRef] [PubMed]
37. Phillips, R.J.; Powley, T. Gastric volume rather than nutrient content inhibits food intake. *Am. J. Physiol. Regul. Integr. Comp. Physiol.* **1996**, *271*, R766–R769. [CrossRef] [PubMed]
38. Read, N.; French, S.; Cunningham, K. The role of the gut in regulating food intake in man. *Nutr. Rev.* **2009**, *52*, 1–10. [CrossRef] [PubMed]
39. Geliebter, A.; Melton, P.M.; Gage, D.; McCray, R.S.; Hashim, S.A. Gastric balloon to treat obesity: A double-blind study in nondieting subjects. *Am. J. Clin. Nutr.* **1990**, *51*, 584–588. [CrossRef]
40. Oesch, S.; Rüegg, C.; Fischer, B.; Degen, L.; Beglinger, C. Effect of gastric distension prior to eating on food intake and feelings of satiety in humans. *Physiol. Behav.* **2006**, *87*, 903–910. [CrossRef]
41. Sturm, K.; Parker, B.; Wishart, J.; Feinle-Bisset, C.; Jones, K.L.; Chapman, I.; Horowitz, M. Energy intake and appetite are related to antral area in healthy young and older subjects. *Am. J. Clin. Nutr.* **2004**, *80*, 656–667. [CrossRef]
42. Distrutti, E.; Azpiroz, F.; Soldevilla, A.; Malagelada, J. Gastric wall tension determines perception of gastric distention. *Gastroenterology* **1999**, *116*, 1035–1042. [CrossRef]
43. Settell, M.L.; Pelot, N.A.; Knudsen, B.E.; Dingle, A.M.; McConico, A.L.; Nicolai, E.N.; Trevathan, J.K.; Ezzell, J.A.; Ross, E.K.; Gustafson, K.J.; et al. Functional vagotopy in the cervical vagus nerve of the domestic pig: Implications for the study of vagus nerve stimulation. *J. Neural Eng.* **2020**, *17*, 026022. [CrossRef]
44. Malbert, C.H.; Horowitz, M. The pig as a model for human digestive motor activity. In *Digestive Physiology in Pigs*; Laplace, J.P., Fevrier, C., Barbeau, A., Eds.; EAAP Publication: Paris, France, 1997; pp. 3–13.
45. Lepionka, L.; Malbert, C. Are fundic receptors sensitive to circumferential wall tension in vivo? *Gastroenterology* **1998**, *114*, A787. [CrossRef]
46. Phillips, R.J.; Powley, T.L. Tension and stretch receptors in gastrointestinal smooth muscle: Re-evaluating vagal mechanoreceptor electrophysiology. *Brain Res. Rev.* **2000**, *34*, 1–26. [CrossRef]
47. Wang, Y.B.; De Lartigue, G.; Page, A.J. Dissecting the role of subtypes of gastrointestinal vagal afferents. *Front. Physiol.* **2020**, *11*, 643. [CrossRef] [PubMed]
48. Browning, K.N.; Verheijden, S.; Boeckxstaens, G.E. The vagus nerve in appetite regulation, mood, and intestinal inflammation. *Gastroenterology* **2017**, *152*, 730–744. [CrossRef] [PubMed]
49. Ladabaum, U.; Minoshima, S.; Hasler, W.L.; Cross, D.; Chey, W.D.; Owyang, C. Gastric distention correlates with activation of multiple cortical and subcortical regions. *Gastroenterology* **2001**, *120*, 369–376. [CrossRef] [PubMed]
50. Ladabaum, U.; Roberts, T.P.L.; Mcgonigle, D.J. Gastric fundic distension activates fronto-limbic structures but not primary somatosensory cortex: A functional magnetic resonance imaging study. *NeuroImage* **2007**, *34*, 724–732. [CrossRef]
51. Wang, G.-J.; Tomasi, D.; Backus, W.; Wang, R.; Telang, F.; Geliebter, A.; Korner, J.; Bauman, A.; Fowler, J.S.; Thanos, P.K.; et al. Gastric distention activates satiety circuitry in the human brain. *NeuroImage* **2008**, *39*, 1824–1831. [CrossRef]
52. Alger, S.E.; Payne, J.D. The differential effects of emotional salience on direct associative and relational memory during a nap. *Cogn. Affect. Behav. Neurosci.* **2016**, *16*, 1150–1163. [CrossRef]
53. McClure, S.M.; York, M.K.; Montague, P.R. The neural substrates of reward processing in humans: The modern role of fMRI. *Neuroscience* **2004**, *10*, 260–268. [CrossRef]
54. Berthoud, H.-R.; Lenard, N.R.; Shin, A.C. Food reward, hyperphagia, and obesity. *Am. J. Physiol. Integr. Comp. Physiol.* **2011**, *300*, R1266–R1277. [CrossRef]
55. Geliebter, A. Neuroimaging of gastric distension and gastric bypass surgery. *Appetite* **2013**, *71*, 459–465. [CrossRef]
56. Berthoud, H.-R.; Neuhuber, W.L. Functional and chemical anatomy of the afferent vagal system. *Auton. Neurosci.* **2000**, *85*, 1–17. [CrossRef]
57. Lapouble, E.; Guérin, S.; Malbert, C.H. Vagal versus non vagal gastric afferent signals processing in the brain. *Gastroenterology* **2007**, *51*, 61–62.
58. Kumbhari, V.; Oberbach, A.; Nimgaonkar, A. Primary endoscopic therapies for obesity and metabolic diseases. *Curr. Opin. Gastroenterol.* **2015**, *31*, 351–358. [CrossRef] [PubMed]
59. Tate, C.M.; Geliebter, A. Intragastric balloon treatment for obesity: Review of recent studies. *Adv. Ther.* **2017**, *34*, 1859–1875. [CrossRef] [PubMed]
60. Layec, S.; Val-Laillet, D.; Heresbach, D.; Malbert, C.-H. Gastric tone, volume and emptying after implantation of an intragastric balloon for weight control. *Neurogastroenterol. Motil.* **2010**, *22*, 1016.e266. [CrossRef] [PubMed]

61. Layec, S.; Lapouble, E.; Val-Laillet, D.; Guérin, S.; Chauvin, A.; Heresbach, D.; Malbert, C.-H. T1805 Chronic but not accute gastric distension activates brain reward circuit. *Gastroenterology* **2009**, *136*, A583. [CrossRef]
62. Sabatinelli, D.; Bradley, M.M.; Lang, P.J.; Costa, V.D.; Versace, F. Pleasure rather than salience activates human nucleus accumbens and medial prefrontal cortex. *J. Neurophysiol.* **2007**, *98*, 1374–1379. [CrossRef] [PubMed]
63. Roura, E.; Fu, M. Taste, nutrient sensing and feed intake in pigs (130 years of research: Then, now and future). *Anim. Feed Sci. Technol.* **2017**, *233*, 3–12. [CrossRef]
64. Maltecca, C.; Bergamaschi, M.; Tiezzi, F. The interaction between microbiome and pig efficiency: A review. *J. Anim. Breed. Genet.* **2020**, *137*, 4–13. [CrossRef]
65. Malbert, C.-H.; Horowitz, M.; Young, R.L. Low-calorie sweeteners augment tissue-specific insulin sensitivity in a large animal model of obesity. *Eur. J. Nucl. Med. Mol. Imaging* **2019**, *46*, 2380–2391. [CrossRef]
66. Malbert, C.H.; Mathis, C. Antro-Pyloric modulation of the transpyloric flow of liquids in pigs. *Gastroenterology* **1994**, *107*, 37–46. [CrossRef]
67. Jones, K.L.; O'Donovan, D.; Horowitz, M.; Russo, A.; Lei, Y.; Hausken, T. Effects of posture on gastric emptying, transpyloric flow, and hunger after a glucose drink in healthy humans. *Dig. Dis. Sci.* **2006**, *51*, 1331–1338. [CrossRef] [PubMed]
68. Malbert, C.-H.; Leitner, L.-M. Mechanoreceptors sensitive to flow at the gastroduodenal junction of the cat. *Am. J. Physiol. Gastrointest. Liver Physiol.* **1993**, *265*, G310–G313. [CrossRef] [PubMed]
69. Vozzo, R.; Su, Y.-C.; Fraser, R.J.; Wittert, G.A.; Horowitz, M.; Malbert, C.-H.; Shulkes, A.; Volombello, T.; Chapman, I.M. Antropyloroduodenal, cholecystokinin and feeding responses to pulsatile and non-pulsatile intraduodenal lipid infusion. *Neurogastroenterol. Motil.* **2002**, *14*, 25–33. [CrossRef] [PubMed]
70. Wölnerhanssen, B.K.; Meyer-Gerspach, A.C.; Peters, T.; Beglinger, C.; Peterli, R. Incretin effects, gastric emptying and insulin responses to low oral glucose loads in patients after gastric bypass and lean and obese controls. *Surg. Obes. Relat. Dis.* **2016**, *12*, 1320–1327. [CrossRef] [PubMed]
71. Lindqvist, A.; Ekelund, M.; Pierzynowski, S.; Groop, L.; Hedenbro, J.; Wierup, N. Gastric bypass in the pig increases GIP levels and decreases active GLP-1 levels. *Peptides* **2017**, *90*, 78–82. [CrossRef]
72. Soty, M.; Gautier-Stein, A.; Rajas, F.; Mithieux, G. Gut-brain glucose signaling in energy homeostasis. *Cell Metab.* **2017**, *25*, 1231–1242. [CrossRef]
73. Sandoval, D.A.; Cota, D.; Seeley, R.J. The integrative role of CNS fuel-sensing mechanisms in energy balance and glucose regulation. *Annu. Rev. Physiol.* **2008**, *70*, 513–535. [CrossRef]
74. Pal, A.; Rhoads, D.B.; Tavakkoli, A. Effect of portal glucose sensing on systemic glucose levels in SD and ZDF rats. *PLoS ONE* **2016**, *11*, e0165592. [CrossRef]
75. Ionut, V.; Castro, A.V.B.; Woolcott, O.O.; Stefanovski, D.; Iyer, M.S.; Broussard, J.L.; Burch, M.; Elazary, R.; Kolka, C.M.; Mkrtchyan, H.; et al. Hepatic portal vein denervation impairs oral glucose tolerance but not exenatide's effect on glycemia. *Am. J. Physiol. Metab.* **2014**, *307*, E644–E652. [CrossRef]
76. Nishizawa, M.; Nakabayashi, H.; Uehara, K.; Nakagawa, A.; Uchida, K.; Koya, D. Intraportal GLP-1 stimulates insulin secretion predominantly through the hepatoportal-pancreatic vagal reflex pathways. *Am. J. Physiol. Metab.* **2013**, *305*, E376–E387. [CrossRef] [PubMed]
77. Eriksson, O.; Rosenström, U.; Selvaraju, R.K.; Eriksson, B.; Velikyan, I. Species differences in pancreatic binding of DO3A-VS-Cys40-Exendin4. *Acta Diabetol.* **2017**, *54*, 1039–1045. [CrossRef] [PubMed]
78. Malbert, C.-H.; Chauvin, A.; Horowitz, M.; Jones, K.L. Glucose-sensing mediated by portal GLP-1 receptor is markedly impaired in insulin-resistant obese animals. *Diabetes* **2021**, *70*, 99–110. [CrossRef] [PubMed]
79. Malbert, C.-H.; Chauvin, A.; Horowitz, M.; Jones, K.L. Pancreatic GLP-1r binding potential is reduced in insulin-resistant pigs. *BMJ Open Diabetes Res. Care* **2020**, *8*, e001540. [CrossRef] [PubMed]
80. Boubaker, J.; Chauvin, A.; Guerin, S.; Malbert, C.-H. *Quantitative Involvement of Duodenal, Portal and Cerebral Nutrient Sensing Towards Food Intake Control*; Karger: Paris, France, 2007; Volume 51, (Suppl. 1).
81. Boubaker, J.; Val-Laillet, D.; Guerin, S.; Malbert, C.-H. Brain processing of duodenal and portal glucose sensing. *J. Neuroendocr.* **2012**, *24*, 1096–1105. [CrossRef] [PubMed]
82. Eklund, A.; Nichols, T.E.; Knutsson, H. Cluster failure: Why fMRI inferences for spatial extent have inflated false-positive rates. *Proc. Natl. Acad. Sci. USA* **2016**, *113*, 7900–7905. [CrossRef] [PubMed]
83. Gortz, L.; Bjorkman, A.-C.; Andersson, H.; Kral, J. Truncal vagotomy reduces food and liquid intake in man. *Physiol. Behav.* **1990**, *48*, 779–781. [CrossRef]
84. Camilleri, M. Peripheral mechanisms in the control of appetite and related experimental therapies in obesity. *Regul. Pept.* **2009**, *156*, 24–27. [CrossRef]
85. Kral, J.G.; Paez, W.; Wolfe, B.M. Vagal nerve function in obesity: Therapeutic implications. *World J. Surg.* **2009**, *33*, 1995–2006. [CrossRef]
86. Sarr, M.G.; The EMPOWER Study Group; Billington, C.J.; Brancatisano, R.; Brancatisano, A.; Toouli, J.; Kow, L.; Nguyen, N.T.; Blackstone, R.; Maher, J.W.; et al. The EMPOWER Study: Randomized, prospective, double-blind, multicenter trial of vagal blockade to induce weight loss in morbid obesity. *Obes. Surg.* **2012**, *22*, 1771–1782. [CrossRef]
87. Bligny, D.; Blat, S.; Chauvin, A.; Guérin, S.; Malbert, C.-H. Reduced mechanosensitivity of duodenal vagal afferent neurons after an acute switch from milk-based to plant-based diets in anaesthetized pigs. *J. Physiol. Pharmacol.* **2005**, *56*, 89–100. [PubMed]

88. De Lartigue, G.; De La Serre, C.B.; Espero, E.; Lee, J.; Raybould, H.E. Diet-induced obesity leads to the development of leptin resistance in vagal afferent neurons. *Am. J. Physiol. Endocrinol. Metab.* **2011**, *301*, E187–E195. [CrossRef] [PubMed]
89. Page, A.J. Vagal afferent dysfunction in obesity: Cause or effect. *J. Physiol.* **2015**, *594*, 5–6. [CrossRef] [PubMed]
90. Kentish, S.J.; Vincent, A.D.; Kennaway, D.J.; Wittert, G.; Page, A.J. High-fat diet-induced obesity ablates gastric vagal afferent circadian rhythms. *J. Neurosci.* **2016**, *36*, 3199–3207. [CrossRef]
91. de Lartigue, G.; Xu, C. Mechanisms of vagal plasticity influencing feeding behavior. *Brain Res.* **2018**, *1693*, 146–150. [CrossRef]
92. Yuan, X.; Huang, Y.; Shah, S.; Wu, H.; Gautron, L. Levels of Cocaine- and Amphetamine-Regulated Transcript in Vagal Afferents in the Mouse Are Unaltered in Response to Metabolic Challenges. *Eneuro* **2016**. [CrossRef]
93. Nunez-Salces, M.; Li, H.; Christie, S.; Page, A.J. The Effect of High-Fat Diet-Induced Obesity on the Expression of Nutrient Chemosensors in the Mouse Stomach and the Gastric Ghrelin Cell. *Nutrients.* **2020**, *12*, 2493. [CrossRef]
94. Hays, S.A.; Rennaker, R.L.; Kilgard, M.P. Targeting plasticity with vagus nerve stimulation to treat neurological disease. *Prog Brain Res.* **2013**, *207*, 275–299. [CrossRef]
95. Gandolfi, D.; Bigiani, A.; Porro, C.A.; Mapelli, J. Inhibitory Plasticity: From Molecules to Computation and Beyond. *Int. J. Mol. Sci.* **2020**, *21*, 1805. [CrossRef]
96. Sobocki, J.; Fourtanier, G.; Estany, J.; Otal, P. Does vagal nerve stimulation affect body composition and metabolism? Experimental study of a new potential technique in bariatric surgery. *Surgery* **2006**, *139*, 209–216. [CrossRef]
97. Laskiewicz, J.; Królczyk, G.; Zurowski, G.; Sobocki, J.; Matyja, A.; Thor, P.J. Effects of vagal neuromodulation and vagotomy on control of food intake and body weight in rats. *J. Physiol. Pharmacol.* **2003**, *54*, 603–610. [PubMed]
98. Bugajski, A.J.; Gil, K.; Ziomber, A.; Zurowski, D.; Zaraska, W.; Thor, P.J. Effect of long-term vagal stimulation on food intake and body weight during diet induced obesity in rats. *J. Physiol. Pharmacol.* **2007**, *58*, 5–12. [PubMed]
99. Val-Laillet, D.; Biraben, A.; Randuineau, G.; Malbert, C.-H. Chronic vagus nerve stimulation decreased weight gain, food consumption and sweet craving in adult obese minipigs. *Appetite* **2010**, *55*, 245–252. [CrossRef] [PubMed]
100. Dali, M.; Picq, C.; Rossel, O.; Maciejasz, P.; Malbert, C.-H.; Guiraud, D. Comparison of the efficiency of chopped and non-rectangular electrical stimulus waveforms in activating small vagus nerve fibers. *J. Neurosci. Methods* **2019**, *320*, 1–8. [CrossRef] [PubMed]
101. Mei, N.; Condamin, M.; Boyer, A. The composition of the vagus nerve of the cat. *Cell Tissue Res.* **1980**, *209*, 423–431. [CrossRef]
102. Guiraud, D.; Andreu, D.; Bonnet, S.; Carrault, G.; Couderc, P.; Hagège, A.; Henry, C.; Hernandez, A.; Karam, N.; Le Rolle, V.; et al. Vagus nerve stimulation: State of the art of stimulation and recording strategies to address autonomic function neuromodulation. *J. Neural Eng.* **2016**, *13*, 041002. [CrossRef]
103. Malbert, C.-H. The brain-gut axis: Insights from the obese pig model. *Bull. Académie Natl. Médecine* **2013**, *197*, 1683–1694. [CrossRef]
104. Malbert, C.-H. Could vagus nerve stimulation have a role in the treatment of diabetes? *Bioelectron. Med.* **2018**, *1*, 13–15. [CrossRef]
105. Helmers, S.L.; Begnaud, J.; Cowley, A.; Corwin, H.M.; Edwards, J.C.; Holder, D.L.; Kostov, H.; Larsson, P.G.; Levisohn, P.M.; De Menezes, M.S.; et al. Application of a computational model of vagus nerve stimulation. *Acta Neurol. Scand.* **2012**, *126*, 336–343. [CrossRef]
106. Conway, C.R.; Chibnall, J.T.; Gebara, M.A.; Price, J.L.; Snyder, A.Z.; Mintun, M.A.; Craig, A.B.; Cornell, M.E.; Perantie, D.C.; Giuffra, L.A.; et al. Association of cerebral metabolic activity changes with vagus nerve stimulation antidepressant response in treatment-resistant depression. *Brain Stimul.* **2013**, *6*, 788–797. [CrossRef]
107. Vonck, K.; De Herdt, V.; Bosman, T.; Dedeurwaerdere, S.; Van Laere, K.; Boon, P. Thalamic and limbic involvement in the mechanism of action of vagus nerve stimulation, a SPECT study. *Seizure* **2008**, *17*, 699–706. [CrossRef] [PubMed]
108. Cao, J.; Lu, K.-H.; Powley, T.L.; Liu, Z. Vagal nerve stimulation triggers widespread responses and alters large-scale functional connectivity in the rat brain. *PLoS ONE* **2017**, *12*, e0189518. [CrossRef] [PubMed]
109. Malbert, C.-H.; Picq, C.; Divoux, J.-L.; Henry, C.; Horowitz, M. Obesity-associated alterations in glucose metabolism are reversed by chronic bilateral stimulation of the abdominal vagus nerve. *Diabetes* **2017**, *66*, 848–857. [CrossRef] [PubMed]
110. Berthoud, H.-R.; Münzberg, H.; Morrison, C.D. Blaming the brain for obesity: Integration of hedonic and homeostatic mechanisms. *Gastroenterology* **2017**, *152*, 1728–1738. [CrossRef]
111. Chen, P.S.; Yang, Y.K.; Yeh, T.L.; Lee, I.-H.; Yao, W.J.; Chiu, N.T.; Lu, R.-B. Correlation between body mass index and striatal dopamine transporter availability in healthy volunteers—A SPECT study. *NeuroImage* **2008**, *40*, 275–279. [CrossRef] [PubMed]
112. Ahren, B.; Taborsky, G.J. The mechanism of vagal nerve stimulation of glucagon and insulin secretion in the dog. *Endocrinology* **1986**, *118*, 1551–1557. [CrossRef]
113. Li, S.; Zhai, X.; Rong, P.; McCabe, M.F.; Wang, X.; Zhao, J.; Ben, H.; Wang, S. Therapeutic effect of vagus nerve stimulation on depressive-like behavior, hyperglycemia and insulin receptor expression in zucker fatty rats. *PLoS ONE* **2014**, *9*, e112066. [CrossRef]
114. Kaneto, A.; Miki, E.; Kosaka, K.; Okinaka, S.; Nakao, K. Effects of stimulation of the cingulate gyrus on insulin secretion. *Endocrinology* **1965**, *77*, 617–624. [CrossRef]
115. Daniele, G.; Iozzo, P.; Molina-Carrion, M.; Lancaster, J.; Ciociaro, D.; Cersosimo, E.; Tripathy, D.; Triplitt, C.; Fox, P.; Musi, N.; et al. Exenatide regulates cerebral glucose metabolism in brain areas associated with glucose homeostasis and reward system. *Diabetes* **2015**, *64*, 3406–3412. [CrossRef]

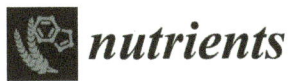

Review

Endocannabinoids and the Gut-Brain Control of Food Intake and Obesity

Nicholas V. DiPatrizio

Division of Biomedical Sciences, School of Medicine, University of California Riverside, Riverside, CA 92521, USA; ndipatri@medsch.ucr.edu; Tel.: +1-951-827-7252

Abstract: Gut-brain signaling controls food intake and energy homeostasis, and its activity is thought to be dysregulated in obesity. We will explore new studies that suggest the endocannabinoid (eCB) system in the upper gastrointestinal tract plays an important role in controlling gut-brain neurotransmission carried by the vagus nerve and the intake of palatable food and other reinforcers. A focus will be on studies that reveal both indirect and direct interactions between eCB signaling and vagal afferent neurons. These investigations identify (*i*) an indirect mechanism that controls nutrient-induced release of peptides from the gut epithelium that directly interact with corresponding receptors on vagal afferent neurons, and (*ii*) a direct mechanism via interactions between eCBs and cannabinoid receptors expressed on vagal afferent neurons. Moreover, the impact of diet-induced obesity on these pathways will be considered.

Keywords: endocannabinoid; CB$_1$ receptor; gut-brain; intestine; food intake; reward

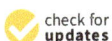

Citation: DiPatrizio, N.V. Endocannabinoids and the Gut-Brain Control of Food Intake and Obesity. *Nutrients* **2021**, *13*, 1214. https://doi.org/10.3390/nu13041214

Academic Editors: Armin Alaedini, Christine Feinle-Bisset and Michael Horowitz

Received: 1 March 2021
Accepted: 2 April 2021
Published: 7 April 2021

Publisher's Note: MDPI stays neutral with regard to jurisdictional claims in published maps and institutional affiliations.

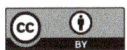

Copyright: © 2021 by the author. Licensee MDPI, Basel, Switzerland. This article is an open access article distributed under the terms and conditions of the Creative Commons Attribution (CC BY) license (https://creativecommons.org/licenses/by/4.0/).

1. Introduction

Gut-brain signaling plays an integral role in food intake, energy homeostasis, and possibly reward [1–3]. Our understanding of the biochemical and molecular pathways involved in these processes and their dysregulation in obesity, however, remains incomplete. Several signals, including gut-derived peptides, have been identified that control neurotransmission from peripheral organs to the brain (see for comprehensive review [4]). These include cholecystokinin (CCK), which is released from subpopulations of enteroendocrine cells in the upper small-intestinal epithelium in response to the presence of nutrients in the lumen and controls food intake and meal size by activating the afferent vagus nerve [1,5–9]. Recent studies in mice suggest that specialized enteroendocrine cells in the intestinal epithelium, termed "neuropods", form functional synapses with gastric afferent vagal fibers and participate in the transduction of signals from food to neural signals carried by vagal afferent neurons to the brain [10]. Neuropods sense nutrients on their luminal side and, in turn, release glutamate and CCK in a coordinated manner that induces rapid or prolonged firing of vagal afferent neurons, respectively [9]. These results highlight neuropods as a key cellular mechanism in nutrient sensing and associated gut-brain signaling. Other studies suggest that vagal afferent neurotransmission recruits brain reward circuits and may participate in food reward [11–14]. For example, optogenetic activation of right gastric vagal afferent neurons increased (i) dopamine release in central reward pathways, (ii) operant responses associated with self-stimulation of brain reward neurons, and (iii) conditioned flavor and place preferences [11]. Specific biochemical and molecular signaling pathways that control these functions, however, remain unclear.

The endocannabinoid (eCB) system is a lipid-derived signaling pathway that controls food intake, energy homeostasis, and reward, and is hijacked by chemicals in the cannabis plant [15–19] (see Figure 1). In general, activating the eCB system increases food intake [20] and inhibiting its activity reduces food intake [21]. The eCB system is located throughout the brain and plays an important role in these functions; however, mounting evidence also suggests that the eCB system in peripheral organs, including the small-intestinal epithelium, serves an integral role [22–36]. Indeed, pharmacological blockade of peripheral cannabinoid subtype-1 receptors (CB_1Rs) reduces food intake and improves metabolic dysfunction associated with obesity in rodents similarly to brain-penetrant CB_1R antagonists [21,23,24,27–30,37]. These studies highlight the peripheral eCB system as a possible target for safe anti-obesity agents that are devoid of psychiatric side-effects associated with drugs that access CB_1Rs in the brain (e.g., rimonabant [38]).

The eCB system in the rodent small-intestinal epithelium becomes activated (*i*) during oral exposure to dietary fats [23,39], (*ii*) during a fast [22,24,40], and (*iii*) after chronic exposure to obesogenic diets [25,40,41]. Moreover, pharmacological inhibition of peripheral CB_1Rs blocked (*i*) cephalic-phase consumption of dietary fats in rats [23,39], (*ii*) refeeding after a fast in rats [40], (*iii*) hyperphagia associated with western diet-induced obesity in mice [25,41], and (*iv*) restored nutrient-induced secretion of satiation peptides in western diet-induced obese mice. These studies suggest a critical role for eCB signaling in the gut in the intake of palatable foods. We will review recent experiments that expand our understanding of roles for the eCB system in the gut in gut-brain neurotransmission associated with food intake, energy homeostasis, and reward. An emphasis will be on studies that reveal both indirect and direct mechanisms of control for CB_1Rs over gut-brain signaling and dysregulation of these pathways in rodent models of diet-induced obesity.

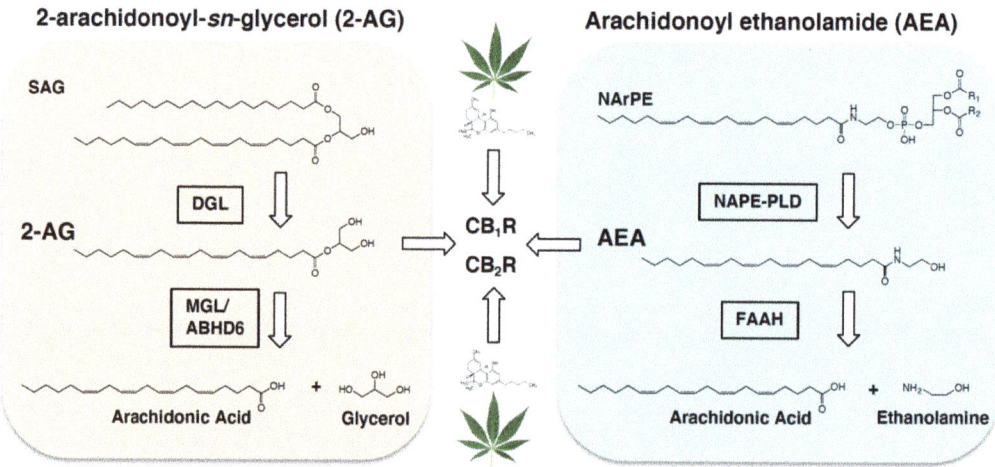

Figure 1. Endocannabinoid metabolic pathways. Biosynthesis of the endocannabinoid, 2-arachidonoyl-*sn*-glycerol (2-AG), is facilitated by diacylglycerol lipase- (DGL) dependent hydrolysis of the 2-AG precursor, 1,stearoyl,2-arachidonoyl-*sn*-glycerol (SAG). 2-AG is degraded by monoacylglycerol lipase (MGL), and to a lesser degree by alpha-beta-hydrolase domain 6 (ABHD6), into arachidonic acid and glycerol. Biosynthesis of the fatty acid ethanolamide, arachidonoyl ethanolamide (AEA, anandamide), is controlled by *N*-acylphosphatidylethanolamine phospholipase D- (NAPE-PLD) dependent hydrolysis of the AEA precursor, *N*-arachidonoylphosphatidylethanolamine (NArPE). AEA is degraded by fatty acid amide hydrolase (FAAH) into arachidonic acid and ethanolamine. 2-AG and AEA activate cannabinoid subtype-1 receptors (CB_1R) and cannabinoid subtype-2 receptors (CB_2R) in cells throughout the body (see for review [42,43]). Alternate endocannabinoid metabolic pathways have also been suggested. The primary intoxicating chemical in the cannabis plant, Δ^9 tetrahydrocannabinol (THC, represented by the green leaf and corresponding THC molecule), hijacks the endocannabioid system and activates cannabinoid receptors in cells throughout the body.

2. Gut-Brain Endocannabinoid Signaling Controls Intake of Palatable Foods

The eCB system is expressed in cells throughout all organs in the body and is comprised of lipid-derived signaling molecules including the primary eCBs, 2-arachidonoyl-*sn*-glycerol (2-AG) and arachidonoyl ethanolamide (anandamide), their metabolic enzymes, and cannabinoid receptor sub-type 1 (CB_1R), cannabinoid receptor sub-type-2 (CB_2Rs), and possibly others [42,43] (see Figure 1). The eCB system in the brain is extensively studied for its roles in controlling the intake and reward value of palatable food [44–60]. In addition to central sites, recent evidence suggests that the eCB system located in cells lining the intestinal epithelium is an integral component of a gut-brain axis that controls the intake of palatable foods [61]. For example, a sham-feeding protocol in rats was utilized to test if eCB signaling in the gut is associated with positive reinforcement that drives intake of food based on its orosensory properties [23]. During sham feeding, rats are allowed to freely consume a liquid diet that drains from a surgically-implanted, reversible, cannulae in the stomach before it reaches the small intestine. Therefore, sham feeding enables isolation of the cephalic phase of food intake and effectively eliminates post-ingestive consequences of food intake. [62]. Separate groups of rats were given access for 30 min to a fixed amount of dietary fats (corn oil emulsion), sucrose, or protein, and levels of 2-AG and anandamide were measured in the upper small-intestinal epithelium by liquid chromatography/mass spectrometry [23]. Tasting dietary fats—but not sucrose or protein—triggered production of eCBs in the upper small-intestinal epithelium, but not in other peripheral organs tested (i.e., tongue, stomach, ileum, pancreas, liver) or in micropunches obtained from brain regions associated with food intake and reward (i.e., ventral striatum, dorsal striatum, lateral regions of hypothalamus, medial regions of the hypothalamus, pontine parabrachial nucleus, or cerebellum). This effect was also specific for mono- and di-unsaturated fats (oleic acid and linoleic acid), but not saturated (stearic acid) or polyunsaturated fats (linolenic acid) [39]. Moreover, production of eCBs in the small-intestinal epithelium was absent in sham feeding rats that received full subdiaphragmatic vagotomy, which suggests that efferent vagal signaling participates in the biosynthesis of eCBs. Furthermore, intra-duodenal administration of a low-dose cannabinoid receptor subtype-1 (CB_1R) inverse agonist or a peripherally-restricted CB_1R antagonist blocked sham feeding of fats. Collectively, these studies suggest that tasting dietary fats recruits an eCB mechanism in the gut that provides positive feedback to the brain and promotes intake of fatty foods.

The aforementioned studies utilized pharmacological, biochemical, and behavioral approaches to identify roles for peripheral CB_1Rs in the intake of palatable food. At the time of these studies, however, appropriate tools were not available to directly ask if CB_1Rs in the intestinal epithelium are required in these processes. To test the necessity for CB_1Rs in the intestinal epithelium in the intake of palatable foods, we developed transgenic mice ($Cnr1^{tm1.1mrl}$/Vil-CRE ERT2) that are conditionally deficient in CB_1Rs in the intestinal epithelium (referred to as IntCB$_1$-/-mice) [63]. Mice were maintained on standard rodent chow low in fats and sugars, then given access for the first time to a palatable western-style diet high in fats and sugars (Research Diets D12079B; 40% kcals from fats and 43% from carbohydrates [64]), and preferences for western diet were measured. This specific western diet was chosen due to its macronutrient composition that more closely matches the human diet (35% kcals from fat and 47% kcals from carbohydrate [46]) when compared to other obesogenic diets routinely used in rodent studies (e.g., Research Diets D12492; 60% kcals from fat and low levels of carbohydrates). Control mice with functional CB_1Rs in the intestinal epithelium displayed large preferences for western diet when compared to chow, with over 90% of total kilocalories consumed from western diet over the testing period. In contrast to controls, preferences for western diet were reduced for up to 12 h in IntCB$_1$-/-mice. These results provide direct evidence that CB_1Rs in the murine intestinal epithelium are required for acute preferences for palatable foods.

Similar to rodents, humans prefer fatty and sweet foods when given a choice [65], and their consumption is associated with elevated levels of eCBs in blood [66]. Moreover, levels of eCBs are increased in blood in both human and rodent obesity [25,67–80]; however, the impact that circulating eCBs may have on gut-brain function associated with food intake, dietary preferences, and obesity is unknown. Nonetheless, it is plausible that circulating eCBs act as a humoral signal that interacts with cannabinoid receptors along the gut-brain axis to facilitate these processes.

3. Endocannabinoids and Gut-Brain Neurotransmission: Indirect Mechanisms

Mounting evidence suggests that eCB signaling in the periphery controls food intake by mechanisms that include both indirect and direct interactions with the afferent vagus nerve (see Figure 2). We will first review evidence of an indirect mechanism for CB_1Rs in the control of gut-brain signaling and its possible dysregulation in diet-induced obesity.

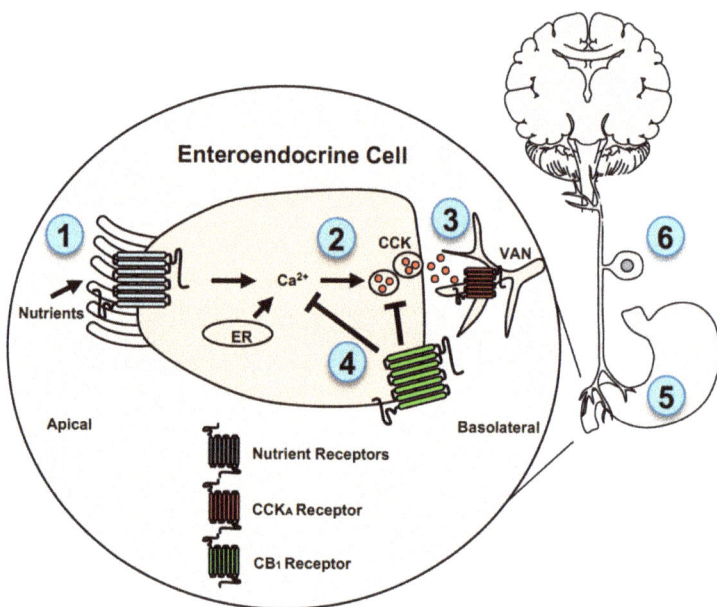

Figure 2. Endocannabinoid system control of gut-brain signaling. CB_1Rs are located on enteroendocrine cells in the small-intestinal epithelium, stomach cells, and vagal afferent neurons (VANs) where they indirectly and directly control gut-brain neurotransmission. CB_1Rs are thought to indirectly interact with VANs by a mechanism that includes controlling nutrient-induced secretion of the satiation peptide, cholecystokinin (CCK), from enteroendocrine cells. Nutrients, including fatty acids and glucose/sweeteners, are sensed by mechanisms that may include several distinct G-protein coupled receptors (GPRCs) located on the apical and/or basolateral membrane of enteroendocrine cells (**1**), which triggers calcium-dependent secretion of CCK (**2**) and other signaling molecules. Glucose sensing is also mediated by a mechanism that requires sodium-glucose linked transporter 1 located on the apical membrane of enteroendocrine cells. CCK activates adjacent CCK_A receptors on VAN fibers (**3**). Levels of eCBs are elevated in the small-intestinal epithelium in rodent models of diet-induced obesity (see [25]), and their increased activity at local CB_1Rs blocks nutrient-induced secretion of CCK (**4**) by a mechanism that is unclear but may include inhibition of Ca^{2+}-mediated vesicular release of CCK (see [41]). Pharmacological inhibition of peripheral CB_1Rs in diet-induced obese mice blocked overeating and restored the ability for nutrients to induce CCK release. Studies also suggest that CB_1Rs on stomach cells (see [81]) may also indirectly interact with VANs by controlling the formation of ghrelin, which can activate ghrelin receptors on VANs (**5**). Together these studies highlight an indirect mechanism for CB1R-mediated control of gut-brain signaling. CB1Rs may also directly control activity of VANs (**6**). CB1Rs are expressed in VANs and their expression is affected by feeding status, pharmacological administration of CCK and ghrelin, and diet-induced obesity (see [82–87]). Moreover, recent studies suggest that CB1Rs control mechanosensitivity of VANs, which may be dysregulated in diet-induced obesity (see [86,88,89]). ER = endoplasmic reticulum.

3.1. Interactions with Satiation Signaling Pathways

Recent studies in mice suggest that CB_1Rs in cells lining the small-intestinal epithelium control food intake by blocking nutrient-induced secretion of the satiation peptide, cholecystokinin (CCK), which leads to increased caloric intake and meal size under conditions of heightened local eCB tone (e.g., diet-induced obesity) [25,41]. Upon arrival of nutrients in the small-intestinal lumen, CCK is released from subpopulations of enteroendocrine cells (i.e., I cells) [4,9,81,82] and controls meal size and satiation by directly activating CCK_A receptors on vagal afferent neurons [1,5–9] and possibly in the brain [90,91]. Immunoreactivity for CB_1Rs was found on CCK-containing cells in the upper small-intestinal epithelium in a CCK-reporter mouse that expresses eGFP selectively in these cells [C57BL/6-Tg(Cck-EGFP)2Mirn/J] [41]. CCK-eGFP cells were then isolated by fluorescence-activated cell sorting (FACS) and expression of messenger RNA (mRNA) for components of the eCB system, including CB_1Rs (Cnr1), was analyzed. CCK-eGFP-positive cells were enriched with mRNA for CB_1Rs when compared to CCK-eGFP-negative cells, which confirms earlier reports of expression of mRNA for CB_1Rs in I cells in another CCK-reporter mouse line [92]. We next asked if pharmacological activation of CB_1Rs with the general cannabinoid receptor agonist, WIN 55,212-2, impacts nutrient-induced release of the bioactive form of CCK, CCK-8. Circulating levels of CCK-8 were increased within 30-min following oral gavage of corn oil, an effect that was completely reversed by pretreatment with WIN 55,212-2. The inhibitory effects of WIN 55,212-2 on corn oil-induced elevations in CCK-8 in blood were blocked by the peripherally-restricted neutral CB_1R antagonist, AM6545, which highlights a role for peripheral CB_1Rs in this response.

The study described above was performed in lean mice fed a low-fat and low-sugar diet, which express low levels of eCBs in the small-intestinal epithelium. Diet-induced obesity is associated with high levels of eCBs in the small-intestinal epithelium, [25,36,40,78], and pharmacological inhibition of this heightened eCB activity at peripheral CB_1Rs blocked overeating resulting from increased meal size and daily caloric intake [25]. These experiments suggest that elevated eCB tone in the small-intestinal epithelium drives the overconsumption of high-energy foods and promotes obesity; however, the mechanism(s) in this response were unclear. Therefore, we tested the hypothesis that heightened eCB signaling at CB_1Rs in the small-intestinal epithelium in our mouse model of western diet-induced obesity drives overeating by blocking nutrient-induced release of CCK-8. Mice were maintained for 60 days on western diet (Research Diets D12079B), which is a time when levels of eCBs are elevated in the intestinal epithelium. Oral gavage of corn oil increased levels of CCK-8 in blood in lean mice with low levels of eCBs in the intestinal epithelium. In contrast to lean mice, corn oil failed to increase levels of CCK-8 in blood in mice fed a western diet for 60 days; however, pretreatment with the peripherally-restricted CB_1R antagonist, AM6545, restored the ability for nutrients to increase levels of CCK-8 in blood. These results suggest that under conditions of heightened eCB activity at CB_1Rs in the small-intestinal epithelium (i.e., diet-induced obesity), CCK-8 release is inhibited, which leads to delayed satiation and overeating. Indeed, inhibition of peripheral CB_1Rs with AM6545 in obese mice attenuated overeating associated with increased meal size and total caloric intake. Moreover, the hypophagic effects of AM6545 were reversed by pretreatment with a low-dose of the CCK_A receptor antagonist, devazepide, which suggests that acute hypophagic effects AM6545 occurs by a mechanism that includes restoring nutrient-induced satiation signaling. Collectively, these studies indicate a key inhibitory role for CB_1Rs in the small-intestinal epithelium in nutrient-induced secretion of satiation peptides. Thus, CB_1Rs in the intestinal epithelium are thought to indirectly control gut-brain neurotransmission via regulating the release of gut-derived peptides that directly interact with the vagal afferent neurons (see Figure 2). Furthermore, these processes become dysregulated in diet-induced obesity, which leads to overeating and possibly obesity. Future studies will be important to elucidate (*i*) specific intracellular signaling pathways (e.g., inhibition of calcium channels) in enteroendocrine cells that link eCB signaling at local CB_1Rs with blockade of secretion of satiation peptides, (*ii*) the impact of eCB activity at CB_1Rs in the intestinal epithelium on activity of gastric vagal afferent neurons, and (*iii*) the impact that this signaling has on recruitment of brain circuits associated with food reward [11,93].

3.2. Interactions with Hunger Signaling Pathways

Recent studies suggest that CB_1Rs in stomach cells influence alcohol intake and preference in mice by controlling local formation of the bioactive appetite-stimulating hormone, ghrelin [81], which directly interacts with growth hormone secretagogue receptor (GHS-R1a) on vagal afferent neurons and the brain (see Figure 2) [82,94,95]. Godlewski and colleagues reported that administration of the peripherally-restricted CB_1R inverse agonist, JD5037, reduced the intake of ethanol in wild-type mice; however, it was ineffective in whole-body CB_1R- and GHS-R1a-null mice. Ethanol-consuming mice also had elevated levels of the eCB, anandamide, in stomach cells, and inhibiting peripheral CB_1Rs with JD5037 blocked formation of the bioactive form of ghrelin, octanoyl-ghrelin. These results suggest that CB_1Rs in stomach cells promote ethanol intake by a mechanism that includes controlling production of ghrelin. Next, a mouse gastric ghrelinoma cell line (MGN3-1)—which contains CB_1Rs and enzymatic machinery for eCB metabolism—was used to identify mechanisms of CB_1R-mediated ghrelin production. Inhibition of CB_1Rs in MGN3-1 cells with JD5037 blocked formation of octanoyl-ghrelin by a mechanism that includes increased oxidative degradation of the ghrelin substrate, octanoyl-carnitine. Moreover, given expression of ghrelin receptors in the brain as well as vagal afferent neurons [82,94,95], the authors aimed to identify if the actions of JD5037 to reduce ethanol intake via changes in ghrelin signaling required gastric vagal afferent neurons. Both JD5037 and the CB_1R inverse agonist, rimonabant, were ineffective at reducing ethanol intake in mice subjected to chemical ablation of sensory afferents by neonatal exposure to capsaicin. Interestingly, mice denervated by capsaicin displayed moderate increases in preference and intake of ethanol. Additionally, mice treated with JD5037 displayed no changes in ad-libitum intake of standard rodent chow under these specific conditions. Together, these studies provide evidence that CB_1Rs in mouse stomach cells control intake and preference for ethanol by a mechanism that includes regulating production of ghrelin and indirect control of gut-brain vagal signaling. Future studies will be important to clarify if activating CB_1Rs stimulates production of ghrelin by increasing conversion of octanoyl-carnitine to octanoyl-ghrelin, and if roles for these pathways extend beyond intake and preference for ethanol to other reinforcers, such as palatable food. In addition, the precise impact that CB_1R-mediated control of ghrelin production has on vagal neurotransmission and associated firing rates remains to be determined.

Notably, ghrelin and CCK inversely affect vagal afferent neural activity, with ghrelin decreasing [94] and CCK increasing activity [6]. Accordingly, it is possible that eCB signaling at CB_1Rs (*i*) on stomach cells that produce ghrelin [81] and (*ii*) on CCK-containing cells in the upper small-intestinal epithelium that inhibit CCK release [41] results in similar reductions in vagal afferent neural activity and increases in food intake. Moreover, these pathways may coordinate vagal afferent neural activity associated with feeding status and become imbalanced in diet-induced obesity. A direct test of these hypotheses, however, remains for future investigations.

4. Endocannabinoids and Gut-Brain Neurotransmission: Direct Mechanisms

In addition to indirect mechanisms, eCBs may also activate CB_1Rs located on the afferent vagus nerve and directly impact gut-brain neurotransmission and food intake (see Figure 2). Indeed, a series of studies by Burdyga and colleagues suggest that expression of CB_1Rs on rat gastric vagal afferent neurons is impacted by feeding status and gut-derived hormones. Immunoreactivity and mRNA for CB_1Rs were identified in the rat and human nodose ganglia [83], and fasting for up to 48 h in rats was associated with time-dependent increases in their expression [83,84]. Refeeding after a 48 h fast led to reductions in expression of mRNA for CB_1Rs in nodose ganglia by 2-hrs after reintroduction of food, an effect mimicked by administration of bioactive CCK-8 in fasted rats. In addition, administration of a CCK$_A$ receptor antagonist blocked refeeding-induced reductions in expression of mRNA for CB$_1$Rs in fasted rats, which suggests a key role for CCK in these processes. Similarly, administration of ghrelin (*i*) blocked refeeding-induced reductions in expression of mRNA for CB$_1$Rs in nodose ganglia and (*ii*) blocked the actions of CCK-8 administration on expression of mRNA for CB$_1$Rs in fasted rats [82,84]. These results highlight the opposing actions that gut-derived satiation (i.e., CCK) and hunger (i.e., ghrelin) signals have on expression of CB$_1$Rs in rodent vagal afferent neurons.

Several studies suggest that expression of CB$_1$Rs in the nodose ganglia is dysregulated in rodent models of diet-induced obesity. Immunoreactivity for CB$_1$Rs was elevated in the nodose ganglia in Zucker or Sprague Dawley rats that were maintained on high-fats diet for 8 weeks when compared to lean controls [85]. Similarly, mRNA for CB$_1$Rs was elevated in nodose ganglia in mice fed a high-fat diet for 12 weeks [86]. In addition, refeeding after a fast [85] or administration of CCK-8 in Wistar rats maintained on a high-fat diet both failed to reduce levels of immunoreactivity for CB$_1$Rs in nodose ganglia [87]. Moreover, levels of mRNA for CB$_1$Rs were elevated in the nucleus of the solitary tract in rats maintained on a high-fat and sugar diet [96]. Collectively, these studies suggest that CB$_1$R expression in rodent vagal afferent neurons is controlled by feeding status, and their meal-related expression is dysregulated by chronic exposure to high-fat diets.

Roles in food intake for CB$_1$Rs expressed in vagal afferent neurons are unclear; however, Elmquist and colleagues reported that genetic deletion of CB$_1$Rs in the afferent and efferent vagus nerve had no impact on food intake, body weight, or energy expenditure in mice maintained on standard rodent chow or a high-fat diet [97]. These results suggest that CB$_1$Rs on vagal afferent neurons may be sufficient to promote food intake but are not required in these processes. With regards to food intake, these findings are also in line with the transient nature of feeding suppression in rodents administered CB$_1$R antagonists, which suggests that CB$_1$Rs may not be required for the long-term maintenance of food intake [21]. Nonetheless, a series of important studies investigated the impact of activating CB$_1$Rs on the neurochemical phenotype of associated neurons and the function of gastric vagal afferent neurons in mice [84]. Similar to CB$_1$Rs, fasting was associated with time-dependent increases in expression of melanin-concentrating hormone 1 receptor (MCH1R) in the nodose ganglia of rats, albeit at later time-points when compared to CB$_1$Rs. In contrast, fasting was associated with time-dependent reductions in expression of neuropeptide Y receptor type 2 (Y2Rs). Administration of CCK-8 reversed the effects of fasting by decreasing expression of CB$_1$Rs and MCH1Rs, and increasing expression of Y2Rs. Notably, administration of the eCB, anandamide, dose-dependently reversed the effects of CCK-8 on expression of CB$_1$Rs, MCH1Rs, and Y2Rs. Moreover, administration of a CB$_1$R inverse agonist reduced expression of CB$_1$Rs and increased expression of Y2Rs with no effect on expression of MCH1Rs in fasted rats. Together, these studies reveal distinct changes in the neurochemical composition of vagal afferents neurons in response to CB$_1$R activation and inactivation, and suggest that CB$_1$Rs may directly modulate activity of vagal afferent neurons in response to food-related signals released from the gut.

Elegant studies conducted by Christie and colleagues suggest that CB$_1$Rs control mechanosensitivity of gastric vagal afferent neurons, which may be dysregulated in diet-induced obesity [86,88,89]. For these studies, a mouse in vitro electrophysiological preparation was utilized that consists of isolated stomach and esophagus with attached vagal fibers and measurement of vagal afferent neural function and mechanosensitivity (see for detailed protocol [98]). Application of methanandamide—a stable analog of anandamide—led to a biphasic effect on activity of vagal fibers in response to stretch, with low doses reducing responses to stretch and high doses increasing responses [88]. These effects were found only in tension sensitive fibers, but not those innervating gastric mucosa. In contrast to mice maintained on standard rodent chow, mice maintained for 12 weeks on a high-fat diet were only responsive to the inhibitory effects of methanandamide on gastric vagal afferent neural activity [86]. To identify receptor signaling pathways mediating these effects, methanandamide was co-incubated with a CB$_1$R inverse agonist, a transient receptor potential vanilloid-1 channel (TRPV1) antagonist, a growth hormone secretagogue receptor (ghrelin receptor, GHSR) antagonist, or several inhibitors of distinct second messenger pathways (i.e., protein kinase A, protein kinase C, G-protein subunits $G\alpha_{io}$ or $G\alpha_q$). The biphasic effects of methanandamide on mechanosensitivity were both inhibited by CB_1R and TRPV1 blockade in mice maintained on standard rodent chow. Furthermore, the excitatory effects of methanandamide may occur via a CB_1R-mediated PKC-TRPV1 second messenger pathway, whereas the inhibitory effects may occur via CB_1R-mediated release of ghrelin from the stomach and its actions on GHSRs on vagal afferent neurons. Together, these studies suggest that endocannabinoids differentially control afferent vagal activity depending upon dose by mechanisms that include distinct interactions between CB_1Rs, TRPV1, and GHSR signaling pathways, which may become dysregulated in diet-induced obesity. Future studies will be important to identify physiological roles in food intake and obesity for CB_1R signaling in distinct populations of gastric vagal afferent neurons (e.g., tension-responsive fibers versus those innervating the gastric mucosa). Moreover, it will be important to delineate how CB_1Rs on sensory vagal terminals in the gut, nodose ganglia, and at terminals in the NTS may participate in distinct or common aspects of vagal afferent neurotransmission.

5. Endocannabinoids and Efferent Autonomic Neurotransmission

Fasting is associated with elevated levels of eCBs in the upper small-intestinal epithelium of rodents, and recent studies suggest that the efferent vagus nerve is required for these processes [22,24,25,40]. The efferent arm of the vagus nerve communicates parasympathetic neurotransmission from the brain to peripheral organs—including the gut—via cholinergic signaling pathways, and participates in a variety of motor functions and possibly food intake. For example, c-Fos expression in the myenteric and submucosal plexus in the rat proximal small intestine was induced by vagal nerve stimulation [99,100], and pharmacological blockade of peripheral muscarinic acetylcholine receptors (mAChRs) with atropine methyl nitrate inhibited both refeeding after a fast [101] and sham feeding of liquid diets in rats [102]. The specific receptor pathways involved in these processes are not fully elucidated. Recent investigations, however, suggest that cholinergic neurotransmission carried by the efferent vagus nerve controls biosynthesis of the eCB, 2-AG, in the proximal small-intestinal epithelium during a fast and participates in refeeding after a fast [24] (see Figure 3). For these studies, rats were fasted for up to 24 h, then levels of 2-AG and its precursor, 1, stearoyl, 2-arachidonoyl-*sn*-glycerol (SAG), were quantified in a variety of peripheral organs by liquid chromatography/tandem mass spectrometry. Levels of 2-AG and SAG were elevated in the upper small-intestinal epithelium by 24 h after fasting; however, no changes were found in stomach, ileum, colon, liver, pancreas, or spleen. This effect was specific for 2-AG, because levels of other common monoacylglycerols in the upper small-intestinal epithelium were unaffected (i.e., 16:0 MAG, 18:0 MAG, 18:1 MAG, 18:2 MAG). Moreover, levels of 2-AG were rapidly normalized by refeeding to levels similar to those in free-feeding animals, an effect mimicked by intra-duodenal infusions of equicaloric quantities of lipid, sucrose, or protein. These results highlight that production of intestinal 2-AG in fasting rats can be rapidly reduced upon refeeding in a manner that is not dependent on macronutrient content.

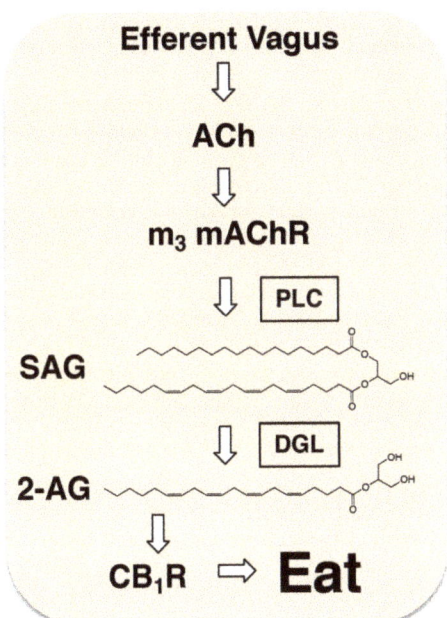

Figure 3. Efferent neurotransmission controls production of 2-AG in the gut. Studies suggest that during a fast, the efferent vagus nerve releases acetylcholine (ACh) into the lining of the small intestine, which in turn, activates local m3-subtype muscarinic acetylcholine receptors (m_3 mAChRs) that trigger production of 2-AG (see [24]). This is thought to happen by a mechanism that includes activation of phospholipase C (PLC) and generation of the diacylglycerol 2-AG precursor, 1, stearoyl,2-arachidonoyl-*sn*-glycerol (SAG). SAG is subsequently hydrolyzed by diacylglycerol lipase (DGL) to ultimately form 2-AG, which activates local CB_1Rs and promotes refeeding after a fast in rodents.

We next aimed to identify if efferent cholinergic activity is required for production of 2-AG in the intestinal epithelium [24]. Rats were given full diaphragmatic vagotomy and fasted for 24 h. When compared to control rats receiving a sham surgery, levels of 2-AG failed to increase in the small-intestinal epithelium after a 24 h fast, which suggests that the efferent vagus may be required for production of 2-AG. We next aimed to identify specific cholinergic receptors involved in vagal-mediated 2-AG production during a fast. The principal neurotransmitter released from the efferent vagus nerve is acetylcholine, which activates a variety of cholinergic receptor subtypes in the periphery, including mAChRs in the intestine [103]. Activation of mAChRs in the brain, including subtype-3 (m3) mAChRs, enhances eCB production that, in turn, participates in the control of synaptic plasticity via CB_1Rs [104–108]. In addition, 2-AG in the brain is formed by a mechanism that includes phospholipase-C-dependent production of SAG, then conversion of SAG to 2-AG by diacylglycerol lipase [109–111]. Notably, m3 mAChRs are G_q-protein coupled receptors that share overlapping downstream pathways as those responsible for biosynthesis of 2-AG, including activation of phospholipase-C and diacylglycerol lipase. Thus, we examined if mAChRs are required for fasting-induced production of 2-AG in the small-intestinal lining. Similar to brain, m3 mAChRs were expressed in the small-intestinal epithelium, and diacylglycerol lipase activity was required for biosynthesis of 2-AG. Systemic administration of a general mAChR antagonist (atropine) or intra-duodenal administration of a selective m3 mAChR antagonist both blocked fasting-induced rises in 2-AG in the small intestine. Moreover, pharmacological inhibition of peripheral CB_1Rs and m3 mAChRs in the intestine equally reduced refeeding after a 24 h fast, with no additive effects when both inhibitors were co-administered. Collectively, these studies suggest that the efferent vagus nerve is recruited during a fast and participates in refeeding after a fast by activating m3 mAChRs in the intestine which, in turn, drives production of 2-AG and activation of local CB_1Rs.

In addition to interactions between efferent parasympathetic neurotransmission and the eCB system, studies also suggest that efferent sympathetic neurotransmission is controlled by CB_1Rs, which may impact food intake through a mechanism that requires the afferent vagus nerve [112]. Feeding suppression associated with a CB_1R inverse agonist was abolished in mice that received (i) a peripheral β-adrenergic inhibitor, (ii) chemical ablation (capsaicin) of afferent sensory fibers, including afferent vagal fibers, and (iii) microinjections of the NMDA glutamatergic receptor antagonist, MK-801, into the nucleus of the solitary tract. Moreover, metabolic benefits of Roux-en-Y gastric bypass in mice were dependent on a mechanism that included interactions between CB_1Rs and sympathetic neurotransmission [113]. Studies will be important to identify possible roles for CB_1Rs in interactions between sympathetic and parasympathetic branches of the autonomic nervous system and their participation in control of food intake and energy metabolism.

6. Targeting the Peripheral ECB System for Treatment of Human Obesity

The pre-clinical studies in rodents discussed above suggest that the eCB system is an integral component of the gut-brain axis that controls food intake and becomes dysregulated in obesity. These investigations provide evidence of specific molecular and cellular mechanisms that underlie eCB-mediated gut-brain signaling, which may inform development of therapeutic strategies for the treatment of human obesity and related metabolic disorders. Indeed, human studies indicate that eCB levels are elevated in blood during consumption of palatable foods and in obesity [66–71,73–77,80,114]. CB_1R antagonists were under development during the 2000s for the treatment of human obesity. In particular, rimonabant—a systemically acting CB_1R antagonist/inverse agonist—showed clinical promise for its anti-obesity effects that included reductions in body weight, waist circumference, and levels of circulating triglycerides, and increases in levels of high-density lipoprotein) [115]. Unfortunately, rimonabant was associated with psychiatric side effects such as increased depression and anxiety, which precluded its approval by the Food and Drug Administration for the treatment of obesity in the Unites States [38]. These effects were likely a result of its ability to access the brain and disrupt cognitive functions. On the other hand, CB_1R antagonists that are designed to have low brain penetrance display similar anti-obesity effects as their brain-penetrant counterparts and may be a useful therapeutic strategy for safe and effective treatment of obesity and related metabolic disorders [21,23,24,27–30,37].

7. Future Considerations

Collectively, these investigations provide evidence that the eCB system in the gastrointestinal tract is a key component of the gut–brain axis that controls food intake and becomes dysregulated in diet-induced obesity. Exciting new studies suggest important interactions between the eCB system and the gut microbiome [35,78,116–121]; however, future investigations will be important to identify molecular and cellular mechanisms in these interactions, and the impact on gut-brain signaling important for food intake and energy metabolism in health and metabolic disease. In addition, studies will be important to elucidate specific intracellular mechanisms that the eCB system recruits to control release of satiation peptides and other signaling molecules from the intestinal epithelium, including those involved in transduction of food-related signals to activation of vagal afferent neurons by "neuropods" [9,10]. It is clear that eCBs have indirect and direct actions on vagal afferent neural signaling; however, it is unclear how gut-brain eCB signaling interacts with brain reward circuits in control of food intake and reward. Moreover, it will be important to identify how gut-brain eCB signaling participates in discrete aspects of food intake and reward, including satiation and satiety versus appetition (i.e., post-oral positive feedback from nutrients that stimulates ingestion and flavor conditioning) [122].

Author Contributions: Conceptualization, methodology, formal analysis, investigation, resources, data curation, writing—original draft preparation, writing—review and editing, project administration, funding acquisition, N.V.D. All authors have read and agreed to the published version of the manuscript.

Funding: This research was funded by the National Institutes of Health, National Institute of Diabetes and Digestive and Kidney Diseases grants DK119498 and DK114978, and the Tobacco-Related Disease Research Program (TRDRP) from the University of California Office of the President grant T29KT0232 to N.V.D.

Conflicts of Interest: The authors declare no conflict of interest.

References

1. Schwartz, G.J. Roles for gut vagal sensory signals in determining energy availability and energy expenditure. *Brain Res.* **2018**, *1693*, 151–153. [CrossRef]
2. Shechter, A.; Schwartz, G.J. Gut-brain nutrient sensing in food reward. *Appetite* **2018**, *122*, 32–35. [CrossRef] [PubMed]
3. Clemmensen, C.; Muller, T.D.; Woods, S.C.; Berthoud, H.R.; Seeley, R.J.; Tschop, M.H. Gut-Brain Cross-Talk in Metabolic Control. *Cell* **2017**, *168*, 758–774. [CrossRef] [PubMed]
4. Steinert, R.E.; Feinle-Bisset, C.; Asarian, L.; Horowitz, M.; Beglinger, C.; Geary, N. Ghrelin, CCK, GLP-1, and PYY(3-36): Secretory Controls and Physiological Roles in Eating and Glycemia in Health, Obesity, and After RYGB. *Physiol. Rev.* **2017**, *97*, 411–463. [CrossRef] [PubMed]
5. Smith, G.P.; Jerome, C.; Cushin, B.J.; Eterno, R.; Simansky, K.J. Abdominal vagotomy blocks the satiety effect of cholecystokinin in the rat. *Science* **1981**, *213*, 1036–1037. [CrossRef]
6. Schwartz, G.J.; Moran, T.H. CCK elicits and modulates vagal afferent activity arising from gastric and duodenal sites. *Ann. N. Y. Acad. Sci.* **1994**, *713*, 121–128. [CrossRef]
7. Raybould, H.E. Mechanisms of CCK signaling from gut to brain. *Curr. Opin. Pharmcol.* **2007**, *7*, 570–574. [CrossRef]
8. Smith, G.P.; Jerome, C.; Norgren, R. Afferent axons in abdominal vagus mediate satiety effect of cholecystokinin in rats. *Am. J. Physiol.* **1985**, *249*, R638–R641. [CrossRef]
9. Kaelberer, M.M.; Buchanan, K.L.; Klein, M.E.; Barth, B.B.; Montoya, M.M.; Shen, X.; Bohorquez, D.V. A gut-brain neural circuit for nutrient sensory transduction. *Science* **2018**, *361*. [CrossRef] [PubMed]
10. Kaelberer, M.M.; Rupprecht, L.E.; Liu, W.W.; Weng, P.; Bohorquez, D.V. Neuropod Cells: The Emerging Biology of Gut-Brain Sensory Transduction. *Ann. Rev. Neurosci.* **2020**, *43*, 337–353. [CrossRef]
11. Han, W.; Tellez, L.A.; Perkins, M.H.; Perez, I.O.; Qu, T.; Ferreira, J.; Ferreira, T.L.; Quinn, D.; Liu, Z.W.; Gao, X.B.; et al. A Neural Circuit for Gut-Induced Reward. *Cell* **2018**, *175*, 665–678.e23. [CrossRef]
12. Han, W.; Tellez, L.A.; Niu, J.; Medina, S.; Ferreira, T.L.; Zhang, X.; Su, J.; Tong, J.; Schwartz, G.J.; van den Pol, A.; et al. Striatal Dopamine Links Gastrointestinal Rerouting to Altered Sweet Appetite. *Cell Metab.* **2016**, *23*, 103–112. [CrossRef] [PubMed]
13. Sclafani, A.; Ackroff, K. Role of gut nutrient sensing in stimulating appetite and conditioning food preferences. *Am. J. Physiol. Regul. Integr. Comp. Physiol.* **2012**, *302*, R1119–R1133. [CrossRef] [PubMed]
14. Sclafani, A. From appetite setpoint to appetition: 50years of ingestive behavior research. *Physiol. Behav.* **2018**, *192*, 210–217. [CrossRef]
15. Wenzel, J.M.; Cheer, J.F. Endocannabinoid Regulation of Reward and Reinforcement through Interaction with Dopamine and Endogenous Opioid Signaling. *Neuropsychopharmacology* **2018**, *43*, 103–115. [CrossRef] [PubMed]
16. DiPatrizio, N.V.; Piomelli, D. The thrifty lipids: Endocannabinoids and the neural control of energy conservation. *Trends Neurosci.* **2012**, *35*, 403–411. [CrossRef]
17. Simon, V.; Cota, D. MECHANISMS IN ENDOCRINOLOGY: Endocannabinoids and metabolism: Past, present and future. *Eur. J. Endocrinol.* **2017**, *176*, R309–R324. [CrossRef] [PubMed]
18. Quarta, C.; Mazza, R.; Obici, S.; Pasquali, R.; Pagotto, U. Energy balance regulation by endocannabinoids at central and peripheral levels. *Trends Mol. Med.* **2011**, *17*, 518–526. [CrossRef]
19. Di Marzo, V.; Goparaju, S.K.; Wang, L.; Liu, J.; Batkai, S.; Jarai, Z.; Fezza, F.; Miura, G.I.; Palmiter, R.D.; Sugiura, T.; et al. Leptin-regulated endocannabinoids are involved in maintaining food intake. *Nature* **2001**, *410*, 822–825. [CrossRef] [PubMed]
20. Jarbe, T.U.; DiPatrizio, N.V. Delta9-THC induced hyperphagia and tolerance assessment: Interactions between the CB1 receptor agonist delta9-THC and the CB1 receptor antagonist SR-141716 (rimonabant) in rats. *Behav. Pharmcol.* **2005**, *16*, 373–380. [CrossRef]
21. Ravinet Trillou, C.; Arnone, M.; Delgorge, C.; Gonalons, N.; Keane, P.; Maffrand, J.P.; Soubrie, P. Anti-obesity effect of SR141716, a CB1 receptor antagonist, in diet-induced obese mice. *Am. J. Physiol. Regul. Integr. Comp. Physiol.* **2003**, *284*, R345–R353. [CrossRef] [PubMed]
22. Gomez, R.; Navarro, M.; Ferrer, B.; Trigo, J.M.; Bilbao, A.; Del Arco, I.; Cippitelli, A.; Nava, F.; Piomelli, D.; Rodriguez de Fonseca, F. A peripheral mechanism for CB1 cannabinoid receptor-dependent modulation of feeding. *J. Neurosci.* **2002**, *22*, 9612–9617. [CrossRef] [PubMed]
23. DiPatrizio, N.V.; Astarita, G.; Schwartz, G.; Li, X.; Piomelli, D. Endocannabinoid signal in the gut controls dietary fat intake. *Proc. Natl. Acad. Sci. USA* **2011**, *108*, 12904–12908. [CrossRef]

24. DiPatrizio, N.V.; Igarashi, M.; Narayanaswami, V.; Murray, C.; Gancayco, J.; Russell, A.; Jung, K.M.; Piomelli, D. Fasting stimulates 2-AG biosynthesis in the small intestine: Role of cholinergic pathways. *Am. J. Physiol. Regul. Integr. Comp. Physiol.* **2015**, *309*, R805–R813. [CrossRef] [PubMed]
25. Argueta, D.A.; DiPatrizio, N.V. Peripheral endocannabinoid signaling controls hyperphagia in western diet-induced obesity. *Physiol. Behav.* **2017**, *171*, 32–39. [CrossRef] [PubMed]
26. Cota, D.; Marsicano, G.; Tschop, M.; Grubler, Y.; Flachskamm, C.; Schubert, M.; Auer, D.; Yassouridis, A.; Thone-Reineke, C.; Ortmann, S.; et al. The endogenous cannabinoid system affects energy balance via central orexigenic drive and peripheral lipogenesis. *J. Clin. Investig.* **2003**, *112*, 423–431. [CrossRef]
27. LoVerme, J.; Duranti, A.; Tontini, A.; Spadoni, G.; Mor, M.; Rivara, S.; Stella, N.; Xu, C.; Tarzia, G.; Piomelli, D. Synthesis and characterization of a peripherally restricted CB1 cannabinoid antagonist, URB447, that reduces feeding and body-weight gain in mice. *Bioorg. Med. Chem. Lett.* **2009**, *19*, 639–643. [CrossRef]
28. Randall, P.A.; Vemuri, V.K.; Segovia, K.N.; Torres, E.F.; Hosmer, S.; Nunes, E.J.; Santerre, J.L.; Makriyannis, A.; Salamone, J.D. The novel cannabinoid CB1 antagonist AM6545 suppresses food intake and food-reinforced behavior. *Pharmcol. Biochem. Behav.* **2010**, *97*, 179–184. [CrossRef]
29. Cluny, N.L.; Vemuri, V.K.; Chambers, A.P.; Limebeer, C.L.; Bedard, H.; Wood, J.T.; Lutz, B.; Zimmer, A.; Parker, L.A.; Makriyannis, A.; et al. A novel peripherally restricted cannabinoid receptor antagonist, AM6545, reduces food intake and body weight, but does not cause malaise, in rodents. *Br. J. Pharmcol.* **2011**, *161*, 629–642. [CrossRef]
30. Tam, J.; Vemuri, V.K.; Liu, J.; Batkai, S.; Mukhopadhyay, B.; Godlewski, G.; Osei-Hyiaman, D.; Ohnuma, S.; Ambudkar, S.V.; Pickel, J.; et al. Peripheral CB1 cannabinoid receptor blockade improves cardiometabolic risk in mouse models of obesity. *J. Clin. Investig.* **2010**, *120*, 2953–2966. [CrossRef]
31. Tam, J.; Cinar, R.; Liu, J.; Godlewski, G.; Wesley, D.; Jourdan, T.; Szanda, G.; Mukhopadhyay, B.; Chedester, L.; Liow, J.S.; et al. Peripheral cannabinoid-1 receptor inverse agonism reduces obesity by reversing leptin resistance. *Cell Metab.* **2012**, *16*, 167–179. [CrossRef]
32. Maccarrone, M.; Bab, I.; Biro, T.; Cabral, G.A.; Dey, S.K.; Di Marzo, V.; Konje, J.C.; Kunos, G.; Mechoulam, R.; Pacher, P.; et al. Endocannabinoid signaling at the periphery: 50 years after THC. *Trends Pharmcol. Sci.* **2015**, *36*, 277–296. [CrossRef]
33. Izzo, A.A.; Sharkey, K.A. Cannabinoids and the gut: New developments and emerging concepts. *Pharmacol. Ther.* **2010**, *126*, 21–38. [CrossRef] [PubMed]
34. Cluny, N.L.; Reimer, R.A.; Sharkey, K.A. Cannabinoid signalling regulates inflammation and energy balance: The importance of the brain-gut axis. *Brain Behav. Immun.* **2012**, *26*, 691–698. [CrossRef]
35. Cani, P.D.; Plovier, H.; Hul, M.V.; Geurts, L.; Delzenne, N.M.; Druart, C.; Everard, A. Endocannabinoids—At the crossroads between the gut microbiota and host metabolism. *Nat. Rev. Endocrinol.* **2016**, *12*, 133–143. [CrossRef] [PubMed]
36. Artmann, A.; Petersen, G.; Hellgren, L.I.; Boberg, J.; Skonberg, C.; Nellemann, C.; Hansen, S.H.; Hansen, H.S. Influence of dietary fatty acids on endocannabinoid and N-acylethanolamine levels in rat brain, liver and small intestine. *Biochim. Biophys. Acta* **2008**, *1781*, 200–212. [CrossRef] [PubMed]
37. Tam, J.; Szanda, G.; Drori, A.; Liu, Z.; Cinar, R.; Kashiwaya, Y.; Reitman, M.L.; Kunos, G. Peripheral cannabinoid-1 receptor blockade restores hypothalamic leptin signaling. *Mol. Metab.* **2017**, *6*, 1113–1125. [CrossRef]
38. Christensen, R.; Kristensen, P.K.; Bartels, E.M.; Bliddal, H.; Astrup, A. Efficacy and safety of the weight-loss drug rimonabant: A meta-analysis of randomised trials. *Lancet* **2007**, *370*, 1706–1713. [CrossRef]
39. DiPatrizio, N.V.; Joslin, A.; Jung, K.M.; Piomelli, D. Endocannabinoid signaling in the gut mediates preference for dietary unsaturated fats. *FASEB J.* **2013**, *27*, 2513–2520. [CrossRef] [PubMed]
40. DiPatrizio, N.V.; Piomelli, D. Intestinal lipid-derived signals that sense dietary fat. *J. Clin. Investig.* **2015**, *125*, 891–898. [CrossRef]
41. Argueta, D.A.; Perez, P.A.; Makriyannis, A.; DiPatrizio, N.V. Cannabinoid CB1 Receptors Inhibit Gut-Brain Satiation Signaling in Diet-Induced Obesity. *Front. Physiol.* **2019**, *10*, 704. [CrossRef] [PubMed]
42. Piomelli, D. The molecular logic of endocannabinoid signalling. *Nat. Rev.* **2003**, *4*, 873–884. [CrossRef] [PubMed]
43. Pertwee, R.G. Endocannabinoids and Their Pharmacological Actions. *Handb. Exp. Pharmcol.* **2015**, *231*, 1–37. [CrossRef]
44. Higuchi, S.; Irie, K.; Yamaguchi, R.; Katsuki, M.; Araki, M.; Ohji, M.; Hayakawa, K.; Mishima, S.; Akitake, Y.; Matsuyama, K.; et al. Hypothalamic 2-arachidonoylglycerol regulates multistage process of high-fat diet preferences. *PLoS ONE* **2012**, *7*, e38609. [CrossRef]
45. Higuchi, S.; Ohji, M.; Araki, M.; Furuta, R.; Katsuki, M.; Yamaguchi, R.; Akitake, Y.; Matsuyama, K.; Irie, K.; Mishima, K.; et al. Increment of hypothalamic 2-arachidonoylglycerol induces the preference for a high-fat diet via activation of cannabinoid 1 receptors. *Behav. Brain Res.* **2011**, *216*, 477–480. [CrossRef] [PubMed]
46. Deshmukh, R.R.; Sharma, P.L. Stimulation of accumbens shell cannabinoid CB(1) receptors by noladin ether, a putative endocannabinoid, modulates food intake and dietary selection in rats. *Pharmcol. Res.* **2012**, *66*, 276–282. [CrossRef] [PubMed]
47. DiPatrizio, N.V.; Simansky, K.J. Activating parabrachial cannabinoid CB1 receptors selectively stimulates feeding of palatable foods in rats. *J. Neurosci.* **2008**, *28*, 9702–9709. [CrossRef]
48. DiPatrizio, N.V.; Simansky, K.J. Inhibiting parabrachial fatty acid amide hydrolase activity selectively increases the intake of palatable food via cannabinoid CB1 receptors. *Am. J. Physiol. Regul. Integr. Comp. Physiol.* **2008**, *295*, R1409–R1414. [CrossRef]
49. Mahler, S.V.; Smith, K.S.; Berridge, K.C. Endocannabinoid hedonic hotspot for sensory pleasure: Anandamide in nucleus accumbens shell enhances 'liking' of a sweet reward. *Neuropsychopharmacology* **2007**, *32*, 2267–2278. [CrossRef]

50. Wei, D.; Lee, D.; Li, D.; Daglian, J.; Jung, K.M.; Piomelli, D. A role for the endocannabinoid 2-arachidonoyl-sn-glycerol for social and high-fat food reward in male mice. *Psychopharmacology* **2016**, *233*, 1911–1919. [CrossRef]
51. Mendez-Diaz, M.; Rueda-Orozco, P.E.; Ruiz-Contreras, A.E.; Prospero-Garcia, O. The endocannabinoid system modulates the valence of the emotion associated to food ingestion. *Addict. Biol.* **2012**, *17*, 725–735. [CrossRef]
52. De Luca, M.A.; Solinas, M.; Bimpisidis, Z.; Goldberg, S.R.; Di Chiara, G. Cannabinoid facilitation of behavioral and biochemical hedonic taste responses. *Neuropharmacology* **2012**, *63*, 161–168. [CrossRef]
53. Jarrett, M.M.; Scantlebury, J.; Parker, L.A. Effect of delta9-tetrahydrocannabinol on quinine palatability and AM251 on sucrose and quinine palatability using the taste reactivity test. *Physiol. Behav.* **2007**, *90*, 425–430. [CrossRef]
54. Melis, T.; Succu, S.; Sanna, F.; Boi, A.; Argiolas, A.; Melis, M.R. The cannabinoid antagonist SR 141716A (Rimonabant) reduces the increase of extra-cellular dopamine release in the rat nucleus accumbens induced by a novel high palatable food. *Neurosci. Lett.* **2007**, *419*, 231–235. [CrossRef] [PubMed]
55. Droste, S.M.; Saland, S.K.; Schlitter, E.K.; Rodefer, J.S. AM 251 differentially effects food-maintained responding depending on food palatability. *Pharmcol. Biochem. Behav.* **2010**, *95*, 443–448. [CrossRef] [PubMed]
56. South, T.; Deng, C.; Huang, X.F. AM 251 and beta-Funaltrexamine reduce fat intake in a fat-preferring strain of mouse. *Behav. Brain Res.* **2007**, *181*, 153–157. [CrossRef] [PubMed]
57. Thornton-Jones, Z.D.; Vickers, S.P.; Clifton, P.G. The cannabinoid CB1 receptor antagonist SR141716A reduces appetitive and consummatory responses for food. *Psychopharmacology* **2005**, *179*, 452–460. [CrossRef]
58. Feja, M.; Leigh, M.P.K.; Baindur, A.N.; McGraw, J.J.; Wakabayashi, K.T.; Cravatt, B.F.; Bass, C.E. The novel MAGL inhibitor MJN110 enhances responding to reward-predictive incentive cues by activation of CB1 receptors. *Neuropharmacology* **2020**, *162*, 107814. [CrossRef]
59. Salamone, J.D.; McLaughlin, P.J.; Sink, K.; Makriyannis, A.; Parker, L.A. Cannabinoid CB1 receptor inverse agonists and neutral antagonists: Effects on food intake, food-reinforced behavior and food aversions. *Physiol. Behav.* **2007**, *91*, 383–388. [CrossRef]
60. Williams, C.M.; Kirkham, T.C. Anandamide induces overeating: Mediation by central cannabinoid (CB1) receptors. *Psychopharmacology* **1999**, *143*, 315–317. [CrossRef]
61. DiPatrizio, N.V. Endocannabinoids in the Gut. *Cannabis Cannabinoid Res.* **2016**, *1*, 67–77. [CrossRef]
62. Greenberg, D.; Smith, G.P. The controls of fat intake. *Psychosom. Med.* **1996**, *58*, 559–569. [CrossRef]
63. Avalos, B.; Argueta, D.A.; Perez, P.A.; Wiley, M.; Wood, C.; DiPatrizio, N.V. Cannabinoid CB1 Receptors in the Intestinal Epithelium Are Required for Acute Western-Diet Preferences in Mice. *Nutrients* **2020**, *12*, 2874. [CrossRef]
64. Centers for Disease Control and Prevention (CDC); National Center for Health Statistics (NCHS). *National Health and Nutrition Examination Survey Data*; U.S. Department of Health and Human: Hyattsville, MD, USA. Available online: https://www.cdc.gov/nchs/nhanes/index.htm (accessed on 6 April 2021).
65. Levine, A.S.; Kotz, C.M.; Gosnell, B.A. Sugars and fats: The neurobiology of preference. *J. Nutr.* **2003**, *133*, 831S–834S. [CrossRef] [PubMed]
66. Monteleone, P.; Piscitelli, F.; Scognamiglio, P.; Monteleone, A.M.; Canestrelli, B.; Di Marzo, V.; Maj, M. Hedonic eating is associated with increased peripheral levels of ghrelin and the endocannabinoid 2-arachidonoyl-glycerol in healthy humans: A pilot study. *J. Clin. Endocrinol. Metab.* **2012**, *97*, E917–E924. [CrossRef] [PubMed]
67. Engeli, S.; Bohnke, J.; Feldpausch, M.; Gorzelniak, K.; Janke, J.; Batkai, S.; Pacher, P.; Harvey-White, J.; Luft, F.C.; Sharma, A.M.; et al. Activation of the peripheral endocannabinoid system in human obesity. *Diabetes* **2005**, *54*, 2838–2843. [CrossRef]
68. Bluher, M.; Engeli, S.; Kloting, N.; Berndt, J.; Fasshauer, M.; Batkai, S.; Pacher, P.; Schon, M.R.; Jordan, J.; Stumvoll, M. Dysregulation of the peripheral and adipose tissue endocannabinoid system in human abdominal obesity. *Diabetes* **2006**, *55*, 3053–3060. [CrossRef] [PubMed]
69. Cote, M.; Matias, I.; Lemieux, I.; Petrosino, S.; Almeras, N.; Despres, J.P.; Di Marzo, V. Circulating endocannabinoid levels, abdominal adiposity and related cardiometabolic risk factors in obese men. *Int. J. Obes.* **2007**, *31*, 692–699. [CrossRef]
70. Di Marzo, V.; Cote, M.; Matias, I.; Lemieux, I.; Arsenault, B.J.; Cartier, A.; Piscitelli, F.; Petrosino, S.; Almeras, N.; Despres, J.P. Changes in plasma endocannabinoid levels in viscerally obese men following a 1 year lifestyle modification programme and waist circumference reduction: Associations with changes in metabolic risk factors. *Diabetologia* **2009**, *52*, 213–217. [CrossRef]
71. Little, T.J.; Cvijanovic, N.; DiPatrizio, N.V.; Argueta, D.A.; Rayner, C.K.; Feinle-Bisset, C.; Young, R.L. Plasma endocannabinoid levels in lean, overweight, and obese humans: Relationships to intestinal permeability markers, inflammation, and incretin secretion. *Am. J. Physiol. Endocrinol. Metab.* **2018**, *315*, E489–E495. [CrossRef]
72. Hillard, C.J. Circulating Endocannabinoids: From Whence Do They Come and Where are They Going? *Neuropsychopharmacology* **2017**. [CrossRef]
73. Lotfi Yagin, N.; Aliasgharzadeh, S.; Alizadeh, M.; Aliasgari, F.; Mahdavi, R. The association of circulating endocannabinoids with appetite regulatory substances in obese women. *Obes. Res. Clin. Pract.* **2020**, *14*, 321–325. [CrossRef] [PubMed]
74. Yagin, N.L.; Hajjarzadeh, S.; Aliasgharzadeh, S.; Aliasgari, F.; Mahdavi, R. The association of dietary patterns with endocannabinoids levels in overweight and obese women. *Lipids Health Dis.* **2020**, *19*, 161. [CrossRef]
75. Tagliamonte, S.; Gill, C.I.R.; Pourshahidi, L.K.; Slevin, M.M.; Price, R.K.; Ferracane, R.; Lawther, R.; O'Connor, G.; Vitaglione, P. Endocannabinoids, endocannabinoid-like molecules and their precursors in human small intestinal lumen and plasma: Does diet affect them? *Eur. J. Nutr.* **2020**. [CrossRef] [PubMed]

76. Depommier, C.; Flamand, N.; Pelicaen, R.; Maiter, D.; Thissen, J.P.; Loumaye, A.; Hermans, M.P.; Everard, A.; Delzenne, N.M.; Di Marzo, V.; et al. Linking the Endocannabinoidome with Specific Metabolic Parameters in an Overweight and Insulin-Resistant Population: From Multivariate Exploratory Analysis to Univariate Analysis and Construction of Predictive Models. *Cells* **2021**, *10*, 71. [CrossRef]
77. Quercioli, A.; Pataky, Z.; Vincenti, G.; Makoundou, V.; Di Marzo, V.; Montecucco, F.; Carballo, S.; Thomas, A.; Staub, C.; Steffens, S.; et al. Elevated endocannabinoid plasma levels are associated with coronary circulatory dysfunction in obesity. *Eur. Heart J.* **2011**, *32*, 1369–1378. [CrossRef]
78. Lacroix, S.; Pechereau, F.; Leblanc, N.; Boubertakh, B.; Houde, A.; Martin, C.; Flamand, N.; Silvestri, C.; Raymond, F.; Di Marzo, V.; et al. Rapid and Concomitant Gut Microbiota and Endocannabinoidome Response to Diet-Induced Obesity in Mice. *mSystems* **2019**, *4*. [CrossRef]
79. Kuipers, E.N.; Kantae, V.; Maarse, B.C.E.; van den Berg, S.M.; van Eenige, R.; Nahon, K.J.; Reifel-Miller, A.; Coskun, T.; de Winther, M.P.J.; Lutgens, E.; et al. High Fat Diet Increases Circulating Endocannabinoids Accompanied by Increased Synthesis Enzymes in Adipose Tissue. *Front. Physiol.* **2018**, *9*, 1913. [CrossRef] [PubMed]
80. Gatta-Cherifi, B.; Matias, I.; Vallee, M.; Tabarin, A.; Marsicano, G.; Piazza, P.V.; Cota, D. Simultaneous postprandial deregulation of the orexigenic endocannabinoid anandamide and the anorexigenic peptide YY in obesity. *Int. J. Obes.* **2012**, *36*, 880–885. [CrossRef] [PubMed]
81. Godlewski, G.; Cinar, R.; Coffey, N.J.; Liu, J.; Jourdan, T.; Mukhopadhyay, B.; Chedester, L.; Liu, Z.; Osei-Hyiaman, D.; Iyer, M.R.; et al. Targeting Peripheral CB1 Receptors Reduces Ethanol Intake via a Gut-Brain Axis. *Cell Metab.* **2019**, *29*, 1320–1333.e8. [CrossRef] [PubMed]
82. Burdyga, G.; Varro, A.; Dimaline, R.; Thompson, D.G.; Dockray, G.J. Ghrelin receptors in rat and human nodose ganglia: Putative role in regulating CB-1 and MCH receptor abundance. *Am. J. Physiol. Gastrointest. Liver Physiol.* **2006**, *290*, G1289–G1297. [CrossRef]
83. Burdyga, G.; Lal, S.; Varro, A.; Dimaline, R.; Thompson, D.G.; Dockray, G.J. Expression of cannabinoid CB1 receptors by vagal afferent neurons is inhibited by cholecystokinin. *J. Neurosci.* **2004**, *24*, 2708–2715. [CrossRef]
84. Burdyga, G.; Varro, A.; Dimaline, R.; Thompson, D.G.; Dockray, G.J. Expression of cannabinoid CB1 receptors by vagal afferent neurons: Kinetics and role in influencing neurochemical phenotype. *Am. J. Physiol. Gastrointest. Liver Physiol.* **2010**, *299*, G63–G69. [CrossRef]
85. de Lartigue, G.; Barbier de la Serre, C.; Espero, E.; Lee, J.; Raybould, H.E. Leptin resistance in vagal afferent neurons inhibits cholecystokinin signaling and satiation in diet induced obese rats. *PLoS ONE* **2012**, *7*, e32967. [CrossRef] [PubMed]
86. Christie, S.; O'Rielly, R.; Li, H.; Nunez-Salces, M.; Wittert, G.A.; Page, A.J. Modulatory effect of methanandamide on gastric vagal afferent satiety signals depends on nutritional status. *J. Physiol.* **2020**, *598*, 2169–2182. [CrossRef] [PubMed]
87. Cluny, N.L.; Baraboi, E.D.; Mackie, K.; Burdyga, G.; Richard, D.; Dockray, G.J.; Sharkey, K.A. High fat diet and body weight have different effects on cannabinoid CB(1) receptor expression in rat nodose ganglia. *Auton. Neurosci.* **2013**, *179*, 122–130. [CrossRef] [PubMed]
88. Christie, S.; O'Rielly, R.; Li, H.; Wittert, G.A.; Page, A.J. Biphasic effects of methanandamide on murine gastric vagal afferent mechanosensitivity. *J. Physiol.* **2020**, *598*, 139–150. [CrossRef] [PubMed]
89. Christie, S.; O'Rielly, R.; Li, H.; Wittert, G.; Page, A. High fat diet induced obesity alters endocannabinoid and ghrelin mediated regulation of components of the endocannabinoid system in nodose ganglia. *Peptides* **2020**, 170371. [CrossRef]
90. Ripken, D.; van der Wielen, N.; van der Meulen, J.; Schuurman, T.; Witkamp, R.F.; Hendriks, H.F.; Koopmans, S.J. Cholecystokinin regulates satiation independently of the abdominal vagal nerve in a pig model of total subdiaphragmatic vagotomy. *Physiol. Behav.* **2015**, *139*, 167–176. [CrossRef]
91. Reidelberger, R.D.; Hernandez, J.; Fritzsch, B.; Hulce, M. Abdominal vagal mediation of the satiety effects of CCK in rats. *Am. J. Physiol. Regul. Integr. Comp. Physiol.* **2004**, *286*, R1005–R1012. [CrossRef] [PubMed]
92. Sykaras, A.G.; Demenis, C.; Case, R.M.; McLaughlin, J.T.; Smith, C.P. Duodenal enteroendocrine I-cells contain mRNA transcripts encoding key endocannabinoid and fatty acid receptors. *PLoS ONE* **2012**, *7*, e42373. [CrossRef] [PubMed]
93. Morales, I.; Berridge, K.C. 'Liking' and 'wanting' in eating and food reward: Brain mechanisms and clinical implications. *Physiol. Behav.* **2020**, *227*, 113152. [CrossRef]
94. Date, Y.; Murakami, N.; Toshinai, K.; Matsukura, S.; Niijima, A.; Matsuo, H.; Kangawa, K.; Nakazato, M. The role of the gastric afferent vagal nerve in ghrelin-induced feeding and growth hormone secretion in rats. *Gastroenterology* **2002**, *123*, 1120–1128. [CrossRef]
95. Zigman, J.M.; Jones, J.E.; Lee, C.E.; Saper, C.B.; Elmquist, J.K. Expression of ghrelin receptor mRNA in the rat and the mouse brain. *J. Comp. Neurol.* **2006**, *494*, 528–548. [CrossRef] [PubMed]
96. Bello, N.T.; Coughlin, J.W.; Redgrave, G.W.; Ladenheim, E.E.; Moran, T.H.; Guarda, A.S. Dietary conditions and highly palatable food access alter rat cannabinoid receptor expression and binding density. *Physiol. Behav.* **2012**, *105*, 720–726. [CrossRef]
97. Vianna, C.R.; Donato, J., Jr.; Rossi, J.; Scott, M.; Economides, K.; Gautron, L.; Pierpont, S.; Elias, C.F.; Elmquist, J.K. Cannabinoid receptor 1 in the vagus nerve is dispensable for body weight homeostasis but required for normal gastrointestinal motility. *J. Neurosci.* **2012**, *32*, 10331–10337. [CrossRef] [PubMed]
98. Page, A.J.; Blackshaw, L.A. An in vitro study of the properties of vagal afferent fibres innervating the ferret oesophagus and stomach. *J. Physiol.* **1998**, *512*, 907–916. [CrossRef]

99. Berthoud, H.R.; Patterson, L.M.; Zheng, H. Vagal-enteric interface: Vagal activation-induced expression of c-Fos and p-CREB in neurons of the upper gastrointestinal tract and pancreas. *Anat. Rec.* **2001**, *262*, 29–40. [CrossRef]
100. Zheng, H.; Berthoud, H.R. Functional vagal input to gastric myenteric plexus as assessed by vagal stimulation-induced Fos expression. *Am. J. Physiol. Gastrointest. Liver Physiol.* **2000**, *279*, G73–G81. [CrossRef]
101. Pradhan, S.N.; Roth, T. Comparative behavioral effects of several anticholinergic agents in rats. *Psychopharmacologia* **1968**, *12*, 358–366. [CrossRef]
102. Lorenz, D.; Nardi, P.; Smith, G.P. Atropine methyl nitrate inhibits sham feeding in the rat. *Pharmcol. Biochem. Behav.* **1978**, *8*, 405–407. [CrossRef]
103. Muise, E.D.; Gandotra, N.; Tackett, J.J.; Bamdad, M.C.; Cowles, R.A. Distribution of muscarinic acetylcholine receptor subtypes in the murine small intestine. *Life Sci.* **2017**, *169*, 6–10. [CrossRef] [PubMed]
104. Rinaldo, L.; Hansel, C. Muscarinic acetylcholine receptor activation blocks long-term potentiation at cerebellar parallel fiber-Purkinje cell synapses via cannabinoid signaling. *Proc. Natl. Acad. Sci. USA* **2013**, *110*, 11181–11186. [CrossRef] [PubMed]
105. Zhao, Y.; Tzounopoulos, T. Physiological activation of cholinergic inputs controls associative synaptic plasticity via modulation of endocannabinoid signaling. *J. Neurosci.* **2011**, *31*, 3158–3168. [CrossRef]
106. Kim, J.; Isokawa, M.; Ledent, C.; Alger, B.E. Activation of muscarinic acetylcholine receptors enhances the release of endogenous cannabinoids in the hippocampus. *J. Neurosci.* **2002**, *22*, 10182–10191. [CrossRef]
107. Ramikie, T.S.; Nyilas, R.; Bluett, R.J.; Gamble-George, J.C.; Hartley, N.D.; Mackie, K.; Watanabe, M.; Katona, I.; Patel, S. Multiple mechanistically distinct modes of endocannabinoid mobilization at central amygdala glutamatergic synapses. *Neuron* **2014**, *81*, 1111–1125. [CrossRef] [PubMed]
108. Straiker, A.; Mackie, K. Metabotropic suppression of excitation in murine autaptic hippocampal neurons. *J. Physiol.* **2007**, *578*, 773–785. [CrossRef]
109. Stella, N.; Schweitzer, P.; Piomelli, D. A second endogenous cannabinoid that modulates long-term potentiation. *Nature* **1997**, *388*, 773–778. [CrossRef] [PubMed]
110. Jung, K.M.; Mangieri, R.; Stapleton, C.; Kim, J.; Fegley, D.; Wallace, M.; Mackie, K.; Piomelli, D. Stimulation of endocannabinoid formation in brain slice cultures through activation of group I metabotropic glutamate receptors. *Mol. Pharmcol.* **2005**, *68*, 1196–1202. [CrossRef]
111. Jung, K.M.; Astarita, G.; Zhu, C.; Wallace, M.; Mackie, K.; Piomelli, D. A key role for diacylglycerol lipase-alpha in metabotropic glutamate receptor-dependent endocannabinoid mobilization. *Mol. Pharmcol.* **2007**, *72*, 612–621. [CrossRef] [PubMed]
112. Bellocchio, L.; Soria-Gomez, E.; Quarta, C.; Metna-Laurent, M.; Cardinal, P.; Binder, E.; Cannich, A.; Delamarre, A.; Haring, M.; Martin-Fontecha, M.; et al. Activation of the sympathetic nervous system mediates hypophagic and anxiety-like effects of CB1 receptor blockade. *Proc. Natl. Acad. Sci. USA* **2013**, *110*, 4786–4791. [CrossRef] [PubMed]
113. Ye, Y.; Abu El Haija, M.; Morgan, D.A.; Guo, D.; Song, Y.; Frank, A.; Tian, L.; Riedl, R.A.; Burnett, C.M.L.; Gao, Z.; et al. Endocannabinoid Receptor-1 and Sympathetic Nervous System Mediate the Beneficial Metabolic Effects of Gastric Bypass. *Cell Rep.* **2020**, *33*, 108270. [CrossRef]
114. Monteleone, A.M.; Di Marzo, V.; Monteleone, P.; Dalle Grave, R.; Aveta, T.; Ghoch, M.E.; Piscitelli, F.; Volpe, U.; Calugi, S.; Maj, M. Responses of peripheral endocannabinoids and endocannabinoid-related compounds to hedonic eating in obesity. *Eur. J. Nutr.* **2016**, *55*, 1799–1805. [CrossRef] [PubMed]
115. Pi-Sunyer, F.X.; Aronne, L.J.; Heshmati, H.M.; Devin, J.; Rosenstock, J. Effect of rimonabant, a cannabinoid-1 receptor blocker, on weight and cardiometabolic risk factors in overweight or obese patients: RIO-North America: A randomized controlled trial. *JAMA* **2006**, *295*, 761–775. [CrossRef]
116. Manca, C.; Boubertakh, B.; Leblanc, N.; Deschenes, T.; Lacroix, S.; Martin, C.; Houde, A.; Veilleux, A.; Flamand, N.; Muccioli, G.G.; et al. Germ-free mice exhibit profound gut microbiota-dependent alterations of intestinal endocannabinoidome signaling. *J. Lipid Res.* **2020**, *61*, 70–85. [CrossRef] [PubMed]
117. Markey, L.; Hooper, A.; Melon, L.C.; Baglot, S.; Hill, M.N.; Maguire, J.; Kumamoto, C.A. Colonization with the commensal fungus Candida albicans perturbs the gut-brain axis through dysregulation of endocannabinoid signaling. *Psychoneuroendocrinology* **2020**, *121*, 104808. [CrossRef]
118. Forte, N.; Fernandez-Rilo, A.C.; Palomba, L.; Di Marzo, V.; Cristino, L. Obesity Affects the Microbiota-Gut-Brain Axis and the Regulation Thereof by Endocannabinoids and Related Mediators. *Int. J. Mol. Sci.* **2020**, *21*, 1554. [CrossRef]
119. Mehrpouya-Bahrami, P.; Chitrala, K.N.; Ganewatta, M.S.; Tang, C.; Murphy, E.A.; Enos, R.T.; Velazquez, K.T.; McCellan, J.; Nagarkatti, M.; Nagarkatti, P. Blockade of CB1 cannabinoid receptor alters gut microbiota and attenuates inflammation and diet-induced obesity. *Sci. Rep.* **2017**, *7*, 15645. [CrossRef]
120. Muccioli, G.G.; Naslain, D.; Backhed, F.; Reigstad, C.S.; Lambert, D.M.; Delzenne, N.M.; Cani, P.D. The endocannabinoid system links gut microbiota to adipogenesis. *Mol. Syst. Biol.* **2010**, *6*, 392. [CrossRef]
121. Ellermann, M.; Pacheco, A.R.; Jimenez, A.G.; Russell, R.M.; Cuesta, S.; Kumar, A.; Zhu, W.; Vale, G.; Martin, S.A.; Raj, P.; et al. Endocannabinoids Inhibit the Induction of Virulence in Enteric Pathogens. *Cell* **2020**. [CrossRef]
122. Sclafani, A. Gut-brain nutrient signaling. Appetition vs. satiation. *Appetite* **2013**, *71*, 454–458. [CrossRef] [PubMed]

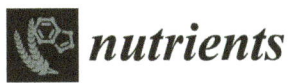

Review

Microbiota's Role in Diet-Driven Alterations in Food Intake: Satiety, Energy Balance, and Reward

Allison W. Rautmann and Claire B. de La Serre *

Department of Nutritional Sciences, University of Georgia, Athens, GA 30605, USA; awr76051@uga.edu
* Correspondence: cdlserre@uga.edu

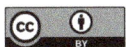

Citation: Rautmann, A.W.; de La Serre, C.B. Microbiota's Role in Diet-Driven Alterations in Food Intake: Satiety, Energy Balance, and Reward. *Nutrients* **2021**, *13*, 3067. https://doi.org/10.3390/nu13093067

Academic Editors: Michael Horowitz and Christine Feinle-Bisset

Received: 18 May 2021
Accepted: 25 August 2021
Published: 31 August 2021

Publisher's Note: MDPI stays neutral with regard to jurisdictional claims in published maps and institutional affiliations.

Copyright: © 2021 by the authors. Licensee MDPI, Basel, Switzerland. This article is an open access article distributed under the terms and conditions of the Creative Commons Attribution (CC BY) license (https://creativecommons.org/licenses/by/4.0/).

Abstract: The gut microbiota plays a key role in modulating host physiology and behavior, particularly feeding behavior and energy homeostasis. There is accumulating evidence demonstrating a role for gut microbiota in the etiology of obesity. In human and rodent studies, obesity and high-energy feeding are most consistently found to be associated with decreased bacterial diversity, changes in main phyla relative abundances and increased presence of pro-inflammatory products. Diet-associated alterations in microbiome composition are linked with weight gain, adiposity, and changes in ingestive behavior. There are multiple pathways through which the microbiome influences food intake. This review discusses these pathways, including peripheral mechanisms such as the regulation of gut satiety peptide release and alterations in leptin and cholecystokinin signaling along the vagus nerve, as well as central mechanisms, such as the modulation of hypothalamic neuroinflammation and alterations in reward signaling. Most research currently focuses on determining the role of the microbiome in the development of obesity and using microbiome manipulation to prevent diet-induced increase in food intake. More studies are necessary to determine whether microbiome manipulation after prolonged energy-dense diet exposure and obesity can reduce intake and promote meaningful weight loss.

Keywords: microbiome; food intake; vagus; CCK; hypothalamus; reward

1. Introduction

The gut microbiota is a collection of over 10^{13} microorganisms, including bacteria and fungi, that inhabit the gastrointestinal (GI) tract and plays a key role in regulating host physiology, particularly GI function and energy homeostasis [1,2]. The microbiome is a relatively stable community of microbes in the individual [3]. In response to the burgeoning obesity epidemic, research has focused on personal and environmental factors that might influence weight status. The discovery that in both humans and rodent models, obese individuals have a distinct microbiome profile compared to their lean counterparts, with an increased capacity to harvest energy from ingested food, has fueled over 15 years of research [2]. Microbiota is vital for proper GI function, as it is implicated in vitamin synthesis, digestion and metabolism of carbohydrate and other dietary components [4], and development and function of the GI immune system [5]. Gut microbes have also been shown to influence the function of other peripheral organs, as well as the central nervous system (CNS), throughout development and the lifespan [6,7]. The importance of the gut microbiota in regulating host biology is evident from gnotobiotic studies: animals born germ-free (GF) present with altered intestinal, metabolic, and neural physiology [8,9].

Recently, advances in sequencing technologies have allowed us to more comprehensively and thoroughly assess microbiota composition and its relation with disease states. Adverse changes in composition have been associated with an array of pathologies, including autoimmune diseases, neurological conditions, and metabolic disorders such as obesity and diabetes [10–13]. It is, however, important to note that any environmental modification is likely to impact microbiome composition, and differences in bacterial makeup associated with pathologies do not equate to a causal link between microbial changes and pathological development.

There is accumulating evidence supporting a role for an individual's microbiota in regulation of food intake through both peripheral and central mechanisms. Peripherally, bacteria and their metabolites interact with vagal afferent neurons (VANs), which transmit information about intestinal contents to the nucleus of the solitary tract (NTS) [14]. The microbiome influences gut–brain satiety signaling via modulation of gut peptide release [15] as well as sensitivity to satiety peptides (such as cholecystokinin, or CCK) and the energy storage hormone leptin [14]. Changes in microbiome composition have also been reported to affect the structural integrity of the gut–brain axis [16]. Centrally, unfavorable microbiome composition is associated with inflammation of key regions involved in the regulation of feeding, particularly the NTS and the hypothalamus [17,18]. Further, there is emerging evidence that certain taxa of bacteria play a role in modulating reward circuitry and motivation [19,20]. The purpose of this review is to describe the microbiota's influence on food intake through the aforementioned mechanisms, including recent developments in the relationship between microbiome, reward, and eating behavior.

2. Energy-Dense Diets Alters Gut–Brain Communication and Regulation of Feeding

Chronic intake of energy-dense food has been linked to excessive weight gain [21]. Despite homeostatic signals that act protectively against food overconsumption, chronic intake of palatable, high-energy diets alters the physiological response to food and favors overeating. Ultimately, this results in increased body weight (BW) and fat deposition. Specifically, sensitivity to hedonic cues is altered, while homeostatic signals of meal termination are dampened [22].

The vagus nerve is a direct pathway that carries post-ingestive feedback from the gut to the brain [23]. Mechano- and chemosensitive VANs respond to the nutrient composition of ingested food to regulate meal size [24]. VANs terminate in the NTS, where postprandial signals increase neuronal activity [25]. In addition, VANs project to limbic brain regions, and this gut–reward circuit is sufficient and necessary for meal termination [23]. Chronic consumption of a high-fat (HF) diet reduces VAN sensitivity to tension [26,27], satiation hormones (e.g., CCK) [26,28–33], and intestinal nutrients [34–37]. As such, diet-induced disruption of vagal signaling coincides with the onset of hyperphagia [38]. In addition, diet-induced obese (DIO) rats also exhibit significantly decreased postprandial neuronal activation in the NTS compared to lean animals [29,37].

Other neuronal networks involved in the regulation of feeding are also altered by chronic HF consumption. Leptin is a key adiposity signal, with amounts produced proportional to the amount of fat stored in the body [39]. Hypothalamic leptin signaling is disrupted during chronic HF feeding [40], with increased expression of suppressor of cytokine signaling 3 (SOCS3) and decreased phosphorylated signal transducer and activator of transcription 3 (STAT3) in the arcuate nucleus [41]. Pro-opiomelanocortin (POMC) neurons in the hypothalamus in a normal physiological state are activated by leptin [42] to ultimately decrease food intake via the production of α-melanocyte-stimulating hormone (α-MSH) [43,44]. Thus, HF-induced disruption of leptin can directly alter hypothalamic inhibition of food intake. Another neuronal system altered by HF intake is the dopaminergic reward system. Food's hedonic value is an important factor in food consumption, and increased motivation for food intake is linked to obesity [45]. Palatable foods initially have a higher reward value [46], while as obesity progresses, reductions in reward signaling emerge and lead to compensatory overeating [47]. Among regions involved in the mesolimbic dopaminergic system, the nucleus accumbens (NAc) and striatum exhibit decreased dopamine release in rodents with long-term exposure to a HF diet [48].

Microbiome Alterations Seen with Energy-Dense Feeding

Dietary intake is a major and easily modifiable determinant of an individual's microbiota composition; other factors include age and genetics [49]. In humans, both short- and long-term intake of specific macronutrients, as well as fibers and other plant foods, are correlated with abundance distribution of specific bacterial taxa present in the GI tract [49]. Obesity is associated with changes in microbiome composition. While the vast majority of the composition is specific to the individual, small-scale studies have found that obesity has been associated with an increased ratio of Firmicutes to Bacteroidetes, the two main phyla present in the GI tract [12]. Conversely, weight loss through caloric restriction has led to an increase in Bacteroidetes abundance, whether that restriction was through a carbohydrate- or fat-restricted diet plan [12]. Similar results are observed in rodent models of DIO, with the addition of a bloom in the pro-inflammatory Proteobacteria sometimes reported in humans with obesity or type 2 diabetes [50]. In rats, 8 weeks of 45% HF-feeding is associated with decreased bacterial α-diversity, a measure of the variety of bacterial taxa colonizing the gut, and increased relative abundances in the Firmicutes orders *Clostridiales* [51], in particular, the *Dorea* genus, and *Erysipelotrichiales* (*Erysipelotrichaceae* family) [52]. Three weeks of 60% HF-feeding has a similar effect on microbiome composition in rats, with increases in relative abundances of several Firmicutes families, including *Streptococcaceae*, *Erysipelotrichaceae*, *Lachnospiraceae* (*Dorea* genus), *Peptococcaceae*, and *Staphylococcaceae*, as well as Proteobacteria families *Desulfovibrionaceae* and *Enterobacteriaceae* [16]. In rats, a mere 7 days of 60% HF-feeding is associated with decreased abundance of the Bacteroidetes orders *Bacteroidales* (*Prevotella* genus) and *Sphingobacteriales*, and increased Firmicutes order *Erysipelotrichales*, and several Proteobacteria orders, including *Rhodocyclales* and *Altermondales*, among others [53]. Diets high in sugars also affect gut microbiome composition, with alterations in the Firmicutes to Bacteroidetes ratio sometimes being reported [17,54], but not always [55]. Different results have also been observed with respect to α-diversity [17,54–56]. In a study comparing high-glucose, high-fructose, and HF diets in mice, researchers found that all three similarly decreased diversity, decreased Bacteroidetes abundance (specifically *Muribaculum* spp.) and increased Proteobacteria abundance (specifically *Desulfovibrio* spp.); however, diets high in sugars led to a significant increase in *Akkermansia muciniphila* abundance compared to a HF diet [54]. When compared to an unrefined chow diet, both refined low-fat, high-sugar (LFHS) and HF, high-sugar (HFHS) diet consumption in rats result in decreased diversity and significant alterations in relative abundances within 1 week of feeding [17]. The LFHS diet increases Firmicutes, particularly *Ruminococcaceae* and *Lachnospiraceae*, as well as Proteobacteria genera *Sutterella* and *Bilophila*, and decreases Bacteroidetes abundances, though changes are more pronounced with HFHS-feeding. [17]. A mere daily 2 h access to HFHS pellets alters gut microbiome composition in chow-fed rats with increased relative abundances of *Lachnospiraceae*, *Ruminoccoceae*, and *Erysipelotrichaceae* families [56].

In humans, specific dietary patterns and components have been reported to affect bacterial taxa relative abundances. Obese humans switched to a strict vegan diet low in fat and high in fiber display an increase in abundance of Bacteroidetes over a 4-week period [57]. Self-classified vegans tend to have lower *Bifidobacterium* spp., *Escherichia coli*, and *Enterobacteriaceae* spp. when compared to vegetarian and omnivorous humans [58]. Two recent studies published in 2021 associated specific dietary components with microbial taxa. In Japanese monozygotic twins, significant associations are found between *Lachnospiraceae* species: *Lachnospira* and *Lachnospiraceae* UCG-008 negatively correlate with protein intake and saturated fat intake, respectively, while the *Lachnospiraceae* ND3007 group correlates positively with total fat intake [59]. A population study of 1920 Chinese adults found that a calculated healthy diet score, based on intakes of fruit, vegetables, seafood, nuts/legumes, refined grains, red meat, and processed meat, is associated with increased abundances within Firmicutes and Actinobacteria, particularly the genera *Coprococcus* and *Bifidobacterium*. Dairy is positively associated with the family *Bifidocacteraceae* and genus *Bifidobacterium*; seafood with families *Alcaligenaceae* and *Desulfovibrionaceae*; and nuts and legumes with the phyla Proteobacteria. Inverse associations are found with processed meat and the family *Lachnospiraceae*, while it was positively associated with *Fusobacteriaceae* and *Acinetobacter* under Proteobacteria [60].

There is evidence that Western-type diet-driven changes in microbiome composition negatively affect host metabolism and energy homeostasis. Studies using microbiota-depleted and GF rodent models have established a relationship between diet-driven dysbiosis and excessive weight gain. GF mice have been shown to exhibit resistance to weight gain when fed a HFHS diet that leads to increased adiposity in a conventional mouse, showing that microbiota is necessary for DIO [61]. Conversely, GF rats and mice colonized with fecal and cecal contents from conventional HFHS-fed animals display a significant increase in BW compared to rodents colonized with chow-fed animal microbiome [16,62]. Similar results have been observed when GF animals are re-colonized with GI contents from a genetically obese donor [2] or from an obese human donor [63]. We have successfully replicated these findings in an antibiotic depletion model [16]. These studies establish that an "obese microbiome" from a host that is obese, or "HF-type microbiome" from a host fed a HF diet, is sufficient to alter energy homeostasis and affect BW regulation, at least in the short term. The GF studies cited here do not extend past 5 weeks post-colonization [2,16,63]. While there is evidence that an individual's microbiota composition may affect energy harvest [2], storage [18], and utilization [64], a major effect on BW may be driven by changes in regulation of energy intake.

Microbiota-depleted rats colonized with a HF-type microbiome have been shown to significantly increase weekly food intake compared to rats colonized with a chow-type microbiome [16]. Conversely, modulation of the microbiome via supplementation of anti-, pro-, or prebiotics impacts weight and intake. In rats fed a 60% HF diet, administration of minocycline, a broad-spectrum antibiotic, lessens microbiome alterations and significantly reduces food intake [53]. In this experiment, 3 weeks of antibiotic administration normalizes HF-fed minocycline-treated rats' intake to that of the control rats. This occurs with restoration of the Firmicutes to Bacteroidetes ratio to a level comparable to that of the chow animals, prevention of the HF-induced decrease in *Bacteroidales* and *Sphingobacteriales*, and significant reduction in *Erysipelotrichales* [53]. Administration of oligofructose, a beneficial prebiotic fermented by intestinal microbes [65], restores populations of *Akkermansia muciniphila* in DIO mice and normalizes BW [66]. In addition to preventing weight gain, probiotics have been found to promote weight loss in mice fed a HF diet for 12 weeks. In these animals, supplementation with a probiotic containing *Lactobacillus rhamnosus*, *Lactobacillus acidophilus*, and *Bifidobacterium bifidum* for 5 weeks decreases BW and food intake [67]. In young men, supplementation with a probiotic along with the initiation of a HF diet (55% kcal from fat, 25% of kcal from saturated fat) reduces the amount of weight gained over 4 weeks [68]. Based on these data, microbiome alterations appear sufficient to alter food intake and necessary for HF-diet-induced increases in intake.

3. Microbiome Composition Influences Peripheral Intake Mechanisms

The presence of food in the GI tract leads to the release of satiety signals, such as CCK, by enteroendocrine cells (EECs) that can signal via the vagus nerve to regulate food intake, particularly meal size [23,24]. There is evidence that GI bacterial makeup modulates several aspects of this gut–brain communication.

3.1. GI Satiety Peptide Expression/Release

An individual's gut microbiota may affect regulation of meal size via modulation of GI satiety peptide expression and release. GF mice, when compared to conventional mice of similar body weight, display decreased intestinal expression of CCK peptide [36]. Further, fructose malabsorption induces microbiome alterations, which, in mice, is associated with changes in CCK expression and secretion [69]. Ketohexokinase (KHK)-knockout mice are a model of fructose malabsorption. KHK catalyzes fructose phosphorylation and KHK deletion prevents the upregulation of GLUT5, a fructose transporter [69]. KHK-KO mice do not absorb most fructose, and feeding these animals a diet of 20% fructose leads to increased fructose concentration in the colon and alterations in microbiome composition, including increased relative abundances of Actinobacteria (families *Coriobacteriaceae* and *Corynebacteri-*

aceae), Bacteroidetes and *Lactobacillaceae* (particularly *Lactobacillus johnsonii*); and decreased Proteobacteria (family *Desulfovibrionaceae*) [69]. These alterations are accompanied by a significant increase in CCK-positive EECs, which can be prevented via antibiotic administration, demonstrating that the microbiota is necessary for fructose malabsorption-induced alterations in CCK release [69]. In addition to modulating CCK expression, microbiome may influence CCK release. In the murine EEC line STC-1, application of certain fatty acid metabolites produced by commensal lactic acid bacteria results in increased CCK release [70].

The microbiota's influence on gut satiety peptides is not limited to CCK. Glucagon-like peptide (GLP) 1 is an incretin released from intestinal L-cells that decreases food intake via a vagally mediated pathway [71]. There is evidence that short chain fatty acids (SCFAs) produced by a healthy microbiome [72] influence GLP-1 release [15]. Application of SCFAs-acetate, propionate, and butyrate-to-mouse colonic cell cultures leads to increased secretion of GLP-1 through activation of the free fatty acid receptor (FFAR) 2, a nutrient-sensing G-protein coupled receptor [15]. This suggests that bacterial metabolites may be able to directly interact with L-cells to regulate GLP-1 release [15]. SCFAs are produced through fermentation of soluble fibers such as inulin, and while most gut bacteria can produce acetate, there are specific taxa that produce propionate and butyrate [73]. Propionate producers include Bacteroides spp., *Salmonella* spp., *Megasphaera elsdenii*, *Coprococcus catus*, and *Ruminococcus obeum*; and butyrate producers include *Anaerostipes* spp., *Roseburia* spp., and *Coprococcus comes, eutactus*, and *catus* (this list is non-exhaustive) [73]. Supplementation of inulin and other prebiotic fibers has been shown to prevent hyperphagia associated with energy-dense diet consumption in rodents [74,75] as well as increased cecal and portal GLP-1 concentrations in rats fed standard chow [76]. Similarly, rats pretreated with 35 days of oligofructose supplementation consumed less food, gained less weight, and had nearly twice the expression of portal and colonic GLP-1 when switched to a HF diet compared to control rats [74]. Oligofructose supplementation for 3 weeks in chow-fed rats leads to a decrease in intake accompanied by increased cecal and portal concentrations of GLP-1 and peptide YY (PYY), another anorexigenic gut peptide [76]. A study in humans found that acute supplementation of inulin-propionate ester increased plasma GLP-1 and PYY and was associated with decreased food intake at a meal post-supplementation when compared to controls [77], showing that propionate has acute effects on food intake. Interestingly, prebiotic supplementation results in increased colon length [75,76] compared to non-supplemented controls, which led the authors to conclude that GLP-1 increase may be due in part to an increased number of secretory cells [76]. However, GF mice with significantly decreased intestinal expression of satiety peptides (CCK, GLP-1, and PYY) exhibit increased cecal and decreased ileal counts of EECs compared to conventional mice [36]. A study found that GF mice have altered ileal expression of genes related to vesicle organization in L cells that was accompanied by increased GLP-1 in ileal L cells, while the colonic transcriptome was not significantly altered [78]. The authors suggest that this is due to the colonic mucus barrier, which prevents bacteria from coming into direct contact with EECs, while microbes in the ileum may come into direct contact with the mucosa [78]. Studies have also found that GF mice have more EECs in the colon compared to conventional mice [36], or mice colonized with *Bacteroides thetaiotaomicron*, which may be due to differences in neurogenesis [79]. Microbiota may influence GLP-1 release through yet another mechanism. Administration of *Akkermansia muciniphila* as a probiotic in obese mice restores levels of acylglycerols in the gut [66]. Acylglycerols are products of fat digestion and components of the endocannabinoid system, and one acylglycerol, 2-oleoylglycerol, stimulates L-cells to secrete gut peptides, including GLP-1, through stimulation of a G-protein-coupled receptor [80] (Table 1).

Table 1. Gastrointestinal (GI) satiety peptides and their association with microbiota.

Satiety Peptide	Association with Microbiota
CCK	VANs exhibit decreased CCK sensitivity when the GI tract is colonized with HF-type microbiome [16].
GLP-1	SCFAs produced when microbiota ferments soluble fibers may promote GLP-1 secretion [15,76].
PYY	Rats fed soluble fiber also exhibit increased PYY levels in the GI tract [76].

3.2. CCK and Leptin Signaling

In addition to affecting gut peptide expression and release [15,69,81], there is evidence that changes in an individual's microbiota composition modulate vagal afferent sensitivity to gut-originating satiety signals, particularly CCK [14]. CCK is released from the proximal GI tract (duodenum and early jejunum) in response to long-chain fatty acids [82] and amino acids [83], and acts on VANs to promote meal termination [84]. Colonization of microbiota-depleted rats with a HF-type microbiome is sufficient to reduce CCK-induced satiety in the receiver animals [16]. Conversely, it has been shown that preventing HF diet-driven dysbiosis through prebiotic supplementation prevents HF diet-induced loss in CCK signaling [52], demonstrating that changes in microbiome composition are also necessary for HF diet-induced alterations in CCK signaling.

VAN sensitivity to CCK may be altered through bacterial metabolites and their effect on leptin signaling. Leptin, an anorexigenic adipokine, is released from adipocytes in proportion to fat mass [39] and enhances CCK signaling [85]. Peripheral leptin resistance has been linked to a reduction in CCK sensitivity and increased intake [14,33]. Lipopolysaccharide (LPS), a pro-inflammatory by-product of Gram-negative bacteria, increases in circulation in DIO rodents [14,86]. Cecal and serum concentrations of LPS are increased in animals fed both LFHS and HFHS diets [17]. In rats, chronic low-dose administration of LPS, resulting in serum levels comparable to those seen in HF-fed animals, leads to VAN leptin resistance and decreased sensitivity to CCK [14]. LPS leads to Toll-like receptor (TLR) 4 activation at the level of the nodose ganglion (NG), where VAN cell bodies are located, which subsequently increases SOCS3 protein levels. SOCS3 inhibits activation of the leptin receptor, potentially abolishing the synergistic effect of leptin on CCK sensitivity and decreasing feeding suppression following CCK injection [14].

3.3. Inflammation

In rats, DIO is characterized by a leaky gut and low-grade inflammation, potentially driven by bacterial products such as LPS [51]. GI-originating inflammation may play a key role in mediating HF diet-associated alterations in post-ingestive gut–brain signaling. Interestingly, HF feeding rapidly activates microglia-like cells in the NG [17,87], and this may be mediated by microbiota. Microglia are the resident macrophages of the CNS [88], and chronic activation of microglia causes inflammation [89]. Colonization of microbiota-depleted rats with a HF-type microbiome leads to an increase in positive staining in the NG for the pan-microglia and monocyte marker-ionized calcium binding adaptor molecule (Iba) 1 [16], while administration of antibiotics [17] or prebiotics [52] prevents Iba1$^+$ cell recruitment along the gut–brain axis. In the CNS, microglia alter synaptic function and axonal growth in response to bacterial products by releasing cytokines [90–92], and HF diet-driven microglial activation is associated with inflammation-mediated neuronal death [93]. It is therefore possible that microbiota-driven recruitment of Iba1$^+$ cells in the NG has a deleterious effect on VAN survival. Co-culture of VANs with Gram-negative bacteria isolated from HF-fed rats (specifically *Proteus mirabilis* of the order *Enterobacteriales* mentioned previously) leads to a dramatic decrease in viable neurons, suggesting that bacterial products can directly influence VAN survival [53]. Further, increased serum LPS and decreased innervation of the cecum was found in rats fed a HF diet [17]. These data would suggest that, in addition to altering vagal afferent signaling, an individual's microbiota composition could also affect the structural integrity of the gut–brain axis. A decrease in VAN number may explain the reduction in c-fibers observed in the NTS of GF rats conventionalized with a HF-type microbiome [16]. At the level of the NTS, c-fibers are predominantly of vagal origin [94]. Conversely, administration of a broad-spectrum antibiotic [17] or prebiotic [52] concomitant with HF diet introduction can prevent both dysbiosis and c-fiber withdrawal from the NTS.

4. Microbiota Influences Central Intake Mechanisms

4.1. Neuroinflammation

Besides altering sensitivity to leptin and CCK, bacterial inflammatory products produced by the obese-type microbiome are linked to inflammation and loss of function in key brain regions involved in food intake—the NTS, as previously discussed, and the hypothalamus [95–97]. The hypothalamus contains key anorexigenic and orexigenic neuronal populations involved in regulating appetite and energy expenditure. Signals related to energy stores within the body, especially leptin, can modulate neuropeptide expression and release within the hypothalamus to regulate energy homeostasis. Inflammation and cytokine signaling interfere with leptin sensitivity in neurons [98]. Conventionally raised mice exhibit increased hypothalamic SOCS3 expression as well as decreased suppression of orexigenic mRNA (*Npy* and *Agrp*) in response to intraperitoneal leptin injection compared to GF mice [99], hinting that the presence of certain bacterial taxa may interfere with hypothalamic leptin sensitivity. Increased bacterial LPS may play a role. Female rats fitted with slow-release pellets set to deliver a daily low (53 μg/day) or high (207 μg/day) dose of LPS were fed a chow or 60% HF diet for 8 weeks [100]. At the end of the study, both LPS groups had gained more weight and consumed more food than the control vehicle pellet group. LPS groups dose-dependently increased expression of IL-1β in the hypothalamus, while increasing the expression of orexin, a neuropeptide that increases food intake, in the low-dose group [100]. In DIO mice, increased TLR4 and IL-6 mRNA expression in the hypothalamus is associated with decreased leptin-induced STAT3 phosphorylation and a failure to decrease food intake in response to intraperitoneal leptin injection [67]. Supplementation with a probiotic containing *Lactobacillus rhamnosus*, *Lactobacillus acidophilus*, and *Bifidobacterium bifidum* results in decreased BW and food intake in DIO animals, as well as normalization of TLR4 and IL-6 mRNA levels in the hypothalamus, and restoration of leptin-induced pSTAT3 expression [67]. Similar preservation of leptin signaling has been observed with *Lactobacillus rhamnosus* supplementation alone [101], demonstrating that the presence or absence of certain bacterial taxa can modulate hypothalamic leptin signaling.

Oxidative stress is another inflammatory measure that is increased in DIO rats and may be related to microbiome composition. In a study by Fouesnard et al., rats were placed on either a chow or high-energy Western diet (WD; 45% fat) for 6 weeks [95]. WD-fed rats exhibited hyperphagia in the first week of feeding, increased weight gain, and adiposity. Metabolomic changes were observed in the hypothalamus within 2 h of diet introduction, and these changes persisted after the first day of feeding [95]. Specific alterations included hypothalamic redox homeostasis (increased oxidized glutathione, among other measures, suggests increased oxidative stress) and cell membrane remodeling processes. Similarly, cecal microbiome composition was significantly altered within hours of diet introduction, with WD feeding leading to decreased α-diversity and increased Proteobacteria relative abundance, particularly the *Desulfovibrionaceae* and *Tannerellaceae* families, as well as decreased *Lactobacillaceae* relative abundance. Cecal metabolites also correlated with hypothalamic metabolites—one notable association was seen between oxidative stress and indices of α-diversity. This demonstrates an immediate pro-inflammatory microbiome shift within 1 day of WD feeding that coincides with alterations in hypothalamic oxidative stress and hyperphagia [95]. Interestingly, in conventionally raised, but not GF, rats, RNA expression of superoxide dismutase 2, glutaredoxin, and IL-6 are increased after 2 days of WD feeding, demonstrating that the microbiota is necessary for the early pro-inflammatory effects of WD in the hypothalamus.

4.2. Reward Pathways

External factors can override homeostatic regulation of intake, including food availability, social and contextual cues, and palatability [71]. The ventral tegmental area (VTA) contains receptors for peripheral energy signals, including ghrelin, insulin, and leptin [102]. It also receives input from the hypothalamus and the NTS [102]. Optogenetic activation of VANs that innervate the upper GI tract stimulates reward-associated behavior such as self-stimulation, place preference, and flavor conditioning, and is sufficient to increase dopamine (DA) levels in the dorsal striatum [23]. Further, ablation of the vagal–parabrachial–nigrostriatal pathway abolishes conditioned preference for gastric infusion of high-calorie nutritive lipids over low-calorie nutritive lipids, while vagal deafferentation alone decreases conditioned preference and avoidance learning in a number of other tests [23]. As microbiota has been found to modulate vagal signaling, changes in bacterial composition are expected to modulate central mechanisms regulating reward.

GF and antibiotic-depleted mice exhibit alterations in dopaminergic reward pathways [19]. GF mice have increased DA turnover in the striatum and lower expression of D1 receptor mRNA in the striatum and NAc [103], a region involved in food-seeking behavior [104], and display increased preference for even low concentrations of intralipid compared to conventional mice [36]. Antibiotic administration has resulted in increased L-3,4-dihydroxyphenylalanine (L-DOPA) in the amygdala of young mice [105] and decreased DA turnover in the amygdala and striatum in rats, suggesting that microbiota modulates DA neurochemistry in rodents. Colonization with fecal contents from mice with chronic ethanol exposure leads to depressive and anxiety-like behaviors similar to those evident in withdrawal [20], and administration of SCFAs to mice previously exposed to a small dose of cocaine abolishes conditioned place preference [106], which suggests that microbiota is directly involved in modulating addiction-like behaviors and may be relevant in food addiction. These data suggest that individual microbiota may affect food intake not only through homeostatic mechanisms, but also through regulation of the reward pathway and hedonic perception. There are studies emerging that support this hypothesis.

In adolescent rats with intermittent daily access to HFHS diet, overall energy intake increases and monoamine gene expression is altered in the hippocampus and prefrontal cortex, and these alterations correlate with bacterial relative abundances [56]. Specifically, prefrontal cortex expression of monoamine oxidase A is positively associated with an unspecified genus of the *Lachnospiraceae* family, while expression in the hippocampus is associated with a number of other families, including unspecified *Bifidobacteriales*, *Bifidobacteriaceae*, unspecified *Bacteroidales*, *Rikenellaceae*, *Lachnospiraceae*, *Ruminococcaceae*, and *Erysipelotrichaceae* [56]. Microbiota may play a role in food preferences as well. Increased preference for sucrose is evident in mice undergoing social stress, and this increased preference is abolished by SCFA supplementation, suggesting that microbiota modulates stress-induced sucrose preference via SCFA production [107]. In rats, chronic consumption of HFHS diets leads to decreased motivation to lever press to receive a sucrose pellet [108]. Fructo-oligosaccharide introduced along with the initiation of HFHS feeding restores motivation for the sucrose pellet; however, supplementation beginning after 10 weeks of HFHS diet exposure is not able to rescue this measure of motivational behavior [108]. Further, supplementation leads to decreased preference for HFHS foods compared to rats without supplementation [108].

Low- and no-calorie artificial sweeteners are another point of contention in terms of their impact on reward and intake, as it has been found that some sweeteners, such as stevia, are metabolized by gut microbiota [109]. While short- and long-term studies in humans do not show that artificial sweetener intake leads to compensatory overeating [110], there is evidence in both humans and rodents that sweetener intake causes alterations in reward pathways. In humans, ingestion of sucralose has significantly different effects in VTA activation compared to glucose or sucrose [111]. Rats exposed to a chronic low dose of rebaudioside A (RebA), a stevia glycoside, exhibit decreased tyrosine hydroxylase and dopamine transporter (DAT) mRNA expression in the NAc [112], which can be rescued by prebiotic oligofructose supplementation [112]. These data suggest that artificial sweeteners that are metabolized by microbiota may alter reward signaling. It should be noted that the evidence is limited as research in this area is still emerging (Table 2).

Table 2. Bacteria associated with food intake alterations. It is important to note that there is currently insufficient evidence to consistently link specific bacterial species to altered intake. Further, these findings have only been demonstrated in rodent models and are not applicable in humans.

Bacteria	Intake Alterations
Lactobacillus rhamnosus, *Lactobacillus acidophilus*, and *Bifidobacteria bifidum*	5 weeks of supplementation decreased hypothalamic inflammation, food intake, and BW compared to DIO animals without the supplement [67]
Akkermansia muciniphila	May promote gut peptide release through increasing acylglycerols in the gut [66]

Gram-negative bacteria	• Produce LPS, which can
	  ○ reduce VAN sensitivity to leptin and CCK [14]
	  ○ hypothalamic inflammation and BW [100]
	• May decrease VAN survival (specifically, *Proteus mirabilis*) [53]

5. Summary

Microbiota exerts an undeniable influence in the regulation of food intake through central and peripheral mechanisms, including satiety peptide release and signaling, inflammation, and modulation of reward pathways. Microbiota-driven changes in gut–brain signaling may be linked to alterations in both homeostatic and hedonic regulation of feeding. Preventing adverse microbial alterations via supplementation of prebiotic fibers and probiotics can successfully prevent hyperphagia in animal models, especially when introduced concomitantly with a dietary challenge. However, changes to the gut–brain axis may have long-term consequences on feeding behavior. HF or HS feeding [17] and HF-type microbiome alone [16] lead to withdrawal of vagal c-fibers from the NTS. This remodeling coincides with onset of weight gain and hyperphagia [38]. Nerve injury-induced [113] or diet-induced [53] vagal withdrawal can be followed by NTS reinnervation (sprouting). Crucially, reinnervation does not appear to restore function in HF-fed rats, as animals remain hyperphagic [38,53], suggesting that gut–brain function may be permanently affected in obesity. It is still unclear if microbiome-based therapy could restore gut–brain signaling in obesity. While weight loss in both humans and rodents is associated with microbiome composition alterations [114,115], there is limited evidence that restoring microbiome in obese individuals can lead to weight loss. Probiotic use may be circumstantially associated with weight loss [116], but no causal link has been established. Most animal studies in the realm of obesity research focus on preventing weight gain when introducing a HF diet and initiate treatments such as pre- and probiotics concomitantly [117–120]. While helpful when flushing out the etiology of obesity, these studies do not determine whether modulation of an individual's microbiota can successfully and effectively decrease food intake and promote clinically meaningful weight loss. More studies should be executed in which pre- or probiotics are supplemented to DIO animals to determine whether microbiome composition can be restored to a pre-obese state, or if modulation is associated with weight loss. Such studies would help determine whether the microbiota is an appropriate target to promote healthy eating behavior and weight loss.

Author Contributions: A.W.R. prepared figures; A.W.R. and C.B.d.L.S. drafted manuscript; A.W.R. and C.B.d.L.S. edited and revised manuscript. Both authors have read and agreed to the published version of the manuscript.

Funding: This research received no external funding.

Conflicts of Interest: The authors declare no conflict of interest.

References

1. Gill, S.R.; Pop, M.; Deboy, R.T.; Eckburg, P.B.; Turnbaugh, P.J.; Samuel, B.S.; Gordon, J.I.; Relman, D.A.; Fraser-Liggett, C.M.; Nelson, K.E. Metagenomic analysis of the human distal gut microbiome. *Science* **2006**, *312*, 1355–1359. [CrossRef]
2. Turnbaugh, P.J.; Ley, R.E.; Mahowald, M.A.; Magrini, V.; Mardis, E.R.; Gordon, J.I. An obesity-associated gut microbiome with increased capacity for energy harvest. *Nature* **2006**, *444*, 1027–1031. [CrossRef] [PubMed]
3. Johnson, A.J.; Vangay, P.; Al-Ghalith, G.A.; Hillmann, B.M.; Ward, T.L.; Shields-Cutler, R.R.; Kim, A.D.; Shmagel, A.K.; Syed, A.N.; Walter, J.; et al. Daily Sampling Reveals Personalized Diet-Microbiome Associations in Humans. *Cell Host Microbe* **2019**, *25*, 789–802.e785. [CrossRef]
4. Rowland, I.; Gibson, G.; Heinken, A.; Scott, K.; Swann, J.; Thiele, I.; Tuohy, K. Gut microbiota functions: Metabolism of nutrients and other food components. *Eur. J. Nutr.* **2018**, *57*, 1–24. [CrossRef] [PubMed]
5. Honda, K.; Littman, D.R. The microbiota in adaptive immune homeostasis and disease. *Nature* **2016**, *535*, 75–84. [CrossRef] [PubMed]
6. Blumberg, R.; Powrie, F. Microbiota, disease, and back to health: A metastable journey. *Sci. Transl. Med.* **2012**, *4*, 137rv7. [CrossRef]
7. Ximenez, C.; Torres, J. Development of Microbiota in Infants and its Role in Maturation of Gut Mucosa and Immune System. *Arch. Med. Res.* **2017**, *48*, 666–680. [CrossRef]
8. Al-Asmakh, M.; Zadjali, F. Use of germ-free animal models in microbiota-related research. *J. Microbiol. Biotechnol.* **2015**, *25*, 1583–1588. [CrossRef]
9. Synowiec, S.; Lu, L.; Yu, Y.; Bretherick, T.; Takada, S.; Yarnykh, V.L.; Caplan, J.; Caplan, M.; Claud, E.C.; Drobyshevsky, A. Microbiota influence the development of the brain and behaviors in C57BL/6J mice. *PLoS ONE* **2018**, *13*, e0201829.
10. De Luca, F.; Shoenfeld, Y. The microbiome in autoimmune diseases. *Clin. Exp. Immunol.* **2019**, *195*, 74–85. [CrossRef]
11. Kallio, K.A.; Hätönen, K.A.; Lehto, M.; Salomaa, V.; Männistö, S.; Pussinen, P.J. Endotoxemia, nutrition, and cardiometabolic disorders. *Acta Diabetol.* **2015**, *52*, 395–404. [CrossRef]
12. Ley, R.E.; Turnbaugh, P.J.; Klein, S.; Gordon, J.I. Microbial ecology: Human gut microbes associated with obesity. *Nature* **2006**, *444*, 1022–1023. [CrossRef]
13. Quigley, E.M.M. Microbiota-Brain-Gut Axis and Neurodegenerative Diseases. *Curr. Neurol. Neurosci. Rep.* **2017**, *17*, 94. [CrossRef]
14. De La Serre, C.B.; de Lartigue, G.; Raybould, H.E. Chronic exposure to low dose bacterial lipopolysaccharide inhibits leptin signaling in vagal afferent neurons. *Physiol. Behav.* **2015**, *139*, 188–194. [CrossRef] [PubMed]
15. Tolhurst, G.; Heffron, H.; Lam, Y.S.; Parker, H.E.; Habib, A.M.; Diakogiannaki, E.; Cameron, J.; Grosse, J.; Reimann, F.; Gribble, F.M. Short-chain fatty acids stimulate glucagon-like peptide-1 secretion via the G-protein–coupled receptor FFAR2. *Diabetes* **2012**, *61*, 364–371. [CrossRef] [PubMed]
16. Kim, J.S.; Kirkland, R.A.; Lee, S.H.; Cawthon, C.R.; Rzepka, K.W.; Minaya, D.M.; de Lartigue, G.; Czaja, K.; de La Serre, C.B. Gut microbiota composition modulates inflammation and structure of the vagal afferent pathway. *Physiol. Behav.* **2020**, *225*, 113082. [CrossRef] [PubMed]
17. Sen, T.; Cawthon, C.R.; Ihde, B.T.; Hajnal, A.; DiLorenzo, P.M.; Claire, B.; Czaja, K. Diet-driven microbiota dysbiosis is associated with vagal remodeling and obesity. *Physiol. Behav.* **2017**, *173*, 305–317. [CrossRef]
18. Heiss, C.N.; Olofsson, L.E. Gut Microbiota-Dependent Modulation of Energy Metabolism. *J. Innate Immun.* **2018**, *10*, 163–171. [CrossRef] [PubMed]
19. González-Arancibia, C.; Urrutia-Piñones, J.; Illanes-González, J.; Martinez-Pinto, J.; Sotomayor-Zárate, R.; Julio-Pieper, M.; Bravo, J.A. Do your gut microbes affect your brain dopamine? *Psychopharmacology* **2019**, *236*, 1611–1622. [CrossRef]
20. Xiao, H.W.; Ge, C.; Feng, G.X.; Li, Y.; Luo, D.; Dong, J.L.; Li, H.; Wang, H.; Cui, M.; Fan, S.J. Gut microbiota modulates alcohol withdrawal-induced anxiety in mice. *Toxicol. Lett.* **2018**, *287*, 23–30. [CrossRef]
21. Ledikwe, J.H.; Blanck, H.M.; Kettel Khan, L.; Serdula, M.K.; Seymour, J.D.; Tohill, B.C.; Rolls, B.J. Dietary energy density is associated with energy intake and weight status in US adults. *Am. J. Clin. Nutr.* **2006**, *83*, 1362–1368. [CrossRef] [PubMed]
22. De Lartigue, G. Role of the vagus nerve in the development and treatment of diet-induced obesity. *J. Physiol.* **2016**, *594*, 5791–5815. [CrossRef]
23. Han, W.; Tellez, L.A.; Perkins, M.H.; Perez, I.O.; Qu, T.; Ferreira, J.; Ferreira, T.L.; Quinn, D.; Liu, Z.W.; Gao, X.B.; et al. A Neural Circuit for Gut-Induced Reward. *Cell* **2018**, *175*, 665–678.e623. [CrossRef]
24. Peters, J.H.; Karpiel, A.B.; Ritter, R.C.; Simasko, S.M. Cooperative activation of cultured vagal afferent neurons by leptin and cholecystokinin. *Endocrinology* **2004**, *145*, 3652–3657. [CrossRef]
25. Moran, T. *Neural and Hormonal Controls of Food Intake and Satiety in Physiology of the Gastrointestinal Tract*, 4th ed.; Johnson, L.R., Ed.; Academic Press: Cambridge, MA, USA, 2006.
26. Daly, D.M.; Park, S.J.; Valinsky, W.C.; Beyak, M.J. Impaired intestinal afferent nerve satiety signalling and vagal afferent excitability in diet induced obesity in the mouse. *J. Physiol.* **2011**, *589*, 2857–2870. [CrossRef] [PubMed]
27. Kentish, S.; Li, H.; Philp, L.K.; O'Donnell, T.A.; Isaacs, N.J.; Young, R.L.; Wittert, G.A.; Blackshaw, L.A.; Page, A.J. Diet-induced adaptation of vagal afferent function. *J. Physiol.* **2012**, *590*, 209–221. [CrossRef] [PubMed]

28. Covasa, M.; Ritter, R.C. Rats maintained on high-fat diets exhibit reduced satiety in response to CCK and bombesin. *Peptides* **1998**, *19*, 1407–1415. [CrossRef]
29. Covasa, M.; Ritter, R.C. Adaptation to high-fat diet reduces inhibition of gastric emptying by CCK and intestinal oleate. *Am. J. Physiol. Regul. Integr. Comp. Physiol.* **2000**, *278*, R166–R170. [CrossRef]
30. Savastano, D.M.; Covasa, M. Adaptation to a high-fat diet leads to hyperphagia and diminished sensitivity to cholecystokinin in rats. *J. Nutr.* **2005**, *135*, 1953–1959. [CrossRef]
31. Swartz, T.D.; Savastano, D.M.; Covasa, M. Reduced sensitivity to cholecystokinin in male rats fed a high-fat diet is reversible. *J. Nutr.* **2010**, *140*, 1698–1703. [CrossRef]
32. Duca, F.A.; Sakar, Y.; Covasa, M. The modulatory role of high fat feeding on gastrointestinal signals in obesity. *J. Nutr. Biochem.* **2013**, *24*, 1663–1677. [CrossRef]
33. De Lartigue, G.; de la Serre, C.B.; Espero, E.; Lee, J.; Raybould, H.E. Leptin resistance in vagal afferent neurons inhibits cholecystokinin signaling and satiation in diet induced obese rats. *PLoS ONE* **2012**, *7*, e32967. [CrossRef] [PubMed]
34. Covasa, M.; Marcuson, J.K.; Ritter, R.C. Diminished satiation in rats exposed to elevated levels of endogenous or exogenous cholecystokinin. *Am. J. Physiol. Regul. Integr. Comp. Physiol.* **2001**, *280*, R331–R337. [CrossRef]
35. Duca, F.A.; Swartz, T.D.; Sakar, Y.; Covasa, M. Decreased intestinal nutrient response in diet-induced obese rats: Role of gut peptides and nutrient receptors. *Int. J. Obes.* **2013**, *37*, 375–381. [CrossRef]
36. Duca, F.A.; Swartz, T.D.; Sakar, Y.; Covasa, M. Increased oral detection, but decreased intestinal signaling for fats in mice lacking gut microbiota. *PLoS ONE* **2012**, *7*, e39748. [CrossRef]
37. Covasa, M.; Grahn, J.; Ritter, R.C. Reduced hindbrain and enteric neuronal response to intestinal oleate in rats maintained on high-fat diet. *Auton. Neurosci. Basic Clin.* **2000**, *84*, 8–18. [CrossRef]
38. De Lartigue, G.; de la Serre, C.B.; Espero, E.; Lee, J.; Raybould, H.E. Diet-induced obesity leads to the development of leptin resistance in vagal afferent neurons. *Am. J. Physiol.-Endocrinol. Metab.* **2011**, *301*, E187–E195. [CrossRef] [PubMed]
39. Friedman, J.M.; Halaas, J.L. Leptin and the regulation of body weight in mammals. *Nature* **1998**, *395*, 763–770. [CrossRef]
40. Townsend, K.L.; Lorenzi, M.M.; Widmaier, E.P. High-fat diet-induced changes in body mass and hypothalamic gene expression in wild-type and leptin-deficient mice. *Endocrine* **2008**, *33*, 176–188. [CrossRef] [PubMed]
41. Münzberg, H.; Flier, J.S.; Bjørbaek, C. Region-specific leptin resistance within the hypothalamus of diet-induced obese mice. *Endocrinology* **2004**, *145*, 4880–4889. [CrossRef]
42. Elias, C.F.; Aschkenasi, C.; Lee, C.; Kelly, J.; Ahima, R.S.; Bjorbaek, C.; Flier, J.S.; Saper, C.B.; Elmquist, J.K. Leptin differentially regulates NPY and POMC neurons projecting to the lateral hypothalamic area. *Neuron* **1999**, *23*, 775–786. [CrossRef]
43. Kim, M.S.; Pak, Y.K.; Jang, P.G.; Namkoong, C.; Choi, Y.S.; Won, J.C.; Kim, K.S.; Kim, S.W.; Kim, H.S.; Park, J.Y.; et al. Role of hypothalamic Foxo1 in the regulation of food intake and energy homeostasis. *Nat. Neurosci.* **2006**, *9*, 901–906. [CrossRef] [PubMed]
44. McMinn, J.E.; Wilkinson, C.W.; Havel, P.J.; Woods, S.C.; Schwartz, M.W. Effect of intracerebroventricular alpha-MSH on food intake, adiposity, c-Fos induction, and neuropeptide expression. *Am. J. Physiol. Regul. Integr. Comp. Physiol.* **2000**, *279*, R695–R703. [CrossRef] [PubMed]
45. La Fleur, S.E.; Vanderschuren, L.J.M.J.; Luijendijk, M.C.; Kloeze, B.M.; Tiesjema, B.; Adan, R.A.H. A reciprocal interaction between food-motivated behavior and diet-induced obesity. *Int. J. Obes.* **2007**, *31*, 1286–1294. [CrossRef]
46. Valdivia, S.; Patrone, A.; Reynaldo, M.; Perello, M. Acute High Fat Diet Consumption Activates the Mesolimbic Circuit and Requires Orexin Signaling in a Mouse Model. *PLoS ONE* **2014**, *9*, e87478. [CrossRef]
47. Kenny, P.J. Reward Mechanisms in Obesity: New Insights and Future Directions. *Neuron* **2011**, *69*, 664–679. [CrossRef]
48. Tellez, L.A.; Medina, S.; Han, W.; Ferreira, J.G.; Licona-Limon, P.; Ren, X.; Lam, T.T.; Schwartz, G.J.; de Araujo, I.E. A gut lipid messenger links excess dietary fat to dopamine deficiency. *Science* **2013**, *341*, 800–802. [CrossRef]
49. Wu, G.D.; Chen, J.; Hoffmann, C.; Bittinger, K.; Chen, Y.-Y.; Keilbaugh, S.A.; Bewtra, M.; Knights, D.; Walters, W.A.; Knight, R. Linking long-term dietary patterns with gut microbial enterotypes. *Science* **2011**, *334*, 105–108. [CrossRef]
50. Shin, N.-R.; Whon, T.W.; Bae, J.-W. Proteobacteria: Microbial signature of dysbiosis in gut microbiota. *Trends Biotechnol.* **2015**, *33*, 496–503. [CrossRef]
51. De La Serre, C.B.; Ellis, C.L.; Lee, J.; Hartman, A.L.; Rutledge, J.C.; Raybould, H.E. Propensity to high-fat diet-induced obesity in rats is associated with changes in the gut microbiota and gut inflammation. *Am. J. Physiol. Gastrointest. Liver Physiol.* **2010**, *299*, G440–G448. [CrossRef]
52. Klingbeil, E.A.; Cawthon, C.; Kirkland, R.; de La Serre, C.B. Potato-Resistant Starch Supplementation Improves Microbiota Dysbiosis, Inflammation, and Gut-Brain Signaling in High Fat-Fed Rats. *Nutrients* **2019**, *11*, 2710. [CrossRef] [PubMed]
53. Vaughn, A.C.; Cooper, E.M.; DiLorenzo, P.M.; O'Loughlin, L.J.; Konkel, M.E.; Peters, J.H.; Hajnal, A.; Sen, T.; Lee, S.H.; de La Serre, C.B.; et al. Energy-dense diet triggers changes in gut microbiota, reorganization of gut-brain vagal communication and increases body fat accumulation. *Acta Neurobiol. Exp.* **2017**, *77*, 18–30. [CrossRef]
54. Do, M.H.; Lee, E.; Oh, M.J.; Kim, Y.; Park, H.Y. High-Glucose or -Fructose Diet Cause Changes of the Gut Microbiota and Metabolic Disorders in Mice without Body Weight Change. *Nutrients* **2018**, *10*, 761. [CrossRef]
55. De Oliveira Neves, V.G.; de Oliveira, D.T.; Oliveira, D.C.; Oliveira Perucci, L.; Dos Santos, T.A.P.; da Costa Fernandes, I.; de Sousa, G.G.; Barboza, N.R.; Guerra-Sá, R. High-sugar diet intake, physical activity, and gut microbiota crosstalk: Implications for obesity in rats. *Food Sci. Nutr.* **2020**, *8*, 5683–5695. [CrossRef]

56. Reichelt, A.C.; Loughman, A.; Bernard, A.; Raipuria, M.; Abbott, K.N.; Dachtler, J.; Van, T.T.H.; Moore, R.J. An intermittent hypercaloric diet alters gut microbiota, prefrontal cortical gene expression and social behaviours in rats. *Nutr. Neurosci.* **2020**, *23*, 613–627. [CrossRef] [PubMed]
57. Kim, M.S.; Hwang, S.S.; Park, E.J.; Bae, J.W. Strict vegetarian diet improves the risk factors associated with metabolic diseases by modulating gut microbiota and reducing intestinal inflammation. *Environ. Microbiol. Rep.* **2013**, *5*, 765–775. [CrossRef] [PubMed]
58. Zimmer, J.; Lange, B.; Frick, J.-S.; Sauer, H.; Zimmermann, K.; Schwiertz, A.; Rusch, K.; Klosterhalfen, S.; Enck, P. A vegan or vegetarian diet substantially alters the human colonic faecal microbiota. *Eur. J. Clin. Nutr.* **2012**, *66*, 53–60. [CrossRef]
59. Matsumoto, N.; Park, J.; Tomizawa, R.; Kawashima, H.; Hosomi, K.; Mizuguchi, K.; Honda, C.; Ozaki, R.; Iwatani, Y.; Watanabe, M.; et al. Relationship between Nutrient Intake and Human Gut Microbiota in Monozygotic Twins. *Medicina* **2021**, *57*, 275. [CrossRef]
60. Yu, D.; Nguyen, S.M.; Yang, Y.; Xu, W.; Cai, H.; Wu, J.; Cai, Q.; Long, J.; Zheng, W.; Shu, X.O. Long-term diet quality is associated with gut microbiome diversity and composition among urban Chinese adults. *Am. J. Clin. Nutr.* **2021**, *113*, 684–694. [CrossRef]
61. Turnbaugh, P.J.; Bäckhed, F.; Fulton, L.; Gordon, J.I. Diet-induced obesity is linked to marked but reversible alterations in the mouse distal gut microbiome. *Cell Host Microbe* **2008**, *3*, 213–223. [CrossRef]
62. Foley, K.P.; Zlitni, S.; Duggan, B.M.; Barra, N.G.; Anhê, F.F.; Cavallari, J.F.; Henriksbo, B.D.; Chen, C.Y.; Huang, M.; Lau, T.C.; et al. Gut microbiota impairs insulin clearance in obese mice. *Mol. Metab.* **2020**, *42*, 101067. [CrossRef]
63. Ridaura, V.K.; Faith, J.J.; Rey, F.E.; Cheng, J.; Duncan, A.E.; Kau, A.L.; Griffin, N.W.; Lombard, V.; Henrissat, B.; Bain, J.R.; et al. Gut microbiota from twins discordant for obesity modulate metabolism in mice. *Science* **2013**, *341*, 1241214. [CrossRef]
64. Huang, W.C.; Chen, Y.H.; Chuang, H.L.; Chiu, C.C.; Huang, C.C. Investigation of the Effects of Microbiota on Exercise Physiological Adaption, Performance, and Energy Utilization Using a Gnotobiotic Animal Model. *Front. Microbiol.* **2019**, *10*, 1906. [CrossRef] [PubMed]
65. Kolida, S.; Tuohy, K.; Gibson, G.R. Prebiotic effects of inulin and oligofructose. *Br. J. Nutr.* **2002**, *87*, S193–S197. [CrossRef]
66. Everard, A.; Belzer, C.; Geurts, L.; Ouwerkerk, J.P.; Druart, C.; Bindels, L.B.; Guiot, Y.; Derrien, M.; Muccioli, G.G.; Delzenne, N.M. Cross-talk between Akkermansia muciniphila and intestinal epithelium controls diet-induced obesity. *Proc. Natl. Acad. Sci. USA* **2013**, *110*, 9066–9071. [CrossRef] [PubMed]
67. Bagarolli, R.A.; Tobar, N.; Oliveira, A.G.; Araújo, T.G.; Carvalho, B.M.; Rocha, G.Z.; Vecina, J.F.; Calisto, K.; Guadagnini, D.; Prada, P.O.; et al. Probiotics modulate gut microbiota and improve insulin sensitivity in DIO mice. *J. Nutr. Biochem.* **2017**, *50*, 16–25. [CrossRef] [PubMed]
68. Osterberg, K.L.; Boutagy, N.E.; McMillan, R.P.; Stevens, J.R.; Frisard, M.I.; Kavanaugh, J.W.; Davy, B.M.; Davy, K.P.; Hulver, M.W. Probiotic supplementation attenuates increases in body mass and fat mass during high-fat diet in healthy young adults. *Obesity* **2015**, *23*, 2364–2370. [CrossRef]
69. Zhang, X.; Grosfeld, A.; Williams, E.; Vasiliauskas, D.; Barretto, S.; Smith, L.; Mariadassou, M.; Philippe, C.; Devime, F.; Melchior, C. Fructose malabsorption induces cholecystokinin expression in the ileum and cecum by changing microbiota composition and metabolism. *FASEB J.* **2019**, *33*, 7126–7142. [CrossRef]
70. Hira, T.; Ogasawara, S.; Yahagi, A.; Kamachi, M.; Li, J.; Nishimura, S.; Sakaino, M.; Yamashita, T.; Kishino, S.; Ogawa, J.; et al. Novel Mechanism of Fatty Acid Sensing in Enteroendocrine Cells: Specific Structures in Oxo-Fatty Acids Produced by Gut Bacteria Are Responsible for CCK Secretion in STC-1 Cells via GPR40. *Mol. Nutr. Food Res.* **2018**, *62*, e1800146. [CrossRef]
71. Riediger, T. The receptive function of hypothalamic and brainstem centres to hormonal and nutrient signals affecting energy balance. *Proc. Nutr. Soc.* **2012**, *71*, 463–477. [CrossRef]
72. Mortensen, P.B.; Clausen, M.R. Short-chain fatty acids in the human colon: Relation to gastrointestinal health and disease. *Scand. J. Gastroenterol.* **1996**, *31*, 132–148. [CrossRef]
73. Koh, A.; De Vadder, F.; Kovatcheva-Datchary, P.; Bäckhed, F. From Dietary Fiber to Host Physiology: Short-Chain Fatty Acids as Key Bacterial Metabolites. *Cell* **2016**, *165*, 1332–1345. [CrossRef] [PubMed]
74. Cani, P.D.; Neyrinck, A.M.; Maton, N.; Delzenne, N.M. Oligofructose promotes satiety in rats fed a high-fat diet: Involvement of glucagon-like Peptide-1. *Obes. Res.* **2005**, *13*, 1000–1007. [CrossRef] [PubMed]
75. Chassaing, B.; Miles-Brown, J.; Pellizzon, M.; Ulman, E.; Ricci, M.; Zhang, L.; Patterson, A.D.; Vijay-Kumar, M.; Gewirtz, A.T. Lack of soluble fiber drives diet-induced adiposity in mice. *Am. J. Physiol. Gastrointest. Liver Physiol.* **2015**, *309*, G528–G541. [CrossRef] [PubMed]
76. Delzenne, N.M.; Cani, P.D.; Daubioul, C.; Neyrinck, A.M. Impact of inulin and oligofructose on gastrointestinal peptides. *Br. J. Nutr.* **2005**, *93*, S157–S161. [CrossRef]
77. Chambers, E.S.; Viardot, A.; Psichas, A.; Morrison, D.J.; Murphy, K.G.; Zac-Varghese, S.E.; MacDougall, K.; Preston, T.; Tedford, C.; Finlayson, G.S.; et al. Effects of targeted delivery of propionate to the human colon on appetite regulation, body weight maintenance and adiposity in overweight adults. *Gut* **2015**, *64*, 1744–1754. [CrossRef]
78. Arora, T.; Akrami, R.; Pais, R.; Bergqvist, L.; Johansson, B.R.; Schwartz, T.W.; Reimann, F.; Gribble, F.M.; Bäckhed, F. Microbial regulation of the L cell transcriptome. *Sci. Rep.* **2018**, *8*, 1207. [CrossRef]
79. Aktar, R.; Parkar, N.; Stentz, R.; Baumard, L.; Parker, A.; Goldson, A.; Brion, A.; Carding, S.; Blackshaw, A.; Peiris, M. Human resident gut microbe Bacteroides thetaiotaomicron regulates colonic neuronal innervation and neurogenic function. *Gut. Microbes* **2020**, *11*, 1745–1757. [CrossRef]

80. Hansen, K.B.; Rosenkilde, M.M.; Knop, F.K.; Wellner, N.; Diep, T.A.; Rehfeld, J.F.; Andersen, U.B.; Holst, J.J.; Hansen, H.S. 2-Oleoyl glycerol is a GPR119 agonist and signals GLP-1 release in humans. *J. Clin. Endocrinol. Metab.* **2011**, *96*, E1409–E1417. [CrossRef]
81. Cherbut, C.; Ferrier, L.; Rozé, C.; Anini, Y.; Blottière, H.; Lecannu, G.; Galmiche, J.-P. Short-chain fatty acids modify colonic motility through nerves and polypeptide YY release in the rat. *Am. J. Physiol. Gastrointest. Liver Physiol.* **1998**, *275*, G1415–G1422. [CrossRef]
82. McLaughlin, J.; Lucà, M.G.; Jones, M.N.; D'Amato, M.; Dockray, G.J.; Thompson, D.G. Fatty acid chain length determines cholecystokinin secretion and effect on human gastric motility. *Gastroenterology* **1999**, *116*, 46–53. [CrossRef]
83. Daly, K.; Al-Rammahi, M.; Moran, A.; Marcello, M.; Ninomiya, Y.; Shirazi-Beechey, S.P. Sensing of amino acids by the gut-expressed taste receptor T1R1-T1R3 stimulates CCK secretion. *Am. J. Physiol. Gastrointest. Liver Physiol.* **2013**, *304*, G271–G282. [CrossRef]
84. Moran, T.H.; Baldessarini, A.R.; Salorio, C.F.; Lowery, T.; Schwartz, G.J. Vagal afferent and efferent contributions to the inhibition of food intake by cholecystokinin. *Am. J. Physiol. Regul. Integr. Comp. Physiol.* **1997**, *272*, R1245–R1251. [CrossRef]
85. Wang, L.; Martínez, V.; Barrachina, M.D.; Taché, Y. Fos expression in the brain induced by peripheral injection of CCK or leptin plus CCK in fasted lean mice. *Brain Res.* **1998**, *791*, 157–166. [CrossRef]
86. Cani, P.D.; Amar, J.; Iglesias, M.A.; Poggi, M.; Knauf, C.; Bastelica, D.; Neyrinck, A.M.; Fava, F.; Tuohy, K.M.; Chabo, C. Metabolic endotoxemia initiates obesity and insulin resistance. *Diabetes* **2007**, *56*, 1761–1772. [CrossRef]
87. Waise, T.M.Z.; Toshinai, K.; Naznin, F.; NamKoong, C.; Md Moin, A.S.; Sakoda, H.; Nakazato, M. One-day high-fat diet induces inflammation in the nodose ganglion and hypothalamus of mice. *Biochem. Biophys. Res. Commun.* **2015**, *464*, 1157–1162. [CrossRef]
88. Aguzzi, A.; Barres, B.A.; Bennett, M.L. Microglia: Scapegoat, saboteur, or something else? *Science* **2013**, *339*, 156–161. [CrossRef] [PubMed]
89. Perry, V.H.; Nicoll, J.A.; Holmes, C. Microglia in neurodegenerative disease. *Nat. Rev. Neurol.* **2010**, *6*, 193. [CrossRef]
90. Sheppard, O.; Coleman, M.P.; Durrant, C.S. Lipopolysaccharide-induced neuroinflammation induces presynaptic disruption through a direct action on brain tissue involving microglia-derived interleukin 1 beta. *J. Neuroinflamm.* **2019**, *16*, 106. [CrossRef] [PubMed]
91. Han, Q.; Lin, Q.; Huang, P.; Chen, M.; Hu, X.; Fu, H.; He, S.; Shen, F.; Zeng, H.; Deng, Y. Microglia-derived IL-1β contributes to axon development disorders and synaptic deficit through p38-MAPK signal pathway in septic neonatal rats. *J. Neuroinflamm.* **2017**, *14*, 52. [CrossRef] [PubMed]
92. Mestre, L.; Carrillo-Salinas, F.J.; Mecha, M.; Feliú, A.; Espejo, C.; Álvarez-Cermeño, J.C.; Villar, L.M.; Guaza, C. Manipulation of Gut Microbiota Influences Immune Responses, Axon Preservation, and Motor Disability in a Model of Progressive Multiple Sclerosis. *Front. Immunol.* **2019**, *10*, 1374. [CrossRef] [PubMed]
93. Thaler, J.P.; Yi, C.-X.; Schur, E.A.; Guyenet, S.J.; Hwang, B.H.; Dietrich, M.O.; Zhao, X.; Sarruf, D.A.; Izgur, V.; Maravilla, K.R.; et al. Obesity is associated with hypothalamic injury in rodents and humans. *J. Clin. Investig.* **2012**, *122*, 153–162. [CrossRef]
94. Hermes, S.M.; Andresen, M.C.; Aicher, S.A. Localization of TRPV1 and P2X3 in unmyelinated and myelinated vagal afferents in the rat. *J. Chem. Neuroanat.* **2016**, *72*, 1–7. [CrossRef]
95. Fouesnard, M.; Zoppi, J.; Petera, M.; Le Gleau, L.; Migné, C.; Devime, F.; Durand, S.; Benani, A.; Chaffron, S.; Douard, V.; et al. Dietary switch to Western diet induces hypothalamic adaptation associated with gut microbiota dysbiosis in rats. *Int. J. Obes.* **2021**, *45*, 1271–1283. [CrossRef] [PubMed]
96. Rorato, R.; Borges, B.C.; Uchoa, E.T.; Antunes-Rodrigues, J.; Elias, C.F.; Elias, L.L.K. LPS-Induced Low-Grade Inflammation Increases Hypothalamic JNK Expression and Causes Central Insulin Resistance Irrespective of Body Weight Changes. *Int. J. Mol. Sci.* **2017**, *18*, 1431. [CrossRef] [PubMed]
97. Maldonado-Ruiz, R.; Cárdenas-Tueme, M.; Montalvo-Martínez, L.; Vidaltamayo, R.; Garza-Ocañas, L.; Reséndez-Perez, D.; Camacho, A. Priming of Hypothalamic Ghrelin Signaling and Microglia Activation Exacerbate Feeding in Rats' Offspring Following Maternal Overnutrition. *Nutrients* **2019**, *11*, 1241. [CrossRef]
98. De Git, K.C.; Adan, R.A. Leptin resistance in diet-induced obesity: The role of hypothalamic inflammation. *Obes. Rev.* **2015**, *16*, 207–224. [CrossRef]
99. Schéle, E.; Grahnemo, L.; Anesten, F.; Hallén, A.; Bäckhed, F.; Jansson, J.-O. The gut microbiota reduces leptin sensitivity and the expression of the obesity-suppressing neuropeptides proglucagon (Gcg) and brain-derived neurotrophic factor (Bdnf) in the central nervous system. *Endocrinology* **2013**, *154*, 3643–3651. [CrossRef]
100. Dudele, A.; Fischer, C.W.; Elfving, B.; Wegener, G.; Wang, T.; Lund, S. Chronic exposure to low doses of lipopolysaccharide and high-fat feeding increases body mass without affecting glucose tolerance in female rats. *Physiol. Rep.* **2015**, *3*, e12584. [CrossRef]
101. Cheng, Y.C.; Liu, J.R. Effect of *Lactobacillus rhamnosus* GG on Energy Metabolism, Leptin Resistance, and Gut Microbiota in Mice with Diet-Induced Obesity. *Nutrients* **2020**, *12*, 2557. [CrossRef] [PubMed]
102. Meye, F.J.; Adan, R.A. Feelings about food: The ventral tegmental area in food reward and emotional eating. *Trends Pharmacol. Sci.* **2014**, *35*, 31–40. [CrossRef] [PubMed]
103. Heijtz, R.D.; Wang, S.; Anuar, F.; Qian, Y.; Björkholm, B.; Samuelsson, A.; Hibberd, M.L.; Forssberg, H.; Pettersson, S. Normal gut microbiota modulates brain development and behavior. *Proc. Natl. Acad. Sci. USA* **2011**, *108*, 3047–3052. [CrossRef]
104. Roitman, M.F.; Stuber, G.D.; Phillips, P.E.; Wightman, R.M.; Carelli, R.M. Dopamine operates as a subsecond modulator of food seeking. *J. Neurosci.* **2004**, *24*, 1265–1271. [CrossRef]

105. Desbonnet, L.; Clarke, G.; Traplin, A.; O'Sullivan, O.; Crispie, F.; Moloney, R.D.; Cotter, P.D.; Dinan, T.G.; Cryan, J.F. Gut microbiota depletion from early adolescence in mice: Implications for brain and behaviour. *Brain Behav. Immun.* **2015**, *48*, 165–173. [CrossRef]
106. Kiraly, D.D.; Walker, D.M.; Calipari, E.S.; Labonte, B.; Issler, O.; Pena, C.J.; Ribeiro, E.A.; Russo, S.J.; Nestler, E.J. Alterations of the Host Microbiome Affect Behavioral Responses to Cocaine. *Sci. Rep.* **2016**, *6*, 35455. [CrossRef]
107. Van de Wouw, M.; Boehme, M.; Lyte, J.M.; Wiley, N.; Strain, C.; O'Sullivan, O.; Clarke, G.; Stanton, C.; Dinan, T.G.; Cryan, J.F. Short-chain fatty acids: Microbial metabolites that alleviate stress-induced brain-gut axis alterations. *J. Physiol.* **2018**, *596*, 4923–4944. [CrossRef]
108. Delbès, A.S.; Castel, J.; Denis, R.G.P.; Morel, C.; Quiñones, M.; Everard, A.; Cani, P.D.; Massiera, F.; Luquet, S.H. Prebiotics Supplementation Impact on the Reinforcing and Motivational Aspect of Feeding. *Front. Endocrinol.* **2018**, *9*, 273. [CrossRef]
109. Magnuson, B.A.; Carakostas, M.C.; Moore, N.H.; Poulos, S.P.; Renwick, A.G. Biological fate of low-calorie sweeteners. *Nutr. Rev.* **2016**, *74*, 670–689. [CrossRef]
110. Pang, M.D.; Goossens, G.H.; Blaak, E.E. The Impact of Artificial Sweeteners on Body Weight Control and Glucose Homeostasis. *Front. Nutr.* **2020**, *7*, 598340. [CrossRef] [PubMed]
111. Van Opstal, A.M.; Kaal, I.; van den Berg-Huysmans, A.A.; Hoeksma, M.; Blonk, C.; Pijl, H.; Rombouts, S.; van der Grond, J. Dietary sugars and non-caloric sweeteners elicit different homeostatic and hedonic responses in the brain. *Nutrition* **2019**, *60*, 80–86. [CrossRef] [PubMed]
112. Nettleton, J.E.; Klancic, T.; Schick, A.; Choo, A.C.; Shearer, J.; Borgland, S.L.; Chleilat, F.; Mayengbam, S.; Reimer, R.A. Low-Dose Stevia (Rebaudioside A) Consumption Perturbs Gut Microbiota and the Mesolimbic Dopamine Reward System. *Nutrients* **2019**, *11*, 1248. [CrossRef]
113. Peters, J.H.; Gallaher, Z.R.; Ryu, V.; Czaja, K. Withdrawal and Restoration of Central Vagal Afferents within the Dorsal Vagal Complex Following Subdiaphragmatic Vagotomy. *J. Comp. Neurol.* **2013**, *521*, 3584–3599. [CrossRef]
114. Santacruz, A.; Marcos, A.; Warnberg, J.; Marti, A.; Martin-Matillas, M.; Campoy, C.; Moreno, L.; Veiga, O.; Redondo-Figuero, C.; Garagorri, J.; et al. Interplay between weight loss and gut microbiota composition in overweight adolescents. *Obesity* **2009**, *17*, 1906–1915. [CrossRef]
115. Liou, A.P.; Paziuk, M.; Luevano, J.-M.; Machineni, S.; Turnbaugh, P.J.; Kaplan, L.M. Conserved Shifts in the Gut Microbiota Due to Gastric Bypass Reduce Host Weight and Adiposity. *Sci. Transl. Med.* **2013**, *5*, 178ra41. [CrossRef]
116. Seganfredo, F.B.; Blume, C.A.; Moehlecke, M.; Giongo, A.; Casagrande, D.S.; Spolidoro, J.V.N.; Padoin, A.V.; Schaan, B.D.; Mottin, C.C. Weight-loss interventions and gut microbiota changes in overweight and obese patients: A systematic review. *Obes. Rev.* **2017**, *18*, 832–851. [CrossRef]
117. Cani, P.D.; Lecourt, E.; Dewulf, E.M.; Sohet, F.M.; Pachikian, B.D.; Naslain, D.; De Backer, F.; Neyrinck, A.M.; Delzenne, N.M. Gut microbiota fermentation of prebiotics increases satietogenic and incretin gut peptide production with consequences for appetite sensation and glucose response after a meal. *Am. J. Clin. Nutr.* **2009**, *90*, 1236–1243. [CrossRef]
118. Cani, P.D.; Neyrinck, A.M.; Fava, F.; Knauf, C.; Burcelin, R.G.; Tuohy, K.M.; Gibson, G.R.; Delzenne, N.M. Selective increases of bifidobacteria in gut microflora improve high-fat-diet-induced diabetes in mice through a mechanism associated with endotoxaemia. *Diabetologia* **2007**, *50*, 2374–2383. [CrossRef]
119. Membrez, M.; Blancher, F.; Jaquet, M.; Bibiloni, R.; Cani, P.D.; Burcelin, R.G.; Corthesy, I.; Mace, K.; Chou, C.J. Gut microbiota modulation with norfloxacin and ampicillin enhances glucose tolerance in mice. *FASEB J.* **2008**, *22*, 2416–2426. [CrossRef]
120. DeFuria, J.; Bennett, G.; Strissel, K.J.; Perfield, J.W.; Milbury, P.E.; Greenberg, A.S.; Obin, M.S. Dietary Blueberry Attenuates Whole-Body Insulin Resistance in High Fat-Fed Mice by Reducing Adipocyte Death and Its Inflammatory Sequelae. *J. Nutr.* **2009**, *139*, 1510–1516. [CrossRef]

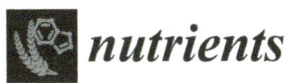

Review

Ghrelin and Glucagon-Like Peptide-1: A Gut-Brain Axis Battle for Food Reward

Lea Decarie-Spain [1] and Scott E. Kanoski [1,2,*]

1. Human & Evolutionary Biology Section, Department of Biological Sciences, University of Southern California, Los Angeles, CA 90089, USA; decaries@usc.edu
2. Neuroscience Graduate Program, University of Southern California, Los Angeles, CA 90089, USA
* Correspondence: kanoski@usc.edu

Abstract: Eating behaviors are influenced by the reinforcing properties of foods that can favor decisions driven by reward incentives over metabolic needs. These food reward-motivated behaviors are modulated by gut-derived peptides such as ghrelin and glucagon-like peptide-1 (GLP-1) that are well-established to promote or reduce energy intake, respectively. In this review we highlight the antagonizing actions of ghrelin and GLP-1 on various behavioral constructs related to food reward/reinforcement, including reactivity to food cues, conditioned meal anticipation, effort-based food-motivated behaviors, and flavor-nutrient preference and aversion learning. We integrate physiological and behavioral neuroscience studies conducted in both rodents and human to illustrate translational findings of interest for the treatment of obesity or metabolic impairments. Collectively, the literature discussed herein highlights a model where ghrelin and GLP-1 regulate food reward-motivated behaviors via both competing and independent neurobiological and behavioral mechanisms.

Keywords: obesity; cue reactivity; GLP-1; meal anticipation; motivation; nutrient preference; flavor; aversion

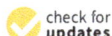

Citation: Decarie-Spain, L.; Kanoski, S.E. Ghrelin and Glucagon-Like Peptide-1: A Gut-Brain Axis Battle for Food Reward. *Nutrients* 2021, 13, 977. https://doi.org/10.3390/nu13030977

Academic Editor: Christine Feinle-Bisset

Received: 24 February 2021
Accepted: 14 March 2021
Published: 17 March 2021

Publisher's Note: MDPI stays neutral with regard to jurisdictional claims in published maps and institutional affiliations.

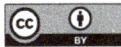

Copyright: © 2021 by the authors. Licensee MDPI, Basel, Switzerland. This article is an open access article distributed under the terms and conditions of the Creative Commons Attribution (CC BY) license (https:// creativecommons.org/licenses/by/ 4.0/).

1. Introduction

The widespread availability of highly palatable and easily affordable food options in the modern era has substantially altered human eating behavior. The decision to eat, not to eat, and/or to select certain food items is largely regulated by hedonic and reward incentives rather than by energetic need. "Food reward" is a poorly defined, yet commonly used concept that generally refers to food-directed behaviors influenced by the potent reinforcing properties of certain food items, often rich in fat and sugar, that are highly palatable but also metabolically maladaptive. The hyper-reinforcing nature of such foods can contribute to the establishment and maintenance of food-motivated habits and lack of impulse control that can lead to metabolic dysfunction and/or obesity over the long term.

Food reward-motivated behaviors are potently influenced by gut-derived peptides that are released by cells of the gastrointestinal (GI) tract. In this review we focus on two such peptides, ghrelin and glucagon-like peptide-1 (GLP-1), that have opposing effects on energy consumption. Ghrelin is a stomach-derived hormone that increases appetite and food intake via its G protein–coupled receptor, type 1a growth hormone secretagogue receptor (GHSR1a) [1]. Circulating ghrelin levels are elevated during energy restriction and in anticipation of eating [2] and are decreased following a meal [3]. Glucagon-like peptide-1 (GLP-1) is a peptide secreted from L cells in the distal intestines and from neurons in the nucleus tractus solitarius (NTS) of the caudal brain stem. In addition to its well-known incretin effects, GLP-1 (and its FDA-approved analogs) potently reduces food intake via its G protein-coupled receptor, GLP-1 receptor (GLP-1R). Both ghrelin and GLP-1 affect food intake and metabolism via multiple biological pathways, including a paracrine vagus nerve pathway [4,5], blood-to-brain signaling, and in the case of GLP-1, projections from the GLP-1-producing preproglucagon neurons in the NTS throughout the neuraxis [6].

Several lines of emerging evidence highlight a role for both ghrelin and GLP-1 signaling in the mediation of food reward-motivated behaviors, and indeed, both systems are pharmaceutical targets for metabolic disorders. The present review addresses the competing influences of ghrelin and GLP-1 on various behavioral and neurocognitive appetitive domains, including reactivity to food cues, learned/conditioned meal anticipation, effort-based food motivated-behaviors, and flavor-nutrient preference and aversion learning. Preclinical rodent model studies reviewed herein emphasize sites of action in the brain mediating the influence of these two peptide systems on various food reward-associated behavioral domains. Studies investigating both endogenous and exogenous ghrelin and GLP-1 signaling in human participants are also reviewed, with an emphasis on the effects of bariatric surgery on these neurobiological processes.

2. Reactivity to Food Cues

Neural reactivity to cues associated with palatable food and the craving and behavioral responses that these cues elicit can be predictive of eating behaviors and propensity for weight gain [7]. Recent rodent model studies discussed herein reveal competing influences of ghrelin and GLP-1 on motivated responses to food reward-conditioned cues.

2.1. Rodent Studies

Results from rodent models reveal that ghrelin promotes food-directed behavior in response to a food-predictive cue. For example, oral gavage with the GHSR antagonist compound 26 in mice abolished food cue-potentiated eating [8]. Another study, however, reported that peripheral administration of a GHSR antagonist impaired the initiation of eating in a cue-potentiated eating procedure, yet had no effect on total sucrose consumed. The ventral subregion of the hippocampus (HPCv) may be a site of action mediating these effects, as rats trained to associate a conditioned stimulus (CS+) with palatable food availability consumed a larger number of meals immediately following CS+ presentation when they received ghrelin administration to the HPCv [9], an outcome that was not observed following presentation of stimuli not associated with food (CS−).

In addition to the HPCv, the VTA may be a brain region mediating ghrelin's effects on food cue-stimulated eating. For example, in rats that had extinguished conditioned lever press responding for chocolate pellets, intra-VTA ghrelin administration facilitated the reinstatement of instrumental responding in response to a food reward-associated stimulus [10]. In contrast, however, another study reported that ghrelin infused directly into the VTA in rats did not influence lever pressing in response to food-associated cue presentation, although this same treatment increased appetitive lever pressing in a context with no stimuli presented [11]. More work is needed to further identify the specific brain regions, neural pathways, and behavioral parameters through which ghrelin potentiates eating and/or motivated responding in response to cues associated with palatable food.

Ghrelin may promote food cue-potentiated eating, in part, by acting as an indicator of fasting and/or food availability itself. For example, in the deprivation intensity discrimination task, where rats discriminate reinforcement outcomes based on food restriction-determined interoceptive state, either peripheral, intracerebroventricular (icv), or direct HPCv administration of ghrelin in food-sated rats mimics their conditioned appetitive behavior as if they had been food deprived for 24 h [12,13]. Ghrelin also alters baseline activity of dopamine neurons projecting from the VTA to the nucleus accumbens (ACB) via intraperitoneal (ip) injection in rats [14] or bath application on rat and mouse brain slices [15], an outcome similar to that occurring during fasting [16,17]. Alternatively, ghrelin signaling may also influence food cue reactivity by acting as a meal initiation signal. For example, neuronal firing patterns in the mediobasal hypothalamus of rats following the presentation of a cue predicting palatable food availability are replicated by an ip injection of ghrelin [18]. Finally, ghrelin may also affect cue-potentiated eating by enhancing the palatability of the reinforcer, an outcome consistent with findings that peripheral administration of a GHSR antagonist reduces sucrose palatability in mice as assessed via licking microstructure analyses [19].

While the effects of GLP-1 signaling on food cue reactivity in rodents have not been investigated as extensively compared to ghrelin, a recent study demonstrated that icv infusion of the GLP-1R agonist exendin-4 inhibits both phasic firing of ACB-projecting VTA dopamine neurons and food anticipatory approach behaviors in response to sucrose-predictive cues in rats [20]. In addition, infusion of exendin-4 into the paraventricular thalamus (PVT) in rats dampened the reinstatement of palatable food cue-induced lever pressing, as well as decreased the excitability of PVT neurons projecting to the ACB [21]. These findings suggest that GLP-1 reduces palatable food cue-induced food-seeking and eating by minimizing VTA and PVT input to the ACB. However, rodent model research on GLP-1 interactions with food cue-associated responses is thus far scarce, thereby highlighting a critical area for future preclinical investigation.

2.2. Human Studies

Functional brain imaging studies in healthy individuals provide additional evidence that ghrelin and GLP-1 have opposing effects on palatable food cue reactivity. For example, endogenous fasting levels of ghrelin predict activation of brain regions involved in reward processing in response to pictures of highly caloric and palatable food, including the caudate, amygdala, anterior cingulate, hippocampus, insula, and orbitofrontal cortex (OFC) [22,23]. In addition to these ghrelin-associated neural responses, plasma ghrelin concentrations can rise in response to viewing food pictures, suggesting a possible bidirectional relationship between ghrelin release and brain activity [24].

In the opposing direction, endogenous circulating concentrations of GLP-1 following consumption of a sugary beverage are negatively associated with dorsal striatum and OFC activation upon visual food cue presentation [25,26]. Further, in overweight participants following a weight loss program, postprandial GLP-1 levels along with dorsolateral prefrontal cortex (PFC) responsiveness to food cues were the best predictors of body mass index reduction [27]. Thus, interventions targeting food cue reactivity via GLP-1 signaling could be of interest for therapies targeting obesity.

In addition to the relationship between endogenous levels of ghrelin and food cue reactivity, administration of exogenous ghrelin modulates brain reactivity to food cues. For instance, subcutaneous (sc) injection of ghrelin in food-sated individuals increased OFC blood -oxygen-level dependent (BOLD) activity upon presentation of high energy food images, to an extent similar to the increased OFC BOLD response following an overnight fast [28]. In another group of healthy participants, intravenous (iv) ghrelin infusion potentiated activity in the ventromedial PFC to in response to abstract images (not food) paired to a food odor [29]. Interestingly, the same study revealed that functional connectivity between the hippocampus and the ventral striatum (containing the ACB) is increased by ghrelin and this is accompanied by improved performance in a reward prediction task. Administration of ghrelin (iv) also enhanced the BOLD responses in the hippocampus, VTA, insula, caudate, and amygdala in response to food cues, with responsiveness of the amygdala and OFC also being positively associated with self-reported hunger [30].

The actions of exogenous GLP-1 on brain reactivity to food cues have been largely investigated in obese and type 2 diabetic populations given the efficacy of long-acting GLP-1 analogs, such as liraglutide, in treating these metabolic conditions. For instance, obesity is characterized by greater insula responsiveness to food cues relative to normal weight individuals and this difference is abolished by acute treatment with the GLP-1R agonist exenatide [31]. Furthermore, the GLP-1-dependent suppression of insula reactivity to food cues predicted both a reduction in caloric intake [31] and lower scores for emotional eating [32]. In addition to the insula, obese individuals with type 2 diabetes show greater activation of the amygdala and OFC upon food cue presentation in a fasted state [32,33]. In a fed state, these effects are replicated by acute injection of the GLP-1R antagonist, exendin-9-39, especially in the type 2 diabetes group [33]. Chronic GLP-1 analog treatment also appears to alter food cue-induced brain activity responses, as 17 days of treatment with liraglutide in diabetic patients is sufficient to reduce insula and putamen responsiveness to highly desirable food cues, in conjunction with a decrease in hunger ratings in response to the food cues [34,35]. Interestingly, these changes occurred prior to any significant reduction in body weight, thus supporting a role for GLP-1 signaling in blunting reactivity to food cues independent of effects on body weight. However, in a subsequent cohort of diabetic patients treated for 5 weeks with liraglutide, activation of the OFC in response to food cues was increased, despite successful weight loss, improved metabolic profile, and reduced fat intake [36]. It remains to be determined whether this compensatory increase in OFC recruitment stems from negative energy balance, and/or whether this outcome impacts long-term weight maintenance.

Various bariatric surgery models are associated with acute improvements in metabolic function even prior to substantial weight loss (for review see [37]). Drastic change in circulating levels and amelioration of sensitivity to gut peptides such as ghrelin and GLP-1 likely contribute to the superiority of bariatric surgeries, such as Roux-en-Y gastric bypass (RYGB) and vertical sleeve gastrectomy (VSG), compared to dietary interventions alone in promoting sustainable weight loss [38,39]. Bariatric and dietary interventions may influence brain function differentially as bariatric surgery decreases resting-state functional connectivity between the precuneus and the insula, whereas dietary interventions increase it [40]. Thus, it may be that bariatric surgery promotes changes in neural activity that favor cognitive control over appetitive processes. For example, VSG surgery enhances resting-state functional connectivity between the hippocampus and the insula [41] and between the dorsolateral PFC and the anterior cingulate, with these outcomes accompanied by dampened cravings for high calorie foods [42] and reduced fasting levels of ghrelin [41,42]. These surgical induced changes in neural activity may influence food cue reactivity, as VSG surgery shifts attention from food to non-food cues, as well as reduces cravings and pleasantness ratings for food items [43]. Further, reductions in dorsolateral PFC BOLD response to food cues correlate with drops in fasting levels of ghrelin [44].

Similarly to the effects of GLP-1R agonism described above, RYGB surgery reduces insula and PFC BOLD signals in response to visual and auditory food cues in fasted obese women [45]. RYGB surgery also increases precuneus BOLD response to low fat/sugar food cues while decreasing response to high fat/sugar food cues [46]. Finally, weight loss and decreased appetite for sweet and fat foods after RYGB surgery coincides with reduced resting-state functional connectivity between the insula and the anterior cingulate as well as improved sensitivity of the default mode network to GLP-1R blockade [47].

2.3. Summary

Preclinical rodent model studies indicate that ghrelin signaling promotes conditioned appetitive behaviors and eating in response to food-associated cues, possibly by contributing to an interoceptive state analogous to fasting, by signaling meal anticipation, and/or by increasing the palatability of food. On the other hand, GLP-1 signaling may prevent cue-induced food-seeking by inhibiting neuronal input from the VTA and PVT to the ACB. These preclinical results are supported by functional neuroimaging analyses in humans revealing that circulating levels of ghrelin predict brain BOLD response to visual food cues while postprandial GLP-1 levels have opposite effects. Further, administration of exogenous ghrelin in food-sated individuals mimics the enhancement of brain BOLD response to food cues induced by fasting, whereas GLP-1R antagonism prevents the reduction of brain reactivity to food cues after consuming a meal. Short-term agonism of GLP-1R (via FDA-approved GLP-1 analog pharmacology) normalizes brain BOLD response to food cues in obese and diabetic individuals, although compensatory mechanisms may occur with longer duration of treatment. Similarly, bariatric surgery influences resting-state brain connectivity and dampens BOLD signal upon food cue presentation and these changes coincide with reduced fasting levels of ghrelin. Altogether, these results highlight the antagonizing actions of ghrelin and GLP-1 on brain reactivity to food cues and the potential therapeutic benefits of modulating these gut peptides.

3. Meal Anticipation

While gut peptide release is directly influenced by both long-term metabolic state and recent energy consumption, the learned anticipation of food availability is also sufficient to influence ghrelin and GLP-1 levels. For example, this is perhaps most dramatically illustrated by work from Woods and colleagues revealing that circulating levels of both GLP-1 and ghrelin are elevated prior to scheduled food access in meal entrained rodents [2,48]. Such endocrine responses may serve as a cephalic physiological primer for nutrient sensing and digestion. Conditioned meal-related factors can also influence postprandial endocrine levels, as meal anticipation potentiates postprandial suppression of circulating ghrelin in healthy men [49]. In this section we review rodent studies exploring the influences of ghrelin and GLP-1 signaling on food anticipatory activity and caloric intake in a scheduled feeding paradigm, as well as research in human participants measuring endocrine and neural outcomes in anticipation of eating.

3.1. Rodent Studies

Rodents on a restricted feeding schedule, with only a few hours of daily access to chow at a consistent time each day, rapidly develop a rise in locomotor activity in the few hours preceding food access, particularly activity directed towards the location of subsequent food access. This type of "food anticipatory activity" (FAA) is dampened in transgenic mice lacking either ghrelin or GHSR [15,50–52], thus supporting a role for ghrelin as a conditioned meal anticipation signal. Blunted FAA in GHSR knock-out (KO) mice is associated with decreased neural activation in the hypothalamus [52], VTA, and ACB shell [53]. Similar to cue-induced eating, the HPCv may be a critical site of action for ghrelin's effects on meal anticipation as HPCv GHSR blockade reduced chow consumption in meal-entrained rats but had no effect on energy intake in non-entrained rats [54].

Ghrelin also appears to influence FAA based on scheduled access to palatable food in otherwise nonrestricted rats. For example, in rats with ad libitum access to chow, but predictable restricted access to high fat/sugar foods for a few hours daily, icv ghrelin increases FAA prior to the high fat/sugar meal and this effect is prevented by treatment with a GHSR antagonist [55]. The VTA may be a site mediating ghrelin effects on FAA for palatable food access, as intra-VTA ghrelin administration in rats entrained with access to a palatable high fat diet increases consumption in a GHSR dependent manner [56]. In contrast, another study reported decreased caloric intake of a high fat diet, but increased consumption of chow, following icv and VTA ghrelin infusion [57]. Although the contribution of ghrelin to FAA for standard chow is well established, additional work is required to further refine the role of ghrelin on FAA for palatable vs. bland/standard food access.

While the role of GLP-1 in food anticipatory behavior has not been as extensively investigated as ghrelin, GLP-1's effects appear to oppose those of ghrelin. For example, infusion of the GLP-1R agonist exendin-4 into the ACB of rats with scheduled access to a high fat/sugar diet prevented the enhanced FAA and food consumption induced by mu opioid receptor agonism [58]. Paradoxically, however, both ghrelin and GLP-1 levels in circulation are increased prior to meal access in meal-entrained rats, as alluded to above in the work from Woods and colleagues. However, the temporal parameters are quite different. GLP-1 levels peak approximately 1 h before meal presentation and return to baseline prior to food presentation. Levels of ghrelin, on the other hand, peak approximately 30 min prior to food access yet remain substantially higher than baseline at the time of meal presentation [2]. GLP-1R antagonism prior to a conditioned spike in GLP-1 release reduced food intake at the subsequent food access period whereas iv infusion of a selective GLP-1R antagonist after the endogenous rise, but before food presentation, had the opposite effect [48]. While collectively these findings suggest that ghrelin and GLP-1 signaling have opposing effects on FAA and conditioned eating, more preclinical rodent work is needed to understand the functional role of premeal GLP-1 release, as well as the larger role of GLP-1 in meal anticipatory behavior.

3.2. Human Studies

Circulating levels of gut peptides in human participants fluctuate in accordance with the timing as well as the composition of an anticipated meal. For example, plasma ghrelin levels peak immediately prior to eating in individuals on a fixed intermeal interval schedule, suggesting that ghrelin primes meal initiation [59]. Interestingly, one's individual habitual meal patterns appear to dictate the timing of a peak in fasting ghrelin prior to eating and this peak of ghrelin does not necessarily precede hunger [60]. These findings suggest ghrelin acts as a conditioned signal for meal anticipation rather than promoting hunger, per se. In addition to timing, preprandial concentrations of ghrelin can be influenced by the hedonic value of a meal. For instance, fasting levels of ghrelin are significantly higher in anticipation of consumption of chocolate versus an isocaloric non-palatable food item in obese male participants [61]. While less is understood about the fluctuation of endogenous GLP-1 level with regards to habitual eating patterns, there is evidence that exogenous GLP-1R agonist administration blunts FAA-associated neural responses. For example, iv infusion of the GLP-1R agonist exenatide dampens the heightened putamen, insula and amygdala BOLD responses in anticipation of chocolate milk delivery in diabetic individuals [62]. Thus, evidence to date is consistent with the notion that ghrelin and GLP-1 signaling have opposing effects on FAA and conditioned food consumption, and that these systems appear to interact with both the temporal and hedonic components of a meal.

3.3. Summary

Ghrelin signaling is strongly tied to FAA in rodent models of scheduled feeding, and these effects may involve signaling to the HPCv and VTA. GLP-1 appears to act via a more complex temporal relationship with conditioned feeding that warrants future studies, although there is evidence that FAA is blunted by ACB GLP-1R activation. In humans, the meal anticipatory rise in circulating ghrelin levels is adapted to both habitual meal patterns and the hedonic value of a meal, whereas GLP-1R agonism provides an avenue to normalize elevated brain reactivity in anticipation of palatable feeding.

4. Food Motivation

Willingness to work to obtain food is not surprisingly enhanced by a negative energy balance, but even under conditions energy repletion or sufficiency, food-motivated behaviors are influenced by gut peptides such as ghrelin and GLP-1. In rodents, motivation to seek out and/or work for food can be assessed in various conditioning tasks. For example, expression of a conditioned place preference (CPP) for a context previously paired with a food reward is indicative of food motivation in rodents, and when CPP compartment preference tests occur without food reinforcement, this procedure can assess food seeking in the absence of consumption. An alternative test is an appetitive operant conditioning task where the animal must press on a lever (or nose poke or other operant response) in order to obtain a food pellet, where the overall number of instrumental responses and the breakpoint (maximal number of presses the animal is willing to perform in order to obtain a reward in a progressive ratio schedule of reinforcement where cost of reward increases across the session) are measures of food motivation/willingness to work for food. Operant responding for food rewards can also be applied to human studies using handgrips or computer mouse clicks, for example.

4.1. Rodent Studies

Peripheral ghrelin administration appears to promote palatable food seeking behavior in rodents. For example, sc injection of ghrelin enhances CPP expression for a high fat diet in mice, whereas CPP expression is absent in GHSR KO mice or wildtype mice receiving acute oral gavage of the GHSR antagonist Compound 26 [63]. Similarly, blocking GHSR signaling with the GHSR antagonist, JMV2959, abolishes the expression of a CPP for chocolate in rats [64]. These effects are not mediated by the lateral parabrachial nucleus (lPBN) as infusion of ghrelin into this region has no impact on CPP for chocolate in rats [65]. Instead, ghrelin may interact with the hypothalamic neuropeptide orexin to drive CPP for palatable food given that CPP expression for a high fat diet is absent in orexin KO mice and in wildtype mice receiving ip injection of the orexin receptor antagonist SB-334867 [63].

In contrast, GLP-1R agonism blunts the expression of a CPP for palatable food in rodents. For example, administration of exendin-4 via ip injection in rats abolishes expression of a CPP for chocolate [66] and this suppression of CPP for palatable food is replicated with infusion of exendin-4 into the NTS [67,68] or the PVT [21], but not the HPCv [69]. This blunting of palatable food-motivated behavior may involve altered dopaminergic signaling as intra-NTS exendin-4 administration, in addition to blocking CPP expression, also increases gene expression levels for the catecholamine synthesis rate-limiting enzyme tyrosine hydroxylase (TH) and dopamine receptor type 2 in the VTA [68].

Ghrelin enhances willingness to work for palatable food in an appetitive operant conditioning task in mice following either sc [63,70] or ip [71] injections. On the other hand, GHSR antagonism via ip injection of JMV2959 reduces lever pressing for a 5% (weight/volume) sucrose solution in rats [72]. Central administration of ghrelin yields similar outcomes to peripheral injections, with an increase in operant responding for sucrose observed in rats following icv ghrelin injections [73,74]. Several pathways likely contribute to the central actions of ghrelin to promote instrumental responses for palatable food, with dopamine signaling from VTA to the ACB at the forefront. For example, VTA-ACB dopamine signaling is a critical for food-motivated behaviors [75], and early work from Abizaid and colleagues revealed that ghrelin binds to VTA neurons, where it increases dopamine turnover in the ACB in a GHSR-dependent manner [15]. Consistent with these results, at the behavioral level intra-VTA ghrelin administration increases lever pressing for sucrose [11,76] and flavored grain-based pellets [77,78]. Further, this influence of intra-VTA ghrelin requires dopamine signaling from the VTA to the ACB [76,78,79]. In addition, the increase in palatable food-motivated behaviors induced by ghrelin is prevented by administration of dopamine receptor type 1 and type 2 antagonists [76,78], thus further highlighting the critical role of downstream dopamine signaling. Ghrelin can also influence food motivation and ACB dopamine activity via sites of action other than the VTA. For example, infusion of ghrelin into the HPCv enhances operant responding for sucrose in rats, as well as increases phosphorylation of the dopamine synthesizing enzyme TH in the ACB [9]. The lateral hypothalamus (LHA) also partakes in the modulation of VTA to ACB dopamine signaling by ghrelin as intra-LHA ghrelin in rats increases lever pressing for sucrose [80] and potentiates dopamine release into the ACB upon pellet retrieval [81]. This could be mediated via interactions with hypothalamic orexin neurons as sc injection of ghrelin has no impact on operant responding for sucrose in orexin KO mice and wildtype animals treated with the orexin receptor antagonist SB-334867 [63]. In addition, infusion of ghrelin into the dorsal lateral septum (LS) increases lever pressing for sucrose in rats, although GHSR blockade into the dorsal LS does not influence operant responding [82]. Finally, the lPBN does not appear to participate in the motivational properties of ghrelin as direct infusion into this nucleus has no impact on lever pressing for sucrose [65].

As opposed to ghrelin, GLP-1 signaling reduces instrumental responding for high fat/sucrose food rewards. Administration of exendin-4 in rats, for example, whether via ip injection [66,83,84] or icv infusion [66,85], dampens motivated lever pressing for sucrose. As a primary CNS node in the gut-to-brain axis, it is not surprising that the NTS contributes to the central effects of GLP-1 signaling on food motivated behaviors.

In fact, the inhibition of lever pressing induced by central administration of exendin-4 is replicated in rats by specific infusion into the NTS [67,68,86], suggesting that the NTS may be mediating the effects of peripheral GLP-1 analog administration on effort-based food-motivated behavior. Several other brain structures also partake in the central actions of GLP-1 signaling on food-motivated operant responding, either via direct projections from the NTS or potentially GLP-1 volume transmission signaling through the cerebrospinal fluid. For example, operant responding for palatable food in rats is reduced by infusion of exendin-4 or GLP-1 into either the VTA or ACB [66,83], PVT [21], HPCv [69], lPBN [87], dorsal LS [88] and supramammillary nucleus (SuM) or LHA [86]. Further, intra-PVT administration blunts the excitability PVT projecting towards the ACB [21], once again evidencing a pivotal role for the ACB and mesolimbic dopamine signaling in GLP-1's role in food motivation. However, dopaminergic activity in other limbic structures can also interact with GLP-1 as, in addition to reducing lever pressing for sucrose, icv exendin-4 enhances dopamine turnover in the amygdala and these effects are partly inhibited by intra-amygdala infusion of a dopamine receptor type 2 antagonist [85].

While there is a consensus in the literature for the opposing effects of ghrelin and GLP-1 signaling on food-motivated behaviors, studies including both male and female rodents shed light on sex-specific mechanisms of action [89]. For example, LHA infusion of ghrelin increases lever pressing for sucrose in both male and female rats, but intra-LHA administration of the GHSR antagonist YIL781 only inhibits operant responding in females [80]. The same group observed that GLP-1R agonism with exendin-4 in the LHA decreases lever pressing for sucrose in both sexes, but GLP-1R blockade enhances operant responding only in male rats [90]. These results suggest that the endogenous relevance of LHA GHSR signaling to palatable food-motivated responding is more prominent in females, whereas the opposite is true for LHA GLP-1 signaling. Additional work highlighted the SuM as a site of action for exendin-4 to diminish lever pressing for sucrose in males only, whereas infusion into the VTA reduced food-directed lever pressing in both sexes, but more potently in females [91]. In addition, the inhibitory effect of intragastric nutrient infusion on food-motivated behaviors may operate via sex-specific pathways as ip injection of the GLP-1R antagonist exendin-9 prevents the reduction in operant responding following nutrient infusion in male but not female rats [92]. Although the general opposing behavioral outcomes related to food-motivated behavior for the GLP-1 and ghrelin systems are similar across sexes, the specific underlying mechanisms mediating neural sites of action can diverge.

Impulsivity, or responding without apparent forethought for the consequences of one's actions, and inhibitory control, or the ability to exert "top-down" control over motivated responses, are key psychological constructs related to food-motivated responding. Ghrelin and GLP-1 have each been associated with impulsivity and inhibitory control. For example, ghrelin can promote food motivated behaviors by driving impulsivity as both icv and VTA infusion of ghrelin increases the rates of impulsive responding in rats assessed in tasks of differential reinforcement of low rates of responding (DRL), go/no-go, and delay discounting [93]. On the other hand, infusion of exendin-4 into the HPCv of rats inhibits impulsive responding for high fat/sucrose pellets in the DRL task [94]. In addition, GLP-1 signaling may limit impulsivity by promoting inhibitory control. For example, daily ip injections with the GLP-1 analog, liraglutide, over 12 days potentiates inhibition of conditioned appetitive responses as rats limit food-seeking behavior in response to a negative feature stimulus that signals when a target stimulus will not be followed by food reinforcement [95]. Thus, food-motivated behavioral responses can be modulated via ghrelin's and GLP-1's influences on impulsivity and inhibitory control. In some cases, impulsive behavior can be observed following treatments that do not also affect food-motivated operant responding [96], and thus it is critical for future work to determine whether the effects of ghrelin and GLP-1 signaling on impulsivity and/or inhibitory control are linked with vs. distinct from the general effects on food-motivated operant responding.

4.2. Human Studies

GLP-1's influence on food-motivated behaviors in human participants can be impaired by metabolic conditions. For example, in an incentive motivation task where participants exert physical strength on a handgrip to obtain food or monetary rewards, sc injection of the GLP-1 analog liraglutide prevents the increase in incentive motivation induced by hunger in participants with high, but not low, insulin sensitivity [97]. Interestingly, RYGB surgery reduces computer mouse clicks for a sweet and fatty candy [98] and this may be related to improvements in GLP-1 signaling. In fact, indirect inhibition of GLP-1 secretion via sc injection of octreotide, a somatostatin analog, enhances computer mouse clicks for chocolate rewards in individuals who underwent RYGB surgery but not in obese non-operated controls, suggesting that RYGB surgery influences the effects of GLP-1 signaling on food-motivated responses [99]. Similarly, patients who underwent esophagectomy for cancer present elevated postprandial levels of GLP-1 relative to healthy control subjects and also present an increase in computer mouse clicks for chocolate following sc injection of octreotide, whereas healthy controls do not [100]. Thus, the extent to which GLP-1 signaling dampens food motivation is influenced by chronic metabolic status. To our knowledge the effects of ghrelin signaling on food-motivated responding has thus far received limited attention, however, based on the wealth of preclinical data discussed above it is highly probable that ghrelin's effects oppose those of GLP-1 in humans as well.

4.3. Summary

Ghrelin and GLP-1 compete to enhance and inhibit the expression of effort-based food-motivated behaviors, respectively. Rodent model studies identify several brain regions through which ghrelin and GLP-1 act to influence CPP expression and operant responding for food, with various neuronal outputs that likely converge onto the ACB. Despite similar behavioral outcomes across sexes, the specific mechanisms and sites of action underlining ghrelin and GLP-1's actions on food motivation can be sex-specific. In addition, food-motivated responding can be modulated by ghrelin and GLP-1, at least in part, via their opposing impacts on impulsivity and inhibitory control. Finally, the contribution of GLP-1 signaling to regulate food motivated behaviors in humans is influenced by metabolic parameters such as insulin resistance and bariatric surgery.

5. Nutrient Preference

Palatable foods are typically rich in fat and/or sugar and tend to be preferred over low fat/sugar items. The magnitude of this preference, however, can be influenced by gut peptides such as ghrelin and GLP-1. In this section, we review studies measuring free intake of palatable foods in rodents and human participants that vary with regards to macronutrient content, palatability, and other factors.

5.1. Rodent Studies

Ghrelin signaling enhances preference for palatable foods, especially sweetened solutions, even if nonnutritive. For example, ip injection of ghrelin enhances consumption of a 0.1% (w/v) saccharin solution in mice [101] and of a 5% (w/v) solution in rats [72], while GHSR antagonism with ip injection of JMV2959 reduces intake of a 2% (w/v) sucrose solution in prairies voles [102] and of a 0.1% (w/v) saccharin beverage in mice [72]. In addition, relative to wildtype controls, preference for a sweetened solution is dampened in transgenic mice lacking ghrelin [103] or GHSR [104]. One study, however, observed that icv infusion of ghrelin does not influence intake of a 5mM saccharin solution in rats [105]. Additional work on the central actions of ghrelin to enhance intake of sugar and other sweet tastants is required in order to elucidate if this finding is related to the route of administration and/or other variables. In contrast, the effects of ghrelin on preference for high fat foods are less consistent across studies. For example, when rats are offered unlimited access to diets enriched in fat, carbohydrate, or protein, intra-VTA infusion of the GHSR antagonist GHRP over 14 days specifically lowers fat intake [77]. Similarly, mice lacking

GHSR and rats injected (ip) with JMV2959 show reduced preference for palatable foods and intra-VTA ghrelin increases intake of peanut butter, but not standard chow [64]. However, rats offered ad libitum access to lard and standard chow increase their intake of both foods following icv infusion of ghrelin, but in contrast to the previous study, only increase their chow intake when ghrelin is infused into the VTA [106]. This specific increase in chow, but not lard intake is also reported in rats receiving ghrelin infusion into the lPBN [65].

In opposite to ghrelin, GLP-1 agonism appears to reduce caloric intake by preferentially targeting consumption of both fat and sugar-rich palatable foods. For example, ip injection of GLP-1 reduces intake of sucrose [107] but not standard chow in mice, at least under the conditions tested in this study [105]. In addition, infusion of exendin-4 into either the VTA or the core subregion of the ACB decreases sucrose intake in rats while consumption of standard chow is unaffected [108]. Similarly, exendin-4 injections into the NTS of rats decreases intake of peanut butter but not standard chow [68] and acute infusion into the 4th ventricle of an inhibitor of the enzyme degrading GLP-1 reduces intake of a high-fat diet and not chow [109]. Interestingly, this preferential reduction of palatable food intake is observed in the few hours following exendin-4 infusion and is followed by a generalized reduction in caloric intake. For example, rats administered exendin-4 into the HPCv only decrease their consumption of a high fat/sugar diet 6h after the infusion, but at the 24h timepoint chow intake is also reduced [69]. This is similar in rats receiving exendin-4 into the SuM, where only sucrose intake is inhibited 1h after treatment, whereas sucrose, fat and standard chow consumption are all lower after 24h [91]. These findings suggest that GLP-1R agonism could acutely preferentially reduce intake of palatable food prior to exerting a generalized decrease in food intake. Consistent with this framework, daily sc injections of liraglutide over 25 days reduce overall caloric intake similarly across macronutrients in rats offered a cafeteria diet [110].

5.2. Human Studies

Ghrelin and GLP-1 are differentially influenced by the consumption of palatable food. For example, postprandial levels of ghrelin are significantly higher after consuming a pleasurable food item, such as a pastry, compared to after eating an isocaloric portion of bread and butter [111,112]. Ghrelin may even contribute to genetic predispositions for sweet taste preference as in a Swedish population cohort, specific haplotypes for the proghrelin gene are associated with an elevated consumption of sucrose, especially in men [72]. In contrast, fasting GLP-1 concentrations negatively predict intake of food rich in simple sugars in a vending machine paradigm [113], which the authors interpreted as evidence that GLP-1 plays a role in reward pathways regulating simple sugar intake. A number of studies also report altered food preferences following gastric bypass surgery, with a shift away from high sugar/fat preference [114–117]. However, the extent to which these surgical-induced changes in food preference are either directly or indirectly influenced by altered post-surgery ghrelin and/or GLP-1 levels requires future investigation.

5.3. Summary

Palatable food intake, especially the consumption sweetened solutions, is enhanced by ghrelin, whereas GLP-1 preferentially reduces intake of high fat and high sugar foods, at least following acute administration. In addition, work in both rodent and humans reveals that preference for fat and sugar can be altered by bariatric surgery and contribute to weight loss, yet linking these effects to altered ghrelin or GLP-1 signaling remain to be established. Finally, circulating levels of ghrelin and GLP-1 can be indicative of palatable food consumption in humans.

6. Flavor

Flavor perception contributes substantially to the reinforcing properties of palatable food and learned associations between flavor and postingestive outcomes can influence future eating behaviors. In this section, we review ghrelin- and GLP-1-relevant rodent model studies assessing licking patterns in response to escalating doses of sucrose solutions or lipid emulsion, as well as orofacial reactions to oral infusions of rewarding or aversive solutions. In addition, we discuss changes in flavor sensitivity and endocrine response to orosensory stimulation in humans.

6.1. Rodent Studies

Work in transgenic mice lacking essential component for ghrelin signaling identify ghrelin's contribution to flavor perception. For example, the distribution of licks in response to increasing concentrations of sodium chloride or citric acid reveals reduced sensitivity to the aversive properties of highly concentrated salty and sour solutions in GHSR KO mice [118]. Similarly, mice lacking ghrelin O-acyltransferase (GOAT), the enzyme generating the active form of ghrelin, display dampened sensitivity to escalating concentrations of sodium chloride, in addition to lower licking responses for high doses of intralipid [119]. These differences in licking responses are associated to altered protein expression for a salt-sensitive subunit in GHSR KO mice [118] and fatty acid receptors in GOAT null mice [119], thus further highlighting the contribution of ghrelin signaling to salty and fatty taste perception.

While genetic ablation of ghrelin signaling appears to make salty tastants less aversive, GLP-1 receptor KO mice on the other hand demonstrate blunted increases in licking for escalating doses of palatable sweet solutions (both sucrose and sucralose solutions) relative to wildtype animals [120–122]. Reduced responsivity to high doses of sucrose is also reported from gustatory nerve recordings in GLP-1R KO mice [122]. In addition to sweet taste, GLP-1 receptor KO mice display greater increases in licking for high doses of umami tastants [121] and a stronger decreased oral response to citric acid [120]. The implication of GLP-1 signaling in the orosensory component of a meal is reinforced by findings that icv infusion of GLP-1 reduces sucrose intake even in rats with gastric cannulas, preventing intestinal nutrient sensing [123]. Interestingly, mice infused with exendin-4 into the dorsal LS present a decrease in licking rate for a 0.25 M sucrose solution whereas licking microstructure is unchanged [88]. In addition, rats receiving ip injection of exendin-4 demonstrate unaltered orofacial reactivity to sucrose, indicating no changes in the hedonic response, yet they also show reduced aversive orofacial responses to a quinine solution [124]. Thus, GLP-1 signaling appears to dampen licking responses to high concentrations of sweet tastant, but not by altering the hedonic properties of sweet taste perception.

6.2. Human Studies

Ghrelin is modulated by orosensory stimulation even in the absence of nutrient absorption. For example, sham feeding studies, where food is smelled, chewed and tasted, but not swallowed, reveal reductions in circulating ghrelin to the same extent as induced by food consumption [125]. Further, despite lack of nutrient sensing in the GI tract, circulating levels of ghrelin are higher after a sham feeding session with a meal enriched in protein rather than carbohydrates or fats [126], solidifying the notion that ghrelin is tied not only to nutrient sensing but also orosensory flavor processing.

Interventions targeting obesity have the potential to alter taste perception, potentially via GLP-1 signaling. For instance, obese women present dampened sweet taste sensitivity when compared to lean individuals [127]. However, taste perception of low concentrations of sucrose is improved following RYGB surgery [128], although these findings are yet to be directly linked to post-surgical changes in circulating GLP-1. In addition, obese subjects chronically treated with liraglutide show a reduction in their preferred concentration of sweet, salty, savory and fatty-flavored solution after 16 weeks, while these preferences remain unchanged in the placebo group [129]. Similarly, GLP-1R agonism over 3 months for the treatment of type 2 diabetes improves sweet taste sensitivity and decreases preferred concentrations for a lipid emulsion [130]. The amplitude of such effects of GLP-1 signaling may be sex-dependent as, in a food choice task based on flavor, women were more likely than men to change their flavor preferences after a GLP-1 iv infusion [131].

6.3. Summary

Ghrelin and GLP-1 signaling contribute to the perception of different flavors, even in the absence of GI nutrient sensing. Enhancement of GLP-1 signaling has the potential to influence food preferences and improve taste sensitivity, especially the detection of low concentrations of sucrose. Consistent with our larger framework that ghrelin and GLP-1 have opposing effects on processes related to food reward, both ghrelin loss of function (transgenic KO models) and GLP-1 gain of function (GLP-1 analog treatment) appear to reduce taste sensitivity to chloride-based solutions, although more research is needed to directly compare the two systems on various domains of flavor processing.

7. Aversion

Eating patterns can be potently shaped by aversive experiences such as malaise, nausea, or emesis that function to discourage future consumption in a flavor-specific manner. Not surprisingly based on their competing influences on gastric motility, ghrelin and GLP-1 appear to distinctively influence GI-associated malaise. Pharmaceutical agents that decrease food intake, including FDA-approved GLP-1 analogs, often concomitantly promote GI discomfort, thus limiting their clinical application by developed tolerance to these aversive effects. In this section, we review rodent model studies examining the impacts of ghrelin and GLP-1 on conditioned flavor avoidance (CFA) where a neutral flavor is paired to an ip injection of some compound that may produce nausea (e.g., lithium chloride), as well as on pica, the consumption of non-nutritive items such as kaolin as a means to relieve nausea. Specifically, we explore the contribution of aversion and nausea to the dampening actions of GLP-1 signaling on food motivation and we discuss the clinical potential for ghrelin to alleviate nausea.

7.1. Rodent Studies

Ghrelin administration attenuates CFA induced by lithium chloride, at least in part, by acting specifically in the lateral amygdala in rats. For example, while ip injection of the GHSR antagonist JMV2959 alone has no impact on CFA [132], infusion of ghrelin directly in the lateral amygdala prevents the acquisition of a lithium chloride-induced CFA in a GHSR-dependent manner [133,134] but also its extinction [135]. In addition, GHSR signaling may provide an avenue to reduce food intake without promoting CFA as treatment with novel GHSR inverse agonists inhibits standard chow intake without promoting CFA in mice [136]. Further, exogenous ghrelin could be beneficial for the relief of nausea associated to medical treatment. Rats receiving the chemotherapy agent cisplatin present dampened ghrelin presence in the hypothalamus [137] and increased gene expression for GHSR in this same region [138], suggesting that these effects could be attenuated by exogenous ghrelin. In fact, ip injection or NTS infusion of ghrelin reduces nausea-related pica by improving gastric motility in rats treated with cisplatin [139,140]. In addition, the GHSR agonist HM01 reduces emesis induced by motion or cisplatin in the shrew [141].

In contrast, GLP-1 signaling delays gastric emptying and the resulting GI discomfort may contribute to GLP-1s capacity to stimulate nausea and conditioned aversion. Pairing an icv infusion of GLP-1 to a neutral flavor is sufficient to induce CFA [142,143] and ip injection of either exendin-4 or liraglutide promotes CFA in a dose-dependent manner in rats [144,145]. The aversive properties of GLP-1 signaling may be dependent on the route of administration, as infusion of GLP-1 into the hepatic portal vein [146], PVN [147], ACB [148], lateral dorsal tegmental nucleus [149] or even the lateral ventricle [150] inhibits food intake without inducing CFA or pica in rats. It has been suggested that the vagus nerve mediates the aversive effects of GLP-1, as ip injection of exendin-4 induces CFA in vagotomised but not sham-operated rats [151]. However, additional work reveals that systemic administration of extendin-4 at various doses induces both CFA and kaolin consumption, and in both vagotomised and sham-operated rats [152]. Further, the authors identify the NTS as the most likely candidate for the malaise induced by GLP-1 signaling [145]. Others, however, have found reductions in CPP expression and lever pressing for palatable food following intra-NTS exendin-4 at doses that do not also produce pica [67,68]. In addition to not assessing CFA, these studies differ from the previous findings by usage of a shorter habituation period to the kaolin pellets [68] or lower dose of intra-NTS exendin-4 [67]. Consistent with a role for NTS GLP-1R signaling in mediating the nausea outcomes induced by this system, GLP-1R blockade attenuates anorexia and weight loss when infused into the NTS of tumor-bearing rats [153], and reduces pica induced by icv infusion in cisplatin-treated rats treated [154].

Although the literature point towards aversive responses to GLP-1, some studies have still found reductions in food reward-motivated behavior by brain site-specific GLP-1R agonists using doses that were not associated with CFA and/or pica. For example, exendin-4 or GLP-1 has been shown to reduced effort-based food-motivated behaviors in rats without influencing CFA or pica when administered into the VTA [66,108], PVT [21], HPCv [69], lPBN [87] and SuM [86]. Infusion of GLP-1R agonists in these brain nuclei possibly targets the neural mechanisms underlying food motivation and bypasses the hindbrain GLP-1 nausea circuitry. These findings overall suggest that GLP-1 signaling can inhibit the palatable food-motivated behaviors by mechanisms other than GI discomfort based on analyses from site-specific brain region application.

7.2. Human Studies

Changes in ghrelin signaling are tied to GI discomfort across various health conditions in humans. In healthy participants, for example, susceptibility to motion sickness is associated to a sudden drop in circulating levels of ghrelin [155]. Patients treated with cisplatin also present lower concentrations of circulating ghrelin [156] and GHSR agonism alleviates nausea and vomiting induced by chemotherapy [157–160]. In addition, GHSR agonists can provide relief to diabetic individuals experiencing nausea and vomiting as a result of gastroparesis [161–164]. Thus, ghrelin signaling may promote food reward-motivated behaviors in humans, in part, by minimizing GI discomfort.

Conversely, the most common side effects associated with treatment for obesity and type 2 diabetes with GLP-1 analogs are nausea and vomiting. These symptoms may be more frequent in women and those also treated with metformin, proton pump inhibitors, and/or anti-histamines [165,166]. While nausea and vomiting associated with weight loss from liraglutide treatment is often transient [167], occurrence of these side effects still limits the therapeutic potential of GLP-1 analogs. A recent study demonstrates that combination of a lower dose of GLP-1 analog with insulin therapy improves glucose homeostasis and reduces the prevalence of GI symptoms, which thus could strengthen treatment adherence [168]. Another therapeutic option is the development of site-specific GLP-1 analogs such as exendin-4 conjugated to vitamin B12 resulting in limited brain penetrance to improve glucose homeostasis without the effects on appetite [169,170]. Moreover, pharmacological targeting of the neural pathways underlining the actions of GLP-1 signaling on food reward without concomitant nausea could promote weight loss and bypass aversive side effects.

7.3. Summary

Ghrelin alleviates GI discomfort while the malaise induced by GLP-1 can drive CFA and pica in rodents. However, rodent model studies reveal that reductions in food reward can be obtained with exendin-4 in the absence of aversive GI effects based on site-specific brain application. The development of improved GLP-1 analogs could ultimately promote weight loss without inducing nausea and vomiting in obese individuals, although clinical use of effective GLP-1 analogs absent of nausea side effects is thus far absent. Overall, the evidence suggests that the opposing effects of ghrelin and GLP-1 on mediating GI-associated malaise may be a driving component of their opposing effects on food reward-motivated behaviors.

8. Future Directions

This review summarizes the antagonizing actions of ghrelin and GLP-1 on distinct food reward-associated behavioral constructs. While basic science knowledge of each of these systems has increased dramatically in the past decade, there are gaps in the literature that, if addressed, could provide a more complete neurobiological and behavioral framework that translates to the clinical setting. For example, additional preclinical work on the role of GLP-1 in reactivity to food cues and meal anticipation would be beneficial given that the majority of rodent model studies focusing on these behavioral domains assessed the contributions of ghrelin and other orexigenic signals (e.g., orexin/hypocretin). In addition, recent advances in real-time in vivo calcium-based neuronal recording in rodents offer an opportunity to bridge findings from human brain imaging studies towards a deeper understanding at the levels of cell type specificity and systems neuroscience. Finally, although the alterations in ghrelin and GLP-1 signaling following bariatric interventions have been widely investigated, the direct causal contributions of these physiological changes to alterations in food reward-associated behaviors remain to be determined.

9. Conclusions

Ghrelin and GLP-1 act as opposing forces on multiple behavioral, physiological, and neural fronts related to obtaining and consuming highly palatable and "rewarding" foods (summarized in Figure 1). For example, prior to feeding, ghrelin promotes whereas GLP-1 dampens brain activity in response to food cues. In addition, meal anticipation is largely driven by endogenous ghrelin, particularly in anticipation of palatable food access. Similar to fasting, ghrelin enhances various palatable food-motivated effort-based responses, whereas GLP-1 has opposing effects via action in multiple sites across the neuraxis. The preference for high fat/sugar foods is also heightened by ghrelin and reduced by GLP-1 signaling. These changes may be attributed, in part, to alterations in flavor perception, and/or modulation of GI-associated nausea and malaise.

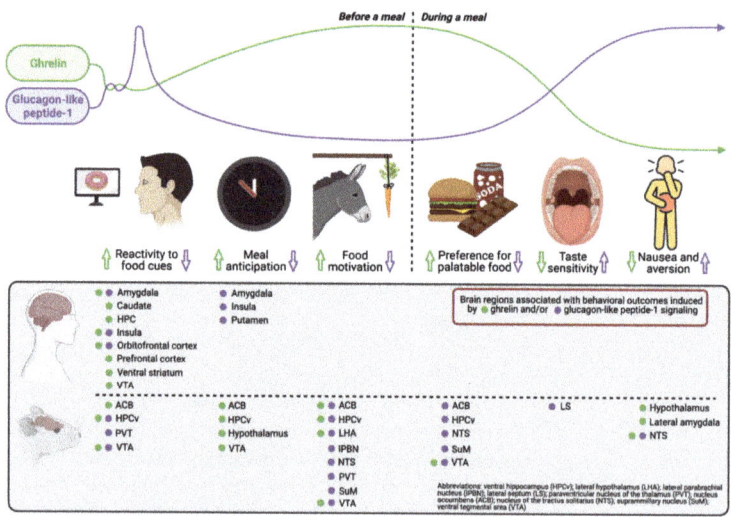

Figure 1. Overview of ghrelin (green) and glucagon-like peptide-1 (purple) circulating levels in relation to a meal (**top row**) and the competing actions (↑increase or ↓decrease) of these systems on distinct behavioral domains related to food reward (**middle row**) and associated sites of actions based on human and rodent model results (**bottom row**).

We conclude by noting that the opposing influences of ghrelin and GLP-1 signaling on these various food reward-associated behavioral constructs (food cue reactivity, meal anticipatory activity, palatable food-motivated responding, altered food preferences, flavor, and/or GI-associated malaise) likely occur with varying degrees of mutual exclusion. In other words, it is likely that modulation of one food reward-associated construct by ghrelin or GLP-1 may be secondary to effects on a separate construct. For example, altered orosensory and retronasal flavor processing, and/or altered GI-malaise processing, is likely to subsequently influence food-motivated responses, reactivity to food cues, nutrient preference, etc. Generally, however, the literature suggests that ghrelin and GLP-1 have opposing effects on these food reward-associated behaviors via both distinct and overlapping neurobiological and behavioral mechanisms. Understanding the extent that these (and other) gut peptide systems concurrently but also independently affect these food reward-associated processes will require sophisticated behavioral analyses to carefully dissect these distinct constructs.

Author Contributions: L.D.-S. and S.E.K. equally contributed to the scholarship and redaction of this manuscript. All authors have read and agreed to the published version of the manuscript.

Funding: S.K. received funding support from the NIH/NIDDK: DK118402.

Acknowledgments: The figure was created with BioRender.com (accessed on 12 Mar 2021).

Conflicts of Interest: The authors declare no conflict of interest.

References

1. Sun, Y.; Wang, P.; Zheng, H.; Smith, R.G. Ghrelin stimulation of growth hormone release and appetite is mediated through the growth hormone secretagogue receptor. *Proc. Natl. Acad. Sci. USA* **2004**, *101*, 4679–4684. [CrossRef]
2. Drazen, D.L.; Vahl, T.P.; D'Alessio, D.A.; Seeley, R.J.; Woods, S.C. Effects of a fixed meal pattern on ghrelin secretion: Evidence for a learned response independent of nutrient status. *Endocrinology* **2006**, *147*, 23–30. [CrossRef] [PubMed]
3. Callahan, H.S.; Cummings, D.E.; Pepe, M.S.; Breen, P.A.; Matthys, C.C.; Weigle, D.S. Postprandial suppression of plasma ghrelin level is proportional to ingested caloric load but does not predict intermeal interval in humans. *J. Clin. Endocrinol. Metab.* **2004**, *89*, 1319–1324. [CrossRef]
4. Davis, E.A.; Wald, H.S.; Suarez, A.N.; Zubcevic, J.; Liu, C.M.; Cortella, A.M.; Kamitakahara, A.K.; Polson, J.W.; Arnold, M.; Grill, H.J.; et al. Ghrelin signaling regulates feeding behavior, metabolism, and memory through the vagus nerve. *Curr. Biol.* **2020**. [CrossRef]
5. Krieger, J.P.; Arnold, M.; Pettersen, K.G.; Lossel, P.; Langhans, W.; Lee, S.J. Knockdown of GLP-1 receptors in vagal afferents affects normal food intake and glycemia. *Diabetes* **2016**, *65*, 34–43. [CrossRef] [PubMed]
6. Kanoski, S.E.; Hayes, M.R.; Skibicka, K.P. GLP-1 and weight loss: Unraveling the diverse neural circuitry. *Am. J. Physiol. Regul. Integr. Comp. Physiol.* **2016**, *310*, R885–R895. [CrossRef]
7. Boswell, R.G.; Kober, H. Food cue reactivity and craving predict eating and weight gain: A meta-analytic review. *Obes. Rev.* **2016**, *17*, 159–177. [CrossRef]
8. Walker, A.K.; Ibia, I.E.; Zigman, J.M. Disruption of cue-potentiated feeding in mice with blocked ghrelin signaling. *Physiol. Behav.* **2012**, *108*, 34–43. [CrossRef] [PubMed]
9. Kanoski, S.E.; Fortin, S.M.; Ricks, K.M.; Grill, H.J. Ghrelin signaling in the ventral hippocampus stimulates learned and motivational aspects of feeding via PI3K-Akt signaling. *Biol. Psychiatry* **2013**, *73*, 915–923. [CrossRef] [PubMed]
10. St-Onge, V.; Watts, A.; Abizaid, A. Ghrelin enhances cue-induced bar pressing for high fat food. *Horm. Behav.* **2016**, *78*, 141–149. [CrossRef]
11. Sommer, S.; Hauber, W. Ghrelin receptor activation in the ventral tegmental area amplified instrumental responding but not the excitatory influence of Pavlovian stimuli on instrumental responding. *Neurobiol. Learn. Mem.* **2016**, *134*, 210–215. [CrossRef]
12. Davidson, T.L.; Kanoski, S.E.; Tracy, A.L.; Walls, E.K.; Clegg, D.; Benoit, S.C. The interoceptive cue properties of ghrelin generalize to cues produced by food deprivation. *Peptides* **2005**, *26*, 1602–1610. [CrossRef] [PubMed]
13. Suarez, A.N.; Liu, C.M.; Cortella, A.M.; Noble, E.E.; Kanoski, S.E. Ghrelin and Orexin Interact to Increase Meal Size Through a Descending Hippocampus to Hindbrain Signaling Pathway. *Biol. Psychiatry* **2020**, *87*, 1001–1011. [CrossRef] [PubMed]
14. Van Der Plasse, G.; Van Zessen, R.; Luijendijk, M.C.M.; Erkan, H.; Stuber, G.D.; Ramakers, G.M.J.; Adan, R.A.H. Modulation of cue-induced firing of ventral tegmental area dopamine neurons by leptin and ghrelin. *Int. J. Obes.* **2015**, *39*, 1742–1749. [CrossRef] [PubMed]
15. Abizaid, A.; Liu, Z.-W.; Andrews, Z.B.; Shanabrough, M.; Borok, E.; Elsworth, J.D.; Roth, R.H.; Sleeman, M.W.; Picciotto, M.R.; Tschöp, M.H.; et al. Ghrelin modulates the activity and synaptic input organization of midbrain dopamine neurons while promoting appetite. *J. Clin. Investig.* **2006**, *116*, 3229–3239. [CrossRef] [PubMed]

16. Roseberry, A.G. Acute fasting increases somatodendritic dopamine release in the ventral Tegmental area. *J. Neurophysiol.* **2015**, *114*, 1072–1082. [CrossRef]
17. Godfrey, N.; Borgland, S.L. Sex differences in the effect of acute fasting on excitatory and inhibitory synapses onto ventral tegmental area dopamine neurons. *J. Physiol.* **2020**, *598*, 5523–5539. [CrossRef]
18. Van Der Plasse, G.; Merkestein, M.; Luijendijk, M.C.M.; Van Der Roest, M.; Westenberg, H.G.M.; Mulder, A.B.; Adan, R.A.H. Food cues and ghrelin recruit the same neuronal circuitry. *Int. J. Obes.* **2013**, *37*, 1012–1019. [CrossRef] [PubMed]
19. Johnson, A.W.; Canter, R.; Gallagher, M.; Holland, P.C. Assessing the Role of the Growth Hormone Secretagogue Receptor in Motivational Learning and Food Intake. *Behav. Neurosci.* **2009**, *123*, 1058–1065. [CrossRef]
20. Konanur, V.R.; Hsu, T.M.; Kanoski, S.E.; Hayes, M.R.; Roitman, M.F. Phasic dopamine responses to a food-predictive cue are suppressed by the glucagon-like peptide-1 receptor agonist Exendin-4. *Physiol. Behav.* **2020**, *215*, 112771. [CrossRef] [PubMed]
21. Ong, Z.Y.; Liu, J.J.; Pang, Z.P.; Grill, H.J. Paraventricular thalamic control of food intake and reward: Role of glucagon-like peptide-1 receptor signaling. *Neuropsychopharmacology* **2017**, *42*, 2387–2397. [CrossRef]
22. Kroemer, N.B.; Krebs, L.; Kobiella, A.; Grimm, O.; Pilhatsch, M.; Bidlingmaier, M.; Zimmermann, U.S.; Smolka, M.N. Fasting levels of ghrelin covary with the brain response to food pictures. *Addict. Biol.* **2013**, *18*, 855–862. [CrossRef] [PubMed]
23. Holsen, L.M.; Lawson, E.A.; Christensen, K.; Klibanski, A.; Goldstein, J.M. Abnormal relationships between the neural response to high- and low-calorie foods and endogenous acylated ghrelin in women with active and weight-recovered anorexia nervosa. *Psychiatry Res. Neuroimaging* **2014**, *223*, 94–103. [CrossRef] [PubMed]
24. Schüssler, P.; Kluge, M.; Yassouridis, A.; Dresler, M.; Uhr, M.; Steiger, A. Ghrelin levels increase after pictures showing food. *Obesity* **2012**, *20*, 1212–1217. [CrossRef]
25. Dorton, H.M.; Luo, S.; Monterosso, J.R.; Page, K.A. Influences of dietary added sugar consumption on striatal food-cue reactivity and postprandial GLP-1 response. *Front. Psychiatry* **2018**, *8*. [CrossRef] [PubMed]
26. Heni, M.; Kullmann, S.; Gallwitz, B.; Häring, H.U.; Preissl, H.; Fritsche, A. Dissociation of GLP-1 and insulin association with food processing in the brain: GLP-1 sensitivity despite insulin resistance in obese humans. *Mol. Metab.* **2015**, *4*, 971–976. [CrossRef] [PubMed]
27. Maurer, L.; Mai, K.; Krude, H.; Haynes, J.D.; Weygandt, M.; Spranger, J. Interaction of circulating GLP-1 and the response of the dorsolateral prefrontal cortex to food-cues predicts body weight development. *Mol. Metab.* **2019**, *29*, 136–144. [CrossRef]
28. Goldstone, A.P.; Prechtl, C.G.; Scholtz, S.; Miras, A.D.; Chhina, N.; Durighel, G.; Deliran, S.S.; Beckmann, C.; Ghatei, M.A.; Ashby, D.R.; et al. Ghrelin mimics fasting to enhance human hedonic, orbitofrontal cortex, and hippocampal responses to food. *Am. J. Clin. Nutr.* **2014**, *99*, 1319–1330. [CrossRef]
29. Han, J.E.; Frasnelli, J.; Zeighami, Y.; Larcher, K.; Boyle, J.; McConnell, T.; Malik, S.; Jones-Gotman, M.; Dagher, A. Ghrelin Enhances Food Odor Conditioning in Healthy Humans: An fMRI Study. *Cell Rep.* **2018**, *25*, 2643–2652. [CrossRef]
30. Malik, S.; McGlone, F.; Bedrossian, D.; Dagher, A. Ghrelin Modulates Brain Activity in Areas that Control Appetitive Behavior. *Cell Metab.* **2008**, *7*, 400–409. [CrossRef] [PubMed]
31. Van Bloemendaal, L.; IJzerman, R.G.; Ten Kulve, J.S.; Barkhof, F.; Konrad, R.J.; Drent, M.L.; Veltman, D.J.; Diamant, M. GLP-1 receptor activation modulates appetite- and reward-related brain areas in humans. *Diabetes* **2014**, *63*, 4186–4196. [CrossRef]
32. Van Bloemendaal, L.; Veltman, D.J.; Ten Kulve, J.S.; Drent, M.L.; Barkhof, F.; Diamant, M.; Ijzerman, R.G. Emotional eating is associated with increased brain responses to food-cues and reduced sensitivity to GLP-1 receptor activation. *Obesity* **2015**, *23*, 2075–2082. [CrossRef]
33. Ten Kulve, J.S.; Veltman, D.J.; van Bloemendaal, L.; Barkhof, F.; Deacon, C.F.; Holst, J.J.; Konrad, R.J.; Sloan, J.H.; Drent, M.L.; Diamant, M.; et al. Endogenous GLP-1 mediates postprandial reductions in activation in central reward and satiety areas in patients with type 2 diabetes. *Diabetologia* **2015**, *58*, 2688–2698. [CrossRef]
34. Farr, O.M.; Li, C.R.; Mantzoros, C.S. Central nervous system regulation of eating: Insights from human brain imaging. *Metabolism* **2016**, *65*, 699–713. [CrossRef]
35. Farr, O.M.; Tsoukas, M.A.; Triantafyllou, G.; Dincer, F.; Filippaios, A.; Ko, B.J.; Mantzoros, C.S. Short-term administration of the GLP-1 analog liraglutide decreases circulating leptin and increases GIP levels and these changes are associated with alterations in CNS responses to food cues: A randomized, placebo-controlled, crossover study. *Metabolism* **2016**, *65*, 945–953. [CrossRef]
36. Farr, O.M.; Upadhyay, J.; Rutagengwa, C.; DiPrisco, B.; Ranta, Z.; Adra, A.; Bapatla, N.; Douglas, V.P.; Douglas, K.A.A.; Nolen-Doerr, E.; et al. Longer-term liraglutide administration at the highest dose approved for obesity increases reward-related orbitofrontal cortex activation in response to food cues: Implications for plateauing weight loss in response to anti-obesity therapies. *Diabetes Obes. Metab.* **2019**, *21*, 2459–2464. [CrossRef]
37. Sinclair, P.; Brennan, D.J.; le Roux, C.W. Gut adaptation after metabolic surgery and its influences on the brain, liver and cancer. *Nat. Rev. Gastroenterol. Hepatol.* **2018**, *15*, 606–624. [CrossRef] [PubMed]
38. Madsbad, S.; Dirksen, C.; Holst, J.J. Mechanisms of changes in glucose metabolism and bodyweight after bariatric surgery. *Lancet Diabetes Endocrinol.* **2014**, *2*, 152–164. [CrossRef]
39. Hutch, C.R.; Sandoval, D. The role of GLP-1 in the metabolic success of bariatric surgery. *Endocrinology* **2017**, *158*, 4139–4151. [CrossRef] [PubMed]
40. Lepping, R.J.; Bruce, A.S.; Francisco, A.; Yeh, H.W.; Martin, L.E.; Powell, J.N.; Hancock, L.; Patrician, T.M.; Breslin, F.J.; Selim, N.; et al. Resting-state brain connectivity after surgical and behavioral weight loss. *Obesity* **2015**. [CrossRef]

41. Zhang, Y.; Ji, G.; Li, G.; Hu, Y.; Liu, L.; Jin, Q.; Meng, Q.; Zhao, J.; Yuan, K.; Liu, J.; et al. Ghrelin reductions following bariatric surgery were associated with decreased resting state activity in the hippocampus. *Int. J. Obes.* **2019**, *43*, 842–851. [CrossRef]
42. Hu, Y.; Ji, G.; Li, G.; Manza, P.; Zhang, W.; Wang, J.; Lv, G.; He, Y.; Zhang, Z.; Yuan, K.; et al. Brain Connectivity, and Hormonal and Behavioral Correlates of Sustained Weight Loss in Obese Patients after Laparoscopic Sleeve Gastrectomy. *Cereb. Cortex* **2021**, *31*, 1284–1295. [CrossRef]
43. Giel, K.E.; Rieber, N.; Enck, P.; Friederich, H.C.; Meile, T.; Zipfel, S.; Teufel, M. Effects of laparoscopic sleeve gastrectomy on attentional processing of food-related information: Evidence from eye-tracking. *Surg. Obes. Relat. Dis.* **2014**. [CrossRef] [PubMed]
44. Li, G.; Ji, G.; Hu, Y.; Liu, L.; Jin, Q.; Zhang, W.; Liu, L.; Wang, Y.; Zhao, J.; von Deneen, K.M.; et al. Reduced plasma ghrelin concentrations are associated with decreased brain reactivity to food cues after laparoscopic sleeve gastrectomy. *Psychoneuroendocrinology* **2019**, *100*, 229–236. [CrossRef]
45. Ochner, C.N.; Laferrère, B.; Afifi, L.; Atalayer, D.; Geliebter, A.; Teixeira, J. Neural responsivity to food cues in fasted and fed states pre and post gastric bypass surgery. *Neurosci. Res.* **2012**, *74*, 138–143. [CrossRef] [PubMed]
46. Zoon, H.F.A.; de Bruijn, S.E.M.; Jager, G.; Smeets, P.A.M.; de Graaf, C.; Janssen, I.M.C.; Schijns, W.; Deden, L.; Boesveldt, S. Altered neural inhibition responses to food cues after Roux-en-Y Gastric Bypass. *Biol. Psychol.* **2018**, *137*, 34–41. [CrossRef] [PubMed]
47. Van Duinkerken, E.; Bernardes, G.; van Bloemendaal, L.; Veltman, D.J.; Barkhof, F.; Mograbi, D.C.; Gerdes, V.E.A.; Deacon, C.F.; Holst, J.J.; Drent, M.L.; et al. Cerebral effects of glucagon-like peptide-1 receptor blockade before and after Roux-en-Y gastric bypass surgery in obese women: A proof-of-concept resting-state functional MRI study. *Diabetes Obes. Metab.* **2020**, *23*, 415–424. [CrossRef]
48. Vahl, T.P.; Drazen, D.L.; Seeley, R.J.; D'Alessio, D.A.; Woods, S.C. Meal-anticipatory glucagon-like peptide-1 secretion in rats. *Endocrinology* **2010**, *151*, 569–575. [CrossRef] [PubMed]
49. Ott, V.; Friedrich, M.; Zemlin, J.; Lehnert, H.; Schultes, B.; Born, J.; Hallschmid, M. Meal anticipation potentiates postprandial ghrelin suppression in humans. *Psychoneuroendocrinology* **2012**, *37*, 1096–1100. [CrossRef]
50. Davis, J.F.; Choi, D.L.; Clegg, D.J.; Benoit, S.C. Signaling through the ghrelin receptor modulates hippocampal function and meal anticipation in mice. *Physiol. Behav.* **2011**, *103*, 39–43. [CrossRef]
51. Lesauter, J.; Hoque, N.; Weintraub, M.; Pfaff, D.W.; Silver, R. Stomach ghrelin-secreting cells as food-entrainable circadian clocks. *Proc. Natl. Acad. Sci. USA* **2009**, *106*, 13582–13587. [CrossRef]
52. Blum, I.D.; Patterson, Z.; Khazall, R.; Lamont, E.W.; Sleeman, M.W.; Horvath, T.L.; Abizaid, A. Reduced anticipatory locomotor responses to scheduled meals in ghrelin receptor deficient mice. *Neuroscience* **2009**, *164*, 351–359. [CrossRef]
53. Lamont, E.W.; Patterson, Z.; Rodrigues, T.; Vallejos, O.; Blum, I.D.; Abizaid, A. Ghrelin-deficient mice have fewer orexin cells and reduced cFOS expression in the mesolimbic dopamine pathway under a restricted feeding paradigm. *Neuroscience* **2012**, *218*, 12–19. [CrossRef]
54. Hsu, T.M.; Hahn, J.D.; Konanur, V.R.; Noble, E.E.; Suarez, A.N.; Thai, J.; Nakamoto, E.M.; Kanoski, S.E. Hippocampus ghrelin signaling mediates appetite through lateral hypothalamic orexin pathways. *Elife* **2015**, *4*. [CrossRef] [PubMed]
55. Merkestein, M.; Brans, M.A.D.; Luijendijk, M.C.M.; De Jong, J.W.; Egecioglu, E.; Dickson, S.L.; Adan, R.A.H. Ghrelin mediates anticipation to a palatable meal in rats. *Obesity* **2012**, *20*, 963–971. [CrossRef]
56. Wei, X.J.; Sun, B.; Chen, K.; Lv, B.; Luo, X.; Yan, J.Q. Ghrelin signaling in the ventral tegmental area mediates both reward-based feeding and fasting-induced hyperphagia on high-fat diet. *Neuroscience* **2015**, *300*, 53–62. [CrossRef]
57. Bake, T.; Hellgren, K.T.; Dickson, S.L. Acute ghrelin changes food preference from a high-fat diet to chow during binge-like eating in rodents. *J. Neuroendocrinol.* **2017**, *29*. [CrossRef] [PubMed]
58. Pierce-Messick, Z.; Pratt, W.E. Glucagon-like peptide-1 receptors modulate the binge-like feeding induced by μ-opioid receptor stimulation of the nucleus accumbens in the rat. *Neuroreport* **2020**, *31*, 1283–1288. [CrossRef]
59. Cummings, D.E.; Purnell, J.Q.; Frayo, R.S.; Schmidova, K.; Wisse, B.E.; Weigle, D.S. A Preprandial Rise in Plasma Ghrelin Levels Suggests a Role in Meal Initiation in Humans. *Diabetes* **2001**, *50*, 1714–1719. [CrossRef] [PubMed]
60. Frecka, J.M.; Mattes, R.D. Possible entrainment of ghrelin to habitual meal patterns in humans. *Am. J. Physiol. Liver Physiol.* **2008**, *294*, G699–G707. [CrossRef]
61. Rigamonti, A.E.; Piscitelli, F.; Aveta, T.; Agosti, F.; De Col, A.; Bini, S.; Cella, S.G.; Di Marzo, V.; Sartorio, A. Anticipatory and consummatory effects of (hedonic) chocolate intake are associated with increased circulating levels of the orexigenic peptide ghrelin and endocannabinoids in obese adults. *Food Nutr. Res.* **2015**, *59*. [CrossRef]
62. Van Bloemendaal, L.; Veltman, D.J.; Ten Kulve, J.S.; Groot, P.F.C.; Ruhé, H.G.; Barkhof, F.; Sloan, J.H.; Diamant, M.; Ijzerman, R.G. Brain reward-system activation in response to anticipation and consumption of palatable food is altered by glucagon-like peptide-1 receptor activation in humans. *Diabetes Obes. Metab.* **2015**, *17*, 878–886. [CrossRef] [PubMed]
63. Perello, M.; Sakata, I.; Birnbaum, S.; Chuang, J.C.; Osborne-Lawrence, S.; Rovinsky, S.A.; Woloszyn, J.; Yanagisawa, M.; Lutter, M.; Zigman, J.M. Ghrelin Increases the Rewarding Value of High-Fat Diet in an Orexin-Dependent Manner. *Biol. Psychiatry* **2010**, *67*, 880–886. [CrossRef] [PubMed]
64. Egecioglu, E.; Jerlhag, E.; Salomé, N.; Skibicka, K.P.; Haage, D.; Bohlooly-Y, M.; Andersson, D.; Bjursell, M.; Perrissoud, D.; Engel, J.A.; et al. Ghrelin increases intake of rewarding food in rodents. *Addict. Biol.* **2010**, *15*, 304–311. [CrossRef] [PubMed]
65. Bake, T.; Le May, M.V.; Edvardsson, C.E.; Vogel, H.; Bergström, U.; Albers, M.N.; Skibicka, K.P.; Farkas, I.; Liposits, Z.; Dickson, S.L. Ghrelin Receptor Stimulation of the Lateral Parabrachial Nucleus in Rats Increases Food Intake but not Food Motivation. *Obesity* **2020**, *28*, 1503–1511. [CrossRef]

66. Dickson, S.L.; Shirazi, R.H.; Hansson, C.; Bergquist, F.; Nissbrandt, H.; Skibicka, K.P. The glucagon-like peptide 1 (GLP-1) analogue, exendin-4, decreases the rewarding value of food: A new role for mesolimbic GLP-1 receptors. *J. Neurosci.* **2012**, *32*, 4812–4820. [CrossRef] [PubMed]
67. Alhadeff, A.L.; Grill, H.J. Hindbrain nucleus tractus solitarius glucagon-like peptide-1 receptor signaling reduces appetitive and motivational aspects of feeding. *Am. J. Physiol. Regul. Integr. Comp. Physiol.* **2014**, *307*. [CrossRef]
68. Richard, J.E.; Anderberg, R.H.; Göteson, A.; Gribble, F.M.; Reimann, F.; Skibicka, K.P. Activation of the GLP-1 receptors in the nucleus of the solitary tract reduces food reward behavior and targets the mesolimbic system. *PLoS ONE* **2015**, *10*. [CrossRef]
69. Hsu, T.M.; Hahn, J.D.; Konanur, V.R.; Lam, A.; Kanoski, S.E. Hippocampal GLP-1 receptors influence food intake, meal size, and effort-based responding for food through volume transmission. *Neuropsychopharmacology* **2015**, *40*, 327–337. [CrossRef] [PubMed]
70. Davis, J.F.; Perello, M.; Choi, D.L.; Magrisso, I.J.; Kirchner, H.; Pfluger, P.T.; Tschoep, M.; Zigman, J.M.; Benoit, S.C. GOAT induced ghrelin acylation regulates hedonic feeding. *Horm. Behav.* **2012**, *62*, 598–604. [CrossRef]
71. Finger, B.C.; Dinan, T.G.; Cryan, J.F. Diet-induced obesity blunts the behavioural effects of ghrelin: Studies in a mouse-progressive ratio task. *Psychopharmacol.* **2012**, *220*, 173–181. [CrossRef]
72. Landgren, S.; Simms, J.A.; Thelle, D.S.; Strandhagen, E.; Bartlett, S.E.; Engel, J.A.; Jerlhag, E. The ghrelin signalling system is involved in the consumption of sweets. *PLoS ONE* **2011**, *6*. [CrossRef] [PubMed]
73. Bake, T.; Edvardsson, C.E.; Cummings, C.J.; Dickson, S.L. Ghrelin's effects on food motivation in rats are not limited to palatable foods. *J. Neuroendocrinol.* **2019**, *31*. [CrossRef] [PubMed]
74. Overduin, J.; Figlewicz, D.P.; Bennett-Jay, J.; Kittleson, S.; Cummings, D.E. Ghrelin increases the motivation to eat, but does not alter food palatability. *Am. J. Physiol. Regul. Integr. Comp. Physiol.* **2012**, *303*, 259–269. [CrossRef]
75. Salamone, J.D.; Correa, M. The Mysterious Motivational Functions of Mesolimbic Dopamine. *Neuron* **2012**, *76*, 470–485. [CrossRef]
76. Skibicka, K.P.; Shirazi, R.H.; Rabasa-Papio, C.; Alvarez-Crespo, M.; Neuber, C.; Vogel, H.; Dickson, S.L. Divergent circuitry underlying food reward and intake effects of ghrelin: Dopaminergic VTA-accumbens projection mediates ghrelin's effect on food reward but not food intake. *Neuropharmacology* **2013**, *73*, 274–283. [CrossRef]
77. King, S.J.; Isaacs, A.M.; O'Farrell, E.; Abizaid, A. Motivation to obtain preferred foods is enhanced by ghrelin in the ventral tegmental area. *Horm. Behav.* **2011**, *60*, 572–580. [CrossRef]
78. Weinberg, Z.Y.; Nicholson, M.L.; Currie, P.J. 6-Hydroxydopamine lesions of the ventral tegmental area suppress ghrelin's ability to elicit food-reinforced behavior. *Neurosci. Lett.* **2011**, *499*, 70–73. [CrossRef]
79. Skibicka, K.P.; Hansson, C.; Alvarez-Crespo, M.; Friberg, P.A.; Dickson, S.L. Ghrelin directly targets the ventral tegmental area to increase food motivation. *Neuroscience* **2011**, *180*, 129–137. [CrossRef] [PubMed]
80. López-Ferreras, L.; Richard, J.E.; Anderberg, R.H.; Nilsson, F.H.; Olandersson, K.; Kanoski, S.E.; Skibicka, K.P. Ghrelin's control of food reward and body weight in the lateral hypothalamic area is sexually dimorphic. *Physiol. Behav.* **2017**, *176*, 40–49. [CrossRef]
81. Cone, J.J.; McCutcheon, J.E.; Roitman, M.F. Ghrelin acts as an interface between physiological state and phasic dopamine signaling. *J. Neurosci.* **2014**, *34*, 4905–4913. [CrossRef]
82. Terrill, S.J.; Wall, K.D.; Medina, N.D.; Maske, C.B.; Williams, D.L. Lateral septum growth hormone secretagogue receptor affects food intake and motivation for sucrose reinforcement. *Am. J. Physiol. Regul. Integr. Comp. Physiol.* **2018**, *315*, R76–R83. [CrossRef] [PubMed]
83. Howell, E.; Baumgartner, H.M.; Zallar, L.J.; Selva, J.A.; Engel, L.; Currie, P.J. Glucagon-like peptide-1 (GLP-1) and 5-hydroxytryptamine 2c (5-HT2c) receptor agonists in the ventral tegmental area (VTA) inhibit ghrelin-stimulated appetitive reward. *Int. J. Mol. Sci.* **2019**, *20*. [CrossRef]
84. Bernosky-Smith, K.A.; Stanger, D.B.; Trujillo, A.J.; Mitchell, L.R.; España, R.A.; Bass, C.E. The GLP-1 agonist exendin-4 attenuates self-administration of sweetened fat on fixed and progressive ratio schedules of reinforcement in rats. *Pharmacol. Biochem. Behav.* **2016**, *142*, 48–55. [CrossRef]
85. Anderberg, R.H.; Anefors, C.; Bergquist, F.; Nissbrandt, H.; Skibicka, K.P. Dopamine signaling in the amygdala, increased by food ingestion and GLP-1, regulates feeding behavior. *Physiol. Behav.* **2014**, *136*, 135–144. [CrossRef] [PubMed]
86. Vogel, H.; Wolf, S.; Rabasa, C.; Rodriguez-Pacheco, F.; Babaei, C.S.; Stöber, F.; Goldschmidt, J.; DiMarchi, R.D.; Finan, B.; Tschöp, M.H.; et al. GLP-1 and estrogen conjugate acts in the supramammillary nucleus to reduce food-reward and body weight. *Neuropharmacology* **2016**, *110*, 396–406. [CrossRef]
87. Alhadeff, A.L.; Baird, J.P.; Swick, J.C.; Hayes, M.R.; Grill, H.J. Glucagon-like peptide-1 receptor signaling in the lateral parabrachial nucleus contributes to the control of food intake and motivation to feed. *Neuropsychopharmacology* **2014**, *39*, 2233–2243. [CrossRef]
88. Terrill, S.J.; Holt, M.K.; Maske, C.B.; Abrams, N.; Reimann, F.; Trapp, S.; Williams, D.L. Endogenous GLP-1 in lateral septum promotes satiety and suppresses motivation for food in mice. *Physiol. Behav.* **2019**, *206*, 191–199. [CrossRef] [PubMed]
89. López-Ferreras, L.; Eerola, K.; Mishra, D.; Shevchouk, O.T.; Richard, J.E.; Nilsson, F.H.; Hayes, M.R.; Skibicka, K.P. GLP-1 modulates the supramammillary nucleus-lateral hypothalamic neurocircuit to control ingestive and motivated behavior in a sex divergent manner. *Mol. Metab.* **2019**, *20*, 178–193. [CrossRef] [PubMed]
90. Richard, J.E.; Anderberg, R.H.; López-Ferreras, L.; Olandersson, K.; Skibicka, K.P. Sex and estrogens alter the action of glucagon-like peptide-1 on reward. *Biol. Sex Differ.* **2016**, *7*, 1–6. [CrossRef]
91. López-Ferreras, L.; Richard, J.E.; Noble, E.E.; Eerola, K.; Anderberg, R.H.; Olandersson, K.; Taing, L.; Kanoski, S.E.; Hayes, M.R.; Skibicka, K.P. Lateral hypothalamic GLP-1 receptors are critical for the control of food reinforcement, ingestive behavior and body weight. *Mol. Psychiatry* **2018**, *23*, 1157–1168. [CrossRef]

92. Maske, C.B.; Loney, G.C.; Lilly, N.; Terrill, S.J.; Williams, D.L. Intragastric nutrient infusion reduces motivation for food in male and female rats. *Am. J. Physiol. Endocrinol. Metab.* **2018**, *315*, E81–E90. [CrossRef] [PubMed]
93. Anderberg, R.H.; Hansson, C.; Fenander, M.; Richard, J.E.; Dickson, S.L.; Nissbrandt, H.; Bergquist, F.; Skibicka, K.P. The Stomach-Derived Hormone Ghrelin Increases Impulsive Behavior. *Neuropsychopharmacology* **2016**, *41*, 1199–1209. [CrossRef] [PubMed]
94. Hsu, T.M.; Noble, E.E.; Liu, C.M.; Cortella, A.M.; Konanur, V.R.; Suarez, A.N.; Reiner, D.J.; Hahn, J.D.; Hayes, M.R.; Kanoski, S.E. A hippocampus to prefrontal cortex neural pathway inhibits food motivation through glucagon-like peptide-1 signaling. *Mol. Psychiatry* **2018**, *23*, 1555–1565. [CrossRef] [PubMed]
95. Jones, S.; Sample, C.H.; Davidson, T.L. The effects of a GLP-1 analog liraglutide on reward value and the learned inhibition of appetitive behavior in male and female rats. *Int. J. Obes.* **2019**, *43*, 1875–1879. [CrossRef]
96. Noble, E.E.; Wang, Z.; Liu, C.M.; Davis, E.A.; Suarez, A.N.; Stein, L.M.; Tsan, L.; Terrill, S.J.; Hsu, T.M.; Jung, A.-H.; et al. Hypothalamus-hippocampus circuitry regulates impulsivity via melanin-concentrating hormone. *Nat. Commun.* **2019**, *10*, 4923. [CrossRef] [PubMed]
97. Hanssen, R.; Kretschmer, A.C.; Rigoux, L.; Albus, K.; Thanarajah, S.E.; Sitnikow, T.; Melzer, C.; Cornely, O.A.; Brüning, J.C.; Tittgemeyer, M. GLP-1 and hunger modulate incentive motivation depending on insulin sensitivity in humans. *Mol. Metab.* **2021**, *45*, 101163. [CrossRef] [PubMed]
98. Miras, A.D.; Jackson, R.N.; Jackson, S.N.; Goldstone, A.P.; Olbers, T.; Hackenberg, T.; Spector, A.C.; Le Roux, C.W. Gastric bypass surgery for obesity decreases the reward value of a sweet-fat stimulus as assessed in a progressive ratio task. *Am. J. Clin. Nutr.* **2012**, *96*, 467–473. [CrossRef] [PubMed]
99. Goldstone, A.P.; Miras, A.D.; Scholtz, S.; Jackson, S.; Neff, K.J.; Pénicaud, L.; Geoghegan, J.; Chhina, N.; Durighel, G.; Bell, J.D.; et al. Link between increased satiety gut hormones and reduced food reward after gastric bypass surgery for obesity. *J. Clin. Endocrinol. Metab.* **2016**, *101*, 599–609. [CrossRef]
100. Elliott, J.A.; Docherty, N.G.; Haag, J.; Eckhardt, H.G.; Ravi, N.; Reynolds, J.V.; Le Roux, C.W. Attenuation of satiety gut hormones increases appetitive behavior after curative esophagectomy for esophageal cancer. *Am. J. Clin. Nutr.* **2019**, *109*, 335–344. [CrossRef]
101. Disse, E.; Bussier, A.L.; Veyrat-Durebex, C.; Deblon, N.; Pfluger, P.T.; Tschöp, M.H.; Laville, M.; Rohner-Jeanrenaud, F. Peripheral ghrelin enhances sweet taste food consumption and preference, regardless of its caloric content. *Physiol. Behav.* **2010**, *101*, 277–281. [CrossRef] [PubMed]
102. Stevenson, J.R.; Francomacaro, L.M.; Bohidar, A.E.; Young, K.A.; Pesarchick, B.F.; Buirkle, J.M.; McMahon, E.K.; O'Bryan, C.M. Ghrelin receptor (GHS-R1A) antagonism alters preference for ethanol and sucrose in a concentration-dependent manner in prairie voles. *Physiol. Behav.* **2016**, *155*, 231–236. [CrossRef]
103. Lockie, S.H.; Dinan, T.; Lawrence, A.J.; Spencer, S.J.; Andrews, Z.B. Diet-induced obesity causes ghrelin resistance in reward processing tasks. *Psychoneuroendocrinology* **2015**, *62*, 114–120. [CrossRef]
104. Pierre, A.; Regin, Y.; Van Schuerbeek, A.; Fritz, E.M.; Muylle, K.; Beckers, T.; Smolders, I.J.; Singewald, N.; De Bundel, D. Effects of disrupted ghrelin receptor function on fear processing, anxiety and saccharin preference in mice. *Psychoneuroendocrinology* **2019**, *110*. [CrossRef] [PubMed]
105. Furudono, Y.; Ando, C.; Yamamoto, C.; Kobashi, M.; Yamamoto, T. Involvement of specific orexigenic neuropeptides in sweetener-induced overconsumption in rats. *Behav. Brain Res.* **2006**, *175*, 241–248. [CrossRef] [PubMed]
106. Schéle, E.; Bake, T.; Rabasa, C.; Dickson, S.L. Centrally administered ghrelin acutely influences food choice in rodents. *PLoS ONE* **2016**, *11*. [CrossRef]
107. Yamaguchi, E.; Yasoshima, Y.; Shimura, T. Systemic administration of anorexic gut peptide hormones impairs hedonic-driven sucrose consumption in mice. *Physiol. Behav.* **2017**, *171*, 158–164. [CrossRef]
108. Alhadeff, A.L.; Rupprecht, L.E.; Hayes, M.R. GLP-1 neurons in the nucleus of the solitary tract project directly to the ventral tegmental area and nucleus accumbens to control for food intake. *Endocrinology* **2012**, *153*, 647–658. [CrossRef]
109. Mietlicki-Baase, E.G.; McGrath, L.E.; Koch-Laskowski, K.; Krawczyk, J.; Pham, T.; Lhamo, R.; Reiner, D.J.; Hayes, M.R. Hindbrain DPP-IV inhibition improves glycemic control and promotes negative energy balance. *Physiol. Behav.* **2017**, *173*, 9–14. [CrossRef]
110. Hyde, K.M.; Blonde, G.D.; le Roux, C.W.; Spector, A.C. Liraglutide suppression of caloric intake competes with the intake-promoting effects of a palatable cafeteria diet, but does not impact food or macronutrient selection. *Physiol. Behav.* **2017**, *177*, 4–12. [CrossRef]
111. Monteleone, P.; Piscitelli, F.; Scognamiglio, P.; Monteleone, A.M.; Canestrelli, B.; Di Marzo, V.; Maj, M. Hedonic eating is associated with increased peripheral levels of ghrelin and the endocannabinoid 2-arachidonoyl-glycerol in healthy humans: A pilot study. *J. Clin. Endocrinol. Metab.* **2012**, *97*. [CrossRef]
112. Monteleone, P.; Scognamiglio, P.; Monteleone, A.M.; Perillo, D.; Canestrelli, B.; Maj, M. Gastroenteric hormone responses to hedonic eating in healthy humans. *Psychoneuroendocrinology* **2013**, *38*, 1435–1441. [CrossRef]
113. Basolo, A.; Heinitz, S.; Stinson, E.J.; Begaye, B.; Hohenadel, M.; Piaggi, P.; Krakoff, J.; Votruba, S.B. Fasting glucagon-like peptide 1 concentration is associated with lower carbohydrate intake and increases with overeating. *J. Endocrinol. Investig.* **2019**, *42*, 557–566. [CrossRef] [PubMed]
114. Hankir, M.K.; Seyfried, F.; Hintschich, C.A.; Diep, T.A.; Kleberg, K.; Kranz, M.; Deuther-Conrad, W.; Tellez, L.A.; Rullmann, M.; Patt, M.; et al. Gastric Bypass Surgery Recruits a Gut PPAR-α-Striatal D1R Pathway to Reduce Fat Appetite in Obese Rats. *Cell Metab.* **2017**, *25*, 335–344. [CrossRef]

115. Søndergaard Nielsen, M.; Rasmussen, S.; Just Christensen, B.; Ritz, C.; le Roux, C.W.; Berg Schmidt, J.; Sjödin, A. Bariatric Surgery Does Not Affect Food Preferences, but Individual Changes in Food Preferences May Predict Weight Loss. *Obesity* **2018**, *26*, 1879–1887. [CrossRef] [PubMed]
116. Kittrell, H.; Graber, W.; Mariani, E.; Czaja, K.; Hajnal, A.; Di Lorenzo, P.M. Taste and odor preferences following roux-en-Y surgery in humans. *PLoS ONE* **2018**, *13*. [CrossRef]
117. Le Roux, C.W.; Bueter, M.; Theis, N.; Werling, M.; Ashrafian, H.; Löwenstein, C.; Athanasiou, T.; Bloom, S.R.; Spector, A.C.; Olbers, T.; et al. Gastric bypass reduces fat intake and preference. *Am. J. Physiol. Regul. Integr. Comp. Physiol.* **2011**, *301*, R1057. [CrossRef]
118. Shin, Y.K.; Martin, B.; Kim, W.; White, C.M.; Ji, S.; Sun, Y.; Smith, R.G.; Sévigny, J.; Tschöp, M.H.; Maudsley, S.; et al. Ghrelin is produced in taste cells and ghrelin receptor null mice show reduced taste responsivity to salty (NaCl) and sour (Citric Acid) tastants. *PLoS ONE* **2010**, *5*, e12729. [CrossRef] [PubMed]
119. Cai, H.; Cong, W.N.; Daimon, C.M.; Wang, R.; Tschöp, M.H.; Sévigny, J.; Martin, B.; Maudsley, S. Altered Lipid and Salt Taste Responsivity in Ghrelin and GOAT Null Mice. *PLoS ONE* **2013**, *8*. [CrossRef]
120. Shin, Y.K.; Martin, B.; Golden, E.; Dotson, C.D.; Maudsley, S.; Kim, W.; Jang, H.J.; Mattson, M.P.; Drucker, D.J.; Egan, J.M.; et al. Modulation of taste sensitivity by GLP-1 signaling. *J. Neurochem.* **2008**, *106*, 455–463. [CrossRef]
121. Martin, B.; Dotson, C.D.; Shin, Y.K.; Ji, S.; Drucker, D.J.; Maudsley, S.; Munger, S.D. Modulation of taste sensitivity by GLP-1 signaling in taste buds. In *Annals of the New York Academy of Sciences*; Wiley-Blackwell: Hoboken, NJ, USA, 2009; Volume 1170, pp. 98–101.
122. Takai, S.; Yasumatsu, K.; Inoue, M.; Iwata, S.; Yoshida, R.; Shigemura, N.; Yanagawa, Y.; Drucker, D.J.; Margolskee, R.F.; Ninomiya, Y. Glucagon-like peptide-1 is specifically involved in sweet taste transmission. *FASEB J.* **2015**, *29*, 2268–2280. [CrossRef]
123. Asarian, L.; Corp, E.S.; Hrupka, B.; Geary, N. Intracerebroventricular glucagon-like peptide-1 (7-36) amide inhibits sham feeding in rats without eliciting satiety. *Physiol. Behav.* **1998**. [CrossRef]
124. Douton, J.E.; Norgren, R.; Grigson, P.S. Effects of a glucagon-like peptide-1 analog on appetitive and consummatory behavior for rewarding and aversive gustatory stimuli in rats. *Physiol. Behav.* **2021**, *229*. [CrossRef] [PubMed]
125. Arosio, M.; Ronchi, C.L.; Beck-Peccoz, P.; Gebbia, C.; Giavoli, C.; Cappiello, V.; Conte, D.; Peracchi, M. Effects of modified sham feeding on ghrelin levels in healthy human subjects. *J. Clin. Endocrinol. Metab.* **2004**, *89*, 5101–5104. [CrossRef] [PubMed]
126. Zhu, Y.; Hsu, W.H.; Hollis, J.H. Modified sham feeding of foods with different macronutrient compositions differentially influences cephalic change of insulin, ghrelin, and NMR-based metabolomic profiles. *Physiol. Behav.* **2014**, *135*, 135–142. [CrossRef]
127. Uygun, B.; Kiyici, S.; Ozmen, S.; Gul, Z.; Sigirli, D.; Cavun, S. The Association between Olfaction and Taste Functions with Serum Ghrelin and Leptin Levels in Obese Women. *Metab. Syndr. Relat. Disord.* **2019**, *17*, 452–457. [CrossRef] [PubMed]
128. Bueter, M.; Miras, A.D.; Chichger, H.; Fenske, W.; Ghatei, M.A.; Bloom, S.R.; Unwin, R.J.; Lutz, T.A.; Spector, A.C.; Le Roux, C.W. Alterations of sucrose preference after Roux-en-Y gastric bypass. *Physiol. Behav.* **2011**, *104*, 709–721. [CrossRef] [PubMed]
129. Kadouh, H.; Chedid, V.; Halawi, H.; Burton, D.D.; Clark, M.M.; Khemani, D.; Vella, A.; Acosta, A.; Camilleri, M. GLP-1 analog modulates appetite, taste preference, gut hormones, and regional body fat stores in adults with obesity. *J. Clin. Endocrinol. Metab.* **2020**, *105*, 1552. [CrossRef] [PubMed]
130. Brindisi, M.C.; Brondel, L.; Meillon, S.; Barthet, S.; Grall, S.; Fenech, C.; Liénard, F.; Schlich, P.; Astruc, K.; Mouillot, T.; et al. Proof of concept: Effect of GLP-1 agonist on food hedonic responses and taste sensitivity in poor controlled type 2 diabetic patients. *Diabetes Metab. Syndr. Clin. Res. Rev.* **2019**, *13*, 2489–2494. [CrossRef]
131. Baretić, M.; Kušec, V.; Uroić, V.; Pavlić-Renar, I.; Altabas, V. Glucagon-like peptide-1 affects taste perception differently in women: A randomized, placebo-controlled crossover study. *Acta Clin. Croat.* **2019**, *58*, 240–248. [CrossRef]
132. Rodriguez, J.A.; Fehrentz, J.A.; Martinez, J.; Ben Haj Salah, K.; Wellman, P.J. The GHR-R antagonist JMV 2959 neither induces malaise nor alters the malaise property of LiCl in the adult male rat. *Physiol. Behav.* **2018**, *183*, 46–48. [CrossRef]
133. Song, L.; Zhu, Q.; Liu, T.; Yu, M.; Xiao, K.; Kong, Q.; Zhao, R.; Li, G.D.; Zhou, Y. Ghrelin Modulates Lateral Amygdala Neuronal Firing and Blocks Acquisition for Conditioned Taste Aversion. *PLoS ONE* **2013**, *8*. [CrossRef]
134. Li, N.; Song, G.; Wang, Y.; Zhu, Q.; Han, F.; Zhang, C.; Zhou, Y. Blocking constitutive activity of GHSR1a in the lateral amygdala facilitates acquisition of conditioned taste aversion. *Neuropeptides* **2018**, *68*, 22–27. [CrossRef] [PubMed]
135. Song, G.; Zhu, Q.; Han, F.; Liu, S.; Zhao, C.; Zhou, Y. Local infusion of ghrelin into the lateral amygdala blocks extinction of conditioned taste aversion in rats. *Neurosci. Lett.* **2018**, *662*, 71–76. [CrossRef] [PubMed]
136. Abegg, K.; Bernasconi, L.; Hutter, M.; Whiting, L.; Pietra, C.; Giuliano, C.; Lutz, T.A.; Riediger, T. Ghrelin receptor inverse agonists as a novel therapeutic approach against obesity-related metabolic disease. *Diabetes Obes. Metab.* **2017**. [CrossRef]
137. Yakabi, K.; Sadakane, C.; Noguchi, M.; Ohno, S.; Ro, S.; Chinen, K.; Aoyama, T.; Sakurada, T.; Takabayashi, H.; Hattori, T. Reduced ghrelin secretion in the hypothalamus of rats due to cisplatin-induced anorexia. *Endocrinology* **2010**, *151*, 3773–3782. [CrossRef]
138. Malik, N.M.; Moore, G.B.T.; Kaur, R.; Liu, Y.L.; Wood, S.L.; Morrow, R.W.; Sanger, G.J.; Andrews, P.L.R. Adaptive upregulation of gastric and hypothalamic ghrelin receptors and increased plasma ghrelin in a model of cancer chemotherapy-induced dyspepsia. *Regul. Pept.* **2008**, *148*, 33–38. [CrossRef]
139. Liu, Y.L.; Malik, N.M.; Sanger, G.J.; Andrews, P.L.R. Ghrelin alleviates cancer chemotherapy-associated dyspepsia in rodents. *Cancer Chemother. Pharmacol.* **2006**, *58*, 326–333. [CrossRef] [PubMed]
140. Gong, Y.L.; Liu, F.; Jin, H.; Xu, L.; Guo, F.F. Involvement of ghrelin in nucleus tractus solitaries on gastric signal afferent and gastric motility in cisplatin-treated rats. *Eur. Rev. Med. Pharmacol. Sci.* **2016**, *20*, 3480–3489.

141. Rudd, J.A.; Chan, S.W.; Ngan, M.P.; Tu, L.; Lu, Z.; Giuliano, C.; Lovati, E.; Pietra, C. Anti-emetic action of the brain-penetrating new ghrelin agonist, HM01, alone and in combination with the 5-HT3 antagonist, palonosetron and with the NK1 antagonist, netupitant, against cisplatin- and motion-induced emesis in Suncus murinus (house musk shr. *Front. Pharmacol.* **2018**, *9*. [CrossRef]
142. Thiele, T.E.; Van Dijk, G.; Campfield, L.A.; Smith, F.J.; Burn, P.; Woods, S.C.; Bernstein, J.L.; Seeley, R.J. Central infusion of GLP-1, but not leptin, produces conditioned taste aversions in rats. *Am. J. Physiol. Regul. Integr. Comp. Physiol.* **1997**, *272*. [CrossRef]
143. Kinzig, K.P.; D'Alessio, D.A.; Seeley, R.J. The diverse roles of specific GLP-1 receptors in the control of food intake and the response to visceral illness. *J. Neurosci.* **2002**, *22*, 10470–10476. [CrossRef] [PubMed]
144. Baraboi, E.D.; St-Pierre, D.H.; Shooner, J.; Timofeeva, E.; Richard, D. Brain activation following peripheral administration of the GLP-1 receptor agonist exendin-4. *Am. J. Physiol. Regul. Integr. Comp. Physiol.* **2011**. [CrossRef]
145. Kanoski, S.E.; Rupprecht, L.E.; Fortin, S.M.; De Jonghe, B.C.; Hayes, M.R. The role of nausea in food intake and body weight suppression by peripheral GLP-1 receptor agonists, exendin-4 and liraglutide. *Neuropharmacology* **2012**. [CrossRef] [PubMed]
146. Punjabi, M.; Arnold, M.; Rüttimann, E.; Graber, M.; Geary, N.; Pacheco-López, G.; Langhans, W. Circulating Glucagon-like Peptide-1 (GLP-1) Inhibits Eating in Male Rats by Acting in the Hindbrain and Without Inducing Avoidance. *Endocrinology* **2014**. [CrossRef] [PubMed]
147. McMahon, L.R.; Wellman, P.J. PVN infusion of GLP-1-(7-36) amide suppresses feeding but does not induce aversion or alter locomotion in rats. *Am. J. Physiol. Regul. Integr. Comp. Physiol.* **1998**, *274*. [CrossRef] [PubMed]
148. Dossat, A.M.; Lilly, N.; Kay, K.; Williams, D.L. Glucagon-like peptide 1 receptors in nucleus accumbens affect food intake. *J. Neurosci.* **2011**, *31*, 14453–14457. [CrossRef] [PubMed]
149. Reiner, D.J.; Leon, R.M.; McGrath, L.E.; Koch-Laskowski, K.; Hahn, J.D.; Kanoski, S.E.; Mietlicki-Baase, E.G.; Hayes, M.R. Glucagon-Like Peptide-1 Receptor Signaling in the Lateral Dorsal Tegmental Nucleus Regulates Energy Balance. *Neuropsychopharmacology* **2018**, *43*, 627–637. [CrossRef] [PubMed]
150. Tang-Christensen, M.; Larsen, P.J.; Göke, R.; Fink-Jensen, A.; Jessop, D.S.; Møller, M.; Sheikh, S.P. Central administration of GLP-1-(7-36) amide inhibits food and water intake in rats. *Am. J. Physiol. Regul. Integr. Comp. Physiol.* **1996**, *271*. [CrossRef] [PubMed]
151. Labouesse, M.A.; Stadlbauer, U.; Weber, E.; Arnold, M.; Langhans, W.; Pacheco-López, G. Vagal Afferents Mediate Early Satiation and Prevent Flavour Avoidance Learning in Response to Intraperitoneally Infused Exendin-4. *J. Neuroendocrinol.* **2012**. [CrossRef]
152. Quigley, K.S.; Kanoski, S.; Grill, W.M.; Barrett, L.F.; Tsakiris, M. Functions of Interoception: From Energy Regulation to Experience of the Self. *Trends Neurosci.* **2021**, *44*, 29–38. [CrossRef]
153. Borner, T.; Liberini, C.G.; Lutz, T.A.; Riediger, T. Brainstem GLP-1 signalling contributes to cancer anorexia-cachexia syndrome in the rat. *Neuropharmacology* **2018**, *131*, 282–290. [CrossRef] [PubMed]
154. De Jonghe, B.C.; Holland, R.A.; Olivos, D.R.; Rupprecht, L.E.; Kanoski, S.E.; Hayes, M.R. Hindbrain GLP-1 receptor mediation of cisplatin-induced anorexia and nausea. *Physiol. Behav.* **2016**, *153*, 109–114. [CrossRef] [PubMed]
155. Farmer, A.D.; Ban, V.F.; Coen, S.J.; Sanger, G.J.; Barker, G.J.; Gresty, M.A.; Giampietro, V.P.; Williams, S.C.; Webb, D.L.; Hellström, P.M.; et al. Visually induced nausea causes characteristic changes in cerebral, autonomic and endocrine function in humans. *J. Physiol.* **2015**, *593*, 1183–1196. [CrossRef] [PubMed]
156. Hiura, Y.; Takiguchi, S.; Yamamoto, K.; Kurokawa, Y.; Yamasaki, M.; Nakajima, K.; Miyata, H.; Fujiwara, Y.; Mori, M.; Doki, Y. Fall in plasma ghrelin concentrations after cisplatin-based chemotherapy in esophageal cancer patients. *Int. J. Clin. Oncol.* **2012**, *17*, 316–323. [CrossRef] [PubMed]
157. Ohno, T.; Yanai, M.; Ando, H.; Toyomasu, Y.; Ogawa, A.; Morita, H.; Ogata, K.; Mochiki, E.; Asao, T.; Kuwano, H. Rikkunshito, a traditional Japanese medicine, suppresses cisplatin-induced anorexia in humans. *Clin. Exp. Gastroenterol.* **2011**, *4*, 291–296. [CrossRef]
158. Hiura, Y.; Takiguchi, S.; Yamamoto, K.; Takahashi, T.; Kurokawa, Y.; Yamasaki, M.; Nakajima, K.; Miyata, H.; Fujiwara, Y.; Mori, M.; et al. Effects of ghrelin administration during chemotherapy with advanced esophageal cancer patients: A prospective, randomized, placebo-controlled phase 2 study. *Cancer* **2012**, *118*, 4785–4794. [CrossRef]
159. Harada, T.; Amano, T.; Ikari, T.; Takamura, K.; Ogi, T.; Fujikane, T.; Fujita, Y.; Taima, K.; Tanaka, H.; Sasaki, T.; et al. Rikkunshito for preventing chemotherapy-induced nausea and vomiting in lung cancer patients: Results from 2 prospective, randomized phase 2 trials. *Front. Pharmacol.* **2018**, *8*. [CrossRef]
160. Hamai, Y.; Yoshiya, T.; Hihara, J.; Emi, M.; Furukawa, T.; Yamakita, I.; Ibuki, Y.; Okada, M. Traditional Japanese herbal medicine rikkunshito increases food intake and plasma acylated ghrelin levels in patients with esophageal cancer treated by cisplatin-based chemotherapy. *J. Thorac. Dis.* **2019**, *11*, 2470–2478. [CrossRef]
161. Wo, J.M.; Ejskjaer, N.; Hellström, P.M.; Malik, R.A.; Pezzullo, J.C.; Shaughnessy, L.; Charlton, P.; Kosutic, G.; McCallum, R.W. Randomised clinical trial: Ghrelin agonist TZP-101 relieves gastroparesis associated with severe nausea and vomiting—Randomised clinical study subset data. *Aliment. Pharmacol. Ther.* **2011**, *33*, 679–688. [CrossRef]
162. Mccallum, R.W.; Lembo, A.; Esfandyari, T.; Bhandari, B.R.; Ejskjaer, N.; Cosentino, C.; Helton, N.; Mondou, E.; Quinn, J.; Rousseau, F. Phase 2b, randomized, double-blind 12-week studies of TZP-102, a ghrelin receptor agonist for diabetic gastroparesis. *Neurogastroenterol. Motil.* **2013**, *25*, e705–e717. [CrossRef]

163. Camilleri, M.; McCallum, R.W.; Tack, J.; Spence, S.C.; Gottesdiener, K.; Fiedorek, F.T. Efficacy and Safety of Relamorelin in Diabetics With Symptoms of Gastroparesis: A Randomized, Placebo-Controlled Study. *Gastroenterology* **2017**, *153*, 1240–1250. [CrossRef]
164. Hong, S.W.; Chun, J.; Kim, J.; Lee, J.; Lee, H.J.; Chung, H.; Cho, S.J.; Im, J.P.; Kim, S.G.; Kim, J.S. Efficacy and safety of ghrelin agonists in patients with diabetic gastroparesis: A systematic review and meta-analysis. *Gut Liver* **2020**, *14*, 589–600. [CrossRef] [PubMed]
165. Bettge, K.; Kahle, M.; Abd El Aziz, M.S.; Meier, J.J.; Nauck, M.A. Occurrence of nausea, vomiting and diarrhoea reported as adverse events in clinical trials studying glucagon-like peptide-1 receptor agonists: A systematic analysis of published clinical trials. *Diabetes Obes. Metab.* **2017**, *19*, 336–347. [CrossRef]
166. Shiomi, M.; Takada, T.; Tanaka, Y.; Yajima, K.; Isomoto, A.; Sakamoto, M.; Otori, K. Clinical factors associated with the occurrence of nausea and vomiting in type 2 diabetes patients treated with glucagon-like peptide-1 receptor agonists. *J. Diabetes Investig.* **2019**, *10*, 408–417. [CrossRef] [PubMed]
167. Lean, M.E.J.; Carraro, R.; Finer, N.; Hartvig, H.; Lindegaard, M.L.; Rössner, S.; Van Gaal, L.; Astrup, A. Tolerability of nausea and vomiting and associations with weight loss in a randomized trial of liraglutide in obese, non-diabetic adults. *Int. J. Obes.* **2014**, *38*, 689–697. [CrossRef] [PubMed]
168. Rayner, C.K.; Wu, T.; Aroda, V.R.; Whittington, C.; Kanters, S.; Guyot, P.; Shaunik, A.; Horowitz, M. Gastrointestinal adverse events with insulin glargine/lixisenatide fixed-ratio combination versus glucagon-like peptide-1 receptor agonists in people with type 2 diabetes mellitus: A network meta-analysis. *Diabetes Obes. Metab.* **2021**, *23*, 136–146. [CrossRef] [PubMed]
169. Mietlicki-Baase, E.G.; Liberini, C.G.; Workinger, J.L.; Bonaccorso, R.L.; Borner, T.; Reiner, D.J.; Koch-Laskowski, K.; McGrath, L.E.; Lhamo, R.; Stein, L.M.; et al. A vitamin B12 conjugate of exendin-4 improves glucose tolerance without associated nausea or hypophagia in rodents. *Diabetes Obes. Metab.* **2018**, *20*, 1223–1234. [CrossRef] [PubMed]
170. Borner, T.; Workinger, J.L.; Tinsley, I.C.; Fortin, S.M.; Stein, L.M.; Chepurny, O.G.; Holz, G.G.; Wierzba, A.J.; Gryko, D.; Nexø, E.; et al. Corrination of a GLP-1 Receptor Agonist for Glycemic Control without Emesis. *Cell Rep.* **2020**, *31*. [CrossRef] [PubMed]

Review

Central Neurocircuits Regulating Food Intake in Response to Gut Inputs—Preclinical Evidence

Kirsteen N. Browning * and Kaitlin E. Carson

Department of Neural and Behavioral Sciences, Penn State College of Medicine, Hershey, PA 17033, USA; kcarson2@pennstatehealth.psu.edu
* Correspondence: akbrowning@pennstatehealth.psu.edu; Tel.: +1-717-531-8267

Abstract: The regulation of energy balance requires the complex integration of homeostatic and hedonic pathways, but sensory inputs from the gastrointestinal (GI) tract are increasingly recognized as playing critical roles. The stomach and small intestine relay sensory information to the central nervous system (CNS) via the sensory afferent vagus nerve. This vast volume of complex sensory information is received by neurons of the nucleus of the tractus solitarius (NTS) and is integrated with responses to circulating factors as well as descending inputs from the brainstem, midbrain, and forebrain nuclei involved in autonomic regulation. The integrated signal is relayed to the adjacent dorsal motor nucleus of the vagus (DMV), which supplies the motor output response via the efferent vagus nerve to regulate and modulate gastric motility, tone, secretion, and emptying, as well as intestinal motility and transit; the precise coordination of these responses is essential for the control of meal size, meal termination, and nutrient absorption. The interconnectivity of the NTS implies that many other CNS areas are capable of modulating vagal efferent output, emphasized by the many CNS disorders associated with dysregulated GI functions including feeding. This review will summarize the role of major CNS centers to gut-related inputs in the regulation of gastric function with specific reference to the regulation of food intake.

Keywords: brainstem; vagus; feeding; gastrointestinal

1. Introduction

Sensory information from the gastrointestinal (GI) tract is relayed centrally via neural and humoral pathways; the central nervous system (CNS) integrates this large volume of sensory afferent information and coordinates a precise series of efferent responses to regulate food and caloric intake including the modulation of gastric motility, tone, and emptying, as well as intestinal motility, transit, secretion and absorption. This efferent output is regulated meticulously in order to maintain homeostasis based on current energy needs and visceral sensory stimuli. The advent of novel and emerging molecular and genetic labeling techniques implies that, as a field, we are in a better position to be able to potentially delineate the exact phenotype of neurons involved in distinct aspects of nutrient signaling, and to interrogate and manipulate those neurocircuits with spatial and temporal precision. Characterizing the central neurocircuits involved following activation of gut inputs, including their phenotypes, activation characteristics, and connectomes, will be important to understand the physiology and pathophysiology of food intake.

1.1. Afferent Inputs

GI sensory information is relayed centrally via both vagal and spinal afferents. Spinal afferents, particularly those within the splanchnic nerves, relay low- or high-threshold mechanical and chemical information centrally and are considered primarily to be involved in nociceptive processing [1,2]. In contrast, the majority of interoceptive information is relayed centrally via vagal afferents, the cell bodies of which reside in the nodose and jugular ganglion. The central terminals of most of the gastrointestinal vagal afferents terminate within the brainstem at the level of the nucleus tractus solitarus (NTS), with a minority of terminals found in the area postrema (AP), the dorsal motor nucleus of the vagus (DMV), and the trigeminal islands [3]. Vagal afferent signaling is critical for the regulation of food intake and selective surgical denervation of GI vagal afferents has been shown to increase meal size and blunt the response to peripheral administration of GI peptides implicating vagal afferent signaling in the regulation of food intake [4] (Figure 1).

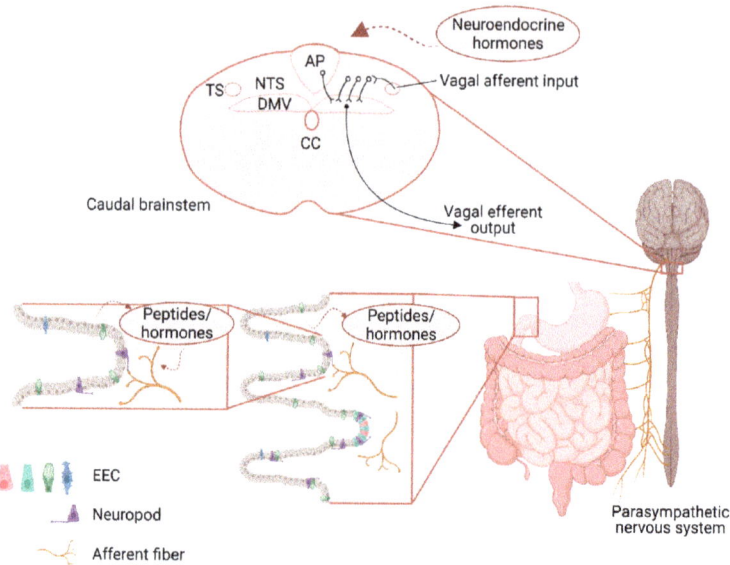

Figure 1. Schematic representation of the neuroanatomical connections between the gastrointestinal (GI) tract and brainstem vagal nuclei involved in the regulation of food intake. Sensory information from the GI tract is relayed centrally via the afferent vagus which responds both directly (via neuropods) and indirectly (via paracrine signaling) to gastrointestinal stimulation. At the level of the dorsal hindbrain, afferent vagal inputs enter the brainstem via the tractus solitarius (TS) and terminate on neurons of the nucleus of the tractus solitarius (NTS). The integrated signal is relayed from the NTS to the adjacent dorsal motor nucleus of the vagus (DMV) via catecholaminergic, glutamatergic, and predominantly gamma aminobutyric acid (GABA)-ergic, synapses. The DMV contains preganglionic parasympathetic motoneurons that relayed the resulting output signal to the GI tract via the efferent motor vagus. EEC—enteroendocrine cells; CC—central canal.

Gastric vagal afferents can be distinguished on the basis of their preferred response modality; mechanosensitive afferents, for example, innervate the GI smooth muscle and are activated by distention and stretch in response to food ingestion (reviewed in [5]). Recent studies have also shown that these tension-sensitive afferents can be further distinguished based upon their neurochemical phenotype, with glucagon-like peptide 1 receptor (GLP-1R) positive afferents innervating the stomach and oxytocin (OXT) positive afferents innervating the intestine [6]. Their distinct neurochemical phenotypes allow for selective experimental manipulation; optogenetic stimulation of these mechanosensitive afferents, for example, mimics central responses to gastric stretch, including the activation of distinct NTS populations and reduced food intake.

Mucosal afferents, in contrast, innervate the mucosal layer but do not make direct contact with the GI lumen. They are responsive to mucosal stroking and chemosensation and may play a role in the detection of food, particularly the size of food particles, within the GI lumen. The mucosal afferents are unresponsive to mechanical distention but are activated by intestinal nutrient infusion, and project to the NTS commisuralis [7]. Mucosal afferents also express distinct neurochemical phenotypes demonstrated by *Gpr65*-expressing neurons that display extensive innervation of the duodenal mucosa and are unresponsive to mechanical distention. Mucosal afferents are in close contact with enteroendocrine cells (EEC), and are respond to released gut endocrine peptides to induce an appropriate response in the vagal afferent neurons, and, subsequently, within the NTS, DMV, and the arcuate nucleus of the hypothalamus, [8] to regulate gastric emptying, pancreatic exocrine signaling, and intestinal fluid secretion, ultimately regulating food and caloric intake [5,9]. The presence of fat and protein within the intestinal lumen, for example, induces the release of cholecystokinin (CCK) from intestinal I-cells which leads to a pronounced vagal afferent-dependent reduction in meal size and is associated with activation of central activity in the hindbrain and hypothalamus [10–12]. The extensive connectivity of the NTS also provides pathways by which higher CNS centers can be activated in response to gut inputs; post-ingestive sucrose, for example, increases in activity in the left nodose ganglion and activates dopaminergic neurons in the ventral tegmental area (VTA) as a mechanism to reinforce food seeking behavior [13].

It should also be noted that recent studies have shown an additional specialized mechanism through which these EEC activate vagal afferents directly [14]. "Neuropods", composed of long, axon-like projections from the basolateral side of the EEC, make direct synaptic connections with vagal afferent terminals (as well as other cells in the GI tract including enteric glia). Sucrose infusion in the distal intestine, for example, induces EEC glutamate release that activates vagal afferents in a synaptic transmission-dependent manner [14]. Subsequent studies have also shown that feeding-dependent neuropod activation induces activation of vagal afferents in the right nodose ganglion and a gut-induced ascending reward pathway via the parabrachial nucleus (PBN) to the Substantia nigra (SN) [13] (Figure 1).

1.2. Nucleus of the Tractus Solitarius (NTS)

The NTS is the major integrative center for various thoracic and abdominal sensory information and contains moderate viscerotropic organization of vagal afferent terminals (reviewed in [1]). Sensory inputs related to taste from the tongue, for example, project to the ventral NTS whereas afferents from the GI tract project to the caudal NTS [15,16]. Subnuclei within the caudal NTS form distinct neural populations relative to afferent inputs from the GI tract; gastric afferents innervate the NTS gelatinosus and commisuralis, while esophageal afferents innervate the NTS centralis [17,18]. Dendritic projections from these afferents have been shown to run the entire rostral-caudal extent of the NTS; however, providing a potential mechanism by which sensory inputs from the GI tract may be integrated with those from other viscera including gustatory areas as well as cardiothoracic and respiratory inputs [19].

Despite displaying immunoreactivity to a variety of neurotransmitters/modulators/ hormones, GI sensory information is relayed principally, if not exclusively, via glutamate release from vagal afferent terminals and the activation of ionotropic glutamate receptors on NTS neurons [20,21]. Interestingly, while many studies have demonstrated that AMPA (and kainite) receptors are activated by vagal afferent-released glutamate, NMDA receptors may also be important in the regulation of food intake. Typically inactive at resting membrane potential due to the prominent Mg^{2+} ion block of the ligand-gated ion channel, NMDA receptors are not normally activated by synaptic release of glutamate [22,23]. Fourth ventricular microinjection of NMDA receptor antagonists, however, increase food intake following overnight fasting and abolish the satiating effects of peripheral CCK administration implying a role for these receptors in physiological feeding patterns [24,25]. Of note, electrophysiological studies investigating afferent-NTS glutamate transmission have shown that NMDA receptors are recruited following even relatively modest afferent stimulation frequencies (>5 Hz) and appear important in maintaining synaptic throughput when AMPA/kainate receptors are desensitized [26]. This implies that vagal activation in response to feeding is sufficient to induce NMDA receptor activation and likely either gates how much information from the viscera is projected to efferent pathways via the NTS or helps maintain reliable transmission across a wide range of stimulation frequencies. Afferent-released glutamate also activates metabotropic glutamate receptors (mGluRs) which have been identified at both pre- and post-synaptic locations, and heterosynaptic crosstalk has also been shown to modulate GABA release from NTS terminals [27,28].

Several studies have shown that spontaneous glutamate release from vagal afferents is modulated in an ongoing and tonic manner by a variety of neurotransmitters/modulators, including several neuropeptides contained within afferent terminals themselves [29]. Glucose, for example, regulates afferent glutamate release in a linear manner over a wide range of extracellular glucose levels via modulation of $5-HT_3$ receptor density [30–34]. The brainstem receives a dense serotonergic innervation from dorsal raphe nuclei, which tonically activates presynaptic $5-HT_3$ receptors; elevated glucose induces the trafficking of internalized $5-HT_3$ receptors to the membrane surface of vagal afferent neurons and their central terminals, increasing glutamate release; decreased glucose levels, in contrast, induces $5-HT_3$ receptor internalization, decreasing glutamate release [29,33–35]. Feeding neuropeptides, including cholecystokinin (CCK), ghrelin, cocaine- and amphetamine-regulated transcript (CART), and melanocortin concentrating hormone (MCH), amongst others, have all been shown to modulate afferent activity, hence regulate NTS neuronal excitation. Leptin, primarily produced by adipocytes [36], but also by gastric epithelial cells [37], has been shown to enhance glutamatergic transmission at the afferent-NTS synapse to reduce food intake [38], while activation of leptin-receptor expression NTS neurons has similar effects [39]. It is important to note that the dorsal vagal complex (DVC, i.e., the NTS, DMV and area postrema (AP)) is essentially a circumventricular organ with a leaky blood brain barrier and fenestrated capillaries [40]. Circulating neuropeptides, are significantly more likely, therefore, to activate central vagal neurocircuits [41,42]. Peripheral CCK, for example, has been shown to activate NTS neurons directly following a vagotomy [43]. "Feeding" neuropeptides released from enteroendocrine cells (EECs) may modulate vagal afferent activity at several discrete peripheral and central sites, therefore, in a prolonged temporal manner [29].

Neurons in the NTS can be identified by their distinct neurochemical phenotypes, principally glutamate, GABA, and norepinephrine (NE), but it should also be noted that many of the neuropeptides that activate vagal afferent terminals, including GLP-1 and CCK, are also expressed by neurons of the NTS and have been linked to the regulation of intake. For example, activation of GLP-1-containing NTS neurons reduces food intake [44,45] and modulates several autonomic responses. Furthermore, CCK- and dopamine beta hydroxylase (DBH)-containing NTS neurons form distinct neuronal populations that are activated by food intake in a vagal afferent-dependent manner, and induce downstream activation of calcitonin gene-related peptide (CGRP)-positive neurons in the PBN [46] to reduce food intake, while NTS neurons that co-express neuropeptide Y (NPY) and epinephrine (Epi) are distinct from those that express NE, and have opposing effects on vagal-afferent-dependent feeding behavior in a fasted state [47]. Taken together, it is clear that functionally-specific populations of NTS neurons play distinct roles in feeding behavior, and interrogation of these pathway-specific neurocircuits may increase our understanding of how such peripheral signals are integrated centrally to regulate energy homeostasis. Because of its projections to, and reciprocal innervation of, many other CNS areas involved in regulation of GI function and food intake the NTS plays a pivotal role in the central integration of gut inputs as well as efferent outputs to control, regulate, and modulate feeding behavior (Figure 1).

1.3. Dorsal Motor Nucleus of the Vagus (DMV)

Located ventral to the NTS, the dorsal motor nucleus of the vagus (DMV) contains the preganglionic parasympathetic motoneurons that provide efferent innervation to the esophagus, stomach, small intestine, and proximal colon. The subdiaphragmatic branches of the vagus nerve (5 branches in rodents: anterior gastric, posterior gastric, hepatic, celiac, and accessory celiac) have a medial-lateral columnar organization within the DMV [16,48,49]. While all DMV neurons are cholinergic, they differ in soma size and extent of dendritic arborization as per their efferent target organ [50–52]. DMV neurons innervating the stomach for example, are smaller and more excitable, hence more responsive to synaptic inputs and neuromodulation, than neurons that innervate the intestine. Vagal efferent DMV neurons that innervate the GI tract synapse onto postganglionic neurons that form one of two pathways; either excitatory cholinergic neurons that mediate smooth muscle contraction via muscarinic receptors or inhibitory neurons that mediate smooth muscle relaxation via nitric oxide (NO) or vasoactive intestinal peptide (VIP) (reviewed in [1,53]). Those involved in the excitatory pathway appear to originate more commonly in the medial and rostral DMV, with those involved in the inhibitory pathway more commonly found in the caudal DMV [54–57]. Through these opposing neural circuits, the DMV is able to exert fine-tuned control over GI functions, including gastric volume, contractile state, and rate of emptying, transit, and absorption, all of which influence feeding behavior.

While intrinsic biophysical properties of DMV neurons renders them spontaneously active pacemakers, firing at approximately 1 Hz [22], their activity is influenced by glutamatergic, catecholaminergic, and predominately tonic GABAergic inputs from the NTS [22,58,59]. Notably, however, the ability of this critical GABAergic synapse to be modulated—its "state of activation"—is controlled by presynaptic group II mGluR, activated by glutamate released from monosynaptic vagal afferent inputs. Tonic activation of these presynaptic receptors decreases cAMP levels, and prevents signaling through neurotransmitter receptors negatively coupled to adenylate cyclase (including μ-opioid, α2 adrenergic, NPY/PYY Y2, 5-HT1A receptors) [1]. Neuromodulators that activate cAMP-PKA signaling, e.g., CCK, GLP-1, corticotropin releasing factor (CRF), and insulin, increase the "state of activation" of this synapse, allowing GABAergic signaling to be inhibited, and increased activity of vagal efferent motoneurons [1]. Interestingly, in pathological states such as obesity where vagal afferent excitability is reduced, activation of the presynaptic mGluR is decreased and GABAergic signaling is enhanced rendering DMV neurons and vagal efferent output less excitable [60]. Leptin has also been shown to have direct inhibitory actions on DMV neurons, providing an additional mechanism in which this critical feeding peptide can alter GI functions, and food intake, via actions at central vagal sites [61].

Short-term neuroplasticity within NTS–DMV synapses has been identified recently as an important means by which food intake and caloric balance is regulated. Rodents respond to a calorically dense, palatable diet with an immediate short (24 h) period of hyperphagia before food intake is reduced after 3–5 days to restore caloric balance. This period of homeostatic regulation is associated with increased activation of synaptic NMDA receptors at the NTS–DMV synapse, leading to a subsequent increase in DMV neuronal excitability that could be driving this change in feeding behavior [23]. While studies have shown that gut peptides, including gastric inhibitor peptide (GIP) can induce central inflammation in pathological nutrient states [62], the increased activation of synaptic NMDA receptors coincides with an increase in neuroinflammatory markers in the brainstem, suggesting astroglia activation, which has been observed in the hypothalamus and nodose ganglion at this time point [62,63]. The full role these astroglia play in these central feeding centers, and how they can affect feeding behavior, in pathological conditions like obesity are the subject of renewed attention and focus, given their profound ability to alter synaptic efficacy and efficiency (Figure 1).

1.4. Area Postrema

The area postrema (AP) is a circumventricular organ situated in the fourth ventricle on the dorsal surface of the medulla, located adjacent to the NTS. As a circumventricular organ, it is highly vascularized with fenestrated capillaries and has dendritic projections that extend to the basal lamina side of the vascular endothelial cells, allowing it to be more exposed to circulating factors than the other regions of the brainstem that are involved in controlling feeding behavior [64]. Known classically as an emetic chemoreceptor trigger zone, AP neurons display receptors for many neuromodulators and immune mediators [65] including CCK, GLP-1, ghrelin, and PYY [64]. Administration of orexigenic gut peptides like CCK, GLP-1 and PYY alter AP neuron activation and excitability with subsequent effects on food intake [66–70] and ghrelin-dependent stimulation of feeding requires an intact AP [71].

In addition to its increased exposure to circulating factors, the AP also projects to, and receives input from, many regions involved in the regulation of nutrient status and feeding behavior. Basal dendrites of AP neurons receive direct inputs from gastric vagal afferents as well as having dense reciprocal connections with the NTS, PBN. AP neurons additionally receive inputs from the parvocellular neurons of the paraventricular and dorsomedial hypothalamus (PVN and DMH, respectively) [49,72], and have minor projections to the nucleus ambiguus, DMV, and cerebellum [49,72–75]. Due to its anatomical location, as well as its neurocircuitry, the AP serves a unique role as major integrative center for peripheral inputs, including from the GI tract, neuromodulatory circulating factors, and central areas involved in feeding control (Figures 1 and 2).

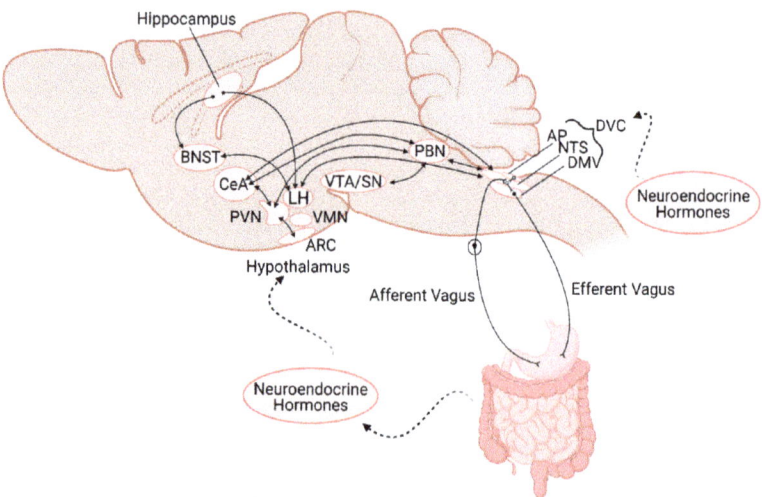

Figure 2. Schematic representation of the neuroanatomical connections between the gastrointestinal (GI) tract and central nervous system nuclei involved in regulation of GI functions and feeding. Note the location of the nuclei are not intended to be anatomically accurate. AP—area postrema; NTS—nucleus of the tractus solitarius, DMV—dorsal motor nucleus of the vagus; DVC—dorsal vagal complex; PBN—parabrachial nucleus; VTA/SN—ventral tegmental area/Substantia Nigra; PVN—paraventricular nucleus of the hypothalamus; VMH—ventromedial hypothalamus; LH—lateral hypothalamus; ARC—arcuate nucleus; CeA—central nucleus of the amygdala; BNST—bed nucleus of the stria terminalis.

1.5. Parabrachial Nucleus

Located in the dorsolateral pons, the PBN is responsible for relaying sensory inputs from the tongue and other viscera inputs from the NTS to forebrain structures involved in autonomic regulation [76]. Mechanical distension of the GI tract activates an NTS-PBN pathway that suppresses food and water intake [77]. In particular, the lateral PBN receives innervation from NE-, GLP-1-, and CCK-containing NTS neurons, and chemogenetic activation of these neurons induces satiation. Meal ingestion activates CCK- and GLP-1-expressing NTS neurons to excite CGRP-positive neurons in the lateral PBN [46,78]. In turn, these CGRP-positive PBN neurons project to, and activate, PKC-δ-positive neurons in the central amygdala (CeA) decreasing appetite [79]. Conversely, silencing of these same lateral PBN neurons delayed meal termination, subsequently increased meal size [80].

Beyond the homeostatic regulation of food intake as a response to the nutrient status of the organism, however, the lateral PBN has also been shown to be involved in a gut-mediated reward pathway. Activation of upper GI tract sensory vagal afferents induce dopamine release in striatal-related reward pathways, and the lateral PBN has been confirmed as the relay link between the DVC and the SN (Figure 2) [81]. Interestingly, it was CGRP- lateral PBN neurons that were activated by this vagal-dependent pathway, implying distinct subpopulations of lateral PBN neurons are responsible for mediating the rewarding response versus the meal termination response to food ingestion [81].

1.6. Cerebellum

The cerebellum, located posterior to and heavily connected with the brainstem, is canonically thought to be involved in motor control. Several lines of evidence, however, show that cerebellum also plays a critical role in the regulation of feeding behavior. Cerebellar lesions have been shown to alter feeding behavior and dysregulate blood glucose and body weight [82]. Although this may be caused by physical and motor impairment, it likely involves the well-established bidirectional links between the fastigial and interposed cerebellar nuclei with various hypothalamic nuclei including the lateral, ventromedial, dorsomedial and paraventricular hypothalamus (LH, VMH, DMH, and PVN, respectively) [83–86]. Interestingly, multiple studies have shown that projections from the cerebellum and the NTS converge on the same hypothalamic neurons, providing a means by which cerebellar signals can be integrated with gut inputs [82,87–89]. These same neurons have also been shown to respond to CCK, glucose, and ghrelin [87]. The cerebellum also innervates the DVC hence is able to modulate output responses to the GI [90,91].

1.7. Hypothalamus

The hypothalamus lies rostral to the brainstem, making up the floor of the third ventricle. Composed of many subnuclei, the hypothalamus has pivotal roles in the autonomic control of thirst, temperature, biological rhythms as well as feeding and glycemic regulation. Focusing on its role in the integration of sensory gut inputs and the regulation of feeding patterns, the hypothalamus receives ascending gut-related projections from the NTS as well as responding directly to circulating feeding-related factors.

Located in the basal hypothalamus adjacent to the arcuate (ARC) nucleus, the median eminence is a circumventricular organ [41,42] that has been shown to be responsive to circulating gut peptides, including ghrelin, which activates orexigenic ARC neurons (expressing Neuropeptide Y (NPY) and agouti-related peptide (AgRP) and inhibits anorexigenic neurons (pro-opiomelanocortin (POMC)- and melanocyte-stimulating hormone (MSH-containing) in order to stimulate feeding behavior [92]. Peripheral administration of Peptide YY (PYY), a gut peptide produce by L-cells in response to luminal contents, reduces food intake, which is at least partially driven by PYY acting on its receptors in the ARC to inhibit NPY/AgRP neurons [93,94]. Thus, circulating gut peptides may modulate feeding behavior by regulating the balance of NPY/AgRP orexigenic and POMC/MSH anorexigenic activation.

Beyond exposure to circulating factors, the ARC receives input from other hypothalamic nuclei as well as the NTS, the locus ceruleus, reticular formation, and bed nucleus of the stria terminalis (BNST; Figure 2 [95,96]. Noradrenergic projections from the NTS have been shown to mediate feeding behavior through direct projections to AgRP neurons in the ARC to stimulate feeding in a hypoglycemic state [97]. Conversely, TH/Prolactin releasing peptide (PrPR)-containing NTS neurons inhibit ARC AgRP neurons in response to high protein meals [98]. In addition to its projections to other hypothalamic and brainstem nuclei, the ARC also sends descending projections to the DVC, which allows for the direct regulation of visceral efferent outputs [95]. This connection with the DVC appears to play an important role in leptin's ability to modulate food intake, as loss of leptin receptor signaling at the DVC reduced the ability of leptin to decrease food intake through its actions at the hypothalamus [99].

The PVN has also been implicated in affecting feeding behavior via gut-dependent inputs. The PVN has reciprocal connections to may central feeding-related nuclei including the ARC, NTS, PBN, BNST, and CeA (reviewed in [100]). Peripheral CCK administration, for example, excites MC4R-containing PVN neurons, subsequent to activation of TH-positive NTS neurons, resulting in rapid satiation [101]. The PVN additionally sends descending projections to the DVC and PBN which have profound effects on GI outcomes, including feeding patterns [100,102,103]. PVN-derived CRF, for example, activate DVC neurons to modulate gastric motility and emptying [104,105], while oxytocin (OXT) released decrease gastric motility through a vagal-dependent pathway [106–108].

A subpopulation of the LH, composed of orexin/hypocretin neurons, has been shown to form synaptic connections with NTS neurons and modulate food intake [109]. This provides an avenue for hypothalamic orexin neurons, classically thought of as mediating attention and arousal, to affect the brain-gut axis [110]. The suprachiasmatic nucleus (SCN), the master clock of the brain, is known to control the daily rhythms of many biological functions. Ablation of the SCN leads to a loss of the feeding-fasting cycle, with no changes in food intake or meal frequency, implicating it in control of meal timing [111]. SCN neurons are also responsive to glucose and ghrelin, implying modulation by nutrients and gut-related signal [112] but it should be noted that the SCN does not appear to become entrained to changes in diet, implying there are other regions (including vagal afferents and the NTS) that are likely to play a larger role in the control of food rhythms [111].

1.8. Hippocampus

Beyond autonomic and homeostatic control, feeding is also regulated by higher cognitive centers. The memory of recent meals can control initiation, frequency, and size of future meals, as well as encoding information regarding where food was available. The hippocampus, split anatomically into dorsal and ventral regions, is known to be involved in these memory formations, placing it as a potentially critical central region for controlling food intake. Indeed, hippocampal neurons are activated by gastric distention [113] in addition displaying receptors for many GI peptides including CCK, GLP-1, ghrelin, and other endocrine factors like insulin, leptin, and amylin [114]. Although monosynaptic inputs from the NTS have not been identified, the hippocampus receives inputs from other brainstem regions including the locus ceruleus and dorsal raphe nuclei that may relay information from the NTS (Figure 2) [114]. The hippocampus has descending projections to other central regions known to be involved in food intake, including the BNST and LH [115–117]. Inactivation of ventral hippocampal neurons decreases inter-meal intervals, increase meal size, frequency, and total intake [116,118–122]. In contrast, the dorsal hippocampus is necessary for the episodic memory of a recently eaten meal, influencing the inter-meal interval and amount eaten at that next meal [123,124].

1.9. Amygdala

The amygdala, located in the temporal lobe, lies adjacent to the inferior horn of the lateral ventricle and medial to the hypothalamus. The amygdala can be broken down into substructures that include the central amygdala (CeA) and the extended amygdala that includes the bed nucleus of the stria terminalis (BNST). The CeA receives projections from the PBN and the PVN and sends descending projections to the hypothalamus and brainstem in order to mediate physiological responses to fear and anxiety (Figure 2) [125]. The CeA has also been suggested to play a more direct role in the regulation of feeding behavior, however. A subpopulation of neurons (PKC-δ-positive) in the lateral CeA are activated by anorexigenic signals from the gut such as CCK, and play a critical role in mediating the subsequent inhibition of food intake [79]. A second population of neurons in the CeA (PKC-δ-negative/5-HTR-positive) have also been shown to promote feeding behavior through inhibitory projections to the PBN. The BNST-LH neurocircuit has also been implicated in controlling feeding behavior [126]. Thus, while inter-amygdala circuits and descending control from the amygdala have shown to mediate feeding behaviors, the exact mechanisms and physiological relevance are still subject to investigation.

2. Pathophysiology

2.1. Obesity, Diabetes, Inflammation

Several studies have highlighted changes in vagal afferent responsiveness and signaling following high fat diet (HFD) exposure and diet-induced obesity (DIO), including a decreased vagal afferent response to mechanical stretch of the stomach and neuroendocrine peptides including CKK, GLP-1, leptin, and serotonin, as well as impaired responses to glucose [31,127,128]. HFD exposure is associated with altered gut peptide secretion, which mimics a perpetual fasting phenotype at the level of the vagal afferents, exacerbating the changes in GI function and food intake seen in the development of obesity [129]. HFD exposure also modulates central neurocircuits, both at the level of the brainstem and hypothalamus. Within vagal neurocircuits, the decrease in vagal afferent sensitivity responsiveness would be reasonably expected to decrease afferent glutamate release centrally. Indeed, HFD is associated with decreased afferent-dependent activation of presynaptic metabotropic glutamate receptors (mGluR) on inhibitory GABAergic NTS–DMV synapses, increasing the inhibitory drive to vagal efferent motoneurons. DMV neurons are also less excitable and less responsive to satiety neuropeptides such as CCK and GLP-1 following DIO [60,130,131]. In fact, these effects can be observed even before the onset of weight gain, suggesting that the HFD itself is responsible for at least some of these neuronal and synaptic changes, independent of the increased adiposity associated with obesity [23,132].

Another interesting phenomenon, well documented by Levin and colleagues, has shown that HFD-fed male Sprague-Dawley rats separate into two populations, one that become hyperphagic and obese, and another that maintain their eating patterns and resist weight gain [133]. Of note, hindbrain catecholaminergic ventrolateral medulla and NTS neurons that relay GI-sensitive inputs to the PVN, DMH, and ARC within the hypothalamus are disrupted in the obesity-prone population, highlighting neurodevelopmental differences that may underlie the propensity to develop DIO [134].

2.2. Developmental Modulation of Central Neurocircuits

Central feeding circuits develop during the embryonic period, but are subject to significant development maturation in the early postnatal period. In rodents, descending autonomic inputs from the hypothalamus, CeA, BNST, and cortex reach the DVC in the first postnatal week, marking this as a critical window during which early life experiences can shape the connectivity of these central feeding nuclei [135]. Several studies have demonstrated that maternal and early postnatal diet affects the development of central feeding-related neurocircuits [136,137]. Offspring exposed to perinatal HFD have increased body weight and an increased risk for developing obesity in adulthood [138]. At the NTS–DMV brainstem synapse, for example, there is a attenuation of the developmental switch in $GABA_A$ receptors subunit composition that alters the channel kinetics and subsequently increases inhibitory drive from the NTS that is associated with decreased gastric motility [139], although the long-term effects of this developmental delay on feeding behavior needs to be determined. Hypothalamic-DVC neurocircuits are also altered by maternal HFD exposure [140]. Elevated levels of orexigenic neuropeptides are present after maternal HFD that resembles the phenotype observed following adult HFD exposure [138], possibly due to transcriptional changes at the neuronal level [141,142]. Postnatal HFD exposure has also been shown decrease, while postnatal undernutrition increases, AgRP ARC fiber density [143,144]. Taken together, postnatal diet has the ability to influence the responsivity and developmental maturation of hypothalamic neurons, including their descending projections to the DVC, which may have long term and persistent consequences on central responses to gut inputs and dysregulated feeding behavior.

2.3. Neurological Disorders

Because of the extensive interconnectivity of brainstem, midbrain, and higher CNS centers with the DVC and brainstem neurocircuitry involved in the regulation of GI functions, several neurological, developmental, and behavioral disorders are associated with alterations in gut functions, including those involved in the regulation of food intake and energy balance.

Stress has been defined as a stimulus or event that challenges the physiological and psychological homeostatic state of an individual [145–147]. Critical to the central stress response is activation of the hypothalamic-pituitary-adrenal (HPA) axis, including activation of descending hypothalamic-DVC projections which modulate GI functions. In fact, functional GI disorders correlate with stress, including function dyspepsia and irritable bowel syndrome, and stress is known to exacerbate GI dysfunction in vulnerable individuals. [148,149]. Of note, while CRF- containing PVN-DVC neurons play a pivotal role in the effects of stress on visceral organs, CRF antagonists do not appear to modulate GI functions in non-stressed individuals. The effects of acute stress to delay gastric emptying and accelerate colonic transit can be mimicked by a temporally restricted exposure to CRF. Adaptation to prolonged stress, however, requires a more profound adaptive neuroplasticity, and several studies have shown that this involves upregulation of descending PVN-DVC OXT inputs, which play a major role in the recovery of GI functions [147,150].

Autism spectrum disorder (ASD) is a neurodevelopmental disorder characterized by behavioral disturbances such as repetitive behaviors and impaired social behaviors. Beyond changes to social behavior, these patients also exhibit altered eating patterns where children with ASD are considered very selective eaters (picky eaters), with aversions to particular food colors, smells, and textures, amongst other characteristics [151,152]. An overall change in total caloric intake is not reported, however, implying that satiety mechanisms may not necessarily be dysfunctional [153]. GI dysfunctions are reported in up to 91% of individuals with ASD, including bloating, constipation, diarrhea, and gastroesophageal reflux [154], indeed, this picky eating has been hypothesized to be an adaptive behavior to avoid GI discomfort [153,155]. Although ASD has been associated with many changes in the gut microbiome, central cranial nerve abnormalities, including motor nuclei in the brainstem and reduced vagal tone, have also been reported [156,157]. Peripheral OXT levels are also disrupted which, as discussed previously, may also contribute to the GI dysregulation and alterations in food intake, in addition to the well-recognized role in impaired social behaviors [158,159].

Parkinson's disease (PD) is a neurodegenerative disorder characterized by severe degeneration of dopaminergic neurons in the substantia nigra pars compacta (SNpc). It is considered a movement disorder marked by bradykinesia, rigidity, tremor, and gait/posture disorders. However, PD patients also experience a wide array of prodromal symptoms that include sleep disorders, orthostatic hypotension, and GI dysfunction [160–162]. Disorders of the GI tract include dysphagia, nausea, delayed gastric emptying, dysmotility, constipation, and fecal incontinence that can be detected in some patients many years before the onset of motor symptoms [163,164]. Interestingly, α-synuclein protein aggregates, known as Lewy bodies, have been shown to be present in the myenteric neurons within the ENS as well as the vagal motor neurons in the DMV, providing a potential explanation of the manifestation of prodromal GI dysfunction [165]. The recent discovery of a monosynaptic nigro-vagal pathway provides a pathway by which dopaminergic projections from the SNpc modulate DMV neuronal activity, hence GI functions [166,167], as well as providing an anatomical means by which an ENS-DVC-SNpc neurocircuit may underlie the pathophysiology of PD [168].

3. Conclusions and Future Directions

The regulation of food intake is a result of a coordinated and intricate series of short- and long-term responses to peripheral and central nervous system signals. Although circulating factors can modulate the activity of circumventricular nuclei directly, sensory inputs from the gut are relayed centrally via the afferent vagus nerve, terminating in a pathway-specific manner predominately within the NTS. Because of its reciprocal connections with other brainstem, midbrain, and forebrain nuclei, the NTS plays a major role in consolidating responses from across the CNS and relaying an integrated signal to the adjacent DMV to control the vagal motor output to the GI tract. This interconnectivity has led to the increased appreciation that many disorders of the CNS are accompanied by dysregulated central control of GI dysfunction, including disruptions in feeding, metabolism, and energy balance which significantly affects many patient's quality of life.

The advent of novel and emerging molecular and genetic techniques has allowed identification of discrete gut–brain neurocircuits involved in particular GI responses, and affirmed that many such neurocircuits are exquisitely specialized as per their physiological response. Using a multi-functional approach, the gut–brain axis has been shown to determine preference for sugar (but not artificial sweetener, hence not sweet-taste) via post-ingestive mechanisms involving afferent vagus nerve-mediated activation of the caudal NTS [169]. While the association of distinct and different neurocircuits for sweet taste in the tongue and gut–brain axis may reinforce the preference for sugar-rich foods, development of an artificial sweetener that can co-activate both pathways may well reduce the drive for sugar consumption [169]. Neuroplasticity is the hallmark of learning, memory, and homeostatic adaptation to ongoing physiological conditions and alterations within the gut–brain axis is no exception. As described above, decreased sensiivity and responsiveness in vagal afferents occurs following high fat diet exposure or the development of diet-induced obesity. Hypersensitivity within vagal afferents, however, may be responsible the unwelcome GI symptoms that result from ingestion of food allergens. The recent finding that bacterial infections cause the breakdown of oral tolerance to food antigens via a histamine H1 receptor-mediated sensitization of visceral afferents may provide a mechanistic basis by which food sensitivies and/or allergies can occur [170]. Furthermore, not only may this provide therapeutic targets by which inappropriate immune responses may be addressed, it may also uncover avenues by which visceral hypersensitivity disorders that are exacerbated by food ingestion (such as irritable bowel syndrome and functional dyspepsia) may be alleviated. Of note, the intestinal EEC are also equipped to function as "sentinels" within the intestinal environment and release cytokines in response to microbial metabolites and pathogens [171]; the direct synaptic connection between EEC and vagal afferent nerve endings suggests an additional role for neuropods in rapid signaling of mucosal immune responses via the gut–brain axis, or even in axon reflex responses to sensory stimulation [172].

Many challenges and barriers still exist to understanding the mechanisms by which central neurociruits regulate food intake in response to gut inputs. The central connectome of the gut–brain axis has yet to be fully elucidated, particularly in regard to pathway-specific neurocircuits. While studies from several groups have provided a great deal of information regarding vagal efferent control of GI functions in both physiological and pathophysiological conditions, there is surprisingly little phenotypic characterization of vagal efferent neurons involved in different visceral functions. Questions still remain regarding the validity of many animal models used to investigate complex human physiologial systems; while the use of transgenic animals has clearly pushed our understanding of nutrition, feeding and the role of the gut–brain axis forward, using such a reductionist approach to answer polygenic pathophysiological problems is not without translational difficulties. Little is known about how the gut–brain axis or the responsiveness of central neurocircuits to visceral inputs vary across the life span or during ageing and, despite strong clinical evidence that the perinatal enviornment is critically important to offspring outcomes, few studies have investigated how early life events alter the development of feeding related neurocircuits. Nevertheless, increasing awareness of the crucial role that the CNS plays in modulating GI sensory and motor functions should encourage continued investigations into the reciprocal 'big brain–little brain' partnership.

Author Contributions: Writing—original draft, K.E.C. and K.N.B.; Writing—Review and Editing, K.E.C. and K.N.B.; Funding Acquisition, K.N.B. All authors have read and agreed to the published version of the manuscript.

Funding: This work was supported by NIH grant DK111667.

Acknowledgments: We thank Courtney Clyburn for helpful critical comments on previous versions of this manuscript. We thank W. Nairn Browning for support and encouragement. Figures prepared with BioRender.com accessed on 3 March 2021.

Conflicts of Interest: The authors declare no conflict of interest.

References

1. Browning, K.N.; Travagli, R.A. Central nervous system control of gastrointestinal motility and secretion and modulation of gastrointestinal functions. *Compr. Physiol.* **2014**, *4*, 1339–1368. [CrossRef]
2. Brookes, S.J.; Spencer, N.J.; Costa, M.; Zagorodnyuk, V.P. Extrinsic primary afferent signalling in the gut. *Nat. Rev. Gastroenterol. Hepatol.* **2013**, *10*, 286–296. [CrossRef]
3. Berthoud, H.R.; Neuhuber, W.L. Functional and chemical anatomy of the afferent vagal system. *Auton. Neurosci.* **2000**, *85*, 1–17. [CrossRef]
4. Moran, T.H.; Ladenheim, E.E. Physiologic and Neural Controls of Eating. *Gastroenterol. Clin. N. Am.* **2016**, *45*, 581–599. [CrossRef] [PubMed]
5. Wang, Y.B.; de Lartigue, G.; Page, A.J. Dissecting the Role of Subtypes of Gastrointestinal Vagal Afferents. *Front. Physiol.* **2020**, *11*, 643. [CrossRef] [PubMed]
6. Bai, L.; Mesgarzadeh, S.; Ramesh, K.S.; Huey, E.L.; Liu, Y.; Gray, L.A.; Aitken, T.J.; Chen, Y.; Beutler, L.R.; Ahn, J.S.; et al. Genetic Identification of Vagal Sensory Neurons That Control Feeding. *Cell* **2019**, *179*, 1129–1143.e1123. [CrossRef] [PubMed]
7. Williams, E.K.; Chang, R.B.; Strochlic, D.E.; Umans, B.D.; Lowell, B.B.; Liberles, S.D. Sensory Neurons that Detect Stretch and Nutrients in the Digestive System. *Cell* **2016**, *166*, 209–221. [CrossRef]
8. Vincent, K.M.; Sharp, J.W.; Raybould, H.E. Intestinal glucose-induced calcium-calmodulin kinase signaling in the gut-brain axis in awake rats. *Neurogastroenterol. Motil.* **2011**, *23*, e282–e293. [CrossRef] [PubMed]
9. Raybould, H.E. Gut chemosensing: Interactions between gut endocrine cells and visceral afferents. *Auton. Neurosci.* **2010**, *153*, 41–46. [CrossRef]
10. Dockray, G.J. Enteroendocrine cell signalling via the vagus nerve. *Curr. Opin. Pharm.* **2013**, *13*, 954–958. [CrossRef] [PubMed]
11. Dockray, G.J. Luminal sensing in the gut: An overview. *J. Physiol. Pharmacol.* **2003**, *54* (Suppl. 4), 9–17. [PubMed]
12. Lassman, D.J.; McKie, S.; Gregory, L.J.; Lal, S.; D'Amato, M.; Steele, I.; Varro, A.; Dockray, G.J.; Williams, S.C.; Thompson, D.G. Defining the role of cholecystokinin in the lipid-induced human brain activation matrix. *Gastroenterology* **2010**, *138*, 1514–1524. [CrossRef]
13. Fernandes, A.B.; Alves da Silva, J.; Almeida, J.; Cui, G.; Gerfen, C.R.; Costa, R.M.; Oliveira-Maia, A.J. Postingestive Modulation of Food Seeking Depends on Vagus-Mediated Dopamine Neuron Activity. *Neuron* **2020**, *106*, 778–788.e776. [CrossRef]
14. Kaelberer, M.M.; Buchanan, K.L.; Klein, M.E.; Barth, B.B.; Montoya, M.M.; Shen, X.; Bohórquez, D.V. A gut-brain neural circuit for nutrient sensory transduction. *Science* **2018**, *361*. [CrossRef]
15. Kalia, M.; Mesulam, M.M. Brain stem projections of sensory and motor components of the vagus complex in the cat: I. The cervical vagus and nodose ganglion. *J. Comp. Neurol.* **1980**, *193*, 435–465. [CrossRef]
16. Norgren, R.; Smith, G.P. Central distribution of subdiaphragmatic vagal branches in the rat. *J. Comp. Neurol.* **1988**, *273*, 207–223. [CrossRef] [PubMed]
17. Altschuler, S.M.; Bao, X.M.; Bieger, D.; Hopkins, D.A.; Miselis, R.R. Viscerotopic representation of the upper alimentary tract in the rat: Sensory ganglia and nuclei of the solitary and spinal trigeminal tracts. *J. Comp. Neurol.* **1989**, *283*, 248–268. [CrossRef]
18. Broussard, D.L.; Altschuler, S.M. Brainstem viscerotopic organization of afferents and efferents involved in the control of swallowing. *Am. J. Med.* **2000**, *108* (Suppl. 4a), 79s–86s. [CrossRef]
19. Jean, A. The nucleus tractus solitarius: Neuroanatomic, neurochemical and functional aspects. *Arch. Int. Physiol. Biochim. Biophys.* **1991**, *99*, A3–A52. [CrossRef]
20. Andresen, M.C.; Yang, M.Y. Non-NMDA receptors mediate sensory afferent synaptic transmission in medial nucleus tractus solitarius. *Am. J. Physiol.* **1990**, *259*, H1307–H1311. [CrossRef] [PubMed]
21. Andresen, M.C.; Kunze, D.L. Nucleus tractus solitarius—Gateway to neural circulatory control. *Annu. Rev. Physiol.* **1994**, *56*, 93–116. [CrossRef]
22. Travagli, R.A.; Gillis, R.A.; Rossiter, C.D.; Vicini, S. Glutamate and GABA-mediated synaptic currents in neurons of the rat dorsal motor nucleus of the vagus. *Am. J. Physiol.* **1991**, *260*, G531–G536. [CrossRef]
23. Clyburn, C.; Travagli, R.A.; Browning, K.N. Acute high-fat diet upregulates glutamatergic signaling in the dorsal motor nucleus of the vagus. *Am. J. Physiol. Gastrointest. Liver Physiol.* **2018**, *314*, G623–G634. [CrossRef]

24. Wright, J.; Campos, C.; Herzog, T.; Covasa, M.; Czaja, K.; Ritter, R.C. Reduction of food intake by cholecystokinin requires activation of hindbrain NMDA-type glutamate receptors. *Am. J. Physiol. Regul. Integr Comp. Physiol.* **2011**, *301*, R448–R455. [CrossRef]
25. Guard, D.B.; Swartz, T.D.; Ritter, R.C.; Burns, G.A.; Covasa, M. Blockade of hindbrain NMDA receptors containing NR2 subunits increases sucrose intake. *Am. J. Physiol. Regul. Integr. Comp. Physiol.* **2009**, *296*, R921–R928. [CrossRef] [PubMed]
26. Zhao, H.; Peters, J.H.; Zhu, M.; Page, S.J.; Ritter, R.C.; Appleyard, S.M. Frequency-dependent facilitation of synaptic throughput via postsynaptic NMDA receptors in the nucleus of the solitary tract. *J. Physiol.* **2015**, *593*, 111–125. [CrossRef]
27. Glaum, S.R.; Miller, R.J. Activation of metabotropic glutamate receptors produces reciprocal regulation of ionotropic glutamate and GABA responses in the nucleus of the tractus solitarius of the rat. *J. Neurosci.* **1993**, *13*, 1636–1641. [CrossRef]
28. Foley, C.M.; Moffitt, J.A.; Hay, M.; Hasser, E.M. Glutamate in the nucleus of the solitary tract activates both ionotropic and metabotropic glutamate receptors. *Am. J. Physiol.* **1998**, *275*, R1858–R1866. [CrossRef] [PubMed]
29. De Lartigue, G. Putative roles of neuropeptides in vagal afferent signaling. *Physiol. Behav.* **2014**, *136*, 155–169. [CrossRef] [PubMed]
30. Babic, T.; Troy, A.E.; Fortna, S.R.; Browning, K.N. Glucose-dependent trafficking of 5-HT3 receptors in rat gastrointestinal vagal afferent neurons. *Neurogastroenterol. Motil.* **2012**, *24*, e476–e488. [CrossRef]
31. Troy, A.E.; Simmonds, S.S.; Stocker, S.D.; Browning, K.N. High fat diet attenuates glucose-dependent facilitation of 5-HT3-mediated responses in rat gastric vagal afferents. *J. Physiol.* **2016**, *594*, 99–114. [CrossRef] [PubMed]
32. Wan, S.; Browning, K.N. D-glucose modulates synaptic transmission from the central terminals of vagal afferent fibers. *Am. J. Physiol. Gastrointest. Liver Physiol.* **2008**, *294*, G757–G763. [CrossRef] [PubMed]
33. Wan, S.; Browning, K.N. Glucose increases synaptic transmission from vagal afferent central nerve terminals via modulation of 5-HT3 receptors. *Am. J. Physiol. Gastrointest. Liver Physiol.* **2008**, *295*, G1050–G1057. [CrossRef] [PubMed]
34. Roberts, B.L.; Zhu, M.; Zhao, H.; Dillon, C.; Appleyard, S.M. High glucose increases action potential firing of catecholamine neurons in the nucleus of the solitary tract by increasing spontaneous glutamate inputs. *Am. J. Physiol. Regul. Integr. Comp. Physiol.* **2017**, *313*, R229–R239. [CrossRef]
35. Hosford, P.S.; Mifflin, S.W.; Ramage, A.G. 5-hydroxytryptamine-mediated neurotransmission modulates spontaneous and vagal-evoked glutamate release in the nucleus of the solitary tract effect of uptake blockade. *J. Pharmacol. Exp. Ther.* **2014**, *349*, 288–296. [CrossRef] [PubMed]
36. Zhang, Y.; Proenca, R.; Maffei, M.; Barone, M.; Leopold, L.; Friedman, J.M. Positional cloning of the mouse obese gene and its human homologue. *Nature* **1994**, *372*, 425–432. [CrossRef]
37. Bado, A.; Levasseur, S.; Attoub, S.; Kermorgant, S.; Laigneau, J.P.; Bortoluzzi, M.N.; Moizo, L.; Lehy, T.; Guerre-Millo, M.; Le Marchand-Brustel, Y.; et al. The stomach is a source of leptin. *Nature* **1998**, *394*, 790–793. [CrossRef] [PubMed]
38. Neyens, D.; Zhao, H.; Huston, N.J.; Wayman, G.A.; Ritter, R.C.; Appleyard, S.M. Leptin Sensitizes NTS Neurons to Vagal Input by Increasing Postsynaptic NMDA Receptor Currents. *J. Neurosci.* **2020**, *40*, 7054–7064. [CrossRef]
39. Cheng, W.; Ndoka, E.; Hutch, C.; Roelofs, K.; MacKinnon, A.; Khoury, B.; Magrisso, J.; Kim, K.S.; Rhodes, C.J.; Olson, D.P.; et al. Leptin receptor-expressing nucleus tractus solitarius neurons suppress food intake independently of GLP1 in mice. *JCI Insight* **2020**, *5*. [CrossRef] [PubMed]
40. Hoyda, T.D.; Smith, P.M.; Ferguson, A.V. Gastrointestinal hormone actions in the central regulation of energy metabolism: Potential sensory roles for the circumventricular organs. *Int. J. Obes.* **2009**, *33* (Suppl. 1), S16–S21. [CrossRef]
41. Cottrell, G.T.; Ferguson, A.V. Sensory circumventricular organs: Central roles in integrated autonomic regulation. *Regul. Pept.* **2004**, *117*, 11–23. [CrossRef] [PubMed]
42. Fry, M.; Ferguson, A.V. The sensory circumventricular organs: Brain targets for circulating signals controlling ingestive behavior. *Physiol. Behav.* **2007**, *91*, 413–423. [CrossRef] [PubMed]
43. Baptista, V.; Browning, K.N.; Travagli, R.A. Effects of cholecystokinin-8s in the nucleus tractus solitarius of vagally deafferented rats. *Am. J. Physiol. Regul. Integr. Comp. Physiol.* **2007**, *292*, R1092–R1100. [CrossRef] [PubMed]
44. Trapp, S.; Richards, J.E. The gut hormone glucagon-like peptide-1 produced in brain: Is this physiologically relevant? *Curr. Opin. Pharmacol.* **2013**, *13*, 964–969. [CrossRef] [PubMed]
45. Browning, K.N.; Travagli, R.A. Central control of gastrointestinal motility. *Curr. Opin. Endocrinol. Diabetes Obes.* **2019**. [CrossRef]
46. Roman, C.W.; Derkach, V.A.; Palmiter, R.D. Genetically and functionally defined NTS to PBN brain circuits mediating anorexia. *Nat. Commun.* **2016**, *7*, 11905. [CrossRef]
47. Chen, R.; Zhang, Y.-Y.; Lan, J.-N.; Liu, H.-M.; Li, W.; Wu, Y.; Leng, Y.; Tang, L.-H.; Hou, J.-B.; Sun, Q.; et al. Ischemic Postconditioning Alleviates Intestinal Ischemia-Reperfusion Injury by Enhancing Autophagy and Suppressing Oxidative Stress through the Akt/GSK-/Nrf2 Pathway in Mice. *Oxidative Med. Cell. Longev.* **2020**, *2020*, 1–14. [CrossRef]
48. Fox, E.A.; Powley, T.L. Longitudinal columnar organization within the dorsal motor nucleus represents separate branches of the abdominal vagus. *Brain Res.* **1985**, *341*, 269–282. [CrossRef]
49. Shapiro, R.E.; Miselis, R.R. The central organization of the vagus nerve innervating the stomach of the rat. *J. Comp. Neurol.* **1985**, *238*, 473–488. [CrossRef]
50. Browning, K.N.; Renehan, W.E.; Travagli, R.A. Electrophysiological and morphological heterogeneity of rat dorsal vagal neurones which project to specific areas of the gastrointestinal tract. *J. Physiol.* **1999**, *517 Pt 2*, 521–532. [CrossRef]

51. Fogel, R.; Zhang, X.; Renehan, W.E. Relationships between the morphology and function of gastric and intestinal distention-sensitive neurons in the dorsal motor nucleus of the vagus. *J. Comp. Neurol.* **1996**, *364*, 78–91. [CrossRef]
52. Valenzuela, I.M.; Browning, K.N.; Travagli, R.A. Morphological differences between planes of section do not influence the electrophysiological properties of identified rat dorsal motor nucleus of the vagus neurons. *Brain Res.* **2004**, *1003*, 54–60. [CrossRef] [PubMed]
53. Travagli, R.A.; Hermann, G.E.; Browning, K.N.; Rogers, R.C. Brainstem circuits regulating gastric function. *Annu. Rev. Physiol.* **2006**, *68*, 279–305. [CrossRef]
54. Cruz, M.T.; Murphy, E.C.; Sahibzada, N.; Verbalis, J.G.; Gillis, R.A. A reevaluation of the effects of stimulation of the dorsal motor nucleus of the vagus on gastric motility in the rat. *Am. J. Physiol. Regul. Integr. Comp. Physiol.* **2007**, *292*, R291–R307. [CrossRef]
55. Krowicki, Z.K.; Sharkey, K.A.; Serron, S.C.; Nathan, N.A.; Hornby, P.J. Distribution of nitric oxide synthase in rat dorsal vagal complex and effects of microinjection of nitric oxide compounds upon gastric motor function. *J. Comp. Neurol.* **1997**, *377*, 49–69. [CrossRef]
56. Rogers, R.C.; Hermann, G.E.; Travagli, R.A. Brainstem pathways responsible for oesophageal control of gastric motility and tone in the rat. *J. Physiol.* **1999**, *514 Pt 2*, 369–383. [CrossRef]
57. Rogers, R.C.; Travagli, R.A.; Hermann, G.E. Noradrenergic neurons in the rat solitary nucleus participate in the esophageal-gastric relaxation reflex. *Am. J. Physiol. Regul. Integr. Comp. Physiol.* **2003**, *285*, R479–R489. [CrossRef]
58. Guo, J.J.; Browning, K.N.; Rogers, R.C.; Travagli, R.A. Catecholaminergic neurons in rat dorsal motor nucleus of vagus project selectively to gastric corpus. *Am. J. Physiol. Gastrointest. Liver Physiol.* **2001**, *280*, G361–G367. [CrossRef]
59. Babic, T.; Browning, K.N.; Travagli, R.A. Differential organization of excitatory and inhibitory synapses within the rat dorsal vagal complex. *Am. J. Physiol. Gastrointest. Liver Physiol.* **2011**, *300*, G21–G32. [CrossRef]
60. Bhagat, R.; Fortna, S.R.; Browning, K.N. Exposure to a high fat diet during the perinatal period alters vagal motoneurone excitability, even in the absence of obesity. *J. Physiol.* **2015**, *593*, 285–303. [CrossRef] [PubMed]
61. Williams, K.W.; Zsombok, A.; Smith, B.N. Rapid inhibition of neurons in the dorsal motor nucleus of the vagus by leptin. *Endocrinology* **2007**, *148*, 1868–1881. [CrossRef] [PubMed]
62. Fu, Y.; Kaneko, K.; Lin, H.Y.; Mo, Q.; Xu, Y.; Suganami, T.; Ravn, P.; Fukuda, M. Gut Hormone GIP Induces Inflammation and Insulin Resistance in the Hypothalamus. *Endocrinology* **2020**, *161*. [CrossRef] [PubMed]
63. Clyburn, C.; Browning, K.N. Role of astroglia in diet-induced central neuroplasticity. *J. Neurophysiol.* **2019**. [CrossRef] [PubMed]
64. Price, C.J.; Hoyda, T.D.; Ferguson, A.V. The area postrema: A brain monitor and integrator of systemic autonomic state. *Neuroscientist* **2008**, *14*, 182–194. [CrossRef] [PubMed]
65. Babic, T.; Browning, K.N. The role of vagal neurocircuits in the regulation of nausea and vomiting. *Eur. J. Pharmacol.* **2014**, *722*, 38–47. [CrossRef] [PubMed]
66. Hill, D.R.; Campbell, N.J.; Shaw, T.M.; Woodruff, G.N. Autoradiographic localization and biochemical characterization of peripheral type CCK receptors in rat CNS using highly selective nonpeptide CCK antagonists. *J. Neurosci.* **1987**, *7*, 2967–2976. [CrossRef] [PubMed]
67. Mercer, L.D.; Beart, P.M. Immunolocalization of CCK1R in rat brain using a new anti-peptide antibody. *Neurosci. Lett.* **2004**, *359*, 109–113. [CrossRef] [PubMed]
68. Covasa, M.; Ritter, R.C. Reduced CCK-induced Fos expression in the hindbrain, nodose ganglia, and enteric neurons of rats lacking CCK-1 receptors. *Brain Res.* **2005**, *1051*, 155–163. [CrossRef] [PubMed]
69. Yamamoto, H.; Kishi, T.; Lee, C.E.; Choi, B.J.; Fang, H.; Hollenberg, A.N.; Drucker, D.J.; Elmquist, J.K. Glucagon-like peptide-1-responsive catecholamine neurons in the area postrema link peripheral glucagon-like peptide-1 with central autonomic control sites. *J. Neurosci.* **2003**, *23*, 2939–2946. [CrossRef] [PubMed]
70. Bonaz, B.; Taylor, I.; Taché, Y. Peripheral peptide YY induces c-fos-like immunoreactivity in the rat brain. *Neurosci. Lett.* **1993**, *163*, 77–80. [CrossRef]
71. Gilg, S.; Lutz, T.A. The orexigenic effect of peripheral ghrelin differs between rats of different age and with different baseline food intake, and it may in part be mediated by the area postrema. *Physiol. Behav.* **2006**, *87*, 353–359. [CrossRef]
72. Van der Kooy, D.; Koda, L.Y. Organization of the projections of a circumventricular organ: The area postrema in the rat. *J. Comp. Neurol.* **1983**, *219*, 328–338. [CrossRef] [PubMed]
73. Menani, J.V.; Thunhorst, R.L.; Johnson, A.K. Lateral parabrachial nucleus and serotonergic mechanisms in the control of salt appetite in rats. *Am. J. Physiol.* **1996**, *270*, R162–R168. [CrossRef] [PubMed]
74. Miura, M.; Takayama, K. Circulatory and respiratory responses to glutamate stimulation of the lateral parabrachial nucleus of the cat. *J. Auton. Nerv. Syst* **1991**, *32*, 121–133. [CrossRef]
75. Vigier, D.; Portalier, P. Efferent projections of the area postrema demonstrated by autoradiography. *Arch. Ital. Biol.* **1979**, *117*, 308–324. [PubMed]
76. Andermann, M.L.; Lowell, B.B. toward a wiring diagram understanding of appetite control. *Neuron* **2017**. [CrossRef] [PubMed]
77. Kim, D.Y.; Heo, G.; Kim, M.; Kim, H.; Jin, J.A.; Kim, H.K.; Jung, S.; An, M.; Ahn, B.H.; Park, J.H.; et al. A neural circuit mechanism for mechanosensory feedback control of ingestion. *Nature* **2020**, *580*, 376–380. [CrossRef]
78. Kreisler, A.D.; Davis, E.A.; Rinaman, L. Differential activation of chemically identified neurons in the caudal nucleus of the solitary tract in non-entrained rats after intake of satiating vs. non-satiating meals. *Physiol. Behav.* **2014**, *136*, 47–54. [CrossRef]

79. Cai, H.; Haubensak, W.; Anthony, T.E.; Anderson, D.J. Central amygdala PKC-δ(+) neurons mediate the influence of multiple anorexigenic signals. *Nat. Neurosci.* **2014**, *17*, 1240–1248. [CrossRef]
80. Campos, C.A.; Bowen, A.J.; Schwartz, M.W.; Palmiter, R.D. Parabrachial CGRP Neurons Control Meal Termination. *Cell Metab.* **2016**, *23*, 811–820. [CrossRef]
81. Han, W.; Tellez, L.A.; Perkins, M.H.; Perez, I.O.; Qu, T.; Ferreira, J.; Ferreira, T.L.; Quinn, D.; Liu, Z.W.; Gao, X.B.; et al. A Neural Circuit for Gut-Induced Reward. *Cell* **2018**, *175*, 665–678.e623. [CrossRef] [PubMed]
82. Zhu, J.N.; Yung, W.H.; Kwok-Chong Chow, B.; Chan, Y.S.; Wang, J.J. The cerebellar-hypothalamic circuits: Potential pathways underlying cerebellar involvement in somatic-visceral integration. *Brain Res. Rev.* **2006**, *52*, 93–106. [CrossRef]
83. Dietrichs, E.; Haines, D.E.; Røste, G.K.; Røste, L.S. Hypothalamocerebellar and cerebellohypothalamic projections—Circuits for regulating nonsomatic cerebellar activity? *Histol. Histopathol.* **1994**, *9*, 603–614. [PubMed]
84. Haines, D.E.; Dietrichs, E.; Mihailoff, G.A.; McDonald, E.F. The cerebellar-hypothalamic axis: Basic circuits and clinical observations. *Int. Rev. Neurobiol.* **1997**, *41*, 83–107. [CrossRef] [PubMed]
85. Cavdar, S.; San, T.; Aker, R.; Sehirli, U.; Onat, F. Cerebellar connections to the dorsomedial and posterior nuclei of the hypothalamus in the rat. *J. Anat.* **2001**, *198*, 37–45. [CrossRef]
86. Cavdar, S.; Onat, F.; Aker, R.; Sehirli, U.; San, T.; Yananli, H.R. The afferent connections of the posterior hypothalamic nucleus in the rat using horseradish peroxidase. *J. Anat.* **2001**, *198*, 463–472. [CrossRef]
87. Li, B.; Zhuang, Q.X.; Gao, H.R.; Wang, J.J.; Zhu, J.N. Medial cerebellar nucleus projects to feeding-related neurons in the ventromedial hypothalamic nucleus in rats. *Brain Struct. Funct.* **2017**, *222*, 957–971. [CrossRef]
88. Zhu, J.N.; Li, H.Z.; Ding, Y.; Wang, J.J. Cerebellar modulation of feeding-related neurons in rat dorsomedial hypothalamus. *J. Neurosci. Res.* **2006**, *84*, 1597–1609. [CrossRef]
89. Zhu, J.N.; Guo, C.L.; Li, H.Z.; Wang, J.J. Dorsomedial hypothalamic nucleus neurons integrate important peripheral feeding-related signals in rats. *J. Neurosci. Res.* **2007**, *85*, 3193–3204. [CrossRef]
90. Li, B.; Guo, C.L.; Tang, J.; Zhu, J.N.; Wang, J.J. Cerebellar fastigial nuclear inputs and peripheral feeding signals converge on neurons in the dorsomedial hypothalamic nucleus. *Neurosignals* **2009**, *17*, 132–143. [CrossRef] [PubMed]
91. Suzuki, T.; Sugiyama, Y.; Yates, B.J. Integrative responses of neurons in parabrachial nuclei to a nauseogenic gastrointestinal stimulus and vestibular stimulation in vertical planes. *Am. J. Physiol. Regul. Integr. Comp. Physiol.* **2012**, *302*, R965–R975. [CrossRef]
92. Mihalache, L.; Gherasim, A.; Niţă, O.; Ungureanu, M.C.; Pădureanu, S.S.; Gavril, R.S.; Arhire, L.I. Effects of ghrelin in energy balance and body weight homeostasis. *Hormones* **2016**, *15*, 186–196. [CrossRef]
93. Teubner, B.J.; Bartness, T.J. PYY(3-36) into the arcuate nucleus inhibits food deprivation-induced increases in food hoarding and intake. *Peptides* **2013**, *47*, 20–28. [CrossRef]
94. Jones, E.S.; Nunn, N.; Chambers, A.P.; Østergaard, S.; Wulff, B.S.; Luckman, S.M. Modified Peptide YY Molecule Attenuates the Activity of NPY/AgRP Neurons and Reduces Food Intake in Male Mice. *Endocrinology* **2019**, *160*, 2737–2747. [CrossRef]
95. Chronwall, B.M. Anatomy and physiology of the neuroendocrine arcuate nucleus. *Peptides* **1985**, *6* (Suppl. 2), 1–11. [CrossRef]
96. DeFalco, J.; Tomishima, M.; Liu, H.; Zhao, C.; Cai, X.; Marth, J.D.; Enquist, L.; Friedman, J.M. Virus-assisted mapping of neural inputs to a feeding center in the hypothalamus. *Science* **2001**, *291*, 2608–2613. [CrossRef]
97. Aklan, I.; Sayar Atasoy, N.; Yavuz, Y.; Ates, T.; Coban, I.; Koksalar, F.; Filiz, G.; Topcu, I.C.; Oncul, M.; Dilsiz, P.; et al. NTS Catecholamine Neurons Mediate Hypoglycemic Hunger via Medial Hypothalamic Feeding Pathways. *Cell Metab.* **2020**, *31*, 313–326.e315. [CrossRef]
98. Tsang, A.H.; Nuzzaci, D.; Darwish, T.; Samudrala, H.; Blouet, C. Nutrient sensing in the nucleus of the solitary tract mediates non-aversive suppression of feeding via inhibition of AgRP neurons. *Mol. Metab.* **2020**, *42*, 101070. [CrossRef]
99. Harris, R.B.S. Loss of leptin receptor-expressing cells in the hindbrain decreases forebrain leptin sensitivity. *Am. J. Physiol. Endocrinol. Metab.* **2020**, *318*, E806–E816. [CrossRef]
100. Swanson, L.W.; Sawchenko, P.E. Hypothalamic integration: Organization of the paraventricular and supraoptic nuclei. *Annu. Rev. Neurosci.* **1983**, *6*, 269–324. [CrossRef]
101. D'Agostino, G.; Lyons, D.J.; Cristiano, C.; Burke, L.K.; Madara, J.C.; Campbell, J.N.; Garcia, A.P.; Land, B.B.; Lowell, B.B.; Dileone, R.J.; et al. Appetite controlled by a cholecystokinin nucleus of the solitary tract to hypothalamus neurocircuit. *Elife* **2016**, *5*. [CrossRef]
102. Luiten, P.G.; ter Horst, G.J.; Karst, H.; Steffens, A.B. The course of paraventricular hypothalamic efferents to autonomic structures in medulla and spinal cord. *Brain Res.* **1985**, *329*, 374–378. [CrossRef]
103. Saper, C.B.; Loewy, A.D.; Swanson, L.W.; Cowan, W.M. Direct hypothalamo-autonomic connections. *Brain Res.* **1976**, *117*, 305–312. [CrossRef]
104. Heymann-Mönnikes, I.; Taché, Y.; Trauner, M.; Weiner, H.; Garrick, T. CRF microinjected into the dorsal vagal complex inhibits TRH analog- and kainic acid-stimulated gastric contractility in rats. *Brain Res.* **1991**, *554*, 139–144. [CrossRef]
105. Lewis, M.W.; Hermann, G.E.; Rogers, R.C.; Travagli, R.A. In vitro and in vivo analysis of the effects of corticotropin releasing factor on rat dorsal vagal complex. *J. Physiol.* **2002**, *543*, 135–146. [CrossRef]
106. Holmes, G.M.; Browning, K.N.; Babic, T.; Fortna, S.R.; Coleman, F.H.; Travagli, R.A. Vagal afferent fibres determine the oxytocin-induced modulation of gastric tone. *J. Physiol.* **2013**, *591*, 3081–3100. [CrossRef]

107. Peters, J.H.; McDougall, S.J.; Kellett, D.O.; Jordan, D.; Llewellyn-Smith, I.J.; Andresen, M.C. Oxytocin enhances cranial visceral afferent synaptic transmission to the solitary tract nucleus. *J. Neurosci.* **2008**, *28*, 11731–11740. [CrossRef]
108. Richard, P.; Moos, F.; Freund-Mercier, M.J. Central effects of oxytocin. *Physiol. Rev.* **1991**, *71*, 331–370. [CrossRef]
109. Zheng, H.; Patterson, L.M.; Berthoud, H.R. Orexin-A projections to the caudal medulla and orexin-induced c-Fos expression, food intake, and autonomic function. *J. Comp. Neurol.* **2005**, *485*, 127–142. [CrossRef]
110. Grill, H.J.; Hayes, M.R. Hindbrain Neurons as an Essential Hub in the Neuroanatomically Distributed Control of Energy Balance. *Cell Metab.* **2012**, *16*, 296–309. [CrossRef]
111. Challet, E. The circadian regulation of food intake. *Nat. Rev. Endocrinol.* **2019**, *15*, 393–405. [CrossRef]
112. Page, A.J.; Christie, S.; Symonds, E.; Li, H. Circadian regulation of appetite and time restricted feeding. *Physiol. Behav.* **2020**, *220*, 112873. [CrossRef] [PubMed]
113. Min, D.K.; Tuor, U.I.; Chelikani, P.K. Gastric distention induced functional magnetic resonance signal changes in the rodent brain. *Neuroscience* **2011**, *179*, 151–158. [CrossRef]
114. Kanoski, S.E.; Grill, H.J. Hippocampus Contributions to Food Intake Control: Mnemonic, Neuroanatomical, and Endocrine Mechanisms. *Biol. Psychiatry* **2017**, *81*, 748–756. [CrossRef] [PubMed]
115. Cenquizca, L.A.; Swanson, L.W. Analysis of direct hippocampal cortical field CA1 axonal projections to diencephalon in the rat. *J. Comp. Neurol.* **2006**, *497*, 101–114. [CrossRef] [PubMed]
116. Hsu, T.M.; Hahn, J.D.; Konanur, V.R.; Noble, E.E.; Suarez, A.N.; Thai, J.; Nakamoto, E.M.; Kanoski, S.E. Hippocampus ghrelin signaling mediates appetite through lateral hypothalamic orexin pathways. *Elife* **2015**, *4*. [CrossRef] [PubMed]
117. Radley, J.J.; Sawchenko, P.E. A common substrate for prefrontal and hippocampal inhibition of the neuroendocrine stress response. *J. Neurosci.* **2011**, *31*, 9683–9695. [CrossRef] [PubMed]
118. Hannapel, R.C.; Henderson, Y.H.; Nalloor, R.; Vazdarjanova, A.; Parent, M.B. Ventral hippocampal neurons inhibit postprandial energy intake. *Hippocampus* **2017**, *27*, 274–284. [CrossRef] [PubMed]
119. Suarez, A.N.; Liu, C.M.; Cortella, A.M.; Noble, E.E.; Kanoski, S.E. Ghrelin and Orexin Interact to Increase Meal Size Through a Descending Hippocampus to Hindbrain Signaling Pathway. *Biol. Psychiatry* **2020**, *87*, 1001–1011. [CrossRef] [PubMed]
120. Davis, E.A.; Wald, H.S.; Suarez, A.N.; Zubcevic, J.; Liu, C.M.; Cortella, A.M.; Kamitakahara, A.K.; Polson, J.W.; Arnold, M.; Grill, H.J.; et al. Ghrelin Signaling Affects Feeding Behavior, Metabolism, and Memory through the Vagus Nerve. *Curr. Biol.* **2020**, *30*, 4510–4518.e4516. [CrossRef] [PubMed]
121. Kanoski, S.E.; Hayes, M.R.; Greenwald, H.S.; Fortin, S.M.; Gianessi, C.A.; Gilbert, J.R.; Grill, H.J. Hippocampal leptin signaling reduces food intake and modulates food-related memory processing. *Neuropsychopharmacology* **2011**, *36*, 1859–1870. [CrossRef] [PubMed]
122. Hsu, T.M.; Noble, E.E.; Liu, C.M.; Cortella, A.M.; Konanur, V.R.; Suarez, A.N.; Reiner, D.J.; Hahn, J.D.; Hayes, M.R.; Kanoski, S.E. A hippocampus to prefrontal cortex neural pathway inhibits food motivation through glucagon-like peptide-1 signaling. *Mol. Psychiatry* **2018**, *23*, 1555–1565. [CrossRef] [PubMed]
123. Henderson, Y.O.; Smith, G.P.; Parent, M.B. Hippocampal neurons inhibit meal onset. *Hippocampus* **2013**, *23*, 100–107. [CrossRef] [PubMed]
124. Parent, M.B. Cognitive control of meal onset and meal size: Role of dorsal hippocampal-dependent episodic memory. *Physiol. Behav.* **2016**, *162*, 112–119. [CrossRef]
125. Van den Burg, E.H.; Stoop, R. Neuropeptide signalling in the central nucleus of the amygdala. *Cell Tissue Res.* **2019**, *375*, 93–101. [CrossRef]
126. Wang, Y.; Kim, J.; Schmit, M.B.; Cho, T.S.; Fang, C.; Cai, H. A bed nucleus of stria terminalis microcircuit regulating inflammation-associated modulation of feeding. *Nat. Commun.* **2019**, *10*, 2769. [CrossRef]
127. De Lartigue, G.; Xu, C. Mechanisms of vagal plasticity influencing feeding behavior. *Brain Res.* **2018**, *1693*, 146–150. [CrossRef]
128. Kentish, S.; Li, H.; Philp, L.K.; O'Donnell, T.A.; Isaacs, N.J.; Young, R.L.; Wittert, G.A.; Blackshaw, L.A.; Page, A.J. Diet-induced adaptation of vagal afferent function. *J. Physiol.* **2012**, *590*, 209–221. [CrossRef] [PubMed]
129. Feinle-Bisset, C. Upper gastrointestinal sensitivity to meal-related signals in adult humans—Relevance to appetite regulation and gut symptoms in health, obesity and functional dyspepsia. *Physiol. Behav.* **2016**, *162*, 69–82. [CrossRef] [PubMed]
130. Daly, D.M.; Park, S.J.; Valinsky, W.C.; Beyak, M.J. Impaired intestinal afferent nerve satiety signalling and vagal afferent excitability in diet induced obesity in the mouse. *J. Physiol.* **2011**, *589*, 2857–2870. [CrossRef]
131. Browning, K.N.; Fortna, S.R.; Hajnal, A. Roux-en-Y gastric bypass reverses the effects of diet-induced obesity to inhibit the responsiveness of central vagal motoneurones. *J. Physiol.* **2013**, *591*, 2357–2372. [CrossRef] [PubMed]
132. Waise, T.M.Z.; Toshinai, K.; Naznin, F.; NamKoong, C.; Md Moin, A.S.; Sakoda, H.; Nakazato, M. One-day high-fat diet induces inflammation in the nodose ganglion and hypothalamus of mice. *Biochem. Biophys. Res. Commun.* **2015**, *464*, 1157–1162. [CrossRef] [PubMed]
133. Levin, B.E.; Triscari, J.; Hogan, S.; Sullivan, A.C. Resistance to diet-induced obesity: Food intake, pancreatic sympathetic tone, and insulin. *Am. J. Physiol.* **1987**, *252*, R471–R478. [CrossRef]
134. Lee, S.J.; Jokiaho, A.J.; Sanchez-Watts, G.; Watts, A.G. Catecholaminergic projections into an interconnected forebrain network control the sensitivity of male rats to diet-induced obesity. *Am. J. Physiol. Regul. Integr. Comp. Physiol.* **2018**, *314*, R811–R823. [CrossRef] [PubMed]

135. Rinaman, L. Postnatal development of hypothalamic inputs to the dorsal vagal complex in rats. *Physiol. Behav.* **2003**, *79*, 65–70. [CrossRef]
136. Levin, B.E. Developmental gene x environment interactions affecting systems regulating energy homeostasis and obesity. *Front. Neuroendocrinol.* **2010**, *31*, 270–283. [CrossRef]
137. Levin, B.E. Metabolic imprinting: Critical impact of the perinatal environment on the regulation of energy homeostasis. *Philos. Trans. R. Soc. Lond. B Biol. Sci.* **2006**, *361*, 1107–1121. [CrossRef]
138. Bocarsly, M.E.; Barson, J.R.; Hauca, J.M.; Hoebel, B.G.; Leibowitz, S.F.; Avena, N.M. Effects of perinatal exposure to palatable diets on body weight and sensitivity to drugs of abuse in rats. *Physiol. Behav.* **2012**, *107*, 568–575. [CrossRef] [PubMed]
139. Clyburn, C.; Howe, C.A.; Arnold, A.C.; Lang, C.H.; Travagli, R.A.; Browning, K.N. Perinatal high-fat diet alters development of GABA A receptor subunits in dorsal motor nucleus of vagus. *Am. J. Physiol. Gastrointest. Liver Physiol.* **2019**, *317*, G40–G50. [CrossRef]
140. Poon, K. Behavioral Feeding Circuit: Dietary Fat-Induced Effects of Inflammatory Mediators in the Hypothalamus. *Front. Endocrinol.* **2020**, *11*, 591559. [CrossRef]
141. Poon, K.; Mandava, S.; Chen, K.; Barson, J.R.; Buschlen, S.; Leibowitz, S.F. Prenatal exposure to dietary fat induces changes in the transcriptional factors, TEF and YAP, which may stimulate differentiation of peptide neurons in rat hypothalamus. *PLoS ONE* **2013**, *8*, e77668. [CrossRef]
142. Stump, M.; Guo, D.F.; Lu, K.T.; Mukohda, M.; Cassell, M.D.; Norris, A.W.; Rahmouni, K.; Sigmund, C.D. Nervous System Expression of PPARγ and Mutant PPARγ Has Profound Effects on Metabolic Regulation and Brain Development. *Endocrinology* **2016**, *157*, 4266–4275. [CrossRef]
143. Sullivan, E.L.; Rivera, H.M.; True, C.A.; Franco, J.G.; Baquero, K.; Dean, T.A.; Valleau, J.C.; Takahashi, D.L.; Frazee, T.; Hanna, G.; et al. Maternal and postnatal high-fat diet consumption programs energy balance and hypothalamic melanocortin signaling in nonhuman primate offspring. *Am. J. Physiol. Regul. Integr. Comp. Physiol.* **2017**, *313*, R169–R179. [CrossRef]
144. Juan De Solis, A.; Baquero, A.F.; Bennett, C.M.; Grove, K.L.; Zeltser, L.M. Postnatal undernutrition delays a key step in the maturation of hypothalamic feeding circuits. *Mol. Metab.* **2016**, *5*, 198–209. [CrossRef]
145. Franklin, T.B.; Saab, B.J.; Mansuy, I.M. Neural mechanisms of stress resilience and vulnerability. *Neuron* **2012**, *75*, 747–761. [CrossRef]
146. Ulrich-Lai, Y.M.; Herman, J.P. Neural regulation of endocrine and autonomic stress responses. *Nat. Rev. Neurosci.* **2009**, *10*, 397–409. [CrossRef] [PubMed]
147. Jiang, Y.; Greenwood-Van Meerveld, B.; Johnson, A.C.; Travagli, R.A. Role of estrogen and stress on the brain-gut axis. *Am. J. Physiol. Gastrointest. Liver Physiol.* **2019**, *317*, G203–G209. [CrossRef] [PubMed]
148. Drossman, D.A. Functional Gastrointestinal Disorders: History, Pathophysiology, Clinical Features and Rome IV. *Gastroenterology* **2016**. [CrossRef] [PubMed]
149. Fukudo, S. Stress and visceral pain: Focusing on irritable bowel syndrome. *Pain* **2013**, *154* (Suppl. 1), S63–S70. [CrossRef] [PubMed]
150. Jiang, Y.; Travagli, R.A. Hypothalamic-vagal oxytocinergic neurocircuitry modulates gastric emptying and motility following stress. *J. Physiol.* **2020**, *598*, 4941–4955. [CrossRef] [PubMed]
151. Horvath, K.; Perman, J.A. Autistic disorder and gastrointestinal disease. *Curr. Opin. Pediatr.* **2002**, *14*, 583–587. [CrossRef]
152. Chistol, L.T.; Bandini, L.G.; Must, A.; Phillips, S.; Cermak, S.A.; Curtin, C. Sensory Sensitivity and Food Selectivity in Children with Autism Spectrum Disorder. *J. Autism Dev. Disord.* **2018**, *48*, 583–591. [CrossRef]
153. Ristori, M.V.; Quagliariello, A.; Reddel, S.; Ianiro, G.; Vicari, S.; Gasbarrini, A.; Putignani, L. Autism, Gastrointestinal Symptoms and Modulation of Gut Microbiota by Nutritional Interventions. *Nutrients* **2019**, *11*, 2812. [CrossRef]
154. Lefter, R.; Ciobica, A.; Timofte, D.; Stanciu, C.; Trifan, A. A Descriptive Review on the Prevalence of Gastrointestinal Disturbances and Their Multiple Associations in Autism Spectrum Disorder. *Medicina* **2019**, *56*, 11. [CrossRef]
155. Horvath, K.; Papadimitriou, J.C.; Rabsztyn, A.; Drachenberg, C.; Tildon, J.T. Gastrointestinal abnormalities in children with autistic disorder. *J. Pediatr.* **1999**, *135*, 559–563. [CrossRef]
156. Rodier, P.M.; Ingram, J.L.; Tisdale, B.; Nelson, S.; Romano, J. Embryological origin for autism: Developmental anomalies of the cranial nerve motor nuclei. *J. Comp. Neurol.* **1996**, *370*, 247–261. [CrossRef]
157. Kushki, A.; Brian, J.; Dupuis, A.; Anagnostou, E. Functional autonomic nervous system profile in children with autism spectrum disorder. *Mol. Autism* **2014**, *5*, 39. [CrossRef]
158. Modahl, C.; Green, L.; Fein, D.; Morris, M.; Waterhouse, L.; Feinstein, C.; Levin, H. Plasma oxytocin levels in autistic children. *Biol. Psychiatry* **1998**, *43*, 270–277. [CrossRef]
159. Fetissov, S.O.; Averina, O.V.; Danilenko, V.N. Neuropeptides in the microbiota-brain axis and feeding behavior in autism spectrum disorder. *Nutrition* **2019**, *61*, 43–48. [CrossRef]
160. Cersosimo, M.G.; Benarroch, E.E. Neural control of the gastrointestinal tract: Implications for Parkinson disease. *Mov. Disord.* **2008**, *23*, 1065–1075. [CrossRef] [PubMed]
161. Grinberg, L.T.; Rueb, U.; Alho, A.T.; Heinsen, H. Brainstem pathology and non-motor symptoms in PD. *J. Neurol. Sci.* **2010**, *289*, 81–88. [CrossRef]
162. Jellinger, K.A. Synuclein deposition and non-motor symptoms in Parkinson disease. *J. Neurol. Sci.* **2011**, *310*, 107–111. [CrossRef] [PubMed]

163. Natale, G.; Pasquali, L.; Ruggieri, S.; Paparelli, A.; Fornai, F. Parkinson's disease and the gut: A well known clinical association in need of an effective cure and explanation. *Neurogastroenterol. Motil.* **2008**, *20*, 741–749. [CrossRef] [PubMed]
164. Travagli, R.A.; Browning, K.N.; Camilleri, M. Parkinson disease and the gut: New insights into pathogenesis and clinical relevance. *Nat. Rev. Gastroenterol. Hepatol.* **2020**. [CrossRef] [PubMed]
165. Braak, H.; Braak, E. Pathoanatomy of Parkinson's disease. *J. Neurol.* **2000**, *247* (Suppl. 2), II3–II10. [CrossRef] [PubMed]
166. Anselmi, L.; Toti, L.; Bove, C.; Hampton, J.; Travagli, R.A. A Nigro-Vagal Pathway Controls Gastric Motility and Is Affected in a Rat Model of Parkinsonism. *Gastroenterology* **2017**, *153*, 1581–1593. [CrossRef] [PubMed]
167. Toti, L.; Travagli, R.A. Gastric dysregulation induced by microinjection of 6-OHDA in the substantia nigra pars compacta of rats is determined by alterations in the brain-gut axis. *Am. J. Physiol. Gastrointest. Liver Physiol.* **2014**, *307*, G1013–G1023. [CrossRef]
168. Bove, C.; Travagli, R.A. Neurophysiology of the brain stem in Parkinson's disease. *J. Neurophysiol.* **2019**, *121*, 1856–1864. [CrossRef]
169. Tan, H.-E.; Sisti, A.C.; Jin, H.; Vignovich, M.; Villavicencio, M.; Tsang, K.S.; Goffer, Y.; Zuker, C.S. The gut-brain axis mediates sugar preference. *Nature* **2020**, *580*, 511–516. [CrossRef]
170. Aguilera-Lizarraga, J.; Florens, M.V.; Viola, M.F.; Jain, P.; Decraecker, L.; Appeltans, I.; Cuende-Estevez, M.; Fabre, N.; Van Beek, K.; Perna, E.; et al. Local immune response to food antigens drives-meal-induced abdominal pain. *Nature* **2021**, *591*, 151–156. [CrossRef]
171. Worthington, J.J.; Reimann, F.; Gribble, F.M. Enteroendocrine cells-sensory sentinels of the intestinal environment and orchestrators of mucosal immunity. *Mucosal Immunol.* **2018**, *11*, 3–20. [CrossRef] [PubMed]
172. Powley, T.L.; Jaffey, D.M.; McAdams, J.; Baronowsky, E.A.; Black, D.; Chesney, L.; Evans, C.; Phillips, R.J. Vagal innervation of the stomach reassessed: Brain-gut connectome uses smart terminals. *Ann. N. Y. Acad. Sci.* **2019**, *1451*, 14–30. [CrossRef] [PubMed]

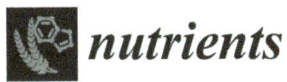

Review

Effects of Oro-Sensory Exposure on Satiation and Underlying Neurophysiological Mechanisms—What Do We Know So Far?

Marlou P. Lasschuijt, Kees de Graaf and Monica Mars *

Division of Human Nutrition and Health, Wageningen University & Research, P.O. Box 17,
NL-6700 AA Wageningen, The Netherlands; marlou.lasschuijt@wur.nl (M.P.L.); kees.degraaf@wur.nl (K.d.G.)
* Correspondence: Monica.Mars@wur.nl

Abstract: The mouth is the first part of the gastrointestinal tract. During mastication sensory signals from the mouth, so-called oro-sensory exposure, elicit physiological signals that affect satiation and food intake. It has been established that a longer duration of oro-sensory exposure leads to earlier satiation. In addition, foods with more intense sweet or salty taste induce earlier satiation compared to foods that are equally palatable, but with lower taste intensity. Oro-sensory exposure to food affects satiation by direct signaling via the brainstem to higher cortical regions involved in taste and reward, including the nucleus accumbens and the insula. There is little evidence that oro-sensory exposure affects satiation indirectly through either hormone responses or gastric signals. Critical brain areas for satiation, such as the brainstem, should be studied more intensively to better understand the neurophysiological mechanisms underlying the process of satiation. Furthermore, it is essential to increase the understanding of how of highly automated eating behaviors, such as oral processing and eating rate, are formed during early childhood. A better understanding of the aforementioned mechanisms provides fundamental insight in relation to strategies to prevent overconsumption and the development of obesity in future generations.

Keywords: satiation; food intake; taste; texture; oro-sensory exposure; sensory science; cephalic responses; brain areas; brain stem; weight management

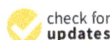

Citation: Lasschuijt, M.P.; de Graaf, K.; Mars, M. Effects of Oro-Sensory Exposure on Satiation and Underlying Neurophysiological Mechanisms—What Do We Know So Far? *Nutrients* **2021**, *13*, 1391.
https://doi.org/10.3390/nu13051391

Academic Editors:
Christine Feinle-Bisset and
Michael Horowitz

Received: 1 February 2021
Accepted: 13 April 2021
Published: 21 April 2021

Publisher's Note: MDPI stays neutral with regard to jurisdictional claims in published maps and institutional affiliations.

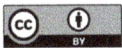

Copyright: © 2021 by the authors. Licensee MDPI, Basel, Switzerland. This article is an open access article distributed under the terms and conditions of the Creative Commons Attribution (CC BY) license (https://creativecommons.org/licenses/by/4.0/).

1. Introduction

Eating is an episodic process, people consume meals or snacks followed by periods of fasting. People eat of a meal until they feel satiated, which translates into satiety, i.e., the period between two eating episodes. The processes of satiation and hunger involve feedback mechanisms that originate from different parts of the gastro-intestinal tract. Ingested and absorbed food components elicit a cascade of physiological and metabolic processes that affect satiety and, consequently, food intake [1,2]. Oral signals and perceived sensory properties of foods have been considered to play a role in the early, pre-absorptive phase of food ingestion. Post-absorptive factors, arising from the stomach and intestines, play a role in satiety and the initiation of the next meal. In this review, we focus on the physiological processes that are initiated as a result of the presence of food in the mouth, i.e., oro-sensory signals. This review addresses how oro-sensory signals relate to earlier satiation and lowering food intake, in the context of weight management and obesity prevention.

In textbooks, food digestion is often referred to as the digestive process that starts in the stomach and continues in the intestines. However, food digestion already starts in the mouth and it has an essential function in food digestion. The mouth has a gate-keeping function as it prevents ingestion of unfamiliar, bad-tasting and potentially dangerous food. Additionally, it prepares the body for food digestion further along the digestive tract. In the mouth, food is masticated to be mechanically broken down into small pieces, which enlarges the surface area. The food is mixed and lubricated with α-amylase containing saliva to form a bolus. This allows for the start of carbohydrate digestion in the mouth and makes the bolus safe to swallow [3]. During this mastication process, food is perceived in the mouth by the senses (mostly taste and retro-nasal smell) and multiple physiological processes are initiated (for reviews see [4,5]). Eating food is potentially a threat to the body's homeostasis, therefore, oral exposure serves as an alarm such that the body can anticipate and prepare incoming nutrients for optimal digestion [6,7].

The role of oral exposure to food (taste, flavor, texture) has been extensively studied in relation to satiety and food intake. One of the most prominent findings in this area is a phenomenon now referred to as "sensory-specific satiety". Sensory-specific satiety was first described by Rolls et al. in 1981, where it was defined as the decrease in pleasantness of the eaten food relative to the pleasantness of foods not eaten [8]. It was found that if people were instructed to eat a certain food until satiation, and then were provided with a series of different tasting foods, the rating of pleasantness of the just eaten foods was decreased more compared to the non-eaten foods. This decrease in pleasantness could be explained primarily by the sensory characteristics of the food, rather than sensory fatigue or the nutrient composition of the food. This observation establishes that sensory exposure to food directly affects its hedonic value while being consumed to satiation.

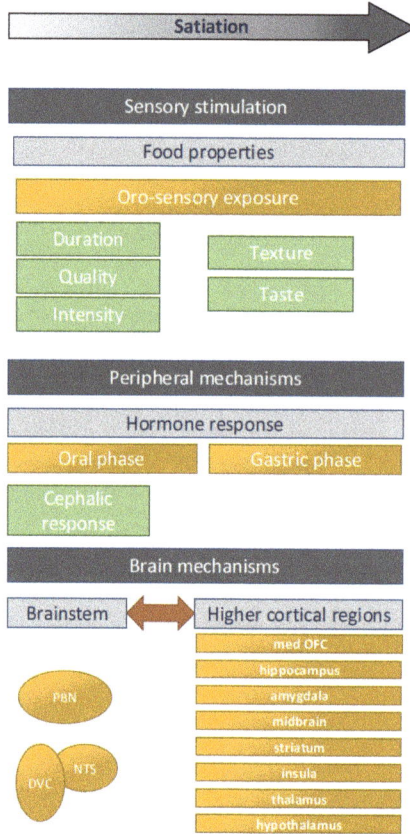

Figure 1. Overview of the factors involved in the relation between oro-sensory exposure and food intake. This figure is based partly on Hopkins and Blundell et al. [1,9]. PBN = parabrachial nuclei, NTS = nuclei of the solitary tract, DVC = dorsal vagal complex, med OFC = medial orbitofrontal cortex.

In this review, we reflect on the scientific evidence that demonstrates the relation between oro-sensory exposure and the regulation of food intake, with a focus on satiation (within meal satiety). In addition to the different components of oro-sensory exposure and their effects on food intake, we discuss hypothesized underlying neuro-physiological mechanisms (Figure 1). We describe main knowledge gaps and directions for future research. Finally, the implications for obesity prevention are discussed.

2. Effects on Satiation
2.1. Factors Affecting Oro-Sensory Exposure

Oro-sensory exposure reflects the overall exposure of the oral cavity to sensory cues during food consumption [10,11]. The level of oro-sensory exposure, also called "in-mouth sensory exposure", is determined by both the sensory properties of a food and its processing in the mouth (oral processing). The magnitude of sensory exposure is determined by (1) the intensity of the stimulus and (2) the duration of exposure to the stimulus (see Figure 2). The duration and intensity of oro-sensory exposure are not two distinct factors, but often interact, especially in food with complex textures where oral processing affects the release of tastants and vice versa. Furthermore, the nature of the stimulus, i.e., the sensory quality or modality of the ingested food, is important. In this review, we focus on texture and taste as being the main qualities of importance for oro-sensory exposure. Taste and texture affect the duration, quality, and intensity of oro-sensory exposure which affects satiation and, consequently, the amount of food consumed. In the following paragraphs, we reflect on the evidence for an effect of oro-sensory exposure on food intake, starting with the duration of oral exposure.

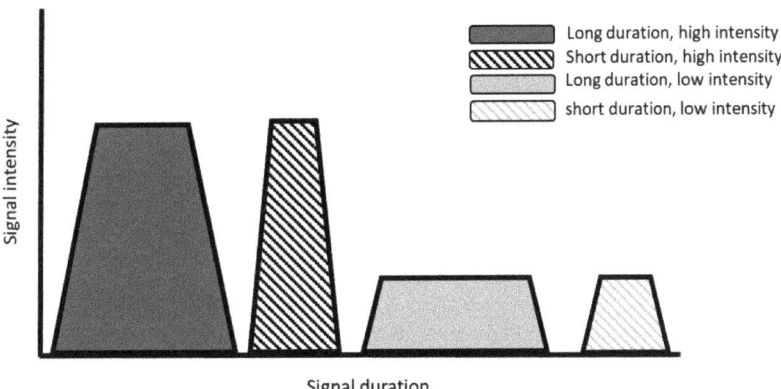

Figure 2. Schematic overview of our hypothesis underlying oro-sensory exposure. The area under the curve represents the level of oro-sensory exposure, which depend on both the intensity and the duration of the sensory signal.

2.2. Oral Exposure Duration

The duration of oral exposure is determined mainly by the texture of food and the rate at which it is eaten. Different textures elicit different oral processing behavior and may therefore affect oro-sensory exposure time to the food. There is a wide variation in eating rate of foods available in our diet [12,13], and in how people process food in mouth [14]. Accordingly, oral processing time is in part determined by individual eating behavior, but for a larger part, by the food's textural properties [13,15].

Texture can be defined as the multimodal sensory experience derived from the structure of food. It can be characterized by terms such as viscous, chewy, elastic, and hard [16]. Food texture may also be classified into broader groups of food form: liquid, semi-solid, soft solid, and hard solid [17]. Furthermore, there are mixed structures, for example hard particles added to semi-solids, can change oral processing behavior [18,19].

In the last 15 years, many experimental studies have shown consistently that food form affects how much people eat, independent of the palatability of the food. Liquids have a lower satiation capacity relative to their energy content compared to semi-solids and solids. This is due to the high eating or drinking rate at which liquids can be consumed which induces short oro-sensory exposure [20]. For example, Zijlstra et al. reported that food intake decreased when the viscosity of chocolate milk was increased to a custard like product [15]. This observation has been replicated several times [21,22]. It has also shown that this effect is mainly due to oral exposure time [15,23]. Eating the same semi-liquid with a food with a straw (short oral exposure) compared to eating with a spoon (longer oral exposure) resulted in a significantly lower intake [23]. Accordingly, eating foods in a way that it yields longer oral exposure leads to earlier satiation and consequently lower food intake.

Within the group of semi-solid and solid foods, there appears to be a window of opportunity to change satiating capacity by changing the food structure and thus oral processing. For example, mashed potatoes are less satiating compared to potatoes with their full structure [24] and hamburgers with crispy hard bread compared to soft bread [25]. However, the changes in oral processing that are elicited by texture changes should be large enough to alter the rate at which the foods are eaten. For example, Zijlstra et al., compared different textures of three solids foods, candies, meat, and meat replacers, and found the changes that were elicited in oral processing were not large enough to result in effects in food intake [26]. Recently Chayadi et al., failed to show an effect between two types of crisps with different textures [27]. In a recent review, Bolhuis and Forde provided an elaborate overview with food structure manipulations that can potentially lead to foods that have a high satiating capacity [28].

In addition to changing oral exposure time indirectly by altering the texture of foods, it has also been shown that manipulating oro-sensory exposure duration directly affects intake. For example, by manipulating sip sizes by using peristaltic pumps, or instructions during eating. For example, Weijzen et al. manipulated sip sizes of sweet orangeades with a peristaltic pump; drinking small sips (5 g) compared to large sips (20 g) resulted in a lower intake [29]. However, this effect was only statistically significant for sugar-sweetened drinks and not when the orangeades were sweetened with non-caloric sweeteners. This indicates that a metabolic reward is involved in this effect. Similarly, Zijlstra et al. did an experiment in which they manipulated bite-size and oral processing time of chocolate milk with a peristaltic pump [21]. Instructing individuals to eat slower and process foods longer in their mouths resulted in smaller intakes, also compared to the "free eating conditions" in which individuals could choose their own bite size and oral processing time. Also, more real-life experiments have also shown this effect. For example, Weijzen et al. instructed individuals to either eat nibble-sized or bar size snacks, and either eat them attentively or without any specific instruction [30]. Subjects ate less of the nibbles compared to the bars. Interestingly, they only found a clear effect of nibbles and bars on food intake but no convincing effect of eating with more attention.

In summary, it has been shown in numerous studies that longer oro-sensory exposure by processing foods longer in the mouth, and thus eating slower, decreases meal size. This effect appears to be independent of palatability or the degree of attention to food.

2.3. Taste Intensity and Quality

The intensity of oro-sensory exposure intensity is reflected by the perceived intensity. The latter is determined by the binding of the tastant to the taste receptors in the oral cavity and tongue. This is dependent on the concentration of the tastant, as well as on the surface availability and its solubility in saliva [31]. Surface availability and the capacity of tastants to dissolve in saliva are both dependent on food texture. For example, two foods with the same amount of sucrose, but differing in texture, (liquid vs. solid), have different sweetness intensities [32]. For a solid food product to be equally sweet to a liquid, twice the amount of sucrose is needed [33,34].

The taste intensity of food affects satiation and subsequent food intake. Accordingly, smaller meals are consumed when foods of higher sweetness when provided *ad libitum* [35–37] even if the rated palatability of the two products before ingestion was the same. This is also the case for salt intensity. Bolhuis conducted a series of experiments in which salt intensity was varied; tomato soups with similar palatability, but slightly higher and lower than ideal salt intensities were provided and intake was measured [11,38]. Subjects consumed less soup in the high compared to the low salt intensity. Therefore it appears that exposure to higher sweetness intensity and higher saltiness intensity leads to earlier meal termination and a reduction in food intake.

It may be argued that this effect is only specific for sweetness and saltiness, and that the magnitude may differ between tastes. However, to our knowledge, there is only one study that investigated whether exposure to different taste qualities has different effects on satiation. Griffioen, et al. offered two equally liked rice meals, with similar structure and macronutrient content, one with sweet taste compared to savory rice meals, and found no difference in *ad libitum* consumption of these two meals, that is they were equally satiating [39].

The concentration of a tastant in a food product does not predict intensity per se as the release of tastes and flavors is also dependent on the structure of the food. It has been shown that a harder structure enhances the effect of intensity, by prolonging the exposure duration (i.e., harder textures require longer oral processing before a bolus is safe to swallow) [24,40]. For example, Forde et al. reported that a higher savory taste, in combination with a harder texture of the food, led to a significant decrease in food intake compared to non-flavored soft food [24]. While Lasschuijt et al. reported that a combination of a harder texture and higher sweetness intensity leads to a reduction in intake. The latter study also showed that the effect of texture was much larger compared to the effect of sweetness intensity [40].

2.4. Discussion Effects of Oro-Sensory Exposure on Satiation

To summarize, it has been established that oro-sensory exposure has an important role in satiation. The taste intensity of foods and how they are processed in the mouth affect the amount of food people consume, independently of the initial palatability of the food. A review by McCrickerd et al. argues that the effect of texture on food intake is approximately 30% and that of taste 10%, depending on the differences in texture hardness and taste intensity between two foods [41].

In this review, we have only focused on within meal satiation. Although we did not discuss the evidence here, we also know that food form (liquid vs. solids) affects appetite and food intake beyond a single meal [42]. Similarly, taste and flavor of a particular meal may also affect appetite and satiety after the meal [43]. For example, after eating a savory meal, there is a preference for sweet food items for the following meal or snack [43]. This effect on satiety may reflect both direct and indirect signaling related to the entry of food entering the stomach and intestines.

The effect of texture on satiation appears to be universal effect, so independent of eating habits, that is familiarity with the food. We have shown in the past that the effect of texture on satiation exists both for familiar as well as unfamiliar foods [44,45]. Moreover, it has also been shown in Western and Asian populations that texture modifies oral processing consistently across different populations or cultures [42,46,47]. Although between population groups (sex, ages, ethnicity) the effect sizes may differ, the direction of the effects is identical within an individual (lower eating rate and lower intake with harder textures) [48].

Equal palatability of the foods is essential in studies investigating oro-sensory exposure and food intake. It is possible to investigate. You can study two suboptimal perceived intensities of sweet and salt taste that are equally liked [11,36]. However, for the other sensory qualities this is much more difficult to control. For example, we do not know whether bitterness, sourness, or sensory sensations such as trigeminal taste (for example pepper, carbonation, mint) have similar effects on food intake, as the capacity to manipulate these sensory sensations is limited, without foods becoming unpalatable. A number of studies have been done on retro-nasal odors, that is the odor released during mastication, and satiation, but have shown little effect on food intake [46,47].

One of the proposed hypotheses to explain these potent effects of oro-sensory exposure on food intake is that taste and texture are strong predictors of the nutrient content of the food, such as sugar and salt [49]. For example, solid foods have low water content and are therefore more energy-dense. Furthermore, low taste intensity signals low nutrient density. Because of this, solid high taste intensity foods may be perceived as being more rewarding and satiating [50]. An alternative mechanism by which the intensity of oro-sensory exposure may affect satiation is though sensory-specific satiety; strong taste intensities may induce this on more rapidly compared to low taste intensities [10]. This decrease in hedonic value of a taste may lead to meal termination. It has been hypothesized that this phenomenon of sensory specific satiety is essential for survival as it stimulates variety in the diet [49].

3. Neurophysiological Mechanisms

The precise physiological mechanisms by which oro-sensory exposure affects satiation has not been elucidated. It has been hypothesized that sensory signals travel from the oral cavity through afferent cranial nerves V VII, IX, X, and XII to the brainstem, and then higher cortical regions, as discussed in Section 3.2. In addition, oro-sensory exposure signals induce a cascade of efferent responses responsible for optimal food digestion, as discussed in Section 3.3 [51]. Ultimately, satiation evolves in the brain (among other regions in the reward center and orbitofrontal cortex) as a result of the integration of direct oro-sensory signals and indirect signals arising from the gastrointestinal tract. The following paragraphs discusses these hypothesized mechanisms in more detail.

3.1. Brain Stem

There have been many neuroimaging studies comparing brain responses in hungry and satiated state, however little is known about the brainstem in relation to sensory cues and satiation. The brainstem is the first part of the brain that processes afferent taste and gastric signals, but only limited research has been done in this area [52–54]. The brainstem is inherently difficult to investigate because it is a complex area and the cluster size of nuclei with the same function is very small ($n = 2$–5). Even within these small nuclei clusters, nuclei may have very distinct roles. For example, a study in monkeys reported that the posterior part of nuclei of the solitary tract (NTS) is most responsive to glucose, whereas the anterior NTS was particularly responsive to NaCl [55]. This shows the heterogeneity of nuclei even within these small brainstem areas.

The brainstem is inherently challenging to study. The current brain stem atlases show lack of detail and do not cover all different nuclei in the brainstem. In addition, the brainstem area is difficult to probe as the current fMRI approaches have only limited resolution. As the brainstem is close to the heart and lungs, fMRI signals are prone to artefacts and confounding by physiological noise.

Due to these technical challenges few human studies have been performed; the majority of evidence is derived from animal studies. Based on this work, the dorsal vagal complex (DVC) in the medulla and the parabrachial nucleus (PBN) in the pons play key roles in satiation. The DVC includes the nucleus of the solitary tract (NTS), the dorsal motor vagal nucleus (DMV), and area postrema (AP). Together with the PBN the DVC is involved in the integration of energy-related peripheral signals and processing of taste and gastric signals [56–60]. These brainstem areas receive satiation-related input at three levels. First, neurons sense circulating metabolites and hormones such as glucose and CCK (DMV). Second, the brainstem receives vagal input from the sensory system and the gastrointestinal tract, such as taste (NTS, PBN) and gastric distention signals (PBN). Finally, the brainstem receives input from the mid- and forebrain, which is integrated together with energy-related signals in the area postrema (AP). The brainstem then projects these signals to hepatic and gastric efferent nerves [61]. An overview of the brainstem areas involved in satiation is shown in Figure 3.

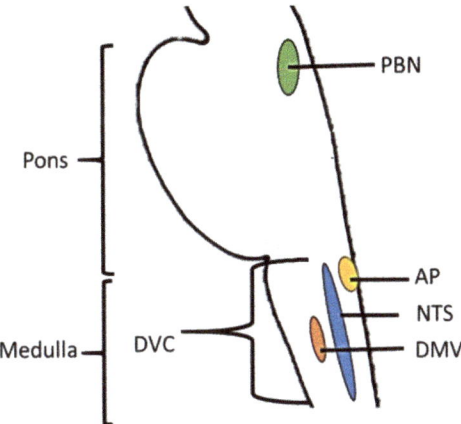

Figure 3. Graphical representation of a sagittal section of the brainstem. Depicted areas are involved in processing taste- and gastric signals and energy-related peripheral signals (hormones and metabolites). AP = Area postrema, DVC = dorsal vagal complex, DMV = Dorsal motor vagus, NTS = nucleus of the solitary tract, PBN = Parabrachial nuclei. Locations of brain areas are based on Duvernoy's Atlas of the human brain stem [62].

As discussed before only a couple of human studies have investigated taste processing and satiation in the brainstem. For example, Small et al. reported that greater taste intensity led to increased activation in the PBN region of the pons [63]. Other studies have found NTS activation after oro-sensory exposure to sour-sweet-salt-bitter mixtures [64] and sucrose solutions [65]. The most convincing evidence for brainstem involvement in the process of satiation comes from a study in rats. Animals that were decerebrated rejected taste stimuli when satiated [66], indicating that despite the absence of functional higher cortical regions, taste signals are still processed in relation to satiation in the brainstem (PBN).

3.2. Higher Cortical Regions

From the brainstem oro-sensory signals diverge into an affective and sensory pathways [61]. The affective pathway includes projections to the hypothalamus, amygdala, parahippocampal gyrus, orbitofrontal cortex (OFC), striatum, and midbrain. The sensory pathway includes the thalamus and insula. Together, these areas regulate the release of hormones involved in digestion and satiety [60,67].

The most prominent region involved in satiation, is the reward system (areas that are part of the affective pathway). With increasing fullness, the reward system is downregulated which lowers the hedonic responses to food (due to direct and indirect signals induced by food intake) leading to meal termination [68].

Other relevant brain regions are the insula and the amygdala. It has been shown that internal state modulates the activation of the insula and that this is associated with a reduction in affective value or pleasantness of the taste stimuli, specific satiation [63,67,69]. The amygdala is associated with the perception of both positive and negative verbal, visual, odor and taste stimuli [70–75]. Therefore, the amygdala may signal both pleasure and aversion of taste stimuli, dependent on the satiated state. This is in line with the observations of La Bar et al. and Morris et al. of enhanced responses to food pictures in a hungry state compared to the satiated state [76,77]. However, observations have shown to be inconsistent as some studies reported that activation of the amygdala reflects odor and taste stimulus intensity, irrespective of liking [63,78].

3.3. Cephalic Phase Responses

In addition to a direct effect on higher cortical regions, oro-sensory exposure also affects food intake indirectly through so-called cephalic phase reflexes, or cephalic phase responses (CPRs) [5,6,8]. As mentioned, these are induced when oro-sensory signals reach the brainstem, and thought to support optimal food digestion.

CPRs are anticipatory and conditioned responses to food cues [5,6]. They occur within minutes after food consumption and are, therefore, not related to nutrient sensing further down in the digestive tract [4,5]. Cephalic responses include increased production of saliva, gastric juice, secretion of bile by the gallbladder, increased gut motility, and gastric and pancreatic hormone secretion [79–82]. Examples of cephalic hormones are insulin, pancreatic polypeptide, and ghrelin [4,5,83]. The supposed function of CPRs is to "prepare" the body for incoming nutrients to optimize digestion [6,84].

Until recently, a reduction in CPRs was thought to be associated with impaired appetite regulation and weight gain [85–87]. Based on this, we hypothesized that a reduction in CPRs from little oro-sensory exposure may represent physiological mechanism underlying reduced satiation—for example, when foods with little taste are eaten quickly [88,89]. Recently, we performed a systematic and quantitative review which investigated the magnitude of the cephalic response of insulin and pancreatic peptide. We concluded that the cephalic insulin and pancreatic responses are almost indistinguishable from normal variation, and exhibit substantial variation in both magnitude and timing of onset. Additionally, only two studies found an effect of a reduced CPRs on subjective appetite ratings [83,90]. Accordingly, it should be questioned whether these CPRs affect satiation and are biologically meaningful in daily life [4]. If cephalic phase responses play an important role in satiation, it is likely to be caused by cephalic phase responses other than insulin and pancreatic polypeptide response, such as early production of saliva and gastric juice [69].

3.4. Discussion Neurophysiological Mechanisms in Satiation

To summarize, the neuro-physiological mechanisms underlying satiation are gradually becoming clearer as research progresses. In particularly, neuroimaging studies have provided insight into the processing of sensory signals in the higher cortical regions of the brain in relation to satiation. However, the precise neurophysiological mechanisms of how oro-sensory signals affect the process of satiation, and the role of the brain stem remains to be elucidated.

As mentioned before, neuroimaging of the brain stem is inherently difficult. To improve research in this area, a brainstem atlas suitable for fMRI and optimized normalization of the brainstem is needed. A brainstem atlas would allow for distinction between sensory responses, physiological processes and movement. For example, discriminating tongue movements from taste perception activation. The development of a brainstem atlas would also allow future studies to measure brainstem areas specifically involved in sensory processing, gastric distention, and satiation.

In addition to neuro-physiology, research in the area of the peripheral physiological mechanisms underlying satiation could progress by having a clear definition of cephalic phase responses. Such a definition should take baseline variation of the cephalic variable into consideration to conclude whether a peak increase reflects the presented food cue or biological fluctuations. Furthermore, the definition should include a strict time range in which the cephalic peak response should occur, for example within 2–5 min after food ingestion. Such a clear definition would be helpful in combining and comparing results of different studies which investigate early responses to food cues in relation to satiation.

In this review we have focused solely on the effects of oro-sensory exposure on satiation. However, as shown in Figure 1, both the oral as well as the gastric phase are important. For example, factors in the gastric phase that contribute to satiation are meal volume, meal weight, and, indirectly, gastro-intestinal hormones that inhibit gastric emptying [91,92]. Also gastric emptying is affected by food texture; it is more difficult for digestive fluids to penetrate hard textured foods and are therefore their biochemical breakdown is much slower [93]. Moreover, larger solid particles require more mechanical breakdown, that is muscle movements of the stomach, to reduce the particle size to a level appropriate for entering the duodenum [94]. When gastric emptying rate is low, stomach distention activates stretch and mechanoreceptors send fullness signals to the brain via vagal afferent nerves to the brainstem [95]. Simultaneously, nutrients that enter the small intestine trigger GI hormones including CCK, PYY, and GLP-1 that reach the brain through the blood brain barrier [96,97]. These postprandial hormonal responses are substantially greater than the before mentioned CPRs. It is believed that postprandial responses to account for 40–70% of the variation in predicted food intake [98,99]. However, as these responses occur are mainly elicited after consumption, they are more likely to affect satiety (i.e., between meal suppression of appetite) than the amount eaten within a meal, i.e., satiation.

4. Recommendations for Future Research

Eating slowly due to food texture, or because of individual eating behavior decreases food intake compared to more rapid food intake [20,100]. Oral processing such as chewing behaviour and eating rate differs not only between food structures, but also between individuals. Eating behavior is dependent on gender, age, ethnicity and body weight status [20,100]. Why some people simply eat faster than others is not fully understood. Although eating rate differs between people, within-subject eating speed is a relatively steady and automated behavior. The same person eating the same food product twice results in a similar eating rate. This constant or fixed eating rate appears to be acquired at a young age. Eating rate is in part inheritable, and acquired through learning as children's eating rate is affected by parental feeding strategies and early exposure to foods with hard texture [101,102]. There is relatively little information on the etiology of children's eating behavior but it is important to better understand how eating behaviour is formed, a more rapid eating rate at a young age is predictive of adult BMI [103–105].

Apart from the etiology of eating behaviour there is little known about the physiology of satiation, i.e., the process of going from a hungry to full state. In particular, information about the brainstem is needed to understand how oro-sensory exposure affects satiation. The brainstem is of particular interest as this is where the sensory signals first arrive in the brain to signal incoming food. To research this area a specific human brainstem atlas needs to be developed.

With respect to the effects of oro-sensory exposure on satiation, the largest body of evidence relates to the effects of texture or eating duration and on the effect of salty and sweet taste. Few studies have investigated other taste effects on satiation, such as bitter, sour, and umami. Taste intensity is difficult to manipulate while maintaining palatability, and energy density-, and macronutrient composition equal. Future research studies should improve the definition of the manipulation of interest while minimizing potential confounding due to changes in other sensory properties or energy density. Chemical and texture analyses, as well as sensory panel evaluations of the study products should be done routinely to better describe the manipulated products.

Besides much controlled 'sensory' studies in healthy individuals, research is required in overweight or obese individuals to determine whether a decrease in food intake leads due to texture manipulations results in actual weight loss. It is possible that overweight or obese individuals may be less sensitive to internal food cues and when eating highly palatable foods the effect of oro-sensory exposure duration on satiation may be overruled by hedonic eating [106]. Another strategy may be to determine whether recommending eating foods with hard texture as part of a low-calorie diet may support weight loss in individuals who are overweight or obese. Such an intervention may potentially be considered successful at 10% weight loss, although 5% sustained weight loss already reduces the risk of cardiovascular diseases and type II diabetes [107–110].

5. Conclusions

Oro-sensory exposure to food has a direct effect on satiation by direct signaling via the brainstem to higher cortical regions involved in taste and reward, including the nucleus accumbens and the insula. So far there is little evidence that oro-sensory exposure affects satiation indirectly through hormone responses and gastric signals (Figure 4). Critical brain areas involved in satiation, such as the brainstem, must be studied more intensively to better understand the neurophysiological mechanisms underlying satiation. Furthermore, it is crucial to better understand how highly automated eating behaviors, such as oral processing and eating rate, develop during early childhood. Insights into the aforementioned mechanisms will provide novel strategies to prevent overconsumption and the further increases in the bodyweights of future generations.

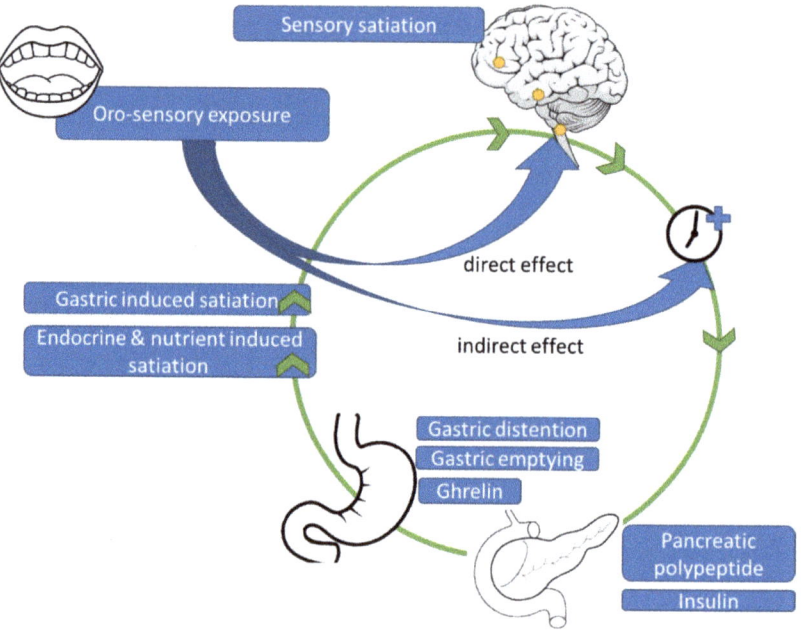

Figure 4. Proposed physiological mechanism underlying effects of oro-sensory exposure on satiation.

6. Implications

Based on the research referred to in this review it appears clear that oro-sensory exposure should play an important role in strategies to maintain healthy body weight. Harder food structures and a slow eating rate can be used as a strategy to prevent overeating due to the high energy density and palatability of the foods in our food environment. It appears that not all calories are the same, foods with the same caloric content can have markedly different satiating capacities. To prevent overeating and consequent weight gain, it may be beneficial to foods that have a high satiation/energy density ratio. For example, calculating the satiation/energy ratio for a standard portion of popcorn (25 g, 75 kcal), with an average eating rate of 5 g per minute the ratio is 75/5 = 15 kcal/min. This is a rather slow ingestion rate of energy due to the high air content of popcorn. Almonds have a much harder texture compared to popcorn but a higher energy density. The satiation ratio of a standard portion of almonds (158 kcal), with an average eating rate of 5 g per minute would be 158/5 = 32 kcal/min. The higher the ratio, the lower the satiation capacity of the food per kcal, the more needs to be ingested of the food item to feel satiated [13].

The knowledge that is gained can also be better exploited by food industries that may develop new (versions of existing) food products with a harder structure relative to their caloric content. This represents a challenge as texture and taste are major drivers of palatability and food acceptance [41,111]. Recently, Bolhuis and Forde provided directions for food technologists to make their foods more satiating by changing food structures [28]. In addition to the prevention of weight gain, this knowledge may be used to develop food products that stimulate food intake in malnourished populations.

Besides direct food manipulations, the way of eating may potentially also be modified to slow the rate of food intake. For example, using a spoon instead of a straw or eating with chopsticks instead of a fork. These relatively simple adjustments have shown to reduce food intake [23]. Digital tools have also been developed to slow eating rate. Such tools provide immediate feed-back on the rate of eating, such as the smart fork or Mandometer [112,113].

Finally, we advocate that foods with a harder texture (relative to their energy content) should be part of dietary guidelines to maintain a healthy body weight. Currently the Dutch Nutrition Center ('Voedingscentrum'), the Dutch equivalent to the US MyPlate, a federal program of the US Department of Agriculture (USDA), already mentions that smoothies and juices should not be counted as a daily portion of fruit given that you feel less satiated after a smoothie compared to eating whole pieces of fruit (hard texture) [114]. Furthermore, in the Dutch dietary guidelines it is stated that sugar containing beverages should be limited as these calories do not satiate [114]. Similarly the HHS recommends fruits, especially whole fruits [115]. An important step in the right direction, however clear recommendations about the consumption of foods with a "low energy intake rate" should be added, that is foods that are relatively low in eating rate given the energy that they provide. Such a recommendation has the potential to contribute to the solution to the prevention of overeating and the consequent development of overweight and obesity.

Author Contributions: Conceptualization, M.P.L., K.d.G. and M.M.; writing—original draft preparation, M.P.L. and M.M.; writing—review and editing, M.P.L., K.d.G. and M.M.; visualization, M.P.L. and M.M. All authors have read and agreed to the published version of the manuscript.

Funding: This work was carried out as part of a public-private partnership funded by the Netherlands Organization for Scientific Research (NWO, grant 057-14-001).

Institutional Review Board Statement: Not applicable.

Informed Consent Statement: Not applicable.

Conflicts of Interest: The authors declare no conflict of interest.

References

1. Blundell, J.; de Graaf, C.; Hulshof, T.; Jebb, S.; Livingstone, B.; Lluch, A.; Mela, D.; Salah, S.; Schuring, E.; van der Knaap, H.; et al. Appetite control: Methodological aspects of the evaluation of foods. *Obes. Rev.* **2010**, *11*, 251–270. [CrossRef] [PubMed]
2. Delzenne, N.; Blundell, J.; Brouns, F.; Cunningham, K.; De Graaf, K.; Erkner, A.; Lluch, A.; Mars, M.; Peters, H.P.; Westerterp-Plantenga, M. Gastrointestinal targets of appetite regulation in humans. *Obes. Rev.* **2010**, *11*, 234–250. [CrossRef]
3. Stieger, M.; van de Velde, F. Microstructure, texture and oral processing: New ways to reduce sugar and salt in foods. *Curr. Opin. Colloid Interface Sci.* **2013**, *18*, 334–348. [CrossRef]
4. Lasschuijt, M.P.; Mars, M.; de Graaf, C.; Smeets, P.A.M. Endocrine cephalic phase responses to food cues: A systematic review. *Adv. Nutr.* **2020**, *11*, 1364–1383. [CrossRef] [PubMed]
5. Smeets, P.A.; Erkner, A.; de Graaf, C. Cephalic phase responses and appetite. *Nutr. Rev.* **2010**, *68*, 643–655. [CrossRef] [PubMed]
6. Power, M.L.; Schulkin, J. Anticipatory physiological regulation in feeding biology: Cephalic phase responses. *Appetite* **2008**, *50*, 194–206. [CrossRef] [PubMed]
7. Woods, S.C. The eating paradox: How we tolerate food. *Psychol. Rev.* **1991**, *98*, 488–505. [CrossRef] [PubMed]
8. Rolls, B.J.; Rolls, E.T.; Rowe, E.A.; Sweeney, K. Sensory specific satiety in man. *Physiol. Behav.* **1981**, *27*, 137–142. [CrossRef]
9. Hopkins, M.; Blundell, J.; Halford, J.; King, N.; Finlayson, G. The Regulation of Food Intake in Humans. In *Endotext*; Feingold, K.R., Anawalt, B., Boyce, A., Chrousos, G., de Herder, W.W., Dhatariya, K., Dungan, K., Grossman, A., Hershman, J.M., Hofland, J., Eds.; MDText.com, Inc.: South Dartmouth, MA, USA, 2000.
10. de Graaf, C. Texture and satiation: The role of oro-sensory exposure time. *Physiol. Behav.* **2012**, *107*, 496–501. [CrossRef] [PubMed]

11. Bolhuis, D.P.; Lakemond, C.M.; de Wijk, R.A.; Luning, P.A.; Graaf, C. Both longer oral sensory exposure to and higher intensity of saltiness decrease ad libitum food intake in healthy normal-weight men. *J. Nutr.* **2011**, *141*, 2242–2248. [CrossRef] [PubMed]
12. Forde, C.G.; Mars, M.; de Graaf, K. Ultra-processing or oral processing? A role for energy density and eating rate in moderating energy intake from processed foods. *Curr. Dev. Nutr.* **2020**, *4*, nzaa019. [CrossRef]
13. van den Boer, J.; Werts, M.; Siebelink, E.; de Graaf, C.; Mars, M. The availability of slow and fast calories in the dutch diet: The current situation and opportunities for interventions. *Foods* **2017**, *6*, 87. [CrossRef] [PubMed]
14. Devezeaux de Lavergne, M.; Derks, J.A.M.; Ketel, E.C.; de Wijk, R.A.; Stieger, M. Eating behaviour explains differences between individuals in dynamic texture perception of sausages. *Food Qual. Pref.* **2015**, *41*, 189–200. [CrossRef]
15. Zijlstra, N.; Mars, M.; de Wijk, R.A.; Westerterp-Plantenga, M.S.; de Graaf, C. The effect of viscosity on ad libitum food intake. *Int. J. Obes.* **2008**, *32*, 676–683. [CrossRef] [PubMed]
16. Szczesniak, A.S. Texture is a sensory property. *Food Qual. Pref.* **2002**, *13*, 215–225. [CrossRef]
17. van Vliet, T.; van Aken, G.A.; de Jongh, H.H.; Hamer, R.J. Colloidal aspects of texture perception. *Adv. Colloid. Interface. Sci.* **2009**, *150*, 27–40. [CrossRef] [PubMed]
18. Mosca, A.C.; Torres, A.P.; Slob, E.; de Graaf, K.; McEwan, J.A.; Stieger, M. Small food texture modifications can be used to change oral processing behaviour and to control ad libitum food intake. *Appetite* **2019**, *142*, 104375. [CrossRef] [PubMed]
19. Lasschuijt, M.; Mars, M.; de Graaf, C.; Smeets, P.A.M. How oro-sensory exposure and eating rate affect satiation and associated endocrine responses-a randomized trial. *Am. J. Clin. Nutr.* **2020**, *111*, 1137–1149. [CrossRef]
20. Robinson, E.; Almiron-Roig, E.; Rutters, F.; de Graaf, C.; Forde, C.G.; Tudur Smith, C.; Nolan, S.J.; Jebb, S.A. A systematic review and meta-analysis examining the effect of eating rate on energy intake and hunger. *Am. J. Clin. Nutr.* **2014**, *100*, 123–151. [CrossRef]
21. Zijlstra, N.; de Wijk, R.A.; Mars, M.; Stafleu, A.; de Graaf, C. Effect of bite size and oral processing time of a semisolid food on satiation. *Am. J. Clin. Nutr.* **2009**, *90*, 269–275. [CrossRef]
22. den Boer, A.; Boesveldt, S.; Lawlor, J.B. How sweetness intensity and thickness of an oral nutritional supplement affects intake and satiety. *Food Qual. Pref.* **2019**, *71*, 406–414. [CrossRef]
23. Hogenkamp, P.S.; Mars, M.; Stafleu, A.; de Graaf, C. Intake during repeated exposure to low- and high-energy-dense yogurts by different means of consumption. *Am. J. Clin. Nutr.* **2010**, *91*, 841–847. [CrossRef] [PubMed]
24. Forde, C.G.; van Kuijk, N.; Thaler, T.; de Graaf, C.; Martin, N. Texture and savoury taste influences on food intake in a realistic hot lunch time meal. *Appetite* **2013**, *60*, 180–186. [CrossRef] [PubMed]
25. Bolhuis, D.P.; Forde, C.G.; Cheng, Y.; Xu, H.; Martin, N.; de Graaf, C. Slow food: Sustained impact of harder foods on the reduction in energy intake over the course of the day. *PLoS ONE* **2014**, *9*, e93370. [CrossRef] [PubMed]
26. Zijlstra, N.; Mars, M.; Stafleu, A.; de Graaf, C. The effect of texture differences on satiation in 3 pairs of solid foods. *Appetite* **2010**, *55*, 490–497. [CrossRef] [PubMed]
27. Cahayadi, J.; Leong, S.Y.; Oey, I.; Peng, M. Textural effects on perceived satiation and ad libitum intake of potato chips in males and females. *Foods* **2020**, *9*, 85. [CrossRef] [PubMed]
28. Bolhuis, D.P.; Forde, C.G. Application of food texture to moderate oral processing behaviors and energy intake. *Trends Food Sci. Technol.* **2020**, *106*, 445–456. [CrossRef]
29. Weijzen, P.L.; Smeets, P.A.; de Graaf, C. Sip size of orangeade: Effects on intake and sensory-specific satiation. *Br. J. Nutr.* **2009**, *102*, 1091–1097. [CrossRef]
30. Weijzen, P.L.; Liem, D.G.; Zandstra, E.H.; de Graaf, C. Sensory specific satiety and intake: The difference between nibble- and bar-size snacks. *Appetite* **2008**, *50*, 435–442. [CrossRef] [PubMed]
31. Cook, D.J.; Hollowood, T.A.; Taylor, A.J. Effects of viscosity on flavor perception: Multi-modal approach. *Abstr. Pap. Am. Chem. Soc.* **2002**, *224*, U75.
32. Hollowood, T.A.; Linforth, R.S.; Taylor, A.J. The effect of viscosity on the perception of flavour. *Chem. Senses* **2002**, *27*, 583–591. [CrossRef] [PubMed]
33. Nishinari, K. Rheology, food texture and mastication. *J. Text. Stud.* **2004**, *35*, 113–124. [CrossRef]
34. Bourne, M. *Food Texture and Viscosity: Concept and Measurement*; Academic Press: Cambridge, MA, USA, 2002.
35. Lucas, F.; Bellisle, F. The measurement of food preferences in humans: Do taste-and-spit tests predict consumption? *Phys. Behav.* **1987**, *39*, 739–743. [CrossRef]
36. Vickers, Z.; Holton, E.; Wang, J. Effect of ideal-relative sweetness on yogurt consumption. *Food Qual. Pref.* **2001**, *12*, 521–526. [CrossRef]
37. Vickers, Z.; Holton, E.; Wang, J. Effect of yogurt sweetness on sensory specific satiety. *J. Sens. Stud.* **1998**, *13*, 377–388. [CrossRef]
38. Bolhuis, D.P.; Lakemond, C.M.; de Wijk, R.A.; Luning, P.A.; de Graaf, C. Effect of salt intensity in soup on ad libitum intake and on subsequent food choice. *Appetite* **2012**, *58*, 48–55. [CrossRef]
39. Griffioen-Roose, S.; Mars, M.; Finlayson, G.; Blundell, J.E.; de Graaf, C. Satiation due to equally palatable sweet and savory meals does not differ in normal weight young adults. *J. Nutr.* **2009**, *139*, 2093–2098. [CrossRef] [PubMed]
40. Lasschuijt, M.P.; Mars, M.; Stieger, M.; Miquel-Kergoat, S.; de Graaf, C.; Smeets, P. Comparison of oro-sensory exposure duration and intensity manipulations on satiation. *Physiol. Behav.* **2017**, *176*, 76–83. [CrossRef] [PubMed]
41. McCrickerd, K.; Forde, C.G. Sensory influences on food intake control: Moving beyond palatability. *Obes. Rev.* **2016**, *17*, 18–29. [CrossRef] [PubMed]

42. Stribitcaia, E.; Evans, C.E.L.; Gibbons, C.; Blundell, J.; Sarkar, A. Food texture influences on satiety: Systematic review and meta-analysis. *Sci. Rep.* **2020**, *10*, 12929. [CrossRef]
43. Griffioen-Roose, S.; Finlayson, G.; Mars, M.; Blundell, J.E.; de Graaf, C. Measuring food reward and the transfer effect of sensory specific satiety. *Appetite* **2010**, *55*, 648–655. [CrossRef] [PubMed]
44. Mars, M.; Hogenkamp, P.S.; Gosses, A.M.; Stafleu, A.; De Graaf, C. Effect of viscosity on learned satiation. *Physiol. Behav.* **2009**, *98*, 60–66. [CrossRef]
45. Hogenkamp, P.S.; Stafleu, A.; Mars, M.; Brunstrom, J.M.; de Graaf, C. Texture, not flavor, determines expected satiation of dairy products. *Appetite* **2011**, *57*, 635–641. [CrossRef] [PubMed]
46. Ruijschop, R.M.; Zijlstra, N.; Boelrijk, A.E.; Dijkstra, A.; Burgering, M.J.; Graaf, C.; Westerterp-Plantenga, M.S. Effects of bite size and duration of oral processing on retro-nasal aroma release—Features contributing to meal termination. *Br. J. Nutr.* **2011**, *105*, 307–315. [CrossRef] [PubMed]
47. Ruijschop, R.M.; Boelrijk, A.E.; de Ru, J.A.; de Graaf, C.; Westerterp-Plantenga, M.S. Effects of retro-nasal aroma release on satiation. *Br. J. Nutr.* **2008**, *99*, 1140–1148. [CrossRef] [PubMed]
48. Ketel, E.C.; Aguayo-Mendoza, M.G.; de Wijk, R.A.; de Graaf, C.; Piqueras-Fiszman, B.; Stieger, M. Age, gender, ethnicity and eating capability influence oral processing behaviour of liquid, semi-solid and solid foods differently. *Food. Res. Int.* **2019**, *119*, 143–151. [CrossRef] [PubMed]
49. de Graaf, C.; Kok, F.J. Slow food, fast food and the control of food intake. *Nat. Rev. Endocrinol.* **2010**, *6*, 290–293. [CrossRef] [PubMed]
50. van Dongen, M.V.; van den Berg, M.C.; Vink, N.; Kok, F.J.; de Graaf, C. Taste-nutrient relationships in commonly consumed foods. *Br. J. Nutr.* **2012**, *108*, 140–147. [CrossRef]
51. Sessle, B.J. Mechanisms of oral somatosensory and motor functions and their clinical correlates. *J. Oral. Rehabil.* **2006**, *33*, 243–261. [CrossRef]
52. Harvey, A.K.; Pattinson, K.T.; Brooks, J.C.; Mayhew, S.D.; Jenkinson, M.; Wise, R.G. Brainstem functional magnetic resonance imaging: Disentangling signal from physiological noise. *J. Magn. Reson. Imaging.* **2008**, *28*, 1337–1344. [CrossRef]
53. Brooks, J.C.; Faull, O.K.; Pattinson, K.T.; Jenkinson, M. Physiological noise in brainstem fmri. *Front. Hum. Neurosci.* **2013**, *7*, 623. [CrossRef] [PubMed]
54. Beissner, F. Functional mri of the brainstem: Common problems and their solutions. *Clin. Neuroradiol.* **2015**, *25* (Suppl. 2), 251–257. [CrossRef]
55. Scott, T.R.; Yaxley, S.; Sienkiewicz, Z.J.; Rolls, E.T. Gustatory responses in the nucleus tractus solitarius of the alert cynomolgus monkey. *J. Neurophysiol.* **1986**, *55*, 182–200. [CrossRef] [PubMed]
56. Alhadeff, A.L.; Baird, J.P.; Swick, J.C.; Hayes, M.R.; Grill, H.J. Glucagon-like peptide-1 receptor signaling in the lateral parabrachial nucleus contributes to the control of food intake and motivation to feed. *Neuropsychopharmacology* **2014**, *39*, 2233–2243. [CrossRef] [PubMed]
57. Baird, J.P.; Travers, S.P.; Travers, J.B. Integration of gastric distension and gustatory responses in the parabrachial nucleus. *Am. J. Physiol. Regul. Integr. Comp. Physiol.* **2001**, *281*, R1581–R1593. [CrossRef] [PubMed]
58. Baird, J.P.; Travers, J.B.; Travers, S.P. Parametric analysis of gastric distension responses in the parabrachial nucleus. *Am. J. Physiol. Regul. Integr. Comp. Physiol.* **2001**, *281*, R1568–R1580. [CrossRef] [PubMed]
59. Blouet, C.; Schwartz, G.J. Brainstem nutrient sensing in the nucleus of the solitary tract inhibits feeding. *Cell Metab.* **2012**, *16*, 579–587. [CrossRef] [PubMed]
60. Schneeberger, M.; Gomis, R.; Claret, M. Hypothalamic and brainstem neuronal circuits controlling homeostatic energy balance. *J. Endocrinol.* **2014**, *220*, T25–T46. [CrossRef]
61. Small, D.M. Taste representation in the human insula. *Brain. Struct. Funct.* **2010**, *214*, 551–561. [CrossRef] [PubMed]
62. Naidich, T.h.P.; Duvernoy, H.M.; Delman, B.N.; Sorensen, A.G.; Kollias, S.S.; Haacke, E.M. *Duvernoy's Atlas of The Human Brain Stem and Cerebellum: High-Field Mri, Surface Anatomy, Internal Structure, Vascularization And 3 D Sectional Anatomy*; Springer Science & Business Media: Berlin/Heidelberg, Germany, 2009.
63. Small, D.M.; Gregory, M.D.; Mak, Y.E.; Gitelman, D.; Mesulam, M.M.; Parrish, T. Dissociation of neural representation of intensity and affective valuation in human gustation. *Neuron* **2003**, *39*, 701–711. [CrossRef]
64. Komisaruk, B.R.; Mosier, K.M.; Liu, W.C.; Criminale, C.; Zaborszky, L.; Whipple, B.; Kalnin, A. Functional localization of brainstem and cervical spinal cord nuclei in humans with fmri. *Am. J. Neuroradiol.* **2002**, *23*, 609–617.
65. Topolovec, J.C.; Gati, J.S.; Menon, R.S.; Shoemaker, J.K.; Cechetto, D.F. Human cardiovascular and gustatory brainstem sites observed by functional magnetic resonance imaging. *J. Comp. Neurol.* **2004**, *471*, 446–461. [CrossRef]
66. Grill, H.J.; Norgren, R. Chronically decerebrate rats demonstrate satiation but not bait shyness. *Science* **1978**, *201*, 267–269. [CrossRef]
67. Small, D.M.; Zatorre, R.J.; Dagher, A.; Evans, A.C.; Jones-Gotman, M. Changes in brain activity related to eating chocolate: From pleasure to aversion. *Brain* **2001**, *124*, 1720–1733. [CrossRef]
68. Devoto, F.; Zapparoli, L.; Bonandrini, R.; Berlingeri, M.; Ferrulli, A.; Luzi, L.; Banfi, G.; Paulesu, E. Hungry brains: A meta-analytical review of brain activation imaging studies on food perception and appetite in obese individuals. *Neurosci. Biobehav. Rev.* **2018**, *94*, 271–285. [CrossRef]

69. Smeets, P.A.; de Graaf, C.; Stafleu, A.; van Osch, M.J.; Nievelstein, R.A.; van der Grond, J. Effect of satiety on brain activation during chocolate tasting in men and women. *Am. J. Clin. Nutr.* **2006**, *83*, 1297–1305. [CrossRef] [PubMed]
70. Winston, J.S.; Gottfried, J.A.; Kilner, J.M.; Dolan, R.J. Integrated neural representations of odor intensity and affective valence in human amygdala. *J. Neurosci.* **2005**, *25*, 8903–8907. [CrossRef] [PubMed]
71. Paton, J.J.; Belova, M.A.; Morrison, S.E.; Salzman, C.D. The primate amygdala represents the positive and negative value of visual stimuli during learning. *Nature* **2006**, *439*, 865–870. [CrossRef] [PubMed]
72. Garavan, H.; Pendergrass, J.C.; Ross, T.J.; Stein, E.A.; Risinger, R.C. Amygdala response to both positively and negatively valenced stimuli. *Neuroreport* **2001**, *12*, 2779–2783. [CrossRef] [PubMed]
73. Hamann, S.; Mao, H. Positive and negative emotional verbal stimuli elicit activity in the left amygdala. *Neuroreport* **2002**, *13*, 15–19. [CrossRef] [PubMed]
74. Jin, J.; Zelano, C.; Gottfried, J.A.; Mohanty, A. Human amygdala represents the complete spectrum of subjective valence. *J. Neurosci.* **2015**, *35*, 15145–15156. [CrossRef] [PubMed]
75. O'Doherty, J.; Rolls, E.T.; Francis, S.; Bowtell, R.; McGlone, F. Representation of pleasant and aversive taste in the human brain. *J. Neurophysiol.* **2001**, *85*, 1315–1321. [CrossRef] [PubMed]
76. Morris, J.S.; Dolan, R.J. Involvement of human amygdala and orbitofrontal cortex in hunger-enhanced memory for food stimuli. *J. Neurosci.* **2001**, *21*, 5304–5310. [CrossRef]
77. LaBar, K.S.; Gitelman, D.R.; Parrish, T.B.; Kim, Y.H.; Nobre, A.C.; Mesulam, M.M. Hunger selectively modulates corticolimbic activation to food stimuli in humans. *Behav. Neurosci.* **2001**, *115*, 493–500. [CrossRef]
78. Anderson, A.K.; Christoff, K.; Stappen, I.; Panitz, D.; Ghahremani, D.G.; Glover, G.; Gabrieli, J.D.; Sobel, N. Dissociated neural representations of intensity and valence in human olfaction. *Nat. Neurosci.* **2003**, *6*, 196–202. [CrossRef] [PubMed]
79. Berthoud, H.R. Vagal and hormonal gut-brain communication: From satiation to satisfaction. *Neurogastroenterol. Motil.* **2008**, *20* (Suppl. 1), 64–72. [CrossRef] [PubMed]
80. Richardson, C.T.; Feldman, M. Salivary response to food in humans and its effect on gastric acid secretion. *Am. J. Physiol.* **1986**, *250*, G85–G91. [CrossRef] [PubMed]
81. Powley, T.L. The ventromedial hypothalamic syndrome, satiety, and a cephalic phase hypothesis. *Psychol. Rev.* **1977**, *84*, 89–126. [CrossRef] [PubMed]
82. Mattes, R.D. Fat taste and lipid metabolism in humans. *Physiol. Behav.* **2005**, *86*, 691–697. [CrossRef] [PubMed]
83. Teff, K.L.; Mattes, R.D.; Engelman, K. Cephalic phase insulin release in normal weight males: Verification and reliability. *Am. J. Physiol.* **1991**, *261*, E430–E436. [CrossRef] [PubMed]
84. Katschinski, M. Nutritional implications of cephalic phase gastrointestinal responses. *Appetite* **2000**, *34*, 189–196. [CrossRef] [PubMed]
85. Zafra, M.A.; Molina, F.; Puerto, A. The neural/cephalic phase reflexes in the physiology of nutrition. *Neurosci. Biobehav. Rev.* **2006**, *30*, 1032–1044. [CrossRef]
86. Yamashita, H.; Iwai, M.; Nishimura, K.; Kobayashi, N.; Shimazu, T. Altered lipid metabolism during enteral or parenteral nutrition in rats: Comparison with oral feeding. *J. Nutr. Sci. Vitaminol.* **1993**, *39*, 151–161. [CrossRef]
87. Sakata, T.; Yoshimatsu, H.; Masaki, T.; Tsuda, K. Anti-obesity actions of mastication driven by histamine neurons in rats. *Exp. Biol. Med.* **2003**, *228*, 1106–1110. [CrossRef]
88. Tucker, R.M.; Mattes, R.D. 10—Satiation, satiety: The puzzle of solids and liquids. In *Satiation, Satiety and the Control of Food Intak*; Blundell, J.E., Bellisle, F., Eds.; Woodhead Publishing: Sawston, UK, 2013; pp. 182–201.
89. Dhillon, J.; Lee, J.Y.; Mattes, R.D. The cephalic phase insulin response to nutritive and low-calorie sweeteners in solid and beverage form. *Physiol. Behav.* **2017**, *181*, 100–109. [CrossRef] [PubMed]
90. Kashima, H.; Eguchi, K.; Miyamoto, K.; Fujimoto, M.; Endo, M.Y.; Aso-Someya, N.; Kobayashi, T.; Hayashi, N.; Fukuba, Y. Suppression of oral sweet taste sensation with gymnema sylvestre affects postprandial gastrointestinal blood flow and gastric emptying in humans. *Chem. Senses* **2017**, *42*, 295–302. [CrossRef]
91. Cecil, J.E.; Francis, J.; Read, N.W. Comparison of the effects of a high-fat and high-carbohydrate soup delivered orally and intragastrically on gastric emptying, appetite, and eating behaviour. *Physiol. Behav.* **1999**, *67*, 299–306. [CrossRef]
92. Mackie, A.R.; Rafiee, H.; Malcolm, P.; Salt, L.; van Aken, G. Specific food structures supress appetite through reduced gastric emptying rate. *Am. J. Physiol. Gastrointest. Liver Physiol.* **2013**, *304*, G1038–G1043. [CrossRef] [PubMed]
93. Deng, R.; Mars, M.; Van Der Sman, R.G.M.; Smeets, P.A.M.; Janssen, A.E.M. The importance of swelling for in vitro gastric digestion of whey protein gels. *Food. Chem.* **2020**, *330*, 127182. [CrossRef] [PubMed]
94. Marciani, L.; Hall, N.; Pritchard, S.E.; Cox, E.F.; Totman, J.J.; Lad, M.; Hoad, C.L.; Foster, T.J.; Gowland, P.A.; Spiller, R.C. Preventing gastric sieving by blending a solid/water meal enhances satiation in healthy humans. *J. Nutr.* **2012**, *142*, 1253–1258. [CrossRef] [PubMed]
95. Ritter, R.C. Gastrointestinal mechanisms of satiation for food. *Physiol. Behav.* **2004**, *81*, 249–273. [CrossRef] [PubMed]
96. Chambers, A.P.; Sandoval, D.A.; Seeley, R.J. Integration of satiety signals by the central nervous system. *Curr. Biol.* **2013**, *23*, R379–R388. [CrossRef] [PubMed]
97. Rasoamanana, R.; Darcel, N.; Fromentin, G.; Tome, D. Nutrient sensing and signalling by the gut. *Proc. Nutr. Soc.* **2012**, *71*, 446–455. [CrossRef]

98. Lemmens, S.G.; Martens, E.A.; Kester, A.D.; Westerterp-Plantenga, M.S. Changes in gut hormone and glucose concentrations in relation to hunger and fullness. *Am. J. Clin. Nutr.* **2011**, *94*, 717–725. [CrossRef] [PubMed]
99. Bellisle, F.; Drewnowski, A.; Anderson, G.H.; Westerterp-Plantenga, M.; Martin, C.K. Sweetness, satiation, and satiety. *J. Nutr.* **2012**, *142*, 1149S–1154S. [CrossRef] [PubMed]
100. Krop, E.M.; Hetherington, M.M.; Nekitsing, C.; Miquel, S.; Postelnicu, L.; Sarkar, A. Influence of oral processing on appetite and food intake—A systematic review and meta-analysis. *Appetite* **2018**, *125*, 253–269. [CrossRef] [PubMed]
101. Llewellyn, C.H.; van Jaarsveld, C.H.; Boniface, D.; Carnell, S.; Wardle, J. Eating rate is a heritable phenotype related to weight in children. *Am. J. Clin. Nutr.* **2008**, *88*, 1560–1566. [CrossRef]
102. Drucker, R.R.; Hammer, L.D.; Agras, W.S.; Bryson, S. Can mothers influence their child's eating behavior? *J. Dev. Behav. Pediatr.* **1999**, *20*, 88–92. [CrossRef] [PubMed]
103. Murakami, K.; Miyake, Y.; Sasaki, S.; Tanaka, K.; Arakawa, M. Self-reported rate of eating and risk of overweight in japanese children: Ryukyus child health study. *J. Nutr. Sci. Vitaminol.* **2012**, *58*, 247–252. [CrossRef]
104. Fogel, A.; Fries, L.R.; McCrickerd, K.; Goh, A.T.; Quah, P.L.; Chan, M.J.; Toh, J.Y.; Chong, Y.S.; Tan, K.H.; Yap, F.; et al. Oral processing behaviours that promote children's energy intake are associated with parent-reported appetitive traits: Results from the gusto cohort. *Appetite* **2018**, *126*, 8–15. [CrossRef]
105. Fogel, A.; Goh, A.T.; Fries, L.R.; Sadananthan, S.A.; Velan, S.S.; Michael, N.; Tint, M.T.; Fortier, M.V.; Chan, M.J.; Toh, J.Y.; et al. Faster eating rates are associated with higher energy intakes during an ad libitum meal, higher bmi and greater adiposity among 4.5-year-old children: Results from the growing up in singapore towards healthy outcomes (gusto) cohort. *Br. J. Nutr.* **2017**, *117*, 1042–1051. [CrossRef] [PubMed]
106. Saper, C.B.; Chou, T.C.; Elmquist, J.K. The need to feed: Homeostatic and hedonic control of eating. *Neuron* **2002**, *36*, 199–211. [CrossRef]
107. Anderson, J.W.; Konz, E.C. Obesity and disease management: Effects of weight loss on comorbid conditions. *Obes. Res.* **2001**, *9* (Suppl. 4), 326S–334S. [CrossRef] [PubMed]
108. Tuomilehto, J.; Lindstrom, J.; Eriksson, J.G.; Valle, T.T.; Hamalainen, H.; Ilanne-Parikka, P.; Keinanen-Kiukaanniemi, S.; Laakso, M.; Louheranta, A.; Rastas, M.; et al. Prevention of type 2 diabetes mellitus by changes in lifestyle among subjects with impaired glucose tolerance. *N. Engl. J. Med.* **2001**, *344*, 1343–1350. [CrossRef] [PubMed]
109. Burke, M.V.; Small, D.M. Physiological mechanisms by which non-nutritive sweeteners may impact body weight and metabolism. *Physiol. Behav.* **2015**, *152*, 381–388. [CrossRef] [PubMed]
110. Katz, D.L.; O'Connell, M.; Yeh, M.C.; Nawaz, H.; Njike, V.; Anderson, L.M.; Cory, S.; Dietz, W.; The Community Preventive Services Task Force. Public health strategies for preventing and controlling overweight and obesity in school and worksite settings: A report on recommendations of the task force on community preventive services. *Morb. Mortal. Wkly. Rep. Recomm. Rep.* **2005**, *54*, 1–12.
111. Jeltema, M.; Beckley, J.; Vahalik, J. Model for understanding consumer textural food choice. *Food. Sci. Nutr.* **2015**, *3*, 202–212. [CrossRef]
112. Hermsen, S.; Mars, M.; Higgs, S.; Frost, J.H.; Hermans, R.C.J. Effects of eating with an augmented fork with vibrotactile feedback on eating rate and body weight: A randomized controlled trial. *Int. J. Behav. Nutr. Phys. Act.* **2019**, *16*, 90. [CrossRef]
113. Ford, A.L.; Bergh, C.; Sodersten, P.; Sabin, M.A.; Hollinghurst, S.; Hunt, L.P.; Shield, J.P. Treatment of childhood obesity by retraining eating behaviour: Randomised controlled trial. *BMJ* **2009**, *340*, b5388. [CrossRef] [PubMed]
114. Gezondheidsraad Onafhankelijk Wetenschappelijk Adviesorgaan voor Regering en Parlement. Available online: https://www.gezondheidsraad.nl/documenten/adviezen/2015/11/04/richtlijnen-goede-voeding-2015 (accessed on 11 April 2021).
115. U.S. Department of Agriculture and hhs, Dietary Guidelines for Americans 2015–2020. Available online: http://health.Gov/dietaryguidelines/2015/ (accessed on 11 April 2021).

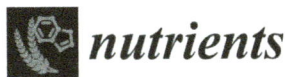

Review

Gastrointestinal Contributions to the Postprandial Experience

Dan M. Livovsky [1,2,3] and Fernando Azpiroz [1,*]

[1] Digestive System Research Unit, University Hospital Vall d'Hebron, Centro de Investigación Biomédica en Red de Enfermedades Hepáticas y Digestivas (Ciberehd), Departament de Medicina, Universitat Autònoma de Barcelona, 08193 Bellaterra, Cerdanyola del Vallès, Spain; danlivo@yahoo.com
[2] Faculty of Medicine, Hebrew University of Jerusalem, Jerusalem 9103102, Israel
[3] ShaareZedek Medical Center, Digestive Diseases Institute, Jerusalem 9103102, Israel
* Correspondence: azpiroz.fernando@gmail.com; Tel.: +34-93-2746259

Abstract: Food ingestion induces homeostatic sensations (satiety, fullness) with a hedonic dimension (satisfaction, changes in mood) that characterize the postprandial experience. Both types of sensation are secondary to intraluminal stimuli produced by the food itself, as well as to the activity of the digestive tract. Postprandial sensations also depend on the nutrient composition of the meal and on colonic fermentation of non-absorbed residues. Gastrointestinal function and the sensitivity of the digestive tract, i.e., perception of gut stimuli, are determined by inherent individual factors, e.g., sex, and can be modulated by different conditioning mechanisms. This narrative review examines the factors that determine perception of digestive stimuli and the postprandial experience.

Keywords: food ingestion; digestion; satiety; digestive well-being; functional gastrointestinal disorders; postprandial symptoms; homeostatic sensations; hedonic sensations

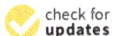

Citation: Livovsky, D.M.; Azpiroz, F. Gastrointestinal Contributions to the Postprandial Experience. *Nutrients* 2021, 13, 893. https://doi.org/10.3390/nu13030893

Academic Editor: Miriam Clegg

Received: 28 January 2021
Accepted: 3 March 2021
Published: 10 March 2021

Publisher's Note: MDPI stays neutral with regard to jurisdictional claims in published maps and institutional affiliations.

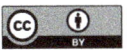

Copyright: © 2021 by the authors. Licensee MDPI, Basel, Switzerland. This article is an open access article distributed under the terms and conditions of the Creative Commons Attribution (CC BY) license (https://creativecommons.org/licenses/by/4.0/).

1. Introduction

Food ingestion activates the digestive system and induces conscious sensations. The digestive tract, in the first place, accommodates the ingested food, digests nutrients by mechanical and chemical actions, absorbs usable elements and disposes of non-absorbable residues. Conscious sensations related to ingestion involve the preingestive period, i.e., the eating experience, and postprandial sensations. This narrative review examines the factors that determine perception of digestive stimuli and the postprandial experience: (a) gut sensitivity; (b) digestive response; (c) composition of the meal, both absorbable nutrients and non-absorbable residues; (d) conditioning factors, e.g., hedonic (palatability), homeostatic (appetite) and cognitive/emotive (attention, beliefs, expectations, education); and (e) constitutive individual factors, e.g., sex (Figure 1). Since factual neurophysiological and molecular experimental evidence is scarce, the current understanding of the postprandial experience relies on studies that examine subjective experiences. Understanding the factors that determine the postprandial experience is key to the development of healthy habits in the general population, the design of beneficial and rewarding foods and for the management of patients with eating disorders or functional digestive symptoms.

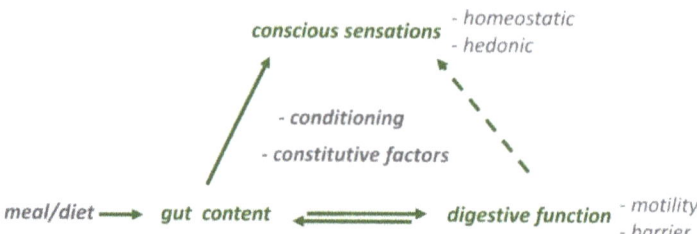

Figure 1. Gastrointestinal contributions to the 'postprandial experience'. Meal-derived stimuli in the gut activate reflex pathways, that regulate digestive function (motility, barrier), homeostatic (satiety, fullness) and hedonic sensations (digestive well-being and mood). Sensations after ingestion are secondary to gut content and to the activity of the digestive tract. The responses to food ingestion are determined by intrinsic characteristics of the individual (constitutive factors) and are modulated by a variety of conditioning mechanisms (homeostatic, hedonic, cognitive/emotive factors).

2. Meal Ingestion and Digestive Sensations

The cephalic phase of digestion, involving both digestive function and sensation before and during the eating process [1], is reviewed in other articles of this special issue. Meal ingestion induces homeostatic sensations involved in the control of food consumption. Ingestion reduces hunger sensation and induces satiation. Hunger and satiety refer to opposite directions of the same sensation and can be measured by analogue scales ranging from a negative value rating maximal hunger (extremely hungry) to a positive end rating at maximal satiation (completely sated). Conceptually, satiation is the homeostatic sensation responsible for meal ending and satiety refers to the homeostatic sensation, that is responsible for the interval between meals, but this distinction in the English language seems more semantic than physiological. Beyond a certain threshold satiety is associated with the sensation of abdominal fullness. Yet, these sensations are different and individuals are able to discriminate between them, such that with increasing meal loads and increasing satiety, individuals begin to report fullness sensation, and with larger meal loads their desire to eat a food of choice diminishes. The intensity of these homeostatic sensations is related to the meal load with different thresholds: increasing meal loads induce first satiation, followed by fullness, and later by progressive reduction in the eating desire of choice. Both the volume and the caloric content of the meal influence postprandial sensations.

Homeostatic sensations have a hedonic dimension revealed by their association with changes in digestive well-being and mood. Depending on the conditions, hedonic sensations may be positive or negative, so that the postprandial experience may have a pleasant/rewarding or an aversive dimension. The relation between homeostatic and hedonic sensations was investigated measuring sensory responses before, during, and after stepwise ingestion of a comfort meal up to full satiation. During stepwise ingestion, homeostatic sensations progressively increased up to full satiation and, hence, exhibit a direct relation to the meal load. Hedonic sensations initially increased up to a peak, and later decreased down to negative sensation of digestive well-being at the point of full satiation [2]. These data indicate that the relation of homeostatic and hedonic responses to a meal is bimodal depending on the meal load.

Homeostatic and hedonic sensations decrease in intensity during the postprandial period: the consummatory reward fades and as satiety exhausts, while rising hunger sensation calls for the next meal. Experimental data suggest that different biological mechanism mediate homeostatic and hedonic components of the postprandial experience [3]. For example, studies combining measurement of sensations and brain activity show that specific changes in brain activity are selectively related to homeostatic or hedonic sensations [3–5]. Some of the changes in blood levels of compounds that originate from the food (e.g., glucose, lipids), from the subject (e.g., gut hormones) or from the microbiota metabolism of meal residues are selectively related to specific postprandial sensations [6,7].

3. Gastrointestinal Responses to Meal Ingestion

Digestive function determines how intraluminal stimuli are perceived, so that a satisfactory postprandial experience depends on adequate digestive responses to the meal [8–11]. A complex network of neuro-hormonal reflex mechanisms, finely regulates the digestive process, allowing the gut to sense and react to intraluminal stimuli, as well as to adapt to a wide range of circumstances [1,12]. The enteric nervous system is a neuronal network located within the gut wall that takes large part of the reflex regulation of gastrointestinal function. The autonomic nervous system, both vagal and sympathetic divisions, participates in the digestive regulation by means of reflex arcs, involving receptors, afferent pathways, relay stations and effector neurons. While the vagus plays a major role in the regulation of gastric accommodation and emptying, the sympathetic nervous system is involved in intestinal peristalsis. The participation of the autonomic nervous system in conveying afferent information leading to conscious sensations, is reviewed in another article of this special issue and is also briefly discussed below.

3.1. Digestive Function

During fasting, the stomach and small intestine exhibit cyclic activity: periods of quiescence alternate with short periods of intense activity featuring powerful gastrointestinal contractions and bouts of gastrointestinal and bilio-pancreatic secretion. This cyclic activity is independent of external stimuli and its proposed function is to clear secretions, cellular debris or remaining residues from the lumen.

After ingestion, meal-related stimuli in the gastrointestinal tract activate specific receptors in the gut wall and release a complex series of reflexes that replace the stereotyped fasting activity pattern by a tightly regulated gastrointestinal motor and barrier function (secretion, absorption) to accomplish the digestive process, such that only non-absorbed residues reach the colon [12]. During the fasting period, the stomach is contracted and virtually collapsed; meal ingestion induces a relaxation of the gastric walls to accommodate the meal load without increases in gastric wall tension. The gastric accommodation reflex is driven by vagal pathways. This relaxation determines the tolerance to meals, because perception of gastric distension depends on tension receptors [13–15]. After ingestion, the stomach gradually re-contracts "squeezing" the liquid chyme through the pyloric channel into the duodenum [14,16]. The arrival of nutrients into the small bowel activates reflexes that influence gastrointestinal activity (motility, secretion, absorption). In response to intraluminal stimuli, the gut secrets large amounts of fluid, electrolytes and enzymes in the form of gastric, bilio-pancreatic and intestinal secretions. Secretions carry out the chemical process of digestion, and are then reabsorbed back into the bloodstream together with digested foodstuffs. The lymphatic circulation takes part in this process carrying larger, mostly lipid, molecules. It is calculated that per liter of ingested fluid (part as solid foods), the digestive tract secretes 8–10 L; the largest part is absorbed in the small bowel, only a small fraction passes into the colon, and finally 100–200 g of residues (largely microbiota) are eliminated by feces [17]. The ultimate fluid, electrolyte and acid-base homeostasis of the organism is controlled by renal function and urine excretion. Intraluminal stimuli also induce the secretion of a host of gut peptides [18]. In the context of the postprandial experience the most important are ghrelin, cholecystokinin, the proglucagon-derived peptides and the pancreatic polypeptide family. Gut hormones in health and disease are discussed in other articles of this special issue; see also reference [18]. Meal ingestion also affects the activity of the colon via reflex pathways (e.g., the gastrocolonic reflex) before the arrival of non-absorbed meal residues; however, the most prominent effect of stimuli related to meal ingestion is exerted down to the ileocecal junction.

Intraluminal stimuli gradually fade as the digestive process (gastric emptying, intestinal absorption and clearance) takes place, and this is associated with a decay of postprandial sensations. Hunger sensation after a meal has been related to the first period of activity of the fasting motor pattern after the end of the digestive process (hunger contractions) [10].

3.2. Somatic Responses to Meal Ingestion

Alteration of digestive function impairs the postprandial experience. For instance, experimental distortion of gastric accommodation produced by distension of the stomach with a balloon, was associated with fullness sensation and impaired hedonic responses to a probe meal [19]. Patients with postprandial symptoms (functional dyspepsia) exhibit impaired gastric accommodation and hypersensitivity of the stomach, so that physiological meal-related stimuli induce abnormal sensations [12,20–22]; see Section 6.2 Functional gut disorders).

Meal ingestion also induces somatic responses that may influence the postprandial experience. In normal conditions, the activity of the muscles of the abdomino-thoracic walls adapt to the volume of content. This phenomenon is known as abdominal accommodation [23,24]. Meal ingestion induces relaxation of the diaphragm allowing an upward expansion of the abdominal cavity and limiting the increment in abdominal girth, and the magnitude of this somatic response is related to the meal load [25]. Postprandial abdominal distention in patients is produced by impaired relaxation of the diaphragm associated with protrusion of the abdominal wall in response to meal ingestion (i.e., abdomino-phrenic dyssynergia) [26–28]. Postprandial objective abdominal distention is frequently associated with a subjective sensation of abdominal fullness/bloating. To examine the relation between the somatic postural tone and digestive sensations, healthy subjects were taught to produce diaphragmatic contraction and visible abdominal distention. A challenge meal up to maximal satiation was administered to induce abdominal fullness/bloating sensation, and under these conditions, intentional abdominal distention was associated with significantly more intense sensation of bloating and impaired sensation of digestive well-being [29]. Conversely, a study in patients with functional gut disorders showed that correction of abdominal distention by biofeedback, improved associated abdominal symptoms [30].

3.3. Gastrointestinal Sensitivity

It has been shown that intraluminal stimuli in the gut activate sensory afferents and elicit conscious sensations. Conscious information from the gut is driven by sympathetic-spinal afferents [14,31]: Peripheral afferents activated by gut stimuli follow splanchnic-sympathetic pathways up to the posterior root ganglia, where the body of the peripheral sensory neuron is located. These neurons project to the central nervous system via ascending spinal pathways [32–34]. Thus, a complex interaction takes place in order to integrate reflexes and behavioral responses [14]. Brain imaging and neurophysiological studies have shown that different modulatory stations at various levels between the sensory receptor in the digestive tract and the brain cortex, tune the information travelling along this neural pathway. The intensity of conscious sensations depends on the balance between facilitatory and inhibitory mechanisms, and impaired modulatory balance has been proposed as an important pathophysiological factor in functional gut disorders with visceral hypersensitivity [35].

Different types of experimental stimuli, including mechanical, thermal, chemical and electrical, induce, in healthy subjects, sensations similar to the symptoms experienced by patients with functional gut disorders, such as abdominal fullness, bloating, cramps, stinging sensation and nausea [36]. It has been shown that gastric balloon distention and intragastric nutrient infusion, induce specific responses in the brain; interestingly, the nutrient infusion has been associated with inactivation of pain-related brain signals, which may constitute an important mechanism to explain the tolerance of normal meal loads in contrast to experimental gastric distension [37].

The intensity of conscious sensations is directly related to the magnitude of stimulation; low magnitude stimuli are barely perceived, and conscious perception progressively increases with stronger stimuli, until it becomes uncomfortable or painful. Perception of mechanical stimuli in the digestive tract depends on activation of tension receptors [13]. Different receptors with low, high and in-between thresholds that detect stomach wall tension have been described [14]. In contrast, the quality of the sensation (e.g., bloating) is not correlated with the magnitude of the stimulus (i.e., the same sensation appears with low or high magnitude stimuli), and the intensity of the sensation progressively increases up to the discomfort/pain threshold [14,38]. Additionally, as shown by inflating balloons of different lengths with the same intraballoon pressure in the small intestine, perception is influenced by the number of receptors activated: longer balloons produce more intense perception [39,40]. Spatial summation phenomena influence the sensations induced by meal ingestion. For instance, a recent study showed that in patients with functional dyspepsia and concomitant constipation, postprandial symptoms improved by correcting evacuation [41].There is no clear evidence that the vagus nerve drives sensory afferents directly eliciting conscious sensations in response to meals; i.e., vagal afferents are primarily involved in reflex control and homeostasis [33–35,42,43]; however, the vagus nerve may modulate the transmission of afferent conscious sensations [38]: vagal afferents activate structures in the central nervous system that have descending influences, both facilitatory and inhibitory, on spinal sensory transmission.

4. Composition of the Meal

As described above, the meal contains components that are digested and absorbed in the small bowel and non-absorbable residues that pass into the colon and are fermented by the microbiota. Meal composition, specifically the type of absorbable components and the content of non-absorbable residues, influence the postprandial experience.

4.1. Absorbable Meal Components

A recent proof-of-concept study explored the role of meal composition on the postprandial experience, by comparing the effect of two types of meals with agreeable flavors: a homogeneous nutrient drink versus a heterogeneous solid-liquid meal (ham and cheese sandwich plus fruit juice meal) [5]. Despite the fact that participants rated both meals as equally palatable; the postprandial experience was distinctively different. Compared to the nutrient drink, and despite higher volume and caloric load, the solid-liquid meal was associated with significantly lower homeostatic sensations (less satiety and fullness) and with stronger hedonic reward (more satisfaction).

The effect of nutrient composition of the meal on postprandial sensations was further explored by comparing the responses to a high-fat versus a low-fat hummus; all other characteristics, presentation, palatability and volume, were identical. The high-fat meal induced more satiety/fullness but less satisfaction (less digestive well-being) than the low-fat meal [44]. Hence, the composition of meals with equal palatability has differential effects on homeostatic and hedonic sensations. Intraluminal lipids induce a gastric relaxation that reduces gastric wall tension and improves the tolerance to gastric filling, but on the other hand, perfusion of lipids at physiological loads within the intestine sensitizes gut mechanoreceptors [45,46] and may increase the perception of large gastric volumes. Hence, the net effect depends on the balance between the motor and sensory effects of lipids and intragastric contents. The gut hormone cholecystokinin appears to be involved in the sensitizing effects that lipids have in the mechanoreceptors [23,24]. The situation is even more complex, because fat is the key element in the hedonic reward to comfort foods [47], but at high doses intraluminal lipids induce discomfort and an aversive sensation [9]. The increase in sensitivity of gut receptors induced by intraluminal nutrients depends on the concentration and the type of nutrient: at physiological loads, lipids have a marked effect, but the influence of carbohydrates is much weaker [46].

During the post-absorption phase of digestion meal components in the internal milieu may also influence the postprandial experience. Little is known about the specific influence of each of the absorbed components on the postprandial experience, and further research is needed. However; the metabolomic response to a comfort meal and the correlation between sensations and circulating metabolites was explored in 32 healthy men. The postprandial experience in this experimental paradigm was characterized by increased homeostatic sensations (satiety and fullness) with a positive hedonic component (well-being and mood) and a robust change in the metabolomic profile. Meal ingestion was associated with an increase in the levels of acetate, alanine, creatinine, formate, glucose and very low-density lipoproteins (VLDL), and a decrease in the levels of acetone, isoleucine, low-density lipoproteins (LDL) and high-density lipoproteins (HDL). The sensation of fullness after the meal correlated with the postprandial increase in glucose and alanine. Furthermore; the increase in glucose correlated with mood improvement and the increase in alanine correlated with postprandial satisfaction. Mood improvement was also positively correlated with medium size HDL particles and inversely correlated with large size HDL particles; large LDL particles exhibited an inverse correlation with digestive well-being [7].

4.2. Non-Absorbable Meal Residues, Colonic Content and Microbiota

In contrast to the virtually empty stomach and small bowel during fasting, in normal conditions a biomass between 500–800 mL permanently sits in the lumen of the colon. With a 100–200 mL faecal output per day, the daily turnover of colonic biomass is about 30% [48]. Colonic biomass is formed by the meal residues cleared from the small intestine and a pool of microorganisms (microbiota) that metabolize the meal residues and produce a series of secondary metabolic products, which in turn serve as substrates for other microorganisms in a chain of reactions. There is a synergistic interaction between microbiota and host: the colon provides an appropriate niche and feeds the microbiota, and the microbiota influences the function of the host, including the function and sensitivity of the digestive tract [49–51]. The messengers and circuits for communication between microbiota and host are not well known, but some data indicate that metabolites derived from the biomass are involved [52]. Fermentation of meal residues releases gas. Gas production increases with the entry of residues into the colon after meals: between 200 and 600 mL are produced for 6 h after ingestion depending on the content of non-absorbable, fermentable residues (e.g., fiber) in the meal [3]. However, gas production persists depending on the availability of fermentable substrates in the colonic biomass [53,54], so that gas production depends on the load of fermentable residues in the diet [55].

Colonic biomass influences digestive sensations by two mechanisms: the volume of colonic content (both gas and faecal content) and the influence of microbiota on gut function. The effect of non-absorbable residues in the diet on gut sensations was investigated by a series of different studies using a method to measure gut content based on abdominal magnetic resonance imaging [56,57]. Using this methodology, it was shown that non-absorbable meal residues that enter the colon, increase the volume of colonic biomass [48]. Low-residue diets reduce colonic content, intestinal gas production and improve bloating sensation in patients with functional gut disorders [58]. Direct intervention on colonic content, by correcting evacuation in patients with constipation, modifies postprandial sensations and improves the meal tolerance in patients with postprandial symptoms [41]. Specific residues, that may be classified as prebiotics, such as inulin [59], fructooligosaccharides [60] and galactooligosaccharides [58] modify colonic microbiota and influence digestive sensations, anxiety and mood. Not only prebiotics, but also specific living microorganisms, classified as probiotics, administered in the diet, improve the tolerance to a challenge diet in healthy subjects [61] and symptoms in patients with functional gut disorders [62–64].

5. Conditioning Factors

The responses to meal ingestion and the way meal-related stimuli in the gut are perceived may be influenced by different conditioning factors related to the meal load (as discussed above), valence (palatability), homeostatic status of the individual (appetite) and cognitive/emotive mechanisms (attention, habits, education, beliefs and expectations).

5.1. Meal Palatability

Palatability of the meal is determined by the organoleptic characteristics of the meal (food flavor) and by the way the individual perceives it [65]. Food flavor involves gustatory (taste) and olfactory sensations (smell), but other senses, including proprioception (food texture), temperature, vision (appearance) and sound (e.g., crispy fries) also play a role [66]. A study was designed to investigate the influence of meal palatability on postprandial sensations in healthy subjects. In order to modify meal palatability without changes in meal composition, two meal courses were prepared: a potato and cream cheese plate and a vanilla cream dessert; both creams were designed to have the same texture, consistency, temperature, and color (by adding a thickener and a color additive to the vanilla cream). Two meals were prepared: the conventional meal was achieved by serving the potato and cream cheese first and the vanilla cream dessert second; the unconventional meal was carried out by mixing the two courses in a single dish, maintaining the same physical characteristics of the individual components. In this way both meals had the same composition and physical characteristics but different palatability. Healthy subjects received the conventional and the unconventional meal in a cross-over design on different days. Both courses of the conventional meal (the potato and cream cheese and the vanilla creams) were found to be palatable, while the mixed meal had negative palatability scores. As compared to the palatable two course meal, the low palatability meal induced more satiety/fullness, but less satisfaction (lower digestive well-being/mood) [67]. These data indicate that meal palatability bears a direct relation with hedonic sensations and an inverse relation with homeostatic sensations.

5.2. Physiological Status

The homeostatic status of the eater influences the responses to meal ingestion and the postprandial experience: internal signals influence perception arising from sensory receptors [68]. In healthy subjects, appetite was experimentally modulated by ingestion of a low-versus a high-calorie breakfast (preload conditioning). A comfort meal eaten 2 h after the high-calorie breakfast induced more satiety and fullness, but lower postprandial satisfaction than when ingested after the low-calorie breakfast. These data indicate that appetite modulation by preload conditioning has differential effects on the cognitive and emotive responses to a meal [69]. Other studies showed that the manner of eating also plays a role: a slower eating rate prolongs oropharyngeal signaling and increases satiation and postprandial fullness [70–73].

5.3. Cognitive/Emotive Conditioning

It is not known whether and to what extent the effect of cognitive/emotive conditioning on postprandial sensations is exerted via modulation of gut function or sensitivity. There is a close interaction between the brain and the gut. Gut stimuli activate receptors in the gut wall and induce conscious sensations. As discussed above, the sensory input is modulated at different levels between the gut wall and the brain and, specifically, the activity of the central nervous system modulates gut perception. On the other hand, under certain conditions emotive/cognitive factors may influence the activity of the digestive system [74,75]. Perception of digestive stimuli is modulated by the level of attention. For instance, intestinal distension produces more intense sensations when the subjects are paying attention (anticipatory knowledge) than when they are distracted [76]. Furthermore, in healthy subjects distracted by playing a computer game, ingestion of a meal induced less postprandial fullness and less desire to eat than when sitting in silence [77]. It has been shown that the way the meal is presented, e.g., environmental conditions and company, influence meal selection and eating behavior [78–82]; although not explored yet, conceivably, these factors may also affect postprandial sensations.

A recent study showed that an educational intervention modified the postprandial experience. The study measured the responses to a probe meal on 2 separate days before and after a single sensory-cognitive educational intervention (taste recognition test of supra- and sub-threshold tastands for real and sham education, respectively). In contrast to sham education, real education enhanced both homeostatic and hedonic responses to the probe meal [83]. These data indicate that education modifies the subjects' receptiveness and influences the responses to a meal: by an educational intervention they learned to enjoy the probe meal more and experienced stronger consummatory reward. However, the contrary may also be true, and associative learning may condition aversive responses to a meal (see below).

Beliefs and expectations play an important role in this context. Some patients complain (and believe) that eating lettuce, gives them gas and abdominal distention. Using computed tomography (CT) scans to measure the amount of intestinal gas and the morphometric configuration of the abdominal cavity, it was shown that during an episode of lettuce-induced distension patients exhibited a real increase in girth, but without a significant increase in the content of colonic gas. Abdominal distension was related to a descent of the diaphragm with redistribution of normal abdominal contents. Using a biofeedback technique [30], patients learned to control the activity of the abdominal walls, and thereby prevented lettuce-induced distension [84]. Thus, abdominal distension in these patients is a somatic behavioral response, but why, in the first place, they acquired their belief and the mechanisms by which lettuce induces the abnormal response are not known.

In healthy subjects, neutral stimuli, may become aversive when paired with painful digestive sensations. This has been shown using painful rectal distension as the unconditioned stimulus and neutral visual stimuli (plain geometric figures) as the conditioned stimulus [85–87]. Similarly, well-liked foods may become aversive by an unpleasant experience after ingestion [88], and this is probably the mechanism by which food ingested just before an episode of gastroenteritis, becomes disgusting and is considered by the patients as responsible for their illness.

These data indicate that associative learning might be a significant factor determining the postprandial experience. This is particularly interesting, since fear of conditioning to innocuous gastrointestinal sensations may be an important mechanism in the pathogenesis of functional gut disorders. For example, in functional dyspepsia the information provided to patients regarding the fat content of a meal is associated with symptom production without direct correlation with the actual fat content [89,90] (Figure 2), and faulty abdominal pain-related fear learning and memory processes have been suggested in irritable bowel syndrome [91].

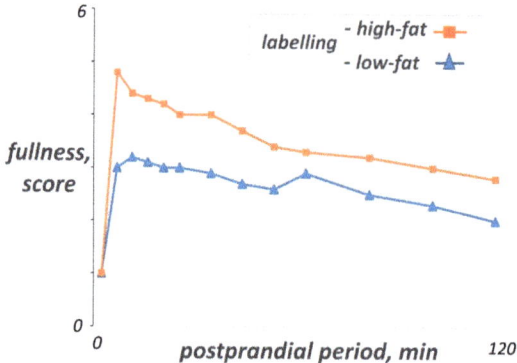

Figure 2. Cognitive conditioning of the postprandial experience. On 2 separate days, the same low-fat yogurt was given to patients with functional dyspepsia correctly presented as low-fat or mislabeled as high-fat; high-fat labeling was associated with significantly more of fullness sensation than the low-fat label. "Adapted by permission from BMJ Publishing Group Limited. [Role of cognitive factors in symptom induction following high and low fat meals in patients with functional dyspepsia, Feinle-Bisset C, Meier B, Fried M, Beglinger C. Gut. 52(10):1414–8. Copyright 2003 by Gut].

6. Other Factors Inherent to the Individual

The data described above show that conditioning influences the sensory response to a meal via inducible factors. However, inherent characteristics of the eater (constitutive factors) also play a role.

6.1. Effect of Sex

A proof-of-concept study investigated the role of sex, as a constitutive factor, on the meal-related experience, comparing the sensations before, during, and after stepwise ingestion of a comfort meal up to full satiation. Satisfaction increased gradually up to a peak, and then decreased to a nadir at the point of full satiation. Compared to men, the meal load consumed at the well-being peak was lower and induced significantly less fullness in women. Consequently, men required larger amounts of food as well as stronger homeostatic sensations to achieve satisfaction. The same pattern was observed at the level of full satiation: men ate more and experienced positive well-being, while in women, well-being scores dropped below pre-meal level [2]. The effect of sex on the ingestion experience suggests that other constitutive factors of the eater may influence the responses to meals.

A subsequent study compared the postprandial responses to a palatable comfort meal in women and men, measuring homeostatic sensations (hunger/satiety, fullness) and hedonic sensations (digestive well-being, mood), vagal tone (by heart rate variability) and the metabolomic profile before and after meal ingestion. Women exhibited a more intense sensory experience, in particular more postprandial fullness, than men, and their vagal tone response was also more pronounced [92]. The study further showed sex differences in the metabolomic response, specifically in relation to the lipoprotein profile.

More intense fullness in women with the same meal load could be explained by a smaller gastric capacity; however, this possibility was ruled out by a study showing no differences in fasting gastric compliance (the pressure volume curve during inflation) between women and men [93]. By contrast, the same distending levels induced more intense sensations in women than men. Higher gastric sensitivity in women has also been detected with water or nutrient drinks up to maximal tolerance when administered at high ingestion rates, but not at low rates [94]. Furthermore, the reflex relaxation of the stomach induced by meal ingestion (gastric accommodation reflex) was more prolonged in women than men [93], and this may be related to sex-differences in the vagal response to ingestion, because gastric accommodation is a vagal reflex [12,14]. Since gradual reversion of the accommodation reflex produces gastric emptying (progressive re-contraction after meal ingestion squeezes gastric chime through the pylorus), more prolonged accommodation of the stomach is concordant with the slower emptying rate reported in women [95,96] and may contribute to more persistent postprandial sensations.

Another study compared the impact of a well-liked meal on brain activity in women and men [97]. In both women and men, the insula showed extensive postprandial reductions in connectivity with sensorimotor and prefrontal cortices, while the thalamus showed increases in connectivity with insular, frontal, and occipital cortices. However, in men, reductions in insular connectivity were more prominent, and only in men, were related to changes in meal-related sensations (satiety and digestive well-being). In contrast, women showed more prominent increases in thalamic connectivity, that were related to changes in satiety and digestive well-being in women only [97]. These data indicate that sex differences in the subjective sensations related to meal ingestion are associated to specific brain responses.

As discussed above, perception of meal-related stimuli in the gut is influenced by conditioning factors. A study investigated the effect of the eating schedule, comparing the responses to a consistent savory lunch-type meal (stewed beans) eaten at the customary afternoon schedule or in the morning. The sensory experience induced by the probe meal, predominantly postprandial satisfaction, was weaker when eaten at an unconventional time (i.e., at breakfast) in women. While men were resilient to the changes in the customary eating schedule and experienced the same sensations regardless of the timing of ingestion; the effect of the eating schedule was significantly more pronounced in women for fullness, digestive well-being and mood. This was not associated todifferences in the physiological responses induced by the afternoon and morning meals both in women or men [98] (Figure 3). Hence, women are more susceptible to conditioning. Functional gut disorders are more frequent in women than men, and sex differences in the response to meal ingestion, particularly the susceptibility to conditioning, may explain the predisposition of women to meal-related complaints. Furthermore, it has been also shown that neural processes mediating aversive visceral learning are different in women and men [99].

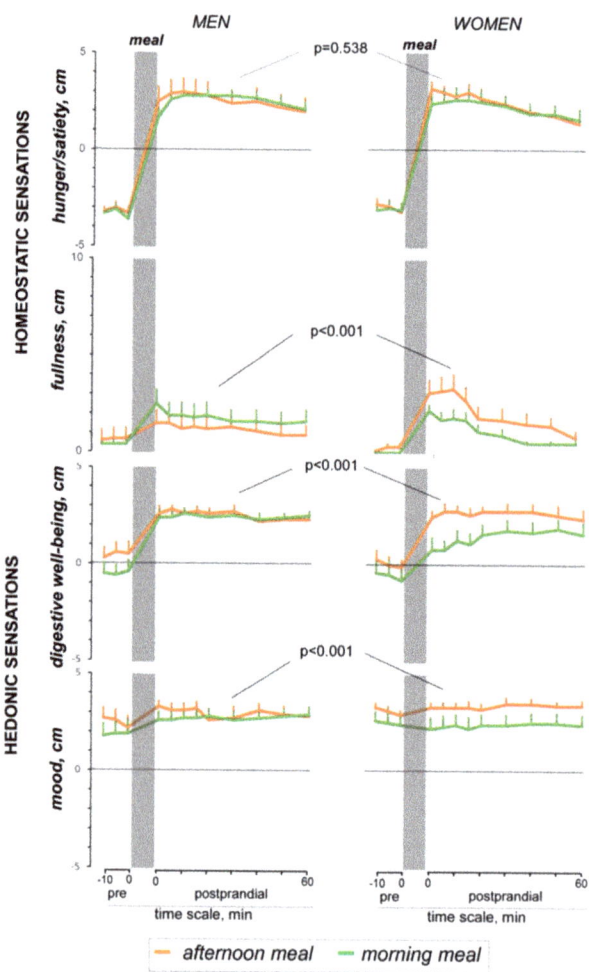

Figure 3. Sex differences in the conditioning by eating habits. Effect of the eating schedule on postprandial sensations in healthy male and women. In women, a consistent savory lunch-type meal eaten at an unconventional time in the morning produced more fullness, but less satisfaction than at the habitual time. Men were resilient to conditioning by eating schedule. "Modified from [Influence of Eating Schedule on the Postprandial Response: Gender Differences, Masihy M, Monrroy H, Borghi G, Pribic T, Galan C, Nieto A, et al., Nutrients. 14;11, Copyright © 2021 by the authors Licensee MDPI, Basel, Switzerland, an open access article distributed under the terms and conditions of the Creative Commons Attribution (CC BY)".

6.2. Functional Gut Disorders

Neurophysiological and brain imaging studies have shown that modulation of visceral sensory input involves a balance between facilitation and inhibition, and this balance is altered in patients with functional gut disorders, leading to visceral hypersensitivity and perception of symptoms in response to physiological stimuli [35]. Specifically, patients with functional gut disorders, especially those with functional dyspepsia, complain of postprandial symptoms in the absence of organic disorders. It has been shown that these patients exhibit increased sensitivity of the stomach to distension during basal (fasting) conditions, and impaired gastric accommodation, i.e., a defective relaxation of the stomach during meal ingestion, which may result in increased gastric wall tension. Both mechanisms (increased wall tension and heightened sensitivity) may have synergistic effects and contribute to their symptoms. Furthermore, they also exhibit distorted responses to intraluminal nutrients, particularly lipids, with: (a) increased sensitivity to lipids (discomfort in response to intraluminal lipids); (b) exaggerated sensitizing effect of lipids on gut mechanoreceptors; and (c) impaired enterogastric reflexes (impaired gastric accommodation) [100–105]. Accordingly, patients with functional gut disorders recognize fatty foods as the most important foodstuff related to their symptoms [100,101]. Other food elements such as fermentable oligosaccharides, disaccharides, monosaccharides and polyols (FOODMAPs) have been shown to induce symptoms in patients with functional gut disorders, particularly irritable bowel syndrome. Conversely, low FOODMAP diets are associated with improved symptoms; however, their effect is similar to that produced by conventional low-residue diets [106]. Low-residue diets reduce the load fermentable substrates reaching the colon and reduce intestinal gas production [107]. However, some non-absorbable components of meals (prebiotics) may exert similar improvement in symptoms, because they induce an adaptation of microbiota activity towards less flatulent fermentative pathways [58]. Abdominal bloating and distension following meal ingestion are frequent and most bothersome complaints in patients with functional gut disorders. Bloating is a subjective sensation of abdominal pressure/fullness, is a subjective sensation of abdominal distension, andinvolves an objective increase in girth [53]. While bloating is a visceral sensation related to hypersensitivity, abdominal distension is a behavioural somatic response, featuring diaphragmatic contraction and descent coupled with relaxation and protrusion of the anterior abdominal wall [28,30,84]. The relation between bloating and distention is not clear, but conceivably, the sensation of bloating triggers the somatic behavioural response leading to distention, and in turn, the somatic response worsens bloating sensation. The mechanisms by which meals, foods and dietary products originate in digestive complaints in patients with functional gastrointestinal disorders are incompletely understood and warrant further investigation [108].

7. Conclusions

The digestive tract has a sensory system that detects intraluminal stimuli; sensory receptors in the gut wall are linked to reflex pathways, that regulate gut function, and to sensory pathways, that elicit conscious sensations. Ingestion of a meal activates the digestive system to accomplish the digestive process. The way gastrointestinal stimuli derived from food ingestion are perceived depends on the meal (amount, composition and palatability) and the response of the digestive system (accommodation, digestion and clearance). Both gastrointestinal sensitivity and function (sensory and reflex responses) depend on intrinsic characteristics of the individual (constitutive factors), but are modulated by a variety of conditioning mechanisms. In normal conditions, meal ingestion induces homeostatic sensations (satiety, fullness) with a rewarding hedonic dimension (satisfaction). In patients with alterations of gastrointestinal sensitivity and/or impaired control of the digestive function (i.e., patients with functional gut disorders) the postprandial experience turns out to be symptomatic with aversive sensations. Understanding the gastrointestinal contributions to the postprandial experience may help in developing healthy habits, planning dietary interventions and in the management of patients with functional gut disorders.

Author Contributions: D.M.L. Review of the literature, manuscript revision. F.A. Review of the literature, manuscript preparation. All authors have read and agreed to the published version of the manuscript.

Funding: This work was supported in part by the Spanish Ministry of Economy and Competitiveness (Dirección General de InvestigaciónCientífica y Técnica, SAF 2016-76648-R). Ciberehd is funded by the Instituto de Salud Carlos III. Dan M. Livovsky received support from the Israeli Medical Association and from Israel Gastroenterological Association 2020 fellowship grants.

Institutional Review Board Statement: Not applicable.

Informed Consent Statement: Not applicable.

Data Availability Statement: Not applicable.

Acknowledgments: The authors thank Gloria Santaliestra for secretarial assistance.

Conflicts of Interest: No competing interests declared.

References

1. Pribic, T.; Azpiroz, F. Biogastronomy: Factors that determine the biological response to meal ingestion. *Neurogastroenterol. Motil.* **2018**, *30*, e13309. [CrossRef]
2. Monrroy, H.; Pribic, T.; Galan, C.; Nieto, A.; Amigo, N.; Accarino, A.; Correig, X.; Azpiroz, F. Meal Enjoyment and Tolerance in Women and Men. *Nutrients* **2019**, *11*, 119. [CrossRef]
3. Simon, J.J.; Wetzel, A.; Sinno, M.H.; Skunde, M.; Bendszus, M.; Preissl, H.; Enck, P.; Herzog, W.; Friederich, H.-C. Integration of homeostatic signaling and food reward processing in the human brain. *JCI Insight* **2017**, *2*. Available online: https://insight.jci.org/articles/view/92970 (accessed on 8 March 2021). [CrossRef]
4. Pribic, T.; Kilpatrick, L.; Ciccantelli, B.; Malagelada, C.; Accarino, A.; Rovira, A.; Pareto, D.; Mayer, E.; Azpiroz, F. Brain networks associated with cognitive and hedonic responses to a meal. *Neurogastroenterol. Motil.* **2017**, *29*, e13031. [CrossRef]
5. Ciccantelli, B.; Pribic, T.; Malagelada, C.; Accarino, A.; Azpiroz, F. Relation between cognitive and hedonic responses to a meal. *Neurogastroenterol. Motil.* **2017**, *29*, e13011. [CrossRef]
6. Malagelada, C.; Barba, I.; Accarino, A.; Molne, L.; Mendez, S.; Campos, E.; Gonzalez, A.; Alonso-Cotoner, C.; Santos, J.; Malagelada, J.-R.; et al. Cognitive and hedonic responses to meal ingestion correlate with changes in circulating metabolites. *Neurogastroenterol. Motil.* **2016**, *28*, 1806–1814. [CrossRef]
7. Malagelada, C.; Pribic, T.; Ciccantelli, B.; Cañellas, N.; Gomez, J.; Amigo, N.; Accarino, A.; Correig, X.; Azpiroz, F. Metabolomic signature of the postprandial experience. *Neurogastroenterol. Motil.* **2018**, *30*, e13447. [CrossRef]
8. Camilleri, M. Peripheral mechanisms in appetite regulation. *Gastroenterology* **2015**, *148*, 1219–1233. [CrossRef]
9. Feinle-Bisset, C. Upper gastrointestinal sensitivity to meal-related signals in adult humans—Relevance to appetite regulation and gut symptoms in health, obesity and functional dyspepsia. *Physiol. Behav.* **2016**, *162*, 69–82. [CrossRef]
10. Tack, J.; Deloose, E.; Ang, D.; Scarpellini, E.; Vanuytsel, T.; Van Oudenhove, L.; Depoortere, I. Motilin-induced gastric contractions signal hunger in man. *Gut* **2016**, *65*, 214–224. [CrossRef]
11. Halawi, H.; Camilleri, M.; Acosta, A.; Vazquez-Roque, M.; Oduyebo, I.; Burton, D.; Busciglio, I.; Zinsmeister, A.R. Relationship of gastric emptying or accommodation with satiation, satiety, and postprandial symptoms in health. *Am. J. Physiol. Gastrointest. Liver Physiol.* **2017**, *313*, G442–G447. [CrossRef] [PubMed]
12. Boeckxstaens, G.; Camilleri, M.; Sifrim, D.; Houghton, L.A.; Elsenbruch, S.; Lindberg, G.; Azpiroz, F.; Parkman, H.P. Fundamentals of Neurogastroenterology: Physiology/Motility—Sensation. *Gastroenterology* **2016**, *150*, 1292–1304.e2. [CrossRef]
13. Distrutti, E.; Azpiroz, F.; Soldevilla, A.; Malagelada, J.R. Gastric wall tension determines perception of gastric distention. *Gastroenterology* **1999**, *116*, 1035–1042. [CrossRef]
14. Azpiroz, F.; Feinle-Bisset, C.; Grundy, D.; Tack, J. Gastric sensitivity and reflexes: Basic mechanisms underlying clinical problems. *J. Gastroenterol.* **2014**, *49*, 206–218. [CrossRef] [PubMed]
15. Notivol, R.; Coffin, B.; Azpiroz, F.; Mearin, F.; Serra, J.; Malagelada, J.R. Gastric tone determines the sensitivity of the stomach to distention. *Gastroenterology* **1995**, *108*, 330–336. [CrossRef]
16. Moragas, G.; Azpiroz, F.; Pavia, J.; Malagelada, J.R. Relations among intragastric pressure, postcibal perception, and gastric emptying. *Am. J. Physiol.* **1993**, *264 Pt 1*, G1112–G1117. [CrossRef] [PubMed]
17. Kiela, P.R.; Ghishan, F.K. Physiology of Intestinal Absorption and Secretion. *Best Pract. Res. Clin. Gastroenterol.* **2016**, *30*, 145–159. [CrossRef] [PubMed]
18. Alhabeeb, H.; AlFaiz, A.; Kutbi, E.; AlShahrani, D.; Alsuhail, A.; AlRajhi, S.; Alotaibi, N.; Alotaibi, K.; AlAmri, S.; Alghamdi, S.; et al. Gut Hormones in Health and Obesity: The Upcoming Role of Short Chain Fatty Acids. *Nutrients* **2021**, *13*, 481. [CrossRef] [PubMed]

19. Malagelada, C.; Accarino, A.; Molne, L.; Mendez, S.; Campos, E.; Gonzalez, A.; Malagelada, J.R.; Azpiroz, F. Digestive, cognitive and hedonic responses to a meal. *Neurogastroenterol Motil.* **2015**, *27*, 389–396. [CrossRef] [PubMed]
20. Coffin, B.; Azpiroz, F.; Guarner, F.; Malagelada, J.R. Selective gastric hypersensitivity and reflex hyporeactivity in functional dyspepsia. *Gastroenterology* **1994**, *107*, 1345–1351. [CrossRef]
21. Caldarella, M.P.; Azpiroz, F.; Malagelada, J.-R. Antro-fundic dysfunctions in functional dyspepsia. *Gastroenterology* **2003**, *124*, 1220–1229. [CrossRef]
22. Enck, P.; Azpiroz, F.; Boeckxstaens, G.; Elsenbruch, S.; Feinle-Bisset, C.; Holtmann, G.; Lackner, J.M.; Ronkainen, J.; Schemann, M.; Stengel, A.; et al. Functional dyspepsia. *Nat. Rev. Dis. Primers.* **2017**, *3*, 17081. [CrossRef]
23. Villoria, A.; Azpiroz, F.; Soldevilla, A.; Perez, F.; Malagelada, J.-R. Abdominal accommodation: A coordinated adaptation of the abdominal wall to its content. *Am. J. Gastroenterol.* **2008**, *103*, 2807–2815. [CrossRef] [PubMed]
24. Burri, E.; Cisternas, D.; Villoria, A.; Accarino, A.; Soldevilla, A.; Malagelada, J.-R.; Azpiroz, F. Accommodation of the abdomen to its content: Integrated abdomino-thoracic response. *Neurogastroenterol. Motil.* **2012**, *24*, 312-e162. [CrossRef]
25. Burri, E.; Cisternas, D.; Villoria, A.; Accarino, A.; Soldevilla, A.; Malagelada, J.-R.; Azpiroz, F. Abdominal accommodation induced by meal ingestion: Differential responses to gastric and colonic volume loads. *Neurogastroenterol. Motil.* **2013**, *25*, 339-e253. [CrossRef]
26. Villoria, A.; Azpiroz, F.; Burri, E.; Cisternas, D.; Soldevilla, A.; Malagelada, J.-R. Abdomino-phrenic dyssynergia in patients with abdominal bloating and distension. *Am. J. Gastroenterol.* **2011**, *106*, 815–819. [CrossRef]
27. Burri, E.; Barba, E.; Huaman, J.W.; Cisternas, D.; Accarino, A.; Soldevilla, A.; Malagelada, J.-R.; Azpiroz, F. Mechanisms of postprandial abdominal bloating and distension in functional dyspepsia. *Gut* **2014**, *63*, 395–400. [CrossRef]
28. Barba, E.; Burri, E.; Accarino, A.; Cisternas, D.; Quiroga, S.; Monclus, E.; Navazo, I.; Malagelada, J.-R.; Azpiroz, F. Abdominothoracic mechanisms of functional abdominal distension and correction by biofeedback. *Gastroenterology* **2015**, *148*, 732–739. [CrossRef]
29. Livovsky, D.M.; Barber, C.; Barba, E.; Accarino, A.; Azpiroz, F. Abdominothoracic Postural Tone Influences the Sensations Induced by Meal Ingestion. *Nutrients* **2021**, *13*, 658. [CrossRef]
30. Barba, E.; Accarino, A.; Azpiroz, F. Correction of Abdominal Distention by Biofeedback-Guided Control of Abdominothoracic Muscular Activity in a Randomized, Placebo-Controlled Trial. *Clin. Gastroenterol. Hepatol.* **2017**, *15*, 1922–1929. [CrossRef] [PubMed]
31. Rayner, C.K.; Hughes, P.A. Small Intestinal Motor and Sensory Function and Dysfunction. In *Sleisenger and Fordtran's Gastrointestinal and Liver Disease*; Pathophysiology, Diagnosis, Management; Elsevier: Philadelphia, PA, USA, 2021; pp. 1580–1594.e3.
32. Furness, J.B.; Kunze, W.A.A.; Clerc, N., II. The intestine as a sensory organ: Neural, endocrine, and immune responses. *Am. J. Physiol. Gastrointest. Liver Physiol.* **1999**, *277*, G922–G928. [CrossRef]
33. Bentley, F.H.; Smithwick, R. Visceral pain produced by balloon distension of the jejunum. *Lancet* **1940**, *236*, 389–391. [CrossRef]
34. Ray, B.S.; Neill, C.L. Abdominal Visceral Sensation in Man. *Ann. Surg.* **1947**, *126*, 709–723. [CrossRef]
35. Wilder-Smith, C.H. The balancing act: Endogenous modulation of pain in functional gastrointestinal disorders. *Gut* **2011**, *60*, 1589–1599. [CrossRef] [PubMed]
36. Azpiroz, F. Intestinal perception: Mechanisms and assessment. *Br. J. Nutr.* **2005**, *93* (Suppl. 1), S7–S12. [CrossRef] [PubMed]
37. Ly, H.G.; Dupont, P.; Van Laere, K.; Depoortere, I.; Tack, J.; Van Oudenhove, L. Differential brain responses to gradual intragastric nutrient infusion and gastric balloon distension: A role for gut peptides? *Neuroimage* **2017**, *144 Pt A*, 101–112. [CrossRef] [PubMed]
38. Accarino, A.M.; Azpiroz, F.; Malagelada, J.R. Symptomatic responses to stimulation of sensory pathways in the jejunum. *Am. J. Physiol.* **1992**, *263 Pt 1*, G673–G677. [CrossRef] [PubMed]
39. Serra, J.; Azpiroz, F.; Malagelada, J.R. Perception and reflex responses to intestinal distention in humans are modified by simultaneous or previous stimulation. *Gastroenterology* **1995**, *109*, 1742–1749. [CrossRef]
40. Serra, J.; Azpiroz, F.; Malagelada, J.R. Modulation of gut perception in humans by spatial summation phenomena. *J. Physiol.* **1998**, *506 Pt 2*, 579–587. [CrossRef]
41. Huaman, J.-W.; Mego, M.; Bendezú, A.; Monrroy, H.; Samino, S.; Accarino, A.; Saperas, E.; Azpiroz, F. Correction of Dyssynergic Defecation, but Not Fiber Supplementation, Reduces Symptoms of Functional Dyspepsia in Patients With Constipation in a Randomized Trial. *Clin. Gastroenterol. Hepatol.* **2020**, *18*, 2463–2470.e1. [CrossRef]
42. Grundy, D. Neuroanatomy of Visceral Nociception: Vagal and Splanchnic Afferent. *Gut* **2002**, *51* (Suppl. 1), i2–i5. [CrossRef]
43. Azpiroz, F. Gastrointestinal perception: Pathophysiological implications. *Neurogastroenterol. Motil.* **2002**, *14*, 229–239. [CrossRef]
44. Pribic, T.; Vilaseca, H.; Nieto, A.; Hernandez, L.; Monrroy, H.; Malagelada, C.; Accarino, A.; Roca, J.; Azpiroz, F. Meal composition influences postprandial sensations independently of valence and gustation. *Neurogastroenterol. Motil.* **2018**, *25*, e13337. [CrossRef]
45. Accarino, A.M.; Azpiroz, F.; Malagelada, J.R. Modification of small bowel mechanosensitivity by intestinal fat. *Gut* **2001**, *48*, 690–695. [CrossRef]
46. Caldarella, M.P.; Azpiroz, F.; Malagelada, J.-R. Selective effects of nutrients on gut sensitivity and reflexes. *Gut* **2007**, *56*, 37–42. [CrossRef]
47. Weltens, N.; Zhao, D.; Van Oudenhove, L. Where is the comfort in comfort foods? Mechanisms linking fat signaling, reward, and emotion. *Neurogastroenterol. Motil.* **2014**, *26*, 303–315. [CrossRef] [PubMed]
48. Bendezú, R.A.; Mego, M.; Monclus, E.; Merino, X.; Accarino, A.; Malagelada, J.R.; Navazo, I.; Azpiroz, F. Colonic content: Effect of diet, meals, and defecation. *Neurogastroenterol. Motil.* **2017**, *29*, e12930. [CrossRef]

49. Simrén, M.; Barbara, G.; Flint, H.J.; Spiegel, B.M.R.; Spiller, R.C.; Vanner, S.; Verdu, E.F.; Whorwell, P.J.; Zoetendal, E.G. Rome Foundation Committee Intestinal Microbiota in Functional Bowel Disorders: A Rome Foundation Report. *Gut* **2013**, *62*, 159–176.
50. Aziz, Q.; Doré, J.; Emmanuel, A.; Guarner, F.; Quigley, E.M.M. Gut microbiota and gastrointestinal health: Current concepts and future directions. *Neurogastroenterol. Motil.* **2013**, *25*, 4–15. [CrossRef] [PubMed]
51. Wu, G.D.; Lewis, J.D. Analysis of the human gut microbiome and association with disease. *Clin. Gastroenterol. Hepatol.* **2013**, *11*, 774–777. [CrossRef]
52. Mayer, E.A.; Hsiao, E.Y. The Gut and Its Microbiome as Related to Central Nervous System Functioning and Psychological Well-being: Introduction to the Special Issue of Psychosomatic Medicine. *Psychosom. Med.* **2017**, *79*, 844–846. [CrossRef]
53. Azpiroz, F. Intestinal gas. In *Sleisenger and Fordtran's Gastrointestinal and Liver Disease*, 10th ed.; Pathophysiology, Diagnosis, Management; Elsevier: Amsterdam, The Netherlands, 2015; pp. 242–250.
54. Manichanh, C.; Eck, A.; Varela, E.; Roca, J.; Clemente, J.C.; González, A.; Knights, D.; Knight, R.; Estrella, S.; Hernandez, C.; et al. Anal gas evacuation and colonic microbiota in patients with flatulence: Effect of diet. *Gut* **2014**, *63*, 401–408. [CrossRef] [PubMed]
55. Mego, M.; Accarino, A.; Malagelada, J.-R.; Guarner, F.; Azpiroz, F. Accumulative effect of food residues on intestinal gas production. *Neurogastroenterol. Motil.* **2015**, *27*, 1621–1628. [CrossRef] [PubMed]
56. Ceballos Inza, V.; MonclúsLahoya, E.; Vázquez Alcocer, P.P.; Bendezú García, Á.; Mego Silva, M.; Merino Casabiel, X.; AzpirozVidaur, F.; Navazo Álvaro, I. Colonic content assessment from MRI imaging using a semi-automatic approach. In *EG VCBM 2019: Eurographics Workshop on Visual Computing for Biology and Medicine: Full and Short Paper Proceedings, Brno, Czech Republic, 4–6 September 2019*; European Association for Computer Graphics (Eurographics): Geneva, Switzerland, 2019; pp. 17–26. Available online: https://upcommons.upc.edu/handle/2117/174469 (accessed on 8 March 2021).
57. Orellana, B.; Monclús, E.; Brunet, P.; Navazo, I.; Bendezú, Á.; Azpiroz, F. A scalable approach to T2-MRI colon segmentation. *Med. Image Anal.* **2020**, *63*, 101697. [CrossRef]
58. Huaman, J.-W.; Mego, M.; Manichanh, C.; Cañellas, N.; Cañueto, D.; Segurola, H.; Jansana, M.; Malagelada, C.; Accarino, A.; Vulevic, J.; et al. Effects of Prebiotics vs a Diet Low in FODMAPs in Patients With Functional Gut Disorders. *Gastroenterology* **2018**, *155*, 1004–1007. [CrossRef]
59. Azpiroz, F.; Molne, L.; Mendez, S.; Nieto, A.; Manichanh, C.; Mego, M.; Accarino, A.; Santos, J.; Sailer, M.; Theis, S.; et al. Effect of Chicory-derived Inulin on Abdominal Sensations and Bowel Motor Function. *J. Clin. Gastroenterol.* **2017**, *51*, 619–625. [CrossRef]
60. Azpiroz, F.; Dubray, C.; Bernalier-Donadille, A.; Cardot, J.-M.; Accarino, A.; Serra, J.; Wagner, A.; Respondek, F.; Dapoigny, M. Effects of scFOS on the composition of fecal microbiota and anxiety in patients with irritable bowel syndrome: A randomized, double blind, placebo controlled study. *Neurogastroenterol. Motil.* **2017**, *29*, e12911. [CrossRef]
61. Le Nevé, B.; de la Torre, A.M.; Tap, J.; Derrien, M.; Cotillard, A.; Barba, E.; Mego, M.; Nieto Ruiz, A.; Hernandez-Palet, L.; Dornic, Q.; et al. A Fermented Milk Product with, B. Lactis CNCM I-2494 and Lactic Acid Bacteria Improves Gastrointestinal Comfort in Response to a Challenge Diet Rich in Fermentable Residues in Healthy Subjects. *Nutrients* **2020**, *12*, 320. [CrossRef] [PubMed]
62. Hungin, A.P.S.; Mitchell, C.R.; Whorwell, P.; Mulligan, C.; Cole, O.; Agréus, L.; Fracasso, P.; Lionis, C.; Mendive, J.; Philippart de Foy, J.-M.; et al. Systematic review: Probiotics in the management of lower gastrointestinal symptoms—An updated evidence-based international consensus. *Aliment. Pharmacol. Ther.* **2018**, *47*, 1054–1070. [CrossRef]
63. Sanders, M.E.; Merenstein, D.J.; Reid, G.; Gibson, G.R.; Rastall, R.A. Probiotics and prebiotics in intestinal health and disease: From biology to the clinic. *Nat. Rev. Gastroenterol. Hepatol.* **2019**, *16*, 605–616. [CrossRef]
64. Guarino, M.P.L.; Altomare, A.; Emerenziani, S.; Di Rosa, C.; Ribolsi, M.; Balestrieri, P.; Iovino, P.; Rocchi, G.; Cicala, M. Mechanisms of Action of Prebiotics and Their Effects on Gastro-Intestinal Disorders in Adults. *Nutrients* **2020**, *12*, 1037. [CrossRef] [PubMed]
65. Sauer, H.; Ohla, K.; Dammann, D.; Teufel, M.; Zipfel, S.; Enck, P.; Mack, I. Changes in Gustatory Function and Taste Preference Following Weight Loss. *J. Pediatr.* **2017**, *182*, 120–126. [CrossRef] [PubMed]
66. Livovsky, D.M.; Pribic, T.; Azpiroz, F. Food, Eating, and the Gastrointestinal Tract. *Nutrients* **2020**, *12*, 986. [CrossRef] [PubMed]
67. Pribic, T.; Hernandez, L.; Nieto, A.; Malagelada, C.; Accarino, A.; Azpiroz, F. Effects of meal palatability on postprandial sensations. *Neurogastroenterol. Motil.* **2018**, *30*, e13248. [CrossRef]
68. Cabanac, M. Physiological role of pleasure. *Science* **1971**, *173*, 1103–1107. [CrossRef] [PubMed]
69. Pribic, T.; Nieto, A.; Hernandez, L.; Malagelada, C.; Accarino, A.; Azpiroz, F. Appetite influences the responses to meal ingestion. *Neurogastroenterol. Motil.* **2017**, *29*, e13072. [CrossRef]
70. de Graaf, C. Texture and satiation: The role of oro-sensory exposure time. *Physiol. Behav.* **2012**, *107*, 496–501. [CrossRef]
71. Andrade, A.M.; Greene, G.W.; Melanson, K.J. Eating slowly led to decreases in energy intake within meals in healthy women. *J. Am. Diet. Assoc.* **2008**, *108*, 1186–1191. [CrossRef]
72. Robinson, E.; Almiron-Roig, E.; Rutters, F.; de Graaf, C.; Forde, C.G.; Tudur Smith, C.; Nolan, S.J.; Jebb, S.A. A systematic review and meta-analysis examining the effect of eating rate on energy intake and hunger. *Am. J. Clin. Nutr.* **2014**, *100*, 123–151. [CrossRef]
73. Viskaal-van Dongen, M.; Kok, F.J.; de Graaf, C. Eating rate of commonly consumed foods promotes food and energy intake. *Appetite* **2011**, *56*, 25–31. [CrossRef] [PubMed]
74. Mearin, F.; Cucala, M.; Azpiroz, F.; Malagelada, J.R. The origin of symptoms on the brain-gut axis in functional dyspepsia. *Gastroenterology* **1991**, *101*, 999–1006. [CrossRef]
75. Khlevner, J.; Park, Y.; Margolis, K.G. Brain–Gut Axis Clinical Implications. *Gastroenterol. Clin. N. Am.* **2018**, *47*, 727–739. [CrossRef]

76. Accarino, A.M.; Azpiroz, F.; Malagelada, J.R. Attention and distraction: Effects on gut perception. *Gastroenterology* **1997**, *113*, 415–422. [CrossRef]
77. Brunstrom, J.M.; Mitchell, G.L. Effects of distraction on the development of satiety. *Br. J. Nutr.* **2006**, *96*, 761–769.
78. Hardcastle, S.J.; Thøgersen-Ntoumani, C.; Chatzisarantis, N.L.D. Food Choice and Nutrition: A Social Psychological Perspective. *Nutrients* **2015**, *7*, 8712–8715. [CrossRef]
79. Péneau, S.; Mekhmoukh, A.; Chapelot, D.; Dalix, A.-M.; Airinei, G.; Hercberg, S.; Bellisle, F. Influence of environmental factors on food intake and choice of beverage during meals in teenagers: A laboratory study. *Br. J. Nutr.* **2009**, *102*, 1854–1859. [CrossRef] [PubMed]
80. Coelho, J.S.; Idler, A.; Werle, C.O.C.; Jansen, A. Sweet temptation: Effects of exposure to chocolate-scented lotion on food intake. *Food Qual. Prefer.* **2011**, *22*, 780–784. [CrossRef]
81. Edwards, J.S.A.; Meiselman, H.L.; Edwards, A.; Lesher, L. The influence of eating location on the acceptability of identically prepared foods. *Food Qual. Prefer.* **2003**, *14*, 647–652. [CrossRef]
82. Guéguen, N.; Petr, C. Odors and consumer behavior in a restaurant. *Int. J. Hosp. Manag.* **2006**, *25*, 335–339. [CrossRef]
83. Pribic, T.; Vilaseca, H.; Nieto, A.; Hernandez, L.; Malagelada, C.; Accarino, A.; Roca, J.; Azpiroz, F. Education of the postprandial experience by a sensory-cognitive intervention. *Neurogastroenterol. Motil.* **2018**, *30*, e13197. [CrossRef]
84. Barba, E.; Sánchez, B.; Burri, E.; Accarino, A.; Monclus, E.; Navazo, I.; Guarner, F.; Margolles, A.; Azpiroz, F. Abdominal distension after eating lettuce: The role of intestinal gas evaluated in vitro and by abdominal CT imaging. *Neurogastroenterol. Motil.* **2019**, *31*, e13703. [CrossRef] [PubMed]
85. Gramsch, C.; Kattoor, J.; Icenhour, A.; Forsting, M.; Schedlowski, M.; Gizewski, E.R.; Elsenbruch, S. Learning pain-related fear: Neural mechanisms mediating rapid differential conditioning, extinction and reinstatement processes in human visceral pain. *Neurobiol. Learn Mem.* **2014**, *116*, 36–45. [CrossRef]
86. Kattoor, J.; Gizewski, E.R.; Kotsis, V.; Benson, S.; Gramsch, C.; Theysohn, N.; Maderwald, S.; Forsting, M.; Schedlowski, M.; Elsenbruch, S. Fear conditioning in an abdominal pain model: Neural responses during associative learning and extinction in healthy subjects. *PLoS ONE* **2013**, *8*, e51149. [CrossRef] [PubMed]
87. Icenhour, A.; Labrenz, F.; Ritter, C.; Theysohn, N.; Forsting, M.; Bingel, U.; Elsenbruch, S. Learning by experience? Visceral pain-related neural and behavioral responses in a classical conditioning paradigm. *Neurogastroenterol. Motil.* **2017**, *29*, e13026. [CrossRef] [PubMed]
88. Yamamoto, T. Central mechanisms of roles of taste in reward and eating. *Acta Physiol. Hung.* **2008**, *95*, 165–186. [CrossRef]
89. Feinle-Bisset, C.; Meier, B.; Fried, M.; Beglinger, C. Role of cognitive factors in symptom induction following high and low fat meals in patients with functional dyspepsia. *Gut* **2003**, *52*, 1414–1418. [CrossRef] [PubMed]
90. Lee, I.-S.; Kullmann, S.; Scheffler, K.; Preissl, H.; Enck, P. Fat label compared with fat content: Gastrointestinal symptoms and brain activity in functional dyspepsia patients and healthy controls. *Am. J. Clin. Nutr.* **2018**, *108*, 127–135. [CrossRef]
91. Icenhour, A.; Langhorst, J.; Benson, S.; Schlamann, M.; Hampel, S.; Engler, H.; Forsting, M.; Elsenbruch, S. Neural circuitry of abdominal pain-related fear learning and reinstatement in irritable bowel syndrome. *Neurogastroenterol. Motil.* **2015**, *27*, 114–127. [CrossRef]
92. Monrroy, H.; Borghi, G.; Pribic, T.; Galan, C.; Nieto, A.; Amigo, N.; Accarino, A.; Correig, X.; Azpiroz, F. Biological Response to Meal Ingestion: Gender Differences. *Nutrients* **2019**, *11*, 702. [CrossRef]
93. Mearadji, B.; Penning, C.; Vu, M.K.; van der Schaar, P.J.; van Petersen, A.S.; Kamerling, I.M.; Masclee, A.A. Influence of gender on proximal gastric motor and sensory function. *Am. J. Gastroenterol.* **2001**, *96*, 2066–2073. [CrossRef]
94. Abid, S.; Anis, M.K.; Azam, Z.; Jafri, W.; Lindberg, G. Satiety drinking tests: Effects of caloric content, drinking rate, gender, age, and body mass index. *Scand J. Gastroenterol.* **2009**, *44*, 551–556. [CrossRef] [PubMed]
95. Hutson, W.R.; Roehrkasse, R.L.; Wald, A. Influence of gender and menopause on gastric emptying and motility. *Gastroenterology* **1989**, *96*, 11–17. [CrossRef]
96. Bennink, R.; Peeters, M.; Van den Maegdenbergh, V.; Geypens, B.; Rutgeerts, P.; De Roo, M.; Mortelmans, L. Comparison of total and compartmental gastric emptying and antral motility between healthy men and women. *Eur. J. Nucl. Med.* **1998**, *25*, 1293–1299. [CrossRef] [PubMed]
97. Kilpatrick, L.; Pribic, T.; Ciccantelli, B.; Malagelada, C.; Livovsky, D.M.; Accarino, A.; Pareto, D.; Azpiroz, F.; Mayer, E.A. Sex Differences and Commonalities in the Impact of a Palatable Meal on Thalamic and Insular Connectivity. *Nutrients* **2020**, *12*, 1627. [CrossRef] [PubMed]
98. Masihy, M.; Monrroy, H.; Borghi, G.; Pribic, T.; Galan, C.; Nieto, A.; Accarino, A.; Azpiroz, F. Influence of Eating Schedule on the Postprandial Response: Gender Differences. *Nutrients* **2019**, *11*, 401. [CrossRef] [PubMed]
99. Benson, S.; Kattoor, J.; Kullmann, J.S.; Hofmann, S.; Engler, H.; Forsting, M.; Gizewski, E.R.; Elsenbruch, S. Towards understanding sex differences in visceral pain: Enhanced reactivation of classically-conditioned fear in healthy women. *Neurobiol. Learn. Mem.* **2014**, *109*, 113–121. [CrossRef]
100. Feinle-Bisset, C.; Azpiroz, F. Dietary and lifestyle factors in functional dyspepsia. *Nat. Rev. Gastroenterol. Hepatol.* **2013**, *10*, 150–157. [CrossRef]
101. Feinle-Bisset, C.; Azpiroz, F. Dietary lipids and functional gastrointestinal disorders. *Am. J. Gastroenterol.* **2013**, *108*, 737–747. [CrossRef]

102. Feinle, C.; Meier, O.; Otto, B.; D'Amato, M.; Fried, M. Role of duodenal lipid and cholecystokinin A receptors in the pathophysiology of functional dyspepsia. *Gut* **2001**, *48*, 347–355. [CrossRef]
103. Fried, M.; Feinle, C. The role of fat and cholecystokinin in functional dyspepsia. *Gut* **2002**, *51* (Suppl. 1), i54–i57. [CrossRef]
104. Barbera, R.; Feinle, C.; Read, N.W. Nutrient-specific modulation of gastric mechanosensitivity in patients with functional dyspepsia. *Dig. Dis. Sci.* **1995**, *40*, 1636–1641. [CrossRef]
105. Pilichiewicz, A.N.; Feltrin, K.L.; Horowitz, M.; Holtmann, G.; Wishart, J.M.; Jones, K.L.; Talley, N.J.; Feinle-Bisset, C. Functional dyspepsia is associated with a greater symptomatic response to fat but not carbohydrate, increased fasting and postprandial CCK, and diminished PYY. *Am. J. Gastroenterol.* **2008**, *103*, 2613–2623. [CrossRef]
106. Böhn, L.; Störsrud, S.; Liljebo, T.; Collin, L.; Lindfors, P.; Törnblom, H.; Simrén, M. Diet low in FODMAPs reduces symptoms of irritable bowel syndrome as well as traditional dietary advice: A randomized controlled trial. *Gastroenterology* **2015**, *149*, 1399–1407.e2. [CrossRef] [PubMed]
107. Azpiroz, F.; Hernandez, C.; Guyonnet, D.; Accarino, A.; Santos, J.; Malagelada, J.-R.; Guarner, F. Effect of a low-flatulogenic diet in patients with flatulence and functional digestive symptoms. *Neurogastroenterol. Motil.* **2014**, *26*, 779–785. [CrossRef] [PubMed]
108. Moayyedi, P.; Simrén, M.; Bercik, P. Evidence-based and mechanistic insights into exclusion diets for IBS. *Nat. Rev. Gastroenterol. Hepatol.* **2020**, *17*, 406–413. [CrossRef] [PubMed]

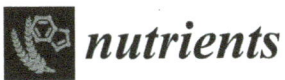

Review

Macronutrient Sensing in the Oral Cavity and Gastrointestinal Tract: Alimentary Tastes

Russell Keast *, Andrew Costanzo and Isabella Hartley

CASS Food Research Centre, School of Exercise and Nutrition Sciences, Deakin University, Burwood, VIC 3125, Australia; andrew.costanzo@deakin.edu.au (A.C.); b.hartley@deakin.edu.au (I.H.)
* Correspondence: russell.keast@deakin.edu.au; Tel.: +31-3-92446944

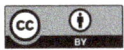

Abstract: There are numerous and diverse factors enabling the overconsumption of foods, with the sense of taste being one of these factors. There are four well established basic tastes: sweet, sour, salty, and bitter; all with perceptual independence, salience, and hedonic responses to encourage or discourage consumption. More recently, additional tastes have been added to the basic taste list including umami and fat, but they lack the perceptual independence and salience of the basics. There is also emerging evidence of taste responses to kokumi and carbohydrate. One interesting aspect is the link with the new and emerging tastes to macronutrients, with each macronutrient having two distinct perceptual qualities that, perhaps in combination, provide a holistic perception for each macronutrient: fat has fat taste and mouthfeel; protein has umami and kokumi; carbohydrate has sweet and carbohydrate tastes. These new tastes can be sensed in the oral cavity, but they have more influence post- than pre-ingestion. Umami, fat, kokumi, and carbohydrate tastes have been suggested as an independent category named alimentary. This narrative review will present and discuss evidence for macronutrient sensing throughout the alimentary canal and evidence of how each of the alimentary tastes may influence the consumption of foods.

Keywords: taste; obesity; fat; protein; carbohydrate

1. Introduction

The alimentary canal comprises various organs including the mouth, throat, esophagus, stomach, intestines, and anus and encompasses a system that is responsible for identifying foods suitable for consumption, preparation for swallowing, digestion, absorption, and finally excretion of waste. Put simply, the alimentary canal can be considered a mouth to anus nutrient (and non-nutrient) recognition and processing system. It appears logical that we have sensing systems that respond to the macronutrients fat, protein, and carbohydrate. For each macronutrient, there are two perceptual outcomes (at least), one for the monomer, one for larger compounds: fat has a fat taste for the monomer fatty acid (FA), and mouthfeel for triacylglycerol (TAG) compounds; protein has umami for the monomer L-glutamate and kokumi for γ-glutamyl peptide compounds; carbohydrate has sweet for the monomer sugar, and carbohydrate for oligosaccharide compounds.

Within the alimentary canal, there are two distinct areas of signaling nutrient composition, the upper alimentary canal, comprising the mouth and pharynx, where recognition of various food chemicals signals basic taste qualities (sweet, sour, salty, and bitter), and the lower alimentary canal comprising the stomach and small intestine where digestion of protein, carbohydrate and fat is completed and the absorption of nutrient occurs. What follows is a brief overview of the taste system, and a narrative review of the non-traditional tastes responding to macronutrients, from pre-ingestion to post-ingestion.

2. Taste

Sensing of foods by the taste system has been critical for species survival, signaling via taste quality (and hedonic response) whether the food is fit for ingestion. As an example, if potential food is excessively bitter or sour, ingestion is discouraged via a negative hedonic response and the food would be rejected. The basic taste system is a robust initial screening protecting the digestive system from foods that may be harmful whereas sweet and salty signals both encourage ingestion via a positive hedonic response. The ability to swiftly assess the suitability of foods for consumption has been vital during the successful evolution of species.

2.1. Basic Taste

Taste research is ever evolving through advancements in psychophysical research and molecular biology, particularly the discovery of taste receptors. Traditionally and throughout history, there have been four tastes considered to be the basics: sweet, sour, salty, and bitter. Due to their perceptual salience, these four tastes have been consistently named in taste lists across several thousands of years and multiple cultures (Greek, Aristotle; ancient Chinese medicine, and Indian medicine, Ayurveda) [1,2]. These basic tastes have an important influence on the nutritional or toxic status of the food when it enters the oral cavity [3–5], and have unmistakable perceptual salience. It is this clear perceptual salience and historical categorization of these four independent tastes that has stood the test of time and solidifies these tastes as the basic tastes [1,2].

2.2. Measuring Taste

In human studies, measures of taste function include detection threshold (DT), the lowest concentration of a stimulus that is perceivable, recognition threshold (RT), the concentration at which the quality of the stimuli can be correctly identified, and the suprathreshold intensity range, which increases with increasing stimuli concentration to a terminal threshold [6]. These three measures are all reflective of taste's perceptual domain, but studies have illustrated that the measures are not necessarily correlated with each other. For example, an individual who has a low detection threshold for sucrose (sweet) is termed hypersensitive, but the same individual may experience low intensity of sweetness at a higher concentration of sucrose and be termed hyposensitive [7]. Therefore, within a basic taste quality, an individual may be classified as more or less sensitive. To further confound, there may be a lack of association in taste sensitivity between compounds that elicit the same quality, for example, an individual may have different taste sensitivity to sucrose and acesulfame K which are both sweet stimuli. The same principle applies across taste qualities, and just because an individual is termed hypersensitive to a bitter compound (e.g., 6-n-propylthiouracil) does not predicate that they will be sensitive to sucrose [8]. That the basic tastes are not correlated may be a reason for the lack of consistency between studies when assessing basic taste sensitivity and dietary consumption [9]. However, the development of taste research beyond the four basic tastes provides many avenues for future research.

3. Beyond Basic Tastes: Alimentary Tastes

Advancements in molecular biology and the discovery of taste receptors that detect specific taste stimuli have begun to broaden the initial four independent tastes to potentially include a myriad of new tastes, which do not have the same perceptual salience as the basic tastes. For example, in the early 2000s, umami taste, and more recently, fat taste, have been added to this basic taste list based on the discovery of receptors specific to umami [10] and fat stimuli [11]. However, due to more recent advancements in technology, the future discovery of taste receptors that respond to other taste stimuli such as γ-glutamyl peptides (kokumi) [12] and oligosaccharides (carbohydrates) is inevitable. Thus, the four basic tastes (sweet, sour, salty, and bitter) that have been solidified across several thousands of years are in a class of their own, and new tastes predominately discovered by molecular and modern psychophysical research should be considered in a new subgroup of tastes, for example, alimentary tastes, which emerging evidence suggests have an influence on diet via post-ingestive consequences [2]. Of main relevance to this topic, the gastrointestinal tract (GIT) can sense nutrients, supported by the discovery of 'taste' receptors throughout the GIT [13–17].

Putative tastes that have been proposed to fit into the alimentary taste classification include umami and fat (Figure 1), with further research required to confirm carbohydrate and kokumi (see [2]). Fat is the most scientifically mature non-traditional taste as illustrated by this review. Kokumi and carbohydrate taste are both emerging areas with more research required to achieve the level of sophistication of knowledge that exists for fat taste.

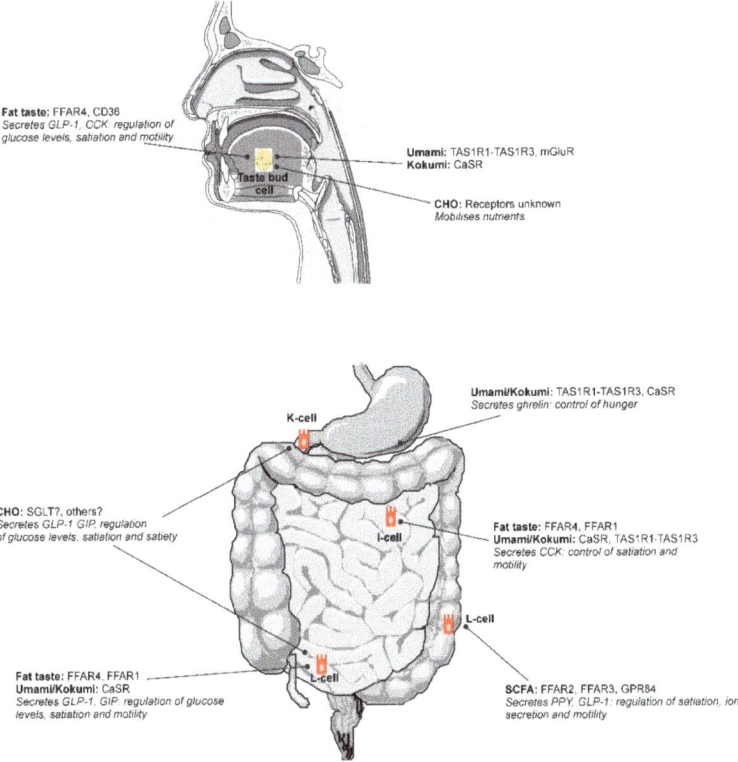

Figure 1. A diagram of putative and potential alimentary taste receptors throughout the alimentary canal. Reproduced from [18].

4. Macronutrient Fat: Fat Taste and Mouthfeel

Fat is one of the essential components of human diet and is necessary for the maintenance and function of many human processes. However, it is well established that overconsumption of fat has negative health implications and is associated with increased risk of obesity and metabolic disease [19]. Dietary fat consumption and energy homeostasis are regulated, in part, by fat sensing mechanisms during and following ingestion. Fat sensing is the ability to detect the presence of dietary fat in ingested foods in the mouth, throat, and GIT, which triggers a multitude of signals and processes to prepare the body for metabolism and satiety.

Fat is a satiating nutrient where, in general, the more fat is consumed, the more satiated an individual will feel [20]. Fat intake is regulated by providing negative feedback to hunger signals or acting as a hunger 'brake', where the initial intake of fat slows subsequent intake until the individual reaches a point of satiation and a meal is ceased. It should be noted that the satiating power of fat does decrease when presented in mixed composition foods [21,22], although this does not undercut the importance of the role of fat in energy regulation. Therefore, it is important to understand the mechanisms involved in fat sensing in facilitating energy overconsumption and the pathogenesis of obesity. There are two main signaling mechanisms for fat sensing. First is the mouthfeel of TAG within the oral cavity where it imparts a textural quality [23]. The other is the detection of FA throughout the alimentary canal via FA sensing receptors [24,25]. It is possible that these sensory modalities complement each other to provide a full sensory perception of fat. It should be noted that fat also harbors odorous properties of foods, although these are usually fat-soluble compounds within the lipid matrix of a food and not necessarily the fats themselves.

Most of the dietary fat that is consumed by humans is made up of TAG. Free fatty acid (FFA) may occur in quantities of less than 1% in most foods of the current food supply [26,27] due to modern refining processes and storage solutions. It is speculated that FFA may have been more abundant in foods in earlier periods of human history, so that the perception of naturally occurring FFA in food was an important gustatory function. Regardless, under normal circumstances, TAG is partially hydrolyzed into diglyceride (DG), monoglyceride (MG), and/or FFA by lingual lipase in the oral cavity, gastric lipase in the stomach, and a range of pancreatic lipases in the small intestine [28]. This demonstrates that even though the dietary fat in food is mostly comprised of TAG, it is still able to activate FA sensing pathways throughout all points of the alimentary canal. Thus, all dietary fat can trigger the satiety cascade upon ingestion, well prior to absorption of FA into the bloodstream via the small intestine.

4.1. Triacylglycerol

TAG mouthfeel is the initial mode of fat sensing that occurs during an eating event as most dietary fat is comprised of TAG [26,27]. The associated textural properties of fat depend on the structure of the fats and the food matrix. These may be perceived as moistness, juiciness, smoothness, thickness, or crispiness depending on the role of fat in the food [29]. While the mechanisms for the sensing of each of these textural attributes may differ, they likely trigger the firing of oral responsive neurons. Unimodal neurons dedicated to the perception of viscosity in foods are present within the oral cavity [30], and more viscous foods are associated with greater feelings of satiety compared to non-viscous foods. For example, Marciani et al. showed that high-viscosity meals are more likely to slow gastric emptying and increase self-reported perception of satiety when nutrient loads are equal [31]. In addition, food with textures that require increased mastication—namely, crispiness and thickness for fatty food—increase the oro-sensory exposure time, thus allowing greater opportunity for sensory stimulation and signaling in the oral cavity [32,33]. However, the neurons involved in texture signaling are not necessarily specific to fat and may be influenced by other textural food components.

Non-hydrolyzed TAG does not aid in the regulation of food intake within the GIT. Matzinger et al. conducted a randomized crossover trial to assess the influence of TAG on appetite when infused directly into the GIT—bypassing the oral cavity and stomach—in 36 healthy male subjects [34]. Infusion of TAG into the duodenum reduced subsequent food intake compared to the control saline infusion. However, when TAG was infused with 120 mg of tetrahydrolipstatin, a lipase inhibitor, subsequent food intake was comparable to that of the control infusion. This highlights that TAG requires hydrolysis into FA via digestion before it can be sensed in the GIT.

4.2. Fatty Acid Sensing

FA sensing is the detection of FFA by FA receptors and the role of fat sensing in the alimentary canal is to signal the body in preparation for fat metabolism and energy homeostasis. This usually occurs subconsciously, particularly in the modern food environment where the proportion of FFA in dietary fat is relatively low compared to TAG [26,27], although recognition as a taste may occur in the oral cavity at slightly higher concentrations than would normally be found in food [25]. Very high concentrations may lead to epithelial irritation [35], although this is independent of FA taste sensing mechanisms.

Multiple receptors have been identified as candidate receptors for FA sensing in the alimentary canal including FA transporter CD36; G-protein coupled receptors (GPR) FFAR1, FFAR2, FFAR3, FFAR4, GPR84; and Delayed Rectifying K+ (DRK) channels [11,36–38]. Most of these receptors are present throughout the entire alimentary canal, although FFAR1 and FFAR3 have not been identified on taste bud cells in the oral cavity and are likely to only be present in the GIT in humans [39]. FA receptors are embedded on taste bud cells (TBC) in the oral cavity—specifically, within fungiform, foliate, and circumvallate papillae [39]—and enteroendocrine cells within the GIT [40].

Activation of FA receptors triggers a complex cascade of cellular events that result in hormone release and gut–brain signals via the vagus nerve, ultimately contributing to satiation and satiety [41]. Each receptor has similar, yet distinct, roles in the regulation of energy homeostasis [40], and there may also be some autocrine signaling between receptors within a cell [42]. FFAR4, previously known as GPR120, binds to medium-chain fatty acid (MCFA) and long-chain fatty acid (LCFA), with a greater affinity for LCFA [43]. The activation of FFAR4 by LCFA or FFAR4 agonists such as potent agonist GSK137657A in isolated mouse circumvallate papillae tissue triggers the release of glucagon-like-peptide (GLP-1) [44]. Similarly, FFAR4 expressed on enteroendocrine cells from mouse small intestine also triggers the release of GLP-1 and peptide tyrosine tyrosine (PYY) when activated [45], and FFAR4 knockout mice have reduced systemic release of GLP-1 following FA exposure [46]. CD36 is a FA translocator, where it transports LCFA through membranes to activate cellular signal cascades. It has a role in the release of oleoylethanolamide (OEA), which is a potent appetite regulator [47], via a cascade of intracellular signaling with peroxisome-proliferator-activated receptor (PPAR)-α [48]. There is also evidence in mice that CD36 may mediate the release of cholecystokinin (CCK), where LCFA infused into the stomach led to a greater release of CCK in wild-type mice compared to CD36 knockout mice [49], which may reflect coordinated crosstalk between CD36 and FFAR4 [42]. FFAR1, embedded within enteroendocrine cells, binds to MCFA and LCFA [43]. Following activation by LCFA, FFAR1 mediates the release of GLP-1 and GIP from L- and K-cells [50], and CCK in I-cells isolated from wildtype, but not FFAR1 knockout, mice [51]. FFAR2 and FFAR3 are involved in the chemoreception of short-chain fatty acid (SCFA) and GPR84 in the chemoreception of MCFA [11]. There is little evidence to support a role in satiety mediated by FA sensing from these receptors. Rather, their purpose seems to more related to the detection of FA that are produced from gut bacteria in regulating inflammation [52].

4.3. Individual Differences in Fatty Acid Sensing and Implications

There is large variation in FA sensing within and between individuals, with demonstrated differences in interindividual ability to detect FA ranging in concentrations up to as large as 1000-fold (0.02 mM to 20 mM) [22,53–57]. A test-retest analysis of fat taste sensitivity tests revealed high within day consistency (ICC = 0.80–0.88), whereas tests conducted at the same time across different days were only moderately consistent (ICC = 0.60–0.69), suggesting that fat taste sensitivity varies from day-to-day within an individual [58]. Variation in FA sensing is largely regulated by acute and habitual intake of dietary fat. Multiple dietary interventions have demonstrated that habitual low-fat intake increases fat taste sensitivity and, conversely, habitual high-fat intake attenuates sensitivity [59,60], even when body weight, gender, age, and genetics are controlled [61]. Following a recent analysis of the latter study, it was proposed that this may be due to the regulation of FA receptor gene expression, where it was found that an average reduction of approximately 20% energy from dietary fat for eight weeks resulted in the upregulation of *FFAR4* expression, the gene that encodes for FFAR4, by approximately 38% [62]. It has been hypothesized that these changes to sensitivity following dietary modification also occur in the GIT, although this has not been studied. Variation of FA sensitivity is an important phenomenon because it mediates how FA sensing influences appetite. Individuals with attenuated FA sensing have reduced signaling and a delayed satiety cascade [25], therefore they are intuitively more likely to consume excess energy and become overweight or obese.

FA sensing occurs in all regions of the alimentary canal and each autonomously trigger the satiety cascade. Research from our group demonstrated that FA sensing in the oral cavity, without exposure in the stomach or GIT, was able to influence self-reported perception of satiety [63]. A FA oral rinse increased the perception of fullness and reduced the perception of hunger compared to the control rinse. As for the GIT, French et al. conducted a study where multiple different FA were infused on separate occasions directly into the small intestine, thus bypassing the oral cavity and stomach [64]. All FA infusions increased self-reported perception of satiety, reduced subsequent meal intake, and triggered a greater release of serum CCK compared to the saline control, with linoleic acid (C18:2) demonstrating the strongest effect. These studies demonstrate the independent ability of tissues throughout the alimentary canal to sense FA and stimulate satiety.

Despite being able to act independently, the chemoreception of FA in the oral cavity and GIT are intrinsically linked [65] with various studies demonstrating an association between oral FA chemoreception and GIT response to FA [60,66,67]. Stewart et al. assessed isolated pyloric pressure waves (IPPWs) during an intraduodenal infusion of oleic acid (C18:1) over 90 min in eight lean and 11 obese males [68]. IPPWs slow gastric emptying and are stimulated by small intestinal exposure to FA, and thus a higher number of IPPWs suggest a gut that is more sensitive and responsive to FA. The study reported a relationship between the total number of IPPWs following C18:1 duodenal infusion and C18:1 taste threshold (Figure 2), suggesting that sensitivity in the oral cavity and GIT are associated. This is currently the strongest evidence to support the concept of the coordinated activity of FA sensing throughout the alimentary canal.

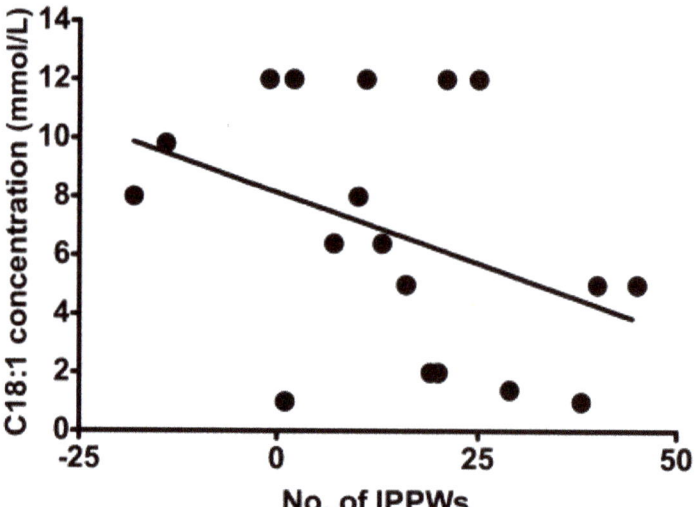

Figure 2. Relation between oral detection thresholds for oleic acid (18:1) and total number of isolated pyloric pressure waves (IPPWs) during 90-min intraduodenal infusions (0.78 kcal/min) of saline and oleic acid (18:1) in lean ($n = 8$) and overweight or obese ($n = 11$) subjects. Taken from [62].

4.4. Fatty Acid Sensing, Satiety, and Diet

The ability of fat to stimulate satiation and satiety is likely to be an important regulator of energy intake and can vary widely depending on circumstance. For example, Keast et al. assessed subsequent intake of an *ad libitum* lunch after consumption of isoenergetic breakfasts of varying macronutrient composition [69]. In 24 participants, the high-protein breakfast caused the greatest level satiety. However, when stratified by fat taste sensitivity, individuals that were hypersensitive to fat taste ($n = 14$) consumed the least *ad libitum* lunch following the high-fat breakfast rather than the high-protein breakfast. This supports the concept that individuals have different satiety responses following food intake, which depend on their ability to sense nutrients in food. This may also change within an individual given that taste sensitivity varies day-to-day depending on recent meal intake [58,60].

Acute feeding studies have shown that intake of a high-fat meal/food leads to a greater release of satiety hormones in the gut and greater perceptions of satiety compared to lower fat meals/foods [66,70–72]. In one crossover trial, 16 overweight and obese participants (11 female) were provided with isoenergetic high-fat or high-carbohydrate breakfasts on separate days, then measured postprandial gut peptides and self-reported appetite over 180 min [71]. The high-fat meal led to a greater rise in GLP-1 and PYY compared to the high-carbohydrate meal, and self-reported ratings of satiety indicated that the high-carbohydrate meal was more satiating, although there was no significant difference between the two meals. Another study compared the effect of carbohydrate and protein meals with additional fat on plasma GIP in eight lean participants (four female, four male) [70]. Both the carbohydrate + fat meal and the protein + fat meal led to a greater rise in plasma GLP compared to the carbohydrate or protein meals without fat, respectively. However, as these meals were not isoenergetic, it does not indicate relative satiation of fat compared to other macronutrients. A study in eight obese females assessed the effect of plasma PYY—specifically a truncated version of PYY, PYY_{3-36}—following intake of a high-fat, high-carbohydrate or high-protein meal over 180 min [72]. The high-fat meal caused the greatest increase in PYY, with at least 30% greater postprandial PYY levels over the other meals at 15–30 min. Another trial on 16 healthy men and 16 obese men was conducted where participants were fed a high-fat, high-carbohydrate, and high-protein meal on separate days, and gut hormone response and perception of satiety were measured over 180 min [66]. The high-fat meal caused greater perceived fullness and reduced perceived hunger compared to the high-carbohydrate meal and was similar to the high-protein meal. There was also a greater release of PYY following the high-fat meal compared to the other meals, but not for CCK. Finally, multiple studies have shown that acute fat intake has a similar or reduced ability to suppress ghrelin compared to other macronutrients [66,71,73,74]. Together, these studies highlight the effective capacity for fat to influence GLP-1, GIP and PYY release and self-reported perception of satiety, but is a relatively weak suppressor of ghrelin.

Sham-feeding studies can be used to expose the oral cavity to fat stimuli while preventing the swallowing of food, thus testing the effect of fat sensing in the oral cavity without the influence of fat sensing in the gut. However, only a few studies have assessed the effect of sham-feeding fats on satiety or food intake. One study compared the effects of sham-feeding and consumption of a modest-fat meal in 10 healthy subjects (six female), and assessed CCK and pancreatic polypeptide (PP) over 90 min [75]. Compared to the control rinse (water), sham-feeding of the meal resulted in a greater release of CCK but not for PP. The consumption of the meal had a far greater effect on CCK and PP than sham-feeding. This shows that sham-feeding does influence some metabolic activity in the gut, but the effect appears to be small compared to actual ingestion. Another study that assessed the effect of sham-feeding of both a solid and liquid high-fat meal on 10 lean and 10 obese females yielded similar results, with a marked increase in plasma CCK and PP following sham-feeding of either meal [76]. However, this study only compared the effect to baseline levels of gut hormones, so there was no control meal for comparison. A randomized crossover trial by Costanzo et al. provided an oleic acid (C18:1) oral rinsing solution to 31 healthy participants and assessed their perception of satiety over 180 min [63]. Compared to the control rinse, the C18:1 oral rinse increased feelings of fullness and decreased feelings of hunger. This demonstrates that FA sensing in the oral cavity is still able to influence satiety, although it should be noted that this was only measured as self-reported satiety and not gut hormones.

There is substantial evidence to demonstrate the role of FA sensing in the oral cavity being associated with dietary habit [7]. Multiple studies have reported an association between fat taste sensitivity and dietary fat intake where, in general, hypersensitive individuals are less likely to consume excess energy—particularly from high-fat foods—compared to hyposensitive individuals [53,54,57,59,60,77–80].

There is also strong evidence to demonstrate the influence of FA sensing in the GIT on dietary intake [81]. A study by Feltrin et al. compared the effect of decanoic acid (C10:0) and lauric acid (C12:0) infusion into the duodenum on *ad libitum* buffet food intake after 90 min in 8 healthy male participants [82]. Energy intake was substantially reduced after the C12:0 infusion compared to the C10:0 and saline control infusions, suggesting that chain lengths of 12 (and above) are necessary for FA sensing in the GIT to trigger the satiety cascade. Another study by Feltrin et al. administered C12:0 and C18:1 infusions into the duodenum of 13 healthy men and measured *ad libitum* buffet food intake after 60 min [83]. Energy intake from the buffet meal was least following the C12:0 infusion compared to the C18:1 and saline control infusions. Interestingly, C18:1 infusion did not reduce food intake compared to the control, even though longer chain length FA are reported to have the greatest satiating effect [34]. A similar study had opposing findings, with C18:1 infusion in the duodenum reducing buffet meal intake after 90 min compared to a saline control infusion in 8 lean males [68]. The difference in meal intake between conditions was less in the 11 overweight or obese male subjects, suggesting that body mass or FA sensing sensitivity might modify the strength of this effect.

Despite strong evidence to suggest that fat sensing regulates satiety and dietary intake, the evidence for the link between attenuated fat sensing and obesity remains contentious. Various human studies that have assessed the link between fat taste sensitivity and body weight have reported that participants who were more sensitive to FA were more likely to have lower BMI than less sensitive individuals [53,55,78–80,84]. On the other hand, some studies have failed to find such associations [54,56,60]. A meta-analysis of 7 studies, conducted to assess the relationship between fat taste sensitivity and body weight [85], reported a minimal difference in fat taste threshold between lean vs. overweight and obese individuals (standard mean difference 0.19 [95% CI: -0.09, 0.47]) suggesting that fat taste sensitivity is not mediated by body mass. However, this analysis was based on a limited number of studies and did not include a wider range of methodologies and conclusions. A number of new studies have been published since the original meta-analysis, so an updated meta-analysis is warranted.

Similarly, the literature suggests that body mass is not associated with attenuated sensitivity throughout the whole alimentary canal. One study compared the effect of a high-fat meal on plasma GLP-1 and GIP between 6 lean and 6 obese women matched for age [86]. They reported no difference in plasma GIP and minimal difference in plasma GLP-1 between lean and obese subjects following high fat meal intake, suggesting that obesity has minimal influence on the effect of fat-mediated release of satiety hormone within the GIT. Another study compared the effect of a high-fat pasta meal matched to 30% of each subject's estimated daily energy requirement between 16 lean and 16 obese men [66]. There were trends for a greater initial reduction in hunger ($p = 0.08$) and increase in fullness ($p = 0.09$) in lean individuals compared to obese individuals following intake of the high-fat meal. Additionally, there were no differences in the AUC for either marker of perceived satiety between the obese and lean subjects. Similarly, no differences were reported in CCK, PYY, or ghrelin between the obese and lean subjects following the high-fat meal. French et al. reported similar findings from a preliminary study. Eight obese and 7 age and sex-matched healthy weight participants were given a high-fat soup (containing 30 g of margarine) and gastric emptying, mouth to caecum transit time (MCTT), plasma CCK, and perception of satiety were assessed [87]. They observed no difference in gastric emptying or MCTT between healthy-weight and obese subjects. Obese subjects did have higher CCK levels than healthy-weight subjects and a reduced feeling of hunger following the high-fat soup ingestion. Together, these studies suggest that the GIT response to dietary fat does not differ substantially between lean and obese individuals. However, it should be noted that these studies did not take sensitivity to satiety hormones into consideration. It is possible that although the hormonal response is comparable in lean and obese individuals, their responsiveness to these hormones may differ.

As discussed above, there is extensive research on the sensing and implications of dietary fat consumption, from pre-ingestion FA sensing in the oral cavity by taste receptors, to post-ingestive signaling by 'taste' receptors throughout the GIT and subsequent hormonal modification and satiety. Fat taste has a prominent role in the regulation of dietary fat intake and future studies should focus on the use of fat stimuli as a potential mechanism for appetite regulation.

5. Macronutrient Protein: Umami and Kokumi Tastes

Proteins are highly diverse in composition, found in all organ systems of animals and plants, and are involved in key functions enabling life. Protein is composed of 20+ amino acids, nine of which are considered essential to humans, and must be obtained via diet. It was a requirement for continued survival that if a species came upon a food source that contained protein, there were sensing mechanisms to identify the protein and encourage consumption of the food. Foods that contain proteins also naturally contain peptides and amino acids, and proteases in saliva start to hydrolyze protein to release peptides and amino acids. It is the peptides and amino acids that allow protein to be sensed and in humans, the two perceptual qualities associated with protein are umami and kokumi, which may enable the regulation of protein intake [88–90].

There has been considerable research on umami taste from the early 2000s, aided by the identification of a glutamate taste receptor [10]. Umami, which is described as savory and delicious, is predominately stimulated by the ionic form of the amino acid glutamic acid, L-glutamate, or more precisely the sodium salt form of L-glutamate. The umami quality is synergistically enhanced by ribonucleotides, inosinate, and guanylate monophosphate (IMP and GMP) [91]. Taste receptors responsible for detecting L-glutamate include the T1R1/T1R3, and metabotropic glutamate receptors (mGluRs) [10,92,93].

Kokumi is a relatively new taste concept following the recognition of γ-glutamyl peptides found in foods including legumes, some cheeses, and fermented foods [94]. In isolation, koku stimuli elicit minimal taste, but instead enhance thickness, mouthfeel, and continuity when mixed with other taste stimuli such as umami, sweet, and salty stimuli [12,95]. Koku compounds (γ-glutamyl peptides) have been shown to activate a calcium-sensing receptor (CaSR) in taste cells on the tongue [12,96,97], however, the mechanisms by which kokumi enhances other basic tastes on a molecular level has not been elucidated.

These proteins signaling mechanisms are first initiated in the oral cavity via the T1R1/T1R3 L-glutamate taste receptor, and the CaSR activation via y-glutamyl peptides; importantly, the same umami taste receptors and the CaSR are found throughout the gastrointestinal tract (GIT), with the post-ingestive activation triggering the release of hormones that play a role in modulating satiation and hunger [98–100].

5.1. Sensing Glutamate and γ-Glutamyl Peptides Throughout the Alimentary Canal

Studies in rats suggest that there is an existing sensing system for glutamate in the gastric mucosa, so that when monosodium glutamate (MSG) is infused into the stomach, there is an increase in the firing of the vagus afferent nerves, which interestingly was not seen in response to the 19 other amino acids, nor sodium chloride [17]. From this, it was hypothesized that the surface of the stomach can sense glutamate [17]. The physiological response to this GIT glutamate sensing includes several hormones that play a role in moderating food intake. The predominant hormones include ghrelin and cholecystokinin (CKK), which are likely to contribute to slowing gastric emptying, moderating motility of the intestine, and stimulating secretions in other organs (i.e., pancreatic and gallbladder secretions) [101,102].

In vitro animal studies have shown that umami and amino acid taste receptors (T1R1-T1R3) detect umami stimuli (MSG) on a gastric ghrelinoma cell line and play a role in the release of ghrelin [101]. T1R1-T1R3 and CaSR receptors are similarly expressed on cells that release CCK, and are involved in CCK release, thus having a satiating effect [14,103]. The T1R1-T1R3 is expressed in intestinal endocrine cells and is activated by a broad range of L-amino acids, which promotes CCK secretion. This activation and CCK secretion is further enhanced with the addition of IMP [14]. Interestingly, enhancement of CCK secretion in the presence of IMP is similar to the synergistic effect on taste perception seen when IMP is applied with L-glutamate in the oral cavity; it may be that a synergistic effect also occurs with CCK secretion in the GIT [14]. Moreover, recent research has shown that kokumi active γ-glu peptides have an in vitro dose response release effect on CCK and GLP-1, providing further evidence that CaSR activation by kokumi active peptides is likely involved in the release of hormones responsible for appetite and food intake regulation [103]. Altogether, these animal studies suggest the umami and koku stimuli play a role in the release of digestive hormones.

It is well known that protein mediates the release of hunger and satiety-related hormones [98], thereby contributing to the regulation of food intake. The effect is enhanced with the addition of umami tasting stimuli (MSG or MSG + IMP) [98,100], although the impact on *ad libitum* food intake and subjective appetite ratings is mixed [98,100,104–107]. A recent study found that the addition of MSG to a soup alone did not affect food intake or blood hormones, however, when consumed in combination with protein, changes in subjective ratings (increased fullness, reduced desire to eat, and reduced appetite) were seen in conjunction with a decrease in blood glucose and increase in plasma insulin and C-peptide [98]. Moreover, the addition of MSG to a carbohydrate-based pre-load soup did not alter post prandial blood glucose levels or appetite ratings in healthy individuals, however, partial energy compensation at the subsequent *ad libitum* lunch was observed between the low energy dense savory pre-load soup in comparison to the sweet pre-load, although the same effect was not seen in the high energy dense pre-load [99]. This suggests that it is energy density, rather than taste perception that may regulate food intake and post prandial glucose release [99]. However, the use of maltodextrin in both sweet and savory soups adds an aspect of carbohydrate content and carbohydrate taste stimulation to both conditions, potentially impacting the outcomes, as sensitivity to maltodextrin (stimuli for carbohydrate taste) has been shown to impact *ad libitum* consumption of complex carbohydrates [108], and is associated with habitual energy intake [109]. In contrast, Hosaka et al. found that following an MSG-containing liquid meal reduced postprandial glucose concentration and increased GLP-1 secretion in comparison to a NaCl control, indicating that MSG may influence satiety by stimulating the release of GIT hormones [100].

Accordingly, the evidence suggests that umami and kokumi receptors exist in the GIT, and the presence of stimuli in the GIT can lead to the release of digestive hormones that play a role in moderating the digestion process, satiety, appetite, and food intake.

5.2. Behavioral and Health Outcomes of Umami/Kokumi Stimuli

Umami and kokumi stimuli have been shown to have beneficial effects on appetite and satiety, particularly when combined with protein, through the potential modulation of digestion and satiety related hormone release post-ingestion, and thus food intake regulation [98–100]. Additionally, umami/kokumi taste perception and hedonic responses may be associated with protein intake regulation [98], because many high protein foods having an umami/savory flavor [110].

Savory (or umami) food liking, and preference is closely tied with the protein content of food, and high protein foods often (but not always) have umami characteristics [110]. The liking and preference of protein foods is also associated with the protein or nutritional status of the individual, however, links with umami and kokumi taste perception require further research [111,112]. Studies have shown that when participants are in a protein deficit or have an overall poor nutritional status, there is a preference for increased concentrations of

MSG [111], and higher intake of savory protein foods [112], thereby regulating their protein intake. Unfortunately, the umami or kokumi taste sensitivity of subjects in these studies was not assessed, so the role of taste perception in protein intake regulation is unclear.

Prolonged consumption of MSG-containing soup decreases umami taste perception, desire for savory foods, and intake of savory foods in healthy populations [107], potentially due to effects on appetite occurring post-ingestion. Interestingly, obese adolescents [113] and obese adult women have a lower sensitivity to MSG and prefer higher concentrations of MSG when compared to healthy weight women [114]. Obese populations have been found to consume a higher proportion of daily energy from salt-, fat-, and umami-dominant foods than healthy weight individuals [115], potentially contributing to their reduced umami sensitivity. This reduced MSG sensitivity is not observed in healthy weight populations, in fact, the inverse has been reported, with healthy participants who are more sensitive to MSG at threshold concentrations having a greater liking and preference for high protein foods in comparison to less sensitive participants [116]. Although further research is required, it appears that obesity is associated with a reduced umami taste perception and preference toward higher concentrations of MSG and umami/savory flavored food. In some cases, this could be attributed to the nutritional status of overweight/obese participants, as poor nutritional status and protein deficits have been associated with the preference of higher concentrations of umami stimuli [111,112]. It may also be that higher concentrations of umami stimuli are required for both taste detection/perception to occur, and for umami GIT receptor activation in order to elicit the same physiological response seen in healthy weight individuals.

Although taste perception and umami/savory food preferences in obese and overweight individuals appear to differ from healthy weight counterparts, there are also studies supporting the concept of using umami stimuli to decrease food intake and enhance satiety. In overweight and obese women, the addition of MSG to a soup pre-load reduced total energy intake and energy intake from high-fat savory foods at a subsequent *ad libitum* lunch and tended to lower energy intake at a further afternoon snack, in comparison to the no MSG control [117]. In support of this, when energy content of a pre-load soup is increased through the addition of protein, participants can adjust their energy consumption at an *ad libitum* meal more precisely than when energy is increased using carbohydrates; this energy compensation effect is enhanced further with the addition of MSG to the protein pre-load, Figure 3 [105]. Interestingly, although energy compensation occurred, this was not associated with an enhancement in satiety or reductions in appetite ratings prior to the *ad libitum* meal [105]. This is supported by a study showing that prolonged MSG consumption leads to a reduction in both desire for, and intake of savory foods without altering subjective appetite and hunger ratings during the *ad libitum* meal [107]. Possibly, this adjustment of energy intake during the *ad libitum* meals reflected post-ingestive appetite regulation, potentially through activation of GIT glutamate receptors promoting the release of digestive hormones, rather than impacting subjective satiety and appetite, as supported in previous studies [14,100,103]. In contrast, the presence of umami flavored food in the oral cavity results in an immediate increase in appetite, followed by an increase in post-ingestive satiety, potentially indicating a biphasic effect of MSG [104], however, this enhancement in satiety has not consistently resulted in subsequent decreased energy intake [106].

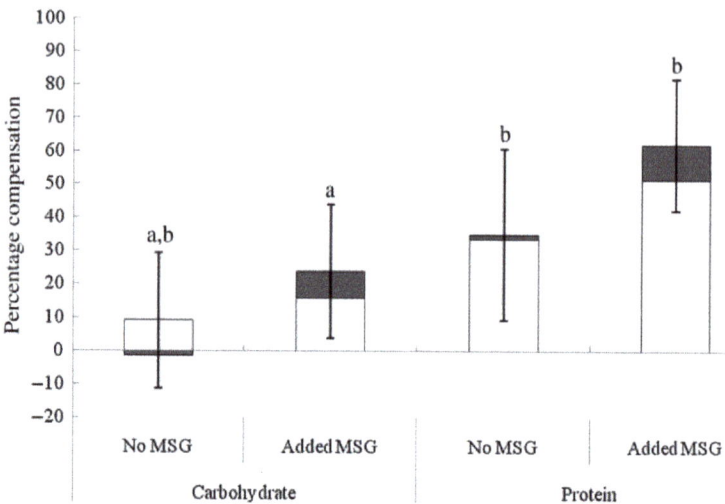

Figure 3. Energy compensation at an *ad libitum* test meal (pasta main course (□) and ice cream dessert (■)) after fixed consumption of high-energy carbohydrates and high-energy protein soup pre-loads with and without added monosodium glutamate (MSG). Values are means, with standard errors represented by vertical bars. [a, b] Mean values with unlike letters were significantly different ($p \leq 0.05$; within-subjects Bonferroni-corrected contrasts). Reproduced from [105].

An alternative health promoting role of umami/kokumi stimuli is to promote health in the elderly, where there are some promising results. A common problem that can favor undernourishment in the elderly is a decline in taste perception, which ultimately contributes to a reduction in appetite and food intake, leading to loss in body weight, predisposition to comorbidities, and reduced quality of life [118]. It is similarly common for the elderly to experience a dry mouth caused by a reduction in salivary output that can contribute to these taste sensation disorders [119]. It has been shown that salivary stimulation by umami stimuli can relieve dry mouth symptoms and improve oral functioning including taste sensation [120], increasing the mucosa to prevent bacterial contamination in the oral cavity [121], and consumption of umami flavored food may enhance overall dietary intake and nutritional status in the elderly [122].

Thus, the use of umami stimuli to alleviate disorders in oral functioning that contribute to malnutrition in the elderly may represent another potential health benefit of umami or kokumi tastants in a nutritionally at-risk population group. Moreover, physiological, and behavioral evidence suggests that the addition of, or the flavor of, MSG and kokumi in food can regulate protein intake, enhance satiety, and potentially moderate food intake through the modulation of digestive hormones. However, further research is required, particularly for use in overweight and obese populations, and other sub-population groups such as those with type 2 diabetes, which would help develop our understanding of the potential clinical application of umami and kokumi stimuli. To further develop our understanding of the clinical applications of MSG and kokumi on long-term food intake, appetite, and satiety regulation (including modulation of digestive hormones), long-term clinical trials assessing these associations are required. Additionally, studies researching associations between umami and kokumi taste perception and these behavioral and physiological outcomes are needed. Finally, as there is little research investigating the role of oral stimulation by umami and kokumi compounds on cephalic phase responses, further investigation is required.

6. Macronutrient Carbohydrate: Sweet and Carbohydrate Taste

There are three main classes of carbohydrate: mono/disaccharides (sugars), oligosaccharides, and polysaccharides, with the chain length of the compound the determining factor for class membership. To add to the complexity, some carbohydrates provide energy, while others cannot be metabolized and are classified as dietary fiber. Some carbohydrates are soluble in aqueous solutions and others remain insoluble. For the purpose of this review (unless otherwise stated), carbohydrate taste stimuli are soluble oligosaccharides, usually maltodextrin. Maltodextrin is a complex carbohydrate that has a variable starch-based structure composed of d-glucose chains linked by glycosidic α-(1–4) and α-(1–6) bonds [123].

As opposed to simple carbohydrates (sugars elicit sweet taste, for review see Trumbo et al. [124]), complex carbohydrate taste research is in its infancy. Indeed, it has long been assumed that maltodextrin is invisible to taste [125,126], and as such has been used as tasteless caloric ingredients in flavor-nutrient conditioning studies [127–129]. However, there is evidence demonstrating that rodents (e.g., rats, mice, gerbils, hamsters) and even some non-human primates are attracted to the taste of maltodextrin [130,131]. Sclafani and Mann [132] found that the preference profiles for five different carbohydrates varied as a function of concentration in three-minute two-bottle choice tests. At low molar concentrations, rats preferred maltodextrin to sugars (maltose, sucrose, glucose, fructose), whereas at higher molar concentrations, rats preferred sucrose and maltose in comparison to maltodextrin [66].

Recent physiological evidence from exercise science suggests that performance is improved after participants rinsed their mouth with solutions containing maltodextrin compared to non-nutritive sweetener (NNS) control solutions [133]. Additionally, Chambers et al. [134] investigated the cortical response to oral maltodextrin and glucose solutions, revealing a similar pattern of brain activation in response to both solutions including brain areas involved in the reward system (i.e., activates brain reward centers in orbitofrontal cortex and striatum similar to oral glucose, which were unresponsive to NNS). Psychophysical research also provides evidence that humans perceive maltodextrins and that sensitivity to simple carbohydrates is independent of that to complex carbohydrates [109,135–138]. Together, these findings provide evidence of taste transduction pathways that respond to maltodextrin independently to those for sweet taste [139]. What follows is an overview of relevant human psychophysical studies using maltodextrin.

6.1. Carbohydrate Taste Psychophysics

Research conducted at Oregon State explored individual differences in the taste perception of carbohydrates, individual differences in activity of salivary alpha-amylase, and the role that salivary α-amylase plays in the taste perception of glucose polymers [135,136]. To assess individual differences in the taste perception of carbohydrates, participants tested six stimuli (three glucose polymers [10% maltodextrin preparations with varying levels of dextrose equivalence (DE of 5, 10, and 20)] and three prototypical stimuli [10% glucose monohydrate, 6% sucrose, and 0.6% sodium chloride]). Maltodextrins were shown to be associated with lower average intensity ratings compared with the sweet and salty stimuli, and the intensity ratings of the maltodextrins highly correlated with one another. Furthermore, the taste responsiveness to the maltodextrins showed greater variability across individuals when compared to the sweet and salty stimuli.

The same research group subsequently investigated taste detection and discrimination of maltodextrins with varying chain length while inhibiting α-amylase activity and additionally explored the effects of a sweet taste inhibitor (lactisole) on taste discrimination. To investigate the taste discrimination of maltodextrins, 22 participants were presented with 6% and 8% samples of two maltodextrins (DP 7 and DP 14) and maltodextrin polymer (DP 44), all spiked with 5 mM of acarbose (an α-amylase activity inhibitor). To investigate the effects of a sweet taste inhibitor (lactisole) on taste discrimination, participants were instructed to taste five samples (75 mM glucose, 75 mM maltose, 0.025 mM sucralose and two maltodextrins [DP 7 and DP 14]). The potentially confounding factor of salivary α-amylase activity was also inhibited by adding 5 mM acarbose to all samples. Controlling for α-amylase is important as the hydrolysis by-products of maltodextrin is glucose, which may activate sweet taste receptors [135,136]. It was found that participants could differentiate between the two maltodextrin oligomer samples, but not the maltodextrin polymer sample [136]. Furthermore, when lactisole was present in the samples, the detectability of the maltodextrin oligomers was not compromised, in contrast to the other samples. This supports the concept that oligomers such as maltodextrin have a taste transduction mechanism independent of the hT1R2/hT1R3 sweet receptor.

Our research group used taste assessment methodology to assess if oral sensitivity to maltodextrin and oligofructose is independent of basic tastes [138]. This taste assessment methodology recruited 34 healthy adult participants to receive 12 samples (two oligosaccharides [maltodextrin, oligofructose], six sweeteners [caloric and NNS], and prototypical stimuli [sour, salty, umami and bitter]) over 28 sessions. Detection and recognition thresholds and intensity ratings were assessed for all stimuli. The outcomes showed that that oligosaccharides can be sensed in the oral cavity and that maltodextrin and oligofructose were highly correlated (r = 0.94–0.95), indicating that the oligomers access the same peripheral receptor mechanism [138]. It was also interesting that at lower concentrations of maltodextrin and oligofructose, there were no associations with sweet taste, but at higher concentrations, there was some overlap with sweet taste. It is unlikely that lingual amylase activity was responsible for increasing free sugars, thereby causing the association between sweet and carbohydrate taste as oligofructose is a fiber and not broken down by oral amylase. Accordingly, there appears to be an independent taste transduction pathway for oligomers at low concentrations, but sweet taste and carbohydrate taste may share some peripheral physiology at higher concentrations [138].

6.2. Behavioral and Health Outcomes of Carbohydrate Taste

Low et al. examined associations between carbohydrate (maltodextrin) taste sensitivity and *ad libitum* consumption of complex carbohydrate foods [108]. In this study, 51 adult females consumed two different iso-caloric pre-load milkshakes followed by an *ad libitum* intake of milkshakes (a sweet glucose-based milkshake and a non-sweet maltodextrin-based milkshake) in a crossover design. Detection threshold and suprathreshold intensity perception ratings for glucose and maltodextrin were collected as well as hedonic (rating of liking) ratings for glucose and maltodextrin and hedonic ratings for various sweet and complex carbohydrate foods. It was found that participants who were more taste sensitive toward maltodextrin consumed more maltodextrin-based milkshake compared to less taste sensitive participants, and this was independent of liking (Figure 4). Although there were variances in intake of maltodextrin-based milkshake, there were no significant differences in appetite ratings (i.e., decrease in hunger and prospective consumption, increase in fullness) between those who were more sensitive and less sensitive to maltodextrin. Maltodextrin sensitivity may be associated with increased consumption of carbohydrate foods although the mechanism remains unknown. The authors speculate that sensing carbohydrates (maltodextrin) may promote unconscious consumption due to the activation of specific brain regions involved with taste and reward [108].

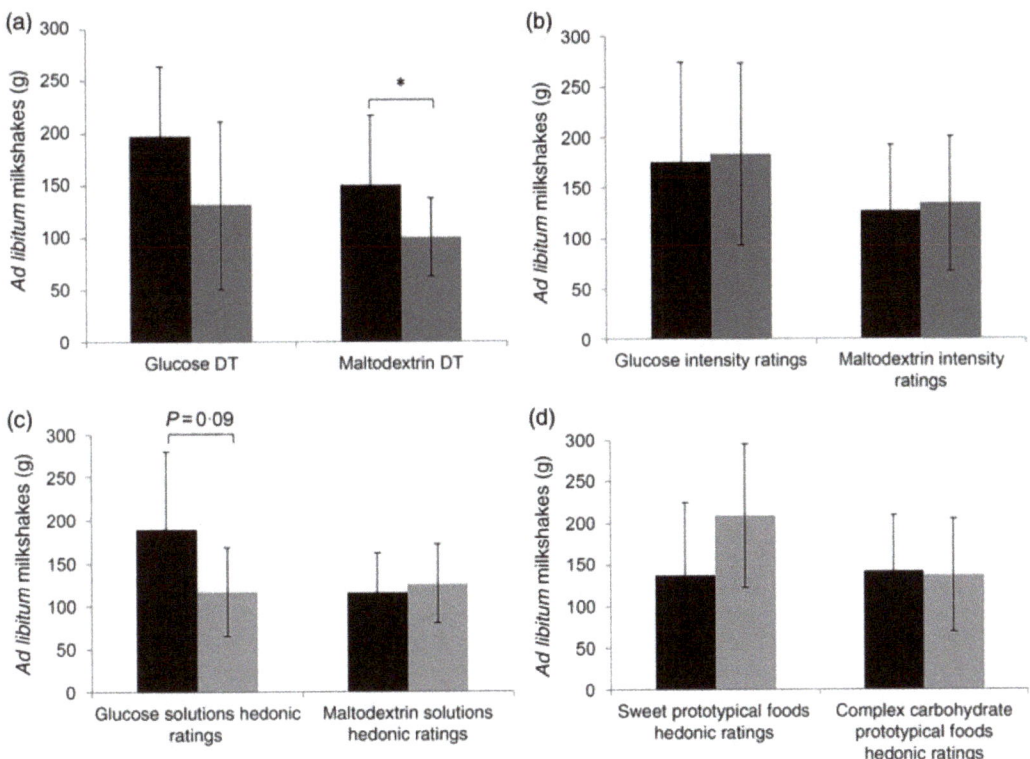

Figure 4. (**a**,**b**) *Ad libitum* milkshake intake means and standard deviations between more sensitive and less sensitive participants or those who experienced high and low intensity ratings. (**c**,**d**) *Ad libitum* milkshake intake means and standard deviations between participants with high hedonic ratings and low hedonic ratings for both sweet and complex carbohydrate solutions and prototypical foods. For sweet taste function and sweet hedonic ratings, comparisons were only made for sweet (glucose) milkshakes, and vice versa for complex carbohydrate (maltodextrin). * $p = 0.01$. DT = Detection threshold (reproduced with permission from the authors [108]).

Further research into the associations of oral complex sensitivity was conducted by Low et al. [109]. Using taste assessment methodology (detection threshold and suprathreshold intensity perception), participants tested two samples (maltodextrin and oligofructose). To determine sensitivity to the carbohydrate compounds, 34 participants (18 female) were grouped into tertiles: tertile 1 (participants experiencing higher sensitivity), tertile 2 (normal sensitivity), and tertile 3 (less sensitivity). This was done through assessing differences between the continuous variables (waist circumference, BMI, and habitual energy intake via quantitative FFQ) and the detection threshold ratings. The outcomes showed an association between carbohydrate taste sensitivity and consumption of complex carbohydrates. Experiencing strong taste intensity or being more sensitive to maltodextrin were associated with a greater energy and starch intake and also a greater waist circumference. The authors suggest that individuals with heightened oral sensitivity responses to maltodextrin may have developed preferences for complex carbohydrate flavors because of post-digestive nutritive cues (conditioned preferences), leading to a greater intake of energy and starch and consequently a larger waist circumference [109]. The body of research from Low et al. established the importance of assessing individual sensitivity to carbohydrates as it may influence other factors including taste intensity, waist circumference, energy intake, and consumption [108,109,138,140].

Carbohydrate taste research is in its infancy, with both animal and human data strongly indicating there are oral peripheral mechanism/s that respond to maltodextrins, that are associated with consumption, and the potential development of overweight and obesity. Future research should look at individual differences in 'taste' sensitivity to maltodextrins and incorporate advanced molecular biology techniques to identify the peripheral mechanisms along with downstream processing. If carbohydrate receptors are an accelerator of consumption when activated, understanding the structure of ligands may provide opportunities for new foods to help populations suffering from wasting, for example, cancer cachexia.

7. Conclusions

Taste receptors originally identified in the oral cavity have subsequently been located through the GIT, indicating that at least at the epithelium of the alimentary canal, there is commonality in peripheral sensing mechanisms. Taking this further, the concept of a coordinated macronutrient sensing throughout the alimentary canal seems logical. This involves multiple perceptual phenomena for each macronutrient, working in combination to tailor liking and preference of foods and regulate consumption through the activation of the satiety cascade. The macronutrient taste qualities working in combination may represent an important focus for future investigations on the links between the taste system and diet, given the variable outcomes of past studies, or qualities like sweet where no associations with diet have often been reported [7].

The extent and sophistication of research for fat, protein, and carbohydrate sensing is variable, with umami and fat tastes being mature fields, while kokumi and carbohydrate are in their relative infancy. A major area of interest is the directional difference in how the sensitivity of alimentary tastes moderate satiety and intake. Those more sensitive to the fat taste consume less fat and have lower BMI, while those who are more sensitive to maltodextrin (carbohydrate) appear to consume more carbohydrate and energy and have increased waist circumference. This indicates that individuals who are less sensitive to fat and more sensitive to carbohydrate may have more difficulty in achieving fullness without overconsuming fat, carbohydrate, and energy. More comprehensive studies are required including alimentary taste directed acute and habitual dietary interventions, satiety protocols, combined with molecular biology to understand the link between alimentary taste sensitivity, satiety hormones, diet, overweight/obesity, and taste receptor expression.

Author Contributions: Conceptualization, R.K.; Writing—original draft preparation, R.K., A.C. and I.H.; Writing—review and editing, R.K., A.C. and I.H. All authors have read and agreed to the published version of the manuscript.

Funding: This research received no external funding.

Conflicts of Interest: The authors declare no conflict of interest.

References

1. Beauchamp, G.K. Basic Taste: A Perceptual Concept. *J. Agric. Food Chem.* **2019**, *67*, 13860–13869. [CrossRef]
2. Hartley, I.E.; Liem, D.G.; Keast, R. Umami as an 'Alimentary' Taste. A New Perspective on Taste Classification. *Nutrients* **2019**, *11*, 182. [CrossRef] [PubMed]
3. Chaudhari, N.; Roper, S.D. The cell biology of taste. *J. Cell Biol.* **2010**, *190*, 285. [CrossRef] [PubMed]
4. Chandrashekar, J.; Hoon, M.A.; Ryba, N.J.P.; Zuker, C.S. The receptors and cells for mammalian taste. *Nature* **2006**, *444*, 288. [CrossRef]
5. Breslin, P.A.S. An Evolutionary Perspective on Food Review and Human Taste. *Curr. Biol.* **2013**, *23*, 409–418. [CrossRef] [PubMed]
6. Keast, R.S.J.; Roper, J. A Complex Relationship among Chemical Concentration, Detection Threshold, and Suprathreshold Intensity of Bitter Compounds. *Chem. Senses* **2007**, *32*, 245–253. [CrossRef]
7. Keast, R. Effects of sugar and fat consumption on sweet and fat taste. *Curr. Opin. Behav. Sci.* **2016**, *9*, 55–60. [CrossRef]
8. Hayes, J.E.; Keast, R.S.J. Two decades of supertasting: Where do we stand? *Physiol. Behav.* **2011**, *104*, 1072–1074. [CrossRef] [PubMed]
9. Webb, J.; Bolhuis, D.P.; Cicerale, S.; Hayes, J.E.; Keast, R. The Relationships Between Common Measurements of Taste Function. *Chemosens. Percept.* **2015**, *8*, 11–18. [CrossRef] [PubMed]

10. Nelson, G.; Chandrashekar, J.; Hoon, M.A.; Feng, L.; Zhao, G.; Ryba, N.J.P.; Zuker, C.S. An amino-acid taste receptor. *Nature* **2002**, *416*, 199. [CrossRef]
11. Liu, D.; Archer, N.; Duesing, K.; Hannan, G.; Keast, R. Mechanism of fat taste perception: Association with diet and obesity. *Prog. Lipid Res.* **2016**, *63*, 41–49. [CrossRef]
12. Ohsu, T.; Amino, Y.; Nagasaki, H.; Yamanaka, T.; Takeshita, S.; Hatanaka, T.; Maruyama, Y.; Miyamura, N.; Eto, Y. Involvement of the Calcium-sensing Receptor in Human Taste Perception. *J. Biol. Chem.* **2010**, *285*, 1016–1022. [CrossRef] [PubMed]
13. San Gabriel, A.; Uneyama, H. Amino acid sensing in the gastrointestinal tract. *Amino Acids* **2013**, *45*, 451–461. [CrossRef]
14. Daly, K.; Al-Rammahi, M.; Moran, A.; Marcello, M.; Ninomiya, Y.; Shirazi-Beechey, S.P. Sensing of amino acids by the gut-expressed taste receptor T1R1-T1R3 stimulates CCK secretion. *Am. J. Physiol. Gastrointest. Liver Physiol.* **2013**, *304*, G271–G282. [CrossRef] [PubMed]
15. Wauson, E.M.; Lorente-Rodríguez, A.; Cobb, M.H. Minireview: Nutrient Sensing by G Protein-Coupled Receptors. *Mol. Endocrinol.* **2013**, *27*, 1188–1197. [CrossRef] [PubMed]
16. Norton, M.; Murphy, K.G. Targeting gastrointestinal nutrient sensing mechanisms to treat obesity. *Curr. Opin. Pharmacol.* **2017**, *37*, 16–23. [CrossRef] [PubMed]
17. Uneyama, H.; Niijima, A.; San Gabriel, A.; Torii, K. Luminal amino acid sensing in the rat gastric mucosa. *Am. J. Physiol. Gastrointest. Liver Physiol.* **2006**, *291*, G1163–G1170. [CrossRef]
18. Depoortere, I. Taste receptors of the gut: Emerging roles in health and disease. *Gut* **2014**, *63*, 179–190. [CrossRef]
19. Hooper, L.; Abdelhamid, A.; Bunn, D.; Brown, T.; Summerbell, C.D.; Skeaff, C.M. Effects of total fat intake on body weight. *Cochrane Database Syst. Rev.* **2015**. [CrossRef]
20. Blundell, J.E.; Macdiarmid, J.I. Fat as a risk factor for overconsumption: Satiation, satiety, and patterns of eating. *J. Am. Diet. Assoc.* **1997**, *97*, S63–S69. [CrossRef]
21. Cotton, J.; Burley, V.; Blundell, J. Fat and satiety: Effect of fat in combination with either protein or carbohydrate. *Int. J. Obes.* **1993**, *17*, 63.
22. Bolhuis, D.P.; Costanzo, A.; Newman, L.P.; Keast, R.S.J. Salt Promotes Passive Overconsumption of Dietary Fat in Humans. *J. Nutr.* **2015**, *146*, 838–845. [CrossRef]
23. Heinze, J.M.; Preissl, H.; Fritsche, A.; Frank, S. Controversies in fat perception. *Physiol. Behav.* **2015**, *152*, 479–493. [CrossRef] [PubMed]
24. Running, C.A.; Craig, B.A.; Mattes, R.D. Oleogustus: The Unique Taste of Fat. *Chem. Senses* **2015**, *40*, 507–516. [CrossRef]
25. Keast, R.; Costanzo, A. Is fat the sixth taste primary? Evidence and implications. *Flavour* **2015**, *4*, 1–7. [CrossRef]
26. Che Man, Y.B.; Haryati, T.; Ghazali, H.M.; Asbi, B.A. Composition and thermal profile of crude palm oil and its products. *J. Am. Oil Chem. Soc.* **1999**, *76*, 237–242. [CrossRef]
27. Koriyama, T.; Wongso, S.; Watanabe, K.; Abe, H. Fatty Acid Compositions of Oil Species Affect the 5 Basic Taste Perceptions. *J. Food Sci.* **2002**, *67*, 868–873. [CrossRef]
28. Mukherjee, M. Human digestive and metabolic lipases—A brief review. *J. Mol. Catal. B Enzym.* **2003**, *22*, 369–376. [CrossRef]
29. Drewnowski, A. Why do we like fat? *J. Am. Diet. Assoc.* **1997**, *97*, S58–S62. [CrossRef]
30. Verhagen, J.V.; Kadohisa, M.; Rolls, E.T. Primate insular/opercular taste cortex: Neuronal representations of the viscosity, fat texture, grittiness, temperature, and taste of foods. *J. Neurophysiol.* **2004**, *92*, 1685–1699. [CrossRef]
31. Marciani, L.; Gowland, P.A.; Spiller, R.C.; Manoj, P.; Moore, R.J.; Young, P.; Fillery-Travis, A.J. Effect of meal viscosity and nutrients on satiety, intragastric dilution, and emptying assessed by MRI. *Am. J. Physiol. Gastrointest. Liver Physiol.* **2001**, *280*. [CrossRef] [PubMed]
32. De Graaf, C. Why liquid energy results in overconsumption. *Proc. Nutr. Soc.* **2011**, *70*, 162–170. [CrossRef]
33. Bolhuis, D.P.; Forde, C.G.; Cheng, Y.; Xu, H.; Martin, N.; de Graaf, C. Slow Food: Sustained Impact of Harder Foods on the Reduction in Energy Intake over the Course of the Day. *PLoS ONE* **2014**, *9*, e93370. [CrossRef] [PubMed]
34. Matzinger, D.; Degen, L.; Drewe, J.; Meuli, J.; Duebendorfen, R.; Ruckstuhl, N.; D'Amato, M.; Rovati, L.; Beglinger, C. The role of long chain fatty acids in regulating food intake and cholecystokinin release in humans. *Gut* **2000**, *46*, 688–693. [CrossRef] [PubMed]
35. Stillman, M.A.; Maibach, H.I.; Shallita, A.R. Relative irritancy of free fatty acids of different chain length. *Contact Dermat.* **1975**, *1*, 65–69. [CrossRef]
36. Colombo, M.; Trevisi, P.; Gandolfi, G.; Bosi, P. Assessment of the presence of chemosensing receptors based on bitter and fat taste in the gastrointestinal tract of young pig1. *J. Anim. Sci.* **2012**, *90*, 128–130. [CrossRef] [PubMed]
37. Galindo, M.M.; Voigt, N.; Stein, J.; van Lengerich, J.; Raguse, J.-D.; Hofmann, T.; Meyerhof, W.; Behrens, M. G Protein-Coupled Receptors in Human Fat Taste Perception. *Chem. Senses* **2012**, *37*, 123–139. [CrossRef]
38. Tanaka, T.; Yano, T.; Adachi, T.; Koshimizu, T.A.; Hirasawa, A.; Tsujimoto, G. Cloning and characterization of the rat free fatty acid receptor GPR120: In vivo effect of the natural ligand on GLP-1 secretion and proliferation of pancreatic β cells. *Naunyn-Schmiedeberg's Arch. Pharmacol.* **2008**, *377*, 515–522. [CrossRef]
39. Liu, D.; Costanzo, A.; Evans, M.D.M.; Archer, N.S.; Nowson, C.; Duesing, K.; Keast, R. Expression of the candidate fat taste receptors in human fungiform papillae and the association with fat taste function. *Br. J. Nutr.* **2018**, *120*, 64–73. [CrossRef] [PubMed]

40. Cvijanovic, N.; Feinle-Bisset, C.; Young, R.L.; Little, T.J. Oral and intestinal sweet and fat tasting: Impact of receptor polymorphisms and dietary modulation for metabolic disease. *Nutr. Rev.* **2015**, *73*, 318–334. [CrossRef]
41. Steinert, R.E.; Beglinger, C. Nutrient sensing in the gut: Interactions between chemosensory cells, visceral afferents and the secretion of satiation peptides. *Physiol. Behav.* **2011**, *105*, 62–70. [CrossRef]
42. Abdoul-Azize, S.; Selvakumar, S.; Sadou, H.; Besnard, P.; Khan, N.A. Ca^{2+} signaling in taste bud cells and spontaneous preference for fat: Unresolved roles of CD36 and GPR120. *Biochimie* **2014**, *96*, 8–13. [CrossRef] [PubMed]
43. Cartoni, C.; Yasumatsu, K.; Ohkuri, T.; Shigemura, N.; Yoshida, R.; Godinot, N.; Le Coutre, J.; Ninomiya, Y.; Damak, S. Taste preference for fatty acids is mediated by GPR40 and GPR120. *J. Neurosci.* **2010**, *30*, 8376–8382. [CrossRef]
44. Martin, C.; Passilly-Degrace, P.; Chevrot, M.; Ancel, D.; Sparks, S.M.; Drucker, D.J.; Besnard, P. Lipid-mediated release of GLP-1 by mouse taste buds from circumvallate papillae: Putative involvement of GPR120 and impact on taste sensitivity. *J. Lipid Res.* **2012**, *53*, 2256–2265. [CrossRef] [PubMed]
45. Hirasawa, A.; Tsumaya, K.; Awaji, T.; Katsuma, S.; Adachi, T.; Yamada, M.; Sugimoto, Y.; Miyazaki, S.; Tsujimoto, G. Free fatty acids regulate gut incretin glucagon-like peptide-1 secretion through GPR120. *Nat. Med.* **2005**, *11*, 90–94. [CrossRef]
46. Ichimura, A.; Hirasawa, A.; Poulain-Godefroy, O.; Bonnefond, A.; Hara, T.; Yengo, L.; Kimura, I.; Leloire, A.; Liu, N.; Iida, K.; et al. Dysfunction of lipid sensor GPR120 leads to obesity in both mouse and human. *Nature* **2012**, *483*, 350–354. [CrossRef] [PubMed]
47. Lo Verme, J.; Gaetani, S.; Fu, J.; Oveisi, F.; Burton, K.; Piomelli, D. Regulation of food intake by oleoylethanolamide. *Cell. Mol. Life Sci.* **2005**, *62*, 708–716. [CrossRef]
48. Schwartz, G.J.; Fu, J.; Astarita, G.; Li, X.; Gaetani, S.; Campolongo, P.; Cuomo, V.; Piomelli, D. The Lipid Messenger OEA Links Dietary Fat Intake to Satiety. *Cell Metab.* **2008**, *8*, 281–288. [CrossRef] [PubMed]
49. Sundaresan, S.; Shahid, R.; Riehl, T.E.; Chandra, R.; Nassir, F.; Stenson, W.F.; Liddle, R.A.; Abumrad, N.A. CD36-dependent signaling mediates fatty acid-induced gut release of secretin and cholecystokinin. *FASEB J.* **2013**, *27*, 1191–1202. [CrossRef]
50. Edfalk, S.; Steneberg, P.; Edlund, H. Gpr40 is expressed in enteroendocrine cells and mediates free fatty acid stimulation of incretin secretion. *Diabetes* **2008**, *57*, 2280–2287. [CrossRef]
51. Liou, A.P.; Lu, X.; Sei, Y.; Zhao, X.; Pechhold, S.; Carrero, R.J.; Raybould, H.E.; Wank, S. The G-protein-coupled receptor GPR40 directly mediates Long-chain fatty acid-induced secretion of cholecystokinin. *Gastroenterology* **2011**, *140*, 903–912. [CrossRef] [PubMed]
52. Kles, K.A.; Chang, E.B. Short-chain fatty acids impact on intestinal adaptation, inflammation, carcinoma, and failure. *Gastroenterology* **2006**, *130*, S100–S105. [CrossRef]
53. Asano, M.; Hong, G.; Matsuyama, Y.; Wang, W.; Izumi, S.; Izumi, M.; Toda, T.; Kudo, T.-a. Association of Oral Fat Sensitivity with Body Mass Index, Taste Preference, and Eating Habits in Healthy Japanese Young Adults. *Tohoku J. Exp. Med.* **2016**, *238*, 93–103. [CrossRef] [PubMed]
54. Costanzo, A.; Orellana, L.; Nowson, C.; Duesing, K.; Keast, R. Fat Taste Sensitivity Is Associated with Short-Term and Habitual Fat Intake. *Nutrients* **2017**, *9*, 781. [CrossRef] [PubMed]
55. Martínez-Ruiz, N.R.; López-Díaz, J.A.; Wall-Medrano, A.; Jiménez-Castro, J.A.; Angulo, O. Oral fat perception is related with body mass index, preference and consumption of high-fat foods. *Physiol. Behav.* **2014**, *129*, 36–42. [CrossRef] [PubMed]
56. Running, C.A.; Mattes, R.D.; Tucker, R.M. Fat taste in humans: Sources of within- and between-subject variability. *Prog. Lipid Res.* **2013**, *52*, 438–445. [CrossRef]
57. Tucker, R.M.; Nuessle, T.M.; Garneau, N.L.; Smutzer, G.; Mattes, R.D. No Difference in Perceived Intensity of Linoleic Acid in the Oral Cavity between Obese and Nonobese Individuals. *Chem. Senses* **2015**, *40*, 557–563. [CrossRef] [PubMed]
58. Newman, L.P.; Keast, R.S.J. The Test-Retest Reliability of Fatty Acid Taste Thresholds. *Chemosens. Percept.* **2013**, *6*, 70–77. [CrossRef]
59. Newman, L.P.; Bolhuis, D.P.; Torres, S.J.; Keast, R.S. Dietary fat restriction increases fat taste sensitivity in people with obesity. *Obesity* **2016**, *24*, 328–334. [CrossRef]
60. Stewart, J.E.; Keast, R.S. Recent fat intake modulates fat taste sensitivity in lean and overweight subjects. *Int. J. Obes.* **2012**, *36*, 834–842. [CrossRef]
61. Costanzo, A.; Nowson, C.; Orellana, L.; Bolhuis, D.; Duesing, K.; Keast, R. Effect of dietary fat intake and genetics on fat taste sensitivity: A co-twin randomized controlled trial. *Am. J. Clin. Nutr.* **2018**, *107*, 683–694. [CrossRef]
62. Costanzo, A.; Liu, D.; Nowson, C.; Duesing, K.; Archer, N.; Bowe, S.; Keast, R. A low-fat diet up-regulates expression of fatty acid taste receptor gene FFAR4 in fungiform papillae in humans: A co-twin randomised controlled trial. *Br. J. Nutr.* **2019**, *122*, 1212–1220. [CrossRef]
63. Costanzo, A.; Russell, C.G.; Lewin, S.; Keast, R. A Fatty Acid Mouth Rinse Decreases Self-Reported Hunger and Increases Self-Reported Fullness in Healthy Australian Adults: A Randomized Cross-Over Trial. *Nutrients* **2020**, *12*, 678. [CrossRef] [PubMed]
64. French, S.J.; Conlon, C.A.; Mutuma, S.T.; Arnold, M.; Read, N.W.; Meijer, G.; Francis, J. The effects of intestinal infusion of long-chain fatty acids on food intake in humans. *Gastroenterology* **2000**, *119*, 943–948. [CrossRef]
65. Mattes, R.D. Fat taste and lipid metabolism in humans. *Physiol. Behav.* **2005**, *86*, 691–697. [CrossRef]
66. Brennan, I.M.; Luscombe-Marsh, N.D.; Seimon, R.V.; Otto, B.; Horowitz, M.; Wishart, J.M.; Feinle-Bisset, C. Effects of fat, protein, and carbohydrate and protein load on appetite, plasma cholecystokinin, peptide YY, and ghrelin, and energy intake in lean and obese men. *Am. J. Physiol. Gastrointest. Liver Physiol.* **2012**, *303*, 129–140. [CrossRef] [PubMed]

67. Pepino, M.Y.; Love-Gregory, L.; Klein, S.; Abumrad, N.A. The fatty acid translocase gene CD36 and lingual lipase influence oral sensitivity to fat in obese subjects. *J. Lipid Res.* **2012**, *53*, 561–566. [CrossRef] [PubMed]
68. Stewart, J.E.; Seimon, R.V.; Otto, B.; Keast, R.S.; Clifton, P.M.; Feinle-Bisset, C. Marked differences in gustatory and gastrointestinal sensitivity to oleic acid between lean and obese men. *Am. J. Clin. Nutr.* **2011**, *93*, 703–711. [CrossRef] [PubMed]
69. Keast, R.S.; Azzopardi, K.M.; Newman, L.P.; Haryono, R.Y. Impaired oral fatty acid chemoreception is associated with acute excess energy consumption. *Appetite* **2014**, *80*, 1–6. [CrossRef]
70. Collier, G.; O'Dea, K. The effect of coingestion of fat on the glucose, insulin, and gastric inhibitory polypeptide responses to carbohydrate and protein. *Am. J. Clin. Nutr.* **1983**, *37*, 941–944. [CrossRef]
71. Gibbons, C.; Caudwell, P.; Finlayson, G.; Webb, D.-L.; Hellström, P.M.; Näslund, E.; Blundell, J.E. Comparison of Postprandial Profiles of Ghrelin, Active GLP-1, and Total PYY to Meals Varying in Fat and Carbohydrate and Their Association With Hunger and the Phases of Satiety. *J. Clin. Endocrinol. Metab.* **2013**, *98*, E847–E855. [CrossRef] [PubMed]
72. Helou, N.; Obeid, O.; Azar, S.T.; Hwalla, N. Variation of Postprandial PYY_{3-36} Response following Ingestion of Differing Macronutrient Meals in Obese Females. *Ann. Nutr. Metab.* **2008**, *52*, 188–195. [CrossRef] [PubMed]
73. Tannous dit El Khoury, D.; Obeid, O.; Azar, S.T.; Hwalla, N. Variations in Postprandial Ghrelin Status following Ingestion of High-Carbohydrate, High-Fat, and High-Protein Meals in Males. *Ann. Nutr. Metab.* **2006**, *50*, 260–269. [CrossRef]
74. Van der Klaauw, A.A.; Keogh, J.M.; Henning, E.; Trowse, V.M.; Dhillo, W.S.; Ghatei, M.A.; Farooqi, I.S. High protein intake stimulates postprandial GLP1 and PYY release. *Obesity* **2013**, *21*, 1602–1607. [CrossRef]
75. Robertson, M.D.; Jackson, K.G.; Williams, C.M.; Fielding, B.A.; Frayn, K.N. Prolonged effects of modified sham feeding on energy substrate mobilization. *Am. J. Clin. Nutr.* **2001**, *73*, 111–117. [CrossRef]
76. Wisén, O.; Björvell, H.; Cantor, P.; Johansson, C.; Theodorsson, E. Plasma concentrations of regulatory peptides in obesity following modified sham feeding (MSF) and a liquid test meal. *Regul. Pept.* **1992**, *39*, 43–54. [CrossRef]
77. Heinze, J.M.; Costanzo, A.; Baselier, I.; Fritsche, A.; Frank-Podlech, S.; Keast, R. Detection thresholds for four different fatty stimuli are associated with increased dietary intake of processed high-caloric food. *Appetite* **2018**, *123*, 7–13. [CrossRef]
78. Kindleysides, S.; Beck, K.; Walsh, D.; Henderson, L.; Jayasinghe, S.; Golding, M.; Breier, B. Fat Sensation: Fatty Acid Taste and Olfaction Sensitivity and the Link with Disinhibited Eating Behaviour. *Nutrients* **2017**, *9*, 879. [CrossRef] [PubMed]
79. Stewart, J.E.; Feinle-Bisset, C.; Golding, M.; Delahunty, C.; Clifton, P.M.; Keast, R.S. Oral sensitivity to fatty acids, food consumption and BMI in human subjects. *Br. J. Nutr.* **2010**, *104*, 145–152. [CrossRef]
80. Stewart, J.E.; Newman, L.P.; Keast, R.S. Oral sensitivity to oleic acid is associated with fat intake and body mass index. *Clin. Nutr.* **2011**, *30*, 838–844. [CrossRef] [PubMed]
81. Little, T. Oral and gastrointestinal sensing of dietary fat and appetite regulation in humans: Modification by diet and obesity. *Front. Neurosci.* **2010**, *1*, 178. [CrossRef] [PubMed]
82. Feltrin, K.L.; Little, T.J.; Meyer, J.H.; Horowitz, M.; Smout, A.J.P.M.; Wishart, J.; Pilichiewicz, A.N.; Rades, T.; Chapman, I.M.; Feinle-Bisset, C. Effects of intraduodenal fatty acids on appetite, antropyloroduodenal motility, and plasma CCK and GLP-1 in humans vary with their chain length. *Am. J. Physiol. Regul. Integr. Comp. Physiol.* **2004**, *287*, 524–533. [CrossRef] [PubMed]
83. Feltrin, K.L.; Little, T.J.; Meyer, J.H.; Horowitz, M.; Rades, T.; Wishart, J.; Feinle-Bisset, C. Comparative effects of intraduodenal infusions of lauric and oleic acids on antropyloroduodenal motility, plasma cholecystokinin and peptide YY, appetite, and energy intake in healthy men. *Am. J. Clin. Nutr.* **2008**, *87*, 1181–1187. [CrossRef]
84. Tucker, R.M.; Edlinger, C.; Craig, B.A.; Mattes, R.D. Associations Between BMI and Fat Taste Sensitivity in Humans. *Chem. Senses* **2014**, *39*, 349–357. [CrossRef]
85. Tucker, R.M.; Kaiser, K.A.; Parman, M.A.; George, B.J.; Allison, D.B.; Mattes, R.D. Comparisons of Fatty Acid Taste Detection Thresholds in People Who Are Lean vs. Overweight or Obese: A Systematic Review and Meta-Analysis. *PLoS ONE* **2017**, *12*, e0169583. [CrossRef] [PubMed]
86. Ranganath, L.R.; Beety, J.M.; Morgan, L.M.; Wright, J.W.; Howland, R.; Marks, V. Attenuated GLP-1 secretion in obesity: Cause or consequence? *Gut* **1996**, *38*, 916–919. [CrossRef]
87. French, S.J.; Murray, B.; Rumsey, R.D.E.; Sepple, C.P.; Read, N.W. Preliminary studies on the gastrointestinal responses to fatty meals in obese people. *Int. J. Obes.* **1993**, *17*, 295–300.
88. van Dongen, M.V.; van den Berg, M.C.; Vink, N.; Kok, F.J.; de Graaf, C. Taste–nutrient relationships in commonly consumed foods. *Br. J. Nutr.* **2012**, *108*, 140–147. [CrossRef]
89. Beauchamp, G.K.; Pearson, P. Human development and umami taste. *Physiol. Behav.* **1991**, *49*, 1009–1012. [CrossRef]
90. Naim, M.; Ohara, I.; Kare, M.R.; Levinson, M. Interaction of MSG taste with nutrition: Perspectives in consummatory behavior and digestion. *Physiol. Behav.* **1991**, *49*, 1019–1024. [CrossRef]
91. Yamaguchi, S. The Synergistic Taste Effect of Monosodium Glutamate and Disodium 5'-Inosinate. *J. Food Sci.* **1967**, *32*, 473–478. [CrossRef]
92. Li, X.; Staszewski, L.; Xu, H.; Durick, K.; Zoller, M.; Adler, E. Human receptors for sweet and umami taste. *Proc. Natl. Acad. Sci. USA* **2002**, *99*, 4692–4696. [CrossRef] [PubMed]
93. Zhao, G.Q.; Zhang, Y.; Hoon, M.A.; Chandrashekar, J.; Erlenbach, I.; Ryba, N.J.P.; Zuker, C.S. The receptors for mammalian sweet and umami taste. *Cell* **2003**, *115*, 255–266. [CrossRef]
94. Yang, J.; Bai, W.; Zeng, X.; Cui, C. Gamma glutamyl peptides: The food source, enzymatic synthesis, kokumi-active and the potential functional properties A review. *Trends Food Sci. Technol.* **2019**, *91*, 339–346. [CrossRef]

95. Rhyu, M.R.; Song, A.Y.; Kim, E.Y.; Son, H.J.; Kim, Y.; Mummalaneni, S.; Qian, J.; Grider, J.R.; Lyall, V. Kokumi taste active peptides modulate salt and umami taste. *Nutrients* **2020**, *12*, 1198. [CrossRef]
96. Maruyama, Y.; Yasuda, R.; Kuroda, M.; Eto, Y. Kokumi substances, enhancers of basic tastes, induce responses in calcium-sensing receptor expressing taste cells. *PLoS ONE* **2012**, *7*, e34489. [CrossRef]
97. Amino, Y.; Nakazawa, M.; Kaneko, M.; Miyaki, T.; Miyamura, N.; Maruyama, Y.; Eto, Y. Structure-CaSR-Activity Relation of Kokumi γ-Glutamyl Peptides. *Chem. Pharm. Bull.* **2016**, *64*, 1181–1189. [CrossRef]
98. Anderson, G.H.; Fabek, H.; Akilen, R.; Chatterjee, D.; Kubant, R. Acute effects of monosodium glutamate addition to whey protein on appetite, food intake, blood glucose, insulin and gut hormones in healthy young men. *Appetite* **2018**, *120*, 92–99. [CrossRef]
99. Tey, S.L.; Salleh, N.; Henry, C.J.; Forde, C.G. Effects of Consuming Preloads with Different Energy Density and Taste Quality on Energy Intake and Postprandial Blood Glucose. *Nutrients* **2018**, *10*, 161. [CrossRef]
100. Hosaka, H.; Kusano, M.; Zai, H.; Kawada, A.; Kuribayashi, S.; Shimoyama, Y.; Nagoshi, A.; Maeda, M.; Kawamura, O.; Mori, M. Monosodium glutamate stimulates secretion of glucagon-like peptide-1 and reduces postprandial glucose after a lipid-containing meal. *Aliment. Pharmacol. Ther.* **2012**, *36*, 895–903. [CrossRef]
101. Vancleef, L.; Van Den Broeck, T.; Thijs, T.; Steensels, S.; Briand, L.; Tack, J.; Depoortere, I. Chemosensory signalling pathways involved in sensing of amino acids by the ghrelin cell. *Sci. Rep.* **2015**, *5*, 15725. [CrossRef]
102. Steinert, R.E.; Feinle-Bisset, C.; Asarian, L.; Horowitz, M.; Beglinger, C.; Geary, N. Ghrelin, CCK, GLP-1, and PYY(3-36): Secretory Controls and Physiological Roles in Eating and Glycemia in Health, Obesity, and After RYGB. *Physiol. Rev.* **2017**, *97*, 411–463. [CrossRef]
103. Yang, J.; Bai, W.; Zeng, X.; Cui, C. γ-[Glu](n=1,2)-Phe/-Met/-Val stimulates gastrointestinal hormone (CCK and GLP-1) secretion by activating the calcium-sensing receptor. *Food Funct.* **2019**, *10*, 4071–4080. [CrossRef] [PubMed]
104. Masic, U.; Yeomans, M.R. Umami flavor enhances appetite but also increases satiety. *Am. J. Clin. Nutr.* **2014**, *100*, 532–538. [CrossRef]
105. Masic, U.; Yeomans, M.R. Monosodium glutamate delivered in a protein-rich soup improves subsequent energy compensation. *J. Nutr. Sci.* **2014**, *3*, e15. [CrossRef]
106. Carter, B.E.; Monsivais, P.; Perrigue, M.M.; Drewnowski, A. Supplementing chicken broth with monosodium glutamate reduces hunger and desire to snack but does not affect energy intake in women. *Br. J. Nutr.* **2011**, *106*, 1441–1448. [CrossRef]
107. Noel, C.A.; Finlayson, G.; Dando, R. Prolonged Exposure to Monosodium Glutamate in Healthy Young Adults Decreases Perceived Umami Taste and Diminishes Appetite for Savory Foods. *J. Nutr.* **2018**, *148*, 980–988. [CrossRef]
108. Low, J.Y.Q.; Lacy, K.E.; McBride, R.L.; Keast, R.S.J. Associations between sweet taste function, oral complex carbohydrate sensitivity, liking and consumption of ad libitum sweet and non-sweet carbohydrate milkshakes among female adults. *Br. J. Nutr.* **2019**, *122*, 829–840. [CrossRef]
109. Low, J.Y.; Lacy, K.E.; McBride, R.L.; Keast, R.S. Carbohydrate Taste Sensitivity Is Associated with Starch Intake and Waist Circumference in Adults. *J. Nutr.* **2017**, *147*, 2235–2242. [CrossRef] [PubMed]
110. Kurihara, K. Umami the Fifth Basic Taste: History of Studies on Receptor Mechanisms and Role as a Food Flavor. *BioMed Res. Int.* **2015**, *2015*, 189402. [CrossRef] [PubMed]
111. Masic, U.; Yeomans, M.R. Does acute or habitual protein deprivation influence liking for monosodium glutamate? *Physiol. Behav.* **2017**, *171*, 79–86. [CrossRef] [PubMed]
112. Griffioen-Roose, S.; Mars, M.; Siebelink, E.; Finlayson, G.; Tomé, D.; de Graaf, C. Protein status elicits compensatory changes in food intake and food preferences. *Am. J. Clin. Nutr.* **2012**, *95*, 32–38. [CrossRef] [PubMed]
113. Overberg, J.; Hummel, T.; Krude, H.; Wiegand, S. Differences in taste sensitivity between obese and non-obese children and adolescents. *Arch. Dis. Child.* **2012**, *97*, 1048. [CrossRef]
114. Pepino, M.Y.; Finkbeiner, S.; Beauchamp, G.K.; Mennella, J.A. Obese Women Have Lower Monosodium Glutamate Taste Sensitivity and Prefer Higher Concentrations Than Do Normal-weight Women. *Obesity* **2010**, *18*, 959–965. [CrossRef]
115. Van Langeveld, A.W.B.; Teo, P.S.; de Vries, J.H.M.; Feskens, E.J.M.; de Graaf, C.; Mars, M. Dietary taste patterns by sex and weight status in the Netherlands. *Br. J. Nutr.* **2018**, *119*, 1195–1206. [CrossRef] [PubMed]
116. Luscombe-Marsh, N.D.; Smeets, A.J.P.G.; Westerterp-Plantenga, M.S. Taste sensitivity for monosodium glutamate and an increased liking of dietary protein. *Br. J. Nutr.* **2008**, *99*, 904–908. [CrossRef] [PubMed]
117. Miyaki, T.; Imada, T.; Shuzhen Hao, S.; Kimura, E. Monosodium l-glutamate in soup reduces subsequent energy intake from high-fat savoury food in overweight and obese women. *Br. J. Nutr.* **2016**, *115*, 176–184. [CrossRef] [PubMed]
118. Imoscopi, A.; Inelmen, E.M.; Sergi, G.; Miotto, F.; Manzato, E. Taste loss in the elderly: Epidemiology, causes and consequences. *Aging Clin. Exp. Res.* **2012**, *24*, 570–579. [CrossRef]
119. Sasano, T.; Satoh-Kuriwada, S.; Shoji, N.; Iikubo, M.; Kawai, M.; Uneyama, H.; Sakamoto, M. Important Role of Umami Taste Sensitivity in Oral and Overall Health. *Curr. Pharm. Des.* **2014**, *20*, 2750–2754. [CrossRef]
120. Sasano, T.; Satoh-Kuriwada, S.; Shoji, N. The important role of umami taste in oral and overall health. *Flavour* **2015**, *4*, 1–5. [CrossRef]
121. Schiffman, S.S.; Miletic, I.D. Effect of taste and smell on secretion rate of salivary IgA in elderly and young persons. *J. Nutr. Health Aging* **1999**, *3*, 158–164. [PubMed]

122. Mathey, M.-F.A.M.; Siebelink, E.; de Graaf, C.; Van Staveren, W.A. Flavor Enhancement of Food Improves Dietary Intake and Nutritional Status of Elderly Nursing Home Residents. *J. Gerontol. Ser. A* **2001**, *56*, M200–M205. [CrossRef]
123. Valenzuela, C.; Aguilera, J.M. Effects of maltodextrin on hygroscopicity and crispness of apple leathers. *J. Food Eng.* **2015**, *144*, 1–9. [CrossRef]
124. Trumbo, P.R.; Appleton, K.M.; de Graaf, K.; Hayes, J.E.; Baer, D.J.; Beauchamp, G.K.; Dwyer, J.T.; Fernstrom, J.D.; Klurfeld, D.M.; Mattes, R.D.; et al. Perspective: Measuring Sweetness in Foods, Beverages, and Diets: Toward Understanding the Role of Sweetness in Health. *Adv. Nutr.* **2020**. [CrossRef]
125. Feigin, M.B.; Sclafani, A.; Sunday, S.R. Species differences in polysaccharide and sugar taste preferences. *Neurosci. Biobehav. Rev.* **1987**, *11*, 231–240. [CrossRef]
126. Hettinger, T.P.; Frank, M.E.; Myers, W.E. Are the tastes of polycose and monosodium glutamate unique? *Chem. Senses* **1996**, *21*, 341–347. [CrossRef]
127. De Araujo, I.E.; Lin, T.; Veldhuizen, M.G.; Small, D.M. Metabolic regulation of brain response to food cues. *Curr. Biol.* **2013**, *23*, 878–883. [CrossRef] [PubMed]
128. Yeomans, M.R.; Leitch, M.; Gould, N.J.; Mobini, S. Differential hedonic, sensory and behavioral changes associated with flavor–nutrient and flavor–flavor learning. *Physiol. Behav.* **2008**, *93*, 798–806. [CrossRef]
129. Yeomans, M.R. Flavour–nutrient learning in humans: An elusive phenomenon? *Physiol. Behav.* **2012**, *106*, 345–355. [CrossRef] [PubMed]
130. Sclafani, A. Starch and sugar tastes in rodents: An update. *Brain Res. Bull.* **1991**, *27*, 383–386. [CrossRef]
131. Sclafani, A. The sixth taste? *Appetite* **2004**, *43*, 1–3. [CrossRef] [PubMed]
132. Sclafani, A.; Mann, S. Carbohydrate taste preferences in rats: Glucose, sucrose, maltose, fructose and polycose compared. *Physiol. Behav.* **1987**, *40*, 563–568. [CrossRef]
133. Brietzke, C.; Franco-Alvarenga, P.E.; Coelho-Junior, H.J.; Silveira, R.; Asano, R.Y.; Pires, F.O. Effects of Carbohydrate Mouth Rinse on Cycling Time Trial Performance: A Systematic Review and Meta-Analysis. *Sports Med.* **2019**, *49*, 57–66. [CrossRef] [PubMed]
134. Chambers, E.; Bridge, M.; Jones, D. Carbohydrate sensing in the human mouth: Effects on exercise performance and brain activity. *J. Physiol.* **2009**, *587*, 1779–1794. [CrossRef] [PubMed]
135. Lapis, T.J.; Penner, M.H.; Lim, J. Evidence that humans can taste glucose polymers. *Chem. Senses* **2014**, *39*, 737–747. [CrossRef]
136. Lapis, T.J.; Penner, M.H.; Lim, J. Humans can taste glucose oligomers independent of the hT1R2/hT1R3 sweet taste receptor. *Chem. Senses* **2016**, *41*, 755–762. [CrossRef]
137. Lim, J.; Pullicin, A.J. Oral carbohydrate sensing: Beyond sweet taste. *Physiol. Behav.* **2019**, *202*, 14–25. [CrossRef]
138. Low, J.Y.Q.; Lacy, K.E.; McBride, R.L.; Keast, R.S.J. Evidence supporting oral sensitivity to complex carbohydrates independent of sweet taste sensitivity in humans. *PLoS ONE* **2017**, *12*, e0188784. [CrossRef]
139. Jeukendrup, A.E.; Chambers, E.S. Oral carbohydrate sensing and exercise performance. *Curr. Opin. Clin. Nutr. Metab. Care* **2010**, *13*, 447–451. [CrossRef]
140. Low, J.Y.Q.; Lacy, K.E.; McBride, R.L.; Keast, R.S.J. The Associations Between Oral Complex Carbohydrate Sensitivity, BMI, Liking, and Consumption of Complex Carbohydrate Based Foods. *J. Food. Sci.* **2018**, *83*, 2227–2236. [CrossRef] [PubMed]

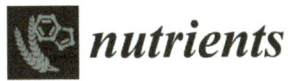

Review

Gastric Sensory and Motor Functions and Energy Intake in Health and Obesity—Therapeutic Implications

Lizeth Cifuentes [1], Michael Camilleri [2] and Andres Acosta [2,*]

[1] Precision Medicine for Obesity Program and Clinical Enteric Neuroscience Translational and Epidemiological Research Program, Department of Medicine, Mayo Clinic, Rochester, MN 55905, USA; Cifuentes.adriana@mayo.edu

[2] Division of Gastroenterology and Hepatology, Mayo Clinic, 200 First Street SW, Rochester, MN 55905, USA; Camilleri.michael@mayo.edu

* Correspondence: acosta.andres@mayo.edu; Tel.: +1-507-266-6931

Abstract: Sensory and motor functions of the stomach, including gastric emptying and accommodation, have significant effects on energy consumption and appetite. Obesity is characterized by energy imbalance; altered gastric functions, such as rapid gastric emptying and large fasting gastric volume in obesity, may result in increased food intake prior to reaching usual fullness and increased appetite. Thus, many different interventions for obesity, including different diets, anti-obesity medications, bariatric endoscopy, and surgery, alter gastric functions and gastrointestinal motility. In this review, we focus on the role of the gastric and intestinal functions in food intake, pathophysiology of obesity, and obesity management.

Keywords: food intake; gastric emptying; gastric accommodation; satiation; satiety

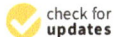

Citation: Cifuentes, L.; Camilleri, M.; Acosta, A. Gastric Sensory and Motor Functions and Energy Intake in Health and Obesity—Therapeutic Implications. *Nutrients* **2021**, *13*, 1158. https://doi.org/10.3390/nu13041158

Academic Editor: Christine Feinle-Bisset

Received: 23 January 2021
Accepted: 26 March 2021
Published: 1 April 2021

Publisher's Note: MDPI stays neutral with regard to jurisdictional claims in published maps and institutional affiliations.

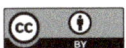

Copyright: © 2021 by the authors. Licensee MDPI, Basel, Switzerland. This article is an open access article distributed under the terms and conditions of the Creative Commons Attribution (CC BY) license (https://creativecommons.org/licenses/by/4.0/).

1. Introduction

Obesity is a chronic and complex disease marked by a body mass index (BMI) greater than 30 kg/m^2 and affects almost 600 million adults worldwide [1]. Obesity complexity is related to a multi-factorial imbalance between energy intake and energy expenditure, leading to excess energy storage [2]. The mechanism of moving from fasting to food-seeking and food intake is closely controlled by homeostatic and hedonic signals that combine to influence eating behavior. This homeostatic regulation involves peripheral organs and the nervous system and is referred to as the gut–brain–adipose axis [3,4]. The behavioral background is essential for explaining normal and disorderly feeding, particularly, excessive overeating, contributing to the obesity crisis. However, the central neural mechanism integrating food reward and gastric sensory and enteroendocrine signals has been adequately reviewed elsewhere [5–9].

In the gut, the stomach plays a significant role in regulating hunger, satiation, and satiety [10]. The stomach can sense mechanical forces, control the rate at which calories reach the duodenum, and trigger gastrointestinal peptide secretion. These functions play an essential role in providing short-term and long-term signals to control food intake [10,11]. Alterations in gastrointestinal motility observed in patients with obesity may contribute to weight gain [12–14]. Therefore, interventions designed to modify gastrointestinal motility or have a secondary impact on gastric physiology are components of obesity treatment.

The present paper is a narrative review based on publications focused on physiological measurements of gastric functions and their potential contribution to obesity. In particular, to understand the effects on gastric sensory and motor functions of different obesity treatments, we considered data from case-control, cross-sectional, cohort, and randomized controlled clinical trials. We excluded data measured by paracetamol drug absorption due to the potential confounding factors. Similarly, we have assessed lifestyle interventions, such as low-calorie diets, on objective measurements of gastric emptying and compared them to subjective scales for appetite. Our assessment included Food and Drug Administration (FDA) approved medications in use for diabetes or obesity. We also examined two meta-analyses that appraised effects of bariatric and surgical procedures on gastric emptying, and we updated the literature search to December 2020.

In this review, we examined the relationship between gastric sensory and motor functions with food intake. We focused first on the regulation of these functions by endocrine and neural pathways on health and discuss the abnormalities observed in obesity. We considered the significance of these functions in the pathophysiology of obesity, the contradictory findings on this topic, and have discussed the contribution of variability in these measurements in interpretation of the data. Finally, we have addressed obesity treatment strategies that target the gastric sensory and motor functions.

2. Regulation of Gastric Emptying and Gastric Accommodation

The stomach accommodates, triturates, and empties food into the duodenum through coordinated motor activities within proximal and distal regions. The proximal region's critical function is to store food, while the distal region generates the mechanical forces for trituration to a particle size <2 mm that facilitates emptying and digestion. Neural and endocrine control mechanisms mediate these functions. For example, the proximal stomach exhibits low sustained contractions responsible for the basal tone. After food reaches the stomach, the vagus nerve coordinates the change in fundic compliance (also called accommodation), which allows the stomach to form a reservoir with only a limited rise in intragastric pressure [15], thereby facilitating food ingestion [16].

The ingestion of a meal is linked to coordinated contractile events in the stomach, especially in the antrum. This series of contractile activities leads to the grinding of solids and the beginning of solid emptying. Moreover, there is a positive relationship between the rate of antral contractions and the emptying of solids [17,18].

When food reaches the stomach, the body and antrum create phasic contractions that are activated by the pacemaker apparatus in the wall of the stomach consisting of interstitial cells of Cajal (ICC) and fibroblast-like cells expressing platelet-derived growth factor-alpha (PDGFR α) receptors [19,20].

Phasic contractions or peristaltic waves originate at the greater curve opposite to the incisura angularis and propagate toward the pylorus. The pylorus relaxes while the contractions increase in frequency and intensity in response to neurotransmitters from enteric neurons released in response to gastric distention [21]. As the pyloric sphincter remains closed, the gastric material is propelled backward where the antral contractions grind and mix the contents, resulting in a viscous pulverized material before being emptied into the duodenum [22]. The stomach empties digestible solids when the particle size has been reduced to about 2 mm or less [23].

Thus, stomach emptying of digestible solids only starts after a lag phase required for trituration; emptying is facilitated by an increase in fundus tone, and the pyloric sphincter opens intermittently as peristaltic waves originating in the body continue to pass into the pylorus. Coordinated antro-pyloric contractions propel chyme into the duodenum [18], which relaxes and allows the well-coordinated chyme distribution. These activities are under the control of neuronal circuits and gastrointestinal hormones (Figure A1 in Appendix A). The enteroendocrine function is closely linked to gastrointestinal motor activity, which determines when and for how long the nutrients interact with enteroendocrine cells. Moreover, the release of hormones, primarily in response to nutrients, provides feedback regulation of gastric emptying.

2.1. Neural Regulation

Interactions between the syncytium formed by smooth muscle, ICCs and PDGFR α cells, the enteric system, and the central nervous system (CNS) involve multiple neurotransmitters [24]. Acetylcholine is the primary excitatory neurotransmitter, and nitric oxide and vasoactive intestinal peptides act as inhibitory neurotransmitters [25,26]. Interneurons integrate information from sensory (e.g., response to distension by food) and motor enteric neurons. The CNS provides extrinsic neural input from parasympathetic and sympathetic pathways. The sympathetic nervous system exerts a direct inhibitory influence on α_1-adrenoceptors and an indirect inhibitory effect on α_2-adrenoceptors. The parasympathetic nervous system exerts both excitatory and inhibitory control through the vagus nerve by activating intrinsic excitatory (e.g., cholinergic) and inhibitory (e.g., nitric oxide, vasoactive intestinal peptide, somatostatin) nerves in the stomach wall [25,27].

The vagus nerves exert both inhibitory and excitatory effects on the stomach [28]. Intraganglionic laminar endings (IGLEs) and intra-muscular arrays (IMAs) serve as sensory end-organs that activate vagal afferents. IGLEs, located between the two smooth muscle layers of the stomach, serve as tension receptors. IMAs, within the smooth muscle layer, function as stretch and length detectors [29]. Smooth muscle tone is also perceived by intrinsic nitrergic nerves and can induce fundic relaxation. The innervation from the extrinsic vagus nerve and the intrinsic nitrergic nerves also control the smooth muscle cells to mediate the postprandial accommodation response [16].

During the filling phase, accommodation maintains low intra-gastric pressure until a critical stretch level is reached and triggers vagal afferents that activate hypothalamic neurons and induce the feeling of fullness and activate tonic contractions of the fundus and peristaltic contractions in the remainder of the stomach [30].

2.2. Hormonal Regulation

Hormones are an effective regulatory mechanism for gastric emptying. The spectrum of hormonal actions ranges from "brake" hormones to accelerating hormones. The brake hormones include cholecystokinin (CCK); the products from pre-proglucagon, glucagon-like peptide-1 (GLP-1), glucagon-like peptide-2 (GLP-2), gastric inhibitory polypeptide (GIP), and oxyntomodulin; the polypeptide-fold family proteins peptide tyrosine-tyrosine (PYY) and pancreatic polypeptide (PP); and leptin.

In the gastrointestinal tract, CCK is released from the duodenal and jejunal mucosa by the enteroendocrine I cells in response to nutrients. Lipids, predominantly long-chain fatty acids, and proteins are the most potent stimuli [31]. CCK activates vagal afferents and thereby relaxes the proximal stomach, reduces antral contractility, and activates pyloric tone, slowing gastric emptying. CCK's effects in gastric motility include tone reduction of the proximal stomach, suppressing antral contractions, and stimulating tonic contraction of the pylorus [32]. CCK, infused at rates to mimic postprandial plasma concentrations, slowed gastric emptying of a liquid meal by 30% and a semisolid meal by 40% [33,34]. Loxiglumide, a potent and highly specific antagonist of CCK, accelerated the gastric emptying rates of a liquid mixed meal and pure glucose meal by about 40% [35].

GLP-1 is a posttranslational product of the proglucagon gene, and it is secreted by L cells in the small intestine and colon, particularly in response to glucose and fat in the intestinal lumen [36]. In addition to a glucose-dependent action, GLP-1 can slow gastric emptying and increase postprandial gastric volume to impact satiety [37]. These actions are mediated via vagal afferent pathways and stimulation of inhibitory nitrergic myenteric neurons [38]. Accordingly, the exogenous administration of GLP-1 delays gastric emptying of liquids and solids, whereas the GLP-1 antagonist, exendin-(9–39), has been proven to accelerate gastric emptying of a mixed nutrient meal [39–42] with even an impact on glycemic responses.

Other proglucagon-derived peptides inhibit gastrointestinal motility to a lesser degree than GLP-1 [43]. Previously, GIP was considered as a component of the brake hormones, delaying gastric emptying [44]; however, physiological concentrations of GIP have failed to affect gastric emptying [45,46]. Therefore, it has not been used as a therapeutic target (e.g., in metabolic syndrome or obesity).

PYY is released from enteroendocrine L cells, both in the ileum and colon, in response to meals [47]. Endogenous PYY was associated with a decreased gastric emptying rate [48], and exogenous PYY_{3-36} resulted in a reduction in food intake without affecting gastric emptying [49]. Amylin is co-secreted with insulin from the β-cells of the pancreas, and it inhibits vagal signaling, slowing gastric emptying and promoting satiety. A decrease in the gastric emptying rate has been replicated with the amylin analog, pramlintide [50].

Leptin is released by the adipocytes around body fat stores and within the gastrointestinal system by the parietal cells of the gastric mucosa [51]. In animal studies, both intraperitoneal and intracerebral administration of leptin decreased the gastric emptying rate. Peripheral administration of leptin increased CCK release and activation of vagal cholinergic receptors, while central administration may affect the dorsal vagal complex [52,53].

Ghrelin is an orexigenic hormone produced by the cells of the gastric oxyntic mucosa and the small intestine [54]. Administration of synthetic ghrelin decreased the autonomic response to gastric distension and accelerated both gastric emptying and small bowel transit [55,56]. The infusion of the ghrelin receptor agonists, relamorelin and ulimorelin, resulted in a dose-dependent acceleration of gastric emptying. Relamorelin accelerated gastric emptying up to 17% from baseline in patients with gastroparesis without inhibiting gastric accommodation in healthy adults [57–59]. Recently, ulimorelin also showed a dose-dependent acceleration of gastric emptying of up to 44% from baseline in healthy adults [60].

2.3. Measurement of Gastric Motor Functions

A variety of tests are available to evaluate gastric motor functions; however, simultaneous assessment of gastric volume, accommodation, and emptying has only been recently reported in healthy adults, not in disease states or in response to pharmacological agents [61]. Gastric volume and accommodation can be invasively measured using an intragastric barostatically-controlled balloon or indirectly using reconstruction of transaxial images acquired with single-photon emission computed tomography (SPECT). Non-invasive imaging techniques (i.e., ultrasound, MRI, and SPECT) allow estimation of gastric volume without evaluating muscle tone [62] (Table 1).

The gold standard for measuring gastric emptying is gamma camera scintigraphy, which is a physiological, non-invasive, and objective assessment of gastric emptying. Scintigraphy comprises a radiolabeled meal, such as with ^{99m}technetium, with subsequent imaging to assess emptying of solids. In 2008, the consensus statement from the American Neurogastroenterology and Motility Society and the Society of Nuclear Medicine recommended a standardized method with a low-fat, egg-white meal of 240 kcal with imaging at 0–2 and 4 h after meal ingestion [63]. Camilleri et al. published data on 314 health adults (210 females and 105 males) from an extensively validated protocol that was introduced into practice in 1991; this meal consisted of a 320 kcal, 30% fat meal with imaging at the same time points after meal ingestion [64,65]. Delayed gastric emptying is classified as >60% of the solid meal being retained at 2 h or more than 10% of the meal being left after 4 h. On the other hand, <70% retention at 30 min or <30% stomach retention at 1 h is indicative of more rapid gastric emptying [63]. Despite the protocol guidelines, several centers continue to perform sub-optimal studies (e.g., imaging for 2 h) that compromises the consistency and usefulness of the research on gastric emptying in disease states, including obesity [66].

Ultrasonography is a widely available bedside approach that quantifies changes in the cross-sectional antral area. Two-dimensional ultrasonography allows inferring gastric emptying and accommodation in various pathologies (e.g., functional dyspepsia, diabetes, gastroesophageal reflux, liver cirrhosis) and correlated antral distension with postprandial satiation in healthy subjects [67–69]. Three-dimensional ultrasonography reproduces the image of the total stomach and shows real-time intragastric meal distribution [70]. The volume changes provide a valid measure of gastric emptying rate in health and disease [71–73]. However, these techniques are difficult to standardize and are operator-dependent, or they are compromised by variation in body habitus, particularly when the proximal stomach is covered by the rib cage.

Table 1. Methods to measure gastric motor functions.

Method	Equipment Required	Principle
Scintigraphy	External gamma camera and isotope-labeled meal	Calculating volume content after ingestion of a isotope-labeled meal, with images obtained with a gamma camera at baseline 1, 2, and 4 h.
Ultrasonography	Ultrasound scanners	Measurement of changes in antral cross-sectional area or diameter over time.
Magnetic Resonance	MRI scanner	Measurement of gastric volume, secretion, emptying, and contractions derived from repetitive scans. Gastric meal volume is calculated by taking into account gastric secretion.
Isotope breath test	Breath collection vials and stable isotope-labeled meal	Measurement of breath excretion of $^{13}CO_2$ after ingestion with a solid meal. After ingestion, it is absorbed in the proximal small intestine, metabolized by the liver, and excreted by the lungs, and results in a rise in expired $^{13}CO_2$.
Drug Absorption	Plasma levels of paracetamol	Measurement of plasma concentrations, assuming that small intestine intestine absorption will reflect the gastric emptying rate.
Wireless pressure and pH capsule	Intraluminal capsule with miniaturized strain gauge and pH measurement.	The simultaneous intragastric measurement of pH and pressure is used to evaluate gastric emptying.
Barostat	Barostatically-controlled balloons.	A polyethylene balloon is inserted via the esophagus, situated in the gastric fundus in apposition with the wall, and distended until an intrabag volume of 30 mL is achieved or until respiratory variation is detected. The volume is calculated based on the changes in pressure and diameter.

A valid alternative approach is the measurement of breath excretion of $^{13}CO_2$ after ingesting a meal containing a stable isotope such as ^{13}C-spirulina or ^{13}C-octanoate [74]. The gastric emptying breath test constitutes an indirect, non-radioactive alternative. The subject consumes a meal with the stable isotope, and this results in a rise in expired $^{13}CO_2$ that is measured [75,76].

Paracetamol absorption was proposed as a surrogate method to measure gastric emptying rate, assuming that the passage time of paracetamol through the stomach is identical to that of the meal. The plasma concentration of paracetamol was later commonly used for gastric emptying assessment [74,77]. However even when administered together with a solid meal, the paracetamol was released from the solid meal, dissolved in the liquid phase of the gastric content, and generally reflected the emptying of liquid from the stomach rather than the emptying of a solid meal. In general, most disease states are associated with normal absorption of Paris eat a mal, and therefore parameters such as the 0–5-h area under the curve of plasma paracetamol concentration is not a good reflection of the potential of a disease or pharmacological agent to modify, particularly delay, the gastric emptying of solids from the stomach. There is, moreover, a lack of consideration of pharmacokinetics in the absorption of paracetamol, which shows strong interindividual variability [78–80]. Using plasma levels of paracetamol for gastric emptying can contribute to incorrect conclusions. This is exemplified by the contradictory information regarding the effects of liraglutide on gastric emptying based on paracetamol absorption versus scintigraphic emptying of a mixed solid and liquid meal [81,82].

Nondigestible wireless capsules are recording devices which move through the gastrointestinal tract to detect pH, pressure, and temperature. The simultaneous intragastric measurement of pH and pressure is used to evaluate gastric emptying [83]. Barostatically-controlled balloons can calculate the gastric volume and estimate gastric accommodation. The volume is calculated based on the changes in pressure and diameter [84]. This procedure is the gold standard, but it is an invasive, non-physiologic, uncomfortable technique with relatively low reliability. However, these techniques have not been widely used in relation to obesity.

In order to assess the association between gastric motor functions and gastrointestinal symptoms or appetite sensations, a physiological test, i.e., a nutrient drink test, has been developed [85–87]. The test was initially designed to correlate symptoms of functional dyspepsia with maximum tolerated volume. It traditionally involved the ingestion of a nutrient drink at a constant rate of 30 mL per minute using a constant-rate perfusion pump. Participants record their sensations at 5-min intervals using a numerical scale from 0 to 5, with 0 being no symptoms, 3 corresponding to fullness sensation after a typical meal to address the volume to fullness (VTF), and 5 corresponding to the maximum tolerated volume (MTV). Nutrient intake is stopped when subjects reach a score of 5 [85]. Vijayvargiya et al. showed that, in 62 obese adults (92% females), a higher fasting gastric volume correlated with the calorie intake to reach comfortable fullness at a single meal and the VTF in the nutrient drink test [88].

3. Gastric Sensory and Motor Functions and Food Intake

Physiological information and external environmental cues regulate food intake and appetite. The steps in the cycle of food consumption have been determined as hunger, satiation, and satiety [89]. Hunger is defined as the desire to eat, usually associated with the duration of fasting. Satiation is the process that controls meal size and leads to meal termination, characterized by the postprandial perception of fullness or symptoms such as nausea and bloating. The number of calories consumed that is associated with these symptoms allows quantification of satiation [10,90]. Satiety denotes the intensity and duration of fullness after reaching satiation, delaying subsequent meal consumption [91]. Therefore, measurements of satiety can be based on subjective feelings or the objective duration of the period of fasting between meals.

Gastric sensory and motor functions are crucial in the regulatory process. During fasting, the stomach releases ghrelin, which induces hunger. At the initiation of the meal, stomach distention induces the sensation of satiation or fullness as originally described by Walter Cannon in 1911 in studies involving inflation of an intragastric balloon [92]. In healthy subjects, liquid preload induced gastric distention (assuming a wider antral area) and decreased both appetite and subsequent food intake [90]. On the other hand, several studies have subsequently found that increased gastric volumes are associated with a higher calorie demand for fullness [88,93]. While normal gastric accommodation facilitates food ingestion, an impaired gastric accommodation can cause gastrointestinal symptoms and gastrointestinal disorders, including functional dyspepsia [94,95].

The stomach signals sensory information for changes in volume (with or without calories) and pressure to the brain. The stomach also controls the rate of content delivered into the small intestine, thus, regulating further nutrient digestion and coordinating the enteroendocrine hormone release [96]. Gastrointestinal motility and food-activated enteroendocrine signals to the brain contribute to satiation and satiety signals. As absorption in the small intestine is highly efficient, gastric emptying is pivotal in the regulation of energy intake and nutrient absorption [97]. There is a correlation between gastric emptying of solids with the calorie intake at subsequent buffet meals and the volume to fullness. Patients with delayed gastric emptying experience fullness with lower calorie intake [90].

In addition to the neural control of food intake, emptying of nutrients from the stomach to the intestine induces neurohormonal responses. Enteroendocrine cells distributed throughout the gastrointestinal tract sense the nutrient content in the lumen and release hormones to coordinate the sensation of appetite and food consumption [10]. These enteroendocrine hormones induce local paracrine effects and distant endocrine effects, mainly in the central nervous system (CNS) [38,42,98]. The transfer of nutrients into the small intestine is essential to stimulate this endocrine control of food intake. The intestinal infusion of macronutrients can regulate appetite, with lipids being the most potent inhibitors of food intake and being highly correlated to hormonal release and gastric motor functions [99–101]. Therefore, the rate of nutrient delivery into the small intestine contributes to the feedback regulation of food intake.

Meal patterns and diet features contribute to the short-term control of food intake mediated by gastric motor functions. For example, four days of fasting promoted a delay in gastric emptying of liquids in patients with normal weight [102]. Timing and meal composition may influence gastric emptying. Whey protein preload has been associated with stimulation of GLP-1 release and slowing of gastric emptying [103–105]. This trend was sustained for four weeks after the intervention, indicating the effect of previous diet on gastric emptying [106]. Other factors such as exogenous fiber added to liquid meals or present in solids produced a small delay in gastric emptying; however, there was no impact on appetite [107–109]. The impact of diet history on gastric emptying highlights the challenge of standardizing results among research participants in studies of gastric functions and food intake.

Basic features such as gender, age, and BMI have been proposed as factors that influence energy intake and alter gastric emptying [110–112]. Gender is the major contributor to differences in gastric motor functions, with gastric emptying being around 15% slower in females and influencing the energy intake in controlled interventions [64,111]. However, the biochemical mechanisms contributing to the variance is uncertain, and research performed to determine the influence of sex hormones has failed to explain the disparity observed in women [113]. Age does not substantially change the rate of solid food emptying from the stomach, and the reported delay in liquid emptying among older participants is relatively minor and not considered clinically relevant. Still, there is an apparent decrease in caloric intake with aging and the mechanism is incompletely understood [114–116].

The majority of available gastric emptying trials using accurate methods have examined Caucasian patients; hence, the possible effect of ethnicity is uncertain. Data shows that some ethnicities, such as Mexican Americans, American Indians, Ethiopian refugees, and Han Chinese, have more rapid gastric emptying [117–121]. Physical activity may also impact gastric emptying. When compared to sedentary participants, long-distance runners had faster gastric emptying at baseline [122]. A similar pattern has been observed in individuals with obesity, where those engaging in physical exercise have demonstrated increased gastric emptying [123]. Furthermore, gastric emptying may change according to exercise intensity. High-intensity exercise may slow gastric emptying, although mild to moderate exercise has little effect or may accelerate gastric emptying [124,125].

Gastric Sensory and Motor Functions in Obesity

The balance between energy intake and energy expenditure is a simplistic way to understand body weight regulation. An imbalance, mainly due to disruptions in food intake, is a contributor to obesity [2]. In patients with obesity, gastric volume and gastric emptying strongly correlate with hunger and fullness scores [126]. This rise in fasting gastric volumes resulted in delayed satiation, and thus a higher caloric intake is required to induce satiation, favoring weight gain [126,127]. Therefore, all processes involved in controlling gastric functions may affect body weight.

In 1975, Hunt et al. observed an accelerated transfer of calories from the stomach to the duodenum in obese patients, which was thought to lead to shorter duration of satiety [12]. Since then, gastric sensory and motor functions have been evaluated with contradictory findings, that is, both sides: rapid [14,128,129] and delayed gastric emptying have been reported [130–132]. These contradictory findings may be due to confounding factors such as participants' comorbidities; concomitant medications; previous weight loss history; smoking; or study design with different criteria for participant selection, sample size, and non-standardized methods to evaluate gastric sensory and motor functions [66,133–136].

Among 328 participants, in the largest cohort reported to date, obesity was associated overall with accelerated gastric emptying, with an acceleration by 24 and 17 min for solids and 9 and 7 min for liquids in class I and class II obesity, respectively [14]. There is also evidence in normal and overweight patients that there is a relationship between weight and gastric emptying [14,137]. Furthermore, young adults with more rapid gastric emptying were shown to be more likely to gain weight [138]. A larger gastric capacity has also been reported in patients with obesity based on maximum tolerated volume during a nutrient drink test or as measured by an intragastric latex balloon [139–141]. SPECT showed increased fasting gastric volume in participants who were overweight or obese [14,142,143]. Successful dietary weight loss was associated with a decrease in gastric volume [141].

In adult patients with obesity, baseline gastric emptying may be associated with weight loss in response to several types of interventions. The BMI change ranged from 9% for dietary interventions to 23% for Roux-Y-gastric bypass (RYGB) (additional details in next section) [82,129,144–146] As weight loss itself, in response to lifestyle interventions, does not seem to affect the gastric emptying rate, we may conclude that gastric emptying facilitates response to treatment [147–152]. As a result, slowing gastric emptying was suggested as one of the pathways for understanding weight loss in response to both pharmacological and endoscopic treatments. This was tested in several randomized, double-blind, placebo-controlled pilot trials with subcutaneous liraglutide and semaglutide and in a randomized, controlled trial with an intragastric balloon where retarding gastric emptying was one significant mechanism of action of those obesity treatments [90,153,154]. There is still insufficient proof of the extent of the impact of gastric emptying changes on weight loss, although it has also been shown that obese patients with accelerated gastric emptying will benefit more from specific gastric motility therapy [155].

Many syndromic and non-syndromic types of obesity provide insights into the crucial and complex role of genetics on energy balance, body weight, and the individual's predisposition to obesity [156–158]. Syndromic obesity describes obesity in the clinical sense of a distinct collection of organ-specific abnormalities and additional phenotypes, such as cognitive retardation, developmental abnormalities and hyperphagia [159]. Prader–Willi syndrome is the most prevalent form of syndromic obesity; it is associated with elevated circulating ghrelin levels that lead to the observed hyperphagia [160]. Despite the hypothesis that elevated ghrelin may accelerate gastric emptying, studies have found that gastric emptying in Prader–Willi syndrome is delayed relative to reference values [161,162]. The role of gastric motor functions in other types of syndromic obesity (e.g., leptin deficiency, melanocortin 4 receptor deficiency, Bardet–Biedl syndrome, Alström syndrome) has not been assessed.

Variations in the glucagon-like peptide-1 receptor gene (*GLP1R*), the melanocortin 4 receptor gene (*MC4R*), Transcription Factor 7 Like 2 (*TCF7L2*) gene, and *CCK* gene have been studied to understand the influence of genes on gastric emptying rate and are still being studied. Several SNPs (*rs742764*, *rs9283907*, *rs2268657*, and *rs2254336*) of the GLP1R gene have been associated with statistically significant differences in gastric emptying in a pilot study [163]. The *MC4R rs17782313* CC polymorphism was associated with a 6.7% slower gastric emptying of solids at 2 h when compared with individuals with the TT genotype [164]. Cremonini et al. found an association between the CCK 779T > C polymorphism and slower gastric emptying rate [165]. The T allele at rs7903146 (*TCF7L2*) was non-significantly associated with faster gastric emptying [166]. Genetic variation presents a plausible area of investigation, with a specific pharmacogenetic implication as shown by Chedid et al., with GLP1R (rs6923761) being associated with more significant delay in gastric emptying T1/2 in response to liraglutide and exenatide [167].

4. Treatments of Obesity and Their Effects on Gastric Sensory and Motor Functions
4.1. Lifestyle Interventions

The first-line treatments for weight management include diet change to achieve substantial caloric deficit, increased exercise to burn calories, and behavioral treatment to improve food and physical activity patterns. Patients do not need to reach a BMI < 25 kg/m^2 in all situations to benefit from weight loss. A sustained weight loss of less than 5% may help prevent and control diabetes, and modest weight loss of 5% to 10% has been associated with substantial improvements in cardiovascular disease risk factors [168,169]. Long-term weight maintenance is therefore essential to reducing the incidence of serious diseases. Exercise has beneficial effects on health besides weight control, but the influence of exercise-induced weight loss on gastric motor function is uncertain [170].

There are limited data available on the impact of diet and exercise-induced weight-loss on gastric motility. Table 2 details the effects of dietary interventions on gastric emptying and energy intake. The main limitations in determining the effects of dietary weight loss on gastric emptying and appetite are variation among subjects, prior dietary patterns, inclusion of patients with poorly regulated diabetes, lack of an effective matched control group, appropriate sample size, complexity in measuring gastric emptying in all settings, and lack of standardization of meals. Despite achieving significant weight-loss, most studies of lifestyle interventions have found no effect on gastric emptying after one month. However, data suggest that a rapid gastric emptying of a solid meal in patients with obesity normalizes after sustained weight loss. Changes in gastric emptying do not appear to correlate with changes in appetite.

Further studies are required to evaluate the impact of fitness programs on gastric emptying.

4.2. Pharmacological Treatment

Since the control of food intake is partly mediated through gastric motor functions, delaying gastric emptying may induce a decrease in calorie intake and contribute to the efficacy of weight loss in a majority of patients in the treatment of obesity. Dexfenfluramine, a discontinued anti-obesity agent, significantly slowed gastric emptying of a solid meal in obese patients following short-term therapy (5 days and 29 days) relative to placebo, leading to its effectiveness on weight loss [171].

There are five FDA-approved medications for long-term obesity care: orlistat, phentermine/topiramate, bupropion/naltrexone, and liraglutide for adults, orlistat and liraglutide for patients ≥12 years of age; and phentermine for adolescents ≥16 years [172–174]. Table 3 summarizes the effects of anti-obesity medications on gastric emptying in adults. The effects of orlistat on gastric emptying have been investigated in normal-weight healthy volunteers and diabetic overweight subjects where lipase inhibition resulted in a faster emptying of fats but may worsen postprandial glycemia [175–178]. However, these results have not been replicated in patients with obesity and successful weight loss after treatment [179]. In a placebo-controlled, 2-week trial of phentermine/topiramate ER, gastric emptying T1/2 accelerated by 20 min, and the drug's effect on satiation was more pronounced, indicating a significant CNS effect on satiation resulting in the predicted weight loss [14]. GLP-1 receptor agonists are a group of GLP-1 drugs that decrease gastric emptying rate and control food intake in patients with obesity [81,98,180]. Animal models have demonstrated a decrease in food consumption with bupropion/naltrexone, but this effect and the additional improvements in gastric emptying have not been tested [181].

Six FDA-approved GLP-1 receptor agonists (i.e., exenatide, lixisenatide, liraglutide, dulaglutide, albiglutide, and semaglutide) are available. GLP-1 receptor agonists or GLP-1 analogs decrease gastric emptying rate and control food intake in patients with obesity [81,98,180]. High-dose liraglutide (3.0 mg) is the only medication in this class approved for long-term obesity treatment. Exenatide was the first to show a weight loss benefit associated with a decrease in gastric emptying [182]. A randomized clinical trial found a correlation between a delay in gastric emptying of solids following treatment with liraglutide 3.0 mg and weight loss [82]. Furthermore, gastric emptying changes may be a biomarker for a response, which may help identify patients for extended therapy [82]. Once-weekly subcutaneous semaglutide, which substantially decreased energy intake, was associated with reducing paracetamol AUC_{0-1h}, strongly suggesting it may slow gastric emptying [183,184].

The short-acting GLP-1RAs (i.e., exenatide twice daily and lixisenatide) [182,185] appear to affect gastric emptying more markedly than longer-acting GLP-1RAs (i.e., exenatide once weekly, liraglutide, dulaglutide, albiglutide, semaglutide) [82,154,184,186,187]. However, it is clear that both groups slow gastric emptying, lower pre-prandial and post-prandial glucose levels, and promote weight loss. Nausea and vomiting are the most frequently reported gastrointestinal adverse events for GLP-1RAs, especially for long-acting formulations, and may contribute to greater weight loss in this group [188,189]. The weight loss achieved with subcutaneous semaglutide is independent of gastrointestinal adverse events though other studies confirm that both weekly and oral semaglutide retard gastric emptying [154,189,190]. Nevertheless, weight loss associated with GLP-1 receptor agonists may be independent of gastric motor changes and related to central appetite regulation [191–193].

Pramlintide, an amylin analog, at 120 ug three-times-daily or 360 ug two-times-daily, resulted in long-term maintenance of weight loss and delayed gastric emptying [194]. The long-acting amylin analog, BZ043, which is under development, has demonstrated a decline in gastric emptying in animal studies [195]. PYY analogs are currently being developed based on past reports of decreased energy intake in overweight and obese people [196–198]. Studies in healthy humans suggest that the effects might be mediated by a decreased gastric emptying rate, among other potential mechanisms [199]. Further studies are needed to understand the role of other approved anti-obesity drugs on gastric function.

4.3. Endoscopic Bariatric Procedures

Endoscopic bariatric therapies (EBT) or procedures have an organ-specific target and mechanism of action [200]. Space-occupying devices are a volume-dependent weight loss therapy that encourages sensation of satiety by promoting gastric distention [141]. Fluid-filled intragastric balloons may also affect gastric emptying to facilitate weight loss [145,153,201,202]. However, most of the studies used longitudinal analysis, and only one study was a randomized controlled trial. None of the studies were able to assess possible confounders such as gender, comorbidities, baseline gastric emptying, diet history, and current use of medications.

On meta-analysis, greater changes in gastric emptying were associated with a higher percentage of total body weight lost at six months [203]. Furthermore, gastric emptying at baseline may be a valuable predictor of intolerance since increased baseline gastric retention is correlated with early balloon removal [155]. Therefore, gastric emptying can also help in selection of the appropriate patient for the procedure. Table 4 summarizes the trials evaluating EBTs and gastric emptying.

Other endoscopic restrictive techniques are likely to induce satiety. Endoscopic sleeve gastroplasty is an endoscopic gastric volume reduction technique intended to operate similarly to sleeve gastrectomy [204]. Botulinum toxin type A, a neurotoxin and inhibitor of smooth muscle contractility, has been studied because of its potential to slow gastric motility to result in earlier satiety [205]. Intragastric administration of botulinum toxin has been related to transient time and dose-dependent changes in gastric emptying [206,207]. However, the delay in gastric emptying was not associated with weight loss [203].

4.4. Bariatric Surgery

Table 4 summarizes the trials evaluating the effects of surgical procedures and gastric emptying.

The principal mechanisms of weight loss after bariatric surgery are malabsorption and gastric restriction. Bariatric surgery may also have beneficial effects on gut hormones, including stimulation of GLP-1 and PYY and modifying gastric motor functions [203,208–211]. These observations are indicative of the potential for other weight loss pathways to be enhanced to induce permanent weight loss.

Sleeve gastrectomy decreases gastric capacity and reduces gastric accommodation, leading to high gastric intraluminal pressure [212]. Changes in the total gastric volume, as well as gut hormones can also affect gastric emptying [213]. In a meta-analysis including 233 patients, sleeve gastrectomy was associated with a mean acceleration of gastric emptying $T/2$ of 29.2 min after three months. However, no significant association was found between weight loss at 1-year post-sleeve gastrectomy and gastric emptying [203,214]. Sleeve gastrectomy reduced fasting ghrelin and increased postprandial GLP-1 and PYY. These hormonal changes may impact appetite and reduce food intake [211,215].

RYGB decreased gastric capacity and accelerated the transfer of nutrients as larger particles to the distal small intestine [216]. Additionally, variations in the emptying rate varied between meals where solid emptying was slower and liquid emptying was faster following gastric bypass surgery [149]. A changes in gastric volume may be the primary determinant of weight loss, but it does not adequately explain the impact on the reward system [211,217]. Studies indicate that gastric emptying is faster following treatment; however, there is a lack of data in longitudinal studies [150,151,203,218]. On the other hand, emptying of solids from the pouch immediately after surgery was associated with increased weight loss [218,219].

Loss of normal accommodation in the gastric remnant and accelerated gastric emptying are likely to play important roles in the effects of RYGB on food intake and glycemic control. Bariatric-surgery procedures have shown, especially in the first months after surgery, to substantially increase GLP-1 secretion, which regulates gastric emptying and is related to the improved meal-related glycemia [220]. These effects might be triggered by directly transferring food to the distal small intestine with higher densities of neuroendocrine L-cells; however, there is still mixed evidence explaining the benefits of surgical procedures [221,222].

Table 2. Effect of low-calorie diets on gastric emptying, energy intake, and appetite in obesity.

Study Design/ Intervention	Methods	Effect on GI Motor Function	Weight Loss BMI, kg/m²	Energy Intake Kcal/Day	Appetite Sensations, VAS	Ref.
RCT, SB in obesity (BMI 37.4 ± 4.0 kg/m²) ($n = 42$) Diet: ETEE-600 kcal (minimum 1200 kcal), exercise and behavioral modification.	Scinti-graphic GE and VAS: Pre and 1-month post-Rx	GE $T_{1/2}$ liquids min: baseline 21.8 ± 10.1 vs. 1-month 24.4 ± 8.7; ns GE solids %/h: baseline 30.3 ± 15.2 vs. 1-month 26.2 ± 15.2; ns	Baseline 37.4 ± 3.9 1-month 36.7 ± 3.9, $\Delta -0.8$ (95% CI $[-1.0, -0.5]$; $p < 0.001$).	$\Delta -599.9$ (95% CI $[-885.6, -315.2]$; $p < 0.001$.	Decrease in: Desire to eat AUC, Hunger AUC, and Fullness AUC	[179]

Table 2. Cont.

Study Design/Intervention	Methods	Effect on GI Motor Function	Weight Loss BMI, kg/m^2	Energy Intake Kcal/Day	Appetite Sensations, VAS	Ref.
RCT, DB in obesity (BMI 37.4 ± 4.0 kg/m^2) (n = 14) Placebo vs. diet Diet: ETEE-600 kcal (minimum 1200 kcal).	Scinti-graphic GE and VAS: Pre, 1- and 12 months post-Rx	GE T$_{1/2}$ liquids min: baseline 25.5 ± 10.7; 1-month 19.3 ± 9.0; 12-months 21.8 ± 10.3; ns GE rate %/h solids: baseline 26.6 ± 16.3 1 month: 35.8 ± 13.8; ns 12-months 17.6 ± 13.0; $p < 0.05$ vs baseline	Baseline: 37.6 ± 3.9; 1-month: 37.2 ± 3.9; 12 months: 34.2 ± 5.4; $p < 0.05$	No effect	No effect	[179]
Case-control study Obese (BMI, kg/m^2: 48 [IQR 45.3–53.8) (n = 10). 4 months of low-calorie diet (800–1000 kcal)	Scinti-graphic GE and VAS: Pre vs. 1-month post-Rx	GE rate for solids %/min: Δ 0.80 (IQR: 0.60–1.15); $p < 0.01$	Weight loss: Δ 9% (0.7–23.66); $p < 0.05$	NA	No effect	[129]
Case-control study 19 Obese (mean BMI = 38.7 kg/m^2): Diet-induced wt loss. Low-calorie diet (1000 kcal/day) for 8 weeks, then energy-restricted (1500 kcal/day) for 8 weeks, then maintenance diet for 8 weeks (ETEE286 kcal)	Scinti-graphic GE: Pre and 24 weeks post-Rx	GE solids % at 30 min: Baseline 24.0 (95% CI (18.4, 29.5)), 24-weeks: 18.3 (95% CI (14.0, 22.6)); $p < 0.02$) GE solids AUC$_{0-60\,min}$ %·min: Baseline 4903 (95% CI (4678, 5127)), 24-wks 4651 (95% CI (4404, 4897)); $p < 0.03$	Baseline 38.7 (95% CI [37.2, 40.1]) vs. 24 weeks 33.0, Δ−14.7 (95% CI [30.9, 35.0]); $p < 0.001$	NA	NA	[223]
Cross-sectional study 8 Obese (Weight: 148.9 kg [IQR 81–240] 3 to 4 weeks of a very-low calorie diet.	Scintigraphic GE: Pre- vs. 1-month post-Rx	GE for liquids, min: Baseline 41.0 ± 7.8 vs. 1-month 48.5 ± 8.7; ns GE for solids, min: Baseline 93.0 ± 11.2 vs. 1-month 100.7 ± 12.6; ns	Weight loss (mean 8.3 kg)	NA	NA	[147]

Abbreviations: AUC: area under the curve; BMI: body mass index; CI: confidence interval; DB double blind; ETEE estimated total energy expenditure; GE: gastric emptying; MIN: minutes; NA: not analyzed; ns: non-significant; VAS: visual analog scale; RCT randomized controlled trial; SB single blind.

Table 3. Effect of anti-obesity medications on gastric emptying and energy intake.

Study Design/ Intervention	Methods	Effect on GI Motor Function	Δ Weight, kg	Energy Intake Ad Libitum meal	Ref.
PC, DB, RCT. 20 obese (BMI 33.9 ± 1 kg/m^2) with accelerated GE at baseline Exenatide SQ, 5 μg BID (n = 10) or placebo (n = 10)	Scintigraphic GE test: Pre vs. 1-month post-Rx	GE % 1 h: Exenatide 12.4% (IQR 8–18.5) vs. placebo 38.2% (IQR 26.6–42.1); $p < 0.001$ GE T$_{1/2}$, min: Exenatide 187 (IQR 141–240) vs. placebo 86 (IQR 73–125); $p < 0.001$	Exenatide −0.95 (IQR −0.7–2.1) vs. placebo 0.55 (IQR 0.3–2.1); $p = 0.23$	No effect	[182]
RCT Healthy participants (BMI 29.6 ± 0.6 kg/m^2 vs. 29.5 ± 1.0 kg/m^2) Exenatide 2.0 mg SQ weekly (n = 16) vs. placebo (n = 16)	Scintigraphic GE test: Pre vs. 2-months post-Rx	GE for solids AUC$_{0-120min}$: Exenatide slowed GE vs. placebo; $p = 0.046$ GE for liquids AUC$_{0-120min}$: Exenatide slowed GE vs. placebo; $p = 0.01$	Exenatide −2.1 ± 0.5 vs. placebo 0.2 ± 0.5; $p = 0.001$	NA	[186]
PC, DB, RCT. 40 obese (BMI: 34.6 kg/m^2 vs. 37.2 kg/m^2) Liraglutide group (n = 19) vs. placebo (n = 21) Liraglutide or placebo dose: 0.6 mg increments to 3.0 mg daily.	Scintigraphic GE test and VAS: Pre vs. 16-weeks post-Rx	GE T$_{1/2}$ 16 weeks, min: Liraglutide 142 (IQR 120–177) vs. placebo 113 min (IQR 101–133); ns GE T$_{1/2}$ 16 weeks vs baseline, min: Liraglutide 30.5 (IQR -11–54) vs. placebo 1 min (IQR −19–7); $p = 0.025$	Liraglutide 5.3 (IQR 5.2–6.8) vs. placebo 2.5 (IQR 0.1–4.2); $p = 0.0009$	No effect	[82, 224]
OL, three-arm, RCT 142 Participants with T2DM (BMI 30.8 ± 0.34 kg/m^2) Rx + insulin glargine for 8 wks: a) Lixisenatide 20 μg SQ daily b) Liraglutide 1.2 mg SQ daily c) Liraglutide 1.8 mg SQ daily	^{13}C-sodium-octanoic acid GE test: Pre vs. 2-months post-Rx	GE T$_{1/2}$ 8 weeks vs. baseline, min: Lixisenatide 20 μg 453.6 ± 58.2; $p < 0.001$ Liraglutide 1.2 mg 175.3 ± 58; $p < 0.05$ Liraglutide 1.8 mg 130.5 ± 60.3; $p < 0.05$	Lixisenatide 20 μg −1.6 ± 0.5; $p < 0.05$ Liraglutide 1.2 mg −1.8 ± 0.5; $p < 0.05$ Liraglutide 1.8 mg −2.4 ± 0.5; $p < 0.001$	NA	[225]
OL, parallel-group, RCT Participants with T2DM Lixisenatide of 20 μg SQ daily (n = 69) vs. Sitagliptin 50 mg oral daily (n = 67) Lixisenatide weekly 5 μg increments: from 10 μg to 20 μg daily.	^{13}C-sodium-octanoic acid GE test: Pre vs. 1-month post-Rx.	Lixisenatide vs. sitagliptin GE AUC$_{0-240min}$ mean change from baseline, ng/mL: −4.8 ± 0.47 vs. 0.9 ± 0.48 (−5.8 [−7.10, −4.44]; $p < 0.0001$)	Lixisenatide −0.41 vs. sitagliptin +0.39 (descriptive statistics only)	NA	[226]

Table 3. Cont.

Study Design/Intervention	Methods	Effect on GI Motor Function	Δ Weight, kg	Energy Intake Ad Libitum meal	Ref.
DB, X-O, RCT 8 obese (BMI 30.3 ± 1.0 kg/m^2) with T2DM Lixisenatide 10-μg SQ for 14 days and 20-μg for additional 14 days	^{13}C-octanoate GE test: 1-month post-Rx	GE AUC$_{1-8h}$: reduced after lixisenatide compared with after placebo; $p = 0.048$	Lixisenatide −2.4 ± 4.73 vs. placebo −1.5 ± 4.24; ns	NA	[227]
PC, DB, RCT. 30 patients with T2DM (BMI 32.1 ± 5.1 kg/m^2) Lixisenatide ($n = 19$) vs. placebo ($n = 21$) Lixisenatide or placebo dose was double weekly from 0.5 μg until a dose of 20 μg daily was reached.	Scintigraphic GE test: Pre- vs. 8-weeks. post-Rx	Gastric retention post-Rx AUC$_{0-240min}$: Adjusted geometric means for lixisenatide vs. placebo 2.19 (95% CI 1.82, 2.64; $p < 0.001$)	Lixisenatide −1.20 ± 5.22 vs. placebo −1.0 ± 6.22; ns	NA	[228]
DB, PC, RCT. 24 obese (BMI 30.3 ± 1.0 kg/m^2) Phentermine/topiramate 3.75 mg and 23 mg, respectively, for the first 5 days, and 7.5 mg and 46 mg for 10 days	Scintigraphic GE test: Pre- vs. 2-weeks. post-Rx	Phentermine/topiramate vs. placebo GE T$_{1/2}$ Phentermine/Topiramate vs. placebo, min: 109.0 ± 7 vs. 88 ± 7; $p = 0.05$	Phentermine/topiramate −1.42 ± 0.4 vs. placebo −0.23 ± 0.4; $p = 0.03$	Phentermine-topiramate vs. placebo Δ-260 (95% CI [−491.6, −28.3]; $p < 0.05$).	[14]

Abbreviations: AUC: area under the curve; BMI: body mass index; CI: confidence interval; DB double blind; GE: gastric emptying; IQR: inter quantile range; MIN: minutes; NA: not analyzed; ns: non-significant; OL open label; RCT randomized controlled trial; RX prescription; SB single blinded; SE: standard error; T2DM: type 2 diabetes mellitus; VAS: visual analog scale; WKS weeks; X-O cross over.

Table 4. Effect of bariatric endoscopy on gastric emptying and energy intake.

Study Design/Intervention	Methods	Effect on GI Motor Function	Weight Loss	Ref.
10 subjects (BMI 32.4 ± 1.53 kg/m^2) IGB filled with 200–229 mL of air for 12 weeks.	Scintigraphic GE test: pre- and 5-wks. post-Tx	GE T$_{1/2}$ for solids, min: baseline 57 ± 27.8 vs. 5-weeks. Post-Tx. 67 ± 27.5; $p < 0.05$	Δ3 months—BL, kg: −2.4 ± 1.04	[229]
15 subjects (BMI 34.4 ± 0.7 kg/m^2) IGB filled with 600 mL of saline for 24 weeks.	^{13}C-octanoate GE test: pre- and 16-wks. post-Tx	GE T$_{1/2}$ for solids, min: BL 92 ± 45 vs. 16-weeks. post-Tx 157 ± 70; $p = 0.052$	Body weight loss, %: 9.4 ± 1.8	[201]
3 subjects (BMI 40.93 ± 8.8 kg/m^2) IGB filled with 500 cc of saline for 24 weeks.	Scintigraphic GE test: pre- and 3-months post-Tx	GE T$_{1/2}$ for solids, min: BL 114 ± 18.5 vs.12-weeks. post-Tx 375.3 ± 207; $p = 0.02$	Δ6 months—BL, kg: −14.67 ± 4.33	[202]
7 subjects (BMI 33.76 ± 1.78 kg/m^2) IGB filled with 500 cc of saline for 24 weeks.	Scintigraphic GE test: pre- and 3-months post-Tx	GE T$_{1/2}$ for liquids, min: BL 38.71 ± 15.91 vs. 12-wks. 318.71 ± 168.07; $p = 0.001$	Δ6 months—BL, kg: −13.14 ± 2.5	[202]

Table 4. Cont.

Study Design/Intervention	Methods	Effect on GI Motor Function	Weight Loss	Ref.
15 subjects (BMI 34.7 ± 3.42 kg/m^2) vs. 14 controls (BMI 35.6 ± 2.84 kg/m^2) IGB + lifestyle (1000–1500 kcal) vs. lifestyle intervention alone IGB filled with 550 cc of saline for 24 weeks. Lifestyle intervention: Diet: (1000–1500 kcal), exercise, behavioral Rx	Scintigraphic GE test: pre- and 8-, 16-wks. post-IGB	Gastric retention at 120 min after 8 weeks, %: IGB 61.4 ± 23.2 vs. controls 25.7 ± 18; $p = 0.003$ Gastric retention at 120 min after 16 weeks, %: IGB 62.1 ± 16.4 vs. controls 18.7 ± 15.6; $p < 0.001$	Δ26 wks—BL, %TBW: IGB −14 ± 7.8 vs. controls −5.4 ± 4; $p = 0.003$	[153]
24 subjects (BMI 35.58 ± 2.79 kg/m^2) IGB filled with 600 cc of saline for 24 weeks.	Scintigraphic GE test: pre- and 2-months post-IGB	GE $T_{1/2}$ for solids, min: BL 117.92 ± 150.23 vs. 12-weeks. post-Tx 281.48 ± 206.49; $p = 0.004$	Δ6 months—BL, kg: −17.09 ± 3.34; $p < 0.001$	[230]
20 subjects (BMI 51.7 kg/m^2) BPD-DS	Scintigraphic GE test: 3.5y postoperatively	GE $T_{1/2}$ for solids, min: BPD-DS 28 ± 16 vs. laboratory control ($n = 160$) 91 ± 20	Δ 3.5 years—BL BMI, kg/m^2: 51.7 vs. 31.3 (IQR 21.8–46.3)	[231]
16 subjects (BMI 47.8 ± 1.7 kg/m^2) Gastric banding	Scintigraphic GE test: pre- and 6-months post-GB	GE rate, %/h: BL 42 (IQR 23.3–59) vs. 24-weeks. post-Tx 38 (IQR 31–71); ns Fundus emptying rate, %/h: BL 59 (IQR 37–91) vs. 24-weeks. post-Tx 70 (IQR 53–89); ns	Δ6 months—BL BMI, kg/m^2: −6.1 ± 0.66; $p < 0.001$	[232]
33 subjects (weight 76 ± 4.0 kg) Gastric banding ($n = 12$) vs. controls ($n = 11$)	Scintigraphic GE test: 12-months post-GB	GE $T_{1/2}$ for liquids, min: GB 7 ± 3 vs. controls 15 ± 2; ($p < 0.005$) GE $T_{1/2}$ for solids: 8 patients showed slower GE $T_{1/2}$ for solids (147 ± 25 min) vs. controls (70 ± 7 min)	Δ6 months—BL, kg: 28 ± 3	[149]
29 subjects Jejunoileal Bypass	Scintigraphic GE test: 2- and 12-months post-surgical	GE $T_{60\,min}$, %: 2 months 70 ± 24 vs. 12 months 89 ± 7; $p < 0.05$	Δ12 months—BL, kg: 42.3 ± 10.9; $p < 0.001$	[233]
11 subjects, BMI 46.8 kg/m^2 (IQR 35.8–62.5) Laparoscopic Gastric Sleeve	Scintigraphic GE test: pre- and 6-months post-LSG	GE $T_{1/2}$, min: BL 94.3 ± 15.4 vs. 6 months 47.6 ± 23.2; $p < 0.01$ GE at 90 min, %: BL 49.2 ± 8.7 vs. 6 months 75.4 ± 14.9; $p < 0.01$	Δ6 months—BL, kg: 42.3 ± 10.9; $p < 0.001$	[234]
21 subjects (BMI 45.09 ± 6.2 kg/m^2) Laparoscopic Gastric Sleeve	Scintigraphic GE test: pre- and 3-months post-LSG	GE $T_{1/2}$, min: BL 62.39 ± 19.83 vs. 3 months 56.79 ± 18.72 ($p = 0.36$, t = −0.92, ns)	Δ3 months—BL, kg: −7.29 ± 1.87; $p < 0.001$	[235]
20 subjects underwent LSG (BMI 38.3 kg/m^2 [IQR 34.5–48.3]) vs. 18 controls (BMI 19.8–23.5 kg/m^2)	Scintigraphic GE test: 3-months post-LSG	GE $T_{1/2}$ for liquids: control vs post-surgical, min: 34.9 ± 24.6 vs. 13.6 ± 11.9; $p < 0.01$ GE $T_{1/2}$ for solids: control vs post-surgical, min: 78 ± 15.01 vs. 38.3 ± 18.77; $p < 0.01$	Weight lost at the first month after surgery was 11.1 ± 2.2 kg and 45.5 ± 5.2 kg in the sixth months	[236]

Table 4. Cont.

Study Design/Intervention	Methods	Effect on GI Motor Function	Weight Loss	Ref.
23 subjects underwent LSG (BMI 40.7 ± 6.6 kg/m^2) vs. 44 controls, 24 lean (BMI 22.2 ± 2.89 kg/m^2) and 20 obese (BMI 37.7 ± 5.4 kg/m^2)	Scintigraphic GE test: 2 years post-LSG	GE T$_{1/2}$ for solids, min: lean 72.8 ± 29.6 vs. post-surgical 52.8 ± 13.5; $p = 0.025$ GE T$_{1/2}$ for solids, min: obese controls 73.7 ± 29.0 vs. post-surgical 52.8 ± 13.5; $p = 0.01$	Δ12 months—BL, kg: −26.80 ± 5.75; $p < 0.001$	[152]
4 subjects underwent LSG, BMI 41.9 kg/m^2 (IQR 38–44.3)	Scintigraphic GE test: pre- and 3 months post-LSG	GE T$_{1/2}$, min: BL 57.5 ± 12.7 vs. 3-months 32.25 ± 17.3; $p = 0.016$ GE at 90 min, %: BL 20.5 vs 3-months 9.5; $p = 0.073$	Δ3 months—BL, kg: −7.29 ± 1.87; $p < 0.001$	[237]
45 subjects underwent LSG (BMI 49.5 kg/m^2)	Scintigraphic GE test: pre- and 3 months post-LSG	GE T$_{1/2}$, min: BL 80.4 ± 33.1 vs. 3-months 64.3 ± 40; $p = 0.06$	Pre-surgical vs. 12 months BMI, kg/m^2: 48.5 vs. 36.8; $p < 0.05$	[238]
21 subjects underwent LSG, BMI 46.8 kg/m^2 (IQR 35.8–62.5)	Scintigraphic GE test: pre- and 4 months post LSG	GE T$_{1/2}$, min: BL 61.7 (IQR 37.0–94.3) vs. 4-months 49.1 (IQR 22.4–92.1); $p < 0.05$	Pre-surgical vs. 6 months BMI, kg/m^2: 46.8 (35.8–62.5) vs. 37.4 (28.2–53.2) ($p < 0.05$)	[239]
20 subjects underwent LSG, BMI 48.7 ± 3.3 kg/m^2	Scintigraphic GE test: pre- and 1–4 weeks post-LSG for liquids.	GE T$_{1/2}$ for liquids, min: BL 25.3 ± 4.4 vs. 1-months 11.8 ± 3.0; $p < 0.001$	Δ1 month—BL BMI, kg/m^2: −8.20 ± 1.03; $p < 0.001$	[240]
20 subjects underwent LSG, BMI 49.1 ± 7.1 kg/m^2	Scintigraphic GE test: Pre- and 4–6 weeks post-LSG for solids	GE T$_{1/2}$ for solids, min: BL 74.9 ± 7.1 vs. 6-weeks 28.4 ± 8.3; $p < 0.001$	Δ6 weeks—BL BMI, kg/m^2: −11.40 ± 1.86; $p < 0.001$	[240]
20 subjects underwent LSG, dichotomize according to postprandial symptoms. Low symptoms score, BMI 45.5 ± 10.7 kg/m^2 ($n = 13$) vs high symptom score, BMI, 40.5 ± 4.5 kg/m^2 ($n = 7$)	Scintigraphic GE test: 2 years post-LSG.	GE T$_{1/2}$ for liquids, min: Low symptoms 10.4 ± 2.9 vs. high symptom 10.6 ± 4.3; $p = 0.27$ GE T$_{1/2}$ for solids, min: Low symptoms 40.6 ± 10.0 vs. high symptom 34.4 ± 9.3; $p = 0.90$	Group I Δ24 months-BL BMI, kg/m^2: −13.00 ± 3.27; $p < 0.05$ Group II Δ24 months-BL BMI, kg/m^2: −10.50 ± 1.37; $p < 0.05$	[241]
20 subjects underwent LSG, BMI 33.4 ± 1.2 kg/m^2	Scintigraphic GE test: pre- and 3-, 6-, 12- and 24-months post-LSG	GE T$_{1/2}$, min: BL 38.4 ± 13 vs. 3- months 20.3 ± 7.6 vs. 6-months 20.7 ± 9.5 vs. 12-months 20.6 ± 4.4; $p < 0.05$	Δ3 months—BL BMI, kg/m^2: −5.5 ± 1.9; $p < 0.05$	[242]
30 subjects underwent LSG, BMI 50.96 ± 5.18 kg/m^2	Scintigraphic GE test: pre- and 6- and 12-months post-LSG	GE T$_{1/2}$, min: BL 96.5 ± 78.9 vs. 6-months 44.3 ± 21.1 vs. 12-months 36.1 ± 10.2; $p < 0.001$	Δ12 months—BL BMI, kg/m^2: −17.28 ± 6.76; $p < 0.05$	[243]
30 subjects underwent LSG, BMI 51.27 ± 7.20 kg/m^2	Scintigraphic GE test: pre- and 6- and 12-months post-LSG	GE T$_{1/2}$, min: BL 99.9 ± 71.4 vs. 6-months 48,1 ± 21.6 vs. 12-months 44.4 ± 15.9; $p < 0.001$	Δ12 months—BL BMI, kg/m^2: −16.79 ± 8.35; $p < 0.05$	[243]
50 subjects underwent LSG, BMI 44.5 ± 8.1 kg/m^2	Scintigraphic GE test: pre- and 3-months post-LSG	GE T$_{1/2}$ for liquids, min: BL 26.7 ± 23 vs. 3-months 15.2 ± 13; $p < 0.05$ GE T$_{1/2}$ for solids, min: BL 68.7 ± 25 vs. 3-months 15.2 ± 13; $p < 0.05$	%EWL after 3 months ($n = 26$): 24.6 ± 12.1 %EWL after 3 months ($n = 26$): 25.1 ± 10.9	[244]

Table 4. Cont.

Study Design/ Intervention	Methods	Effect on GI Motor Function	Weight Loss	Ref.
38 subjects underwent LSG, 12 with antrum resection-2 cm from the pylorus vs. 13 with antrum preservation-5 cm from the pylorus	Scintigraphic GE test: pre- and 2-months and 1-year post-LSG	AR pre vs. 2 months post LSG $GE_{60\text{-min}}$ for semi-solids, %: 55.8 ± 22 vs. 69.7 ± 18; ns AR pre vs. 12 months post LSG $GE_{60\text{-min}}$ for semi-solids, %: 55.8 ± 22 vs. 66.5 ± 21; ns AP pre vs. 2 months post LSG $GE_{60\text{-min}}$ for semi-solids, %: 52.7 ± 24 vs. 72.8 ± 20; $p = 0.024$ AP pre vs. 12 months post LSG $GE_{60\text{-min}}$ for semi-solids, %: 52.7 ± 24 vs. 74.2 ± 16; $p = 0.010$	AR pre vs. 12 months post-LSG BMI, kg/m^2: 43.01 vs. 31.43 AP pre vs. 12 months post-LSG BMI, kg/m^2: 45.3 vs. 31.88	[214]
23 subjects underwent LSG, BMI 41.9 ± 5.3 kg/m^2	Scintigraphic GE test: pre- and 3-months post-LSG	GE $T_{1/2}$ for solids, min: BL 52.7 ± 20.5 vs. 3-months 33.6 ± 3.0; $p < 0.001$	$\Delta 3$ months—BL BMI, kg/m^2: -7 ± 7.35; $p < 0.001$	[245]
21 subjects underwent LSG, BMI 38.89 ± 7.55 kg/m^2	Scintigraphic GE test: pre- and 3-months post-LSG	GE $T_{1/2}$ for solids, min: BL 67.1 ± 33.43 vs. 3-months 20.71 ± 12.81; $p < 0.05$	$\Delta 3$ months—BL BMI, kg/m^2: -8 ± 9.80; $p < 0.05$	[246]
100 subjects underwent LSG, BMI 43.43 ± 3.8 kg/m^2	Scintigraphic GE test: pre- and 3-months post-LSG	Retention, %: 1 h: 64 ± 13 vs. 54.5 ± 15; $p < 0.0001$ 2 h: 45 ± 12 vs. 35.5 ± 13); $p < 0.0001$ 4 h: 6 ± 3 vs. 4 ± 2; $p < 0.0001$	$\Delta 3$ months—BL BMI, kg/m^2: -8.83 ± 4.54; $p < 0.001$	[247]
23 subjects underwent LSG, BMI 42.4 ± 5.8 kg/m^2	MRI GE test: pre- and after 40% of EBW loss post-LSG	Total gastric volume, mL: BL 467 (95% CI (455, 585)) vs. post-Tx 139 (95% CI (121, 185)); $p < 0.0001$) Early-phase GE, mL/min: 1.9 (95% CI (1.1, 4.0)) vs. 2.69 (95% CI [1.6, 3.4]; $p = 0.001$) Late-phase GE, mL/min: 2.5 (95% CI (2.0, 2.9)) vs. 1.4 (95% CI (1.1, 1.7); $p = 0.001$)	$\Delta 7$ months—BL BMI, kg/m^2: -9.6 ± 7.28; $p < 0.001$	[213]
26 subjects underwent LSG, BMI 47.5 ± 6.6 kg/m^2	Scintigraphic GE test: after >20% TBWL post-LSG	GE $T_{1/2}$ for solids, min: BL 24.4 ± 11.4 vs. post-Tx 75.80 ± 45.19; $p < 0.001$	$\Delta 8$ months—BL BMI, kg/m^2: -12.60 ± 9.99; $p < 0.01$	[248]
10 SG (BMI 33.4 ± 2.4 kg/m^2), 10 RYGB (BMI 33.5 ± 2.1 kg/m^2), and 10 controls (BMI 33.4 ± 1.7 kg/m^2)	Scintigraphic GE test: SG vs. RYGB vs. controls	GE $T_{1/2}$ for solids, min: RYGB 11 ± 2; SG 56 ± 11; controls 113 ± 8; $p < 0.01$	BMI loss %: SG: 60 ± 8 vs. RYGB: 61 ± 7	[249]

Table 4. Cont.

Study Design/ Intervention	Methods	Effect on GI Motor Function	Weight Loss	Ref.
17 RYGB (BMI 45.8 ± 4.7 kg/m^2), and 9 controls (BMI 23.5 ± 1.9 kg/m^2)	Scintigraphic GE test: Between 15- and 21-months post-RYGB	Emptying of pouch or stomach (fraction of total meal x hours): Liquid marker, RYGB vs. controls: 0.19 (IQR 0.07–0.26) vs. 0.49 (IQR 0.47–0.64); $p < 0.001$ Solid marker, RYGB vs. controls: 0.45 (IQR 0.31–1.04) vs. 1.33 (IQR 1.15–1.65); $p = 0.004$	Δ18 months—BL BMI, kg/m^2: −11.20 ± 5.32; $p = 0.04$	[250]
10 RYGB (BMI 29.9 ± 1.9 kg/m^2), and 10 controls (BMI 24.3 ± 0.9 kg/m^2)	Scintigraphic GE test: 5 years post-surgical	RYGB vs. controls Pouch/GE T$_{1/2}$, min: faster un RYGB; $p < 0.001$ RYGB Sitting vs. supine position Pouch/GE T$_{1/2}$, min: 2.5 ± 0.7 vs. 16.6 ± 5.3 min; $p = 0.02$	Δ18 months—BL BMI, kg/m^2: −12.9 ± 3.4 kg/m^2	[221]
8 RYGB, and 24 controls (12 lean controls vs. 12 obese controls)	^{13}C-acetate breath test GE test: RYGB 10 weeks post-surgical	Gastric emptying in lean controls and obese controls was significantly slower vs. RYGB; $p < 0.001$)	Post-surgical BMI, kg/m^2: 38.6 ± 1.7	[251]
10 RYGB, divided according TBWL: poor weight loss (< 25%) ($n = 5$) vs. and Successful weight loss (> 25%) ($n = 5$)	Scintigraphic GE test: 2 years post-surgical	Poor weight loss vs. Successful weight loss Pouch/GE T$_{1/2}$, min: 5.1 ± 1.3 vs. 34 ± 32 ($p = 0.12$) Poor weight loss vs. Successful weight loss PER$_{max}$, %/min: 17 ± 4.7 vs. 5.6 ± 3.4; $p = 0.002$	Poor weight loss vs. Successful weight loss pre-surgical BMI, kg/m^2: 43 ± 4.3 vs. 45 ± 3.8 Poor weight loss vs. Successful weight loss at scintigraphy, %: 17 ± 4.1 vs. 44 ± 5.7	[219]
94 subjects underwent surgery: 47 RYGB BMI 42.4 kg/m^2 (IQR 36.0–54.9) and 47 BRYGB BMI 44.3 kg/m^2 (IQR 21.8–52.5)	Scintigraphic GE test: Between 6 months and 2 years post-surgical	GE T$_{1/2}$ for solids, min: RYGB 65.9 (IQR 40.6–183.0) vs. BRYGB 79.4 (IQR 41.1–390.9); $p = 0.031$	RYGB BMI, kg/m^2: 42.4 (IQR 36.0–54.9) vs. 30.9 (IQR 23.7–43.8) BRYGB BMI, kg/m^2: 44.3 (IQR 37.5–60.8) vs. 29.8 (IQR 21.8–52.5)	[146]

Abbreviations: AP: antral preservation; AR: Antral resection; AUC: area under the curve; BMI: body mass index; BPD-DS: biliopancreatic diversion with duodenal switch; BRYGB: Banded Roux-en-Y Gastric Bypass; CI: confidence interval; EWL: excess weight loss; GE: gastric emptying; IQR: inter quantile range; LGS: laparoscopic gastric sleeve; MIN: minutes; ns: non-significant; PER: pouch emptying rate; RYGB: Roux-en-Y Gastric Bypass; SE: standard error; TBWL: total body weight loss.

5. Conclusions

The effect of the stomach on food intake regulation is mediated by gastric motor and sensory functions, the former controlled by an interconnected net of intrinsic and extrinsic neuroendocrine signals. Gastric emptying and gastric accommodation are associated with appetite sensations, satiation, and satiety signals in health. These functions have been investigated as quantitative traits in relation to the pathophysiology of obesity. Despite advances in the technologies to measure gastric functions, the interpretation and standardization of studies remain challenging, which compromises the analysis of the outcomes. The variability of gastric motor and sensory functions may be influenced but not fully explained by essential characteristics such as gender, age, and weight. In the goal of fully understanding changes in gastric emptying, these variables must be taken into consideration.

Accelerated gastric emptying frequently occurs in patients with obesity. Although the magnitude of weight gain that induces acceleration remains contentious, it is appropriate to consider that gastric emptying may be one abnormal quantitative trait in obesity. Delaying gastric emptying by medications, particularly GLP-1 agonists, is a possible successful target for weight loss; however, the extent of the delay to induce weight loss remains controversial. Changes in gastric motility achieved with weight loss diets or surgical procedures may account for improvements in the gut hormone profiles, inducing release of satiety hormones and, thereby, reducing energy intake. On the road towards more personalized management of obesity, identifying patients with this specific trait may allow prediction of those who could most benefit from medications or procedures that retard gastric emptying. Future studies in treating obesity would be enhanced by optimized controlled trials that follow adequate protocols to measure gastric motility, that is, emptying and accommodation, as well as mechanisms controlling appetite, satiation, and satiety.

Author Contributions: All authors have contributed to writing, review, editing, and approval of the final version of the manuscript. All authors have read and agreed to the published version of the manuscript.

Funding: Acosta is supported by NIH (NIH K23-DK114460, C-Sig P30DK84567), ANMS Career Development Award, Mayo Clinic Center for Individualized Medicine-Gerstner Career Development Award. Camilleri receives funding related to obesity from National Institutes of Health (NIH RO1-DK67071).

Institutional Review Board Statement: Not applicable.

Informed Consent Statement: Not applicable.

Data Availability Statement: Not applicable.

Acknowledgments: Figures were created with BioRender.com (accessed on 30 March 2021).

Conflicts of Interest: Acosta is a stockholder in Gila Therapeutics, Phenomix Sciences; he serves as a consultant for Rhythm Pharmaceuticals, General Mills. Camilleri is a stockholder in Phenomix Sciences and Enterin and serves as a consultant to Takeda, Allergan, Rhythm, Kallyope, and Arena with compensation to his employer, Mayo Clinic.

Appendix A

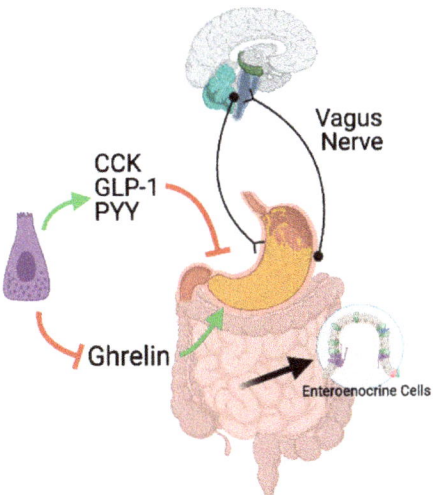

Figure A1. Neural and hormonal regulation of gastric emptying and gastric accommodation in response to meals. The neural regulation of gastric motor functions is commanded by the vagus nerve. The vagus nerve exerts both inhibitory and excitatory effects on the stomach. In response to nutrients, enteroendocrine cells along the gastrointestinal tract secrete CCK, GLP-1, and PYY, which inhibit gastric emptying. In response to the meal, ghrelin secretion, an orexigenic hormone known to stimulate gastric emptying, is blocked.

References

1. WHO. *Obesity and Overweight. Fact Sheet No 311*; WHO Media Centre: 2015. Available online: http://www.who.int/mediacentre/factsheets/fs311/en/ (accessed on 24 December 2015).
2. Hill, J.O.; Wyatt, H.R.; Peters, J.C. Energy balance and obesity. *Circulation* **2012**, *126*, 126–132. [CrossRef] [PubMed]
3. Blundell, J.; de Graaf, C.; Hulshof, T.; Jebb, S.; Livingstone, B.; Lluch, A.; Mela, D.; Salah, S.; Schuring, E.; van der Knaap, H.; et al. Appetite control: Methodological aspects of the evaluation of foods. *Obes. Rev.* **2010**, *11*, 251–270. [CrossRef] [PubMed]
4. Acosta, A.; Dayyeh, B.K.A.; Port, J.D.; Camilleri, M. Recent advances in clinical practice challenges and opportunities in the management of obesity. *Gut* **2014**, *63*, 687–695. [CrossRef] [PubMed]
5. Alhadeff, A.L.; Rupprecht, L.E.; Hayes, M.R. GLP-1 neurons in the nucleus of the solitary tract project directly to the ventral tegmental area and nucleus accumbens to control for food intake. *Endocrinology* **2012**, *153*, 647–658. [CrossRef] [PubMed]
6. Dickson, S.L.; Shirazi, R.H.; Hansson, C.; Bergquist, F.; Nissbrandt, H.; Skibicka, K.P. The glucagon-like peptide 1 (GLP-1) analogue, exendin-4, decreases the rewarding value of food: A new role for mesolimbic GLP-1 receptors. *J. Neurosci.* **2012**, *32*, 4812–4820. [CrossRef] [PubMed]
7. Horner, K.M.; Finlayson, G.; Byrne, N.M.; King, N.A. Food reward in active compared to inactive men: Roles for gastric emptying and body fat. *Physiol. Behav.* **2016**, *160*, 43–49. [CrossRef] [PubMed]
8. Williams, D.L. Neural integration of satiation and food reward: Role of GLP-1 and orexin pathways. *Physiol. Behav.* **2014**, *136*, 194–199. [CrossRef]
9. Rinaman, L. Ascending projections from the caudal visceral nucleus of the solitary tract to brain regions involved in food intake and energy expenditure. *Brain Res.* **2010**, *1350*, 18–34. [CrossRef] [PubMed]
10. Camilleri, M. Peripheral mechanisms in appetite regulation. *Gastroenterology* **2015**, *148*, 1219–1233. [CrossRef]
11. Hussain, S.S.; Bloom, S.R. The regulation of food intake by the gut-brain axis: Implications for obesity. *Int. J. Obes.* **2012**, *37*, 625–633. [CrossRef]
12. Hunt, J.; Cash, R.; Newland, P. Energy density of food, gastric emptying, and obesity. *Lancet* **1975**, *306*, 905–906. [CrossRef]
13. Park, M.I.; Camilleri, M. Gastric motor and sensory functions in obesity. *Obes. Res.* **2005**, *13*, 491–500. [CrossRef] [PubMed]
14. Acosta, A.; Camilleri, M.; Shin, A.; Vazquez-Roque, M.I.; Iturrino, J.; Burton, D.; O'Neill, J.; Eckert, D.; Zinsmeister, A.R. Quantitative Gastrointestinal and Psychological Traits Associated With Obesity and Response to Weight-Loss Therapy. *Gastroenterol.* **2015**, *148*, 537–546.e4. [CrossRef] [PubMed]
15. Jahnberg, T.; Martinson, J.; Hultén, L.; Fasth, S. Dynamic Gastric Response to Expansion before and after Vagotomy. *Scand. J. Gastroenterol.* **1975**, *10*, 593–598. [CrossRef] [PubMed]
16. Kuiken, S.D.; Vergeer, M.; Heisterkamp, S.H.; Tytgat, G.N.J.; Boeckxstaens, G.E.E. Role of nitric oxide in gastric motor and sensory functions in healthy subjects. *Gut* **2002**, *51*, 212–218. [CrossRef] [PubMed]
17. Camilleri, M.; Malagelada, J.R.; Brown, M.L.; Becker, G.; Zinsmeister, A.R. Relation between antral motility and gastric emptying of solids and liquids in humans. *Am. J. Physiol. Liver Physiol.* **1985**, *249*, G580–G585. [CrossRef] [PubMed]
18. Houghton, L.; Read, N.; Heddle, R.; Horowitz, M.; Collins, P.; Chatterton, B.; Dent, J. Relationship of the motor activity of the antrum, pylorus, and duodenum to gastric emptying of a solid-liquid mixed meal. *Gastroenterol.* **1988**, *94*, 1285–1291. [CrossRef]
19. Zhang, R.-X.; Wang, X.-Y.; Chen, D.; Huizinga, J.D. Role of interstitial cells of Cajal in the generation and modulation of motor activity induced by cholinergic neurotransmission in the stomach. *Neurogastroenterol. Motil.* **2011**, *23*, e356–e371. [CrossRef] [PubMed]
20. Ward, S.M.; Sanders, K.M.; Hirst, G.D.S. Role of interstitial cells of Cajal in neural control of gastrointestinal smooth muscles. *Neurogastroenterol. Motil.* **2004**, *16*, 112–117. [CrossRef]
21. Sanders, K.M.; Koh, S.D.; Ro, S.; Ward, S.M. Regulation of gastrointestinal motility—insights from smooth muscle biology. *Nat. Rev. Gastroenterol. Hepatol.* **2012**, *9*, 633–645. [CrossRef]
22. Kong, F.; Singh, R. Disintegration of Solid Foods in Human Stomach. *J. Food Sci.* **2008**, *73*, R67–R80. [CrossRef]
23. Meyer, J.; Ohashi, H.; Jehn, D.; Thomson, J. Size of liver particles emptied from the human stomach. *Gastroenterol.* **1981**, *80*, 1489–1496. [CrossRef]
24. Goyal, R.K.; Hirano, I. The Enteric Nervous System. *New Engl. J. Med.* **1996**, *334*, 1106–1115. [CrossRef] [PubMed]
25. Hunt, R.H.; Camilleri, M.; E Crowe, S.; Elomar, E.M.; Fox, J.G.; Kuipers, E.J.; Malfertheiner, P.; McColl, K.E.L.; Pritchard, D.; Rugge, M.; et al. The stomach in health and disease. *Gut* **2015**, *64*, 1650–1668. [CrossRef] [PubMed]
26. Furness, J.B. The enteric nervous system and neurogastroenterology. *Nat. Rev. Gastroenterol. Hepatol.* **2012**, *9*, 286–294. [CrossRef] [PubMed]
27. Akhavan, T.; Luhovyy, B.L.; Brown, P.H.; E Cho, C.; Anderson, G.H. Effect of premeal consumption of whey protein and its hydrolysate on food intake and postmeal glycemia and insulin responses in young adults. *Am. J. Clin. Nutr.* **2010**, *91*, 966–975. [CrossRef]
28. Goyal, R.K.; Guo, Y.; Mashimo, H. Advances in the physiology of gastric emptying. *Neurogastroenterol. Motil.* **2019**, *31*, e13546. [CrossRef]
29. Powley, T.L.; Jaffey, D.M.; McAdams, J.; Baronowsky, E.A.; Black, D.; Chesney, L.; Evans, C.; Phillips, R.J. Vagal innervation of the stomach reassessed: Brain–gut connectome uses smart terminals. *Ann. N. Y. Acad. Sci.* **2019**, *1454*, 14–30. [CrossRef]
30. Burton, M.; Rolls, E.; Mora, F. Effects of hunger on the responses of neurons in the lateral hypothalamus to the sight and taste of food. *Exp. Neurol.* **1976**, *51*, 668–677. [CrossRef]

31. Matzinger, D.; Degen, L.; Drewe, J.; Meuli, J.; Duebendorfer, R.; Ruckstuhl, N.; D'Amato, M.; Rovati, L.; Beglinger, C. The role of long chain fatty acids in regulating food intake and cholecystokinin release in humans. *Gut* **2000**, *46*, 689–694. [CrossRef] [PubMed]
32. Beglinger, C. Effect of Cholecystokinin on Gastric Motility in Humans. *Ann. N. Y. Acad. Sci.* **1994**, *713*, 219–225. [CrossRef] [PubMed]
33. A Liddle, R.; Morita, E.T.; Conrad, C.K.; A Williams, J. Regulation of gastric emptying in humans by cholecystokinin. *J. Clin. Investig.* **1986**, *77*, 992–996. [CrossRef]
34. Chey, W.; Hitanant, S.; Hendricks, J.; Lorber, S. Effect of Secretin and Cholecystokinin on Gastric Emptying and Gastric Secretion in Man. *Gastroenterology* **1970**, *58*, 820–827. [CrossRef]
35. Fried, M.; Erlacher, U.; Schwizer, W.; Löchner, C.; Koerfer, J.; Beglinger, C.; Jansen, J.B.; Lamers, C.B.; Harder, F.; Bischof-Delaloye, A. Role of cholecystokinin in the regulation of gastric emptying and pancreatic enzyme secretion in humans: Studies with the cholecystokinin-receptor antagonist loxiglumide. *Gastroenterology* **1991**, *101*, 503–511. [CrossRef]
36. Holst, J.J.; Ørskov, C.; Hartmann, B.; Deacon, C.F. Posttranslational Processing of Proglucagon and Postsecretory Fate of Proglucagon Products. *Front. Diabetes* **1997**, *13*, 24–48. [CrossRef]
37. Williams, D.L.; Baskin, D.G.; Schwartz, M.W. Evidence that Intestinal Glucagon-Like Peptide-1 Plays a Physiological Role in Satiety. *Endocrinol.* **2008**, *150*, 1680–1687. [CrossRef] [PubMed]
38. I˙meryüz, N.; Yeğen, B.C.; Bozkurt, A.; Coşkun, T.; Villanueva-Peñacarrillo, M.L.; Ulusoy, N.B. Glucagon-like peptide-1 inhibits gastric emptying via vagal afferent-mediated central mechanisms. *Am. J. Physiol. Gastrointest. Liver Physiol.* **1997**, *273*, G920–G927. [CrossRef] [PubMed]
39. Deane, A.M.; Nguyen, N.Q.; Stevens, J.E.; Fraser, R.J.L.; Holloway, R.H.; Besanko, L.K.; Burgstad, C.; Jones, K.L.; Chapman, M.J.; Rayner, C.K.; et al. Endogenous Glucagon-Like Peptide-1 Slows Gastric Emptying in Healthy Subjects, Attenuating Postprandial Glycemia. *J. Clin. Endocrinol. Metab.* **2010**, *95*, 215–221. [CrossRef] [PubMed]
40. Chakraborty, S.; Halland, M.; Burton, D.; Desai, A.; Neja, B.; Low, P.; Singer, W.; Camilleri, M.; Zinsmeister, A.R.; E Bharucha, A. GI Dysfunctions in Diabetic Gastroenteropathy, Their Relationships With Symptoms, and Effects of a GLP-1 Antagonist. *J. Clin. Endocrinol. Metab.* **2018**, *104*, 1967–1977. [CrossRef] [PubMed]
41. Näslund, E.; Gutniak, M.; Skogar, S.; Rössner, S.; Hellström, P.M. Glucagon-like peptide 1 increases the period of postprandial satiety and slows gastric emptying in obese men. *Am. J. Clin. Nutr.* **1998**, *68*, 525–530. [CrossRef] [PubMed]
42. Nauck, M.A.; Niedereichholz, U.; Ettler, R.; Holst, J.J.; Ørskov, C.; Ritzel, R.; Schmiegel, W.H. Glucagon-like peptide 1 inhibition of gastric emptying outweighs its insulinotropic effects in healthy humans. *Am. J. Physiol. Metab.* **1997**, *273*, E981–E988. [CrossRef] [PubMed]
43. Nagell, C.; Wettergren, A.; Pedersen, J.F.; Mortensen, D.; Holst, J.J. Glucagon-like peptide-2 inhibits antral emptying in man, but is not as potent as glucagon-like peptide-1. *Scand. J. Gastroenterol.* **2004**, *39*, 353–358. [CrossRef] [PubMed]
44. Miki, T.; Minami, K.; Shinozaki, H.; Matsumura, K.; Saraya, A.; Ikeda, H.; Yamada, Y.; Holst, J.J.; Seino, S. Distinct Effects of Glucose-Dependent Insulinotropic Polypeptide and Glucagon-Like Peptide-1 on Insulin Secretion and Gut Motility. *Diabetes* **2005**, *54*, 1056–1063. [CrossRef] [PubMed]
45. Edholm, T.; Degerblad, M.; Grybäck, P.; Hilsted, L.; Holst, J.J.; Jacobsson, H.; Efendic, S.; Schmidt, P.; Hellström, P.M. Differential incretin effects of GIP and GLP-1 on gastric emptying, appetite, and insulin-glucose homeostasis. *Neurogastroenterol. Motil.* **2010**, *22*, 1191-e315. [CrossRef] [PubMed]
46. Kar, P.; Jones, K.L.; Horowitz, M.; Chapman, M.J.; Deane, A.M. Measurement of gastric emptying in the critically ill. *Clin. Nutr.* **2015**, *34*, 557–564. [CrossRef]
47. Adrian, T.; Ferri, G.-L.; Bacarese-Hamilton, A.; Fuessl, H.; Polak, J.; Bloom, S. Human distribution and release of a putative new gut hormone, peptide YY. *Gastroenterology* **1985**, *89*, 1070–1077. [CrossRef]
48. Pironi, L.; Stanghellini, V.; Miglioli, M.; Corinaldesi, R.; de Giorgio, R.; Ruggeri, E.; Tosetti, C.; Poggioli, G.; Morselliˆlabate, A.M.; Monetti, N.; et al. Fat-induced heal brake in humans: A dose-dependent phenomenon correlated to the plasma levels of peptide YY. *Gastroenterology* **1993**, *105*, 733–739. [CrossRef]
49. Batterham, R.L.; Cowley, M.A.; Small, C.J.; Herzog, H.; Cohen, M.A.; Dakin, C.L.; Wren, A.M.; Brynes, A.E.; Low, M.J.; Ghatei, M.A.; et al. Gut hormone PYY3-36 physiologically inhibits food intake. *Nat. Cell Biol.* **2002**, *418*, 650–654. [CrossRef]
50. Samsom, M.; Szarka, L.A.; Camilleri, M.; Vella, A.; Zinsmeister, A.R.; Rizza, R.A. Pramlintide, an amylin analog, selectively delays gastric emptying: Potential role of vagal inhibition. *Am. J. Physiol. Liver Physiol.* **2000**, *278*, G946–G951. [CrossRef] [PubMed]
51. Bado, A.; Levasseur, S.; Attoub, S.; Kermorgant, S.; Laigneau, J.-P.; Bortoluzzi, M.-N.; Moizo, L.; Lehy, T.; Guerre-Millo, M.; Le Marchand-Brustel, Y.; et al. The stomach is a source of leptin. *Nat. Cell Biol.* **1998**, *394*, 790–793. [CrossRef]
52. Martínez, V.; Barrachina, M.-D.; Wang, L.; Taché, Y. Intracerebroventricular leptin inhibits gastric emptying of a solid nutrient meal in rats. *Neuro Rep.* **1999**, *10*, 3217–3221. [CrossRef] [PubMed]
53. Cakir, B.; Kasimay, O.; Devseren, E.; Yeğen, B.C. Leptin inhibits gastric emptying in rats: Role of CCK receptors and vagal afferent fibers. *Physiol. Res.* **2006**, *56*, 315–322. [PubMed]
54. Sanger, G.J.; Hellström, P.M.; Näslund, E. The hungry stomach: Physiology, disease, and drug development opportunities. *Front. Pharmacol.* **2011**, *1*, 145. [CrossRef] [PubMed]
55. Druce, M.R.; Wren, A.M.; Park, A.J.; E Milton, J.; Patterson, M.; Frost, G.; A Ghatei, M.; Small, C.; Bloom, S.R. Ghrelin increases food intake in obese as well as lean subjects. *Int. J. Obes.* **2005**, *29*, 1130–1136. [CrossRef]

56. Meleine, M.; Mounien, L.; Atmani, K.; Ouelaa, W.; Bôle-Feysot, C.; Guérin, C.; Depoortere, I.; Gourcerol, G. Ghrelin inhibits autonomic response to gastric distension in rats by acting on vagal pathway. *Sci. Rep.* **2020**, *10*, 1–10. [CrossRef]
57. Camilleri, M.; McCallum, R.W.; Tack, J.; Spence, S.C.; Gottesdiener, K.; Fiedorek, F.T. Efficacy and Safety of Relamorelin in Diabetics With Symptoms of Gastroparesis: A Randomized, Placebo-Controlled Study. *Gastroenterology* **2017**, *153*, 1240–1250.e2. [CrossRef]
58. Lembo, A.; Camilleri, M.; McCallum, R.; Sastre, R.; Breton, C.; Spence, S.; White, J.; Currie, M.; Gottesdiener, K.; Stoner, E. Relamorelin Reduces Vomiting Frequency and Severity and Accelerates Gastric Emptying in Adults With Diabetic Gastroparesis. *Gastroenterology* **2016**, *151*, 87–96.e6. [CrossRef] [PubMed]
59. Nelson, A.D.; Camilleri, M.; Acosta, A.; Busciglio, I.; Nord, S.L.; Boldingh, A.; Rhoten, D.; Ryks, M.; Burton, D. Effects of ghrelin receptor agonist, relamorelin, on gastric motor functions and satiation in healthy volunteers. *Neurogastroenterol. Motil.* **2016**, *28*, 1705–1713. [CrossRef]
60. James, J.; Mair, S.; Doll, W.; Sandefer, E.; Wurtman, D.; Maurer, A.; Deane, A.M.; Harris, M.S. The effects of ulimorelin, a ghrelin agonist, on liquid gastric emptying and colonic transit in humans. *Neurogastroenterol. Motil.* **2019**, *32*, e13784. [CrossRef] [PubMed]
61. Wang, X.J.; Burton, D.D.; Breen-Lyles, M.; Camilleri, M. Gastric Accommodation Influences Proximal Gastric and Total Gastric Emptying in Concurrent Measurements Conducted in Healthy Volunteers. *Am. J. Physiol. Liver Physiol.* **2021**. [CrossRef]
62. Schwizer, W.; Maecke, H.; Michael, F. Measurement of gastric emptying by magnetic resonance imaging in humans. *Gastroenterology* **1992**, *103*, 369–376. [CrossRef]
63. Abell, T.L.; Camilleri, M.; Donohoe, K.; Hasler, W.L.; Lin, H.C.; Maurer, A.H.; McCallum, R.W.; Nowak, T.; Nusynowitz, M.L.; Parkman, H.P.; et al. Consensus Recommendations for Gastric Emptying Scintigraphy: A Joint Report of the American Neurogastroenterology and Motility Society and the Society of Nuclear Medicine. *J. Nucl. Med. Technol.* **2008**, *36*, 44–54. [CrossRef] [PubMed]
64. Camilleri, M.; Iturrino, J.; Bharucha, A.E.; Burton, D.; Shin, A.; Jeong, I.-D.; Zinsmeister, A.R. Performance characteristics of scintigraphic measurement of gastric emptying of solids in healthy participants. *Neurogastroenterol. Motil.* **2012**, *24*, 1076-e562. [CrossRef] [PubMed]
65. Camilleri, M.; Zinsmeister, A.R.; Greydanus, M.P.; Brown, M.L.; Proano, M. Towards a less costly but accurate test of gastric emptying and small bowel transit. *Dig. Dis. Sci.* **1991**, *36*, 609–615. [CrossRef]
66. Wise, J.L.; Vazquez-Roque, M.I.; McKinney, C.J.; Zickella, M.A.; Crowell, M.D.; Lacy, B.E. Gastric Emptying Scans: Poor Adherence to National Guidelines. *Dig. Dis. Sci.* **2020**, 1–10. [CrossRef] [PubMed]
67. Hveem, K.; Jones, K.L.; E Chatterton, B.; Horowitz, M. Scintigraphic measurement of gastric emptying and ultrasonographic assessment of antral area: Relation to appetite. *Gut* **1996**, *38*, 816–821. [CrossRef] [PubMed]
68. Gilja, O.H.; Hausken, T.; Ødegaard, S.; Berstad, A. Gastric emptying measured by ultrasonography. *World J. Gastroenterol.* **1999**, *5*, 93–94. [CrossRef] [PubMed]
69. Gilja, O.H.; Lunding, J.; Hausken, T.; Gregersen, H. Gastric accommodation assessed by ultrasonography. *World J. Gastroenterol.* **2006**, *12*, 2825–2829. [CrossRef]
70. Gilja, O.; Detmer, P.R.; Jong, J.M.; Leotta, D.F.; Li, X.N.; Beach, K.; Martin, R.; Strandness Jr, D. Intragastric distribution and gastric emptying assessed by three-dimensional ultrasonography. *Gastroenterology* **1997**, *113*, 38–49. [CrossRef]
71. Stevens, J.E.; Gilja, O.H.; Gentilcore, D.; Hausken, T.; Horowitz, M.; Jones, K.L. Measurement of gastric emptying of a high-nutrient liquid by 3D ultrasonography in diabetic gastroparesis. *Neurogastroenterol. Motil.* **2010**, *23*, 220-e114. [CrossRef]
72. Tefera, S.; Gilja, O.H.; Olafsdottir, E.; Hausken, T.; Hatlebakk, J.G.; Berstad, A. Intragastric maldistribution of a liquid meal in patients with reflux oesophagitis assessed by three dimensional ultrasonography. *Gut* **2002**, *50*, 153–158. [CrossRef] [PubMed]
73. Gentilcore, D.; Hausken, T.; Horowitz, M.; Jones, K. Measurements of gastric emptying of low-and high-nutrient liquids using 3D ultrasonography and scintigraphy in healthy subjects. *Neurogastroenterol. Motil.* **2006**, *18*, 1062–1068. [CrossRef]
74. Medhus, A.W.; Lofthus, C.M.; Bredesen, J.; Husebye, E. Gastric emptying: The validity of the paracetamol absorption test adjusted for individual pharmacokinetics. *Neurogastroenterol. Motil.* **2001**, *13*, 179–185. [CrossRef] [PubMed]
75. Szarka, L.A.; Camilleri, M.; Vella, A.; Burton, D.; Baxter, K.; Simonson, J.; Zinsmeister, A.R. A Stable Isotope Breath Test With a Standard Meal for Abnormal Gastric Emptying of Solids in the Clinic and in Research. *Clin. Gastroenterol. Hepatol.* **2008**, *6*, 635–643.e1. [CrossRef] [PubMed]
76. Bluemel, S.; Menne, D.; Fried, M.; Schwizer, W.; Steingoetter, A. On the validity of the13C-acetate breath test for comparing gastric emptying of different liquid test meals: A validation study using magnetic resonance imaging. *Neurogastroenterol. Motil.* **2015**, *27*, 1487–1494. [CrossRef] [PubMed]
77. Heading, R.C.; Nimmo, J.; Prescott, L.F.; Tothill, P. The dependence of paracetamol absorption on the rate of gastric emptying. *Br. J. Pharmacol.* **1973**, *47*, 415–421. [CrossRef]
78. Willems, M.; Quartero, A.O.; Numans, M.E. How Useful Is Paracetamol Absorption as a Marker of Gastric Emptying? A Systematic Literature Study. *Dig. Dis. Sci.* **2001**, *46*, 2256–2262. [CrossRef]
79. Bartholome, R.; Salden, B.; Vrolijk, M.F.; Troost, F.J.; Masclee, A.; Bast, A.; Haenen, G.R. Paracetamol as a Post Prandial Marker for Gastric Emptying, A Food-Drug Interaction on Absorption. *PLoS ONE* **2015**, *10*, e0136618. [CrossRef] [PubMed]
80. Horowitz, M.; Rayner, C.K.; Marathe, C.S.; Wu, T.; Jones, K.L. Glucagon-like peptide-1 receptor agonists and the appropriate measurement of gastric emptying. *Diabetes, Obes. Metab.* **2020**, *22*, 2504–2506. [CrossRef] [PubMed]

81. Van Can, J.; Sloth, B.; Jensen, C.B.; Flint, A.; E Blaak, E.; Saris, W.H.M. Effects of the once-daily GLP-1 analog liraglutide on gastric emptying, glycemic parameters, appetite and energy metabolism in obese, non-diabetic adults. *Int. J. Obes.* **2014**, *38*, 784–793. [CrossRef]
82. Halawi, H.; Khemani, D.; Eckert, D.; O'Neill, J.; Kadouh, H.; Grothe, K.; Clark, M.M.; Burton, D.D.; Vella, A.; Acosta, A.; et al. Effects of liraglutide on weight, satiation, and gastric functions in obesity: A randomised, placebo-controlled pilot trial. *Lancet Gastroenterol. Hepatol.* **2017**, *2*, 890–899. [CrossRef]
83. Maqbool, S.; Parkman, H.P.; Friedenberg, F.K. Wireless Capsule Motility: Comparison of the SmartPill®GI Monitoring System with Scintigraphy for Measuring Whole Gut Transit. *Dig. Dis. Sci.* **2009**, *54*, 2167–2174. [CrossRef] [PubMed]
84. Schwizer, W.; Steingotter, A.; Fox, M.; Zur, T.; Thumshirn, M.; Bosiger, P.; Fried, M. Non-invasive measurement of gastric accommodation in humans. *Gut* **2002**, *51*, i59–i62. [CrossRef] [PubMed]
85. Chial, H.J.; Camilleri, M.; Delgado-Aros, S.; Burton, D.; Thomforde, G.; Ferber, I. A nutrient drink test to assess maximum tolerated volume and postprandial symptoms: Effects of gender, body mass index and age in health. *Neurogastroenterol. Motil.* **2002**, *14*, 249–253. [CrossRef] [PubMed]
86. Kindt, S.; Coulie, B.; Wajs, E.; Janssens, J.; Tack, J. Reproducibility and symptomatic predictors of a slow nutrient drinking test in health and in functional dyspepsia. *Neurogastroenterol. Motil.* **2008**, *20*, 320–329. [CrossRef] [PubMed]
87. Tack, J.; Caenepeel, P.; Piessevaux, H.; Cuomo, R.; Janssens, J. Assessment of meal induced gastric accommodation by a satiety drinking test in health and in severe functional dyspepsia. *Gut* **2003**, *52*, 1271–1277. [CrossRef] [PubMed]
88. Vijayvargiya, P.; Chedid, V.; Wang, X.J.; Atieh, J.; Maselli, D.; Burton, D.D.; Clark, M.M.; Acosta, A.; Camilleri, M. Associations of gastric volumes, ingestive behavior, calorie and volume intake, and fullness in obesity. *Am. J. Physiol. Liver Physiol.* **2020**, *319*, G238–G244. [CrossRef] [PubMed]
89. Blundell, J.E.; Halford, J.C.G. Regulation of nutrient supply: The brain and appetite control. *Proc. Nutr. Soc.* **1994**, *53*, 407–418. [CrossRef] [PubMed]
90. Halawi, H.; Camilleri, M.; Acosta, A.; Vazquez-Roque, M.; Oduyebo, I.; Burton, D.; Busciglio, I.; Zinsmeister, A.R. Relationship of gastric emptying or accommodation with satiation, satiety, and postprandial symptoms in health. *Am. J. Physiol. Liver Physiol.* **2017**, *313*, G442–G447. [CrossRef]
91. Cannon, W.B.; Washburn, A.L. An Explanation of Hunger 1. *Obes. Res.* **1993**, *1*, 494–500. [CrossRef]
92. Cannon, W.B. *The Mechanical Factors of Digestion*; Longmans, Green & Company: New York, NY, USA, 1911.
93. Delgado-Aros, S.; Cremonini, F.; Castillo, J.E.; Chial, H.J.; Burton, D.D.; Ferber, I.; Camilleri, M. Independent influences of body mass and gastric volumes on satiation in humans. *Gastroenterology* **2004**, *126*, 432–440. [CrossRef]
94. Park, S.-Y.; Acosta, A.; Camilleri, M.; Burton, D.; Harmsen, S.W.; Fox, J.; A Szarka, L. Gastric Motor Dysfunction in Patients With Functional Gastroduodenal Symptoms. *Am. J. Gastroenterol.* **2017**, *112*, 1689–1699. [CrossRef] [PubMed]
95. Tack, J.; Piessevaux, H.; Coulie, B.; Caenepeel, P.; Janssens, J. Role of impaired gastric accommodation to a meal in functional dyspepsia. *Gastroenterology* **1998**, *115*, 1346–1352. [CrossRef]
96. Blundell, J.E.; Gillett, A. Control of Food Intake in the Obese. *Obes. Res.* **2001**, *9*, 263S–270S. [CrossRef] [PubMed]
97. Cummings, D.E.; Overduin, J. Gastrointestinal regulation of food intake. *J. Clin. Investig.* **2007**, *117*, 13–23. [CrossRef] [PubMed]
98. Flint, A.; Raben, A.; Rehfeld, J.; Holst, J.; Astrup, A. The effect of glucagon-like peptide-1 on energy expenditure and substrate metabolism in humans. *Int. J. Obes.* **2000**, *24*, 288–298. [CrossRef] [PubMed]
99. Chapman, I.M.; A Goble, E.; A Wittert, G.; Horowitz, M. Effects of small-intestinal fat and carbohydrate infusions on appetite and food intake in obese and nonobese men. *Am. J. Clin. Nutr.* **1999**, *69*, 6–12. [CrossRef]
100. Feinle-Bisset, C.; Christen, M.; Grundy, D.; Faas, H.; Meier, O.; Otto, B.; Fried, M. Effects of duodenal fat, protein or mixed-nutrient infusions on epigastric sensations during sustained gastric distension in healthy humans. *Neurogastroenterol. Motil.* **2002**, *14*, 205–213. [CrossRef] [PubMed]
101. Matzinger, D.; Gutzwiller, J.-P.; Drewe, J.; Orban, A.; Engel, R.; D'Amato, M.; Rovati, L.; Beglinger, C. Inhibition of food intake in response to intestinal lipid is mediated by cholecystokinin in humans. *Am. J. Physiol. Content* **1999**, *277*, R1718–R1724. [CrossRef]
102. Corvilain, B.; Abramowicz, M.; Féry, F.; Schoutens, A.; Verlinden, M.; Balasse, E.; Horowitz, M. Effect of short-term starvation on gastric emptying in humans: Relationship to oral glucose tolerance. *Am. J. Physiol. Liver Physiol.* **1995**, *269*, G512–G517. [CrossRef] [PubMed]
103. Ma, J.; Stevens, J.E.; Cukier, K.; Maddox, A.F.; Wishart, J.M.; Jones, K.L.; Clifton, P.M.; Horowitz, M.; Rayner, C.K. Effects of a Protein Preload on Gastric Emptying, Glycemia, and Gut Hormones After a Carbohydrate Meal in Diet-Controlled Type 2 Diabetes. *Diabetes Care* **2009**, *32*, 1600–1602. [CrossRef] [PubMed]
104. Watson, L.E.; Phillips, L.K.; Wu, T.; Bound, M.J.; Checklin, H.; Grivell, J.; Jones, K.L.; Horowitz, M.; Rayner, C.K. Title: Differentiating the effects of whey protein and guar gum preloads on postprandial glycemia in type 2 diabetes. *Clin. Nutr.* **2019**, *38*, 2827–2832. [CrossRef]
105. Watson, L.E.; Phillips, L.K.; Wu, T.; Bound, M.J.; Checklin, H.L.; Grivell, J.; Jones, K.L.; Clifton, P.M.; Horowitz, M.; Rayner, C.K. A whey/guar "preload" improves postprandial glycaemia and glycated haemoglobin levels in type 2 diabetes: A 12-week, single-blind, randomized, placebo-controlled trial. *Diabetes Obes. Metab.* **2019**, *21*, 930–938. [CrossRef] [PubMed]
106. Ma, J.; Jesudason, D.R.; Stevens, J.E.; Keogh, J.B.; Jones, K.L.; Clifton, P.M.; Horowitz, M.; Rayner, C.K. Sustained effects of a protein 'preload' on glycaemia and gastric emptying over 4 weeks in patients with type 2 diabetes: A randomized clinical trial. *Diabetes Res. Clin. Pract.* **2015**, *108*, e31–e34. [CrossRef] [PubMed]

107. Holt, S.; Carter, D.; Tothill, P.; Heading, R.; Prescott, L. Effect of gel fibre on gastric emptying and absorption of glucose and paracetamol. *Lancet* **1979**, *313*, 636–639. [CrossRef]
108. French, S.J.; Read, N.W. Effect of guar gum on hunger and satiety after meals of differing fat content: Relationship with gastric emptying. *Am. J. Clin. Nutr.* **1994**, *59*, 87–91. [CrossRef] [PubMed]
109. Benini, L.; Castellani, G.; Brighenti, F.; Heaton, K.W.; Brentegani, M.T.; Casiraghi, M.C.; Sembenini, C.; Pellegrini, N.; Fioretta, A.; Minniti, G. Gastric emptying of a solid meal is accelerated by the removal of dietary fibre naturally present in food. *Gut* **1995**, *36*, 825–830. [CrossRef] [PubMed]
110. Rolls, B.J.; Fedoroff, I.C.; Guthrie, J.F. Gender differences in eating behavior and body weight regulation. *Health Psychol.* **1991**, *10*, 133–142. [CrossRef] [PubMed]
111. Giezenaar, C.; Luscombe-Marsh, N.D.; Hutchison, A.T.; Lange, K.; Hausken, T.; Jones, K.L.; Horowitz, M.; Chapman, I.; Soenen, S. Effect of gender on the acute effects of whey protein ingestion on energy intake, appetite, gastric emptying and gut hormone responses in healthy young adults. *Nutr. Diabetes* **2018**, *8*, 1–12. [CrossRef]
112. Giezenaar, C.; Lange, K.; Hausken, T.; Jones, K.L.; Horowitz, M.; Chapman, I.; Soenen, S. Effects of Age on Acute Appetite-Related Responses to Whey-Protein Drinks, Including Energy Intake, Gastric Emptying, Blood Glucose, and Plasma Gut Hormone Concentrations—A Randomized Controlled Trial. *Nutrients* **2020**, *12*, 1008. [CrossRef]
113. Gonenne, J.; Esfandyari, T.; Camilleri, M.; Burton, D.D.; Stephens, D.A.; Baxter, K.L.; Zinsmeister, A.R.; Bharucha, A.E. Effect of female sex hormone supplementation and withdrawal on gastrointestinal and colonic transit in postmenopausal women. *Neurogastroenterol. Motil.* **2006**, *18*, 911–918. [CrossRef]
114. Hellmig, S.; Von Schöning, F.; Gadow, C.; Katsoulis, S.; Hedderich, J.; Fölsch, U.R.; Stüber, E. Gastric emptying time of fluids and solids in healthy subjects determined by 13C breath tests: Influence of age, sex and body mass index. *J. Gastroenterol. Hepatol.* **2006**, *21*, 1832–1838. [CrossRef]
115. Moore, J.G.; Tweedy, C.; Christian, P.E.; Datz, F.L. Effect of age on gastric emptying of liquid-solid meals in man. *Dig. Dis. Sci.* **1983**, *28*, 340–344. [CrossRef] [PubMed]
116. Weindruch, R.; Sohal, R.S. Caloric Intake and Aging. *N. Engl. J. Med.* **1997**, *337*, 986–994. [CrossRef]
117. Schwartz, J.G.; Mcmahan, C.A.; Green, G.M.; Phillips, W.T. Gastric emptying in Mexican Americans compared to non-Hispanic whites. *Dig. Dis. Sci.* **1995**, *40*, 624–630. [CrossRef] [PubMed]
118. Schwartz, J.; Salman, U.; Mcmahan, C.; Phillips, W. Gastric emptying of beer in Mexican-Americans compared with non-hispanic whites. *Metabolism* **1996**, *45*, 1174–1178. [CrossRef]
119. Cohen, M.P.; Stern, E.; Rusecki, Y.; Zeidler, A. High prevalence of diabetes in young adult Ethiopian immigrants to Israel. *Diabetes* **1988**, *37*, 824–828. [CrossRef]
120. Howard, B.V.; Bogardus, C.; Ravussin, E.; E Foley, J.; Lillioja, S.; Mott, D.M.; Bennett, P.H.; Knowler, W.C. Studies of the etiology of obesity in Pima Indians. *Am. J. Clin. Nutr.* **1991**, *53*, 1577S–1585S. [CrossRef] [PubMed]
121. Wang, X.; Xie, C.; Marathe, C.S.; Malbert, C.-H.; Horowitz, M.; Jones, K.L.; Rayner, C.K.; Sun, Z.; Wu, T. Disparities in gastric emptying and postprandial glycaemia between Han Chinese and Caucasians with type 2 diabetes. *Diabetes Res. Clin. Pract.* **2020**, *159*, 107951. [CrossRef] [PubMed]
122. Carrio, I.; Estorch, M.; Serra-Grima, R.; Ginjaume, M.; Notivol, R.; Calabuig, R.; Vilardell, F. Gastric emptying in marathon runners. *Gut* **1989**, *30*, 152–155. [CrossRef] [PubMed]
123. Davis, J.; Camilleri, M.; Eckert, D.; Burton, D.; Joyner, M.; Acosta, A. Physical activity is associated with accelerated gastric emptying and increased ghrelin in obesity. *Neurogastroenterol. Motil.* **2020**, *32*, e13879. [CrossRef] [PubMed]
124. Horner, K.M.; Schubert, M.M.; Desbrow, B.; Byrne, N.M.; King, N.A. Acute Exercise and Gastric Emptying: A Meta-Analysis and Implications for Appetite Control. *Sports Med.* **2015**, *45*, 659–678. [CrossRef] [PubMed]
125. Mateos, A.M.C.; Roa-Colomo, A.; Vílchez, B.V. Changes in gastric emptying of digestible solids in professional cyclists: Relationship with exercise intensity. *Revista Española de Enfermedades Digestivas* **2020**. [CrossRef]
126. Delgado-Aros, S.; Camilleri, M.; Castillo, E.J.; Cremonini, F.; Stephens, D.; Ferber, I.; Baxter, K.; Burton, D.; Zinsmeister, A.R. Effect of Gastric Volume or Emptying on Meal-Related Symptoms After Liquid Nutrients in Obesity: A Pharmacologic Study. *Clin. Gastroenterol. Hepatol.* **2005**, *3*, 997–1006. [CrossRef]
127. Roque, M.I.V.; Camilleri, M.; Stephens, D.A.; Jensen, M.D.; Burton, D.D.; Baxter, K.L.; Zinsmeister, A.R. Gastric Sensorimotor Functions and Hormone Profile in Normal Weight, Overweight, and Obese People. *Gastroenterology* **2006**, *131*, 1717–1724. [CrossRef] [PubMed]
128. Wright, R.A.; Krinsky, S.; Fleeman, C.; Trujillo, J.; Teague, E. Gastric emptying and obesity. *Gastroenterology* **1983**, *84*, 747–751. [CrossRef]
129. Tosetti, C.; Corinaldesi, R.; Stanghellini, V.; Pasquali, R.; Corbelli, C.; Zoccoli, G.; Di Febo, G.; Monetti, N.; Barbara, L. Gastric emptying of solids in morbid obesity. *Int. J. Obes. Relat. Metab. Disord. J. Int. Assoc. Study Obes.* **1996**, *20*, 200.
130. Maddox, A.; Horowitz, M.; Wishart, J.; Collins, P. Gastric and Oesophageal Emptying in Obesity. *Scand. J. Gastroenterol.* **1989**, *24*, 593–598. [CrossRef] [PubMed]
131. Jackson, S.J.; Leahy, F.E.; McGowan, A.A.; Bluck, L.J.C.; Coward, W.A.; Jebb, S.A. Delayed gastric emptying in the obese: An assessment using the non-invasive 13C-octanoic acid breath test. *Diabetes Obes. Metab.* **2004**, *6*, 264–270. [CrossRef]
132. Horowitz, M.; Collins, P.J.; Cook, D.J.; E Harding, P.; Shearman, D.J. Abnormalities of gastric emptying in obese patients. *Int. J. Obes.* **1983**, *7*, 415–421. [CrossRef]

133. Phillips, L.K.; Deane, A.M.; Jones, K.L.; Rayner, C.K.; Horowitz, M. Gastric emptying and glycaemia in health and diabetes mellitus. *Nat. Rev. Endocrinol.* **2015**, *11*, 112–128. [CrossRef]
134. Parkman, H.P.; Urbain, J.-L.C.; Knight, L.C.; Brown, K.L.; Trate, D.M.; A Miller, M.; Maurer, A.H.; Fisher, R.S. Effect of gastric acid suppressants on human gastric motility. *Gut* **1998**, *42*, 243–250. [CrossRef] [PubMed]
135. Cunningham, K.M.; Daly, J.; Horowitz, M.; Read, N.W. Gastrointestinal adaptation to diets of differing fat composition in human volunteers. *Gut* **1991**, *32*, 483–486. [CrossRef] [PubMed]
136. Miller, G.; Palmer, K.R.; Smith, B.; Ferrington, C.; Merrick, M.V. Smoking delays gastric emptying of solids. *Gut* **1989**, *30*, 50–53. [CrossRef] [PubMed]
137. Johansson, C.; Ekelund, K. Relation between body weight and the gastric and intestinal handling of an oral caloric load. *Gut* **1976**, *17*, 456–462. [CrossRef]
138. Pajot, G.; Camilleri, M.; Calderon, G.; Davis, J.; Eckert, D.; Burton, D.; Acosta, A. Association between gastrointestinal phenotypes and weight gain in younger adults: A prospective 4-year cohort study. *Int. J. Obes.* **2020**, *44*, 2472–2478. [CrossRef] [PubMed]
139. Geliebter, A.; Schachter, S.; Lohmann-Walter, C.; Feldman, H.; A Hashim, S. Reduced stomach capacity in obese subjects after dieting. *Am. J. Clin. Nutr.* **1996**, *63*, 170–173. [CrossRef]
140. Granström, L.; Backman, L. Stomach distension in extremely obese and in normal subjects. *Acta Chir. Scand.* **1985**, *151*, 367–370.
141. Geliebter, A. Gastric distension and gastric capacity in relation to food intake in humans. *Physiol. Behav.* **1988**, *44*, 665–668. [CrossRef]
142. Bagger, J.I.; Holst, J.J.; Hartmann, B.; Andersen, B.; Knop, F.K.; Vilsbøll, T. Effect of Oxyntomodulin, Glucagon, GLP-1, and Combined Glucagon +GLP-1 Infusion on Food Intake, Appetite, and Resting Energy Expenditure. *J. Clin. Endocrinol. Metab.* **2015**, *100*, 4541–4552. [CrossRef]
143. Schjoldager, B.; Mortensen, P.E.; Myhre, J.; Christiansen, J.; Holst, J.J. Oxyntomodulin from distal gut. *Dig. Dis. Sci.* **1989**, *34*, 1411–1419. [CrossRef] [PubMed]
144. Naslund, E.; Grybäck, P.; Bäckman, L.; Jacobsson, H.; Holst, J.J.; Theodorsson, H.E.; Hellstrom, P.M.; Juul, J. Distal Small Bowel Hormones (Correlation with Fasting Antroduodenal Motility and Gastric Emptying). *Dig. Dis. Sci.* **1998**, *43*, 945–952. [CrossRef]
145. Bonazzi, P.; Petrelli, M.D.; Lorenzini, I.; Peruzzi, E.; Nicolai, A.; Galeazzi, R. Gastric emptying and intragastric balloon in obese patients. *Eur. Rev. Med Pharmacol. Sci.* **2006**, *9*, 15–21.
146. Reis, G.M.F.; Malheiros, C.A.; Savassi-Rocha, P.R.; Júnior, O.L.C.; Thuler, F.R.; Faria, M.L.; Filho, V.G. Gastric Emptying and Food Tolerance Following Banded and Non-banded Roux-en-Y Gastric Bypass. *Obes. Surg.* **2018**, *29*, 560–568. [CrossRef] [PubMed]
147. Hutson, W.R.; Wald, A. Obesity and weight reduction do not influence gastric emptying and antral motility. *Am. J. Gastroenterol.* **1993**, *88*, 88.
148. Torra, S.; Ilzarbe, L.; Malagelada, J.R.; Negre, M.; Mestre-Fusco, A.; Aguadé-Bruix, S.; Florensa, E.; Suñé, P.; Gras, B.; Hernandez, J.J.; et al. Meal size can be decreased in obese subjects through pharmacological acceleration of gastric emptying (The OBERYTH trial). *Int. J. Obes.* **2010**, *35*, 829–837. [CrossRef] [PubMed]
149. Horowitz, M.; Cook, D.J.; Collins, P.J.; Harding, P.E.; Hooper, M.J.; Walsh, J.F.; Shearman, D.J.C. Measurement of gastric emptying after gastric bypass surgery using radionuclides. *BJS* **1982**, *69*, 655–657. [CrossRef] [PubMed]
150. Morínigo, R.; Moizé, V.; Musri, M.; Lacy, A.M.; Navarro, S.; Marín, J.L.; Delgado, S.; Casamitjana, R.; Vidal, J. Glucagon-Like Peptide-1, Peptide YY, Hunger, and Satiety after Gastric Bypass Surgery in Morbidly Obese Subjects. *J. Clin. Endocrinol. Metab.* **2006**, *91*, 1735–1740. [CrossRef] [PubMed]
151. Falkén, Y.; Hellström, P.M.; Holst, J.J.; Näslund, E. Changes in glucose homeostasis after Roux-en-Y gastric bypass surgery for obesity at day three, two months, and one year after surgery: Role of gut peptides. *J. Clin. Endocrinol. Metab.* **2011**, *96*, 2227–2235. [CrossRef]
152. Shah, S.; Shah, P.; Todkar, J.; Gagner, M.; Sonar, S.; Solav, S. Prospective controlled study of effect of laparoscopic sleeve gastrectomy on small bowel transit time and gastric emptying half-time in morbidly obese patients with type 2 diabetes mellitus. *Surg. Obes. Relat. Dis.* **2010**, *6*, 152–157. [CrossRef]
153. Gómez, V.; Woodman, G.; Abu Dayyeh, B.K. Delayed gastric emptying as a proposed mechanism of action during intragastric balloon therapy: Results of a prospective study. *Obesity* **2016**, *24*, 1849–1853. [CrossRef] [PubMed]
154. Friedrichsen, M.; Breitschaft, A.; Tadayon, S.; Wizert, A.; Skovgaard, D. The effect of semaglutide 2.4 mg once weekly on energy intake, appetite, control of eating and gastric emptying in subjects with obesity. *Diabetes Obes. Metab.* **2021**, *23*, 754–762. [CrossRef]
155. Lopez-Nava, G.; Jaruvongvanich, V.; Storm, A.C.; Maselli, D.B.; Bautista-Castaño, I.; Vargas, E.J.; Matar, R.; Acosta, A.; Abu Dayyeh, B.K. Personalization of Endoscopic Bariatric and Metabolic Therapies Based on Physiology: A Prospective Feasibility Study with a Single Fluid-Filled Intragastric Balloon. *Obes. Surg.* **2020**, *30*, 3347–3353. [CrossRef] [PubMed]
156. Locke, A.E.; Kahali, B.; Berndt, S.I.; Justice, A.E.; Pers, T.H.; Day, F.R.; Powell, C.; Vedantam, S.; Buchkovich, M.L.; Yang, J.; et al. Genetic studies of body mass index yield new insights for obesity biology. *Nature* **2015**, *518*, 197–206. [CrossRef]
157. Loos, R.J. Genetic determinants of common obesity and their value in prediction. *Best Pr. Res. Clin. Endocrinol. Metab.* **2012**, *26*, 211–226. [CrossRef] [PubMed]
158. Pulit, S.L.; Stoneman, C.; Morris, A.P.; Wood, A.R.; Glastonbury, C.A.; Tyrrell, J.; Yengo, L.; Ferreira, T.; Marouli, E.; Ji, Y.; et al. Meta-analysis of genome-wide association studies for body fat distribution in 694 649 individuals of European ancestry. *Hum. Mol. Genet.* **2019**, *28*, 166–174. [CrossRef] [PubMed]
159. Farooqi, I.S.; O'Rahilly, S. Monogenic Obesity in Humans. *Annu. Rev. Med.* **2005**, *56*, 443–458. [CrossRef] [PubMed]

160. Haqq, A.M.; Farooqi, I.S.; O'Rahilly, S.; Stadler, D.D.; Rosenfeld, R.G.; Pratt, K.L.; LaFranchi, S.H.; Purnell, J.Q. Serum Ghrelin Levels Are Inversely Correlated with Body Mass Index, Age, and Insulin Concentrations in Normal Children and Are Markedly Increased in Prader-Willi Syndrome. *J. Clin. Endocrinol. Metab.* **2003**, *88*, 174–178. [CrossRef] [PubMed]
161. Arenz, T.; Schwarzer, A.; Pfluger, T.; Koletzko, S.; Schmidt, H. Delayed gastric emptying in patients with Prader Willi Syndrome. *J. Pediatr. Endocrinol. Metab.* **2010**, *23*, 867–871. [CrossRef] [PubMed]
162. Choe, Y.H.; Jin, D.-K.; Kim, S.E.; Song, S.Y.; Paik, K.H.; Park, H.Y.; Oh, Y.J.; Kim, A.H.; Kim, J.S.; Kim, C.W.; et al. Hyperghrelinemia Does Not Accelerate Gastric Emptying in Prader-Willi Syndrome Patients. *J. Clin. Endocrinol. Metab.* **2005**, *90*, 3367–3370. [CrossRef]
163. Yau, A.M.W.; McLaughlin, J.; Maughan, R.J.; Gilmore, W.; Ashworth, J.J.; Evans, G.H. A Pilot Study Investigating the Influence of Glucagon-Like Peptide-1 Receptor Single Nucleotide Polymorphisms on Gastric Emptying Rate in Caucasian Men. *Front. Physiol.* **2018**, *9*, 1331. [CrossRef]
164. Acosta, A.; Camilleri, M.; Shin, A.; Carlson, P.; Burton, D.; O'Neill, J.; Eckert, D.; Zinsmeister, A.R. Association of melanocortin 4 receptor gene variation with satiation and gastric emptying in overweight and obese adults. *Genes Nutr.* **2014**, *9*, 384. [CrossRef] [PubMed]
165. Cremonini, F.; Camilleri, M.; McKinzie, S.; Carlson, P.; E Camilleri, C.; Burton, D.D.; Thomforde, G.M.; Urrutia, R.; Zinsmeister, A.R. Effect of CCK-1 Antagonist, Dexloxiglumide, in Female Patients with Irritable Bowel Syndrome: A Pharmacodynamic and Pharmacogenomic Study. *Am. J. Gastroenterol.* **2005**, *100*, 652–663. [CrossRef] [PubMed]
166. Anderson, B.; Carlson, P.; Laurenti, M.; Vella, A.; Camilleri, M.; Desai, A.; Feuerhak, K.; Bharucha, A.E. Association between allelic variants in the glucagon-like peptide 1 and cholecystokinin receptor genes with gastric emptying and glucose tolerance. *Neurogastroenterol. Motil.* **2020**, *32*, e13724. [CrossRef] [PubMed]
167. Chedid, V.; Vijayvargiya, P.; Carlson, P.; Van Malderen, K.; Acosta, A.; Zinsmeister, A.; Camilleri, M. Allelic variant in the glucagon-like peptide 1 receptor gene associated with greater effect of liraglutide and exenatide on gastric emptying: A pilot pharmacogenetics study. *Neurogastroenterol. Motil.* **2018**, *30*, e13313. [CrossRef] [PubMed]
168. Ryan, D.H.; Yockey, S.R. Weight Loss and Improvement in Comorbidity: Differences at 5%, 10%, 15%, and Over. *Curr. Obes. Rep.* **2017**, *6*, 187–194. [CrossRef]
169. Wing, R.R.; Lang, W.; Wadden, T.A.; Safford, M.; Knowler, W.C.; Bertoni, A.G.; Hill, J.O.; Brancati, F.L.; Peters, A.; Wagenknecht, L.; et al. Benefits of Modest Weight Loss in Improving Cardiovascular Risk Factors in Overweight and Obese Individuals With Type 2 Diabetes. *Diabetes Care* **2011**, *34*, 1481–1486. [CrossRef]
170. A King, N.; Hopkins, M.; Caudwell, P.; Stubbs, R.J.; E Blundell, J. Beneficial effects of exercise: Shifting the focus from body weight to other markers of health. *Br. J. Sports Med.* **2009**, *43*, 924–927. [CrossRef] [PubMed]
171. Horowitz, M.; Maddox, A.; Wishart, J.; Vernon-Roberts, J.; Chatterton, B.; Shearman, D. Effect of dexfenfluramine on gastric emptying of a mixed solid-liquid meal in obese subjects. *Br. J. Nutr.* **1990**, *63*, 447–455. [CrossRef]
172. Pilitsi, E.; Farr, O.M.; Polyzos, S.A.; Perakakis, N.; Nolen-Doerr, E.; Papathanasiou, A.-E.; Mantzoros, C.S. Pharmacotherapy of obesity: Available medications and drugs under investigation. *Metabolism* **2019**, *92*, 170–192. [CrossRef] [PubMed]
173. Czepiel, K.S.; Perez, N.P.; Reyes, K.J.C.; Sabharwal, S.; Stanford, F.C. Pharmacotherapy for the Treatment of Overweight and Obesity in Children, Adolescents, and Young Adults in a Large Health System in the US. *Front. Endocrinol.* **2020**, *11*, 290. [CrossRef] [PubMed]
174. Kelly, A.S.; Auerbach, P.; Barrientos-Perez, M.; Gies, I.; Hale, P.M.; Marcus, C.; Mastrandrea, L.D.; Prabhu, N.; Arslanian, S. A Randomized, Controlled Trial of Liraglutide for Adolescents with Obesity. *N. Engl. J. Med.* **2020**, *382*, 2117–2128. [CrossRef] [PubMed]
175. Schwizer, W.; Asal, K.; Kreiss, C.; Mettraux, C.; Borovicka, J.; Remy, B.; Guzelhan, C.; Hartmann, D.; Fried, M. Role of lipase in the regulation of upper gastrointestinal function in humans. *Am. J. Physiol. Content* **1997**, *273*, G612–G620. [CrossRef] [PubMed]
176. Borovicka, J.; Schwizer, W.; Guttmann, G.; Hartmann, D.; Kosinski, M.; Wastiel, C.; Bischof-Delaloye, A.; Fried, M. Role of lipase in the regulation of postprandial gastric acid secretion and emptying of fat in humans: A study with orlistat, a highly specific lipase inhibitor. *Gut* **2000**, *46*, 774–781. [CrossRef] [PubMed]
177. Pilichiewicz, A.; O'Donovan, D.; Feinle, C.; Lei, Y.; Wishart, J.M.; Bryant, L.; Meyer, J.H.; Horowitz, M.; Jones, K.L. Effect of Lipase Inhibition on Gastric Emptying of, and the Glycemic and Incretin Responses to, an Oil/Aqueous Drink in Type 2 Diabetes Mellitus. *J. Clin. Endocrinol. Metab.* **2003**, *88*, 3829–3834. [CrossRef] [PubMed]
178. O'Donovan, D.; Horowitz, M.; Russo, A.; Feinle-Bisset, C.; Murolo, N.; Gentilcore, D.; Wishart, J.M.; Morris, H.A.; Jones, K.L. Effects of lipase inhibition on gastric emptying of, and on the glycaemic, insulin and cardiovascular responses to, a high-fat/carbohydrate meal in type 2 diabetes. *Diabetologia* **2004**, *47*, 2208–2214. [CrossRef]
179. Mathus-Vliegen, E.M.H.; Leeuwen, M.L.V.I.-V.; Bennink, R.J. Influences of fat restriction and lipase inhibition on gastric emptying in obesity. *Int. J. Obes.* **2006**, *30*, 1203–1210. [CrossRef] [PubMed]
180. Flint, A.; Raben, A.; Ersbøll, A.; Holst, J.; Astrup, A. The effect of physiological levels of glucagon-like peptide-1 on appetite, gastric emptying, energy and substrate metabolism in obesity. *Int. J. Obes.* **2001**, *25*, 781–792. [CrossRef] [PubMed]
181. Clapper, J.R.; Athanacio, J.; Wittmer, C.; Griffin, P.S.; D'Souza, L.; Parkes, D.G.; Roth, J.D. Effects of amylin and bupropion/naltrexone on food intake and body weight are interactive in rodent models. *Eur. J. Pharmacol.* **2013**, *698*, 292–298. [CrossRef]

182. Acosta, A.; Camilleri, M.; Burton, D.; O'Neill, J.; Eckert, D.; Carlson, P.; Zinsmeister, A.R. Exenatide in obesity with accelerated gastric emptying: A randomized, pharmacodynamics study. *Physiol. Rep.* **2015**, *3*, 12610. [CrossRef] [PubMed]
183. Blundell, J.; Finlayson, G.; Axelsen, M.; Flint, A.; Gibbons, C.; Kvist, T.; Hjerpsted, J.B. Effects of once-weekly semaglutide on appetite, energy intake, control of eating, food preference and body weight in subjects with obesity. *Diabetes Obes. Metab.* **2017**, *19*, 1242–1251. [CrossRef]
184. Hjerpsted, J.B.; Flint, A.; Brooks, A.; Axelsen, M.B.; Kvist, T.; Blundell, J. Semaglutide improves postprandial glucose and lipid metabolism, and delays first-hour gastric emptying in subjects with obesity. *Diabetes Obes. Metab.* **2017**, *20*, 610–619. [CrossRef] [PubMed]
185. Linnebjerg, H.; Park, S.; Kothare, P.A.; Trautmann, M.E.; Mace, K.; Fineman, M.; Wilding, I.; Nauck, M.; Horowitz, M. Effect of exenatide on gastric emptying and relationship to postprandial glycemia in type 2 diabetes. *Regul. Pept.* **2008**, *151*, 123–129. [CrossRef] [PubMed]
186. Jones, K.L.; Huynh, L.Q.; Hatzinikolas, S.; Rigda, R.S.; Phillips, L.K.; Pham, H.T.; Marathe, C.S.; Wu, T.; Malbert, C.H.; Stevens, J.E.; et al. Exenatide once weekly slows gastric emptying of solids and liquids in healthy, overweight people at steady-state concentrations. *Diabetes, Obes. Metab.* **2020**, *22*, 788–797. [CrossRef] [PubMed]
187. Maselli, D.B.; Camilleri, M. Effects of GLP-1 and Its Analogs on Gastric Physiology in Diabetes Mellitus and Obesity. *Adv. Exp. Med. Biol.* **2021**, *1307*, 171–192. [PubMed]
188. Horowitz, M.; Aroda, V.R.; Han, J.; Hardy, E.; Rayner, C.K. Upper and/or lower gastrointestinal adverse events with glucagon-like peptide-1 receptor agonists: Incidence and consequences. *Diabetes Obes. Metab.* **2017**, *19*, 672–681. [CrossRef] [PubMed]
189. Lingvay, I.; Hansen, T.; Macura, S.; Marre, M.; A Nauck, M.; De La Rosa, R.; Woo, V.; Yildirim, E.; Wilding, J. Superior weight loss with once-weekly semaglutide versus other glucagon-like peptide-1 receptor agonists is independent of gastrointestinal adverse events. *BMJ Open Diabetes Res. Care* **2020**, *8*, e001706. [CrossRef] [PubMed]
190. Dahl, K.; Brooks, A.; Almazedi, F.; Hoff, S.T.; Boschini, C.; Bækdal, T.A. Oral semaglutide improves postprandial glucose and lipid metabolism, and delays gastric emptying, in subjects with type 2 diabetes. *Diabetes Obes. Metab.* **2021**. [CrossRef]
191. Holst, J.J. Incretin hormones and the satiation signal. *Int. J. Obes.* **2013**, *37*, 1161–1168. [CrossRef] [PubMed]
192. Farr, O.M.; Sofopoulos, M.; Tsoukas, M.A.; Dincer, F.; Thakkar, B.; Sahin-Efe, A.; Filippaios, A.; Bowers, J.; Srnka, A.; Gavrieli, A.; et al. GLP-1 receptors exist in the parietal cortex, hypothalamus and medulla of human brains and the GLP-1 analogue liraglutide alters brain activity related to highly desirable food cues in individuals with diabetes: A crossover, randomised, placebo-controlled trial. *Diabetologia* **2016**, *59*, 954–965. [CrossRef] [PubMed]
193. Jalleh, R.; Pham, H.; Marathe, C.S.; Wu, T.; Buttfield, M.D.; Hatzinikolas, S.; Malbert, C.H.; Rigda, R.S.; Lange, K.; Trahair, L.G.; et al. Acute Effects of Lixisenatide on Energy Intake in Healthy Subjects and Patients with Type 2 Diabetes: Relationship to Gastric Emptying and Intragastric Distribution. *Nutrients* **2020**, *12*, 1962. [CrossRef]
194. Smith, S.R.; Aronne, L.J.; Burns, C.M.; Kesty, N.C.; Halseth, A.E.; Weyer, C. Sustained Weight Loss Following 12-Month Pramlintide Treatment as an Adjunct to Lifestyle Intervention in Obesity. *Diabetes Care* **2008**, *31*, 1816–1823. [CrossRef] [PubMed]
195. Nascimento, C.V.M.; Sinezia, C.; Sisnande, T.; Lima, L.M.T.; Lacativa, P.G. BZ043, a novel long-acting amylin analog, reduces gastric emptying, food intake, glycemia and insulin requirement in streptozotocin-induced diabetic rats. *Peptides* **2019**, *114*, 44–49. [CrossRef] [PubMed]
196. Batterham, R.L.; Cohen, M.A.; Ellis, S.M.; Le Roux, C.W.; Withers, D.J.; Frost, G.S.; Ghatei, M.A.; Bloom, S.R. Inhibition of Food Intake in Obese Subjects by Peptide YY3–36. *N. Engl. J. Med.* **2003**, *349*, 941–948. [CrossRef] [PubMed]
197. CllinicalTrials.gov. A Research Study of NNC0165-1562 and Semaglutide in People Who Are Overweight or Obese. 2020. Available online: https://clinicaltrials.gov/ct2/show/NCT03574584 (accessed on 22 December 2020).
198. R Mattin, L.; J McIver, V.; Yau, A.M.W.; J James, L.; H Evans, G. A comparison of intermittent and continuous exercise bouts at different intensities on appetite and postprandial metabolic responses in healthy men. *Nutrients* **2020**, *12*, 2370. [CrossRef] [PubMed]
199. Witte, A.-B.; Grybäck, P.; Holst, J.J.; Hilsted, L.; Hellström, P.M.; Jacobsson, H.; Schmidt, P. Differential effect of PYY1-36 and PYY3-36 on gastric emptying in man. *Regul. Pept.* **2009**, *158*, 57–62. [CrossRef] [PubMed]
200. Izundegui, D.G.; Singh, S.; Acosta, A. Food intake regulation: Relevance to bariatric and metabolic endoscopic therapies. *Tech. Innov. Gastrointest. Endosc.* **2020**, *22*, 100–108. [CrossRef]
201. Mion, F.; Napoléon, B.; Roman, S.; Malvoisin, E.; Trepo, C.; Pujol, B.; Lefort, C.; Bory, R.-M. Effects of Intragastric Balloon on Gastric Emptying and Plasma Ghrelin Levels in Non-morbid Obese Patients. *Obes. Surg.* **2005**, *15*, 510–516. [CrossRef] [PubMed]
202. Su, H.-J.; Kao, C.-H.; Chen, W.-C.; Chang, T.-T.; Lin, C.-Y. Effect of Intragastric Balloon on Gastric Emptying Time in Humans for Weight Control. *Clin. Nucl. Med.* **2013**, *38*, 863–868. [CrossRef] [PubMed]
203. Vargas, E.J.; Bazerbachi, F.; Calderon, G.; Prokop, L.J.; Gomez, V.; Murad, M.H.; Acosta, A.; Camilleri, M.; Abu Dayyeh, B.K. Changes in Time of Gastric Emptying After Surgical and Endoscopic Bariatrics and Weight Loss: A Systematic Review and Meta-Analysis. *Clin. Gastroenterol. Hepatol.* **2020**, *18*, 57–68.e5. [CrossRef]
204. Abu Dayyeh, B.K.; Rajan, E.; Gostout, C.J. Endoscopic sleeve gastroplasty: A potential endoscopic alternative to surgical sleeve gastrectomy for treatment of obesity. *Gastrointest. Endosc.* **2013**, *78*, 530–535. [CrossRef] [PubMed]
205. James, A.N.; Ryan, J.P.; Parkman, H.P. Inhibitory effects of botulinum toxin on pyloric and antral smooth muscle. *Am. J. Physiol. Liver Physiol.* **2003**, *285*, G291–G297. [CrossRef] [PubMed]

206. Topazian, M.; Camilleri, M.; De La Mora-Levy, J.; Enders, F.B.; Foxx-Orenstein, A.E.; Levy, M.J.; Nehra, V.; Talley, N.J. Endoscopic ultrasound-guided gastric botulinum toxin injections in obese subjects: A pilot study. *Obes. Surg.* **2008**, *18*, 401–407. [CrossRef] [PubMed]
207. Topazian, M.; Camilleri, M.; Enders, F.T.; Clain, J.E.; Gleeson, F.C.; Levy, M.J.; Rajan, E.; Nehra, V.; Dierkhising, R.A.; Collazo–Clavell, M.L.; et al. Gastric antral injections of botulinum toxin delay gastric emptying but do not reduce body weight. *Clin. Gastroenterol. Hepatol.* **2013**, *11*, 145–150.e1. [CrossRef] [PubMed]
208. Trostler, N.; Mann, A.; Zilberbush, N.; Avinoach, E.; Charuzi, I. Weight Loss and Food Intake 18 Months following Vertical Banded Gastroplasty or Gastric Bypass for Severe Obesity. *Obes. Surg.* **1995**, *5*, 39–51. [CrossRef] [PubMed]
209. Cummings, D.E.; Weigle, D.S.; Frayo, R.S.; Breen, P.A.; Ma, M.K.; Dellinger, E.P.; Purnell, J.Q. Plasma Ghrelin Levels after Diet-Induced Weight Loss or Gastric Bypass Surgery. *N. Engl. J. Med.* **2002**, *346*, 1623–1630. [CrossRef] [PubMed]
210. Le Roux, C.W.; Aylwin, S.J.B.; Batterham, R.L.; Borg, C.M.; Coyle, F.; Prasad, V.; Shurey, S.; Ghatei, M.A.; Patel, A.G.; Bloom, S.R. Gut Hormone Profiles Following Bariatric Surgery Favor an Anorectic State, Facilitate Weight Loss, and Improve Metabolic Parameters. *Ann. Surg.* **2006**, *243*, 108–114. [CrossRef] [PubMed]
211. Gu, L.; Lin, K.; Du, N.; Ng, D.M.; Lou, D.; Chen, P. Differences in the effects of laparoscopic sleeve gastrectomy and laparoscopic Roux-en-Y gastric bypass on gut hormones: Systematic and meta-analysis. *Surg. Obes. Relat. Dis.* **2021**, *17*, 444–455. [CrossRef]
212. Yehoshua, R.T.; Eidelman, L.A.; Stein, M.; Fichman, S.; Mazor, A.; Chen, J.; Bernstine, H.; Singer, P.; Dickman, R.; Shikora, S.A.; et al. Laparoscopic Sleeve Gastrectomy—Volume and Pressure Assessment. *Obes. Surg.* **2008**, *18*, 1083–1088. [CrossRef] [PubMed]
213. Fiorillo, C.; Quero, G.; Dallemagne, B.; Curcic, J.; Fox, M.; Perretta, S. Effects of Laparoscopic Sleeve Gastrectomy on Gastric Structure and Function Documented by Magnetic Resonance Imaging Are Strongly Associated with Post-operative Weight Loss and Quality of Life: A Prospective Study. *Obes. Surg.* **2020**, *30*, 1–10. [CrossRef] [PubMed]
214. Garay, M.; Balagué, C.; Rodríguez-Otero, C.; Gonzalo, B.; Domenech, A.; Pernas, J.C.; Gich, I.J.; Miñambres, I.; Fernández-Ananín, S.; Targarona, E.M. Influence of antrum size on gastric emptying and weight-loss outcomes after laparoscopic sleeve gastrectomy (preliminary analysis of a randomized trial). *Surg. Endosc.* **2018**, *32*, 2739–2745. [CrossRef] [PubMed]
215. Mccarty, T.R.; Jirapinyo, P.; Thompson, C.C. 1128 Effect of Sleeve Gastrectomy on Ghrelin, GLP-1, PYY, and GIP Gut Hormones: A Systematic Review and Meta-Analysis. *Am. J. Gastroenterol.* **2019**, *114*, S633–S634. [CrossRef]
216. Wittgrove, A.C.; Clark, G.W. Laparoscopic Gastric Bypass, Roux en-Y—500 Patients: Technique and Results, with 3-60 month follow-up. *Obes. Surg.* **2000**, *10*, 233–239. [CrossRef] [PubMed]
217. Xu, H.-C.; Pang, Y.-C.; Chen, J.-W.; Cao, J.-Y.; Sheng, Z.; Yuan, J.-H.; Wang, R.; Zhang, C.-S.; Wang, L.-X.; Dong, J. Systematic Review and Meta-analysis of the Change in Ghrelin Levels After Roux-en-Y Gastric Bypass. *Obes. Surg.* **2019**, *29*, 1343–1351. [CrossRef] [PubMed]
218. Akkary, E.; Sidani, S.; Boonsiri, J.; Yu, S.; Dziura, J.; Duffy, A.J.; Bell, R.L. The paradox of the pouch: Prompt emptying predicts improved weight loss after laparoscopic Roux-Y gastric bypass. *Surg. Endosc.* **2008**, *23*, 790–794. [CrossRef] [PubMed]
219. Deden, L.N.; Cooiman, M.I.; Aarts, E.O.; Janssen, I.M.; Gotthardt, M.; Hendrickx, B.W.; Berends, F.J. Gastric pouch emptying of solid food in patients with successful and unsuccessful weight loss after Roux-en-Y gastric bypass surgery. *Surg. Obes. Relat. Dis.* **2017**, *13*, 1840–1846. [CrossRef] [PubMed]
220. E Cummings, D. Endocrine mechanisms mediating remission of diabetes after gastric bypass surgery. *Int. J. Obes.* **2009**, *33*, S33–S40. [CrossRef] [PubMed]
221. Nguyen, N.Q.; Debreceni, T.L.; Burgstad, C.M.; Wishart, J.M.; Bellon, M.; Rayner, C.K.; Wittert, G.A.; Horowitz, M. Effects of Posture and Meal Volume on Gastric Emptying, Intestinal Transit, Oral Glucose Tolerance, Blood Pressure and Gastrointestinal Symptoms After Roux-en-Y Gastric Bypass. *Obes. Surg.* **2014**, *25*, 1392–1400. [CrossRef] [PubMed]
222. Miras, A.D.; Kamocka, A.; Pérez-Pevida, B.; Purkayastha, S.; Moorthy, K.; Patel, A.; Chahal, H.; Frost, G.; Bassett, P.; Castagnetto-Gissey, L.; et al. The Effect of Standard Versus Longer Intestinal Bypass on GLP-1 Regulation and Glucose Metabolism in Patients With Type 2 Diabetes Undergoing Roux-en-Y Gastric Bypass: The Long-Limb Study. *Diabetes Care* **2020**, dc200762. [CrossRef] [PubMed]
223. Verdich, C.; Madsen, J.L.; Toubro, S.; Buemann, B.; Holst, J.; Astrup, A. Effect of obesity and major weight reduction on gastric emptying. *Int. J. Obes.* **2000**, *24*, 899–905. [CrossRef] [PubMed]
224. Kadouh, H.; Chedid, V.; Halawi, H.; Burton, D.D.; Clark, M.M.; Khemani, D.; Vella, A.; Acosta, A.; Camilleri, M. GLP-1 Analog Modulates Appetite, Taste Preference, Gut Hormones, and Regional Body Fat Stores in Adults with Obesity. *J. Clin. Endocrinol. Metab.* **2019**, *105*, 1552–1563. [CrossRef] [PubMed]
225. Meier, J.J.; Rosenstock, J.; Hincelin-Méry, A.; Roy-Duval, C.; Delfolie, A.; Coester, H.-V.; Menge, B.A.; Forst, T.; Kapitza, C. Contrasting Effects of Lixisenatide and Liraglutide on Postprandial Glycemic Control, Gastric Emptying, and Safety Parameters in Patients With Type 2 Diabetes on Optimized Insulin Glargine With or Without Metformin: A Randomized, Open-Label Trial. *Diabetes Care* **2015**, *38*, 1263–1273. [CrossRef] [PubMed]
226. Yamada, Y.; Senda, M.; Naito, Y.; Tamura, M.; Watanabe, D.; Shuto, Y.; Urita, Y. Reduction of postprandial glucose by lixisenatide vs sitagliptin treatment in Japanese patients with type 2 diabetes on background insulin glargine: A randomized phase IV study (NEXTAGE Study). *Diabetes, Obes. Metab.* **2017**, *19*, 1252–1259. [CrossRef] [PubMed]

227. Whyte, M.B.; Shojaee-Moradie, F.; E Sharaf, S.; Jackson, N.C.; Fielding, B.; Hovorka, R.; Mendis, J.; Russell-Jones, D.; Umpleby, A.M. Lixisenatide Reduces Chylomicron Triacylglycerol by Increased Clearance. *J. Clin. Endocrinol. Metab.* **2019**, *104*, 359–368. [CrossRef] [PubMed]
228. Rayner, C.K.; Watson, L.E.; Phillips, L.K.; Lange, K.; Bound, M.J.; Grivell, J.; Wu, T.; Jones, K.L.; Horowitz, M.; Ferrannini, E.; et al. Effects of Sustained Treatment With Lixisenatide on Gastric Emptying and Postprandial Glucose Metabolism in Type 2 Diabetes: A Randomized Controlled Trial. *Diabetes Care* **2020**, *43*, 1813–1821. [CrossRef] [PubMed]
229. Velchik, M.G.; Kramer, F.M.; Stunkard, A.J.; Alavi, A. Effect of the Garren-Edwards gastric bubble on gastric emptying. *J. Nucl. Med.* **1989**, *30*, 692–696.
230. Barrichello, S.; Badurdeen, D.; Hedjoudje, A.; Neto, M.G.; Yance, R.; Veinert, A.; Fayad, L.; Simsek, C.; Grecco, E.; De Souza, T.F.; et al. The Effect of the Intra-gastric Balloon on Gastric Emptying and the DeMeester Score. *Obes. Surg.* **2019**, *30*, 38–45. [CrossRef] [PubMed]
231. Hedberg, J.; Hedenström, H.; Karlsson, F.A.; Edén-Engström, B.; Sundbom, M. Gastric Emptying and Postprandial PYY Response After Biliopancreatic Diversion with Duodenal Switch. *Obes. Surg.* **2010**, *21*, 609–615. [CrossRef]
232. De Jong, J.R.; Van Ramshorst, B.; Gooszen, H.G.; Smout, A.J.P.M.; Buul, M.M.C.T.-V. Weight Loss after Laparoscopic Adjustable Gastric Banding is not Caused by Altered Gastric Emptying. *Obes. Surg.* **2008**, *19*, 287–292. [CrossRef]
233. Näslund, I.; Beckman, K.-W. Gastric Emptying Rate after Gastric Bypass and Gastroplasty. *Scand. J. Gastroenterol.* **1987**, *22*, 193–201. [CrossRef] [PubMed]
234. Melissas, J.; Koukouraki, S.; Askoxylakis, J.; Stathaki, M.; Daskalakis, M.; Perisinakis, K.; Karkavitsas, N. Sleeve gastrectomy—A restrictive procedure? *Obes. Surg.* **2007**, *17*, 57. [CrossRef] [PubMed]
235. Bernstine, H.; Tzioni-Yehoshua, R.; Groshar, D.; Beglaibter, N.; Shikora, S.; Rosenthal, R.J.; Rubin, M. Gastric Emptying is not Affected by Sleeve Gastrectomy—Scintigraphic Evaluation of Gastric Emptying after Sleeve Gastrectomy without Removal of the Gastric Antrum. *Obes. Surg.* **2008**, *19*, 293–298. [CrossRef] [PubMed]
236. Braghetto, I.; DaVanzo, C.; Korn, O.; Csendes, A.; Valladares, H.; Herrera, E.; Gonzalez, P.; Papapietro, K. Scintigraphic Evaluation of Gastric Emptying in Obese Patients Submitted to Sleeve Gastrectomy Compared to Normal Subjects. *Obes. Surg.* **2009**, *19*, 1515–1521. [CrossRef] [PubMed]
237. Michalsky, D.; Dvorak, P.; Belacek, J.; Kasalicky, M. Radical Resection of the Pyloric Antrum and Its Effect on Gastric Emptying After Sleeve Gastrectomy. *Obes. Surg.* **2013**, *23*, 567–573. [CrossRef]
238. Pilone, V.; Tramontano, S.; Di Micco, R.; Monda, A.; Hasani, A.; Izzo, G.; Vitiello, A.; Caprio, M.; Cuocolo, A.; Forestieri, P. Gastric emptying after sleeve gastrectomy: Statistical evidence of a controlled prospective study with gastric scintigraphy (180 visite). *Minerva Chir.* **2013**, *68*, 385–392. [PubMed]
239. Melissas, J.; Leventi, A.; Klinaki, I.; Perisinakis, K.; Koukouraki, S.; de Bree, E.; Karkavitsas, N. Alterations of global gastrointestinal motility after sleeve gastrectomy: A prospective study. *Ann. Surg.* **2013**, *258*, 976–982. [CrossRef] [PubMed]
240. Kandeel, A.A.; Sarhan, M.D.; Hegazy, T.; Mahmoud, M.M.; Ali, M.H. Comparative assessment of gastric emptying in obese patients before and after laparoscopic sleeve gastrectomy using radionuclide scintigraphy. *Nucl. Med. Commun.* **2015**, *36*, 854–862. [CrossRef]
241. Burgerhart, J.S.; Van Rutte, P.W.J.; Edelbroek, M.A.L.; Wyndaele, D.N.J.; Smulders, J.F.; Van De Meeberg, P.C.; Siersema, P.D.; Smout, A.J.P.M. Association Between Postprandial Symptoms and Gastric Emptying After Sleeve Gastrectomy. *Obes. Surg.* **2014**, *25*, 209–214. [CrossRef] [PubMed]
242. Vigneshwaran, B.; Wahal, A.; Aggarwal, S.; Priyadarshini, P.; Bhattacharjee, H.; Khadgawat, R.; Yadav, R. Impact of Sleeve Gastrectomy on Type 2 Diabetes Mellitus, Gastric Emptying Time, Glucagon-Like Peptide 1 (GLP-1), Ghrelin and Leptin in Non-morbidly Obese Subjects with BMI 30–35.0 kg/m^2: A Prospective Study. *Obes. Surg.* **2016**, *26*, 2817–2823. [CrossRef] [PubMed]
243. Vives, M.; Molina, A.; Danús, M.; Rebenaque, E.; Blanco, S.; París, M.; Sánchez, A.; Sabench, F.; Del Castillo, D. Analysis of Gastric Physiology After Laparoscopic Sleeve Gastrectomy (LSG) With or Without Antral Preservation in Relation to Metabolic Response: A Randomised Study. *Obes. Surg.* **2017**, *27*, 2836–2844. [CrossRef] [PubMed]
244. Sista, F.; Abruzzese, V.; Clementi, M.; Carandina, S.; Cecilia, M.; Amicucci, G. The effect of sleeve gastrectomy on GLP-1 secretion and gastric emptying: A prospective study. *Surg. Obes. Relat. Dis.* **2017**, *13*, 7–14. [CrossRef] [PubMed]
245. Yang, P.-J.; Cheng, M.-F.; Yang, W.-S.; Tsai, M.-S.; Lee, P.-C.; Chen, C.-N.; Lin, M.-T.; Tseng, P.-H. A Higher Preoperative Glycemic Profile Is Associated with Rapid Gastric Emptying After Sleeve Gastrectomy for Obese Subjects. *Obes. Surg.* **2018**, *29*, 569–578. [CrossRef] [PubMed]
246. Li, M.; Liu, Y.; Jin, L.; Wang, W.; Zeng, N.; Wang, L.; Zhao, K.; Xu, W.; Zhang, Z.; Yang, J. Alterations of Gastric Emptying Features Following Laparoscopic Sleeve Gastrectomy in Chinese Patients with Obesity: A Self-Controlled Observational Study. *Obes. Surg.* **2018**, *29*, 617–625. [CrossRef] [PubMed]
247. Salman, M.A.; Mikhail, H.M.S.; Abdelsalam, A.; Abdallah, A.; Elshafey, H.E.; Abouelregal, T.E.; Omar, M.G.; ElKassar, H.; Ahmed, R.A.; Atallah, M.; et al. Acceleration of Gastric Emptying and Improvement of GERD Outcome After Laparoscopic Sleeve Gastrectomy in Non-diabetic Obese Patients. *Obes. Surg.* **2020**, *30*, 2676–2683. [CrossRef] [PubMed]
248. Johari, Y.; Wickremasinghe, A.; Kiswandono, P.; Yue, H.; Ooi, G.; Laurie, C.; Hebbard, G.; Beech, P.; Yap, K.; Brown, W.; et al. Mechanisms of Esophageal and Gastric Transit Following Sleeve Gastrectomy. *Obes. Surg.* **2021**, *31*, 725–737. [CrossRef]

249. Svane, M.S.; Bojsen-Møller, K.N.; Martinussen, C.; Dirksen, C.; Madsen, J.L.; Reitelseder, S.; Holm, L.; Rehfeld, J.F.; Kristiansen, V.B.; van Hall, G.; et al. Postprandial Nutrient Handling and Gastrointestinal Hormone Secretion After Roux-en-Y Gastric Bypass vs Sleeve Gastrectomy. *Gastroenterology* **2019**, *156*, 1627–1641. [CrossRef] [PubMed]
250. Dirksen, C.; Damgaard, M.; Bojsen-Møller, K.; Jørgensen, N.; Kielgast, U.; Jacobsen, S.; Naver, L.; Worm, D.; Holst, J.J.; Madsbad, S. Fast pouch emptying, delayed small intestinal transit, and exaggerated gut hormone responses after Roux-en-Y gastric bypass. *Neurogastroenterol. Motil.* **2013**, *25*, 346-e255. [CrossRef]
251. Wölnerhanssen, B.K.; Meyer-Gerspach, A.C.; Peters, T.; Beglinger, C.; Peterli, R. Incretin effects, gastric emptying and insulin responses to low oral glucose loads in patients after gastric bypass and lean and obese controls. *Surg. Obes. Relat. Dis.* **2016**, *12*, 1320–1327. [CrossRef] [PubMed]

Review

Review on the Regional Effects of Gastrointestinal Luminal Stimulation on Appetite and Energy Intake: (Pre)clinical Observations

Jennifer Wilbrink [1], Gwen Masclee [1], Tim Klaassen [1], Mark van Avesaat [1], Daniel Keszthelyi [1,2] and Adrian Masclee [1,2,*]

1. Division of Gastroenterology-Hepatology, Maastricht University Medical Center, 6229 HX Maastricht, The Netherlands; jawilbrink@hotmail.com (J.W.); gwen.masclee@mumc.nl (G.M.); tim.klaassen@mumc.nl (T.K.); mark.van.avesaat@mumc.nl (M.v.A.); daniel.keszthelyi@maastrichtuniversity.nl (D.K.)
2. NUTRIM School of Nutrition and Translational Research in Metabolism, 6229 ER Maastricht, The Netherlands
* Correspondence: a.masclee@mumc.nl; Tel.: +31-43-3875021

Abstract: Macronutrients in the gastrointestinal (GI) lumen are able to activate "intestinal brakes", feedback mechanisms on proximal GI motility and secretion including appetite and energy intake. In this review, we provide a detailed overview of the current evidence with respect to four questions: (1) are regional differences (duodenum, jejunum, ileum) present in the intestinal luminal nutrient modulation of appetite and energy intake? (2) is this "intestinal brake" effect macronutrient specific? (3) is this "intestinal brake" effect maintained during repetitive activation? (4) can the "intestinal brake" effect be activated via non-caloric tastants? Recent evidence indicates that: (1) regional differences exist in the intestinal modulation of appetite and energy intake with a proximal to distal gradient for inhibition of energy intake: ileum and jejunum > duodenum at low but not at high caloric infusion rates. (2) the "intestinal brake" effect on appetite and energy appears not to be macronutrient specific. At equi-caloric amounts, the inhibition on energy intake and appetite is in the same range for fat, protein and carbohydrate. (3) data on repetitive ileal brake activation are scarce because of the need for prolonged intestinal intubation. During repetitive activation of the ileal brake for up to 4 days, no adaptation was observed but overall the inhibitory effect on energy intake was small. (4) the concept of influencing energy intake by intra-intestinal delivery of non-caloric tastants is intriguing. Among tastants, the bitter compounds appear to be more effective in influencing energy intake. Energy intake decreases modestly after post-oral delivery of bitter tastants or a combination of tastants (bitter, sweet and umami). Intestinal brake activation provides an interesting concept for preventive and therapeutic approaches in weight management strategies.

Keywords: intestinal brake; duodenal jejunal and ileal brake; tastants; energy intake; appetite; satiety; satiation; carbohydrate; protein; fat

1. Introduction

After ingestion of food, the gastrointestinal (GI) tract is activated to facilitate transport, digestion and absorption of nutrients. Regional differences exist within the GI tract with respect to the modulation of these processes. Entry of nutrients into the small bowel activates so-called "intestinal brakes", negative feedback mechanisms that not only affect motility and secretion but also appetite and energy intake.

Recent studies indicate that all macronutrients are able to activate these "intestinal brakes", although to a different extent and through various mechanisms. In this review we provide a detailed overview of the current evidence with respect to four research questions:

1. Are regional differences (duodenum, jejunum, ileum) present in the intestinal luminal modulation of appetite and energy intake?

2. Is the "intestinal brake" effect on appetite and energy intake macronutrient specific?
3. Is the "intestinal brake" effect that is observed in acute intervention studies maintained during repetitive activation?
4. Can the "intestinal brake" effect on appetite and energy intake be activated via non-caloric tastants?

2. Nutrient Sensing in the Gut

Signals mediating satiety and satiation arise from various locations within the luminal gastrointestinal tract including the stomach, duodenum, jejunum, ileum and colon [1]. Ingestion of food results in mechanical stimulation by distension of the stomach and small intestine and in chemical stimulation via activation of nutrient receptors on enteroendocrine cells (EECs). These EECs play a pivotal role in the gastrointestinal and central regulation of not only of gastrointestinal (GI) motility and secretion but also of food intake. ECCs are scattered as single cells throughout the intestinal tract, located within the intestinal crypts and villi, and comprise about 1% of the total epithelial cell population. EECs act as sensors of luminal content, especially of nutrients, and function as trans-epithelial signal transduction conduits with apical physiochemical signals resulting in basolateral release and exocytosis of biological mediators. Nutrients or their breakdown products interact with G-protein coupled receptors (GPCRs) on EECs resulting in the secretion of gastrointestinal peptides such as cholecystokinin (CCK), peptide YY (PYY) and glucagon-like peptide-1 (GLP-1). These mediators either act in a classical endocrine fashion or by a paracrine effect on adjacent cells, including vagal afferent fibers. Non-nutrient chemical factors also regulate EEC activity, for example via sensing of tastants such as bitter, sweet, salt, sour and umami.

EECs carry specific receptors that upon sensing activate intracellular pathways either through direct gating of ion channels such as the sodium-dependent glucose co-transporter 1 (SGLT-1) or via activation of GPCRs. In recent years, various GPCRs have been identified such as sweet taste receptors (TAS1R/TAS2R), fatty acid-sensing receptors (GPR40, GPR43, GPR119 and GPR120) and various other types including PPAR, melanocortin, TRP family and opioids [2–5].

G-protein coupled taste receptors are expressed not only on the human tongue but also in stomach, proximal and distal small intestine and colon. Bitter taste is sensed by the TAS2R receptor while the TAS1R receptor family is triggered by sweet and umami. Taste receptors are able to "taste" luminal content and transmit signals that induce the release of GI peptides, thereby influencing satiety and food intake in humans [6].

3. Gastric Satiation Signals

Apart from its function to store food, to mix and grind stomach content and initiate the process of digestion, the stomach is able to monitor "food ingestion". Consensus exists on the important role of gastric mechano-sensation in the regulation of satiety and food intake. In contrast to intestinal satiation, which is merely nutrient-induced, gastric satiation is merely volume-dependent. This has been shown for the first time in pyloric cuff experiments in rats [7]. In these experiments, saline or nutrient solutions were infused into the stomach but the pyloric cuffs prevented the infusate from entering the duodenum. Both the saline and nutrient infusate resulted in a similar reduction in food intake, showing that the nutritive effect did not add to the volumetric effect [7]. The satiating effect of gastric distension has been confirmed in human studies employing intragastric balloons. Prolonged distension of gastric balloons is known to result in reduction of food intake and subsequent weight loss [8].

4. Intestinal Satiation Signals

Exposure of the small intestinal lumen to nutrients induces satiety and a reduction in food intake. This was first observed in animal studies using gastric fistulas to exclude ingested food from entering the small intestine [9]. The animals would eat continuously when food was drained from the stomach. When the gastric fistula was closed and food entered the small intestine, the animals rapidly stopped eating, pointing to the pivotal role of the intestine in inducing satiety and satiation. Later, in vivo human intubation studies revealed that intestinal perfusion of proteins, carbohydrates or lipids, all resulted in a significant increase in satiety and decrease in food intake [10–13].

The GI peptides CCK, GLP-1 and PYY, secreted from EECs are known as mediators of intestinal satiation. These peptides induce their effects either via entering the bloodstream, acting as hormones (endocrine effect), via activation of vagal afferents (neuronal effect) or via an effect on neighboring cells (paracrine effect). Ghrelin is produced from the stomach and currently is the only GI peptide known to increase food intake by accelerating gastric emptying [1,6,13–15].

5. Intestinal Brakes

The process of motility, secretion, digestion and absorption is activated upon ingestion of food and its transport into stomach and duodenum. Thereafter, the appearance of nutrients further downward in the small intestine, during the process of digestion, results in activation of the so-called "intestinal brakes": feedback mechanisms from different parts of the intestine to the stomach, to the more proximal parts of the small intestine and also to the central nervous system.

Entry of nutrients into duodenum or jejunum activates the "duodenal brake" or "jejunal brake" while infusion of nutrients into the ileum activates the more distal "ileal brake".

The "duodenal brake" has been well documented as feedback from the duodenum to regulate gastric physiology, that is gastric acid secretion and gastric emptying. Inhibition of gastric emptying is a crucial "brake" against delivery of nutrients to the intestine in excess of digestive and absorptive capacity. In humans, gastric emptying is slowed in proportion to the energy density of the meal, thus leveling the rate of energy delivery to the duodenum [1,7,8,11].

The "ileal brake" is a negative feedback mechanism from the more distal to the proximal gastrointestinal (GI) tract that brings the process of transport, digestion and absorption of nutrients to an end (Figure 1). Activation of the "ileal brake" results in a reduction of gastric acid, biliary and pancreatic secretion, with inhibition of gastric emptying, intestinal motility and transport [14]. This concept of more distal intestinal brake activation with proximal inhibition of motility and secretion was derived from ileal transposition studies in rats. Koopmans and Sclafani were the first to show that transposing a segment of ileum to more proximal regions of the small intestine (i.e., duodenum) also resulted in a significant reduction in food intake and was associated with weight reduction in rats [15]. It was hypothesized that the hormonal changes induced by ileal transposition may have resulted in the observed reduction in food intake and increase in weight loss. Indeed, Strader et al. [16] observed that ileal transposition resulted in 3–4 times higher serum GLP-1 and PYY levels with an increase in satiety and weight loss that was proportional to the measured serum levels of GLP-1 and PYY.

Such a feedback inhibitory mechanism from the distal to the proximal GI tract has repeatedly been demonstrated in animal models. In the 1980s, the first human studies showed that infusion of fat or protein in the ileum delayed gastric emptying and intestinal transport and also increased feelings of satiety and reduced food intake. Welch et al., Read et al. and Spiller et al. [10–13] were among the first to point to the potent anorexic effect of "ileal brake" activation in humans through intestinal nutrient infusion. Welch et al. showed that an ileal lipid infusion of 370 kcal resulted in a decrease in food intake of 575 kcal, resulting in a net reduction in intake of 205 kcal. In a subsequent study comparing jejunal fat versus ileal fat infusion, the anorexic effect was more pronounced when fat was infused into the jejunum instead of the ileum [10]. One should consider that in these studies very high amounts of fat of up to 41 g were administered intestinally. These supraphysiologic amounts may have caused spilling of fat to more distal intestinal regions resulting in larger areas with activated nutrient receptors.

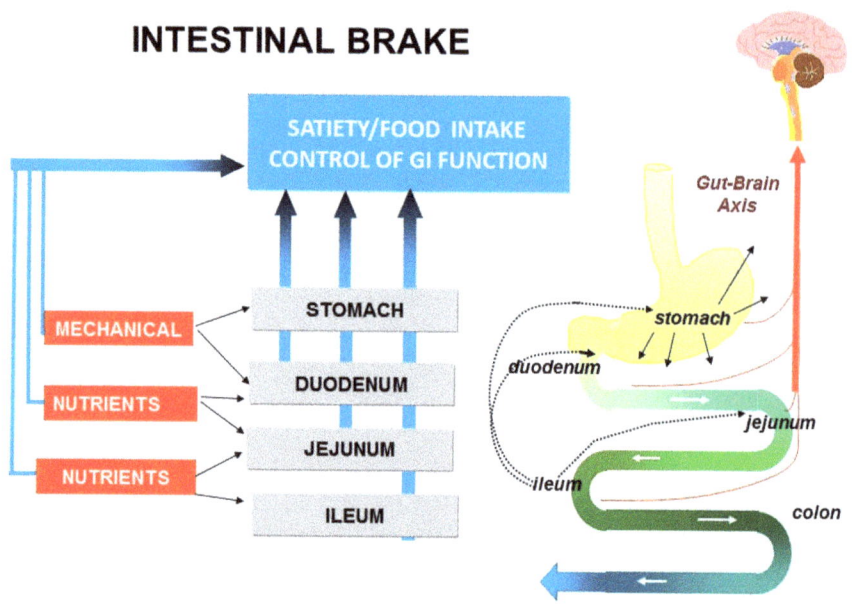

Figure 1. Intestinal brake: effect of luminal stimulation in stomach, duodenum, jejunum and ileum on neurohormonal control of gastrointestinal function, food intake and satiety.

6. Topics in Intestinal Brake, Appetite and Energy Intake

Several questions arise with respect to "intestinal brake" mechanisms and eating behavior:

(1) Are regional differences (duodenum, jejunum, ileum) present in the intestinal luminal modulation of appetite and energy intake?
(2) Is the "intestinal brake" effect on appetite and energy macronutrient specific? Are differences present between fat, carbohydrates and proteins?
(3) Is the "intestinal brake" effect observed in acute intervention studies, maintained during repetitive activation?
(4) Can the "intestinal brake" effect on appetite and energy intake be activated via non-caloric tastants?

6.1. Methods

Relevant studies for this review were identified by a PubMed search using search terms including duodenal, jejunal or ileal brake; duodenal, jejunal or ileal infusion; satiety, energy/food intake, or tastants. Only original articles involving human intervention studies and written in the English language were reviewed and selected. Additionally, reference lists of the original articles were reviewed for other relevant studies in order to be most complete in the current review. The included studies all relate to acute or short-term (single day to several days experiments) intervention studies in humans with either duodenal or jejunal or ileal intubation with intestinal perfusion of nutrients. In the reported publications, young, healthy volunteers, usually of male gender and aged 20–30 years with BMI in the normal range (20–25 kg/m^2) have been studied. In the current review, we specifically report if studied participants were different (obese versus non-obese and younger versus older participants). Different types of stimuli have been used: long-chain fats and fatty acids, protein or amino acids and carbohydrates. The type of stimuli that have been used are listed in Tables 1–3 and for each study separately in the Appendix A: Tables A1–A3.

Table 1. Effect of infusion of fat or fatty acids into duodenum, jejunum or ileum on energy intake and satiety.

Location	Infusate and Infusion Rate: Kcal per min	Energy Intake % Reduction	Energy Intake ↑↓	Satiety ↑↓	References
Fat					
Duodenum	1.1 (0.25–1.5) Corn oil, safflower oil, Intralipid	3% (0–8)	=	=-↑	[17–19]
	3.3 (2.0–4.9) corn oil, Intralipid	21% (10–32)	↓↓	↑	[10,17,18,20–25]
Jejunum	4.9 corn oil	12%	↓↓	↑↑	[26]
	4.9 corn oil	50%	↓↓↓	↑↑	[10]
Ileum	0.5–0.6 rapeseed, safflower oil	18% (15–21)	↓↓	↑	[19,27–29]
	1.8–4.9, corn oil, safflower oil	31% (30–32)	↓↓↓	↑↑	[10,13,28]
Fatty acids					
Duodenum	0.2–0.3 lauric acid	0–4%	=-↓	=	[30,31]
	0.4–0.75 lauric, LCFA	10–15% (60%) *	↓↓	↑	[30,32–34]
Jejunum	-	-	-	-	-
Ileum	-	-	-	-	-

Energy intake in % reduction in caloric intake: = no reduction or increase ↓ 0–10% reduction, ↓↓ 10–25% reduction, ↓↓↓ >25%. reduction versus control condition; ↑ 0–10% increase, ↑↑ 10–25% increase * = in one study (19) a reduction in energy intake of 60% was observed, but subjects were severely nauseated. Data on net intake are not corrected for caloric content of the nutrient infusate. LCFA: long-chain fatty acids. Energy intake reduction is presented as percentage reduction of energy intake as compared to control condition.

Table 2. Effect of infusion of protein or amino acids into duodenum, jejunum or ileum on energy intake and satiety.

Location	Infusate and Infusion Rate Kcal per min	Energy Intake % Reduction	Energy Intake ↑↓	Satiety	References
Protein					
Duodenum	0.5–1.5 whey, casein	8%	↓	=	[35–37]
	3.0 whey, casein	21%	↓↓	=	[24,35,36]
Jejunum	0.85 casein	9%	↓	=	[37]
Ileum	0.19 casein	9.9%	↓	=	[29]
	0.57–0.85 casein	14–22%	↓↓	↑↑	[29,37]
Amino acids					
Duodenum	0.07–0.15 tryptophan	5%	↓	↑	[31,38]
	0.2–0.4 tryptophan, leucine	13%	↓↓	=	[38,39]
Jejunum	-	-	-	-	-
Ileum	-	-	-	-	-

Energy intake in % reduction in caloric intake: = no reduction or increase, ↓ 0–10% reduction, ↓↓ 10–25% reduction. Satiety: = no reduction or in-crease, ↑ 0–10% increase, ↑↑ 10–25% increase. Energy intake reduction is presented as percentage reduction of energy intake as compared to control condition.

Table 3. Effect of infusion of carbohydrate (glucose or sucrose) into duodenum, jejunum or ileum on energy intake and satiety.

Location	Infusate and Infusion Rate Kcal per min	Energy Intake		Satiety	References
		% Reduction	↑↓		
Duodenum	0.6–2.0 glucose	10% (5–13)	↓	↑	[40–42]
	2.9–4.0 glucose	17% (11–26)	↓↓	↑↑	[21–23,40–45]
Jejunum	1.0 glucose	+11% *	↑↑	=	[42]
Ileum	0.19 sucrose	21%	↓↓	=	[29]
	0.57 sucrose	32%	↓↓↓	=	[29]
	0.66 glucose	10%	↓	=	[44]

Energy intake in % reduction in caloric intake: = no reduction or increase, ↓ 0–10% reduction, ↓↓ 10–25% reduction, ↓↓↓ >25% reduction; + 11% * = increase in intake jejunal compared to duodenal infusion [42]. Energy intake reduction is presented as percentage reduction of energy intake as compared to control condition. Satiety: = no reduction or increase, ↑ 0–10% increase, ↑↑ 10–25% increase in satiety.

6.2. Topic 1: Site Specific Effects on Food Intake and Satiety: Duodenum-Jejunum-Ileum

The human studies evaluating the intestinal brake effects have used intubation techniques to isolate the intestinal effects from oral or intragastric effects. Most studies with intestinal nutrient administration have focused on duodenal delivery. Duodenal positioning of an intestinal tube is more easily performed and more convenient compared to intubation of jejunum or ileum. Satiety and reduction in energy intake of a meal during and after intestinal nutrient infusion are the two relevant outcome parameters. The energy content of the nutrient infusate has also been taken into account. The net effect on energy intake has been calculated as the reduction in energy intake of the meal minus the energy intake via the infusate. In case of more distal delivery of nutrients, digestion and absorption may not be complete so that the net reduction in energy intake may have been underestimated in the conditions of the currently included studies.

6.2.1. Dietary Fat: Site Specific Effects?

Compared to oral fat intake, ileal infusion of the same amount of fat (6 g) has a significantly more pronounced effect on food intake resulting in a 15% reduction in caloric intake of a subsequent meal [27]. Maljaars et al. repeated this experiment with 3 g fat and confirmed the observation of an ileal feedback of fat on eating behavior to be operative even at very low doses of fat [28]. It is not only the amount of fat but also the physicochemical properties of fat that affect the magnitude of the inhibitory effect on food intake and satiety. The effect on satiety parameters appears to be more pronounced with smaller fat droplet sizes, in the duodenum but also in the ileum. The reduction in food intake was 9% higher after fine versus coarse droplet infusion, both for duodenal and ileal fat delivery [32]. The reduction in hunger scores and food intake was more pronounced with increasing fatty acid chain length of intraduodenally administered fatty acids [46,47]. Maljaars et al. showed that intra-ileal triacylglycerols with unsaturated fatty acids resulted in a more pronounced increase in satiety compared to triacylglycerols with saturated fatty acids [47].

Data of studies on intestinal site-specific effects of dietary fat on eating behavior are shown in Table 1. After *duodenal* administration of fat at low infusion rates of 0.25 to 1.5 kcal per min, the inhibitory effect on energy intake is very small (mean 3%, range 0–8%) without a significant effect on fullness or satiety. At higher fat infusion rates of 2–4.9 kcal per min, a reduction in energy intake of 21% (range 10–32%) with a significant increase in satiety parameters was observed.

Infusion of fat into the *jejunum* at a high dose of fat of almost 5 kcal per min leads to a mean reduction in energy intake of 31% (range 12–50%) and a significant increase in satiety that at an equicaloric load is more pronounced in the *jejunum* compared to the *duodenum*.

For *ileal* fat administration, low fat infusion rates of around 0.5 kcal per min result in significant reductions in subsequent energy intake of 18% (range 15–21%) and increases in satiety. At higher *ileal* fat infusion rates of up to 5 kcal per min the effect on energy intake is even more pronounced with 31% reduction (range 30–32%).

These studies reveal that at low infusion rates the inhibitory effect of fat on energy intake is more pronounced in the ileum compared to jejunum and duodenum. When the infusion rate of fat is high, at doses of 5 kcal per min, the inhibitory effect on energy intake is in the same range for duodenal, jejunal and ileal fat delivery.

With respect to appetite: in the study of Maljaars et al. [28] the lower and higher dose of ileal fat of 3 and 9 g respectively, resulted in a similar reduction in appetite and increase in satiety, without any evidence for dose dependency, in contrast to intraduodenal fat. This difference between duodenum and ileum may be related to lipolytic capacity that is much smaller in the ileum compared to the duodenum. Digestion of triacylglycerol to fatty acids is considered a necessary step for fat to induce its satiety-inducing effects [48].

Concerning infusion of fatty acids, only data for duodenal perfusion are available. At equicaloric infusion rates, the inhibitory effect on food intake is more pronounced with fatty acids compared to fat: infusion ranges 0.4–0.75 and 0.3–0.9 kcal per min respectively result in reductions in food intake of 10–15% with fatty acids and 0% with fat.

With respect to reduction of energy intake, it is essential to take into account the energy content of the nutrients perfused. In the Table A1, we provide individual study data on the caloric content of the fat and fatty acid nutrients infused and of the change in energy intake (kcal) of the meal compared to control condition, per study [10,13,19,20,22,24,26,27,29–37]. The net effect is the reduction in energy intake of the meal minus the energy intake via the infusate.

6.2.2. Dietary Proteins: Site Specific Effects?

In general, proteins are known to be more satiating at an equicaloric basis compared to either lipids or carbohydrates. Proteins are therefore considered to be the most anorectic of the three macronutrients. Data of studies on intestinal site-specific effects of dietary proteins on eating behavior are shown in Table 2. Several groups have evaluated the effects of *intraduodenal* protein administration on food intake and satiety. Ryan et al. and Soenen et al. [24,35,36] have performed *intraduodenal* perfusion studies with whey protein. A dose-response effect was observed with respect to reductions of energy intake. Infusion doses of 0.5, 1.5 kcal and 3 kcal per min resulted in stepwise dose-dependent inhibitions in subsequent energy intake of 6%, 12.5% and 21% respectively. *Jejunal* and *ileal* protein infusion resulted in reductions in energy intake of respectively 9% and 22% at a dose of 0.85 kcal/min. In the *ileum* lower infusion rates of 0.19–0.57 kcal per min already resulted in a reduction in energy intake of 9.9–14%. Thus, also for proteins an inhibitory, dose-dependent, effect of intestinal protein infusion on energy intake has been demonstrated with a proximal to distal gradient.

Remarkably, no significant effect on fullness, hunger or satiety during or after *intraduodenal* protein infusion was observed (Table 2). Only during *ileal* protein infusion, a significant reduction of hunger was noted. An explanation for the lack of effect of intestinal proteins on satiety parameters may be related to differences in the appetite suppressing effects within different sources of proteins [49].

Concerning amino acids: at low *duodenal* infusion rates of 0.07–0.15 kcal per min and of 0.2–0.4 kcal per min, the reductions in energy intake were small, respectively 5% and 13%. All studies included a 90 min duration of infusion. At equicaloric infusion rates, the inhibitory effect on energy intake of proteins and amino acids was in the same range. Amino acids studied included L-tryptophan [31,38] and leucine [39]. Across studies, the inhibitory effect on energy intake between the different amino acids showed similar effect sizes (net reduction 175 ± 89 kcal [31]; 206 ± 68 kcal [38]; 170 ± 48 kcal [39], however direct comparison of the effect on energy intake reduction between different amino acids has not been studied yet.

In the Table A2 we provide individual study data on the caloric content of the protein and amino acid nutrients infused and of the change in energy intake (kcal) of the meal compared to control condition, per study [29,32,35,39–43]. The net effect is the reduction in energy intake minus the energy intake via the infusate.

6.2.3. Dietary Carbohydrates: Site Specific Effects?

The existence of a "duodenal brake" for carbohydrates with satiating effects has been well established. Lavin et al. [43] observed a significant reduction in energy intake and suppression of hunger when glucose was infused into the *duodenum* compared to the same amount of glucose administered intravenously.

Data of studies on intestinal site-specific effects of dietary carbohydrates on eating behavior are shown in Table 3. Infusion of glucose into the *duodenum* at doses of 0.66 to 2 kcal per min reduced energy intake non-significantly by 10% (range 5–13%). At higher *duodenal* infusion rates a significant inhibition of energy intake was found starting from a caloric load of 2.86 kcal glucose per min resulting in a mean 17% reduction (range 11–26%) in energy intake.

Starting from an *intraduodenal* caloric glucose load of 2.0 kcal per min the "desire to eat" and hunger were suppressed. As shown in Table 3, a dose-dependent effect of intestinal glucose on both satiety and energy intake has been observed. Changes in blood glucose concentrations have significant impact on gastric emptying. A delay in gastric emptying may increase satiation and reduce energy intake. Thus, blood glucose levels should be monitored and adjusted in patients with pronounced hyperglycemia as in diabetes mellitus.

Infusion of glucose at a 1 kcal per min rate into the *jejunum* did not reduce but increased energy intake compared to infusion of the same amount of glucose to the *duodenum*. In the *intrajejunal* experiment, food intake was 11% higher compared to the *duodenal* experiment [42]. Possibly in the duodenal experiment, a larger intestinal area has been exposed to glucose and may have resulted in a more pronounced reduction in energy intake.

Infusion of glucose in the *ileum* at a dose of 0.66 kcal per min induced a reduction of energy intake of 10%, a result that is in line with the reduction of energy intake when the same amount of glucose is administered into the *duodenum*. When instead of glucose, sucrose is administered in low doses of 0.19 to 0.57 kcal per min the inhibitory effect on energy intake is even more pronounced: 21% and 32% respectively. Satiation and fullness were not affected, neither by sucrose nor by glucose.

In the Table A3 we provide individual study data on the caloric content of the carbohydrate nutrients infused and of the change in energy intake (kcal) of the meal compared to control condition, per study [23,26–28,32,45,46,48,49]. The net effect is the reduction in energy intake minus the energy intake via the infusate.

6.3. Topic 2: Is the Intestinal Brake Effect on Appetite and Energy Intake Macronutrient Specific?

This question was addressed in a study by van Avesaat et al. [29] directly comparing isocaloric infusion of fat, protein and carbohydrate with safflower oil, casein and sucrose respectively into the ileum. A significant reduction in energy intake was observed with all three macronutrients: for sucrose 32%, for fat 21% and for casein 22% (differences between macronutrients: n.s.) These results indicate that equicaloric amounts of macronutrients induce an ileal brake inhibition of energy intake and affect eating behavior to the same extent.

In Table 4 we present summarized data from all the studies that are presented in Tables 1–3. We specify in Table 4 energy intake in response to fat, carbohydrates and protein but now compared for each location of perfusion: duodenum, jejunum and ileum. Note that the reduction in energy intake is presented as percentage reduction of energy intake as compared to control conditions and does not represent the absolute difference in caloric intake, as the caloric load by infusion of the macronutrient has not been taken into account in this calculation.

Table 4. Comparison of Energy Intake reduction (EI-red) in response to infusion of equicaloric amounts of fat, protein or carbohydrate (infusion rate in kcal/min) per location: duodenum, jejunum or ileum. Combined results of data obtained from published studies (see references).

Location	Fat		Carbohydrate		Protein	
	kcal/min	EI-Red	kcal/min	EI-Red	kcal/min	EI-Red
Duodenum	0.25–1.5	0–15%	0.6–2	5–13%	0.5–1.5	6–13%
	2–5	10–32%	2.86–4	11–26%	3.0	21%
Jejunum	4.9	12–50%	1	+11%	0.85	9%
Ileum	0.5–0.6	15–21%	0.19–0.66	10–32%	0.19–0.85	14–22%
	1.8–4.9	30–32%				

For duodenum, jejunum, ileum: equicaloric intake reduction: fat = carbohydrate = protein Duode-num/jejunum: infusion rate < 1 kcal/min: intake reduction < 10%, Duodenum/jejunum: infusion rate > 3 kcal/min: intake reduction > 20%, Ileum: infusion rate < 1 kcal/min: intake reduction 10–32%, ileum: infusion rate > 3 kcal/min: intake reduction > 30%. Reference: Duodenum: Fat: [10,17–25,30–34]. Protein: [23,31,35–39]. Carbohydrate: [21–23,40–45]. Jejunum: Fat [10,26]. Protein [37]. Carbohydrate: [42]. Ileum: Fat: [10,13,19,27–29]. Protein: [29,37]. Carbohydrate: [29,44]. Note that + under EI-red means an increase in energy intake. Energy intake reduction is presented as percentage reduction of energy intake as compared to control condition.

For *duodenal* perfusion, the responses to the three macronutrients, when based on caloric perfusion rate, were of the same magnitude: at caloric loads of 0–1 kcal per min, the energy intake was reduced by max 10% while at caloric loads of around 3 kcal per min the energy intake was reduced more than 20%.

For *jejunal* perfusion: only few data are available. The magnitude of energy intake reduction of a subsequent meal was more pronounced after high kcal infusion of fat compared to low kcal dose of protein while in the glucose infusion experiment at 1 kcal per min jejunal infusion resulted in a higher energy intake compared duodenal infusion of the same glucose load.

With respect to the *ileum*, it appears that even at low infusion rates of up to 1 kcal per min the reduction in energy intake is more pronounced with 10–30% inhibition compared to a maximum of 10% for *duodenal* brake and max 9% for *jejunal* brake. At doses > 3 kcal per min the magnitude of energy intake reduction is comparable for duodenal, jejunal and ileal brake with 20–30% reductions in energy intake. Taken together, these data point to brake effects that appear to be not so much macronutrient specific but more dependent on caloric loads.

With respect to location, the data point towards more pronounced brake effects for the ileum compared to jejunum and duodenum (Table 4): a distal to proximal gradient that is equal for the three macronutrients. We separately analyzed the studies [10,19,32,37,42,44] that directly compared the effect of region of infusion of a macronutrient on energy intake within the same study (Table 5) because this represents the most valid comparison. The results of these separately analyzed six studies are not different from the results of the combined data of all published studies together listed in Tables 1–4.

Additionally, an analysis has been performed considering the net energy intake reduction, that is, the reduction in energy intake (kcal) of the meal minus the caloric content of the nutrient infusion. This means that energy intake reduction resembles the absolute reduction in intake of energy from a meal, thus the amount of meal not eaten, while taking the amount of infusion into account. For this analysis, the data from all the individual studies presented in the Tables A1–A3 have been used. These data are presented in Table 6 at an aggregated level. In the studies with duodenal delivery of nutrients high caloric nutrient loads have been used, much higher compared to jejunal or ileal delivery of nutrients. While a reduction in energy intake was observed after duodenal infusion of carbohydrates, fat and proteins as shown in Table 4, when taking into account the high caloric load of the perfused duodenal nutrients, no net reduction was observed but an increase in the amount of calories ingested (Table 6) for duodenal delivery of fat and carbohydrates. For duodenal protein infusion, the net reduction in energy intake remains substantial. When comparing net intake reduction after ileal infusion, the reduction is in the same range for fat, protein and carbohydrate based on caloric load. Future studies on intestinal brake mechanisms should take into account more systematically the caloric load delivered with intestinal nutrient infusion. In case of more distal delivery, digestion and absorption may not be complete so that the net reduction in energy intake may have been underestimated in the conditions of the currently included studies.

Table 5. Comparison of net effect of energy intake reduction: reduction in energy intake of a meal minus energy content of infusate of fat, proteins or carbohydrates with comparison per location within the same study.

Reference	Location	Infusate		Reduction in Energy Intake (EI) of Meal	Net Effect: Reduction EI Meal-EI Infusate
		Type	Energy Content of Infusate		
41	Duodenum	casein	60 kcal	+20 kcal	−
	Jejunum	casein	60 kcal	40 kcal	−
	Ileum	casein	60 kcal	80 kcal	+
47	Duodenum	glucose	90 kcal	+160 kcal	−
	Jejunum	glucose	90 kcal		−
48	Duodenum	glucose	56 kcal	58 kcal	=
	Ileum	glucose	56 kcal	119 kcal	+
10	Jejunum	corn oil	370 kcal	1100 kcal	++
	Ileum	corn oil	370 kcal	650 kcal	++
33	Duodenum	rapeseed oil	54 kcal	14 kcal	−
	Ileum	rapeseed oil	54 kcal	18 kcal	−
19	Duodenum	canola oil	54 kcal	ileum vs. duo: 76 kcal	+
	Ileum	canola oil	54 kcal		

− means reduction EI meal < EI infusate. = means reduction EI meal = EI infusate. +/++/+++ means reduction EI meal > EI infusate. +: 0–100 kcal; ++100–300 kcal; +++: > 300 kcal.

Table 6. Comparison of net energy intake reduction in response to infusion of fat, fatty acids, proteins, amino acids or carbohydrate per location: duodenum, jejunum or ileum.

Location	Infusate	Infusate	Infusate	Infusate	Infusate
	LCT fat	LC fatty acids	Proteins	Amino acids	Carbohydrates
Duodenum	−	+	+	+	−
Jejunum	++	NA	+	NA	−
Ileum	++	NA	++	NA	++

Combined results of data obtained from published studies listed in Tables 1–3 and individual data from Tables A1–A3. NA: not assessed. Net reduction: reduction in energy intake of meal minus energy content of infusate. − means net reduction in energy intake is negative: increase in the amount of calories ingested. = means no net reduction in energy intake, reduction in energy intake of meal = energy content of infusate. +/++/+++ means net reduction in energy intake: reduction in energy intake of meal > energy content of infusate + net reduction 0–100 kcal ++ net reduction 100–300 kcal +++ net reduction > 300 kcal.

Lin et al. and Meyer et al. [50,51] have shown that increasing the small intestinal area exposed to nutrients resulted in more potent brake effects on gastric emptying and on satiety. Maljaars et al. [27] have investigated in more detail whether exposure of larger intestinal areas to nutrients causes a more potent effect on satiety and food intake. In three different experiments the same amount of fat (6 g in total) was administered at equal perfusion rates of 0.6 kcal per min for 90 min into (a) ileum only (6g) (b) duodenum (2g) jejunum (2g) and ileum (2g) simultaneously or (c) duodenum (2g) jejunum (2g) and ileum (2g) sequentially. Compared to control condition with oral fat, inhibition of food intake was 8% and 4% resp. for the simultaneous and sequential perfusion of larger intestinal areas while perfusion of the ileum resulted in the most pronounced and statistically significant reduction in food intake of 16%. Thus, increasing the small intestinal area did not result in larger reduction of food intake. Compared to control condition, hunger was significantly reduced during all three experiments.

6.4. Topic 3: Is the Acute "Intestinal Brake" Effect Maintained during Repetitive Activation?

Most of the studies performed so far have evaluated acute intestinal brake interventions on energy intake and satiety but did not explore whether the observed reductions in food intake in the acute experiments persist after repetitive activation. Data on chronic, prolonged jejunal-ileal brake activation have been obtained with bariatric surgery especially with malabsorptive procedures such as Roux-en-Y Gastric Bypass (RYGB). In this combined restrictive and malabsorptive bariatric procedure the proximal small intestine is bypassed and food is delivered to the more distal small intestine resulting in significant food intake reduction and weight loss on the long term [52].

Avesaat et al. [53] were among the first to investigate the effect of repeated, four days, activation of the "ileal brake" with ileal protein infusion on energy intake and satiety but also on gut peptide secretion and gastric emptying. Compared to control condition, energy intake during brake activation with proteins was lower: respectively 7%, 9%, 17% and 10% at days 1, 2, 3, and 4 compared to control (differences versus control condition: n.s.). While food intake was not significantly affected, satiety parameters were significantly increased and gastric emptying was delayed. These effects did not change during the four days of repetitive ileal brake activation.

6.5. Topic 1–3: Intestinal Brake to Nutrients: Summary of Findings and Perspectives

Compared to the duodenal brake, activation of the jejunal and ileal brake results in a somewhat more pronounced effect on energy intake and satiety, pointing to a distal to proximal gradient in intestinal brake efficacy. This distal to proximal gradient effect remained after correction for the caloric load of the nutrients infused. Thus, the net effect of ileal and jejunal brake activation on energy intake reduction is larger compared to duodenal brake effects (Table 6). During repetitive activation of the ileal brake for a maximum of four days, no adaptation or reduction in brake efficacy was observed.

Several limitations of the human studies with brake activation should be mentioned. First, all intestinal brake activation studies in humans have been performed with intestinal intubation that causes discomfort and inconvenience and may negatively affect eating behavior. On the other hand, the intervention and control experiments all have been performed during intestinal intubation so that conditions were equal. Second, one should realize that the magnitude of the brake effect on food intake is rather small. At lower infusion rates an intake reduction of a subsequent meal of about 10% is reached. Although this effect is not significantly different from control condition it is very consistently reported in all studies and it is clinically relevant as this may help in subsequent desired weight loss. Third, future studies should take into account more systematically the caloric load of the nutrients perfused.

The question arises whether the "ileal brake" can be activated without the need for intestinal intubation. In this respect encapsulation of nutrients or use of slow-release formulas are interesting alternatives. In order to reach the ileum before being digested and absorbed, nutrients should be protected by a structure that not only survives the acidic conditions of the stomach but also protects against the action of digestive enzymes and bile in the proximal small intestine. A prerequisite is that lipolysis and proteolysis should not be completely inhibited in the small intestine, but are delayed to prevent early absorption as degradation products of lipid, protein or carbohydrate digestion. When considering whether one specific macronutrient would be most suitable for encapsulation one should keep in mind the effect on energy intake reduction from the different nutrients (Tables 4 and 6). The effect of reduction of energy intake is dependent on the location of release (ileal versus duodenal) rather than on a specific nutrient, as for ileal release all nutrients appear to have similar effects.

With Fabuless, an emulsion of fractionated palm and oat oils dispersed in water thought to active the jejunal-ileal brake, initially a reduction in energy intake was observed [54], but subsequent studies failed to substantiate this effect [55]. Corstens et al. [56,57] have applied food graded micro-encapsulation systems to study ileal brake activation and satiety induction via delayed lipolysis. A human intervention study was performed using encapsulated lipid as emulsion-alginate beads or an equicaloric mixture of the same non-encapsulated nutrients with similar sensory properties as control condition [56]. Food intake of a subsequent meal was significantly reduced (intake 770 ± 38 kcal versus 821 ± 40 kcal; $p = 0.016$) and satiety was significantly increased after intake of the active substance [56]. Again, the reduction in caloric intake was only small, 6–7%, but may be clinically relevant. Alleleyn et al. [58] have studied the effect of an encapsulated carbohydrate-protein mixture on meal intake in healthy volunteers. A small but significant reduction of 6% in caloric meal intake was observed. These first human intervention studies need confirmation and the application of beads to modulate food intake should be evaluated in larger scale and longer-term intervention studies. With respect to encapsulated carbohydrates in the form of sugar: more distal (ileal) delivery of sugars (glucose) will lead to an increase in GLP-1 release with subsequent insulin release and increase in insulin sensitivity, factors that are beneficial in overweight and type 2 diabetes mellitus. In general, for encapsulation, the more "energy-dense" compounds (fat, fatty acids) are of particular interest.

Several questions arise: Can this reduction in caloric intake be repeated over the day during every meal? Is it affecting in-between meal snacking? Is the effect maintained over a longer period of time? What is the overall effect on weight regulation? These questions, including safety issues, need to be addressed in future studies.

6.6. Topic 4: Can the "Intestinal Brake" Effect on Appetite and Energy Intake Be Activated via Non-Caloric Tastants?

The five prototypical basic tastes sweet, salt, sour, bitter and umami are sensed by taste buds present on the tongue. Ion channels mediate the sensing of salty and sour taste while sensing sweet, bitter and umami taste is mediated by two families of taste receptors. Taste receptor family 1 (TAS1R) generally senses sweet and umami taste and taste receptor family 2 (TAS2R) primarily senses bitter taste [6]. It has been stated that these prototypical tastes exist in order to predict the type of food that will be ingested (i.e., sweet for saccharides, umami for glutamate, and bitter for potentially toxic substances). However, it is well known that negative affective responses to bitter can be uncoupled and converted into positive responses, as for caffeine [59,60]. Taste receptors are not only present on the tongue but are expressed throughout the entire human gut [61,62], in particular on EECs. Activation of taste receptors can result in the release of GI peptides such as CCK, PYY and GLP-1, known to influence satiety and eating behavior. Thus, activation of taste receptors can be elicited using non-caloric tastants. This concept of non-caloric modulation of satiety and eating behavior via intestinal taste receptors deserves further evaluation. Recently several smaller-scale clinical studies have been published on this topic focusing on gastrointestinal delivery of tastants. In these studies, the hypothesis was tested that post-oral delivery of non-caloric tastants will result in a net decreased energy intake compared with placebo. Klaassen et al. recently published a systematic review and meta-analysis on this topic [63]. These authors report on the effects of gastrointestinal administration of tastants on eating behavior. For sweet taste, aspartame and rebaudioside A have been used (Table 7) and a reduction in energy intake varying from 0–10% was observed.

The effect of gastrointestinal delivery of bitter tastants has been studied more extensively. Seven studies showed, small to moderate, non-significant reductions in food intake of a subsequent meal varying from 5 to 11%. In one study with repetitive intraduodenal administration of a bitter mixture, overall daily food intake was significantly reduced by 22% (340 kcal).

Table 7. Effect of tastants after duodenal, jejunal or ileal delivery on energy intake.

Taste	Tastant	Administration	Energy Intake Reduction kcal	Energy Intake Reduction %	Reference
Sweet	aspartame	gastric capsule		10%	[64]
	aspartame	gastric capsule		0%	[65]
	rebaudioside A	duodenal tube	26 kcal	5%	[66]
Bitter	quinine	acid resistant capsule			[67]
	quinine	duodenal tube	44 kcal	9%	[66]
	secoiridoids	micro encapsulation	88 kcal / 340 kcal (day)	11% / 22%	[68]
	bitter mixture	gastric capsule	109 kcal	7%	[69]
	denatonium bezoate	gastric tube	76 kcal	9.5%	[70]
	quinine 600 mg	gastric tube	53 kcal	5%	[71]
	quinine 275 mg	gastric tube	+26 kcal	+3%	[71]
	quinine	gastric tube	68 kcal	9%	[72]
	quinine 37.5 mg	duodenal tube	31 kcal	3%	[73]
	quinine 75 mg	duodenal tube	59 kcal	5%	[73]
	quinine 225 mg	duodenal tube	11 kcal	1%	[73]
Umami	monosodium glutamate	duodenal tube	+5 kcal	+1%	[66]
Combination: sweet, bitter and umami	Reb A, quinine and MSG	duodenal tube	64 kcal	14%	[66]
		duodenal tube	17 kcal	+2%	[72]
	Reb A, quinine and MSG	ileal tube	28 kcal	+4%	[74]
		duodenal+ ileal tube	31 kcal	+4%	[74]

RebA: rebaudioside A, MSG: monosodium glutamate. Note that + means an increase in energy intake. Energy intake reduction is presented as percentage reduction of energy intake as compared to control conditions.

Umami after intraduodenal administration of monosodium glutamate, did not affect intake of the subsequent meal compared to placebo. When sweet, bitter and umami tastants were infused simultaneously, subsequent caloric food intake was significantly impaired by 14%, compared to control condition [66]. None of these tastants when administered separately, had a significant effect on caloric intake. In a subsequent study, with duodenal and ileal infusion of the same combination of sweet, bitter and umami, these findings could not be confirmed [74].

The currently available data show that, among tastants, bitter compounds appear to be the most effective in influencing eating behavior. Energy intake, in the acute setting, decreased modestly after post-oral delivery of bitter tastants. Future studies should focus on dosing of tastants and on potential mechanisms of action. In this respect, effects on GI motility and on systemic and local GI peptide secretion have been observed [70,72,75,76]. Current knowledge on the effects of tastants on energy intake and satiety is limited. The most appropriate location(s) for tastant delivery to modulate eating behavior remains to be established. More research investigating the delivery of various tastants to different locations in the GI tract is needed.

7. Conclusions

In this study, we have reviewed the current literature with respect to human intervention studies of intestinal feedback mechanisms on appetite and energy intake. Most human studies have been performed with intestinal intubations and infusion of nutrients. Recent evidence indicates that:

(1) Regional differences exist in the intestinal modulation of appetite and energy intake with a distal to proximal gradient for inhibition of energy intake: ileum and jejunum > duodenum. This distal to proximal gradient effect remains after correction for the caloric load of the nutrients infused.

(2) The "intestinal brake" effect on appetite and energy appears not to be macronutrient specific. At equicaloric amounts, the inhibition on energy intake and appetite is in the same range for fat, protein and carbohydrate.
(3) Data on repetitive ileal brake activation are scarce because of the need for prolonged intestinal intubation. During repetitive activation of the ileal brake for up to 4 days, no adaptation was observed but overall, the inhibitory effect on energy intake was small.
(4) The concept of influencing energy intake by intra-intestinal delivery of non-caloric tastants is intriguing. Thus far, the available data show that, among tastants, bitter compounds appear to be more effective in influencing energy intake. Energy intake, in the acute setting, decreased modestly after post-oral delivery of bitter tastants or a combination of tastants (bitter, sweet and umami). An advantage is that tastants are non-caloric, in contrast to nutrients. Future studies should focus on optimal dosing and delivery of tastants and their mechanisms of action.

Intestinal brake activation provides an interesting concept for preventive and therapeutic approaches in future weight management strategies.

Author Contributions: Conceptualization, J.W., G.M., D.K. and A.M.; Methodology, J.W., G.M., T.K., M.v.A., D.K., A.M.; Formal analysis, G.M., A.M.; Investigation, J.W., G.M., A.M.; Resources, J.W., G.M., A.M.; Writing-original draft preparation, J.W., G.M., A.M.; Writing-review and editing, J.W., G.M., T.K., M.v.A., D.K., A.M.; Supervision, G.M., A.M.; Project administration, J.W., A.M. All authors have read and agreed to the published version of the manuscript.

Funding: No funding was obtained to write or publish this review.

Institutional Review Board Statement: Ethical review and approval were waived for this study, due to the retrospective nature of the study with use of published data, available in the public domain.

Informed Consent Statement: Not applicable.

Data Availability Statement: Data for this review have been obtained from published studies regarding the topics, not from databases.

Conflicts of Interest: Previously T.K. received a salary from Will Pharma BV as part of the 'Subsidie MKB Innovatiestimulering Topsectoren' (MIT) to study effects of tastants on eating behavior. A.M. has received grants for other purposes from: Grunenthal, ZonMw, Will Pharma, Dutch Cancer Society and Pentax. D.K. has received grants from Will Pharma, Allergan, Grunenthal, ZonMw, Maag-Lever-Darmstichting, United Europe Gastroenterology, EU Horizon 2020, outside the submitted work.

Appendix A

Table A1. Net effect of infusion of fat or fatty acids into duodenum, jejunum or ileum on energy intake, taking into account the reduction in energy intake of meal minus energy content of the infusate.

Reference	Location	Infusate		Reduction in Energy Intake (EI) of Meal	Net Effect: Reduction EI Meal-EI Infusate
		Type	Energy Content of Infusate		
10	Jejunum	corn oil	370 kcal	1100 kcal	+++
10	Ileum	corn oil	370 kca	650 kcal	++
13	Ileum	corn oil	358 kcal	570 kcal	++
19	Ileum	canola oil	54 kcal	60 kcal	=
22	Duodenum	corn oil	75 kcal	55 kcal	−
22	Duodenum	corn oil	200 kcal	150 kcal	−
24	Duodenum	Intralipid	200 kcal	100 kcal	−
26	Duodenum	Intralipid	360 kcal	204 kcal	− (obese: BMI 30–40 kg/m^2)

Table A1. Cont.

Reference	Location	Infusate Type	Energy Content of Infusate	Reduction in Energy Intake (EI) of Meal	Net Effect: Reduction EI Meal-EI Infusate
26	Duodenum	Intralipid	360 kcal	214 kcal	− (lean: BMI 19–26 kg/m^2)
27	Duodenum	Intralipid	343 kcal	200 kcal	−
29	Duodenum	Intralipid	270 kcal	170 kcal	−
30	Duodenum	Intralipid	270 kcal	250 kcal	=
31	Jejunum	corn oil	370 kcal	200 kcal	−
32	Ileum	safflower oil	52 kcal	120 kcal	+
33	Duodenum	rapeseed oil	54 kcal	14 kcal	−
33	Ileum	rapeseed oil	54 kcal	18 kcal	−
20	Duodenum	lauric acid	33 kcal	714 kcal	+++
34	Duodenum	lauric acid	36 kcal	270 kcal	++
35	Duodenum	lauric acid	9 kcal	52 kcal	+
36	Duodenum	lauric acid	24 kcal	130 kcal	+
37	Duodenum	LCT	370 kcal	325 kcal	−
37	Duodenum	LCFA	46 kcal	370 kcal	++

LCT: long chain triglycerides; LCFA: long chain fatty acids. − means reduction EI meal < EI infusate. = means reduction EI meal = EI infusate. +/++/+++ means reduction EI meal > EI infusate. +: 0–100 kcal; ++100–300 kcal; +++: > 300 kcal. Energy intake reduction is presented as percentage reduction of energy intake as compared to control conditions.

Table A2. Net effect of infusion of proteins or amino acids into duodenum, jejunum or ileum on energy intake, taking into account the reduction in energy intake of meal minus energy content of the infusate.

Reference	Location	Infusate: Type	Energy Content of Infusate	Reduction in Energy Intake (EI) of Meal	Net Effect: Reduction EI Meal-EI Infusate
29	Duodenum	whey	270 kcal	210 kcal	−
39	Duodenum	whey	30 kcal	46 kcal	+
			90 kcal	160 kcal	+
			180 kcal	315 kcal	++
32	Ileum	casein	17 kcal	60 kcal	+
			52 kcal	130 kcal	+
35	Duodenum	tryptophan	9 kcal	+37 kcal	−
40 Δ young men, mean age 23 (19–29) yrs	Duodenum	whey	30 kcal	147 kcal	++
			90 kcal	240 kcal	++
			180 kcal	419 kcal	++
40 Δ older men, mean age 74 (68–81) yrs	Duodenum	whey	30 kcal	+60 kcal	−
			90 kcal	+55 kcal	−
			180 kcal	180 kcal	=
41	Duodenum	casein	60 kcal	+20 kcal	−
	Jejunum		60 kcal	40 kcal	−
	Ileum		60 kcal	84 kcal	+
42	Duodenum	tryptophan	7 kcal	60 kcal	+
			14 kcal	220 kcal	++
43	Duodenum	leucine	13 kcal	59 kcal	+
			40 kcal	170 kcal	++

Net effect: − means reduction EI meal < EI infusate. = means reduction EI meal = EI infusate. +/++/+++ means reduction EI meal > EI infusate. +: 0–100 kcal; ++100–300 kcal; +++: > 300 kcal. Note that + in the section Reduction in Energy Intake (EI) of meal means an increase in energy intake compared to control condition. Energy intake reduction is presented as percentage reduction of energy intake as compared to control conditions.

Table A3. Net effect of infusion of carbohydrates into duodenum, jejunum or ileum on energy intake, taking into account the reduction in energy intake of meal minus energy content of the infusate.

Reference	Location	Infusate		Reduction in Energy Intake (EI) of Meal	Net Effect: Reduction EI Meal-EI Infusate
		Type	Energy Content of Infusate		
23	Duodenum	glucose	120 kcal	+128 kcal	−
			240 kcal	+135 kcal	−
			480 kcal	119 kcal	−
26	Duodenum	glucose	342 kcal	98 kcal (BMI 30–40 kg/m^2)	−
			342 kcal	63 kcal (BMI 19–29 kg/m^2)	−
27	Duodenum	glucose	342 kcal	140 kcal	−
28	Duodenum	glucose	348 kcal	350 kcal	=
32	Ileum	sucrose	17 kcal	95 kcal	+
			52 kcal	187 kcal	++
45	Duodenum	glucose	287 kcal	402 kcal	+
46	Duodenum	glucose	180 kcal	30 kcal	−
		fructose	180 kcal	200 kcal	+
48	Duodenum	glucose	56 kcal	58 kcal	=
	Ileum	glucose	56 kcal	119 kcal	+
49	Duodenum	glucose	288 kcal	184 kcal	−

Net effect: − means that reduction energy intake (EI) meal < EI infusate. = means reduction EI meal = EI infusate. +/++/+++ means reduction EI meal > EI infusate. +: 0–100 kcal; ++100–300 kcal; +++: > 300 kcal Note that + in the section Reduction in Energy Intake (EI) of meal means an increase in energy intake compared to control condition. Energy intake reduction is presented as percentage reduction of energy intake as compared to control conditions.

References

1. Cummings, D.E.; Overduin, J. Gastrointestinal regulation of food intake. *J. Clin. Investig.* **2007**, *117*, 13–23. [CrossRef]
2. Burdyga, G.; Lal, S.; Varro, A.; Dimaline, R.; Thompson, D.G.; Dockray, G.J. Expression of Cannabinoid CB1 Receptors by Vagal Afferent Neurons Is Inhibited by Cholecystokinin. *J. Neurosci.* **2004**, *24*, 2708–2715. [CrossRef]
3. Hirasawa, A.; Tsumaya, K.; Awaji, T.; Katsuma, S.; Adachi, T.; Yamada, M.; Sugimoto, Y.; Miyazaki, S.; Tsujimoto, G. Free fatty acids regulate gut incretin glucagon-like peptide-1 secretion through GPR120. *Nat. Med.* **2005**, *11*, 90–94. [CrossRef]
4. Lauffer, L.M.; Iakoubov, R.; Brubaker, P.L. GPR119 Is Essential for Oleoylethanolamide-Induced Glucagon-Like Peptide-1 Secretion from the Intestinal Enteroendocrine L-Cell. *Diabetes* **2009**, *58*, 1058–1066. [CrossRef] [PubMed]
5. Tanaka, T.; Katsuma, S.; Adachi, T.; Koshimizu, T.-A.; Hirasawa, A.; Tsujimoto, G. Free fatty acids induce cholecystokinin secretion through GPR120. *Naunyn Schmiedeberg's Arch. Pharmacol.* **2007**, *377*, 523–527. [CrossRef] [PubMed]
6. Depoortere, I. Taste receptors of the gut: Emerging roles in health and disease. *Gut* **2014**, *63*, 179–190. [CrossRef]
7. Phillips, R.J.; Powley, T.L. Gastric volume rather than nutrient content inhibits food intake. *Am. J. Physiol.* **1996**, *271*, R766–R769. [CrossRef] [PubMed]
8. Powley, T.L.; Phillips, R.J. Gastric satiation is volumetric, intestinal satiation is nutritive. *Physiol. Behav.* **2004**, *82*, 69–74. [CrossRef] [PubMed]
9. Gibbs, J.; Young, R.C.; Smith, G.P. Cholecystokinin elicits satiety in rats with open gastric fistulas. *Nature* **1973**, *245*, 323–325. [CrossRef]
10. Welch, I.M.; Sepple, C.P.; Read, N.W. Comparisons of the effects on satiety and eating behaviour of infusion of lipid into the different regions of the small intestine. *Gut* **1988**, *29*, 306–311. [CrossRef]
11. Read, N.W.; McFarlane, A.; Kinsman, R.I.; Bates, T.E.; Blackhall, N.W.; Farrar, G.B.; Hall, J.C.; Moss, G.; Morris, A.P.; O'Neill, B.; et al. Effect of infusion of nutrient solutions into the ileum on gastrointestinal transit and plasma levels of neurotensin and enteroglucagon. *Gastroenterology* **1984**, *86*, 274–280. [CrossRef]
12. Spiller, R.C.; Trotman, I.F.; Higgins, B.E.; Ghatei, M.A.; Grimble, G.K.; Lee, Y.C.; Bloom, S.R.; Misiewicz, J.J.; Silk, D.B. The ileal brake inhibition of jejunal motility after ileal fat perfusion in man. *Gut* **1984**, *25*, 365–374. [CrossRef]
13. Welch, I.; Saunders, K.; Read, N. Effect of ileal and intravenous infusions of fat emulsions on feeding and satiety in human volunteers. *Gastroenterology* **1985**, *89*, 1293–1297. [CrossRef]
14. Layer, P.; Peschel, S.; Schlesinger, T.; Goebell, H. Human pancreatic secretion and intestinal motility: Effects of ileal nutrient perfusion. *Am. J. Physiol. Liver Physiol.* **1990**, *258*, G196–G201. [CrossRef]
15. Koopmans, H.S.; Sclafani, A. Control of body weight by lower gut signals. *Int. J. Obes.* **1981**, *5*, 491–495. [PubMed]
16. Strader, A.D.; Vahl, T.P.; Jandacek, R.J.; Woods, S.C.; D'Alessio, D.A.; Seeley, R.J. Weight loss through ileal transposition is accompanied by increased ileal hormone secretion and synthesis in rats. *Am. J. Physiol. Metab.* **2005**, *288*, E447–E453. [CrossRef] [PubMed]

17. Pilichiewicz, A.N.; Papadopoulos, P.; Brennan, I.M.; Little, T.J.; Meyer, J.H.; Wishart, J.M.; Horowitz, M.; Feinle-Bisset, C. Load-dependent effects of duodenal lipid on antropyloroduodenal motility, plasma CCK and PYY, and energy intake in healthy men. *Am. J. Physiol. Integr. Comp. Physiol.* **2007**, *293*, R2170–R2178. [CrossRef]
18. Pilichiewicz, A.N.; Little, T.J.; Brennan, I.M.; Meyer, J.H.; Wishart, J.M.; Otto, B.; Horowitz, M.; Feinle-Bisset, C. Effects of load, and duration, of duodenal lipid on antropyloroduodenal motility, plasma CCK and PYY, and energy intake in healthy men. *Am. J. Physiol. Integr. Comp. Physiol.* **2006**, *290*, R668–R677. [CrossRef]
19. Maljaars, P.W.; Masclee, A.A.M. Both intestinal site and timing of fat delivery affect appetite in humans. In *Intestinal Fat and Eating Behavior: Role of the Ileal Brake*; Datawyse/Universitaire PersMaastricht: Maastricht, The Netherland, 2010; pp. 109–126.
20. Castiglione, E.K.; Read, N.W.; French, S.J. Food Intake Responses to Upper Gastrointestinal Lipid Infusions in Humans. *Physiol. Behav.* **1998**, *64*, 141–145. [CrossRef]
21. Chapman, I.M.; Goble, E.A.; Wittert, G.A.; Horowitz, M. Effects of small-intestinal fat and carbohydrate infusions on appetite and food intake in obese and nonobese men. *Am. J. Clin. Nutr.* **1999**, *69*, 6–12. [CrossRef]
22. MacIntosh, C.G.; Horowitz, M.; Verhagen, M.A.; Smout, A.J.; Wishart, J.; Morris, H.; Goble, E.; Morley, J.E.; Chapman, I.M. Effect of Small Intestinal Nutrient Infusion on Appetite, Gastrointestinal Hormone Release, and Gastric Myoelectrical Activity in Young and Older Men. *Am. J. Gastroenterol.* **2001**, *96*, 997–1007. [CrossRef]
23. Cook, C.G.; Andrews, J.M.; Jones, K.L.; Wittert, G.A.; Chapman, I.M.; Morley, J.E.; Horowitz, M. Effects of small intestinal nutrient infusion on appetite and pyloric motility are modified by age. *Am. J. Physiol. Content* **1997**, *273*, R755–R761. [CrossRef]
24. Ryan, A.T.; Luscombe-Marsh, N.D.; Saies, A.A.; Little, T.J.; Standfield, S.; Horowitz, M.; Feinle-Bisset, C. Effects of intraduodenal lipid and protein on gut motility and hormone release, glycemia, appetite, and energy intake in lean men. *Am. J. Clin. Nutr.* **2013**, *98*, 300–311. [CrossRef] [PubMed]
25. Seimon, R.V.; Feltrin, K.L.; Meyer, J.H.; Brennan, I.M.; Wishart, J.M.; Horowitz, M.; Feinle-Bisset, C. Effects of varying combinations of intraduodenal lipid and carbohydrate on antropyloroduodenal motility, hormone release, and appetite in healthy males. *Am. J. Physiol. Integr. Comp. Physiol.* **2009**, *296*, R912–R920. [CrossRef]
26. Drewe, J.; Gadient, A.; Rovati, L.C.; Beglinger, C. Role of circulating cholecystokinin in control of fat-induced inhibition of food intake in humans. *Gastroenterology* **1992**, *102*, 1654–1659.
27. Maljaars, P.W.J.; Peters, H.P.F.; Kodde, A.; Geraedts, M.; Troost, F.J.; Haddeman, E.; Masclee, A.A.M. Length and site of the small intestine exposed to fat influences hunger and food intake. *Br. J. Nutr.* **2011**, *106*, 1609–1615. [CrossRef] [PubMed]
28. Maljaars, P.W.J.; Symersky, T.; Kee, B.C.; Haddeman, E.; Peters, H.P.F.; Masclee, A.A.M. Effect of ileal fat perfusion on satiety and hormone release in healthy volunteers. *Int. J. Obes.* **2008**, *32*, 1633–1639. [CrossRef]
29. Van Avesaat, M.; Troost, F.J.; Ripken, D.; Hendriks, H.F.; Masclee, A.A.M. Ileal brake activation: Macronutrient-specific effects on eating behavior? *Int. J. Obes.* **2014**, *39*, 235–243. [CrossRef]
30. Feltrin, K.L.; Little, T.J.; Meyer, J.H.; Horowitz, M.; Rades, T.; Wishart, J.; Feinle-Bisset, C. Effects of lauric acid on upper gut motility, plasma cholecystokinin and peptide YY, and energy intake are load, but not concentration, dependent in humans. *J. Physiol.* **2007**, *581*, 767–777. [CrossRef]
31. McVeay, C.; Fitzgerald, P.C.E.; Ullrich, S.S.; E Steinert, R.; Horowitz, M.; Feinle-Bisset, C. Effects of intraduodenal administration of lauric acid and L-tryptophan, alone and combined, on gut hormones, pyloric pressures, and energy intake in healthy men. *Am. J. Clin. Nutr.* **2019**, *109*, 1335–1343. [CrossRef] [PubMed]
32. Maljaars, P.J.; van der Wal, R.J.; Wiersma, T.; Peters, H.P.; Haddeman, E.; Masclee, A.A. The effect of lipid droplet size on satiety and peptide secretion is intestinal site-specific. *Clin. Nutr.* **2012**, *31*, 535–542. [CrossRef]
33. Feltrin, K.L.; Little, T.J.; Meyer, J.H.; Horowitz, M.; Rades, T.; Wishart, J.; Feinle-Bisset, C. Comparative effects of intraduodenal infusions of lauric and oleic acids on antropyloroduodenal motility, plasma cholecystokinin and peptide YY, appetite, and energy intake in healthy men. *Am. J. Clin. Nutr.* **2008**, *87*, 1181–1187. [CrossRef]
34. Matzinger, D.; Degen, L.; Drewe, J.; Meuli, J.; Duebendorfer, R.; Ruckstuhl, N.; D'Amato, M.; Rovati, L.; Beglinger, C. The role of long chain fatty acids in regulating food intake and cholecystokinin release in humans. *Gut* **2000**, *46*, 689–694. [CrossRef] [PubMed]
35. Ryan, A.T.; Feinle-Bisset, C.; Kallas, A.; Wishart, J.M.; Clifton, P.M.; Horowitz, M.; Luscombe-Marsh, N.D. Intraduodenal protein modulates antropyloroduodenal motility, hormone release, glycemia, appetite, and energy intake in lean men. *Am. J. Clin. Nutr.* **2012**, *96*, 474–482. [CrossRef]
36. Soenen, S.; Giezenaar, C.; Hutchison, A.T.; Horowitz, M.; Chapman, I.; Luscombe-Marsh, N.D. Effects of intraduodenal protein on appetite, energy intake, and antropyloroduodenal motility in healthy older compared with young men in a randomized trial. *Am. J. Clin. Nutr.* **2014**, *100*, 1108–1115. [CrossRef] [PubMed]
37. Van Avesaat, M.; Ripken, D.; Hendriks, H.F.J.; Masclee, A.A.M.; Troost, F.J. Small intestinal protein infusion in humans: Evidence for a location-specific gradient in intestinal feedback on food intake and GI peptide release. *Int. J. Obes.* **2016**, *41*, 217–224. [CrossRef] [PubMed]
38. Steinert, R.E.; Luscombe-Marsh, N.D.; Little, T.J.; Standfield, S.; Otto, B.; Horowitz, M.; Feinle-Bisset, C. Effects of Intraduodenal Infusion of L-Tryptophan on ad Libitum Eating, Antropyloroduodenal Motility, Glycemia, Insulinemia, and Gut Peptide Secretion in Healthy Men. *J. Clin. Endocrinol. Metab.* **2014**, *99*, 3275–3284. [CrossRef]

39. Steinert, E.R.; Landrock, M.F.; Ullrich, S.S.; Standfield, S.; Otto, B.; Horowitz, M.; Feinle-Bisset, C. Effects of intraduodenal infusion of the branched-chain amino acid leucine on ad libitum eating, gut motor and hormone functions, and glycemia in healthy men. *Am. J. Clin. Nutr.* **2015**, *102*, 820–827. [CrossRef] [PubMed]
40. Pilichiewicz, A.N.; Chaikomin, R.; Brennan, I.M.; Wishart, J.M.; Rayner, C.K.; Jones, K.L.; Smout, A.J.P.M.; Horowitz, M.; Feinle-Bisset, C. Load-dependent effects of duodenal glucose on glycemia, gastrointestinal hormones, antropyloroduodenal motility, and energy intake in healthy men. *Am. J. Physiol. Metab.* **2007**, *293*, E743–E753. [CrossRef] [PubMed]
41. Rayner, C.K.; Park, H.S.; Wishart, J.M.; Kong, M.-F.; Doran, S.M.; Horowitz, M. Effects of intraduodenal glucose and fructose on antropyloric motility and appetite in healthy humans. *Am. J. Physiol. Integr. Comp. Physiol.* **2000**, *278*, R360–R366. [CrossRef] [PubMed]
42. Chaikomin, R.; Wu, K.-L.; Doran, S.; Meyer, J.H.; Jones, K.L.; Feinle-Bisset, C.; Horowitz, M.; Rayner, C.K. Effects of mid-jejunal compared to duodenal glucose infusion on peptide hormone release and appetite in healthy men. *Regul. Pept.* **2008**, *150*, 38–42. [CrossRef]
43. Lavin, J.H.; Wittert, G.A.; Andrews, J.; Yeap, B.; Wishart, J.M.; Morris, H.A.; Morley, J.E.; Horowitz, M.; Read, N.W. Interaction of insulin, glucagon-like peptide 1, gastric inhibitory polypeptide, and appetite in response to intraduodenal carbohydrate. *Am. J. Clin. Nutr.* **1998**, *68*, 591–598. [CrossRef] [PubMed]
44. Poppitt, S.D.; Shin, H.S.; McGill, A.-T.; Budgett, S.C.; Lo, K.; Pahl, M.; Duxfield, J.; Lane, M.; Ingram, J.R. Duodenal and ileal glucose infusions differentially alter gastrointestinal peptides, appetite response, and food intake: A tube feeding study. *Am. J. Clin. Nutr.* **2017**, *106*, 725–735. [CrossRef] [PubMed]
45. Lavin, J.H.; Wittert, G.; Sun, W.M.; Horowitz, M.; Morley, J.E.; Read, N.W. Appetite regulation by carbohydrate: Role of blood glucose and gastrointestinal hormones. *Am. J. Physiol. Metab.* **1996**, *271*, E209–E214. [CrossRef]
46. Feltrin, K.L.; Little, T.J.; Meyer, J.H.; Horowitz, M.; Smout, A.J.P.M.; Wishart, J.; Pilichiewicz, A.N.; Rades, T.; Chapman, I.M.; Feinle-Bisset, C. Effects of intraduodenal fatty acids on appetite, antropyloroduodenal motility, and plasma CCK and GLP-1 in humans vary with their chain length. *Am. J. Physiol. Integr. Comp. Physiol.* **2004**, *287*, R524–R533. [CrossRef]
47. Maljaars, J.; Romeyn, E.A.; Haddeman, E.; Peters, H.P.F.; Masclee, A.A.M. Effect of fat saturation on satiety, hormone release, and food intake. *Am. J. Clin. Nutr.* **2009**, *89*, 1019–1024. [CrossRef] [PubMed]
48. Feinle, C.; O'Donovan, D.; Doran, S.; Andrews, J.M.; Wishart, J.; Chapman, I.; Horowitz, M. Effects of fat digestion on appetite, APD motility, and gut hormones in response to duodenal fat infusion in humans. *Am. J. Physiol. Liver Physiol.* **2003**, *284*, G798–G807. [CrossRef] [PubMed]
49. Anderson, G.H.; Tecimer, S.N.; Shah, D.; Zafar, T.A. Protein Source, Quantity, and Time of Consumption Determine the Effect of Proteins on Short-Term Food Intake in Young Men. *J. Nutr.* **2004**, *134*, 3011–3015. [CrossRef]
50. Lin, H.C.; Doty, J.E.; Reedy, T.J.; Meyer, J.H. Inhibition of gastric emptying by acids depends on pH, titratable acidity, and length of intestine exposed to acid. *Am. J. Physiol. Liver Physiol.* **1990**, *259*, G1025–G1030. [CrossRef]
51. Meyer, J.H.; Tabrizi, Y.; Dimaso, N.; Hlinka, M.; Raybould, H.E. Length of intestinal contact on nutrient-driven satiety. *Am. J. Physiol. Integr. Comp. Physiol.* **1998**, *275*, R1308–R1319. [CrossRef] [PubMed]
52. Lutz, T.A.; Bueter, M. The physiology underlying Roux-en-Y gastric bypass: A status report. *Am. J. Physiol. Integr. Comp. Physiol.* **2014**, *307*, R1275–R1291. [CrossRef] [PubMed]
53. van Avesaat, M.; Troost, F.T.; Ripken, D.; Hendriks, H.F.J.; Masclee, A.A.M. Repeated ileal brake activation: Sustained re-sponses on eating behavior, gastrointestinal motility and peptide release? In *Doctoral Thesis: Nutrient sensing in the gut: Appe-Tite Regulation in Health and Obesity*; Datawyse/Universitaire PersMaastricht: Maastricht, The Netherlands; pp. 150–164. Available online: https://cris.maastrichtuniversity.nl/en/publications/nutrient-sensing-in-the-gut-appetite-regulation-in-health-and-obe (accessed on 8 April 2020).
54. Burns, A.; Livingstone, M.; Welch, R.; Dunne, A.; Reid, C.; Rowland, I. The effects of yoghurt containing a novel fat emulsion on energy and macronutrient intakes in non-overweight, overweight and obese subjects. *Int. J. Obes.* **2001**, *25*, 1487–1496. [CrossRef]
55. Poppitt, S.D.; Han, S.; Strik, C.M.; Kindleysides, S.; Chan, Y.-K. Investigating acute satiation and meal termination effects of a commercial lipid emulsion: A breakfast meal study. *Physiol. Behav.* **2015**, *152*, 20–25. [CrossRef] [PubMed]
56. Corstens, M.N.; Troost, F.J.; Alleleyn, A.M.; Klaassen, T.; Berton-Carabin, C.C.; Schroën, K.; Masclee, A.A. Encapsulation of lipids as emulsion-alginate beads reduces food intake: A randomized placebo-controlled cross-over human trial in overweight adults. *Nutr. Res.* **2019**, *63*, 86–94. [CrossRef]
57. Corstens, M.N.; Berton-Carabin, C.C.; de Vries, R.; Troost, F.J.; Masclee, A.A.; Schroën, K. Food-grade micro-encapsulation systems that may induce satiety via delayed lipolysis: A review. *Crit. Rev. Food. Sci. Nutr.* **2017**, *57*, 2218–2244. [CrossRef] [PubMed]
58. Alleleyn, A.M.E.; Van Avesaat, M.; Ripken, D.; Bleiel, S.B.; Keszthelyi, D.; Wilms, E.; Troost, F.J.; Hendriks, H.F.J.; Masclee, A.A.M. The Effect of an Encapsulated Nutrient Mixture on Food Intake and Satiety: A Double-Blind Randomized Cross-Over Proof of Concept Study. *Nutrients* **2018**, *10*, 1787. [CrossRef]
59. Cines, B.M.; Rozin, P. Some aspects of the liking for hot coffee and coffee flavor. *Appetite* **1982**, *3*, 23–34. [CrossRef]
60. Chambers, L.; Mobini, S.; Yeomans, M.R. Caffeine Deprivation State Modulates Expression of Acquired Liking for Caffeine-Paired Flavours. *Q. J. Exp. Psychol.* **2007**, *60*, 1356–1366. [CrossRef] [PubMed]

61. Van Der Wielen, N.; Van Avesaat, M.; De Wit, N.J.W.; Vogels, J.T.W.E.; Troost, F.; Masclee, A.; Koopmans, S.J.; Van Der Meulen, J.; Boekschoten, M.V.; Müller, M.; et al. Cross-Species Comparison of Genes Related to Nutrient Sensing Mechanisms Expressed along the Intestine. *PLoS ONE* **2014**, *9*, e107531. [CrossRef] [PubMed]
62. Gu, F.; Liu, X.; Liang, J.; Chen, J.; Chen, F.; Li, F. Bitter taste receptor mTas2r105 is expressed in small intestinal villus and crypts. *Biochem. Biophys. Res. Commun.* **2015**, *463*, 934–941. [CrossRef]
63. Klaassen, T.; Keszthelyi, D.; Troost, F.J.; Bast, A.; Masclee, A.A.M. Effects of gastrointestinal delivery of non-caloric tastants on energy intake: A systematic review and meta-analysis. *Eur. J. Nutr.* **2021**, 1–25. [CrossRef]
64. Rogers, P.J.; Pleming, H.C.; Blundell, J.E. Aspartame ingested without tasting inhibits hunger and food intake. *Physiol. Behav.* **1990**, *47*, 1239–1243. [CrossRef]
65. Black, R.M.; Leiter, L.A.; Anderson, G. Consuming aspartame with and without taste: Differential effects on appetite and food intake of young adult males. *Physiol. Behav.* **1993**, *53*, 459–466. [CrossRef]
66. Van Avesaat, M.; Troost, F.J.; Ripken, D.; Peters, J.; Hendriks, H.F.; Masclee, A.A. Intraduodenal infusion of a combination of tastants decreases food intake in humans. *Am. J. Clin. Nutr.* **2015**, *102*, 729–735. [CrossRef]
67. Andreozzi, P.; Sarnelli, G.; Pesce, M.; Zito, F.P.; Alessandro, A.D.; Verlezza, V.; Palumbo, I.; Turco, F.; Esposito, K.; Cuomo, R. The Bitter Taste Receptor Agonist Quinine Reduces Calorie Intake and Increases the Postprandial Release of Cholecystokinin in Healthy Subjects. *J. Neurogastroenterol. Motil.* **2015**, *21*, 511–519. [CrossRef]
68. Mennella, I.; Fogliano, V.; Ferracane, R.; Arlorio, M.; Pattarino, F.; Vitaglione, P. Microencapsulated bitter compounds (from Gentiana lutea) reduce daily energy intakes in humans. *Br. J. Nutr.* **2016**, *116*, 1841–1850. [CrossRef] [PubMed]
69. Peters, H.P.; Koppenol, W.; Schuring, E.A.; Gouka, R.; Mela, D.J.; Blom, W.A. The effect of two weeks ingestion of a bitter tastant mixture on energy intake in overweight females. *Appetite* **2016**, *107*, 268–273. [CrossRef]
70. Deloose, E.; Janssen, P.; Corsetti, M.; Biesiekierski, J.; Masuy, I.; Rotondo, A.; Van Oudenhove, L.; Depoortere, I.; Tack, J. Intragastric infusion of denatonium benzoate attenuates interdigestive gastric motility and hunger scores in healthy female volunteers. *Am. J. Clin. Nutr.* **2017**, *105*, 580–588. [CrossRef]
71. Bitarafan, V.; Fitzgerald, P.C.E.; Little, T.J.; Meyerhof, W.; Jones, K.L.; Wu, T.; Horowitz, M.; Feinle-Bisset, C. Intragastric administration of the bitter tastant quinine lowers the glycemic response to a nutrient drink without slowing gastric emptying in healthy men. *Am. J. Physiol. Integr. Comp. Physiol.* **2020**, *318*, R263–R273. [CrossRef]
72. Iven, J.; Biesiekierski, J.R.; Zhao, D.; Deloose, E.; O'Daly, O.G.; Depoortere, I.; Tack, J.; Van Oudenhove, L. Intragastric quinine administration decreases hedonic eating in healthy women through peptide-mediated gut-brain signaling mechanisms. *Nutr. Neurosci.* **2018**, *22*, 850–862. [CrossRef]
73. Bitarafan, V.; Fitzgerald, P.C.E.; Little, T.J.; Meyerhof, W.; Wu, T.; Horowitz, M.; Feinle-Bisset, C. Effects of Intraduodenal Infusion of the Bitter Tastant, Quinine, on Antropyloroduodenal Motility, Plasma Cholecystokinin, and Energy Intake in Healthy Men. *J. Neurogastroenterol. Motil.* **2019**, *25*, 413–422. [CrossRef] [PubMed]
74. Klaassen, T.; Alleleyn, A.M.E.; Van Avesaat, M.; Troost, F.J.; Keszthelyi, D.; Masclee, A.A.M. Intraintestinal Delivery of Tastants Using a Naso-Duodenal-Ileal Catheter Does Not Influence Food Intake or Satiety. *Nutrients* **2019**, *11*, 472. [CrossRef]
75. Deloose, E.; Corsetti, M.; Van Oudenhove, L.; Depoortere, I.; Tack, J. Intragastric infusion of the bitter tastant quinine suppresses hormone release and antral motility during the fasting state in healthy female volunteers. *Neurogastroenterol. Motil.* **2017**, *30*, e13171. [CrossRef] [PubMed]
76. Tack, J.; Deloose, E.; Ang, D.; Scarpellini, E.; Vanuytsel, T.; Van Oudenhove, L.; Depoortere, I. Motilin-induced gastric contractions signal hunger in man. *Gut* **2016**, *65*, 214–224. [CrossRef] [PubMed]

Review

Effects of Bitter Substances on GI Function, Energy Intake and Glycaemia-Do Preclinical Findings Translate to Outcomes in Humans?

Peyman Rezaie †, Vida Bitarafan †, Michael Horowitz and Christine Feinle-Bisset *

Adelaide Medical School and Centre of Research Excellence in Translating Nutritional Science to Good Health, Faculty of Health and Medical Sciences, University of Adelaide, Adelaide 5005, Australia; peyman.rezaie@adelaide.edu.au (P.R.); vida.bitarafan@adelaide.edu.au (V.B.); michael.horowitz@adelaide.edu.au (M.H.)
* Correspondence: christine.feinle@adelaide.edu.au; Tel.: +61-8-8313-6053
† These authors contributed equally to this work.

Abstract: Bitter substances are contained in many plants, are often toxic and can be present in spoiled food. Thus, the capacity to detect bitter taste has classically been viewed to have evolved primarily to signal the presence of toxins and thereby avoid their consumption. The recognition, based on preclinical studies (i.e., studies in cell cultures or experimental animals), that bitter substances may have potent effects to stimulate the secretion of gastrointestinal (GI) hormones and modulate gut motility, via activation of bitter taste receptors located in the GI tract, reduce food intake and lower postprandial blood glucose, has sparked considerable interest in their potential use in the management or prevention of obesity and/or type 2 diabetes. However, it remains to be established whether findings from preclinical studies can be translated to health outcomes, including weight loss and improved long-term glycaemic control. This review examines information relating to the effects of bitter substances on the secretion of key gut hormones, gastric motility, food intake and blood glucose in preclinical studies, as well as the evidence from clinical studies, as to whether findings from animal studies translate to humans. Finally, the evidence that bitter substances have the capacity to reduce body weight and/or improve glycaemic control in obesity and/or type 2 diabetes, and potentially represent a novel strategy for the management, or prevention, of obesity and type 2 diabetes, is explored.

Keywords: bitter substances; gut hormones; gastric emptying; gastric motor function; food intake; postprandial blood glucose; preclinical studies; human studies; obesity; type 2 diabetes

1. Introduction

There has been increasing interest in the capacity of bitter substances to regulate energy intake and improve glycaemic control, based on reports from preclinical models (i.e., studies in cell cultures or animals) [1–3] that bitter substances have potent effects to secrete gastrointestinal (GI) hormones and slow gastric emptying. It is now well established that these gut functions play important roles in the regulation of both acute energy intake and postprandial glycaemia [4–7]. Thus, bitter substances may potentially represent a novel approach to the management or prevention of obesity and its comorbidities, particularly type 2 diabetes. This is an important issue, given that the efficacy of the majority of currently available treatments for obesity is limited. While lifestyle changes (reduction in energy intake, increased physical activity) lead to weight loss, which, even when modest, is associated with meaningful reductions in the risk of type 2 diabetes, long-term adherence to such interventions is usually poor [8]. The critical importance of the gut is attested to by the efficacy of bariatric surgery in producing sustained weight loss in the morbidly obese and marked improvement in glycaemic control in patients with type 2 diabetes, the latter even before major weight loss occurs [5]. Pharmacological options for the management of obesity are limited. Their use is often associated with adverse effects, particularly nausea, and their effects on body weight are usually limited, possibly because longer-term effective suppression of energy intake is dependent on the interaction of a number of mechanisms. The use of agonists of glucagon-like peptide-1 (GLP-1) in the management of type 2 diabetes and, more recently in higher dosage, obesity is now widespread [9–12]. Weight loss may be greater with higher-dose GLP-1 agonists, but as with all anti-obesity medication, the cost is substantial, particularly as sustained use may be required to prevent weight regain. Thus, there remains an urgent need to identify novel and inexpensive strategies that stimulate these gut functions without adverse effects, to promote the longer-term suppression of energy intake, clinically meaningful weight loss and, in type 2 diabetes, improved glycaemic control.

In studies on both cell lines and experimental animals bitter agonists have been shown to potently stimulate cholecystokinin (CCK), GLP-1 and ghrelin [3,13]. Furthermore, bitter tastants modulate contractility in mouse gastric muscle strips and slow gastric emptying [14,15]. These findings in preclinical studies have triggered considerable interest in the investigation of the effects of bitter agonists in clinical studies, to determine whether their effects can be reproduced in humans and, if so, if they are associated with reductions in energy intake and/or postprandial glycaemic excursions. As will be discussed, while some clinical studies have reported effects of bitter substances to stimulate GLP-1 and CCK [16,17], suppress ghrelin [14,18], modulate gastric motility [19] and/or suppress energy intake [16,18,19], the observed effects are inconsistent and often modest. Moreover, only two studies have, to date, reported effects to lower postprandial blood glucose in humans [17,20].

This review provides a brief summary of key aspects of the GI sensing of bitter substances by luminal bitter receptors. The focus is the evaluation of information relating to the effects of bitter substances on the secretion of gut hormones, gastric emptying and GI motility, energy intake and blood glucose in preclinical and clinical studies. Finally, we explore the question as to whether there is evidence to support the concept that bitter substances have the capacity to reduce body weight and/or improve glycaemic control in obesity and/or type 2 diabetes, with the inherent potential for their use in the prevention and/or management of these disorders.

2. Sensing of Bitter Substances in the GI Lumen

In contrast to sweet, umami or 'fat' tastes (which indicate nutrient availability), bitter taste is inherently aversive and has been viewed traditionally as having evolved primarily to warn against the presence of toxins, particularly in plants, or signal spoiled food [21]. Many foods and other substances taste bitter and are, therefore, unpleasant to ingest. However, bitter receptors, like receptors for nutrients [22,23], are present not only in the oral cavity [24], but throughout the GI tract on enteroendocrine cells [23,25,26]. The recognition that their GI sensing may trigger beneficial metabolic effects, has, in recent years, fuelled substantial interest in a better understanding of GI bitter sensing and the investigation of the GI effects of bitter tastants. Unlike dietary macronutrients, bitter substances are devoid of energy and, accordingly, do not contribute to overall caloric intake, which represents an inherent advantage.

2.1. Sources of Bitter Compounds

Natural bitter-tasting compounds are contained in many foods that provide nutrition and contribute to health, including extracts of many plants (e.g., *Hoodia gordonii, Gentiana scabra, Humulus lupulus* L. flower, bark of the cinchona tree) as well as plant-based foods (e.g., *Brassica* vegetables and certain fruit), and processed dairy products, and include phenols, flavonoids and glucosinolates, amongst many others. They can also be found in animal-derived foods or generated during the process of food aging or spoilage [27,28]. Furthermore, Maillard and fermentation reactions can generate bitter compounds. Many chemically synthesised compounds, including denatonium benzoate, phenylthiocarbamide or 6-n-propylthiouracil (the latter two are often used to determine bitter taste sensitivity experimentally), as well as many drugs, have a strong bitter taste [29–33]. Bitter compounds are not only numerous (the number has been estimated to be in the tens of thousands [34]), but are also each characterised by a unique and diverse structure, consisting of phenols, esters, fatty acids, hydroxy fatty acids, amines, flavonoids, amongst many others, indicative of a broad range of bitter chemotypes [31,34].

2.2. Bitter Taste Receptors

Bitter tastants are detected by taste 2 receptors (TAS2Rs), which are members of the GPCR superfamily of receptors [34,35]. A large number of receptor subtypes has been identified in various species, including current totals of 25 in humans and >30 in rodents [36]. While some bitter compounds activate a single TAS2R subtype, the majority activates a range of TAS2R subtypes, although the combination of subtypes varies [34]. For example, salicin, from willow bark, activates TAS2R16, and both phenylthiocarbamide and propylthiouracil interact only with TAS2R38 [34]. In contrast, quinine, an extract from the bark of the cinchona tree, activates nine (TAS2R4, 7, 10, 14, 39, 40, 43, 44, 46) and denatonium benzoate eight (TAS2R4, 8, 10, 13, 39, 43, 46, 47) subtypes, of which five are in common with quinine. Quassin, an extract of the tropical quassia tree, activates five subtypes (TAS2R4, 10, 14, 46, 47) [34], of which four are in common with both quinine and denatonium benzoate. Bitter substances that activate differing combinations of receptor subtypes include sodium cyclamate, which activates TAS2R1 and 38, and sinigrin, found in cruciferous plants, which activates TAS2R16 and 38 [34]. That bitter substances activate different combinations of receptor subtypes (with varying overlap between individual compounds) may account for why only a limited number of TAS2Rs have the capacity to detect so many bitter compounds. In the absence of a comprehensive understanding of either the function(s) of each receptor subtype or the location and distribution of receptor subtypes on specific cells (e.g., enteroendocrine cells), the variability in receptor activation across bitter substances represents a major challenge to the clarification of their physiological roles and therapeutic potential.

Single nucleotide polymorphisms have also been described in TAS2Rs and shown to be associated with individual differences in bitter taste perception, food preferences and/or food consumption [32,33,37,38]. Thus, while bitter taste perception is reproducible in a given individual, the effects of bitter substances also vary between individuals. A well-documented example of a polymorphism is the ability to taste phenylthiocarbamide and 6-n-propylthiouracil, which is genetically determined by the TAS2R38 gene [39]. Based on the molecular structure of this receptor, individuals can be categorised into two common phenotypes, i.e., those that can taste these compounds and those that are 'non-tasters' [38,39]. The effect(s) of gene polymorphisms on the sensitivity to bitter compounds in extra-oral locations, including the GI tract, and how genetic variations may modify these effects remain to be clarified.

In contrast to knowledge relating to the characteristics of nutrient receptors, including their localisation and distribution along the GI tract, which has been reviewed in detail elsewhere [22,40–48], information regarding the regional distribution of TAS2Rs, and the functions of specific subtypes, is limited. Evaluation of the putative TAS2Rs 1 to 12 gene transcripts (except 11, which is not a functional gene) from rat antral, fundic and duodenal mucosa demonstrated a greater number of bitter receptor subtypes in the duodenum than the stomach [25]. In another study, which investigated locations of TAS2Rs by RNA sequencing on intestinal cells of rhesus macaques, only TAS2R1, 3, 4, 5, 19, 20, 38 and 46 were expressed in the duodenum, ileum and colon, with greater expression of TAS2R38 in the small, than the large, intestine [49]. Based on these observations, targeted administration of bitter compounds directly into the small intestine may potentially be associated with greater potency. However, an important caveat is that animal receptor subtypes may not correspond to those in humans. Knowledge relating to the functions of individual receptor subtypes is limited, but recent studies have defined roles for specific receptor subtypes in the regulation of gut hormones. For example, TAS2R5 and 38 may be involved in the release of GLP-1 from human L-cells and HuTu-80 cells, respectively [50,51], and TAS2R5 and 6 in ghrelin secretion [52]. An improved understanding of the distribution of TAS2Rs along the GI tract in humans, and the specific functions of individual receptor subtypes, will be critical to effective targeting of the administration of bitter substances to optimise bitter agonist-gut interactions.

3. Effects of Bitter Substances on Gut Hormone Release

A large number of gut hormones have been identified and many, including CCK, PYY, GLP-1, glucose-dependent insulinotropic polypeptide (GIP), ghrelin, motilin, oxyntomodulin, are pivotal to the regulation of gut motor function, energy intake and/or blood glucose [53–58]. CCK, PYY, GLP-1 and ghrelin are probably the best characterised. CCK, PYY and GLP-1 all have potent effects to modulate gastropyloroduodenal motility and slow gastric emptying, and reduce energy intake [5]. The critical involvement of endogenous hormones in these effects was confirmed by studies, in which administration of specific hormone receptor antagonists was shown to attenuate the suppression of energy intake [59–61]. These hormones also have potent effects to reduce energy intake when administered intravenously [62–64]. In contrast to CCK, PYY and GLP-1, ghrelin, whose circulating concentrations are high in the fasting state and thought to play a role in the initiation of eating, is suppressed by nutrients [57]. Once released, gut hormones exert their effects in part by activating specific receptors on vagal afferents [65,66], but may also have direct effects in brain centres involved in appetite regulation [5]. GLP-1, which is one of the two 'incretin' hormones (the other being GIP), is a physiological modulator of postprandial glycaemia, stimulating insulin and suppressing glucagon in a glucose-dependent manner [67], and slowing gastric emptying [11,53,68,69]. GLP-1 agonists and dipeptidyl peptidase-4 (DPP-4) inhibitors, which prevent degradation of endogenously secreted active GLP-1, are now used extensively in the management of type 2 diabetes to improve blood glucose control [10,12].

The presence of bitter substances in the GI lumen, following oral consumption or direct luminal administration, initiates a cascade of intracellular events culminating in the release of a number of gut hormones [3,70,71]. A substantial number of studies have evaluated the effects of bitter substances on gut hormone secretion in preclinical studies (Table 1). A range of bitter substances appear to have potent stimulatory effects, particularly on CCK and GLP-1, as well as ghrelin, in the models used. In contrast, effects on PYY are poorly defined. Only a small number of studies has been performed in humans [16–20,72–76] (Table 2). These studies have yielded inconsistent outcomes and, perhaps surprisingly in view of the preclinical outcomes, if positive, the observed effects have been modest. The following sections will review evidence on the effects of bitter substances on the secretion of CCK, GLP-1, PYY and ghrelin, based on studies in both preclinical models and humans.

3.1. Cholecystokinin

3.1.1. Outcomes of Preclinical Studies

The effects of bitter substances on CCK secretion have only been investigated in animal or human cell lines, and gut tissues ex vivo [2,13,77–79]. In mouse STC-1 or Caco-2 cells, matured hop bitter acids (MHBA, an oxidised bitter extract from the hops flower, *Humulus lupulus* L.), denatonium benzoate and phenylthiocarbamide all stimulated CCK release dose-dependently, MHBA 20- to 80-fold and denatonium benzoate 100- to 300-fold, while phenylthiocarbamide only resulted in a 1.5-fold increase [2,77,78]. In both ex cised rat intestinal tissue and the human enteroendocrine cell line, HuTu-80, steroid glycosides (extracted from the succulent plant, Hoodia gordonii), an agonist for hTAS2R7 and 14, stimulated CCK 1.5- to 3-fold, respectively, effects abolished by administration of the TAS2R14 antagonist, compound 03A3 [13]. Moreover, 1,10-phenanthroline, which selectively activates TAS2R5, stimulated CCK, from rat duodenal segments; in contrast, the TAS2R14-specific agonist, flufenamic acid, apparently decreased CCK release [74].

Table 1. Effects of bitter substances on gut hormone secretion in preclinical models.

Bitter Tastant	Model	Doses Given/Location of Delivery	Approx. Equivalent Dose in a 70-kg Human [1]	Observed Effect	Ref #
Berberine	STC-1 cells	1, 10, 100, 200 µM	-	↑ GLP-1	[80]
	NCI-H716 cells	1, 10, 100, 200 µM	-	↑ GLP-1	[81]
Chloroquine	Human fundic cells	0.3–10 mM	-	↑ Ghrelin	[52]
Denatonium benzoate	STC-1 cells	1–10 mM	-	↑ CCK	[2]
	NCI-H716 cells	2, 10 mM	-	↑ GLP-1, PYY	[3]
	Human fundic mucosa	0.5, 1, 5 mM	-	↑ Ghrelin	[52]
	Mice	1 mg/kg/oral	≈70 mg	↑ GLP-1	[3]
	Mice	60 µmol/kg/IG	≈1.8 g	↑ GLP-1	[1]
Epicatechin gallate	MGN3-1 cells	10 µM	-	↓ Ghrelin	[82]
		500 µM	-	↑ Ghrelin	
Erythromycin A	Human fundic mucosa	0.03, 0.3, 1 mmol/L	-	↑ Ghrelin	[52]
Flufenamic acid	Rat ex-vivo segments:				[79]
	- duodenal	10 µM	-	↓ CCK	
	- ileal	10 µM	-	↑ GLP-1 ↔ PYY	
Gallic acid	MGN3-1 cells	10 µM	-	↓ Ghrelin	[82]
Gentiana scabra extract	NCI-H716 cells	100–750 µg/mL	-	↑ GLP-1	[83]
Hoodia gordonii	HuTu-80 cells	10 mM	-	↑ CCK	[13]
KDT501	STC-1 cells	10 µM	-	↑ GLP-1	[84]
	Mice	150 mg/kg/oral	≈10 g	↑ GLP-1	[84]
Mature hop bitter acids	STC-1 cells	50, 100, 200 µg/mL	-	↑ CCK, GLP-1 ↔ PYY	[78]
Ofloxacin	NCI-H716 cells	10, 50, 100 mM	-	↑ GLP-1	[85]
1,10-Phenanthroline	NCI-H716 cells	10–500 µM	-	↑ GLP-1	[51]
	Human fundic mucosa	0.1, 1 mM	-	↑ Ghrelin	[52]
	Rat ex-vivo segments:				[79]
	- duodenal	150 µM	-	↑ CCK	
	- ileal	150 µM	-	↑ GLP-1 ↔ PYY	
Phenylthiocarbamide	STC-1 cells	2, 5, 10 mM	-	↑ CCK	[2]
	Caco-2 cells	10 mM	-	↑ CCK	[77]
	Human fundic cells	0.3–10 mM	-	↑ Ghrelin	[52]
Propylthiouracil	Human fundic cells	0.3–10 mM	-	↑ Ghrelin	[52]
	Mice	200 mg/kg/IG	≈14 g	↑ GLP-1	[50]
Qing-Hua granules	Mice	3.75, 7.5, 15 g/kg/d/IG	≈263–1050 g	↑ GLP-1	[86]
Quinine hydrochloride	NCI-H716 cells	0.5, 1, 2 mM	-	↑ GLP-1	[3]
	Mice	160 µmol/kg/IG	≈4 g	↔ GLP-1, ghrelin	[1]
Vanillic acid	Rat ileal segments	151.17 µM	-	↑ GLP-1	[79]
Wild bitter gourd	STC-1 cells	100, 500, 1000 µg/mL	-	↑ GLP-1	[87]
	Mice	5 g/kg/IG	≈350 g	↑ GLP-1	[87]

CCK, cholecystokinin; GLP-1, glucagon-like peptide-1; IG, intragastric; PYY, peptide YY. [1] Only calculated for whole-animal studies, [2] bitter compound derived from isohumulone, an extract from the hops plant.

3.1.2. Outcomes of Studies in Healthy Humans

In healthy males, administration of amarasate™ (a supercritical CO_2 extract from New Zealand native hops), in a dose of 500 mg, given either in an acid-resistant capsule (to target small intestinal bitter receptors) or a standard capsule (to release its content in the stomach) was reported to stimulate CCK in response to a subsequent lunch, consumed 60 min and 30 min after intestinal- and gastric-targetted administration, respectively, as well as a snack, consumed 120 min after lunch [72], although the magnitude of the effect was not reported. In contrast, in healthy males and females, 18 mg quinine hydrochloride, ingested orally in an acid-resistant capsule did not increase absolute plasma CCK concentrations, although the change in plasma CCK relative to baseline was slightly greater 30 min after consumption of an ad-libitum standardised buffet meal (~0.9 ± 0.6 vs. 0.5 ± 0.8 ng/mL) [16]. Moreover, 60-min intraduodenal infusions of quinine hydrochloride, providing 75 mg [74], or 37.5 mg, 75 mg and 225 mg [76], had no effect on plasma CCK in healthy, lean men. In these latter studies the relatively low infusion rate may have been insufficient to reach a critical threshold for activation of TAS2Rs [20].

Table 2. Effects of bitter substances on gut hormone secretion in healthy humans.

Bitter tastant	Model	Doses Given/Location of Delivery	Observed Effect	Ref #
Amarasate™ [1]	Males	500 mg in acid-resistant or standard capsules/oral	↑ CCK, GLP-1, PYY	[72]
Denatonium benzoate	Females	1 µmol/kg bolus/IG [≈32 mg] [2]	↔ Ghrelin	[19]
Quinine hydrochloride	Males	10 µmol/kg bolus/IG [≈270 mg]	↓ Ghrelin	[18]
	Males and females	18 mg in acid-resistant capsule/oral	↑ CCK	[16]
	Males and females	75 mg/ID over 60 min	↔ CCK, GLP-1, PYY	[74]
	Females	10 µmol/kg bolus/IG [≈270 mg]	↓ Ghrelin	[75]
	Males	37.5, 75, 225 mg/ID over 60 min	↔ CCK	[76]
	Males	275, 600 mg bolus/IG 30 min before meal	↑ GLP-1	[17]
	Males	600 mg bolus/IG 60 min before meal, ID 30 min before meal	↑ GLP-1	[20]
Secoiridoids [3]	Males and females	100 mg/oral (microencapsulated) incorporated in custard	↑ GLP-1 ↔ PYY, ghrelin	[73]

CCK, cholecystokinin; GLP-1, glucagon-like peptide-1; ID, intraduodenal; IG, intragastric; PYY, peptide YY. [1] Supercritical CO_2 extract from New Zealand native hops, [2] approximately equivalent dose in a 70-kg human, [3] bitter compound derived from of *Gentiana lutea* plant.

3.2. Glucagon-Like Peptide-1

3.2.1. Outcomes of Preclinical Studies

The effects of bitter compounds on GLP-1 secretion have been studied extensively [1,3,50,51,78–81,83–87]. A number of bitter compounds have been shown to stimulate GLP-1 in both cell line and animal studies. For example, berberine, found in several bitter plants, stimulated GLP-1 in human enteroendocrine NCI-H716 cells, and phenylthiourea in HuTu-80 cells around 1.5- to 2-fold, by activating TAS2R38 [50,80,81]. The latter effect was diminished, but not abolished, by silencing the TAS2R38 using non-coding small interfering RNA [50], indicating that while this receptor is involved in phenylthiourea-induced GLP-1 release, other mechanisms also contribute. In NCI-H716 cells, 1,10-phenanthroline stimulated GLP-1 via activation of TAS2R5, and denatonium benzoate via a range of TAS2R subtypes, including TAS2R4, 43, and 46 [3,51]. In mouse SCT-1 cells, application of the bitter compounds, MHBA and KDT501, pure derivatives of isohumulone, extracted from hops, stimulated GLP-1 release 1.5- to 2.5-fold [78,84], and the effect of KDT501 was attenuated by silencing the TAS2R108 with small hairpin RNA, implicating a role for this receptor [84]. Moreover, 1,10-phenanthroline, as well as the selective TAS2R14 agonists, vanillic acid and flufenamic acid, stimulated GLP-1 release from ileal segments from rat ~1.5-fold [79].

In mice, oral administration of 1 mg/kg denatonium benzoate and 5 g/kg wild bitter gourd, prior to glucose gavage, or 200 mg/kg propylthiouracil, stimulated GLP-1 secretion ~2–3 fold in all studies [3,50,87]. These doses were equivalent to ~70 mg, ~350 g and ~14 g in a 70 kg person, and were, accordingly, high. In diet-induced obese mice, acute oral gavage of KDT501, in the dose of 150 mg/kg, prior to an oral glucose load (1 g/kg), stimulated GLP-1 levels 3-fold within 15 min, while chronic treatment (150 mg/kg daily) for 17 weeks resulted in a more than 10-fold increase in plasma GLP-1 within four days, with the effect sustained over the treatment period [84]. Moreover, in obese mice, intragastric administration of denatonium benzoate (60 µmol/kg), but not quinine hydrochloride (160 µmol/kg), for four weeks also stimulated plasma GLP-1 ~1.5-fold [1].

3.2.2. Outcomes of Studies in Healthy Humans

Amarasate™, in a dose of 500 mg, also stimulated GLP-1, however, no information was provided about the magnitude of the effect [72]. Two studies that evaluated the effects of quinine (given as quinine hydrochloride) provided evidence that the timing of administration influenced the effect on GLP-1 [17,20]. In the first study, intragastric administration of quinine, in doses of 275 mg and 600 mg, 30 min before a 350-mL mixed-nutrient drink (500 kcal, 74 g carbohydrates) did not stimulate plasma GLP-1 during the first 30 min (i.e., in response to quinine alone), but increased GLP-1 modestly (by ~15 pmol/L) following the drink [17]. In the second study [20], 600 mg quinine was administered either intragastrically 60 min before, or intraduodenally 30 min before, a nutrient drink, and in both conditions plasma GLP-1 was increased modestly, by quinine alone, and further following the drink (Figure 1). These observations suggest that intragastric administration may require a longer time to achieve a comparable effect to that of intraduodenal administration, implying that exposure of small intestinal bitter receptors to quinine may be necessary for stimulation of GLP-1. In contrast to these observations, continuous intraduodenal infusion of quinine, in a dose of 75 mg, over 60 min had no effect on GLP-1 [74], perhaps because a threshold concentration was not achieved at the location of the receptors. The 600-mg dose of quinine hydrochloride in the above studies [17,20] is comparable to the acute therapeutic dose of quinine (500 mg) used for malaria treatment.

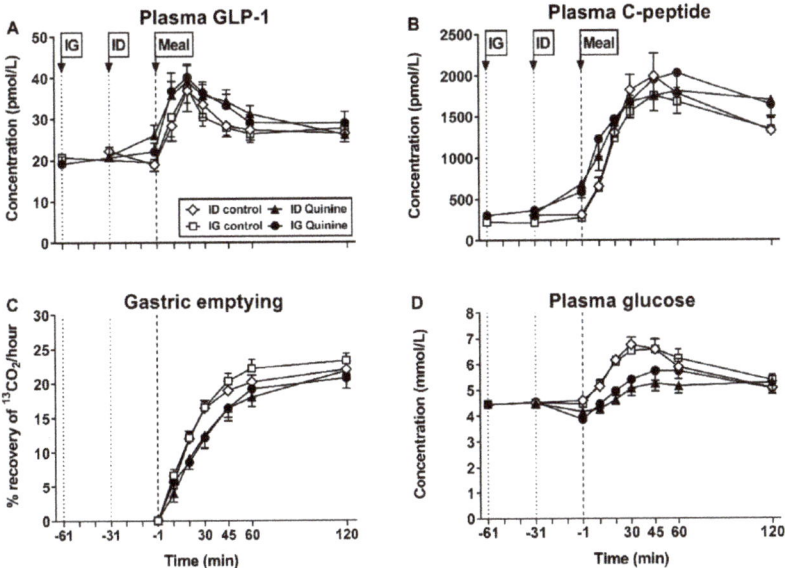

Figure 1. Effects of quinine on (**A**) plasma glucagon-like peptide-1 (GLP-1), (**B**) plasma C-peptide, (**C**) gastric emptying (measured using a ^{13}C-acetate breath test) and (**D**) plasma glucose in 14 healthy men. Quinine, given as quinine hydrochloride in a dose of 600 mg, or control, was administered either intragastrically (IG, at t = −61 min), or intraduodenally (ID, at t = −31 min), before a mixed-nutrient drink (500 kcal, 74 g carbohydrates), consumed at t = −1 min. IG and ID administration of quinine comparably (**A**) increased plasma GLP-1 concentration before, and in response to, the drink, (**B**) increased plasma C-peptide, before, and during the first 10 min in response to, the drink, (**C**) slowed gastric emptying of the drink, and (**D**) reduced plasma glucose before, and particularly following, the drink (Reprinted with permission from ref. [20]. Copyright 2021 Oxford University Press).

3.3. Peptide YY

3.3.1. Outcomes of Preclinical Studies

Information relating to the effects of bitter compounds on PYY secretion is both limited and inconsistent [3,78,79]. While, in murine NCI-H716 cells, denatonium benzoate (2 mmol/L) stimulated PYY release ~2.3 fold [3], in murine STC-1 cells, administration of MHBA was reported to have no effect [78]. Since PYY is co-localised with GLP-1 in enteroendocrine L-cells [88], the effects of bitter substances on PYY would be expected to be comparable to those on GLP-1. It is, accordingly, surprising that this has not been investigated, particularly, given the important role of PYY in the regulation of energy intake [54].

3.3.2. Outcomes of Studies in Healthy Humans

While amarasate™ was reported to stimulate plasma PYY [72], small intestinal administration of 100 mg bitter secoiridoids [73] and a 60-min intraduodenal infusion of quinine, in the dose of 75 mg [74], were found to be ineffective.

3.4. Ghrelin

3.4.1. Outcomes of Preclinical Studies

The effects of bitter compounds on ghrelin secretion have been investigated in a number of studies in both cell and rodent models; the majority of these have been performed by one research group [1,14,52,82]. Denatonium benzoate (0.5, 1 and 5 mmol/L), chloroquine (0.5, 1 and 5 mmol/L), 1,10-phenanthroline (0.1, 1 mmol/L), a selective agonist for TAS2R5, and erythromycin A (0.03, 0.3, 1 mmol/L), a TAS2R10-specific agonist, all stimulate ghrelin secretion in cultures of human fundic mucosa ~2-fold [52]. In a study, which evaluated the effects of phenolic extracts from grape seed, effects varied substantially between compounds, depending on the study conditions [82]. For example, epicatechin gallate, an agonist of mTAS2R14 and mTAS2R39, inhibited ghrelin secretion in a mouse gastric ghrelinoma cell line, MGN3-1, at the low dose of 10 µM by ~20%, while stimulating ghrelin 2-fold at a high dose (500 µM) [82]. Gallic acid also inhibited ghrelin release from MGN3-1 cells by ~20% (although only a 10 µM dose was tested), and by ~33% in rats pre-treated with gallic acid for 8 days [82]. In wild-type mice, intragastric administration of a mixture of bitter compounds containing denatonium benzoate, quinine hydrochloride, phenylthiocarbamide, propylthiouracil and D-salicin, stimulated plasma ghrelin ~2-fold [14]. In contrast, in obese mice on a high-fat diet, daily gavage with quinine (160 µmol/kg) had no effect on plasma ghrelin [1]. Thus, a range of bitter compounds stimulate ghrelin secretion in-vitro, while the outcomes of animal studies are inconsistent.

3.4.2. Outcomes of Studies in Healthy Humans

Intragastric administration of quinine, in a dose of 10 µmol/kg, suppressed plasma ghrelin in males [18] and females [75] modestly, and intragastric administration of denatonium benzoate, in a dose of 1 µmol/kg in healthy females [19], or administration of 100 mg bitter secoiridoids into the small intestine in healthy males and females [73], had no effect. Thus, evidence for a ghrelin-suppressant effect of bitter substances is limited.

Taken together, there is persuasive evidence that bitter substances have the capacity to stimulate gut hormones via a number of specific bitter receptor subtypes, and that subtypes vary between compounds and hormones, however, much more work is required to characterise their involvement. Identification of the specific role of specific receptor subtypes will facilitate targeted use of bitter compounds for defined outcomes. The doses used, particularly in the animal models have, in many cases, been very high, as assessed by calculating equivalent doses in humans. Thus, whether such doses could be used safely in humans, and/or whether lower doses have substantial effects, remains to be determined. The possibility that, because of the high doses used, some of the observed effects may reflect 'non-specific' effects of bitter compounds, requires clarification. For example, some bitter agonists used in these studies (e.g., phenylthiocarbamide), at the doses administered, have, in other studies, been shown to induce potent Ca^{2+} responses in control cells devoid of bitter receptors [89]. It should also be appreciated that because no studies have included positive controls, e.g., dietary nutrients, interpretation of the relative magnitude, and the relevance, of the observed effects on hormone release is confounded. Finally, there is a lack of information about the tolerability of bitter compounds, and the possibility that, at least some of, the observed effects reflect an aversive response, requires investigation.

In contrast to preclinical studies, the effects of bitter substances on gut hormone secretion in humans are largely inconclusive, moreover, the range of bitter compounds studied is limited. While it appears that, in line with preclinical studies, certain bitter compounds are associated with stimulation of GLP-1 in humans, the particular receptor subtype(s) involved remain to be identified. For example, whether stimulation of TAS2R38, which has been identified as a potent mediator of GLP-1 in in-vitro studies using human tissue [50], plays a role or other receptor subtypes (e.g., TAS2R5 or 14) are involved, given that quinine does not stimulate TAS2R38. Studies are required to systematically evaluate the effects of specifically selected compounds (e.g., those activating only specific single receptor subtypes) including targeting specific GI regions (e.g., the duodenum). Given that frequently much higher doses were used in preclinical studies, it will also be important to determine whether pharmacological doses are, indeed, necessary to achieve substantial effects and, if so, whether these occur in the absence of adverse effects.

4. Effects of Bitter Substances on Gastric Emptying and Gastrointestinal Motility

Gastric emptying regulates the transfer of chyme, and, therefore, the rate of nutrient entry, to the small intestine. Slowing of gastric emptying reflects closely coordinated changes in the motor function of the stomach and small intestine, which include relaxation of the proximal stomach, tonic and phasic pyloric contractions and suppression of antral and duodenal pressures [90,91]. As gastric emptying progresses, food components, particularly dietary nutrients, interact with specialised receptors located on the surface of enteroendocrine cells, triggering the secretion of gut hormones [22,40,42–44,48], which, at least in part, mediate nutrient-induced slowing of gastric emptying. The latter prolongs gastric distension and, thereby, enhances the feeling of fullness after a meal [92,93]. While both proximal and distal gastric filling contribute to the perception of fullness [93–95], antral content has been shown to be related closely to energy intake [95], and is, therefore, likely to be a major 'intragastric' mechanism.

Gastric emptying also plays a key role in the postprandial glycaemic response; in this context, regulation of the small intestinal delivery, and subsequent absorption, of glucose, as well as the release of glucoregulatory hormones, including GLP-1 and GIP, are of particular relevance. Thus, gastric emptying accounts for ~35% of the variance in the early (approximately first 30–45 min) rise in postprandial glucose in healthy individuals and those with diabetes [96,97]. It is now also recognised that the primary action of GLP-1 to lower blood glucose probably occurs via slowing of gastric emptying [98,99].

4.1. Outcomes of Preclinical Studies

Preclinical studies suggest that bitter compounds slow gastric emptying and modulate gastric motility [14,15,100,101] (Table 3). For example, in normal-weight mice, intragastric administration of phenylthiocarbamide (30 μmol/kg) or denatonium benzoate (60 μmol/kg) slowed gastric emptying [15], while in another study intragastric administration of denatonium benzoate in the higher dose of 10 mM had no effect [14]. The reason(s) for the discrepancy between the two studies are not clear. In the former study [15], the effect of denatonium benzoate, but not phenylthiocarbamide, was abolished by probenecid (50 mg/kg), an inhibitor of the TAS2R16, 38 and 43 subtypes, suggesting that the effect of denatonium benzoate may be mediated via TAS2R43 (denatonium benzoate does not activate TAS2R16 and 38), while raising the possibility that the effect of phenylthiocarbamide, which only activates TAS2R38, on gastric emptying does not involve bitter receptor activation. The mixture of denatonium benzoate, quinine hydrochloride, phenylthiocarbamide, propylthiouracil and D-salicin, described above, also slowed gastric emptying, which was unaffected by co-administration of the CCK antagonist, devazepide, or the GLP-1 antagonist, exendin (9–39) [14], indicating that slowing of gastric emptying induced by this mixture, and in the doses administered, was not mediated by CCK or GLP-1, but, as evidenced by the inhibition of the electrical field stimulation-induced activity in both antral and duodenal smooth-muscle strips, was likely to reflect a direct inhibitory effect on gastric smooth muscle cells [14,15]. In contrast, in mice, oral administration of swertiamarin, an extract from the *Swertia japonica* plant, in doses of 250 or 500 mg/kg, was reported to accelerate gastric emptying [100].

A few studies have evaluated the effect of bitter compounds on gastric contractile activity, and the reported effects vary substantially among the various compounds, as well as across species. For example, in mouse fundic and antral smooth-muscle strips, denatonium benzoate triggered concentration-dependent tonic fundic contraction (maximal at 100 μM) and antral phasic activity, but at higher concentrations (1 mM) induced fundic relaxation and inhibited antral activity [15]. In contrast, phenylthiocarbamide only induced dose-related relaxation of fundic muscle, while completely inhibiting activity in antral muscle, and salicin was ineffective [15]. These fundus-relaxing and antrum-inhibitory effects would be consistent with the observed slowing of gastric emptying in the in-vivo investigations [15]. In contrast to the effects observed in mouse tissue [15], in guinea pigs, oral (0.2 nmol/mL) and intragastric (0.1 and 1 nmol/kg) administration of denatonium benzoate increased gastric accommodation, consistent with gastric relaxation, while the higher dose of 30 µmol/kg inhibited accommodation [101]. Finally, in mice, oral administration of swertiamarin, in doses of 250 or 500 mg/kg, increased small intestinal motility [100]. The observed differences between some of the bitter compounds (and between species) are likely to be attributable to a number of factors, including the differential involvement of specific bitter taste receptor subtypes and variations in the sensitivity to different compounds.

There is, accordingly, evidence that bitter substances slow gastric emptying and modulate aspects of GI motility, although how some of the observed effects on motility (e.g., increased fundic tone) can be reconciled with the slowing of gastric emptying observed in vivo remains to be determined.

Table 3. Effects of bitter substances on gastric emptying and gastric motor function in preclinical models.

Bitter Tastants	Model	Doses Given/Location of Delivery	Approx. Equivalent Dose in a 70-kg Human [1]	Observed Effect	Ref #
Chloroquine	Mouse fundic and antral smooth-muscle strips	10–100 µM >1mM	–	↑ Phasic antral activity ↔ Tonic fundic contraction ↓ Phasic antral activity ↑ Fundic relaxation	[15]
Denatonium benzoate	Mouse fundic and antral smooth-muscle strips	10–100 µM >1 mM	–	↑ Tonic fundic contraction and phasic antral activity ↑ Fundic relaxation ↓ Phasic antral activity	[15]
	Mice	60 µmol/kg/IG	≈1.8 g	↓ Gastric emptying ↓ Fundic and antral motility	[15]
	Mice	10 mM/IG	≈0.04 g	↔ Gastric emptying	[14]
	Rats	10 mM/IG	≈0.04 g	↓ Gastric emptying	[102]
	Guinea pigs	0.2 nmol/mL/oral 0.1, 1 nmol/kg/IG 30 µmol/kg/IG	≈0.003 mg ≈0.003–0.03 mg ≈0.98 g	↑ Gastric accommodation ↓ Gastric accommodation	[101]
Phenylthiocarbamide	Mouse fundic and antral smooth-muscle strips	10 µM–10 mM	–	↑ Fundic relaxation ↓ Antral activity	[15]
	Mice	30 µmol/kg/IG	≈3.2 g	↓ Gastric emptying ↓ Fundic and antral motility	[15]
Salicin	Mouse fundic and antral smooth-muscle strips	10 µM–10 mM	–	↔ Fundic and antral contractility	[15]
Swertiamarin	Mice	250, 500 mg/kg/oral	≈17.5 and 35 g	↑ Gastric emptying ↑ Small intestinal motility	[100]
Mixture of DB, PTC, PTU, quinine HCl, D-salicin	Mice	DB 10 mM; PTC 10 mM; PTU 5 mM; quinine 1.5 mM; D-salicin 5 mM/IG	DB ≈ 46 mg; PTC ≈ 15 mg; PTU ≈8 mg; quinine ≈ 5 mg; D-salicin ≈ 15 mg	↓ Gastric emptying	[14]

DB, denatonium benzoate; HCl, hydrochloride; IG, intragastric; PTC, phenylthiocarbamide; PTU, propylthiouracil. [1] Only calculated for whole-animal studies.

4.2. Outcomes of Studies in Healthy Humans

A number of studies have evaluated the effect of bitter compounds on gastric emptying [16,17,19,20,103,104], with the majority reporting no effects [16,17,19,103] (Table 4). For example, in healthy males and females, 18 mg quinine hydrochloride, ingested orally in an acid-resistant capsule (to target release in the duodenum) did not affect gastric emptying of a 480-kcal solid meal [16]. Moreover, in healthy females, intragastric administration of 1 µmol/kg denatonium benzoate had no effect on gastric emptying of a 500-kcal pancake [19]. Finally, in healthy males, intragastric administration of quinine hydrochloride, in doses of 275 and 600 mg, had no effect on gastric emptying of a mixed-nutrient drink (350 mL; 500 kcal) consumed 30 min later [17]. In contrast, when the higher dose of quinine (600 mg) was administered either intragastrically 60 min, or intraduodenally 30 min, before the nutrient-drink, gastric emptying was slowed, with no difference between the two routes of administration (Figure 1) [20], providing evidence that intestinal exposure to bitter substances may be critical.

Table 4. Effects of bitter substances on gastric emptying and gastroduodenal motor function in healthy humans.

Bitter Tastants	Model	Doses Given/Location of Delivery	Observed Effect	Ref #
Denatonium benzoate	Females	1 µmol/kg bolus/IG (≈30 mg) [1]	↔ Gastric emptying	[19]
	Males and females	1 µmol/kg bolus/IG	↓ Fundic relaxation	[15]
Naringin	Males and females	1 mM bolus (≈580 mg)/IG	↔ Gastric emptying	[103]
Quinine hydrochloride	Males and females	18 mg in acid-resistant capsule/oral	↔ Gastric emptying	[16]
	Females	10 µmol/kg bolus/IG [≈270 mg]	↓ 'Fluctuations' in antral motility	[75]
			↔ Duodenal motility	
	Males and females	0.198 mM [≈72 mg]/IG	↔ Gastric emptying	[103]
	Males	37.5, 75, 225 mg/ID over 60 min	↔ Antropyloroduodenal motility	[76]
	Males	275, 600 mg bolus/IG 30 min before meal	↔ Gastric emptying	[17]
	Males	600 mg bolus/IG 60 min before meal, ID 30 min before meal	↓ Gastric emptying	[20]
Quinine sulphate	Females	10 mg bolus/oral	↓ Gastric emptying	[104]

ID, intraduodenal; IG, intragastric. [1] Approximately equivalent dose in a 70-kg human.

Information relating to the effect of bitter substances on gastroduodenal motility is also limited and inconsistent. In healthy males and females, intragastric administration of denatonium benzoate attenuated fundic relaxation after a nutrient drink [15], while, in healthy females, intragastric administration of quinine hydrochloride was reported to reduce 'fluctuations' in fasting antral motility, without affecting duodenal motility [75], and, in healthy males, a 60-min intraduodenal infusion of quinine, delivering overall doses of 37.5 mg, 75 mg or 225 mg, did not affect antral, pyloric or duodenal pressures [76].

Thus, while animal studies demonstrate an effect of bitter substances to slow gastric emptying, the effects on gastric emptying in humans, as well as any contributing contractile mechanisms, remain uncertain. Both the timing and location of delivery may be important.

5. Effects of Bitter Substances on Energy Intake

Based on the findings in preclinical studies of potent modulation by bitter substances of key GI factors, i.e., gut hormones and gastric emptying, involved in the acute regulation of food intake, there has been considerable interest in evaluating the effects of bitter substances on eating. This section will discuss studies that have investigated effects on caloric intake.

5.1. Outcomes of Preclinical Studies

A number of preclinical studies have evaluated the effects of bitter compounds on food intake [1,14,79,105–109] (Table 5). For example, in rats, oral gavage of an extract from *Hoodia gordonii* (in doses of 6.25–50 mg/kg) for three days suppressed intake from an ad libitum standard laboratory diet for eight days post-administration, and reduced body weight [107]. In rats with impaired glucose tolerance, oral administration of berberin (doses: 93.75, 187.5 or 562.5 mg/kg) for eight weeks reduced food intake from an ad libitum high-fat laboratory chow and also attenuated weight gain [108]. Moreover, in rats, ad-libitum consumption of a powdered chow diet containing quinine sulphate (0.75% by weight) for 32 days was associated with a reduction in food intake and body weight during the first two days of treatment, although food intake returned to control levels within 2 weeks [109]. While these observations suggest that these bitter compounds have an intake-suppressant effect, the bitter taste associated with oral consumption may have been offensive and discouraged food intake. However, the fact that bitter substances also reduce food intake when administered directly into the stomach argues against this possibility. For example, in mice, acute intragastric administration of a mixture of bitter compounds, including denatonium benzoate, quinine hydrochloride, phenylthiocarbamide, propylthiouracil and D-salicin, while increasing food intake during the first 30 min post-administration, suppressed intake during the subsequent 4 h [14]. The initial increase may potentially reflect stimulation of ghrelin, while the subsequent inhibition was interpreted as reflecting slowing of gastric emptying (despite continued elevation of ghrelin) [14].

Table 5. Effects of bitter substances on food intake and body weight in preclinical models.

Bitter Tastants	Model	Doses Given/Location of Delivery	Approx. Equivalent Dose in a 70-kg Human	Type of Meal or Diet	Observed Effects	Ref #
Berberine	Rats	93.75, 187.5, 562.5 mg/kg/oral	≈6.5, 13, 39 g	Ad libitum high-fat chow	↓ Food intake ↓ Weight gain	[108]
Denatonium benzoate	Mice	60 µmol/kg/IG	≈1.8 g	Mixed-nutrient liquid meal	↓ Food intake ↓ Weight gain	[1]
Epicatechin	Rats	300 mg/kg/IG	≈21 g	Ad libitum standard chow diet	↓ Food intake	[79]
Hoodia gordonii extract	Rats	6.25–50 mg/kg/oral	≈0.4–3.5 g	Ad libitum standard diet (55% CHO, 15% Prot, 3% F)	↓ Food intake ↓ Body weight	[107]
Humulus lupulus L. extract	Mice	2–5% of diet/oral	-	Ad libitum standard (77% CHO, 9.7% F, 13.9% Prot) or high-fat diet (546 kcal/100 g)	↓ Food intake ↔ Weight gain	[105]
	Rodents	0.2–1.2% of diet/oral	-	Ad libitum standard diet (77% CHO, 9.7% F, 13.9% Prot) or high-fat diet (60% F, 14% CHO, 26% Prot)	↓ Food intake ↓ Weight gain	[106]
1,10-Phenanthroline	Rats	200 mg/kg/IG	≈14 g	Ad libitum standard chow diet	↓ Food intake	[79]
Quinine hydrochloride	Mice	160 µmol/kg/IG	≈4 g	Mixed-nutrient liquid meal	↔ Food intake ↓ Weight gain	[1]
Quinine sulphate	Rats	0.75% of diet/oral	-	Ad libitum powdered chow diet	↓ Food intake ↓ Body weight	[109]
Vanillic acid	Rats	252 mg/kg/IG	≈17 g	Ad libitum standard chow diet	↓ Food intake	[79]
Mixture of DB, PTC, PTU, quinine HCl, D-salicin	Mice	DB 10 mM; PTC 10 mM; PTU 5 mM; quinine 1.5 mM; D-salicin 5 mM/IG	DB ≈ 46 mg; PTC ≈ 15 mg; PTU, ≈8 mg; quinine ≈ 5 mg; Salicin ≈ 15 mg	Ad libitum food	↑ Food intake (first 30 min) ↓ Food intake (next 4 h)	[14]

CHO, carbohydrate; DB, denatonium benzoate; F, fat; HCl, hydrochloride; IG, intragastric; Prot, protein; PTC, phenylthiocarbamide; PTU, propylthiouracil.

Moreover, in diet-induced obese mice, intragastric administration of 60 µmol/kg denatonium benzoate for 4 weeks reduced food intake from a liquid meal [1], an effect associated with GLP-1 stimulation. Interestingly, intragastric administration of quinine, in a dose of 160 µmol/kg and using the same study protocol [1], failed to either stimulate GLP-1 or reduce food intake. Furthermore, despite apparent discrepant effects on food intake, both denatonium benzoate and quinine reduced weight gain in mice [1], suggesting that the effect of quinine on body weight may be mediated by other mechanisms. In support of this concept, some bitter substances, including bitter orange extracts [110] and a mixture of salicin and naringin [111], have been reported to increase resting energy expenditure and diet-induced thermogenesis in the absence of a reduction in food intake, associated with weight loss. Finally in rats, intragastric administration of agonists of hTAS2R5 (e.g., 1,10-phenanthroline in a dose of 200 mg/kg) and hTAS2R14 (e.g., vanillic acid in a dose of 252 mg/kg), but not hTAS2R39 agonists, reduced food intake from an ad-libitum standard chow diet 3, 12 and 20 h post-administration [74]. The food intake-suppressant effect of 1,10-phenanthroline was associated with CCK and GLP-1 stimulation, and the effect of vanillic acid with GLP-1 stimulation, as measured using excised intestinal tissue [74].

5.2. Outcomes of Studies in Healthy Humans

There is little information about the effects of bitter compounds on appetite or energy intake in humans, and the reported outcomes are inconclusive [16–19,72–74,76] (Table 6). For example, in healthy females, while intragastric administration of denatonium benzoate (1 µmol/kg) increased 'satiety' and reduced hunger after a standardised meal, there was no significant suppression of energy intake from a subsequent ad-libitum buffet meal [19]. In contrast, in healthy males and females, ingestion of 18 mg quinine hydrochloride in an acid-resistant capsule modestly reduced energy intake from an ad-libitum meal 60 min later by ~82 kcal [16], and an intragastric bolus of 10 µmol/kg (~250 mg) quinine hydrochloride, in healthy females, modestly reduced energy intake from a highly palatable chocolate milk shake, by ~67 kcal [18]. The latter effect was associated with ghrelin suppression and an increased activity of brain centres involved in the control of feeding, including the hypothalamus and hedonic regions [18]. On the other hand, intraduodenal infusion of 75 mg quinine hydrochloride, in healthy volunteers (6 men, 9 women) [74], or doses of 37.5, 75 and 225 mg over 60 min [76], or intragastric bolus administration, in doses 275 and 600 mg [17], in healthy males, did not affect energy intake from ad libitum meals. Only two studies have reported more substantial reductions in energy intake. In one study, including healthy males and females, consumption of a microencapsulated extract of bitter compounds, derived from Gentiana lutea root, incorporated in a standardised custard breakfast (314 kcal), decreased total energy intake on that day by a substantial 22% (~340 kcal) [73]. In the second study in healthy males, administration of amarasate™, in a dose of 500 mg, reduced energy intake from an ad-libitum lunch by 277 kcal, and from a snack, provided 2 h after lunch, by 225 kcal [72].

Taken together, preclinical studies indicate consistent effects of bitter substances to suppress food intake, associated with a reduction in body weight. In contrast, information about the effects of bitter substances on energy intake in healthy humans remains limited, and findings are inconsistent, although there is evidence that some bitter compounds appear to have a potent suppressive effect.

Table 6. Effects of bitter substances on energy intake in healthy humans.

Bitter Tastants	Model	Doses Given/Location of Delivery	Type of Meal or Diet	Observed Effects	Ref #
Amarasate™ [1]	Males	500 mg in acid-resistant or standard capsules/oral	Ad libitum lunch and snack	↓ Energy intake	[72]
Denatonium benzoate	Females	1 μmol/kg bolus/IG (≈30 mg) [2]	Ad libitum meal (2330 kcal, 291 g CHO, 94 g F, 55 g Prot)	Trend for ↓ energy intake	[19]
Quinine hydrochloride	Males and Females	18 mg in acid-resistant capsule/oral	Ad-libitum meal (50% CHO, 31% F, 19% Prot)	↓ Energy intake	[16]
	Males and Females	75 mg/ID over 60 min	Ad libitum meal (160 kcal/100 g; 7.1 g Prot, 11 g CHO, 9.4 g F)	↔ Energy intake	[74]
	Females	10 μmol/kg bolus/IG (≈250 mg)	Ad libitum palatable chocolate milkshake	↓ Energy intake	[18]
	Males	37.5, 75, 225 mg/ID over 60 min	Ad libitum meal (2300 kcal, 52% CHO, 27% F, 21% Prot)	↔ Energy intake	[76]
	Males	275, 600 mg bolus/IG 30 min before meal	Ad libitum meal (2300 kcal, 52% CHO, 27% F, 21% Prot)	↔ Energy intake	[17]
Secoiridoids [3]	Males and females	100 mg/oral (micro-encapsulated) incorporated in custard	Ad libitum meal (3 h later)	↔ Energy intake	[73]

CHO, carbohydrate; F, fat; ID, intraduodenal; IG, intragastric; Prot, protein. [1] Supercritical CO_2 extract of New Zealand native hops plant, [2] approx. equivalent dose in a 70-kg human, [3] bitter compound derived from the *Gentiana lutea* plant.

6. Effects of Bitter Substances on Postprandial Blood Glucose

The potent effects of bitter substances to stimulate glucoregulatory hormones, particularly GLP-1, and slow gastric emptying (a major determinant of postprandial blood glucose), have provided a rationale for the investigation of the capacity of these compounds to reduce postprandial blood glucose levels. The latter is of major clinical relevance, since it is now appreciated that in type 2 diabetes postprandial glycaemic excursions are the major, and in many cases dominant, determinant of average glycaemic control, as assessed by measurement of glycated haemoglobin (HbA1c).

6.1. Outcomes of Preclinical Studies

A consistent effect of bitter compounds to lower postprandial blood glucose has been reported [3,83,87,110] (Table 7). For example, in db/db mice, oral administration of denatonium benzoate, in a dose of 1 mg/kg, reduced blood glucose levels by ~2 mg/dL, 20–40 min after glucose gavage (5 g/kg) [3]. Similarly, in db/db mice, oral administration of an extract from the root of the Gentia scabra plant immediately before an oral glucose load (5 g/kg), reduced blood glucose—the dose of 100 mg/kg by ~1 mg/dL within 90 min, and the 300 mg/kg dose by ~2 mg/dL within 40 min [83]. Moreover, in mice, a high-fat diet containing 5% extract of bitter gourd for 5 weeks reduced blood glucose AUC during a 90-min oral glucose tolerance test (2 g/kg) by ~350 mg/dL·min [87]. The glucose-lowering effects of denatonium benzoate, and Gentia scabra root and bitter gourd extracts, were associated with stimulation of GLP-1 and insulin [3,83,87]. Moreover, the glucose-lowering effect of bitter gourd extract was attenuated by co-administration of the GLP-1 receptor antagonist, exendin (9–39)amide [87], supporting a role for GLP-1 in glucose-lowering.

The effect of bitter compounds to improve glycaemia may also relate to effects on insulin sensitivity [110]. For example, in diabetic KK-A^y mice, the substantial postprandial glucose-lowering effect of a diet containing 0.18% of either isohumulone or isocohumulone (two major bitter acids derived from hops), fed for 14 days, was associated with activation of peroxisome proliferator activated receptors, PPARα and PPRAγ, intranuclear transcription factors known to improve insulin resistance [110]. Moreover, in C57BL/6N high-fat diet-fed mice, administration of isocohumulone (in doses of 10 and 100 mg/kg) for 14 days, reduced the plasma glucose response to an oral glucose load (1 g/kg body weight), associated with an improvement in insulin sensitivity [110].

Table 7. Effects of bitter substances on postprandial blood/plasma glucose in preclinical models and healthy humans.

Bitter Tastants	Model	Doses Given/Location of Delivery	Approx. Equivalent Dose in a 70-kg Human	Type of Meal	Observed Effects	Ref #
(A) Preclinical models						
Denatonium benzoate	Mice	1 mg/kg/oral	≈70 mg	OGTT (5 g glucose/kg BW)	↓ Blood glucose	[3]
Gentiana scabra extract	Mice	100, 300 mg/kg/oral	≈7–21 g	OGTT (5 g glucose/kg BW)	↓ Blood glucose	[83]
Isocohumulone [1]	Mice	10, 100 mg/kg/oral	≈0.7–7 g	OGTT (1 g glucose/kg BW)	↓ Plasma glucose	[110]
Wild bitter gourd	Mice	High-fat diet containing 5% extract/oral	-	OGTT (2 g glucose/kg BW)	↓ Blood glucose	[87]
(B) Healthy humans						
Quinine hydrochloride	Males	37.5, 75, 225 mg/ID over 60 min		N/A [2]	↔ Blood glucose (fasting)	[76]
	Males	275, 600 mg/IG 30 min before meal		Mixed-nutrient drink (500 kcal, 74 g CHO)	↓ Plasma glucose	[17]
	Males	600 mg/IG 60 min before meal, ID 30 min before meal		Mixed-nutrient drink (500 kcal, 74 g CHO)	↓ Plasma glucose	[20]
Secoiridoids [3]	Males and females	100 mg/oral (micro-encapsulated) incorporated in custard		Custard + biscuits (314 kcal, 45.1 g CHO)	↔ Blood glucose	[73]

BW, body weight; CHO, carbohydrate; ID, intraduodenal; IG, intragastric; N/A, not applicable; OGTT, oral glucose tolerance test. [1] bitter acid derived from hops plant, [2] blood glucose was measured in the fasting state, [3] bitter compound derived from the *Gentiana lutea* plant.

Accordingly, a number of bitter substances have potent effects to lower postprandial blood glucose, although evidence to support the involvement of specific receptor subtypes or the role of hormones, particularly GLP-1, is limited. No studies have hitherto evaluated the relationship between the effects on blood glucose with slowing of gastric emptying.

6.2. Outcomes of Studies in Healthy Humans

The effects of bitter substances on postprandial blood glucose have been evaluated in three studies in humans [17,20,73] (Table 7). Intragastric administration of quinine, in doses of 275 and 600 mg, reduced the glucose response to a mixed-nutrient drink containing 74 g carbohydrate in healthy males, associated with enhanced stimulation of GLP-1 and insulin after the drink, but without any effect on gastric emptying [17]. In a subsequent study, 600 mg quinine given either intragastrically 60 min, or intraduodenally 30 min, before a nutrient-drink also reduced blood glucose substantially, with no difference between the two routes of administration (Figure 1) [20]. Moreover, quinine stimulated both plasma GLP-1 and C-peptide (a measure of insulin secretion) immediately before the meal, and also slowed gastric emptying. In this study, the early postprandial plasma glucose response was shown to be related directly to gastric emptying, and inversely to plasma C-peptide immediately before the drink [20], suggesting that both slowing of gastric emptying, as well as insulin stimulation, contributed to glucose lowering. The role of GLP-1 in the observed glucose-lowering is uncertain, given that GLP-1-induced insulin secretion is glucose-dependent requiring plasma concentrations to be elevated above ~7 mmol/L [111]. Thus, it is possible that the glucose-lowering effect of quinine reflects a direct action of quinine on pancreatic beta cells to stimulate insulin [112]. In contrast, the lack of effect of a 60-min intraduodenal in-fusion of quinine, delivering overall doses of 37.5, 75 and 225 mg, in the absence of a carbohydrate source [76], is not surprising. Finally, in healthy males and females, consumption of 100 mg microencapsulated of *Gentiana lutea* plant extract in a custard and biscuit breakfast did not affect blood glucose over the subsequent 180 min [73]. However, only one dose was studied.

Taken together, the available studies, although limited, suggest a substantial effect of quinine, when administered into the upper GI lumen, to lower postprandial blood glucose.

7. Is There Evidence That Bitter Substances Reduce Body Weight and Improve Blood Glucose Control in Obesity and Type 2 Diabetes?

While observations from preclinical studies have provided evidence for potent effects of bitter substances to reduce food intake and lower postprandial blood glucose, in part related to gut hormone secretion, leading to weight loss, observations in healthy humans are less clear-cut, and, for the main part, effects, if any, were modest. Despite the latter, conclusions are frequently drawn as to the major implications of these findings for the development of novel management strategies for obesity and type 2 diabetes. We now address whether this concept is supported adequately by studies in people with obesity and/or type 2 diabetes.

A number of studies have reported associations between oral bitterness perception and body mass index (BMI) [113–117]. For example, higher body weights have been reported to be associated with reduced bitter perception in both adults (i.e., BMI > 28 kg/m^2 vs. BMI < 28 kg/m^2) [116] and children and adolescents (i.e., body weight > 97th percentile vs. body weight < 90th percentile) [117]. While impaired perception of sweet taste has been reported in people with type 2 diabetes [118,119], findings relating to bitter taste perception are less consistent. Some [119,120], but not all [121], studies have reported reduced oral bitter perception in type 2 diabetes. For example, only ~57% of males and females with well-controlled type 2 diabetes, compared with 72% of healthy individuals, were able to identify a bitter stimulus correctly in a taste identification task, independent of gender, disease duration or chronic glycaemic control, in one study [120], while another study found no difference [121], although perception of other tastes, including sweet, sour and salty was reduced.

GI morphological alterations, e.g., reduced numbers of enteroendocrine cells, both in the stomach and duodenum, have been reported in morbidly obese, compared with lean, people [122], which may potentially affect bitter sensing in the GI lumen, with consequences for gut hormone release, food intake and/or blood glucose control. There is evidence that the GI expression of some bitter taste receptor subtypes may be altered in obesity [52,123]. For example, expression of TAS2R38 has been reported to be augmented in colonic enteroendocrine cells producing CCK, GLP-1 and PYY in overweight and obese people [123], although the effect on hormone release by bitter substances was not evaluated. Moreover, in cultures of human gut mucosa, expression of TAS2R10 in ghrelin cells, which was found in both gastric and jejunal tissue, was greater in obese individuals in the stomach, but not the jejunum [52]. This was associated with differential effects on ghrelin stimulation by denatonium benzoate; thus, while denatonium benzoate stimulated ghrelin release from the fundus in both lean and obese, the effect was reduced in the obese, and in the jejunum, ghrelin stimulation only occurred in lean individuals [52], suggesting that sensitivity of ghrelin-secretory cells to this bitter agonist may be altered.

There is limited information regarding the effects of bitter sensing on glucose homeostasis [85,124]. While associations have been found between genetic variants of subtypes, including TAS2R9 and TAS2R38, with the glucose response to an oral glucose tolerance test [124] or GLP-1 and insulin release [85], the effects of bitter substances on blood glucose control have, to date, not been investigated in clinical studies.

No studies have investigated the effects of bitter substances on gut hormone release and gastric emptying in obesity and type 2 diabetes, and whether such effects, if any, are associated with a reduction in energy intake, weight loss and long-term improvement in blood glucose control.

8. Summary and Future Directions

In preclinical models bitter substances unequivocally have potent effects on upper GI functions, particularly the secretion of gut hormones, including CCK, GLP-1 and ghrelin, associated with reductions in food intake and body weight, and a reduction in postprandial blood glucose excursions, including in models of obesity and type 2 diabetes. In contrast, the limited clinical studies have yielded much more inconsistent outcomes and only been performed in healthy humans. These studies are indicative of an effect of bitter compounds to stimulate GLP-1 and to lower postprandial glucose, and to reduce energy intake modestly (Figure 2).

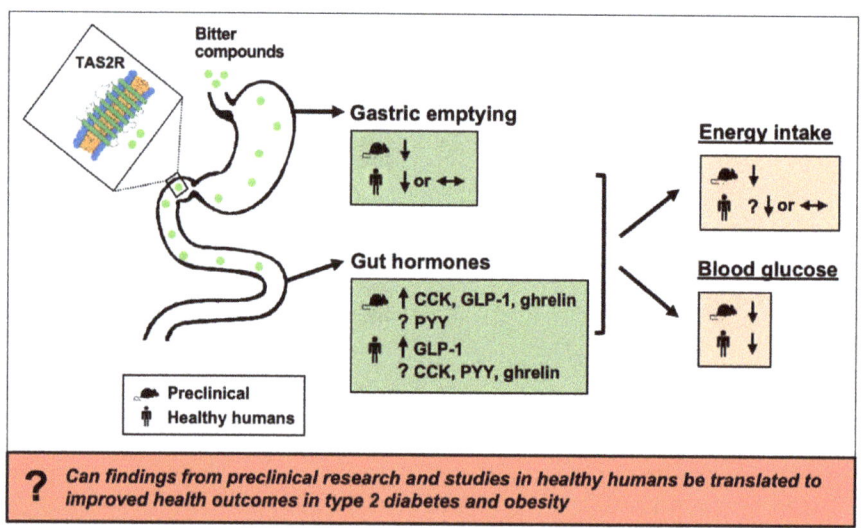

Figure 2. Schematic summarising current knowledge of effects of bitter substances on the secretion of gut hormones, including cholecystokinin (CCK), glucagon-like peptide-1 (GLP-1), peptide YY (PYY) and ghrelin, gastric emptying, energy intake and blood glucose, based on the outcomes of both preclinical studies (cell and animal models) and studies in healthy humans. TAS2R, bitter taste receptor.

There are a number of important issues that need to be addressed. The range of available bitter substances, activating a large variety of combinations of bitter receptor subtypes, not all of which may be relevant to outcomes, represents a major challenge to the systematic evaluation and comprehensive understanding of their effects. At least some of the inconsistencies in findings between humans and preclinical studies may be because the latter have often applied high doses of bitter compounds. Thus, evaluation of a wide range of bitter compounds, including a broad range of doses is required to determine efficacy, as well as tolerability. Moreover, no studies have directly compared the effects of different bitter compounds, administered intestinally, when adjusted for their bitterness, i.e., at identical intensities, to assess their effects independent of bitterness intensity. There is evidence that rats cannot discriminate orally between equibitter solutions of quinine and denatonium benzoate [125]. Characterisation of the specific bitter receptor subtypes involved in the regulation of GI functions, particularly the release of gut hormones, as well as their regional distribution along the human GI tract, may be pivotal to targeted use of specific bitter agonists to achieve defined outcomes, e.g., the release of specific gut hormones and/or slowing of gastric emptying, as well as potency of these effects. The roles of gut hormones and gastric emptying in the effects of bitter substances on energy intake and blood glucose require additional investigation to define whether these are causal or coincidental. Moreover, clarification of the role of genetic variations of receptor subtypes in interindividual differences in bitterness perception, and their relationships with effects on GI functions, energy intake and blood glucose control, is desirable.

A major omission is the absence of studies relating to the effects of bitter substances in people with obesity and/or type 2 diabetes. Such studies, which would initially evaluate acute effects, represent a priority. If the outcomes are positive, longer-term trials to establish whether acute effects translate to sustained weight loss and long-term improvements in glycaemic control will be warranted. Only then will it be known whether the encouraging findings from laboratory-based studies can be translated into innovative strategies for the management, treatment or prevention of obesity and type 2 diabetes.

Author Contributions: All authors contributed to writing, review and editing of the manuscript. All authors have read and agreed to the published version of the manuscript.

Funding: PR and VB were supported by Adelaide Scholarships International provided by the University of Adelaide (VB: 2017-20, PR: 2018-21) and CF-B by a Senior Research Fellowship from the National Health and Medical Research Council of Australia (grant number 1103020, 2016-21).

Conflicts of Interest: The authors declare no conflict of interest.

References

1. Avau, B.; Bauters, D.; Steensels, S.; Vancleef, L.; Laermans, J.; Lesuisse, J.; Buyse, J.; Lijnen, H.R.; Tack, J.; Depoortere, I. The Gustatory Signaling Pathway and Bitter Taste Receptors Affect the Development of Obesity and Adipocyte Metabolism in Mice. *PLoS ONE* **2015**, *10*, e0145538. [CrossRef]
2. Chen, M.C.; Wu, S.V.; Reeve, J.R.; Rozengurt, E. Bitter Stimuli Induce Ca^{2+} Signaling and CCK Release in Enteroendocrine STC-1 Cells: Role of L-Type Voltage-Sensitive Ca^{2+} Channels. *Am. J. Physiology-Cell Physiol.* **2006**, *291*, C726–C739. [CrossRef]
3. Kim, K.-S.; Egan, J.M.; Jang, H.-J. Denatonium Induces Secretion of Glucagon-Like Peptide-1 through Activation of Bitter Taste Receptor Pathways. *Diabetologia* **2014**, *57*, 2117–2125. [CrossRef]
4. Marathe, C.S.; Rayner, C.K.; Jones, K.L.; Horowitz, M. Relationships between Gastric Emptying, Postprandial Glycemia, and Incretin Hormones. *Diabetes Care* **2013**, *36*, 1396–1405. [CrossRef]
5. Steinert, R.E.; Feinle-Bisset, C.; Asarian, L.; Horowitz, M.; Beglinger, C.; Geary, N. Ghrelin, CCK, GLP-1, and PYY(3-36): Secretory Controls and Physiological Roles in Eating and Glycemia in Health, Obesity, and After RYGB. *Physiol. Rev.* **2017**, *97*, 411–463. [CrossRef]
6. Murphy, K.G.; Bloom, S.R. Gut Hormones and the Regulation of Energy Homeostasis. *Nat. Cell Biol.* **2006**, *444*, 854–859. [CrossRef] [PubMed]
7. Seimon, R.V.; Lange, K.; Little, T.J.; Brennan, I.M.; Pilichiewicz, A.N.; Feltrin, K.L.; Smeets, A.J.; Horowitz, M.; Feinle-Bisset, C. Pooled-Data Analysis Identifies Pyloric Pressures and Plasma Cholecystokinin Concentrations as Major Determinants of Acute Energy Intake in Healthy, Lean Men. *Am. J. Clin. Nutr.* **2010**, *92*, 61–68. [CrossRef] [PubMed]
8. Unick, J.L.; Beavers, D.; Bond, D.S.; Clark, J.M.; Jakicic, J.M.; Kitabchi, A.E.; Knowler, W.C.; Wadden, T.A.; Wagenknecht, L.E.; Wing, R.R.; et al. The Long-Term Effectiveness of a Lifestyle Intervention in Severely Obese Individuals. *Am. J. Med.* **2013**, *126*, 236–242. [CrossRef]
9. Bhat, S.P.; Sharma, A. Current Drug Targets in Obesity Pharmacotherapy-A Review. *Curr. Drug Targets* **2017**, *18*, 1. [CrossRef] [PubMed]
10. Drucker, D.J.; Nauck, M.A. The Incretin System: Glucagon-Like Peptide-1 Receptor Agonists and Dipeptidyl Peptidase-4 Inhibitors in Type 2 Diabetes. *Lancet* **2006**, *368*, 1696–1705. [CrossRef]
11. Müller, T.; Finan, B.; Bloom, S.; D'Alessio, D.; Drucker, D.; Flatt, P.; Fritsche, A.; Gribble, F.; Grill, H.; Habener, J.; et al. Glucagon-Like Peptide 1 (GLP-1). *Mol. Metab.* **2019**, *30*, 72–130. [CrossRef] [PubMed]
12. Deacon, C.F.; Mannucci, E.; Ahrén, B. Glycaemic Efficacy of Glucagon-Like Peptide-1 Receptor Agonists and Dipeptidyl Peptidase-4 Inhibitors as Add-on Therapy to Metformin in Subjects with Type 2 Diabetes-a Review and Meta Analysis. *Diabetes Obes. Metab.* **2012**, *14*, 762–767. [CrossRef] [PubMed]
13. Le Nevé, B.; Foltz, M.; Daniel, H.; Gouka, R. The Steroid Glycoside H.g.-12 from Hoodia Gordonii Activates the Human Bitter Receptor TAS2R14 and Induces CCK Release from HuTu-80 cells. *Am. J. Physiol. Liver Physiol.* **2010**, *299*, G1368–G1375. [CrossRef]
14. Janssen, S.; Laermans, J.; Verhulst, P.-J.; Thijs, T.; Tack, J.; Depoortere, I. Bitter Taste Receptors and α-Gustducin Regulate the Secretion of Ghrelin with Functional Effects on Food Intake and Gastric Emptying. *Proc. Natl. Acad. Sci. USA* **2011**, *108*, 2094–2099. [CrossRef]
15. Avau, B.; Rotondo, A.; Thijs, T.; Andrews, C.N.; Janssen, P.; Tack, J.; Depoortere, I. Targeting Extra-Oral Bitter Taste Receptors Modulates Gastrointestinal Motility with Effects on Satiation. *Sci. Rep.* **2015**, *5*, 15985. [CrossRef] [PubMed]
16. Andreozzi, P.; Sarnelli, G.; Pesce, M.; Zito, F.P.; Alessandro, A.D.; Verlezza, V.; Palumbo, I.; Turco, F.; Esposito, K.; Cuomo, R. The Bitter Taste Receptor Agonist Quinine Reduces Calorie Intake and Increases the Postprandial Release of Cholecystokinin in Healthy Subjects. *J. Neurogastroenterol. Motil.* **2015**, *21*, 511–519. [CrossRef]
17. Bitarafan, V.; Fitzgerald, P.C.E.; Little, T.J.; Meyerhof, W.; Jones, K.L.; Wu, T.; Horowitz, M.; Feinle-Bisset, C. Intragastric Administration of the Bitter Tastant Quinine Lowers the Glycemic Response to a Nutrient Drink without Slowing Gastric Emptying in Healthy Men. *Am. J. Physiol. Integr. Comp. Physiol.* **2020**, *318*, R263–R273. [CrossRef] [PubMed]
18. Iven, J.; Biesiekierski, J.R.; Zhao, D.; Deloose, E.; O'Daly, O.G.; Depoortere, I.; Tack, J.; Van Oudenhove, L. Intragastric Quinine Administration decreases Hedonic Eating in Healthy Women through Peptide-Mediated Gut-Brain Signaling Mechanisms. *Nutr. Neurosci.* **2018**, *22*, 850–862. [CrossRef] [PubMed]

19. Deloose, E.; Janssen, P.; Corsetti, M.; Biesiekierski, J.; Masuy, I.; Rotondo, A.; Van Oudenhove, L.; Depoortere, I.; Tack, J. Intragastric Infusion of Denatonium Benzoate Attenuates Interdigestive Gastric Motility and Hunger Scores in Healthy Female Volunteers. *Am. J. Clin. Nutr.* **2017**, *105*, 580–588. [CrossRef]
20. Rose, B.D.; Bitarafan, V.; Rezaie, P.; Fitzgerald, P.C.E.; Horowitz, M.; Feinle-Bisset, C. Comparative Effects of Intragastric and Intraduodenal Administration of Quinine on the Plasma Glucose Response to a Mixed-Nutrient Drink in Healthy Men: Relations with Gluoregulatory Hormones and Gastric Emptying. *J. Nutr.* **2021**. [CrossRef]
21. Bachmanov, A.A.; Beauchamp, G.K. Taste Receptor Genes. *Annu. Rev. Nutr.* **2007**, *27*, 389–414. [CrossRef]
22. Depoortere, I. Taste Receptors of the Gut: Emerging Roles in Health and Disease. *Gut* **2014**, *63*, 179–190. [CrossRef] [PubMed]
23. Lu, P.; Zhang, C.-H.; Lifshitz, L.M.; Zhuge, R. Extraoral Bitter Taste Receptors in Health and Disease. *J. Gen. Physiol.* **2017**, *149*, 181–197. [CrossRef] [PubMed]
24. Adler, E.; Hoon, M.A.; Mueller, K.L.; Chandrashekar, J.; Ryba, N.J.; Zuker, C.S. A Novel Family of Mammalian Taste Receptors. *Cell* **2000**, *100*, 693–702. [CrossRef]
25. Wu, S.V.; Rozengurt, N.; Yang, M.; Young, S.H.; Sinnett-Smith, J.; Rozengurt, E. Expression of Bitter Taste Receptors of the T2R Family in the Gastrointestinal Tract and Enteroendocrine STC-1 cells. *Proc. Natl. Acad. Sci. USA* **2002**, *99*, 2392–2397. [CrossRef] [PubMed]
26. Behrens, M.; Meyerhof, W. *Oral and Extraoral Bitter Taste Receptors*; Meyerhof, W., Beisiegel, U., Joost, H.-G., Eds.; Springer: Berlin, Heidelberg, 2010; pp. 87–99.
27. Drewnowski, A.; Gomez-Carneros, C. Bitter Taste, Phytonutrients, and the Consumer: A Review. *Am. J. Clin. Nutr.* **2000**, *72*, 1424–1435. [CrossRef] [PubMed]
28. Maehashi, K.; Huang, L. Bitter Peptides and Bitter Taste Receptors. *Cell. Mol. Life Sci.* **2009**, *66*, 1661–1671. [CrossRef] [PubMed]
29. Hofmann, T. Taste-Active Maillard Reaction Products: The "Tasty" World of Nonvolatile Maillard Reaction Products. *Ann. N. Y. Acad. Sci.* **2005**, *1043*, 20–29. [CrossRef]
30. Dubois, G.; DeSimone, J.; Lyall, V. *Chemistry of Gustatory Stimuli*; Elsevier BV: Amsterdam, The Netherlands, 2020; pp. 24–64.
31. Belitz, H.; Wieser, H. Bitter Compounds: Occurrence and Structure-Activity Relationships. *Food Rev. Int.* **1985**, *1*, 271–354. [CrossRef]
32. Duffy, V.B.; Davidson, A.C.; Kidd, J.R.; Kidd, K.K.; Speed, W.C.; Pakstis, A.J.; Reed, D.R.; Snyder, D.J.; Bartoshuk, L.M. Bitter Receptor Gene (TAS2R38), 6-n-Propylthiouracil (PROP) Bitterness and Alcohol Intake. *Alcohol. Clin. Exp. Res.* **2004**, *28*, 1629–1637. [CrossRef]
33. Keller, K.L.; Adise, S. Variation in the Ability to Taste Bitter Thiourea Compounds: Implications for Food Acceptance, Dietary Intake, and Obesity Risk in Children. *Annu. Rev. Nutr.* **2016**, *36*, 157–182. [CrossRef] [PubMed]
34. Meyerhof, W.; Batram, C.; Kuhn, C.; Brockhoff, A.; Chudoba, E.; Bufe, B.; Appendino, G.; Behrens, M. The Molecular Receptive Ranges of Human TAS2R Bitter Taste Receptors. *Chem. Senses* **2010**, *35*, 157–170. [CrossRef]
35. Li, F. Taste Perception: From the Tongue to the Testis. *Mol. Hum. Reprod.* **2013**, *19*, 349–360. [CrossRef] [PubMed]
36. Shi, P.; Zhang, J. Extraordinary Diversity of Chemosensory Receptor Gene Repertoires among Vertebrates. In *Chemistry and Biology of Pteridines and Folates*; Springer: Köln, Germany, 2009; Volume 47, pp. 57–75. [CrossRef]
37. Kim, U.; Wooding, S.; Ricci, D.; Jorde, L.B.; Drayna, D. Worldwide Haplotype Diversity and Coding Sequence Variation at Human Bitter Taste Receptor Loci. *Hum. Mutat.* **2005**, *26*, 199–204. [CrossRef]
38. Bufe, B.; Breslin, P.A.; Kuhn, C.; Reed, D.R.; Tharp, C.D.; Slack, J.P.; Kim, U.-K.; Drayna, D.; Meyerhof, W. The Molecular Basis of Individual Differences in Phenylthiocarbamide and Propylthiouracil Bitterness Perception. *Curr. Biol.* **2005**, *15*, 322–327. [CrossRef]
39. Kim, U.-K.; Jorgenson, E.; Coon, H.; Leppert, M.; Risch, N.; Drayna, D. Positional Cloning of the Human Quantitative Trait Locus Underlying Taste Sensitivity to Phenylthiocarbamide. *Science* **2003**, *299*, 1221–1225. [CrossRef]
40. Cvijanovic, N.; Feinle-Bisset, C.; Young, R.L.; Little, T.J. Oral and Intestinal Sweet and Fat Tasting: Impact of Receptor Polymorphisms and Dietary Modulation for Metabolic Disease. *Nutr. Rev.* **2015**, *73*, 318–334. [CrossRef] [PubMed]
41. Hajishafiee, M.; Bitarafan, V.; Feinle-Bisset, C. Gastrointestinal Sensing of Meal-Related Signals in Humans, and Dysregulations in Eating-Related Disorders. *Nutrients* **2019**, *11*, 1298. [CrossRef] [PubMed]
42. Latorre, R.; Sternini, C.; de Giorgio, R.; Meerveld, B.G.-V. Enteroendocrine Cells: A Review of their Role in Brain-Gut Communication. *Neurogastroenterol. Motil.* **2016**, *28*, 620–630. [CrossRef]
43. Psichas, A.; Reimann, F.; Gribble, F.M. Gut Chemosensing Mechanisms. *J. Clin. Investig.* **2015**, *125*, 908–917. [CrossRef]
44. Rasoamanana, R.; Darcel, N.; Fromentin, G.; Tomé, D. Nutrient Sensing and Signalling by the Gut. *Proc. Nutr. Soc.* **2012**, *71*, 446–455. [CrossRef]
45. Vella, A.; Camilleri, M. The Gastrointestinal Tract as an Integrator of Mechanical and Hormonal Response to Nutrient Ingestion. *Diabetes* **2017**, *66*, 2729–2737. [CrossRef]
46. Symonds, E.L.; Peiris, M.; Page, A.J.; Chia, B.; Dogra, H.; Masding, A.; Galanakis, V.; Atiba, M.; Bulmer, D.; Young, R.L.; et al. Mechanisms of Activation of Mouse and Human Enteroendocrine Cells by Nutrients. *Gut* **2015**, *64*, 618–626. [CrossRef] [PubMed]
47. Gribble, F.M.; Reimann, F. Function and Mechanisms of Enteroendocrine Cells and Gut Hormones in Metabolism. *Nat. Rev. Endocrinol.* **2019**, *15*, 226–237. [CrossRef] [PubMed]
48. Sternini, C.; Anselmi, L.; Rozengurt, E. Enteroendocrine Cells: A Site of 'Taste' in Gastrointestinal Chemosensing. *Curr. Opin. Endocrinol. Diabetes Obes.* **2008**, *15*, 73–78. [CrossRef] [PubMed]

49. Imai, H.; Hakukawa, M.; Hayashi, M.; Iwatsuki, K.; Masuda, K. Expression of Bitter Taste Receptors in the Intestinal Cells of Non-Human Primates. *Int. J. Mol. Sci.* **2020**, *21*, 902. [CrossRef] [PubMed]
50. Pham, H.; Hui, H.; Morvaridi, S.; Cai, J.; Zhang, S.; Tan, J.; Wu, V.; Levin, N.; Knudsen, B.; Goddard, W.A.; et al. A Bitter Pill for Type 2 Diabetes? The Activation of Bitter Taste Receptor TAS2R38 can Stimulate GLP-1 Release from Enteroendocrine L-Cells. *Biochem. Biophys. Res. Commun.* **2016**, *475*, 295–300. [CrossRef] [PubMed]
51. Park, J.; Kim, K.-S.; Kim, K.-H.; Lee, I.-S.; Jeong, H.-S.; Kim, Y.; Jang, H.-J. GLP-1 Secretion is Stimulated by 1,10-Phenanthroline via Colocalized T2R5 Signal Transduction in Human Enteroendocrine L Cell. *Biochem. Biophys. Res. Commun.* **2015**, *468*, 306–311. [CrossRef]
52. Wang, Q.; Liszt, K.I.; Deloose, E.; Canovai, E.; Thijs, T.; Farré, R.; Ceulemans, L.J.; Lannoo, M.; Tack, J.; Depoortere, I. Obesity Alters Adrenergic and Chemosensory Signaling Pathways that Regulate Ghrelin Secretion in the Human Gut. *FASEB J.* **2019**, *33*, 4907–4920. [CrossRef]
53. Holst, J.J.; Gribble, F.; Horowitz, M.; Rayner, C.K. Roles of the Gut in Glucose Homeostasis. *Diabetes Care* **2016**, *39*, 884–892. [CrossRef]
54. Suzuki, K.; Jayasena, C.N.; Bloom, S.R. The Gut Hormones in Appetite Regulation. *J. Obes.* **2011**, *2011*, 1–10. [CrossRef]
55. Deloose, E.; Verbeure, W.; Depoortere, I.; Tack, J. Motilin: From Gastric Motility Stimulation to Hunger Signalling. *Nat. Rev. Endocrinol.* **2019**, *15*, 238–250. [CrossRef]
56. Cummings, D.E.; Overduin, J. Gastrointestinal Regulation of Food Intake. *J. Clin. Investig.* **2007**, *117*, 13–23. [CrossRef] [PubMed]
57. Cummings, D.E. Roles for Ghrelin in the Regulation of Appetite and Body Weight. *Arch. Surg.* **2003**, *138*, 389–396. [CrossRef]
58. Field, B.C.T.; Chaudhri, O.B.; Bloom, S.R. Bowels Control Brain: Gut Hormones and Obesity. *Nat. Rev. Endocrinol.* **2010**, *6*, 444–453. [CrossRef]
59. Abbott, C.R.; Small, C.J.; Kennedy, A.R.; Neary, N.M.; Sajedi, A.; Ghatei, M.A.; Bloom, S.R. Blockade of the Neuropeptide Y Y2 Receptor with the Specific Antagonist BIIE0246 Attenuates the Effect of Endogenous and Exogenous Peptide YY(3–36) on Food Intake. *Brain Res.* **2005**, *1043*, 139–144. [CrossRef]
60. Beglinger, C.; Degen, L.; Matzinger, D.; D'Amato, M.; Drewe, J. Loxiglumide, a CCK-A Receptor Antagonist, Stimulates Calorie Intake and Hunger Feelings in Humans. *Am. J. Physiol. Integr. Comp. Physiol.* **2001**, *280*, R1149–R1154. [CrossRef]
61. Steinert, R.E.; Schirra, J.; Meyer-Gerspach, A.C.; Kienle, P.; Fischer, H.; Schulte, F.; Goeke, B.; Beglinger, C. Effect of Glucagon-Like Peptide-1 Receptor Antagonism on Appetite and Food Intake in Healthy Men. *Am. J. Clin. Nutr.* **2014**, *100*, 514–523. [CrossRef]
62. Degen, L.; Oesch, S.; Casanova, M.; Graf, S.; Ketterer, S.; Drewe, J.; Beglinger, C. Effect of Peptide YY3–36 on Food Intake in Humans. *Gastroenterology* **2005**, *129*, 1430–1436. [CrossRef]
63. Gutzwiller, J.-P.; Göke, B.; Drewe, J.; Hildebrand, P.; Ketterer, S.; Handschin, D.; Winterhalder, R.; Conen, D.; Beglinger, C. Glucagon-Like Peptide-1: A Potent Regulator of Food Intake in Humans. *Gut* **1999**, *44*, 81–86. [CrossRef]
64. MacIntosh, C.G.; Morley, J.E.; Wishart, J.; Morris, H.; Jansen, J.B.M.J.; Horowitz, M.; Chapman, I.M. Effect of Exogenous Cholecystokinin (CCK)-8 on Food Intake and Plasma CCK, Leptin, and Insulin Concentrations in Older and Young Adults: Evidence for Increased CCK Activity as a Cause of the Anorexia of Aging. *J. Clin. Endocrinol. Metab.* **2001**, *86*, 5830–5837. [CrossRef]
65. De Lartigue, G.; Diepenbroek, C. Novel Developments in Vagal Afferent Nutrient Sensing and its Role in Energy Homeostasis. *Curr. Opin. Pharmacol.* **2016**, *31*, 38–43. [CrossRef]
66. Dockray, G.J. Enteroendocrine Cell Signalling via the Vagus Nerve. *Curr. Opin. Pharmacol.* **2013**, *13*, 954–958. [CrossRef]
67. Meloni, A.R.; Deyoung, M.B.; Lowe, C.; Parkes, D.G. GLP-1 Receptor Activated Insulin Secretion from Pancreatic β-Cells: Mechanism and Glucose Dependence. *Diabetes Obes. Metab.* **2012**, *15*, 15–27. [CrossRef]
68. Holst, J.J. The Physiology of Glucagon-like Peptide 1. *Physiol. Rev.* **2007**, *87*, 1409–1439. [CrossRef]
69. Kim, W.; Egan, J.M. The Role of Incretins in Glucose Homeostasis and Diabetes Treatment. *Pharmacol. Rev.* **2008**, *60*, 470–512. [CrossRef]
70. Margolskee, R.F. Molecular Mechanisms of Bitter and Sweet Taste Transduction. *J. Biol. Chem.* **2002**, *277*, 1–4. [CrossRef] [PubMed]
71. Xie, C.; Wang, X.; Young, R.L.; Horowitz, M.; Rayner, C.K.; Wu, T. Role of Intestinal Bitter Sensing in Enteroendocrine Hormone Secretion and Metabolic Control. *Front. Endocrinol.* **2018**, *9*, 576. [CrossRef]
72. Ingram, J.R.; Walker, E.G.; Pahl, M.C.; Lo, K.R.; Shin, H.S.; Lang, C.; Wohlers, M.W.; Poppitt, S.; Sutton, K.H. Activation of Gastrointestinal Bitter Taste Receptors Suppresses Food Intake and Stimulates Secretion of Gastrointestinal Peptide Hormones in Healthy Men. *Obes. Facts* **2016**, *9* (Suppl. 1), 46.
73. Mennella, I.; Fogliano, V.; Ferracane, R.; Arlorio, M.; Pattarino, F.; Vitaglione, P. Microencapsulated Bitter Compounds (from Gentiana Lutea) Reduce Daily Energy Intakes in Humans. *Br. J. Nutr.* **2016**, *116*, 1841–1850. [CrossRef]
74. Van Avesaat, M.; Troost, F.J.; Ripken, D.; Peters, J.; Hendriks, H.F.; Masclee, A.A. Intraduodenal Infusion of a Combination of Tastants Decreases Food Intake in Humans. *Am. J. Clin. Nutr.* **2015**, *102*, 729–735. [CrossRef] [PubMed]
75. Deloose, E.; Corsetti, M.; Van Oudenhove, L.; Depoortere, I.; Tack, J. Intragastric Infusion of the Bitter Tastant Quinine Suppresses Hormone Release and Antral Motility during the Fasting State in Healthy Female Volunteers. *Neurogastroenterol. Motil.* **2017**, *30*, e13171. [CrossRef] [PubMed]
76. Bitarafan, V.E.; Fitzgerald, P.C.; Little, T.J.; Meyerhof, W.; Wu, T.; Horowitz, M.; Feinle-Bisset, C. Effects of Intraduodenal Infusion of the Bitter Tastant, Quinine, on Antropyloroduodenal Motility, Plasma Cholecystokinin, and Energy Intake in Healthy Men. *J. Neurogastroenterol. Motil.* **2019**, *25*, 413–422. [CrossRef] [PubMed]

77. Jeon, T.-I.; Seo, Y.-K.; Osborne, T.F. Gut Bitter Taste Receptor Signalling induces ABCB1 through a Mechanism Involving CCK. *Biochem. J.* **2011**, *438*, 33–37. [CrossRef]
78. Yamazaki, T.; Morimoto-Kobayashi, Y.; Koizumi, K.; Takahashi, C.; Nakajima, S.; Kitao, S.; Taniguchi, Y.; Katayama, M.; Ogawa, Y. Secretion of a Gastrointestinal Hormone, Cholecystokinin, by Hop-Derived Bitter Components Activates Sympathetic Nerves in Brown Adipose Tissue. *J. Nutr. Biochem.* **2019**, *64*, 80–87. [CrossRef]
79. Grau-Bové, C.; Miguéns-Gómez, A.; González-Quilen, C.; Fernández-López, J.-A.; Remesar, X.; Torres-Fuentes, C.; Ávila-Román, J.; Rodríguez-Gallego, E.; Beltrán-Debón, R.; Blay, M.T.; et al. Modulation of Food Intake by Differential TAS2R Stimulation in Rat. *Nutrients* **2020**, *12*, 3784. [CrossRef]
80. Yue, X.; Liang, J.; Gu, F.; Du, D.; Chen, F. Berberine Activates Bitter Taste Responses of Enteroendocrine STC-1 Cells. *Mol. Cell. Biochem.* **2018**, *447*, 21–32. [CrossRef]
81. Yu, Y.; Hao, G.; Zhang, Q.; Hua, W.; Wang, M.; Zhou, W.; Zong, S.; Huang, M.; Wen, X. Berberine Induces GLP-1 Secretion through Activation of Bitter Taste Receptor Pathways. *Biochem. Pharmacol.* **2015**, *97*, 173–177. [CrossRef]
82. Serrano, J.; Casanova-Martí, À.; Depoortere, I.; Blay, M.T.; Terra, X.; Pinent, M.; Ardévol, A. Subchronic Treatment with Grape-Seed Phenolics Inhibits Ghrelin Production despite a Short-Term Stimulation of Ghrelin Secretion Produced by Bitter-Sensing Flavanols. *Mol. Nutr. Food Res.* **2016**, *60*, 2554–2564. [CrossRef]
83. Suh, H.-W.; Lee, K.-B.; Kim, K.-S.; Yang, H.J.; Choi, E.-K.; Shin, M.H.; Park, Y.S.; Na, Y.-C.; Ahn, K.S.; Jang, Y.P.; et al. A Bitter Herbal Medicine Gentiana Scabra Root Extract Stimulates Glucagon-Like Peptide-1 Secretion and Regulates Blood Glucose in db/db Mouse. *J. Ethnopharmacol.* **2015**, *172*, 219–226. [CrossRef]
84. Kok, B.P.; Galmozzi, A.; Littlejohn, N.K.; Albert, V.; Godio, C.; Kim, W.; Kim, S.M.; Bland, J.S.; Grayson, N.; Fang, M.; et al. Intestinal Bitter Taste Receptor Activation Alters Hormone Secretion and Imparts Metabolic Benefits. *Mol. Metab.* **2018**, *16*, 76–87. [CrossRef] [PubMed]
85. Dotson, C.D.; Zhang, L.; Xu, H.; Shin, Y.-K.; Vigues, S.; Ott, S.H.; Elson, A.E.T.; Choi, H.J.; Shaw, H.; Egan, J.M.; et al. Bitter Taste Receptors Influence Glucose Homeostasis. *PLoS ONE* **2008**, *3*, e3974. [CrossRef] [PubMed]
86. Li, J.; Xu, J.; Hou, R.; Jin, X.; Wang, J.; Yang, N.; Yang, L.; Liu, L.; Tao, F.; Lu, H. Qing-Hua Granule induces GLP-1 Secretion via Bitter Taste Receptor in db/db Mice. *Biomed. Pharmacother.* **2017**, *89*, 10–17. [CrossRef] [PubMed]
87. Huang, T.-N.; Lu, K.-N.; Pai, Y.-P.; Hsu, C.; Huang, C.-J. Role of GLP-1 in the Hypoglycemic Effects of Wild Bitter Gourd. *Evidence-Based Complement. Altern. Med.* **2013**, *2013*, 1–13. [CrossRef]
88. Habib, A.M.; Richards, P.; Rogers, G.J.; Reimann, F.; Gribble, F.M. Co-Localisation and Secretion of Glucagon-Like Peptide 1 and Peptide YY from Primary Cultured Human L Cells. *Diabetologia* **2013**, *56*, 1413–1416. [CrossRef] [PubMed]
89. Lossow, K.; Hübner, S.; Roudnitzky, N.; Slack, J.P.; Pollastro, F.; Behrens, M.; Meyerhof, W. Comprehensive Analysis of Mouse Bitter Taste Receptors Reveals Different Molecular Receptive Ranges for Orthologous Receptors in Mice and Humans. *J. Biol. Chem.* **2016**, *291*, 15358–15377. [CrossRef] [PubMed]
90. Azpiroz, F.; Malagelada, J.R. Intestinal Control of Gastric Tone. *Am. J. Physiol. Liver Physiol.* **1985**, *249*, G501–G509. [CrossRef] [PubMed]
91. Houghton, L.; Read, N.; Heddle, R.; Horowitz, M.; Collins, P.; Chatterton, B.; Dent, J. Relationship of the Motor Activity of the Antrum, Pylorus, and Duodenum to Gastric Emptying of a Solid-Liquid Mixed Meal. *Gastroenterology* **1988**, *94*, 1285–1291. [CrossRef]
92. Brookes, S.J.; Spencer, N.J.; Costa, M.; Zagorodnyuk, V.P. Extrinsic Primary Afferent Signalling in the Gut. *Nat. Rev. Gastroenterol. Hepatol.* **2013**, *10*, 286–296. [CrossRef]
93. Feinle, C.; Grundy, D.; Read, N.W. Effects of Duodenal Nutrients on Sensory and Motor Responses of the Human Stomach to Distension. *Am. J. Physiol. Content* **1997**, *273*, G721–G726. [CrossRef]
94. Kissileff, H.R.; Carretta, J.C.; Geliebter, A.; Pi-Sunyer, F.X. Cholecystokinin and Stomach Distension Combine to Reduce Food Intake in Humans. *Am. J. Physiol. Integr. Comp. Physiol.* **2003**, *285*, R992–R998. [CrossRef] [PubMed]
95. Sturm, K.; Parker, B.; Wishart, J.; Feinle-Bisset, C.; Jones, K.L.; Chapman, I.; Horowitz, M. Energy Intake and Appetite are Related to Antral Area in Healthy Young and Older Subjects. *Am. J. Clin. Nutr.* **2004**, *80*, 656–667. [CrossRef] [PubMed]
96. Horowitz, M.; Edelbroek, M.A.L.; Wishart, J.M.; Straathof, J.W. Relationship between Oral Glucose Tolerance and Gastric Emptying in Normal Healthy Subjects. *Diabetologia* **1993**, *36*, 857–862. [CrossRef] [PubMed]
97. Jones, K.L.; Horowitz, M.I.; Carney, B.; Wishart, J.M.; Guha, S.; Green, L. Gastric Emptying in Early Noninsulin-Dependent Diabetes Mellitus. *J. Nucl. Med.* **1996**, *37*, 1643–1648.
98. Little, T.J.; Pilichiewicz, A.N.; Russo, A.; Phillips, L.; Jones, K.L.; Nauck, M.A.; Wishart, J.; Horowitz, M.; Feinle-Bisset, C. Effects of Intravenous Glucagon-Like Peptide-1 on Gastric Emptying and Intragastric Distribution in Healthy Subjects: Relationships with Postprandial Glycemic and Insulinemic Responses. *J. Clin. Endocrinol. Metab.* **2006**, *91*, 1916–1923. [CrossRef] [PubMed]
99. Nauck, M.A.; Niedereichholz, U.; Ettler, R.; Holst, J.J.; Ørskov, C.; Ritzel, R.; Schmiegel, W.H. Glucagon-Like Peptide 1 Inhibition of Gastric Emptying Outweighs its Insulinotropic Effects in Healthy Humans. *Am. J. Physiol. Metab.* **1997**, *273*, E981–E988. [CrossRef] [PubMed]
100. Kimura, Y.; Sumiyoshi, M. Effects of Swertia Japonica Extract and its Main Compound Swertiamarin on Gastric Emptying and Gastrointestinal Motility in Mice. *Fitoterapia* **2011**, *82*, 827–833. [CrossRef]
101. Harada, Y.; Koseki, J.; Sekine, H.; Fujitsuka, N.; Kobayashi, H. Role of Bitter Taste Receptors in Regulating Gastric Accommodation in Guinea Pigs. *J. Pharmacol. Exp. Ther.* **2019**, *369*, 466–472. [CrossRef]

102. Glendinning, J.I.; Yiin, Y.-M.; Ackroff, K.; Sclafani, A. Intragastric Infusion of Denatonium Conditions Flavor Aversions and Delays Gastric Emptying in Rodents. *Physiol. Behav.* **2008**, *93*, 757–765. [CrossRef]
103. Little, T.J.; Gupta, N.; Case, R.M.; Thompson, D.G.; McLaughlin, J.T. Sweetness and Bitterness Taste of Meals Per se does not Mediate Gastric Emptying in Humans. *Am. J. Physiol. Integr. Comp. Physiol.* **2009**, *297*, R632–R639. [CrossRef]
104. Wicks, D.; Wright, J.; Rayment, P.; Spiller, R. Impact of Bitter Taste on Gastric Motility. *Eur. J. Gastroenterol. Hepatol.* **2005**, *17*, 961–965. [CrossRef]
105. Sumiyoshi, M.; Kimura, Y. Hop (Humulus Lupulus L.) Extract Inhibits Obesity in Mice Fed a High-Fat Diet over the Long Term. *Br. J. Nutr.* **2013**, *109*, 162–172. [CrossRef]
106. Yajima, H.; Noguchi, T.; Ikeshima, E.; Shiraki, M.; Kanaya, T.; Tsuboyama-Kasaoka, N.; Ezaki, O.; Oikawa, S.; Kondo, K. Prevention of Diet-Induced Obesity by Dietary Isomerized Hop Extract Containing Isohumulones, in Rodents. *Int. J. Obes.* **2005**, *29*, 991–997. [CrossRef]
107. Van Heerden, F.R.; Horak, R.M.; Maharaj, V.J.; Vleggaar, R.; Senabe, J.V.; Gunning, P.J. An Appetite Suppressant from Hoodia Species. *Phytochemistry* **2007**, *68*, 2545–2553. [CrossRef]
108. Leng, S.-H.; Lu, F.-E.; Xu, L.-J. Therapeutic Effects of Berberine in Impaired Glucose Tolerance Rats and its Influence on Insulin Secretion. *Acta Pharmacol. Sin.* **2004**, *25*, 496–502. [PubMed]
109. Kratz, C.M.; Levitsky, D.; Lustick, S.L. Long Term Effects of Quinine on Food Intake and Body Weight in the Rat. *Physiol. Behav.* **1978**, *21*, 321–324. [CrossRef]
110. Yajima, H.; Ikeshima, E.; Shiraki, M.; Kanaya, T.; Fujiwara, D.; Odai, H.; Tsuboyama-Kasaoka, N.; Ezaki, O.; Oikawa, S.; Kondo, K. Isohumulones, Bitter Acids Derived from Hops, Activate Both Peroxisome Proliferator-Activated Receptor α and γ and Reduce Insulin Resistance. *J. Biol. Chem.* **2004**, *279*, 33456–33462. [CrossRef] [PubMed]
111. Nauck, M.A.; Kleine, N.; Holst, J.J.; Willms, B.; Creutzfeldt, W. Normalization of Fasting Hyperglycaemia by Exogenous Glucagon-Like Peptide 1 (7-36 Amide) in Type 2 (Non-Insulin-Dependent) Diabetic Patients. *Diabetologia* **1993**, *36*, 741–744. [CrossRef] [PubMed]
112. Henquin, J.; Horemans, B.; Nenquin, M.; Verniers, J.; Lambert, A. Quinine-Induced Modifications of Insulin Release and Glucose Metabolism by Isolated Pancreatic Islets. *FEBS Lett.* **1975**, *57*, 280–284. [CrossRef]
113. Vignini, A.; Borroni, F.; Sabbatinelli, J.; Pugnaloni, S.; Alia, S.; Taus, M.; Ferrante, L.; Mazzanti, L.; Fabri, M. General Decrease of Taste Sensitivity Is Related to Increase of BMI: A Simple Method to Monitor Eating Behavior. *Dis. Markers* **2019**, *2019*, 1–8. [CrossRef]
114. Bianchi, L.L.; Galmarini, M.; García-Burgos, D.; Zamora, M. Time-Intensity and Reaction-Time Methodology Applied to the Dynamic Perception and Liking of Bitterness in Relation to Body Mass Index. *Food Res. Int.* **2018**, *109*, 606–613. [CrossRef]
115. Garcia-Burgos, D.; Zamora, M. Facial Affective Reactions to Bitter-Tasting Foods and Body Mass Index in Adults. *Appetite* **2013**, *71*, 178–186. [CrossRef] [PubMed]
116. Simchen, U.; Koebnick, C.; Hoyer, S.; Issanchou, S.; Zunft, H.-J.F. Odour and Taste Sensitivity is Associated with Body Weight and Extent of Misreporting of Body Weight. *Eur. J. Clin. Nutr.* **2006**, *60*, 698–705. [CrossRef]
117. Overberg, J.; Hummel, T.; Krude, H.; Wiegand, S. Differences in Taste Sensitivity between Obese and Non-obese Children and Adolescents. *Arch. Dis. Child.* **2012**, *97*, 1048–1052. [CrossRef]
118. De Carli, L.; Gambino, R.; Lubrano, C.; Rosato, R.; Bongiovanni, D.; Lanfranco, F.; Broglio, F.; Ghigo, E.; Bo, S. Impaired Taste Sensation in Type 2 Diabetic Patients without Chronic Complications: A Case–Control Study. *J. Endocrinol. Investig.* **2017**, *41*, 765–772. [CrossRef] [PubMed]
119. Matsugasumi, M.; Hashimoto, Y.; Okada, H.; Tanaka, M.; Kimura, T.; Kitagawa, N.; Tanaka, Y.; Fukuda, Y.; Sakai, R.; Yamazaki, M.; et al. The Association between Taste Impairment and Serum Zinc Concentration in Adult Patients with Type 2 Diabetes. *Can. J. Diabetes* **2018**, *42*, 520–524. [CrossRef] [PubMed]
120. Pugnaloni, S.; Alia, S.; Mancini, M.; Santoro, V.; Di Paolo, A.; Rabini, R.A.; Fiorini, R.; Sabbatinelli, J.; Fabri, M.; Mazzanti, L.; et al. A Study on the Relationship between Type 2 Diabetes and Taste Function in Patients with Good Glycemic Control. *Nutrients* **2020**, *12*, 1112. [CrossRef] [PubMed]
121. Gondivkar, S.M.; Indurkar, A.; Degwekar, S.; Bhowate, R. Evaluation of Gustatory Function in Patients with Diabetes Mellitus Type 2. *Oral Surg. Oral Med. Oral Pathol. Oral Radiol. Endodontol.* **2009**, *108*, 876–880. [CrossRef]
122. Wölnerhanssen, B.K.; Moran, A.W.; Burdyga, G.; Meyer-Gerspach, A.C.; Peterli, R.; Manz, M.; Thumshirn, M.; Daly, K.; Beglinger, C.; Shirazi-Beechey, S.P. Deregulation of Transcription Factors Controlling Intestinal Epithelial Cell Differentiation; a Predisposing Factor for Reduced Enteroendocrine Cell Number in Morbidly Obese Individuals. *Sci. Rep.* **2017**, *7*, 1–13. [CrossRef]
123. Latorre, R.; Huynh, J.; Mazzoni, M.; Gupta, A.; Bonora, E.; Clavenzani, P.; Chang, L.; Mayer, E.A.; de Giorgio, R.; Sternini, C. Expression of the Bitter Taste Receptor, T2R38, in Enteroendocrine Cells of the Colonic Mucosa of Overweight/Obese vs. Lean Subjects. *PLoS ONE* **2016**, *11*, e0147368. [CrossRef]
124. Keller, M.; Liu, X.; Wohland, T.; Rohde, K.; Gast, M.-T.; Stumvoll, M.; Kovacs, P.; Tönjes, A.; Böttcher, Y. TAS2R38 and Its Influence on Smoking Behavior and Glucose Homeostasis in the German Sorbs. *PLoS ONE* **2013**, *8*, e80512. [CrossRef] [PubMed]
125. Spector, A.C.; Kopka, S.L. Rats Fail to Discriminate Quinine from Denatonium: Implications for the Neural Coding of Bitter-Tasting Compounds. *J. Neurosci.* **2002**, *22*, 1937–1941. [CrossRef] [PubMed]

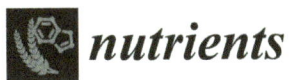

Review

Role of Bile Acids in the Regulation of Food Intake, and Their Dysregulation in Metabolic Disease

Cong Xie [1,†], Weikun Huang [1,2,†], Richard L. Young [1,3], Karen L. Jones [1,4], Michael Horowitz [1,4], Christopher K. Rayner [1,5] and Tongzhi Wu [1,4,6,*]

1. Adelaide Medical School, Center of Research Excellence (CRE) in Translating Nutritional Science to Good Health, The University of Adelaide, Adelaide 5005, Australia; c.xie@adelaide.edu.au (C.X.); weikun.huang@adelaide.edu.au (W.H.); richard.young@adelaide.edu.au (R.L.Y.); karen.jones@adelaide.edu.au (K.L.J.); michael.horowitz@adelaide.edu.au (M.H.); chris.rayner@adelaide.edu.au (C.K.R.)
2. The ARC Center of Excellence for Nanoscale BioPhotonics, Institute for Photonics and Advanced Sensing, School of Physical Sciences, University of Adelaide, Adelaide 5005, Australia
3. Nutrition, Diabetes & Gut Health, Lifelong Health Theme South Australian Health & Medical Research Institute, Adelaide 5005, Australia
4. Endocrine and Metabolic Unit, Royal Adelaide Hospital, Adelaide 5005, Australia
5. Department of Gastroenterology and Hepatology, Royal Adelaide Hospital, Adelaide 5005, Australia
6. Institute of Diabetes, School of Medicine, Southeast University, Nanjing 210009, China
* Correspondence: tongzhi.wu@adelaide.edu.au
† These authors contributed to the review equally.

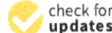

Citation: Xie, C.; Huang, W.; Young, R.L.; Jones, K.L.; Horowitz, M.; Rayner, C.K.; Wu, T. Role of Bile Acids in the Regulation of Food Intake, and Their Dysregulation in Metabolic Disease. *Nutrients* 2021, 13, 1104. https://doi.org/10.3390/nu13041104

Academic Editor: Satoshi Nagaoka

Received: 28 February 2021
Accepted: 25 March 2021
Published: 28 March 2021

Publisher's Note: MDPI stays neutral with regard to jurisdictional claims in published maps and institutional affiliations.

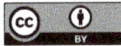

Copyright: © 2021 by the authors. Licensee MDPI, Basel, Switzerland. This article is an open access article distributed under the terms and conditions of the Creative Commons Attribution (CC BY) license (https://creativecommons.org/licenses/by/4.0/).

Abstract: Bile acids are cholesterol-derived metabolites with a well-established role in the digestion and absorption of dietary fat. More recently, the discovery of bile acids as natural ligands for the nuclear farnesoid X receptor (FXR) and membrane Takeda G-protein-coupled receptor 5 (TGR5), and the recognition of the effects of FXR and TGR5 signaling have led to a paradigm shift in knowledge regarding bile acid physiology and metabolic health. Bile acids are now recognized as signaling molecules that orchestrate blood glucose, lipid and energy metabolism. Changes in FXR and/or TGR5 signaling modulates the secretion of gastrointestinal hormones including glucagon-like peptide-1 (GLP-1) and peptide YY (PYY), hepatic gluconeogenesis, glycogen synthesis, energy expenditure, and the composition of the gut microbiome. These effects may contribute to the metabolic benefits of bile acid sequestrants, metformin, and bariatric surgery. This review focuses on the role of bile acids in energy intake and body weight, particularly their effects on gastrointestinal hormone secretion, the changes in obesity and T2D, and their potential relevance to the management of metabolic disorders.

Keywords: bile acids; TGR-5; FXR; gastrointestinal hormones; energy intake; body weight; obesity; type 2 diabetes

1. Introduction

Bile acids are synthesized in the liver, where cholesterol is converted via 7α-hydroxylase (CYP7A1) and, to a lesser extent, 27α-hydroxylase (CYP27A1) and 24-hydroxylase (CYP46A1), to the primary bile acids cholic acid (CA) and chenodeoxycholic acid (CDCA) in humans (CA and muricholic acid in rodents). These are then conjugated to glycine or taurine, prior to their secretion into bile [1]. Following meal ingestion, bile acids are released into the gut upon gallbladder emptying, and about 95% of intestinal bile acids is absorbed in the ileum via the apical sodium bile acid co-transporter (ASBT), returning to the liver for re-secretion—a highly efficient process known as "enterohepatic circulation". A small fraction of bile acids reach the large intestine, where they are modified (through de-conjugation and dihydroxylation) by gut bacteria to secondary bile acids such as deoxycholic acid (DCA), lithocholic acid (LCA), and ursodeoxycholic acid (UDCA, a secondary bile acid in humans, but a primary bile acid in rodents), and absorbed passively into the circulation or excreted in the feces [2] (Figure 1). Bile acids lost to the large intestine are replenished by de novo hepatic synthesis, which is regulated by fibroblast growth factor-19 (FGF19) signaling in the small intestine in humans (or FGF15 in rodents). Thus, bile acids are found in high concentrations in the liver [3], bile [4], and small intestine [5].

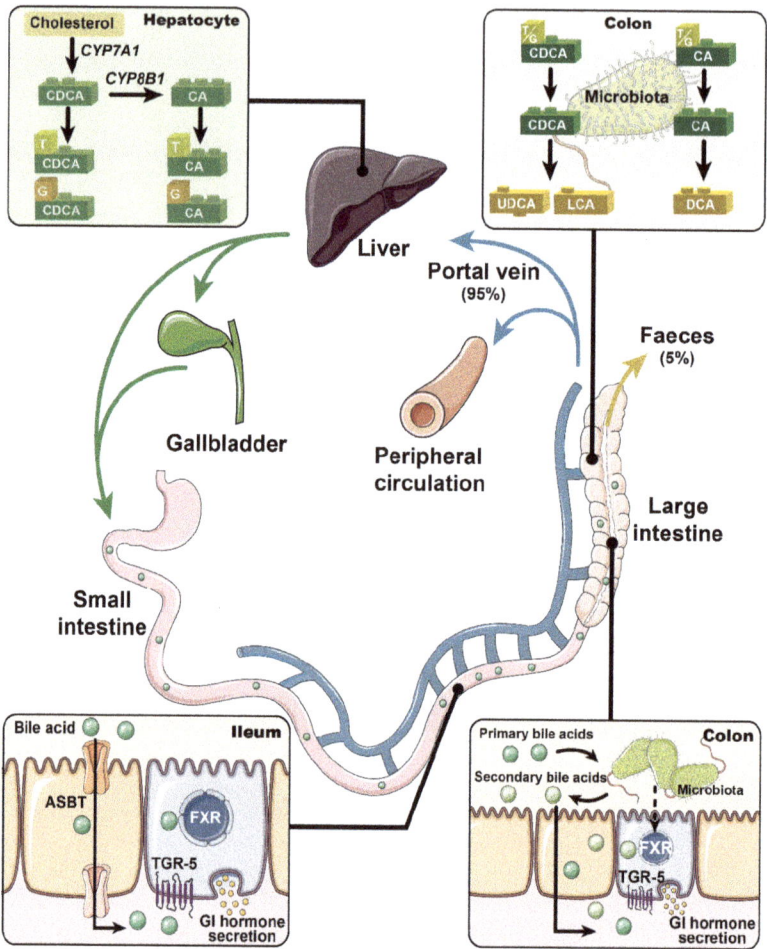

Figure 1. Primary bile acids (i.e., chenodeoxycholic acid (CDCA) and cholic acid (CA)) are synthesized from cholesterol in the liver, and conjugated to glycine and taurine prior to their secretion into bile. In response to meals, bile acids are discharged into the intestine. Approximately 95% of the intestinal bile acids are absorbed in the ileum via apical sodium bile acid co-transporter (ASBT) and return to the liver for re-secretion (i.e., the enterohepatic circulation). Only ~5% of bile acids escape into the large intestine and are modified by gut microbiota into secondary bile acids (e.g., deoxycholic acid (DCA), lithocholic acid (LCA), and ursodeoxycholic acid (UDCA)). Bile acids are now recognized as pivotal signaling molecules that participate in the regulation of metabolic homeostasis through regulating the secretion of gastrointestinal hormones. This complex process has been linked to activation of the nuclear farnesoid X receptor (FXR) and/or the membrane Takeda G-protein-coupled receptor 5 (TGR5). Accordingly, modulation of FXR and/or TGR5 signaling has been actively pursued for the management of metabolic disorders.

For more than a century, bile acids have been regarded solely as "intestinal detergents" that emulsify dietary fat for digestion and transport. The recognition that bile acids are also pivotal signaling molecules orchestrating glucose, lipid and energy metabolism is recent.

Bile acids also bind to numerous nuclear and cytoplasmic receptors such as the vitamin D receptor [6], pregnane X receptor [7], and constitutive androstane receptor [8]. However, it was the identification of the bile acid-specific nuclear farnesoid X receptor (FXR) in 1999 and membrane Takeda G-protein-coupled receptor 5 (TGR5) in 2002 that provided a mechanistic framework for a role of BA signaling in the context of metabolism [9,10]. FXR and TGR5 are present in numerous tissues including the central and peripheral nervous systems; bile acid signaling in the latter has been shown to regulate energy intake [11], as supported by the observation that suppression of energy intake induced by intravenous injection of DCA is attenuated when TGR5 was silenced in the vagal nodose ganglia in rats [12]. However, the clinical relevance of this concept is unclear, particularly given that plasma bile acid concentrations are low and that in obese individuals, relative elevation in plasma bile acid levels are not associated with reduced energy intake. In line with the high turnover of bile acids in the enterohepatic circulation, both FXR and TGR5 are expressed abundantly in the liver and the intestine. Signaling through both receptors has been linked to the secretion of gastrointestinal hormones, known to be integral to the maintenance of metabolic homeostasis (Figure 1). For example, the release of ghrelin from gastric G-cells during fasting appears pivotal to sensations of hunger, and stimulation of energy intake. After meals, the secretion of cholecystokinin (CCK) from enteroendocrine I-cells located in the upper gut, and glucagon-like peptide-1 (GLP-1) and peptide YY (PYY) from L-cells located most abundantly in the distal gut, form an integrated signaling system that slows gastrointestinal motility and transit, drives the secretion of insulin to regulate postprandial glucose metabolism (via GLP-1) and suppresses appetite and energy intake [13]. The role of bile acids in the control of blood glucose and lipid metabolism has been reviewed in detail [14–17], but their potential to impact on the regulation of energy intake has received less attention, despite the recognition, since 1968, that oral administration of CDCA and DCA stimulated PYY secretion and suppressed appetite in obese individuals [18]. The current review addresses the effects of bile acids on gastrointestinal hormone secretion, energy intake, and body weight as well as the relevance of bile acid dysregulation in obesity and type 2 diabetes (T2D).

2. Effects of Bile Acids on Gastrointestinal Hormone Secretion

The last two decades have witnessed a substantial effort to increase the understanding of the effects of bile acids on gastrointestinal hormone secretion and the consequent impact on metabolism. In healthy individuals, postprandial plasma bile acid concentrations have been reported to correlate negatively with ghrelin, and positively with GLP-1 and PYY [19]. Similar relationships have also been observed in obese patients following bariatric surgery [20]. However, bile acids per se do not appear to affect ghrelin secretion in rats; intestinal infusion of a mixture of physiological bile acids did not affect portal ghrelin levels [21]. In contrast, small intestinal sensing of bile acids has been reported to inhibit CCK secretion in both rodents and humans [22,23], supporting the existence of a negative feedback loop between the two. In contrast, the effects on GLP-1 and PYY release from L-cells have been studied extensively in preclinical and clinical models [24–26], stimulating the potential development of bile acid-based interventions for metabolic disorders. While bile acid-induced release of GLP-1 and PYY has been linked to signaling via FXR and TGR5, the data are inconsistent, which may relate to differences in the binding affinity of individual bile acids at FXR and TGR5 (Table 1) and/or complex interactions between the two signaling pathways.

2.1. FXR

FXR is expressed abundantly in the liver and the intestine, and the binding affinity of individual bile acids is variable (CDCA > DCA > LCA > CA > UDCA, Table 1). FXR was initially identified as a regulator of bile acid metabolism [14], and subsequently as a modulator of L-cell secretion. Indeed, FXR is expressed by the murine L-cell line, GLUTag. However, the FXR agonist GW4064 and CDCA (which preferentially binds FXR) were shown to suppress glucose-induced proglucagon expression and GLP-1 secretion in this cell line by decreasing glycolysis, whereas silencing FXR abolished these effects [27]. These observations have been replicated in studies with different L-cell lines (i.e., NCI-H736 [28] and STC-1 [29]). In a similar manner, GW4064 blunted the GLP-1 response to short-chain fatty acids (SCFA) in both GLUTag and NCI-H716 cell lines [30]. Consistent with these observations, FXR-deficient mice exhibited increased GLP-1 secretion in response to both dietary fiber, which increases colonic SCFA [30], and oral glucose [31]. Oral intake of GW4064 (10 mg/kg, 2 doses over 12 h) also decreased active GLP-1 levels in the plasma of mini-pigs [28]. However, in an isolated perfusion model of rat intestine, both luminal and vascular perfusion of GW4064 failed to affect the GLP-1 response to a physiological mixture of bile acids in rats [21]. In mice, diversion of bile acids from the gallbladder to the ileum was shown to modestly increase GLP-1 secretion, improve glucose tolerance, and induce weight loss [32]. The reductions in postprandial blood glucose and body weight induced by this procedure were abolished in intestinal FXR-knockout mice, suggesting that intestinal FXR-signaling can potentially promote GLP-1 secretion. Unfortunately, the study failed to determine whether the rise in GLP-1 was specifically induced by FXR-activation [32]. Of note, oral administration of the intestine-restricted FXR agonist, fexaramine, in mice was reported to increase the abundance of LCA-producing gut bacteria to activate TGR5-signaling indirectly, leading to enhanced GLP-1 secretion and improvement in insulin sensitivity and lipid profile as well as the promotion of adipose tissue browning [33]. Accordingly, outcomes derived from ex vivo and in vivo experiments are, by and large, inconsistent, although the intestine-restricted FXR signaling appears to have an overall favorable effect on metabolic health.

2.2. TGR5

TGR5, also known as GPBAR1, is a G-protein coupled receptor that is expressed widely in the gastrointestinal tract, pancreas, liver, gallbladder, and adipose tissue. Like FXR, its binding affinity for individual bile acids varies substantially (LCA > DCA > CDCA > CA > UDCA, Table 1) [34]. TGR5 activation has been reported to suppress hepatic macrophages, induce gallbladder relaxation and refilling, and promote intestinal motility [14]. TGR5 is also expressed on L-cells. Unlike FXR, stimulation of TGR5 by LCA and DCA was shown to potently stimulate GLP-1 secretion from STC-1 cells in a dose-dependent manner, an effect suppressed by downregulation of TGR5 expression [35]. The stimulatory effect of TGR5 on GLP-1 secretion required the closure of ATP-sensitive potassium (KATP) channels and elevated intracellular concentrations of cAMP and Ca^{2+} [36,37]. A major observation in relation to TGR5 signaling was the demonstration of its basolateral location on L-cells. Thus, to activate TGR5, it is necessary for bile acids or other TGR5 ligands to be transported through the epithelial layer [38]. However, the readily absorbed TGR5 agonist SB-756050 failed to stimulate GLP-1 secretion significantly, or improve glycemic control at various doses compared with the placebo in acute studies involving patients with T2D [39]. It is noteworthy that L-cells are distributed most densely in the distal gut regions [13]. It would therefore be of interest to investigate whether delivery of TGR5 agonists should be targeted at the distal gut.

PYY is co-released with GLP-1 from L-cells, and it was initially noted that perfusion of DCA (1–25 mM) into the isolated rabbit colon increased PYY secretion substantially in a dose-dependent manner [18]. Intracolonic administration of DCA or TCA in humans has also been shown to induce a rapid and substantial rise in plasma PYY [40–42]. Similar to TGR5-mediated GLP-1 secretion, the outcomes of studies using isolated rat colon indicate that bile acid-induced PYY secretion is dependent on bile acid translocation from the luminal to basolateral side [43]. That PYY secretion is less evident in response to bile acids with poor affinity to TGR5, and attenuated in TGR5-knockout models, attests to the fundamental relevance of TGR5-signaling to bile acid-induced PYY secretion [44].

Table 1. Binding affinities of bile acids to human TGR5 and FXR.

Bile Acid	TGR5			FXR		
	Subjects	Indicator	EC_{50}	Subjects	Indicator	EC_{50}
Primary Bile Acids						
CA	CHO cells/HEK293	Intracellular cAMP	7.72 μM [34]/ >10 μM [10]	CV-1 cells	Reporter gene activation	No effect [45]
CDCA	CHO cells/HEK293	Intracellular cAMP	4.43 μM [34]/ 4 μM [10]	HepG2 cells /CV-1 cells	Reporter gene activation	10 μM [9]/ 50 μM [45]
	CHO cells	Reporter gene activation	6.71 μM [46]	Cell-free	Ligand-sensing assay	4.5 μM [47]
Conjugated Primary Bile Acids						
TCA/GCA	CHO cells	Reporter gene activation	4.95 μM/ 13.6 μM [46]	Cell-free	Ligand-sensing assay	No effect [47]
TCDCA/ GCDCA	CHO cells	Reporter gene activation	1.92 μM/ 3.88 μM [46]	Cell-free	Ligand-sensing assay	10 μM [47]
HCA				Cell-free	TR-FRET FXR coactivator assay	70.06 μM (IC_{50}) [28]
Secondary bile acids						
DCA	CHO cells	Intracellular cAMP	1.01 μM [34]	HepG2 cells	Reporter gene activation	100 μM [9]
	HEK293	Intracellular cAMP	575 nM [10]	CV-1 cells	Reporter gene activation	50 μM [45]
LCA	CHO cells	Intracellular cAMP	0.53 μM [34]	CV-1 cells	Reporter gene activation	50 μM [45]
	HEK293	Intracellular cAMP	35 nM [10]	Cell-free	Ligand-sensing assay	25 μM [6]
UDCA	CHO cells	Reporter gene activation/Intracellular cAMP	36.4 μM [46]/ No effect [34]	CV-1 cells	Reporter gene activation	No effect [45]
HDCA	CHO cells	Reporter gene activation	31.6 μM [46]	Cell-free	TR-FRET FXR coactivator assay	62.43 μM [28] (IC_{50})
Conjugated Secondary Bile Acids						
TDCA/ GDCA	CHO cells	Reporter gene activation	0.79 μM /1.18 μM [46]	Cell-free	Ligand-sensing assay	500 μM [47] (IC_{50})
TLCA/ GLCA	CHO cells	Reporter gene activation	0.29 μM /0.54 μM [46]	Cell-free	Ligand-sensing assay	3.8 μM/4.7 μM [47] (IC_{50})
TUDCA/ GUDCA	CHO cells	Reporter gene activation	30.0 μM /33.9 μM [46]	Cell-free	Ligand-sensing assay	No effect [47]
THDCA/GHDCA	CHO cells	Reporter gene activation	24.2 μM/36.7 μM [46]			

Note: EC50: the concentration for a half maximal effect; IC50: the concentration for a half maximal inhibitory effect; CHO: Chinese hamster ovary cells; HepG2 cells: Human hepatoma cell line; CV-1 cells: Monkey kidney fibroblast cells (CV-1 line); HEK293: human embryonic kidney cell line 293; TR-FRET FXR coactivator assay: commercial assay kit for screening ligand for FXR.

In summary, there is compelling evidence for a role of bile acids in the modulation of GLP-1 and PYY secretion in both animals and humans. Stimulation of TGR5 on L-cells induces the secretion of both hormones, while effects of FXR signaling remain controversial. The interactions between FXR and TGR5 signaling remain poorly characterized and an

3. Effects of Bile Acid Signaling on Energy Intake and Body Weight

In light of the effects of bile acids on appetite regulation, particularly via the secretion of gastrointestinal hormones, it is intuitively likely that modulating bile acid signaling affects energy balance. Genetic ablation of the bile acid synthesis enzyme CYP8B1, leading to a deficiency of 12α-hydroxylated bile acids (e.g., CA), has been shown to be associated with reduced energy intake and subsequent weight gain in mice fed a fat enriched diet [48,49]. However, these effects appeared to be secondary to impaired fat hydrolysis and the increased exposure of unabsorbed fat to the distal gut, as in these mice, there was an increase in energy intake when fed a fat-free diet [49]. Nevertheless, this study supports the fundamental role of endogenous bile acids in fat digestion and absorption, which may influence energy intake and body weight indirectly.

The outcomes of preclinical and clinical studies involving administration of various bile acids have been equivocal in relation to effects on energy intake and body weight (Table 2). For example, supplementation with CA or UDCA prevented weight gain in mice fed a high-fat diet [50–52], possibly reflecting a TGR5-related increase in energy expenditure [50]. Moreover, a number of other bile acid species with high affinity for TGR5 including hyocholic acid (HCA), hyodeoxycholic acid (HDCA), DCA, and TCA failed to affect energy intake or body weight in rodents with or without diabetes [28,53,54]. Information relating to the effects of bile acids on appetite and energy intake in humans are limited. In healthy individuals, rectal administration of TCA substantially stimulated GLP-1 and PYY secretion and suppressed hunger in a dose-dependent manner [42]. Similarly, in obese individuals with T2D, rectally administered TCA significantly suppressed energy intake dose-dependently [41]. However, these observations could be confounded by the concurrent urge for defecation induced by rectal TCA perfusion (Figure 2) [42]. More recently, a double-blind, randomized, placebo-controlled 4-week trial that delivered a mixture of encapsulated bile acids (1000mg/day) designed for release in the ileum and colon (to provide dual agonism of FXR and TGR5) showed little effect on body weight in patients with T2D, despite increases in plasma GLP-1 and serum and intestinal bile acids [55].

Table 2. Reported effects of bile acids on energy intake and body weight in preclinical and clinical models.

	Bile Acid	Model	Dose	Method	Effect	Ref
		Conjugated Bile Acid				
Primary	TCA	HFD Sprague-Dawley rat + streptozotocin	0.05% or 0.3%	Fed with high-fat diet for 12 weeks	Body weight − Energy intake −	[54]
		Patients with T2DM	0.66, 2, 6.66, or 20 mmol	Rectal administration	Energy intake ↓ (~47% at 20 mmol)	[41]
	HCA	db/db mice; HFD C57BL/6J mice + streptozotocin; C57BL/6J mice	100 mg/kg/day	Oral gavage for 28 days	Body weight − Energy intake −	[28]
	TUDCA	db/db mice; HFD C57BL/6J mice + streptozotocin; C57BL/6J mice	100 mg/kg/day	Oral gavage for 28 days	Body weight − Energy intake −	[28]
Secondary	HDCA	db/db mice; HFD C57BL/6J mice + streptozotocin; C57BL/6J mice	100 mg/kg/day	Oral gavage for 28 days	Body weight − Energy intake −	[28]

Table 2. Cont.

Bile Acid		Model	Dose	Method	Effect	Ref
			Unconjugated Bile Acid			
Primary	CA	C57BL/6J mice	0.5%	High-fat diet fed for 47 days	Body weight ↓ (24%) Energy expenditure ↑ (~50%) Energy intake —	[50]
			0.5%	High-fat diet fed for 9 weeks	Body weight ↓ (6g, ~18%) Energy expenditure ↑ (29%) Energy intake ↑ (20%)	[52]
	UDCA		0.5%	High-fat diet fed for 8 weeks	Body weight ↓ (15%)	[51]
Secondary	DCA	C57BL/6J mice	0.1%	High-fat diet fed for 3 weeks	Body weight — Energy intake —	[53]

Note: Both ursodeoxycholic acid (UDCA) and tauroursodeoxycholic acid (TUDCA) are primary bile acids in rodents, but secondary bile acids in humans. Given the effects of TUDCA and UDCA on energy intake and body weight were shown in rodents, they are grouped into the primary bile acids in the table.

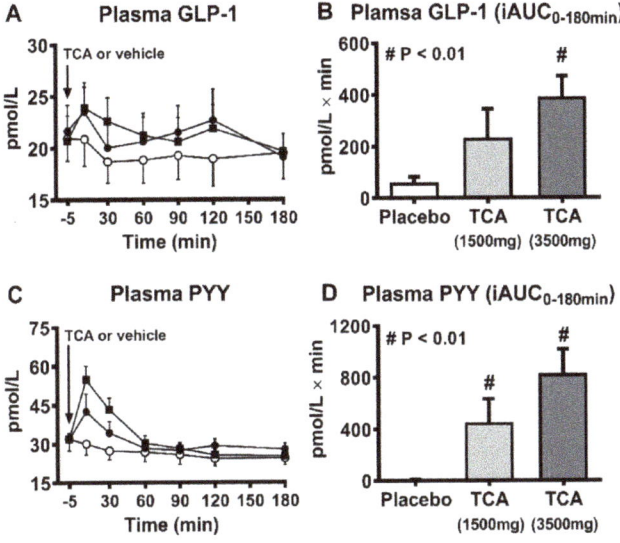

Figure 2. Plasma glucagon-like peptide-1 (GLP-1) (A,B), and peptide YY (PYY) (C,D) (means ± sem.) after rectal taurocholic acid (TCA) enema in 10 healthy humans. (B) $p = 0.019$ for incremental area under the curves (iAUC); $r = 0.48$, $p = 0.004$ for dose-dependent effect; (D) $p = 0.0005$ for iAUC; $r = 0.56$, $p = 0.001$ for dose-dependent effect. Reproduced with permission from [42] © (2013).

As discussed, physiological bile acids often activate both FXR and TGR5, but with preferential affinity depending on their molecular structure. Selective FXR- and TGR5-knockout mice, or specific FXR and TGR agonists, have been pivotal to delineation of the respective signaling pathways to the metabolic effects of bile acids. However, outcomes remain inconclusive. Administration of the intestinal FXR agonist, fexaramine, for five weeks to mice fed a high-fat-diet was reported to prevent weight gain. However, this may have reflected an increase in metabolic rate, rather than a reduction in energy intake [56]. In contrast, GW4064 had no effect on either energy intake or body weight in diabetic or obese mice [50,57]. Notably, mice with FXR deficiency (either whole body or intestine-specific knockout) fed a high-fat diet also exhibited reductions in energy intake and body weight compared with wild-type mice [31,58]. Similarly, TGR5 agonism (e.g., by INT-777) was associated with reduced weight gain, apparently by augmenting energy expenditure, without affecting energy intake [36], whereas knockout of TGR5 had no significant effect on body weight or energy intake in mice fed a high-fat diet [36,59]. Clinical outcomes relating to TGR5 or FXR agonism have been disappointing. As discussed, the TGR5 agonist, SB-756050, failed to stimulate GLP-1 secretion or improve glycemic control in individuals with T2D [39]. The effects of TGR5 agonists on energy intake and body weight in humans have not been reported. Treatment with the semi-synthetic FXR agonist, obeticholic acid, over 72 weeks only achieved a modest reduction in body weight (~2 kg) in patients with non-alcoholic fatty liver disease (NAFLD), with or without, T2D [60]. In another 24-week double-blind, randomized, placebo-controlled trial, the non-bile acid FXR agonist, cilofexor, had no effect on body weight in patients with non-alcoholic steatohepatitis [61]. Accordingly, the concept of supplementing bile acids or targeting BA signaling pathways to reduce energy intake and body weight is currently not supported by current clinical evidence.

4. Bile Acid Dysregulation in Obesity and T2D

The emerging link between bile acid signaling and the regulation of metabolic homeostasis has stimulated substantial interest in potential phenotypical changes in bile acid profiles in metabolic disorders, particularly obesity and T2D. Although bile acids are present at high concentrations in the liver, bile, and small intestine, bile acid profiles have hitherto been compared in peripheral blood and fecal samples predominantly due to their easy accessibility. Accordingly, processes in relation to small intestinal bile acid transport and absorption are poorly characterized, although gallbladder emptying can be readily assessed using ultrasound.

There is a substantial variation in circulating bile acid levels both between and within individuals [62]. In the context of obesity, most studies have reported that fasting serum/plasma bile acid levels are increased as a result of augmented bile acid synthesis (reflected by an increase in 7α-hydroxy-4-cholesten-3-one (C4)) [63–65]. There is evidence that the expression of both hepatic Na+-taurocholate co-transporting polypeptide (NTCP) [66] (responsible for the uptake of bile acids from the portal vein to the liver) and intestinal ASBT is lower in obese individuals [67], and intestinal FGF-19 secretion is also decreased [67,68]. It is, therefore, conceivable that the augmented hepatic bile acid secretion observed during fasting represents a compensatory response to deficiencies in the enterohepatic circulation. In support of this concept, the postprandial increase in circulating bile acids is significantly blunted in obesity [66,69,70] and restored after Roux-en-Y gastric bypass [70]. In addition, the production and fecal excretion of secondary bile acids (e.g., DCA) are increased in obese individuals [71,72], which may be secondary, or contribute to, alterations in gut microbiota ("dysbiosis") [73], leading to impaired energy metabolism in the host [74]. Obesity-related increases in fasting bile acid levels primarily reflect increases in 12α-hydroxylated bile acids (e.g., CA) [64,66], which are more effective in emulsifying dietary fat than non-12α-hydroxylated bile acids [49]. The shift in the bile acid composition in obesity may, therefore, favor improved fat digestion. Although fasting plasma unconjugated primary bile acids (CA and CDCA) and numerous conjugated primary and secondary bile acids (TCA, GCA, GCDCA, TDCA, and GLCA) are related positively with insulin resistance in obesity [75,76], it remains to be determined whether changes in plasma bile acids represent a manifestation, or the drivers, of obesity.

T2D individuals, with or without obesity, exhibit higher fasting bile acid concentrations in the peripheral circulation compared with non-diabetic controls, mainly due to increased unconjugated and glycine-conjugated DCA and UDCA [64,77–80]. This rise in plasma secondary bile acids may reflect increased bile acid delivery and a relative abundance of bile acid de-conjugating bacteria in the large intestine [81,82]. Interestingly, the expression of ASBT has been reported to be increased in diabetic rats [83], which would favor enhanced ileal bile acid resorption. However, this does not necessarily lead to increased FGF-19 secretion [77,79,80], or suppression of bile acid synthesis in T2D. Hepatic bile acid synthesis, particularly CA, is, in fact, known to be increased in patients with T2D [80]. In a small group of individuals with T2D (n = 15), the plasma BA responses to oral glucose or fat-containing mixed nutrients were reported to be modestly elevated [77]. Gallbladder emptying in this group of patients was similar to healthy controls [84]. However, in this study, T2D patients had relatively poor glycemic control (mean HbA1c = 7.5%) and a long duration of diabetes (6–20 years), with the majority receiving medication (e.g., metformin [85]) known to affect bile acid metabolism.

The magnitude of the increase in fasting bile acids in plasma or serum has been shown to correlate positively with fasting and 2 h-postprandial glucose levels and HbA1c in T2D, and with the degree of insulin resistance in individuals, regardless of the presence of diabetes [79,86]. In a recently reported longitudinal study, 23 bile acid species were analyzed to evaluate their baseline association with incident T2D during a median 3-year follow-up in a large cohort of individuals with normal glucose tolerance [87]. Serum fasting unconjugated primary and secondary bile acids (CA, CDCA, and DCA) were reported to be negatively associated with the risk of T2D, while conjugated primary and secondary bile acids (GCA, TCA, GCDCA, TCDCA, and TUDCA) were positively associated. Moreover, the ratios of conjugated to unconjugated bile acids (TCA/CA, GCA/CA, TCDCA/CDCA, and GCDCA/CA) were positively associated with the development of T2D. These observations support the concept that impaired catalysis of conjugated bile acids by the hepatic bile acid-CoA:amino acid N-acyltransferase (BAAT) [88] and/or intestinal resorption of unconjugated bile acids contribute to the development of T2D. The relevance of postprandial bile acid levels, particularly in the small intestine and liver, to the risk of T2D, however, remains unknown. Further studies are, therefore, required to clarify how bile acid metabolism changes with the progression of glucose dysregulation.

5. Relevance of Bile Acids to Therapies for Metabolic Disorders

As discussed, it remains to be clarified whether alterations in bile acids underpin the pathogenesis, or represent a consequence of metabolic derangement. However, there is increasing persuasive evidence to support a role for bile acids in mediating the metabolic benefits of therapies used to treat metabolic disorders including bile acid sequestrants, ASBT inhibitors, metformin, and bariatric surgery.

5.1. Bile Acid Sequestrants

Bile acid sequestrants are resins that bind to intestinal bile acids to disrupt their enterohepatic circulation and increase hepatic bile acid synthesis from cholesterol to reduce intestinal secretion of FGF19 (or FGF15 in rodents) [89,90], elevate plasma C4 levels [91], and augment expression of hepatic CYP7A1 [89,91,92]. The increase in de novo bile acid synthesis is sufficient to maintain the size of the total bile acid, but often changes its composition [80,93]. For example, in T2D patients, treatment with colesevelam (3.75 g/day) over eight weeks increased CA, but decreased CDCA and DCA [80], shifting the bile acid pool toward a more hydrophilic phenotype. Due to their effects on the enterohepatic circulation, bile acid sequestrants were initially developed to treat hypercholesterolemia. Surprisingly, they were also shown to be associated with a substantial improvement in glycemic control in patients with T2D, leading to potential re-purposing for the management of T2D [94], although the mechanism of their glucose-lowering action remains elusive. Several preclinical and clinical studies have reported a significant increase in GLP-1 secretion, associated with the use of bile acid sequestrants [89,93,95], although some studies have reported minimal [96,97], or the opposite effect [97,98]. Similarly, evidence for the effects of bile acid sequestrants on energy intake and energy expenditure is also inconsistent. In high-fat fed C57BL/6J mice, the bile acid sequestrant, colestimide, was reported to increase energy expenditure in brown adipose tissue and prevent diet-induced obesity, without affecting energy intake or lipid absorption [90]. In a similar study of hyperlipidemic transgenic mice, colestilan was reported to reduce body weight, accompanied by an increase in energy intake, a reduction in total energy expenditure, and enhanced carbohydrate catabolism [99]. In clinical trials of healthy individuals and patients with obesity and/or T2D, bile acid sequestrants have been found to be weight-neutral [93,100–102]. While further studies are required to clarify the glucose-lowering mechanisms of bile acid sequestrants, the latter do not appear to be an effective treatment for obesity.

5.2. Apical Sodium Bile Acid Co-Transporter (ASBT) Inhibitors

Similar to bile acid sequestrants, ASBT inhibitors impair intestinal bile acid resorption, leading to increased delivery of bile acids to the large intestine and decreased bile acid concentrations in the circulation [103–106]. These agents were first developed to treat hypercholesterolemia, but were subsequently applied to the management of functional constipation and non-alcoholic steatohepatitis [107]. While inhibition of ASBT remarkedly increases GLP-1 secretion in both rodents [108] and humans [109], ASBT inhibitors have not affected the energy intake or body weight in animals [104,106]. Their effect on energy intake in humans has not been reported.

5.3. Metformin

Metformin remains the first-line therapy for glucose-lowering in T2D [85], but also suppresses appetite and reduces body weight modestly [110–113]. The potential for metformin to increase plasma GLP-1 and PYY levels has been widely recognized in both preclinical and clinical studies [114–117]. There is evidence that the latter may be attributable, at least in part, to the inhibition of intestinal bile acid resorption by metformin. Indeed, metformin substantially decreases serum FGF-19, and increases fecal bile acid excretion and serum C4 levels in T2D [118]. In high-fat-fed mice, metformin was also shown to prevent weight gain, apparently by increasing energy expenditure through upregulation of the thermogenic gene (Ucp1) in white adipose tissue, without affecting energy intake [118]. That the effect on body weight was abolished in mice with intestinal-specific FXR knockout supports an important role for intestinal FXR signaling in metformin-induced weight loss in mice [118]. Moreover, metformin modifies the gut microbiota [119]; metformin therapy (1700 mg/day) over four months results in major shifts in over 50 bacterial strains, which may account for glucose-lowering in T2D [113]. In mice, weight loss induced by metformin may be attributable to a reduction in intestinal Bacteroides fragilis and resultant increases in GUDCA; the latter antagonizes FXR signaling to improve glucose metabolism and reduce body weight [118]. In this context, delayed-released metformin (of minimal intestinal absorption) may be desirable to maximize the interaction between metformin and the gut microbiota for the management of T2D.

5.4. Bariatric Surgery

Despite emerging pharmaceutical treatments, bariatric surgery remains the most effective intervention for obesity and T2D. Relative to adjustable gastric banding and sleeve gastrectomy, procedures that bypass segments of the small intestine (e.g., Roux-en-Y gastric bypass, duodenal-jejunal bypass, and biliopancreatic diversion) are in general more effective [120,121]. While the underlying mechanisms remain incompletely understood, emerging evidence suggests that the expedited flow of bile acids to the distal gut may be important. Indeed, bile acid diversion from the duodenum to distal ileum increases GLP-1 [122], decreases blood glucose [32,122,123], and reduces body weight substantially [32,123] in rodents with diet-induced obesity. While the expression of bile acid receptors (i.e., TGR5 and FXR) in the distal gut is not affected by bariatric surgery [123], increased delivery of bile acids into the large intestine may alter the composition of the gut microbiome after bariatric surgery (or vice versa) [32,123,124], thereby influencing host energy metabolism [125]. That FXR-knockout abolishes [32,58], while TGR5 knock-out preserves [32], the weight loss effect of Roux-en-Y gastric bypass or ileal biliary diversion in high-fat-fed mice, suggests that FXR, but not TGR5, signaling is indispensable for weight loss induced by the diversion of bile acids to the distal small intestine. However, the significance of FXR signaling in humans is questionable, since the administration of the FXR agonist, obeticholic acid, over 72 weeks, showed little effect on body weight in patients with NAFLD [60].

6. Concluding Comments

The recognition of bile acids as important signaling molecules that orchestrate metabolic homeostasis through specialized receptors (FXR and TGR5) has stimulated active research to determine their relevance to the pathogenesis of, and therapeutic potential for the management of, metabolic disorders. Recent studies, focusing on the enterohepatic circulation and bile acid sensing, are indicative of major shifts in plasma and fecal bile acid profiles in obesity and T2D, and of the potent effects of bile acids on GLP-1 and PYY secretion from enteroendocrine L-cells. Accordingly, assessment of the bile acid profile may be of relevance to predict the risk of obesity and T2D, while targeting bile acid signaling pathways may represent an attractive strategy for the prevention and management of these metabolic disorders. The efficacy of bile acids to stimulate gut hormone secretion is related to their affinity for TGR5 and FXR; activation of TGR5 (expressed on the basolateral side of the L-cells) mediates bile acid-induced GLP-1 and PYY secretion, whereas FXR signaling has been shown to suppress these actions, or modify TGR5 signaling indirectly, while studies of physiological bile acids or agonists of TGR5 and FXR have yielded inconsistent outcomes on blood glucose, energy intake, and body weight changes in both animal and human studies. However, several interventions with proven benefits on metabolic health are clearly associated with disrupted, or potentially accelerated, enterohepatic circulation. Studies are now warranted to determine whether there are causal links between the bile acid profile and metabolic outcomes and, if so, the underlying mechanisms. Finally, it would also be of interest to explore whether bile acids have additive or synergistic effects with other (dietary or pharmaceutical) interventions to promote weight loss and glycemic control.

Author Contributions: C.X.: W.H., R.L.Y., K.L.J., M.H., C.K.R., and T.W. were all involved in the conception, design, and writing of the manuscript. All authors have read and agreed to the published version of the manuscript.

Funding: The authors' work in this area is supported by the Australia National Health and Medical Research Council (NHMRC ID: 1147333), Diabetes Australia (ID: Y20G-WUTO) and the National Natural Science Foundation of China (81870561). C.X. is supported by a postgraduate scholarship from the China Scholarship Council. KLJ is supported by a University of Adelaide William T Southcott Research Fellowship. TW is supported by a Mid-Career Fellowship from the Hospital Research Foundation.

Acknowledgments: The Centre of Research Excellence (CRE) in Translating Nutritional Science to Good Health has been supported by the Hospital Research Foundation.

Conflicts of Interest: The authors declare no conflict of interests relevant to this work.

References

1. Russell, D.W. The enzymes, regulation, and genetics of bile acid synthesis. *Annu. Rev. Biochem.* **2003**, *72*, 137–174. [CrossRef]
2. Thomas, C.; Pellicciari, R.; Pruzanski, M.; Auwerx, J.; Schoonjans, K. Targeting bile-acid signalling for metabolic diseases. *Nat. Rev. Drug Discov.* **2008**, *7*, 678–693. [CrossRef]
3. Setchell, K.D.; Rodrigues, C.M.; Clerici, C.; Solinas, A.; Morelli, A.; Gartung, C.; Boyer, J. Bile acid concentrations in human and rat liver tissue and in hepatocyte nuclei. *Gastroenterology* **1997**, *112*, 226–235. [CrossRef]
4. Shiffman, M.L.; Sugerman, H.J.; Kellum, J.M.; Moore, E.W. Changes in gallbladder bile composition following gallstone formation and weight reduction. *Gastroenterology* **1992**, *103*, 214–221. [CrossRef]
5. Northfield, T.C.; McColl, I. Postprandial concentrations of free and conjugated bile acids down the length of the normal human small intestine. *Gut* **1973**, *14*, 513–518. [CrossRef]

6. Makishima, M.; Lu, T.T.; Xie, W.; Whitfield, G.K.; Domoto, H.; Evans, R.M.; Haussler, M.R.; Mangelsdorf, D.J. Vitamin D receptor as an intestinal bile acid sensor. *Science* **2002**, *296*, 1313–1316. [CrossRef] [PubMed]
7. Ihunnah, C.A.; Jiang, M.; Xie, W. Nuclear receptor PXR, transcriptional circuits and metabolic relevance. *Biochim. Biophys. Acta* **2011**, *1812*, 956–963. [CrossRef]
8. Wagner, M.; Halilbasic, E.; Marschall, H.U.; Zollner, G.; Fickert, P.; Langner, C.; Zatloukal, K.; Denk, H.; Trauner, M. CAR and PXR agonists stimulate hepatic bile acid and bilirubin detoxification and elimination pathways in mice. *Hepatology* **2005**, *42*, 420–430. [CrossRef] [PubMed]
9. Makishima, M.; Okamoto, A.Y.; Repa, J.J.; Tu, H.; Learned, R.M.; Luk, A.; Hull, M.V.; Lustig, K.D.; Mangelsdorf, D.J.; Shan, B. Identification of a nuclear receptor for bile acids. *Science* **1999**, *284*, 1362–1365. [CrossRef] [PubMed]
10. Maruyama, T.; Miyamoto, Y.; Nakamura, T.; Tamai, Y.; Okada, H.; Sugiyama, E.; Nakamura, T.; Itadani, H.; Tanaka, K. Identification of membrane-type receptor for bile acids (M-BAR). *Biochem. Biophys. Res. Commun.* **2002**, *298*, 714–719. [CrossRef]
11. Mertens, K.L.; Kalsbeek, A.; Soeters, M.R.; Eggink, H.M. Bile acid signaling pathways from the enterohepatic circulation to the central nervous system. *Front. Neurosci.* **2017**, *11*, 617. [CrossRef]
12. Wu, X.; Li, J.-Y.; Lee, A.; Lu, Y.-X.; Zhou, S.-Y.; Owyang, C. Satiety induced by bile acids is mediated via vagal afferent pathways. *JCI Insight* **2020**, *5*. [CrossRef] [PubMed]
13. Xie, C.; Jones, K.L.; Rayner, C.K.; Wu, T. Enteroendocrine hormone secretion and metabolic control: Importance of the region of the gut stimulation. *Pharmaceutics* **2020**, *12*, 790. [CrossRef] [PubMed]
14. Lefebvre, P.; Cariou, B.; Lien, F.; Kuipers, F.; Staels, B. Role of bile acids and bile acid receptors in metabolic regulation. *Physiol. Rev.* **2009**, *89*, 147–191. [CrossRef]
15. Fiorucci, S.; Mencarelli, A.; Palladino, G.; Cipriani, S. Bile-acid-activated receptors: Targeting TGR5 and farnesoid-X-receptor in lipid and glucose disorders. *Trends Pharmacol. Sci.* **2009**, *30*, 570–580. [CrossRef]
16. Kuipers, F.; Bloks, V.W.; Groen, A.K. Beyond intestinal soap—Bile acids in metabolic control. *Nat. Rev. Endocrinol.* **2014**, *10*, 488–498. [CrossRef] [PubMed]
17. Ahmad, T.R.; Haeusler, R.A. Bile acids in glucose metabolism and insulin signalling–mechanisms and research needs. *Nat. Rev. Endocrinol.* **2019**. [CrossRef]
18. Bray, G.A.; Gallagher, T.F., Jr. Suppression of appetite by bile acids. *Lancet* **1968**, *1*, 1066–1067. [CrossRef]
19. Roberts, R.E.; Glicksman, C.; Alaghband-Zadeh, J.; Sherwood, R.A.; Akuji, N.; le Roux, C.W. The relationship between postprandial bile acid concentration, GLP-1, PYY and ghrelin. *Clin. Endocrinol.* **2011**, *74*, 67–72. [CrossRef]
20. Nakatani, H.; Kasama, K.; Oshiro, T.; Watanabe, M.; Hirose, H.; Itoh, H. Serum bile acid along with plasma incretins and serum high-molecular weight adiponectin levels are increased after bariatric surgery. *Metabolism* **2009**, *58*, 1400–1407. [CrossRef]
21. Kuhre, R.E.; Wewer Albrechtsen, N.J.; Larsen, O.; Jepsen, S.L.; Balk-Moller, E.; Andersen, D.B.; Deacon, C.F.; Schoonjans, K.; Reimann, F.; Gribble, F.M.; et al. Bile acids are important direct and indirect regulators of the secretion of appetite- and metabolism-regulating hormones from the gut and pancreas. *Mol. Metab.* **2018**, *11*, 84–95. [CrossRef] [PubMed]
22. Gomez, G.; Upp, J.R., Jr.; Lluis, F.; Alexander, R.W.; Poston, G.J.; Greeley, G.H., Jr.; Thompson, J.C. Regulation of the release of cholecystokinin by bile salts in dogs and humans. *Gastroenterology* **1988**, *94*, 1036–1046. [CrossRef]
23. Koop, I.; Schindler, M.; Bosshammer, A.; Scheibner, J.; Stange, E.; Koop, H. Physiological control of cholecystokinin release and pancreatic enzyme secretion by intraduodenal bile acids. *Gut* **1996**, *39*, 661–667. [CrossRef] [PubMed]
24. Sonne, D.P.; Hansen, M.; Knop, F.K. Bile acid sequestrants in type 2 diabetes: Potential effects on GLP1 secretion. *Eur. J. Endocrinol.* **2014**, *171*, R47–R65. [CrossRef]
25. Guida, C.; Ramracheya, R. PYY, a therapeutic option for type 2 diabetes? *Clin. Med. Insights Endocrinol. Diabetes* **2020**, *13*, 1179551419892985. [CrossRef]
26. Wu, T.; Bound, M.J.; Standfield, S.D.; Jones, K.L.; Horowitz, M.; Rayner, C.K. Effects of taurocholic acid on glycemic, glucagon-like peptide-1, and insulin responses to small intestinal glucose infusion in healthy humans. *J. Clin. Endocrinol. Metab.* **2013**, *98*, E718–E722. [CrossRef]
27. Trabelsi, M.S.; Daoudi, M.; Prawitt, J.; Ducastel, S.; Touche, V.; Sayin, S.I.; Perino, A.; Brighton, C.A.; Sebti, Y.; Kluza, J.; et al. Farnesoid X receptor inhibits glucagon-like peptide-1 production by enteroendocrine L cells. *Nat. Commun.* **2015**, *6*, 7629. [CrossRef]
28. Zheng, X.; Chen, T.; Jiang, R.; Zhao, A.; Wu, Q.; Kuang, J.; Sun, D.; Ren, Z.; Li, M.; Zhao, M.; et al. Hyocholic acid species improve glucose homeostasis through a distinct TGR5 and FXR signaling mechanism. *Cell Metab.* **2020**. [CrossRef]
29. Li, P.; Zhu, L.; Yang, X.; Li, W.; Sun, X.; Yi, B.; Zhu, S. Farnesoid X receptor interacts with cAMP response element binding protein to modulate glucagon-like peptide-1 (7-36) amide secretion by intestinal L cell. *J. Cell Physiol.* **2019**, *234*, 12839–12846. [CrossRef]
30. Ducastel, S.; Touche, V.; Trabelsi, M.S.; Boulinguiez, A.; Butruille, L.; Nawrot, M.; Peschard, S.; Chavez-Talavera, O.; Dorchies, E.; Vallez, E.; et al. The nuclear receptor FXR inhibits Glucagon-Like Peptide-1 secretion in response to microbiota-derived Short-Chain Fatty Acids. *Sci. Rep.* **2020**, *10*, 174. [CrossRef]
31. Xie, C.; Jiang, C.; Shi, J.; Gao, X.; Sun, D.; Sun, L.; Wang, T.; Takahashi, S.; Anitha, M.; Krausz, K.W.; et al. An intestinal farnesoid X receptor-ceramide signaling axis modulates hepatic gluconeogenesis in mice. *Diabetes* **2017**, *66*, 613–626. [CrossRef] [PubMed]
32. Albaugh, V.L.; Banan, B.; Antoun, J.; Xiong, Y.; Guo, Y.; Ping, J.; Alikhan, M.; Clements, B.A.; Abumrad, N.N.; Flynn, C.R. Role of bile acids and GLP-1 in mediating the metabolic improvements of bariatric surgery. *Gastroenterology* **2019**, *156*, 1041–1051.e1044. [CrossRef] [PubMed]

33. Pathak, P.; Xie, C.; Nichols, R.G.; Ferrell, J.M.; Boehme, S.; Krausz, K.W.; Patterson, A.D.; Gonzalez, F.J.; Chiang, J.Y.L. Intestine farnesoid X receptor agonist and the gut microbiota activate G-protein bile acid receptor-1 signaling to improve metabolism. *Hepatology* **2018**, *68*, 1574–1588. [CrossRef] [PubMed]
34. Kawamata, Y.; Fujii, R.; Hosoya, M.; Harada, M.; Yoshida, H.; Miwa, M.; Fukusumi, S.; Habata, Y.; Itoh, T.; Shintani, Y.; et al. A G protein-coupled receptor responsive to bile acids. *J. Biol. Chem.* **2003**, *278*, 9435–9440. [CrossRef]
35. Katsuma, S.; Hirasawa, A.; Tsujimoto, G. Bile acids promote glucagon-like peptide-1 secretion through TGR5 in a murine enteroendocrine cell line STC-1. *Biochem. Biophys. Res. Commun.* **2005**, *329*, 386–390. [CrossRef] [PubMed]
36. Thomas, C.; Gioiello, A.; Noriega, L.; Strehle, A.; Oury, J.; Rizzo, G.; Macchiarulo, A.; Yamamoto, H.; Mataki, C.; Pruzanski, M.; et al. TGR5-mediated bile acid sensing controls glucose homeostasis. *Cell Metab.* **2009**, *10*, 167–177. [CrossRef]
37. Parker, H.E.; Wallis, K.; le Roux, C.W.; Wong, K.Y.; Reimann, F.; Gribble, F.M. Molecular mechanisms underlying bile acid-stimulated glucagon-like peptide-1 secretion. *Br. J. Pharmacol.* **2012**, *165*, 414–423. [CrossRef]
38. Brighton, C.A.; Rievaj, J.; Kuhre, R.E.; Glass, L.L.; Schoonjans, K.; Holst, J.J.; Gribble, F.M.; Reimann, F. Bile acids trigger GLP-1 release predominantly by accessing basolaterally located G protein-coupled bile acid receptors. *Endocrinology* **2015**, *156*, 3961–3970. [CrossRef]
39. Hodge, R.J.; Lin, J.; Vasist Johnson, L.S.; Gould, E.P.; Bowers, G.D.; Nunez, D.J.; Team, S.B.P. Safety, pharmacokinetics, and pharmacodynamic effects of a selective TGR5 agonist, SB-756050, in type 2 diabetes. *Clin. Pharmacol. Drug Dev.* **2013**, *2*, 213–222. [CrossRef]
40. Adrian, T.; Ballantyne, G.; Longo, W.; Bilchik, A.; Graham, S.; Basson, M.; Tierney, R.; Modlin, I. Deoxycholate is an important releaser of peptide YY and enteroglucagon from the human colon. *Gut* **1993**, *34*, 1219–1224. [CrossRef]
41. Adrian, T.E.; Gariballa, S.; Parekh, K.A.; Thomas, S.A.; Saadi, H.; Al Kaabi, J.; Nagelkerke, N.; Gedulin, B.; Young, A.A. Rectal taurocholate increases L cell and insulin secretion, and decreases blood glucose and food intake in obese type 2 diabetic volunteers. *Diabetologia* **2012**, *55*, 2343–2347. [CrossRef]
42. Wu, T.; Bound, M.J.; Standfield, S.D.; Gedulin, B.; Jones, K.L.; Horowitz, M.; Rayner, C.K. Effects of rectal administration of taurocholic acid on glucagon-like peptide-1 and peptide YY secretion in healthy humans. *Diabetes Obes. Metab.* **2013**, *15*, 474–477. [CrossRef]
43. Tough, I.R.; Schwartz, T.W.; Cox, H.M. Synthetic G protein-coupled bile acid receptor agonists and bile acids act via basolateral receptors in ileal and colonic mucosa. *Neurogastroenterol. Motil.* **2020**, *32*, e13943. [CrossRef]
44. Christiansen, C.B.; Trammell, S.A.J.; Wewer Albrechtsen, N.J.; Schoonjans, K.; Albrechtsen, R.; Gillum, M.P.; Kuhre, R.E.; Holst, J.J. Bile acids drive colonic secretion of glucagon-like-peptide 1 and peptide-YY in rodents. *Am. J. Physiol. Gastrointest. Liver Physiol.* **2019**, *316*, G574–G584. [CrossRef]
45. Wang, H.; Chen, J.; Hollister, K.; Sowers, L.C.; Forman, B.M. Endogenous bile acids are ligands for the nuclear receptor FXR/BAR. *Mol. Cell* **1999**, *3*, 543–553. [CrossRef]
46. Sato, H.; Macchiarulo, A.; Thomas, C.; Gioiello, A.; Une, M.; Hofmann, A.F.; Saladin, R.; Schoonjans, K.; Pellicciari, R.; Auwerx, J. Novel potent and selective bile acid derivatives as TGR5 agonists: Biological screening, structure-activity relationships, and molecular modeling studies. *J. Med. Chem.* **2008**, *51*, 1831–1841. [CrossRef] [PubMed]
47. Parks, D.J.; Blanchard, S.G.; Bledsoe, R.K.; Chandra, G.; Consler, T.G.; Kliewer, S.A.; Stimmel, J.B.; Willson, T.M.; Zavacki, A.M.; Moore, D.D.; et al. Bile acids: Natural ligands for an orphan nuclear receptor. *Science* **1999**, *284*, 1365–1368. [CrossRef]
48. Bertaggia, E.; Jensen, K.K.; Castro-Perez, J.; Xu, Y.; Di Paolo, G.; Chan, R.B.; Wang, L.; Haeusler, R.A. Cyp8b1 ablation prevents Western diet-induced weight gain and hepatic steatosis because of impaired fat absorption. *Am. J. Physiol. Endocrinol. Metab.* **2017**, *313*, E121–E133. [CrossRef] [PubMed]
49. Higuchi, S.; Ahmad, T.R.; Argueta, D.A.; Perez, P.A.; Zhao, C.; Schwartz, G.J.; DiPatrizio, N.V.; Haeusler, R.A. Bile acid composition regulates GPR119-dependent intestinal lipid sensing and food intake regulation in mice. *Gut* **2020**, *69*, 1620–1628. [CrossRef]
50. Watanabe, M.; Houten, S.M.; Mataki, C.; Christoffolete, M.A.; Kim, B.W.; Sato, H.; Messaddeq, N.; Harney, J.W.; Ezaki, O.; Kodama, T.; et al. Bile acids induce energy expenditure by promoting intracellular thyroid hormone activation. *Nature* **2006**, *439*, 484–489. [CrossRef] [PubMed]
51. Wei, M.; Huang, F.; Zhao, L.; Zhang, Y.; Yang, W.; Wang, S.; Li, M.; Han, X.; Ge, K.; Qu, C.; et al. A dysregulated bile acid-gut microbiota axis contributes to obesity susceptibility. *EBioMedicine* **2020**, *55*, 102766. [CrossRef]
52. Zietak, M.; Kozak, L.P. Bile acids induce uncoupling protein 1-dependent thermogenesis and stimulate energy expenditure at thermoneutrality in mice. *Am. J. Physiol. Endocrinol. Metab.* **2016**, *310*, E346–E354. [CrossRef]
53. Zaborska, K.E.; Lee, S.A.; Garribay, D.; Cha, E.; Cummings, B.P. Deoxycholic acid supplementation impairs glucose homeostasis in mice. *PLoS ONE* **2018**, *13*, e0200908. [CrossRef] [PubMed]
54. Cheng, Z.; Liu, G.; Zhang, X.; Bi, D.; Hu, S. Improvement of glucose metabolism following long-term taurocholic acid gavage in a diabetic rat model. *Med. Sci. Monit.* **2018**, *24*, 7206–7212. [CrossRef] [PubMed]
55. Calderon, G.; McRae, A.; Rievaj, J.; Davis, J.; Zandvakili, I.; Linker-Nord, S.; Burton, D.; Roberts, G.; Reimann, F.; Gedulin, B.; et al. Ileo-colonic delivery of conjugated bile acids improves glucose homeostasis via colonic GLP-1-producing enteroendocrine cells in human obesity and diabetes. *EBioMedicine* **2020**, *55*, 102759. [CrossRef]

56. Fang, S.; Suh, J.M.; Reilly, S.M.; Yu, E.; Osborn, O.; Lackey, D.; Yoshihara, E.; Perino, A.; Jacinto, S.; Lukasheva, Y.; et al. Intestinal FXR agonism promotes adipose tissue browning and reduces obesity and insulin resistance. *Nat. Med.* **2015**, *21*, 159–165. [CrossRef] [PubMed]
57. Zhang, Y.; Lee, F.Y.; Barrera, G.; Lee, H.; Vales, C.; Gonzalez, F.J.; Willson, T.M.; Edwards, P.A. Activation of the nuclear receptor FXR improves hyperglycemia and hyperlipidemia in diabetic mice. *Proc. Natl. Acad. Sci. USA* **2006**, *103*, 1006–1011. [CrossRef] [PubMed]
58. Li, K.; Zou, J.; Li, S.; Guo, J.; Shi, W.; Wang, B.; Han, X.; Zhang, H.; Zhang, P.; Miao, Z.; et al. Farnesoid X receptor contributes to body weight-independent improvements in glycemic control after Roux-en-Y gastric bypass surgery in diet-induced obese mice. *Mol. Metab.* **2020**, *37*, 100980. [CrossRef]
59. McGavigan, A.K.; Garibay, D.; Henseler, Z.M.; Chen, J.; Bettaieb, A.; Haj, F.G.; Ley, R.E.; Chouinard, M.L.; Cummings, B.P. TGR5 contributes to glucoregulatory improvements after vertical sleeve gastrectomy in mice. *Gut* **2017**, *66*, 226–234. [CrossRef]
60. Neuschwander-Tetri, B.A.; Loomba, R.; Sanyal, A.J.; Lavine, J.E.; Van Natta, M.L.; Abdelmalek, M.F.; Chalasani, N.; Dasarathy, S.; Diehl, A.M.; Hameed, B.; et al. Farnesoid X nuclear receptor ligand obeticholic acid for non-cirrhotic, non-alcoholic steatohepatitis (FLINT): A multicentre, randomised, placebo-controlled trial. *Lancet* **2015**, *385*, 956–965. [CrossRef]
61. Patel, K.; Harrison, S.A.; Elkhashab, M.; Trotter, J.F.; Herring, R.; Rojter, S.E.; Kayali, Z.; Wong, V.W.; Greenbloom, S.; Jayakumar, S.; et al. Cilofexor, a nonsteroidal FXR agonist, in patients with noncirrhotic NASH: A phase 2 randomized controlled trial. *Hepatology* **2020**, *72*, 58–71. [CrossRef]
62. Steiner, C.; Othman, A.; Saely, C.H.; Rein, P.; Drexel, H.; von Eckardstein, A.; Rentsch, K.M. Bile acid metabolites in serum: Intraindividual variation and associations with coronary heart disease, metabolic syndrome and diabetes mellitus. *PLoS ONE* **2011**, *6*, e25006. [CrossRef]
63. Prinz, P.; Hofmann, T.; Ahnis, A.; Elbelt, U.; Goebel-Stengel, M.; Klapp, B.F.; Rose, M.; Stengel, A. Plasma bile acids show a positive correlation with body mass index and are negatively associated with cognitive restraint of eating in obese patients. *Front. Neurosci.* **2015**, *9*, 199. [CrossRef]
64. Cariou, B.; Chetiveaux, M.; Zair, Y.; Pouteau, E.; Disse, E.; Guyomarc'h-Delasalle, B.; Laville, M.; Krempf, M. Fasting plasma chenodeoxycholic acid and cholic acid concentrations are inversely correlated with insulin sensitivity in adults. *Nutr. Metab.* **2011**, *8*, 48. [CrossRef]
65. Straniero, S.; Rosqvist, F.; Edholm, D.; Ahlstrom, H.; Kullberg, J.; Sundbom, M.; Riserus, U.; Rudling, M. Acute caloric restriction counteracts hepatic bile acid and cholesterol deficiency in morbid obesity. *J. Intern. Med.* **2017**, *281*, 507–517. [CrossRef] [PubMed]
66. Haeusler, R.A.; Camastra, S.; Nannipieri, M.; Astiarraga, B.; Castro-Perez, J.; Xie, D.; Wang, L.; Chakravarthy, M.; Ferrannini, E. Increased Bile Acid Synthesis and Impaired Bile Acid Transport in Human Obesity. *J. Clin. Endocrinol. Metab.* **2016**, *101*, 1935–1944. [CrossRef] [PubMed]
67. Renner, O.; Harsch, S.; Matysik, S.; Lutjohann, D.; Schmitz, G.; Stange, E.F. Upregulation of hepatic bile acid synthesis via fibroblast growth factor 19 is defective in gallstone disease but functional in overweight individuals. *United Eur. Gastroenterol. J.* **2014**, *2*, 216–225. [CrossRef] [PubMed]
68. Gomez-Ambrosi, J.; Gallego-Escuredo, J.M.; Catalan, V.; Rodriguez, A.; Domingo, P.; Moncada, R.; Valenti, V.; Salvador, J.; Giralt, M.; Villarroya, F.; et al. FGF19 and FGF21 serum concentrations in human obesity and type 2 diabetes behave differently after diet- or surgically-induced weight loss. *Clin. Nutr.* **2017**, *36*, 861–868. [CrossRef] [PubMed]
69. Glicksman, C.; Pournaras, D.J.; Wright, M.; Roberts, R.; Mahon, D.; Welbourn, R.; Sherwood, R.; Alaghband-Zadeh, J.; le Roux, C.W. Postprandial plasma bile acid responses in normal weight and obese subjects. *Ann. Clin. Biochem.* **2010**, *47*, 482–484. [CrossRef] [PubMed]
70. Ahmad, N.N.; Pfalzer, A.; Kaplan, L.M. Roux-en-Y gastric bypass normalizes the blunted postprandial bile acid excursion associated with obesity. *Int. J. Obes.* **2013**, *37*, 1553–1559. [CrossRef]
71. Aleman, J.O.; Bokulich, N.A.; Swann, J.R.; Walker, J.M.; De Rosa, J.C.; Battaglia, T.; Costabile, A.; Pechlivanis, A.; Liang, Y.; Breslow, J.L.; et al. Fecal microbiota and bile acid interactions with systemic and adipose tissue metabolism in diet-induced weight loss of obese postmenopausal women. *J. Transl. Med.* **2018**, *16*, 244. [CrossRef]
72. Kudchodkar, B.J.; Sodhi, H.S.; Mason, D.T.; Borhani, N.O. Effects of acute caloric restriction on cholesterol metabolism in man. *Am. J. Clin. Nutr.* **1977**, *30*, 1135–1146. [CrossRef]
73. Gomes, A.C.; Hoffmann, C.; Mota, J.F. The human gut microbiota: Metabolism and perspective in obesity. *Gut Microbes* **2018**, *9*, 308–325. [CrossRef]
74. Fiorucci, S.; Distrutti, E. Bile acid-activated receptors, intestinal microbiota, and the treatment of metabolic disorders. *Trends Mol. Med.* **2015**, *21*, 702–714. [CrossRef] [PubMed]
75. Legry, V.; Francque, S.; Haas, J.T.; Verrijken, A.; Caron, S.; Chavez-Talavera, O.; Vallez, E.; Vonghia, L.; Dirinck, E.; Verhaegen, A.; et al. Bile acid alterations are associated with insulin resistance, but not with NASH, in obese subjects. *J. Clin. Endocrinol. Metab.* **2017**, *102*, 3783–3794. [CrossRef] [PubMed]
76. De Vuono, S.; Ricci, M.A.; Nulli Migliola, E.; Monti, M.C.; Morretta, E.; Boni, M.; Ministrini, S.; Carino, A.; Fiorucci, S.; Distrutti, E.; et al. Serum bile acid levels before and after sleeve gastrectomy and their correlation with obesity-related comorbidities. *Obes. Surg.* **2019**, *29*, 2517–2526. [CrossRef]
77. Sonne, D.P.; van Nierop, F.S.; Kulik, W.; Soeters, M.R.; Vilsboll, T.; Knop, F.K. Postprandial plasma concentrations of individual bile acids and FGF-19 in patients with type 2 diabetes. *J. Clin. Endocrinol. Metab.* **2016**, *101*, 3002–3009. [CrossRef] [PubMed]

78. Haeusler, R.A.; Astiarraga, B.; Camastra, S.; Accili, D.; Ferrannini, E. Human insulin resistance is associated with increased plasma levels of 12alpha-hydroxylated bile acids. *Diabetes* **2013**, *62*, 4184–4191. [CrossRef]
79. Wewalka, M.; Patti, M.E.; Barbato, C.; Houten, S.M.; Goldfine, A.B. Fasting serum taurine-conjugated bile acids are elevated in type 2 diabetes and do not change with intensification of insulin. *J. Clin. Endocrinol. Metab.* **2014**, *99*, 1442–1451. [CrossRef]
80. Brufau, G.; Stellaard, F.; Prado, K.; Bloks, V.W.; Jonkers, E.; Boverhof, R.; Kuipers, F.; Murphy, E.J. Improved glycemic control with colesevelam treatment in patients with type 2 diabetes is not directly associated with changes in bile acid metabolism. *Hepatology* **2010**, *52*, 1455–1464. [CrossRef]
81. Bennion, L.J.; Grundy, S.M. Effects of diabetes mellitus on cholesterol metabolism in man. *N. Engl. J. Med.* **1977**, *296*, 1365–1371. [CrossRef]
82. Wu, H.; Tremaroli, V.; Schmidt, C.; Lundqvist, A.; Olsson, L.M.; Kramer, M.; Gummesson, A.; Perkins, R.; Bergstrom, G.; Backhed, F. The gut microbiota in prediabetes and diabetes: A population-based cross-sectional study. *Cell Metab.* **2020**, *32*, 379–390.e373. [CrossRef]
83. Annaba, F.; Ma, K.; Kumar, P.; Dudeja, A.K.; Kineman, R.D.; Shneider, B.L.; Saksena, S.; Gill, R.K.; Alrefai, W.A. Ileal apical Na+-dependent bile acid transporter ASBT is upregulated in rats with diabetes mellitus induced by low doses of streptozotocin. *Am. J. Physiol. Gastrointest. Liver Physiol.* **2010**, *299*, G898–G906. [CrossRef]
84. Sonne, D.P.; Rehfeld, J.F.; Holst, J.J.; Vilsboll, T.; Knop, F.K. Postprandial gallbladder emptying in patients with type 2 diabetes: Potential implications for bile-induced secretion of glucagon-like peptide 1. *Eur. J. Endocrinol.* **2014**, *171*, 407–419. [CrossRef]
85. Sansome, D.J.; Xie, C.; Veedfald, S.; Horowitz, M.; Rayner, C.K.; Wu, T. Mechanism of glucose-lowering by metformin in type 2 diabetes: Role of bile acids. *Diabetes Obes. Metab.* **2020**, *22*, 141–148. [CrossRef] [PubMed]
86. Lee, S.G.; Lee, Y.H.; Choi, E.; Cho, Y.; Kim, J.H. Fasting serum bile acids concentration is associated with insulin resistance independently of diabetes status. *Clin. Chem. Lab. Med.* **2019**, *57*, 1218–1228. [CrossRef]
87. Lu, J.; Wang, S.; Li, M.; Gao, Z.; Xu, Y.; Zhao, X.; Hu, C.; Zhang, Y.; Liu, R.; Hu, R.; et al. Association of serum bile acids profile and pathway dysregulation with the risk of developing diabetes among normoglycemic chinese adults: Findings from the 4C study. *Diabetes Care* **2021**, *44*, 499–510. [CrossRef]
88. Chiang, J.Y. Bile acid metabolism and signaling. *Compr. Physiol.* **2013**, *3*, 1191–1212. [CrossRef] [PubMed]
89. Fuchs, C.D.; Paumgartner, G.; Mlitz, V.; Kunczer, V.; Halilbasic, E.; Leditznig, N.; Wahlstrom, A.; Stahlman, M.; Thuringer, A.; Kashofer, K.; et al. Colesevelam attenuates cholestatic liver and bile duct injury in Mdr2(−/−) mice by modulating composition, signalling and excretion of faecal bile acids. *Gut* **2018**, *67*, 1683–1691. [CrossRef] [PubMed]
90. Watanabe, M.; Morimoto, K.; Houten, S.M.; Kaneko-Iwasaki, N.; Sugizaki, T.; Horai, Y.; Mataki, C.; Sato, H.; Murahashi, K.; Arita, E.; et al. Bile acid binding resin improves metabolic control through the induction of energy expenditure. *PLoS ONE* **2012**, *7*, e38286. [CrossRef] [PubMed]
91. Schadt, H.S.; Wolf, A.; Mahl, J.A.; Wuersch, K.; Couttet, P.; Schwald, M.; Fischer, A.; Lienard, M.; Emotte, C.; Teng, C.H.; et al. Bile acid sequestration by cholestyramine mitigates FGFR4 inhibition-induced ALT elevation. *Toxicol. Sci.* **2018**, *163*, 265–278. [CrossRef]
92. Herrema, H.; Meissner, M.; van Dijk, T.H.; Brufau-Dones, G.; Boverhof, R.; Müller, M.; Stellaard, F.; Kuipers, F. Bile salt sequestration induces the hepatic lipogenic pathway without altering bile salt pool size and transhepatic bile salt flux in mice. *Chem. Phys. Lipids* **2008**, *154*, S59. [CrossRef]
93. Beysen, C.; Murphy, E.J.; Deines, K.; Chan, M.; Tsang, E.; Glass, A.; Turner, S.M.; Protasio, J.; Riiff, T.; Hellerstein, M.K. Effect of bile acid sequestrants on glucose metabolism, hepatic de novo lipogenesis, and cholesterol and bile acid kinetics in type 2 diabetes: A randomised controlled study. *Diabetologia* **2012**, *55*, 432–442. [CrossRef]
94. Karhus, M.L.; Bronden, A.; Sonne, D.P.; Vilsboll, T.; Knop, F.K. Evidence connecting old, new and neglected glucose-lowering drugs to bile acid-induced GLP-1 secretion: A review. *Diabetes Obes. Metab.* **2017**, *19*, 1214–1222. [CrossRef] [PubMed]
95. Shang, Q.; Saumoy, M.; Holst, J.J.; Salen, G.; Xu, G. Colesevelam improves insulin resistance in a diet-induced obesity (F-DIO) rat model by increasing the release of GLP-1. *Am. J. Physiol. Gastrointest. Liver Physiol.* **2010**, *298*, G419–G424. [CrossRef] [PubMed]
96. Smushkin, G.; Sathananthan, M.; Piccinini, F.; Dalla Man, C.; Law, J.H.; Cobelli, C.; Zinsmeister, A.R.; Rizza, R.A.; Vella, A. The effect of a bile acid sequestrant on glucose metabolism in subjects with type 2 diabetes. *Diabetes* **2013**, *62*, 1094–1101. [CrossRef] [PubMed]
97. Hansen, M.; Scheltema, M.J.; Sonne, D.P.; Hansen, J.S.; Sperling, M.; Rehfeld, J.F.; Holst, J.J.; Vilsboll, T.; Knop, F.K. Effect of chenodeoxycholic acid and the bile acid sequestrant colesevelam on glucagon-like peptide-1 secretion. *Diabetes Obes. Metab.* **2016**, *18*, 571–580. [CrossRef] [PubMed]
98. Bronden, A.; Alber, A.; Rohde, U.; Gasbjerg, L.S.; Rehfeld, J.F.; Holst, J.J.; Vilsboll, T.; Knop, F.K. The bile acid-sequestering resin sevelamer eliminates the acute GLP-1 stimulatory effect of endogenously released bile acids in patients with type 2 diabetes. *Diabetes Obes. Metab.* **2018**, *20*, 362–369. [CrossRef]
99. Sugimoto-Kawabata, K.; Shimada, H.; Sakai, K.; Suzuki, K.; Kelder, T.; Pieterman, E.J.; Cohen, L.H.; Havekes, L.M.; Princen, H.M.; van den Hoek, A.M. Colestilan decreases weight gain by enhanced NEFA incorporation in biliary lipids and fecal lipid excretion. *J. Lipid Res.* **2013**, *54*, 1255–1264. [CrossRef]
100. Fonseca, V.A.; Rosenstock, J.; Wang, A.C.; Truitt, K.E.; Jones, M.R. Colesevelam HCl improves glycemic control and reduces LDL cholesterol in patients with inadequately controlled type 2 diabetes on sulfonylurea-based therapy. *Diabetes Care* **2008**, *31*, 1479–1484. [CrossRef]
101. Goldberg, R.B.; Fonseca, V.A.; Truitt, K.E.; Jones, M.R. Efficacy and safety of colesevelam in patients with type 2 diabetes mellitus and inadequate glycemic control receiving insulin-based therapy. *Arch. Intern. Med.* **2008**, *168*, 1531–1540. [CrossRef]

102. Bays, H.E.; Goldberg, R.B.; Truitt, K.E.; Jones, M.R. Colesevelam hydrochloride therapy in patients with type 2 diabetes mellitus treated with metformin: Glucose and lipid effects. *Arch. Intern. Med.* **2008**, *168*, 1975–1983. [CrossRef] [PubMed]
103. Graffner, H.; Gillberg, P.G.; Rikner, L.; Marschall, H.U. The ileal bile acid transporter inhibitor A4250 decreases serum bile acids by interrupting the enterohepatic circulation. *Aliment. Pharmacol. Ther.* **2016**, *43*, 303–310. [CrossRef]
104. Kitayama, K.; Nakai, D.; Kono, K.; van der Hoop, A.G.; Kurata, H.; de Wit, E.C.; Cohen, L.H.; Inaba, T.; Kohama, T. Novel non-systemic inhibitor of ileal apical Na+-dependent bile acid transporter reduces serum cholesterol levels in hamsters and monkeys. *Eur. J. Pharmacol.* **2006**, *539*, 89–98. [CrossRef]
105. Wu, Y.; Aquino, C.J.; Cowan, D.J.; Anderson, D.L.; Ambroso, J.L.; Bishop, M.J.; Boros, E.E.; Chen, L.; Cunningham, A.; Dobbins, R.L.; et al. Discovery of a highly potent, nonabsorbable apical sodium-dependent bile acid transporter inhibitor (GSK2330672) for treatment of type 2 diabetes. *J. Med. Chem.* **2013**, *56*, 5094–5114. [CrossRef] [PubMed]
106. Rao, A.; Kosters, A.; Mells, J.E.; Zhang, W.; Setchell, K.D.; Amanso, A.M.; Wynn, G.M.; Xu, T.; Keller, B.T.; Yin, H.; et al. Inhibition of ileal bile acid uptake protects against nonalcoholic fatty liver disease in high-fat diet-fed mice. *Sci. Transl. Med.* **2016**, *8*, 357ra122. [CrossRef] [PubMed]
107. Al-Dury, S.; Marschall, H.U. Ileal bile acid transporter inhibition for the treatment of chronic constipation, cholestatic pruritus, and NASH. *Front. Pharmacol.* **2018**, *9*, 931. [CrossRef]
108. Chen, L.; Yao, X.; Young, A.; McNulty, J.; Anderson, D.; Liu, Y.; Nystrom, C.; Croom, D.; Ross, S.; Collins, J.; et al. Inhibition of apical sodium-dependent bile acid transporter as a novel treatment for diabetes. *Am. J. Physiol. Endocrinol. Metab.* **2012**, *302*, E68–E76. [CrossRef] [PubMed]
109. Rudling, M.; Camilleri, M.; Graffner, H.; Holst, J.J.; Rikner, L. Specific inhibition of bile acid transport alters plasma lipids and GLP-1. *BMC Cardiovasc. Disord.* **2015**, *15*, 75. [CrossRef]
110. Day, E.A.; Ford, R.J.; Smith, B.K.; Mohammadi-Shemirani, P.; Morrow, M.R.; Gutgesell, R.M.; Lu, R.; Raphenya, A.R.; Kabiri, M.; McArthur, A.G.; et al. Metformin-induced increases in GDF15 are important for suppressing appetite and promoting weight loss. *Nat. Metab.* **2019**, *1*, 1202–1208. [CrossRef] [PubMed]
111. Coll, A.P.; Chen, M.; Taskar, P.; Rimmington, D.; Patel, S.; Tadross, J.A.; Cimino, I.; Yang, M.; Welsh, P.; Virtue, S.; et al. GDF15 mediates the effects of metformin on body weight and energy balance. *Nature* **2020**, *578*, 444–448. [CrossRef] [PubMed]
112. Adeyemo, M.A.; McDuffie, J.R.; Kozlosky, M.; Krakoff, J.; Calis, K.A.; Brady, S.M.; Yanovski, J.A. Effects of metformin on energy intake and satiety in obese children. *Diabetes Obes. Metab.* **2015**, *17*, 363–370. [CrossRef]
113. Wu, H.; Esteve, E.; Tremaroli, V.; Khan, M.T.; Caesar, R.; Manneras-Holm, L.; Stahlman, M.; Olsson, L.M.; Serino, M.; Planas-Felix, M.; et al. Metformin alters the gut microbiome of individuals with treatment-naive type 2 diabetes, contributing to the therapeutic effects of the drug. *Nat. Med.* **2017**, *23*, 850–858. [CrossRef] [PubMed]
114. Wu, T.; Thazhath, S.S.; Bound, M.J.; Jones, K.L.; Horowitz, M.; Rayner, C.K. Mechanism of increase in plasma intact GLP-1 by metformin in type 2 diabetes: Stimulation of GLP-1 secretion or reduction in plasma DPP-4 activity? *Diabetes Res. Clin. Pract.* **2014**, *106*, e3–e6. [CrossRef]
115. Bahne, E.; Sun, E.W.L.; Young, R.L.; Hansen, M.; Sonne, D.P.; Hansen, J.S.; Rohde, U.; Liou, A.P.; Jackson, M.L.; de Fontgalland, D.; et al. Metformin-induced glucagon-like peptide-1 secretion contributes to the actions of metformin in type 2 diabetes. *JCI Insight* **2018**, *3*. [CrossRef] [PubMed]
116. Borg, M.J.; Bound, M.; Grivell, J.; Sun, Z.; Jones, K.L.; Horowitz, M.; Rayner, C.K.; Wu, T. Comparative effects of proximal and distal small intestinal administration of metformin on plasma glucose and glucagon-like peptide-1, and gastric emptying after oral glucose, in type 2 diabetes. *Diabetes Obes. Metab.* **2019**, *21*, 640–647. [CrossRef]
117. Sun, E.W.; Martin, A.M.; Wattchow, D.A.; de Fontgalland, D.; Rabbitt, P.; Hollington, P.; Young, R.L.; Keating, D.J. Metformin triggers PYY secretion in human gut mucosa. *J. Clin. Endocrinol. Metab.* **2019**, *104*, 2668–2674. [CrossRef]
118. Sun, L.; Xie, C.; Wang, G.; Wu, Y.; Wu, Q.; Wang, X.; Liu, J.; Deng, Y.; Xia, J.; Chen, B.; et al. Gut microbiota and intestinal FXR mediate the clinical benefits of metformin. *Nat. Med.* **2018**, *24*, 1919–1929. [CrossRef]
119. Forslund, K.; Hildebrand, F.; Nielsen, T.; Falony, G.; Le Chatelier, E.; Sunagawa, S.; Prifti, E.; Vieira-Silva, S.; Gudmundsdottir, V.; Pedersen, H.K.; et al. Disentangling type 2 diabetes and metformin treatment signatures in the human gut microbiota. *Nature* **2015**, *528*, 262–266. [CrossRef]
120. Fruhbeck, G. Bariatric and metabolic surgery: A shift in eligibility and success criteria. *Nat. Rev. Endocrinol.* **2015**, *11*, 465–477. [CrossRef]
121. Rubino, F.; Schauer, P.R.; Kaplan, L.M.; Cummings, D.E. Metabolic surgery to treat type 2 diabetes: Clinical outcomes and mechanisms of action. *Annu. Rev. Med.* **2010**, *61*, 393–411. [CrossRef]
122. Zhang, X.; Liu, T.; Wang, Y.; Zhong, M.; Zhang, G.; Liu, S.; Wu, T.; Rayner, C.K.; Hu, S. Comparative effects of bile diversion and duodenal-jejunal bypass on glucose and lipid metabolism in male diabetic rats. *Obes. Surg.* **2016**, *26*, 1565–1575. [CrossRef]
123. Flynn, C.R.; Albaugh, V.L.; Cai, S.; Cheung-Flynn, J.; Williams, P.E.; Brucker, R.M.; Bordenstein, S.R.; Guo, Y.; Wasserman, D.H.; Abumrad, N.N. Bile diversion to the distal small intestine has comparable metabolic benefits to bariatric surgery. *Nat. Commun.* **2015**, *6*, 7715. [CrossRef] [PubMed]
124. Wang, W.; Cheng, Z.; Wang, Y.; Dai, Y.; Zhang, X.; Hu, S. Role of bile acids in bariatric surgery. *Front. Physiol.* **2019**, *10*, 374. [CrossRef] [PubMed]
125. Nicholson, J.K.; Holmes, E.; Kinross, J.; Burcelin, R.; Gibson, G.; Jia, W.; Pettersson, S. Host-gut microbiota metabolic interactions. *Science* **2012**, *336*, 1262–1267. [CrossRef] [PubMed]

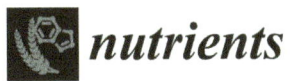

Review

The Function of Gastrointestinal Hormones in Obesity—Implications for the Regulation of Energy Intake

Mona Farhadipour and Inge Depoortere *

Translational Research in Gastrointestinal Disorders, Gut Peptide Research Lab, University of Leuven, Gasthuisberg, 3000 Leuven, Belgium; mona.farhadipour@kuleuven.be
* Correspondence: inge.depoortere@kuleuven.be

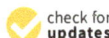

Citation: Farhadipour, M.; Depoortere, I. The Function of Gastrointestinal Hormones in Obesity—Implications for the Regulation of Energy Intake. *Nutrients* 2021, *13*, 1839. https://doi.org/10.3390/nu13061839

Academic Editors: Christine Feinle-Bisset and Michael Horowitz

Received: 20 January 2021
Accepted: 24 May 2021
Published: 27 May 2021

Publisher's Note: MDPI stays neutral with regard to jurisdictional claims in published maps and institutional affiliations.

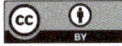

Copyright: © 2021 by the authors. Licensee MDPI, Basel, Switzerland. This article is an open access article distributed under the terms and conditions of the Creative Commons Attribution (CC BY) license (https://creativecommons.org/licenses/by/4.0/).

Abstract: The global burden of obesity and the challenges of prevention prompted researchers to investigate the mechanisms that control food intake. Food ingestion triggers several physiological responses in the digestive system, including the release of gastrointestinal hormones from enteroendocrine cells that are involved in appetite signalling. Disturbed regulation of gut hormone release may affect energy homeostasis and contribute to obesity. In this review, we summarize the changes that occur in the gut hormone balance during the pre- and postprandial state in obesity and the alterations in the diurnal dynamics of their plasma levels. We further discuss how obesity may affect nutrient sensors on enteroendocrine cells that sense the luminal content and provoke alterations in their secretory profile. Gastric bypass surgery elicits one of the most favorable metabolic outcomes in obese patients. We summarize the effect of different strategies to induce weight loss on gut enteroendocrine function. Although the mechanisms underlying obesity are not fully understood, restoring the gut hormone balance in obesity by targeting nutrient sensors or by combination therapy with gut peptide mimetics represents a novel strategy to ameliorate obesity.

Keywords: obesity; gastrointestinal hormones; nutrient sensing; circadian clock; gastric bypass surgery

1. Introduction

Obesity has increased dramatically over the past decades and reached epidemic proportions in adults and in children worldwide [1]. The rising prevalence and increased risk of developing chronic diseases exemplify the need for further research to improve understanding of the molecular mechanisms that are involved in the pathogenesis of obesity. Obesity is defined by the World Health Organization as "abnormal or excessive fat accumulation that may impair health" and is classified by a body mass index (BMI) $\geq 30 \text{ kg/m}^2$, which is a simple index of weight-for-height [2]. Obesity reflects a high dietary intake relative to a low energy expenditure, which causes a disturbed energy balance [3]. However, obesity is a multi-factorial disorder and arises from the complex interaction between genetic, environmental, behavioral and psychological factors [4]. Genetic research has led to the recognition of rare monogenic and more common polygenic forms of obesity with different genes, each contributing to the relative risk of developing obesity [5]. This genetic predisposition is associated with genes that control eating behavior and appetite [6,7].

2. Regulation of Energy Homeostasis

The nuclei of the hypothalamus and brain stem play an important role in the regulation of energy homeostasis [8,9]. These central circuits integrate signals from the periphery to coordinate a response to a change in nutritional status. These signals act on two distinct populations in the arcuate nucleus that have projections to second order neuronal signalling pathways, which transform these inputs into behavioral responses to modify food intake and metabolic rate [9]. In general, peripheral signals can be divided into either long or short acting that communicate the energy status to the arcuate nucleus of the hypothalamus [10].

Long-term peripheral signals relay information about the extent of adipose tissue. These adiposity signals include the satiety hormone leptin, secreted by adipocytes, and insulin secreted by the pancreas. Their plasma levels are proportional to body fat and they can reach their receptors through an incomplete blood brain barrier at the level of the arcuate nucleus [11,12]. Short-term peripheral signals regulate energy homeostasis through the release of a number of peptide hormones that are secreted from enteroendocrine cells (EECs) in response to feeding and fasting [9]. In general, gut hormones are divided into hunger, orexigenic hormones and satiety, anorexigenic hormones. Ghrelin is the main hormone that is released from the stomach in response to fasting and triggers the onset of eating, thus regulating meal frequency [13]. There is also evidence that motilin is a hunger signal in humans through its stimulatory effect on gastric contractions in the fasted state that signal hunger via a cholinergic pathway [14,15]. The other hormones, including cholecystokinin (CCK), glucagon-like peptide 1 (GLP-1), gastric inhibitory peptide (GIP), peptide YY (PYY) and oxyntomodulin are satiety signals released after a meal and determine meal size [16–18]. However, a study in rats showed that non-nutrient driven GLP-1 release was possible prior to a meal after training the rats with time restricted feeding. The rats secreted GLP-1 cephalically in anticipation of a meal [19]. However, cephalic phase secretion in humans elicited by modified sham feeding was not observed for GLP-1 or ghrelin [20].

Brain regions may be activated either directly via the bloodstream or indirectly via activation of their receptors on the vagal nerve [9]. In addition, the vagus nerve induces satiety in response to nutrients through distension. This distention activates mechanoreceptors on intraganglionic laminar endings, which are present throughout the intestine, and contribute to stretch-induced meal termination [21,22]. Using single-cell RNA sequencing, Bai et al. provided a genetic map of vagal afferents innervating the gastrointestinal tract [23]. Food intake was most potently inhibited by vagal afferents that innervate the intestine. Stimulation of these mechanoreceptors activated satiety-promoting pathways in the brainstem to inhibit the hunger-promoting agouti-related protein (AgRP) neurons in the hypothalamus [23]. Furthermore, increasing intestinal volume was sufficient to inhibit food intake and AgRP activation even in the absence of nutrients.

In high-fat diet (HFD) induced obese mice, gastric and jejunal vagal afferents exhibit a reduced response to stretch which may lead to overconsumption of food and maintenance of the obese state [22].

3. Gut Hormones and Enteroendocrine Cell Plasticity

EECs begin as proliferating pluripotent stem cells in the crypt that commit to the secretory EEC lineage upon migration to the villi. EECs represent only 1% of the epithelial cell population [24]. There are several subtypes of EECs that have been classified based on their morphology and hormone production, e.g., P/D1-cells (ghrelin), L-cells (GLP-1, PYY, oxyntomodulin), I-cells (CCK), K-cells (GIP). However, the one cell-one hormone dogma was abandoned when it was shown, using flow cytometry and microarray-based transcriptomics, that some EEC subtypes were bi- or trihormonal and express members of functionally related peptides. It appeared that some EECs contain only 10% of their primary hormone (L-cells), while other EECs, such as the P/D1-cells, express more than 70% of their primary hormone, ghrelin [25,26]. This made the classification more complicated with up to 20 different cell types. These findings were further refined in a mouse single cell transcriptomic study which provided a clear description of the EEC hierarchy and its sub-lineages, identified regulators of lineage specification and showed that EECs display hormonal plasticity in the course of their maturation [27]. Recently, Beumer et al. provided a high-resolution mRNA and secretome atlas of human EECs using an organoid-based platform [28]. Key differences to murine EECs were found with respect to hormones, sensory receptors and transcription factors. For example, although motilin EECs do not exist in mice, in humans they identified a cluster of cells producing motilin and ghrelin with a gradient from predominantly motilin to mainly ghrelin expressing cells [29]. The authors speculated that these might represent different states of the same cell type that can undergo a bone morphogenic protein (BMP)-controlled switch in hormone expression [28]. Another study from this group showed that upon activation of BMP signalling L-cells lose GLP-1 and increase secretin, neurotensin and PYY expression [30]. Therefore, BMP inhibitors have the potential to boost GLP-1 producing cells to improve glycaemic control in the management of type 2 diabetes mellitus (T2DM) [30].

4. Altered Gut Hormone Levels in Obesity

Obesity is known to affect the expression of many hormones. Defects in the long-acting peripheral signals can be due to mutations in the leptin gene or leptin receptor, and have been observed in a limited number of patients [31]. Leptin deficiency is entirely treatable with daily subcutaneous injections of recombinant human leptin. However, the majority of obese patients have high circulating leptin levels and in these patients administration of recombinant leptin failed to decrease body weight and food intake due to leptin resistance [32]. The latter contributes to the maintenance of obesity. Several mechanisms have been identified as potentially underlying leptin resistance, including changes in transport across the blood brain barrier, endoplasmatic reticulum stress and impaired leptin receptor function and STAT3 signalling [33]. A recent study in aged mice even showed that the leptin sensitizer, celastrol, restored sensitivity and induced decreases in fat mass and body weight, but not in young mice [34]. In addition, the vagal afferent pathway plays an important role in signalling of the nutrient content from the gut to the brain through sensing of the gut hormones [35]. De Lartigue et al. found that leptin resistance by the vagal afferent pathway causes hyperphagia, which contributes to the onset of obesity [36]. The sensitivity of gastric vagal afferents that convey satiety signals is decreased in HFD-induced obese mice. In contrast to lean mice, leptin released from gastric epithelial cells further inhibited the response of vagal afferents to mechanical stimuli in HFD-induced obese mice, thereby worsening the situation [37].

Obesity also alters the short-term meal-related signalling of gut hormones. It is tempting to speculate that changes in the gut hormone balance may contribute to hyperphagia in obese patients. Table 1 summarizes the meal-related fluctuations in gut hormone levels and their alterations in obese and T2DM patients.

Table 1. An overview of the meal-related fluctuations in gut hormone levels and their alterations in obesity and type 2 diabetes patients.

Hormone	Localisation	Meal-Related Fluctuations	Effect on Food Intake	Dysregulation in Obesity and Type 2 Diabetes			
				Release	↓	↑	=
Ghrelin (GHRL)	P/D1 cells (stomach)	Preprandial rise	Orexigenic	Fasting	[38–43]		
Motilin (MLN)	M cells (small intestine)	Preprandial rise	Orexigenic	Fasting		[44]	
Cholecystokinin (CCK)	I cells (small intestine)	Postprandial rise	Anorexigenic	Postprandial	[43,45]	[46]	[47]
Glucagon-like-peptide-1 (GLP-1)	L cells (small intestine)	Postprandial rise	Anorexigenic	Postprandial	[48–52]	[53]	[54–56]
Peptide-YY (PYY)	L cells (colon)	Postprandial rise	Anorexigenic	Postprandial	[43,57,58]		

4.1. Orexigenic Hormones

4.1.1. Ghrelin

Ghrelin is a 28-amino acid peptide that is activated upon octanoylation of serine on the third N-terminal amino acid position, a posttranslational modification initiated by ghrelin O-acyl-transferase (GOAT) [59,60]. Ghrelin binds to the growth hormone secretagogue receptor (GHSR1a) on NPY/AgRP neurons in the arcuate nucleus of the hypothalamus to stimulate food intake [61]. However, ghrelin also stimulates many brain regions that are involved in reward and motivation, including the ventral tegmental area and hippocampus [62]. Ghrelin favors hedonic food consumption by enhancing reward signalling [62–64].

Ghrelin is secreted from the P/D1 cells during the preprandial state and influences the frequency of meals [13]. Secretion of ghrelin involves the sympathetic nervous system and is mediated via β1 receptors on the ghrelin cell [65,66]. The magnitude of the postprandial fall is dependent on the macronutrient composition of the meal and caloric content [67,68]. Plasma ghrelin levels are lower in obese patients [38–43]. This decrease is thought to be compensatory rather than causal and to represent a physiological adaptation to the positive energy balance. The only exception is patients with Prader–Willi syndrome, who are characterized by high ghrelin levels long before the onset of hyperphagia [69]. At an early age, these patients suffer from persistent cravings, which lead to increased food intake and childhood obesity. In addition, these patients not only show endocrine dysfunctions such as growth hormone deficiency hypogonadism, hypothyroidism and several others, but also behavior problems, social/learning disabilities, mental issues and comorbidities [70].

Furthermore, obese patients have almost no postprandial decline in response to food intake, and the lack of meal-related fluctuations may continuously stimulate appetite [39]. There are inconsistent findings on the effect of obesity on the number of ghrelin-positive cells and ghrelin mRNA expression in biopsies [40,71,72]. In resection specimens, region-dependent differences in ghrelin mRNA expression were observed in the stomach of lean versus obese subjects, with higher expression levels in the distal stomach of obese subjects compared to lean [73]. Studies in human primary fundic cultures revealed that obesity decreased the production of ghrelin at the protein level in the cell, resulting in a decreased secretion in the cell supernatant without affecting steady state secretory mechanisms [74]. Altered responsiveness to noradrenaline has been observed in primary crypt cultures from obese subjects, as well as from diet-induced obese mice, suggesting that a reduced sympathetic drive may contribute to the disturbed ghrelin regulation [74,75].

Studies in diet-induced obese (DIO) mice suggest that the hypothalamic circuitry, which controls food intake, becomes resistant to ghrelin during obesity [76]. Several mechanisms have been suggested, including hyperleptinemia and inflammation in the hypothalamus and nodose ganglion. Recently, it has been hypothesized that high levels of liver-enriched antimicrobial peptide-2, the endogenous ghrelin receptor antagonist produced in the small intestine, prevent acylated ghrelin from activating ghrelin receptors in the arcuate nucleus in obese individuals [77].

Obese patients may potentially only benefit from treatments with GHSR antagonists or treatments that neutralize ghrelin (e.g., GOAT inhibitors) after diet-induced weight loss, which restores ghrelin sensitivity and is accompanied by an increase in plasma ghrelin levels. Nevertheless, low dose infusion of ghrelin still increased ad libitum energy intake at a buffet meal in obese patients [78]. Therefore, the concept of ghrelin resistance remains to be shown in obese patients.

4.1.2. Motilin

Motilin is a 22-amino acid peptide released by the M-cells in the small intestine that stimulates gastrointestinal motility [79]. It is structurally related to ghrelin, which was originally named motilin-related peptide [80]. Plasma motilin levels fluctuate with the phases of the migrating motor complex (MMC), initiating in the distal stomach or small intestine a pattern of strong contractions during the interdigestive phase that clean the intestine of food remnants [81]. More recently, motilin was identified as a key hunger signal in humans. It was shown that motilin-induced gastric phase III contractions during the MMC signal hunger in the fasting state via a cholinergic pathway [14,15].

Deloose et al. reported higher plasma motilin levels with less fluctuations in the fasting state in obese patients [44]. The lack of elevation in plasma motilin levels before the start of gastric phase III contractions was in line with the switch in origin of phase III contractions from the stomach to the duodenum, initially described by Pieramico et al. [82]. This may explain the reduced hunger observed in obese patients during phase III that was restored by pharmacological induction of gastric phase III contractions with the motilin receptor agonist, erythromycin [44].

4.2. Anorexigenic Hormones

4.2.1. Cholecystokinin

Cholecystokinin (CCK) is secreted mainly by duodenal and jejunal I-cells in response to feeding, particularly fat and protein [83]. It is posttranslationally processed to yield various truncated circulating forms including CCK-8, CCK-33 and CCK-58, that can bind to the CCK1 receptor or CCK2 receptor to exert its biological effects. CCK inhibits food intake by acting on vagal afferents, especially in the duodenum [84]. Slowing of gastric emptying is another mechanism of CCK-induced appetite suppression [85]. In pharmacological concentrations, CCK also stimulates insulin secretion [86].

It remains controversial whether obesity affects CCK secretion; both a reduction [43,45], an increase [46] and unaltered [47] postprandial CCK levels have been reported in obese subjects. Furthermore, the responses to macronutrients have been variable [47]. Defects in CCK signalling have been reported to contribute to obesity, since genetic mutations in CCK1 receptor result in increased meal size and food intake [87,88].

Obese humans are still sensitive to the satiating action of CCK [89]. However, in humans the efficacy of molecule CCK1 receptor agonists has been variable [90]. Furthermore, these molecules suffer from lack of specificity and have off-target effects. Novel strategies are needed to target CCK1 receptors more effectively and to dissociate disease activity from undesirable effects [91].

4.2.2. Glucagon-Like-Peptide 1

Glucagon-like peptide-1 (GLP-1) is a proglucagon-derived hormone that is secreted by L-cells in the small intestine and colon in response to nutrients [16]. L-cells are in direct contact with luminal nutrients and GLP-1 levels increase rapidly upon food intake. The low number of L-cells in the proximal intestine probably accounts, at least in part, for the early postprandial rise in GLP-1 levels, but it has been suggested that neuronal and/or humoral mechanisms contribute as well. GLP-1 is a satiety signal that mainly acts via vagal, rather than, central GLP-1 receptors [16,92]. Once GLP-1 is taken up by capillaries, it is rapidly broken down by dipeptidyl peptidase (DPP4). This limits the amount of GLP-1 reaching the systemic circulation and hence, its endocrine activities. GLP-1 is an important incretin hormone that stimulates glucose-dependent insulin secretion by binding to GLP-1 receptors on β-cells [93].

A study in a large cohort of obese patients showed a ~20% reduction in GLP-1 response to oral glucose compared with normal weight individuals [48]. However, when comparing GLP-1 secretion during an oral glucose tolerance test or meal-tolerance test in subjects with obesity or T2DM, increased [53], decreased [48–52] or unchanged [54–56] GLP-1 responses have been found. In some studies, patients with T2DM were treated with metformin or DPP4 inhibitors, which enhance GLP-1 secretion, and in others insulin resistance was more pronounced, a factor related to impaired GLP-1 release [94]. If the cohorts are not matched closely to the healthy participants, factors such as age, sex and rate of gastric emptying, may all influence the secretion of GLP-1.

Indeed, the pathology of obesity may change according to age and gender, and therefore affect the changes in the levels of the gut hormones. For example, pre-menopausal women may have higher GLP-1 levels relative to their control groups (post-menopausal women and men of the same age), which may provide premenopausal women with relative protection against metabolic diseases and the associated comorbidities [95,96].

Since reduced GLP-1 levels are not representative for all patients, it remains to be further investigated in longitudinal studies whether a decrease in intestinal GLP-1 secretion contributes to obesity in humans. Studies in animal models are also inconsistent with reports of higher GLP-1 levels in diet-induced obese rats than in control rats [97].

Nevertheless, although obesity may affect postprandial GLP-1 secretion, obese patients are still sensitive to systematically administered GLP-1 with consequent reduced hunger ratings and slowed gastric emptying. In fact, GLP-1 receptor agonists and DPP4 inhibitors are widely used classes of anti-diabetic and/or anti-obesity agents [98,99].

4.2.3. Peptide YY

PYY is a 36-amidated amino acid peptide that is secreted by L-cells in the distal gut together with GLP-1, GLP-2 and oxyntomodulin following a meal [100]. Proteins provide the most potent stimuli for the release of PYY [57]. Immediately after an oral nutrient load, PYY levels start to rise even before the nutrients reach the distal gut, implying the involvement of a neural reflex pathway [101]. PYY_{1-36} is cleaved to PYY_{3-36} by the enzyme DPP4 immediately after secretion. PYY_{3-36} acts at Y2 receptors in the arcuate nucleus to inhibit food intake [102]. Meal-induced PYY_{3-36} release tends to be lower in obese than in lean individuals [43,57,58]. Whether peripheral PYY_{3-36} acts as a satiety signal in rodents remains controversial [102,103]. After the initial report by Batterham et al. that peripheral injection of PYY_{3-36} inhibited food intake and reduced body weight in mice but not in Y2R-null mice, several other labs (data from 1000 rodents obtained in 12 labs) failed to replicate these findings [103,104]. Stress was suggested to be a confounding factor. Nevertheless, a follow-up report showed the PYY_{3-36} reduced appetite by 30% in 12 obese and 12 lean volunteers [58].

There are currently two PYY_{3-36} compounds, PYY 1875 (Novo Nordisk) and GT-001 (Gila Therapeutics) in phase 1 trials for the treatment of obesity.

5. Altered Nutrient Sensing in Obesity

Nutrient-sensing G-protein-coupled receptors (GPCRs), similar to those in the lingual system, are present on epithelial cells in the gut and respond to luminal compounds (nutrients, bile acids, bacterial metabolites, toxins etc.) to induce a variety of biological functions [105,106]. Chemoreceptors on EECs in the gut tune the balance of appetite-regulating hormones in response to a meal. Both in vitro studies (cell lines, mucosal segments and isolated crypts) and in vivo studies (taste receptor knockout mice) have been used to demonstrate a role for taste receptors in gut hormone release [106]. For example, in the stomach protein breakdown products are sensed by the umami receptor (TAS1R1–TAS1R3) and other amino acid sensors (CaSR and GPRC6A) on P/D1-cells, to regulate the release of ghrelin [73,107]. Carbohydrate sensing (TAS1R2-TAS1R3, Na^+-glucose cotransporter type 1 (SGLT1)) occurs mainly in L-cells which secrete GLP-1 [108,109]. In addition, bitter taste receptors on EECs may represent an important target to reduce appetite [110].

The nutrient-sensing mechanisms of EECs may be affected by obesity and influence meal-related gut hormone fluctuations. The expression of amino acid sensors and bitter taste receptors in the mucosa of the human stomach and small intestine is affected by obesity in a region-dependent manner [73,74]. Similar findings were reported in HFD induced obese mice [111]. The effect of a casein hydrolysate on ghrelin release was reduced in mucosal segments of the human fundus, whereas the effect of the broadly tuned bitter agonist denatonium benzoate was apparently selectively blunted by obesity in human small intestinal—but not in fundic— segments [73,74]. Nguyen et al. showed that in morbid obesity, proximal intestinal glucose absorption is accelerated and related to increased expression of SGLT1, and may predispose to T2DM [112]. In patients with T2DM the expression of sweet taste receptors has proven to be dysregulated during acute hyperglycemia, and this may contribute to postprandial hyperglycemia [113]. Stewart et al. showed that the sensing of oleic acid by lingual and also intestinal receptors is compromised in obese patients [45]. Furthermore, the increase in plasma CCK levels in response to oleic acid tended to be reduced in the obese population.

A loss of function mutation has been observed in the long chain fatty acid receptor, FFAR4, in obese individuals that increased the risk of obesity and T2DM [114].

Thus, changes in the nutrient sensing mechanisms of EECs have been observed in obesity. The effects are region- and nutrient-specific and may, therefore, also be influenced by the diet of the obese patients. This may contribute to some of the inconsistent findings related to the effect of obesity on meal-related fluctuations in gut hormone levels.

6. Obesity Alters the Circadian Clock and the Diurnal Fluctuations in Gut Hormone Levels

Apart from meal-related fluctuations, gut hormones also show diurnal fluctuations that are regulated by the circadian clock in the hypothalamic suprachiasmatic nucleus. The most important entrainment signal of the master clock in mammals is the light–dark cycle, which inevitably determines the feeding–fasting cycle, which in turn indirectly entrains peripheral clocks via local zeitgebers such as nutrients and hormones [115]. A mismatch between the intrinsic circadian clock and behavior, as occurs during shift-work, leads to chronodisruption and is associated with several diseases including metabolic syndrome and obesity. A HFD alters the phase and amplitude of clock genes that regulate the circadian rhythm and contributes to chronodisruption [115,116]. In obese patients, the nocturnal rise in plasma ghrelin levels is blunted while the amplitude of the diurnal rhythm in leptin levels is increased [117]. GLP-1 levels peak during the day in humans, but the rhythmicity was also lost in obese patients [118]. These alterations in the dynamics of appetite-regulating hormones in obesity may alter the relationship among complex systems that regulate energy homeostasis. In humans intermittent fasting has gained popularity as a weight loss diet. Food is then only consumed within a consistent time window during the normal feeding period, thereby lengthening the daily fasting period. Enforcing nutrient utilization rhythms during chronodisruption leads to rhythmic activation of clock genes that amplify nutrient response mechanisms [119]. A recent randomized controlled trial in obese patients reported that time-restricted eating during eight weeks reduced body weight, insulin resistance and oxidative stress versus a control group that had no meal timing restrictions [120]. A similar randomized, isocaloric trial (five weeks) in men with prediabetes reported that time-restricted eating improved insulin sensitivity, blood pressure and oxidative stress even without weight loss in men [121]. It remains to be investigated whether intermittent fasting also results in a restoration of the gut hormone balance.

7. Strategies for the Management of Obesity: Role of Gut Hormones

7.1. Diet-Induced Weight Loss

Caloric restriction induces weight loss in obese individuals and restores the preprandial rise in ghrelin plasma levels [41]. Evidence from animal studies suggests that this increase in ghrelin levels may resensitize the brain and overcome ghrelin resistance to induce rebound weight gain [122]. Thus, ghrelin may act as a survival hormone to prevent further weight loss during a negative energy balance.

The effect of caloric restriction on plasma motilin levels has not been studied and has been hampered by the fact that motilin does not exist in rodents [29].

In obese patients, lower postprandial levels of GLP-1 and PYY were observed along with increased appetite scores, following an 8-week low-energy intake diet and a 2–3 week refeeding period [123]. Similarly, reductions in leptin, PYY and CCK were observed following a weight loss program with a very low energy diet which was accompanied by an increase in subjective appetite scores [124,125]. Importantly, one year after initial weight reduction, levels did not revert to levels recorded before weight loss, suggesting that alterations in gut hormone levels may facilitate regain of lost weight [124].

Interest in prebiotic supplementation with oligofructose or inulin for weight management stems from studies in rodents that reported reductions in body weight and altered gut hormone levels [126,127]. Prebiotic fibers are fermented by the gut microbiota to short chain fatty acids (SCFAs) that act on enteroendocrine cells via FFAR2 or FFAR3 to affect gut hormone release [106]. In a randomized, double-blind placebo controlled trial, oligofructose supplementation for 12 weeks reduced body weight in overweight and obese adults [128]. Ghrelin levels were reduced and PYY, but not GLP-1 levels were increased. Targeted delivery of the SCFA propionate to the colon of overweight patients with an inulin-propionate ester reduced energy intake and increased postprandial plasma PYY and GLP-1 levels in overweight patients [129]. Supplementation for 24 weeks reduced weight gain and prevented the deterioration in insulin sensitivity observed in the inulin control group. However, the rise in PYY and GLP-1 levels was not observed in the long-term study, indicating that desensitization may have occurred. A recent randomized clinical trial investigated the impact of modulation of the microbiome with isoenergetic diets that differed in their concentrations of prebiotics. The high-fiber diet selectively promoted a group of SCFA producers as the major active producers. When the SCFA producers were present in greater diversity and abundance, the improvement in haemoglobin A1c levels was greater, possibly reflecting in part increased GLP-1 production [130]. Evidence of crosstalk between the gut microbiome is also derived from studies with administration of *Akkermansia muciniphila*, known to prevent diet-induced obesity [131]. This commensal bacterium increased levels of 2-acylglycerols, endogenous cannabinoids, known to stimulate GLP-1 levels via GPR119 [132].

7.2. Roux-en-Y Gastric Bypass Surgery Restores the Gut Hormone Balance

A Roux-en-Y gastric bypass (RYGB) surgery, where the pouch of the stomach is bypassed to the small intestine, is an effective way of inducing and maintaining weight loss in morbidly obese patients. After RYGB surgery, the contact of nutrients with much of the stomach and duodenum is bypassed, resulting in a rapid delivery of undigested nutrients to the jejunum. This rerouting has been shown to affect the expression of nutrient sensors in the gut that together with other intestinal adaptations, such as changes in morphology and altered bacterial fermentation, contribute to alterations in gut hormone profiles [133–135].

Indeed, the reported weight loss with ensuing improvement in glucose homeostasis in patients undergoing RYGB surgery or sleeve gastrectomy is associated with elevated postprandial PYY and GLP-1 levels, even one year after surgery [136,137]. CCK-secreting cells are mainly located in the bypassed duodenum. In two studies, where the effect of RYGB on CCK was investigated, a faster and higher peak response towards a meal was found [137,138]. In addition, there is a possible association between the higher plasma levels of these satiety hormones and the reduced food reward system in patients after a RYGB surgery, these patients exhibit a modified behavioral and brain reward response to food [139,140].

The reported effects of RYGB surgery on plasma ghrelin levels are inconsistent with a decrease, no change or an increase reported [136]. The size of the created pouch and difficulties inherent to the measurement of biological active octanoylated ghrelin levels have contributed to this. It is therefore unlikely that ghrelin is responsible for the post-surgical metabolic improvements. Regarding the other orexigenic hormone, motilin, Deloose et al. reported decreased motilin plasma levels in parallel with hedonic hunger scores after RYGB [44]. Figure 1 summarizes the differences in gut hormone levels in obese individuals before and after RYGB surgery.

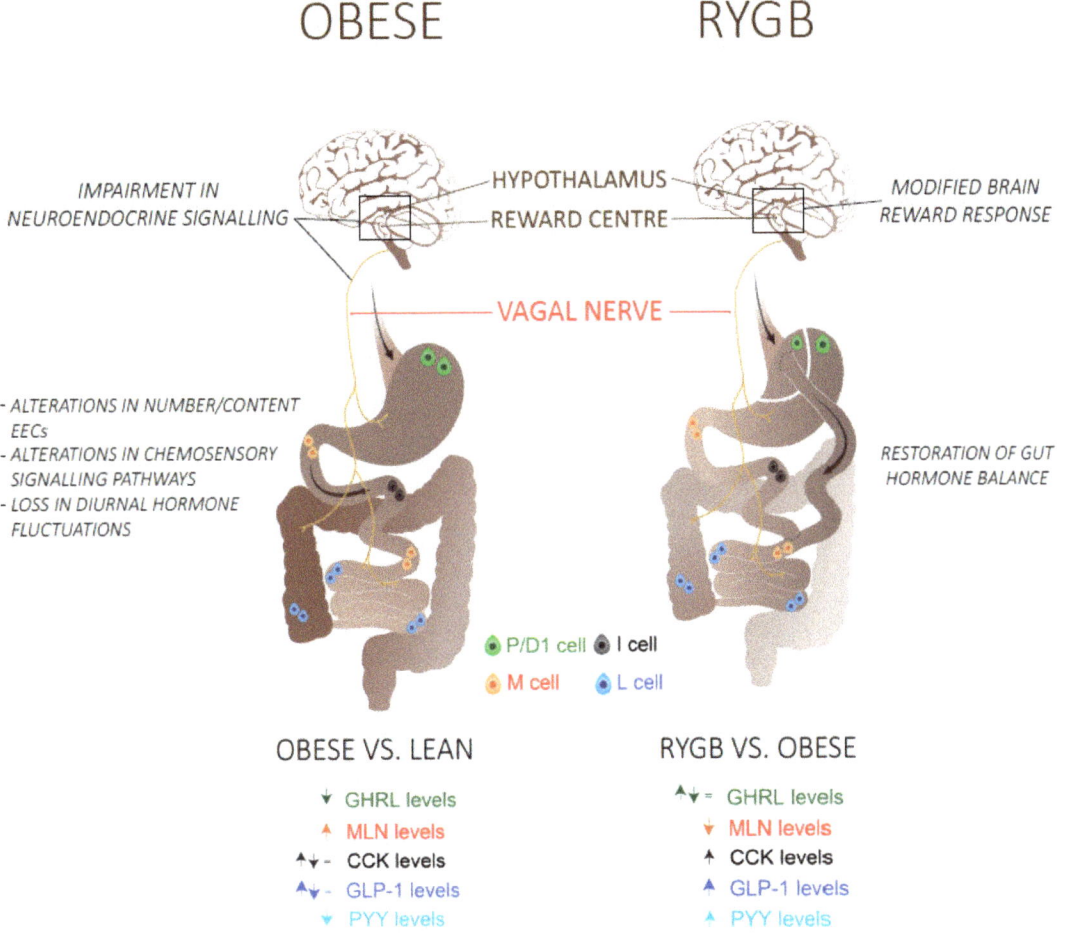

Figure 1. An overview of the mechanisms and the differences in fasting (GHRL, MLN) and postprandial (CCK, GLP-1, PYY) gut hormone plasma levels in obese/type 2 diabetes patients before and after a Roux-en-Y gastric bypass (RYGB) surgery. Abbreviations: GHRL: Ghrelin; MLN: Motilin; CCK: Cholecystokinin; GLP-1: glucagon-like peptide 1; peptide YY.

7.3. Combination Therapy

GLP-1R agonists are used widely to treat T2DM. Liraglutide, which is administered once a day, was until now the only GLP-1 receptor (GLP-1R) agonist to be approved for weight management [141]. Recently, Semaglutide, a long acting GLP-1R agonist, has proven to be effective in weight management as an adjunct to lifestyle by inducing 14.9% weight loss from baseline in overweight and obese individuals [142]. Combined agonism, mostly by combining GLP-1 analogues with other food intake-inhibiting and/or glucose-lowering hormones, may cause a synergistic pharmacological action in obese individuals and patients with T2DM. Therefore, combination therapy is currently considered as the way to go to mimic the beneficial effects of RYGB surgery in a non-surgical manner [143]. Table 2 gives an overview of several combinations with GLP-1R analogues that are currently in clinical trial.

Table 2. An overview of several combination therapies with GLP-1R agonists that are currently in clinical trials.

Combination Therapy	Physiological Effect	Drug Candidates		
GLP-1–GIP	Insulinotropic effect Decrease food intake cardiovascular protection	Drug	Company	Status
		Tirzepatide	Eli Lilly	Phase II
GLP-1–GCG	Insulinotropic effect cardiovascular protection Decrease food intake Increase energy expenditure	Drug	Company	Status
		Cotadutide	Astrazeneca	Phase II
		Efinopegdutide	Hanmi Pharmaceuticals	Phase II
GLP-1–GCG-GIP	Insulinotropic effect Increase energy expenditure cardiovascular protection Decrease food intake	Drug	Company	Status
		MAR423	Novo-nordisk/Marcadia	Phase I
		HM15211	Hanmi Pharmacueticals	Phase II

Glucagon-like-peptide 1 (GLP-1), glucose-dependent insulinotropic peptide (GIP), glucagon (GCG).

7.3.1. GLP-1 and GIP

Glucose-dependent insulinotropic peptide (GIP) is an incretin hormone that is secreted by K-cells in response to nutrients to stimulate insulin secretion through activation of GIP receptors on pancreatic beta cells, and acts as a blood glucose stabilising hormone by regulating insulin and glucagon secretion [144,145]. GIP also exerts direct actions on lipid metabolism, promoting lipogenesis and weight gain, and GIPR agonists have been demonstrated to exacerbate the postprandial glucagon excursion in individuals with T2DM [146]. Therefore, GIP receptor (GIPR) antagonists were initially developed to induce weight loss and to control glycaemia levels in obesity and individuals with T2DM [147]. Even though individuals with T2DM have a decreased insulinotropic effect of GIP, due to impaired responsiveness by beta cells, the loss of GIP has been shown to enhance GLP-1R activity [55,148]. Evidence suggests that GIPR agonism can also positively impact body weight. A recent study showed that injection of a peripherally long acting, selective mouse GIPR agonist in DIO mice, lowered body weight due to reduced food intake [149]. Therefore, dual agonism of GLP-1R, which exerts glycaemic control, and GIPR represents a strategy in treating obesity and T2DM. Coadministration of the selective GIP receptor agonist, ZP4165, together with the GLP-1R agonist, liraglutide, in DIO mice resulted in superior body weight loss and improved blood glucose and plasma cholesterol levels [150]. Currently, tirzepatide, a dual-incretin peptide from Eli Lilly, has reached multi-dose clinical trials and shows promise in the treatment of obesity and T2DM [151].

7.3.2. GLP-1 and GCG

The use of glucagon (GCG) with GLP-1 may intuitively appear contradictory since it antagonizes the effect of insulin and increases glucose levels, evoking hyperglycaemia. Nevertheless, glucagon also induces thermogenesis, increases energy expenditure and has hypolipidemic effects, which are beneficial for weight management in obese individuals [152]. Moreover, while chronic GCG stimulation exhibits glucose intolerance, acute GCG agonism at a lower dose, which is not able to evoke hyperglycaemia, enhances glucose tolerance and improves insulin sensitivity [153]. This suggests the use of GLP1-GCG dual agonists in not only obesity, but also in T2DM. Many preclinical studies have demonstrated the body weight and glucose lowering effects of GLP-1R/GCGR agonists. For example, a single high-dose or multiple low-dose injections of a GLP-1R/GCGR dual agonist induced body weight loss which was associated with increased energy expenditure and thermogenesis [154]. However, the effect of GLP-1R/GCGR dual agonists on body weight in human studies has not yet been found as effective as in animal studies. Cotadutide, a novel dual agonist by AstraZeneca, demonstrated superior results in body weight reduction relative to the GLP-1R agonist liraglutide during preclinical studies in DIO mice and normal weight cynomolgus monkeys [155]. Currently, results from Phase II clinical trials with cotadutide demonstrated beneficial effects on blood glucose levels, changes in liver fat and glycogen stores in patients with T2DM [156].

Oxyntomodulin (OXM) is a naturally occurring GLP1R/GCGR dual agonist that is secreted by L-cells after food intake to induce satiety and increase energy expenditure [157]. As native OXM has a very short half-life due to degradation by DPP4 and fast renal clearance, OXM analogues are being developed as a therapeutic candidate to treat obesity and T2DM. Recently, a PEGylated analogue showed a 27.1% body weight reduction at a high dose in DIO mice, which was significantly higher than the weight loss effect with liraglutide [158].

7.3.3. GLP-1 and PYY$_{3-36}$

The combination of GLP-1 analogue with PYY$_{3-36}$ mainly has a role in body weight management. Co-infusion of PYY$_{3-36}$ and GLP-1 reduced energy intake by 30% compared to placebo in overweight men, which was not achieved when a mono-infusion was administered of PYY$_{3-36}$ or GLP-1 [159]. In addition, co-administration of PYY$_{3-36}$ with oxyntomodulin reduced energy intake by 42.7% in overweight and obese volunteers, and the effect was more pronounced than when either hormone was infused separately [160]. No drugs are yet in clinical trials for combinations with PYY$_{3-36}$.

7.3.4. GLP-1, GCG and GIP

The combination of three gut hormones, triagonists, have emerged as new way of inducing multiple metabolic improvements. An acylated GLP-1R/GCGR/GIPR triagonist exerted in vivo and in vitro receptor activity in rodents with superior metabolic effects, improved glycaemic control and body weight loss, relative to their co-agonists [161]. HM15211 (Hanmi Pharmaceuticals) is a triagonist with high GCG activity for obesity treatment and a balanced GLP-1 and GIP activity, to neutralize the hyperglycemic risk of GCG. Preclinical studies with HM15211 have shown improved weight loss, reduced liver fat and possibly inflammation, and may be effective for the treatment of non-alcoholic fatty liver disease as well [162]. HM15211 is currently in phase II clinical trials with a 30% reduction of liver fat in comparison to placebo after a 12-month treatment [163].

Multi-agonists are the next generation of therapies to treat patients with T2DM and obesity. They avoid the adverse effects of surgery (malnutrition, post-prandial hypoglycaemia, bowel obstruction, etc.) and GLP1R agonists (gastrointestinal symptoms). Multi-agonists can therefore be a solution for these individuals as a way to manage body weight.

8. Conclusions

Gut hormones are important players in the regulation of appetite. Obesity has a clear impact on fasted and meal-related fluctuations in gut hormone release but the effect on some hormones remains controversial. The mechanisms involved are complex and multifactorial, relating to changes in the number/content of EECs, effect of age and gender, alterations in nutrients' sensing mechanisms that regulate postprandial responses, alterations in diurnal fluctuations, and may also involve alterations in the central responsiveness to gut hormones. Further exploration of the crosstalk between the gut microbiome and EECs is of interest. Restoring the disordered gut hormone balance in obesity by targeting nutrient sensors in selective regions of the gut or by combined administration of gut peptide mimetics represent a major potential therapeutic targets to improve the prevention and management of obesity.

Funding: This work was supported by a Methusalem grant from the KU Leuven. The funder of the study had no role in writing of the review.

Conflicts of Interest: The authors declare no conflict of interest.

References

1. Ng, M.; Fleming, T.; Robinson, M.; Thomson, B.; Graetz, N.; Margono, C.; Mullany, E.C.; Biryukov, S.; Abbafati, C.; Abera, S.F.; et al. Global, regional, and national prevalence of overweight and obesity in children and adults during 1980–2013: A systematic analysis for the global burden of disease study 2013. *Lancet* **2014**, *384*, 766–781. [CrossRef]
2. World Health Organization. Obesity. Obesity and Overweight. 2020. Available online: who.int (accessed on 1 January 2021).
3. Spiegelman, B.M.; Flier, J.S. Obesity and the regulation of energy balance. *Cell* **2001**, *104*, 531–543. [CrossRef]
4. Weinsier, R.L.; Hunter, G.R.; Heini, A.F.; Goran, M.I.; Sell, S.M. The etiology of obesity: Relative contribution of metabolic factors, diet, and physical activity. *Am. J. Med.* **1998**, *105*, 145–150. [CrossRef]
5. Rohde, K.; Keller, M.; Poulsen, L.L.C.; Blüher, M.; Kovacs, P.; Böttcher, Y. Genetics and epigenetics in obesity. *Metabolism* **2019**, *92*, 37–50. [CrossRef] [PubMed]
6. Montague, C.T.; Farooqi, I.S.; Whitehead, J.; Soos, M.A.; Rau, H.; Wareham, N.J.; Sewter, C.P.; Digby, J.E.; Mohammed, S.N.; Hurst, J.A.; et al. Congenital leptin deficiency is associated with severe early-onset obesity in humans. *Nature* **1997**, *387*, 903–908. [CrossRef]
7. Cuevas-Sierra, A.; Ramos-Lopez, O.; Riezu-Boj, J.I.; Milagro, F.I.; Martinez, J.A. Diet, gut microbiota, and obesity: Links with host genetics and epigenetics and potential applications. *Adv. Nutr.* **2019**, *10*, S17–S30. [CrossRef]
8. Neary, N.M.; Goldstone, A.P.; Bloom, S.R. Appetite regulation: From the gut to the hypothalamus. *Clin. Endocrinol.* **2004**, *60*, 153–160. [CrossRef] [PubMed]
9. Suzuki, K.; Simpson, K.A.; Minnion, J.; Shillito, J.C.; Bloom, S.R. The role of gut hormones and the hypothalamus in appetite regulation. *Endocr. J.* **2010**, *57*, 359–372. [CrossRef] [PubMed]
10. Owyang, C.; Heldsinger, A. Vagal control of satiety and hormonal regulation of appetite. *J. Neurogastroenterol. Motil.* **2011**, *17*, 338–348. [CrossRef] [PubMed]
11. Niswender, K.D.; Schwartz, M.W. Insulin and leptin revisited: Adiposity signals with overlapping physiological and intracellular signaling capabilities. *Front. Neuroendocrinol.* **2003**, *24*, 1–10. [CrossRef]
12. Quan, W.; Kim, H.-K.; Moon, E.-Y.; Kim, S.S.; Choi, C.S.; Komatsu, M.; Jeong, Y.T.; Lee, M.-K.; Kim, K.-W.; Kim, M.-S.; et al. Role of hypothalamic proopiomelanocortin neuron autophagy in the control of appetite and leptin response. *Endocrinology* **2012**, *153*, 1817–1826. [CrossRef] [PubMed]
13. Cummings, D.E.; Purnell, J.Q.; Frayo, R.S.; Schmidova, K.; Wisse, B.E.; Weigle, D.S. A preprandial rise in plasma ghrelin levels suggests a role in meal initiation in humans. *Diabetes* **2001**, *50*, 1714–1719. [CrossRef]
14. Deloose, E.; Verbeure, W.; Depoortere, I.; Tack, J. Motilin: From gastric motility stimulation to hunger signalling. *Nat. Rev. Endocrinol.* **2019**, *15*, 238–250. [CrossRef]
15. Tack, J.; Deloose, E.; Ang, D.; Scarpellini, E.; Vanuytsel, T.; Van Oudenhove, L.; Depoortere, I. Motilin-induced gastric contractions signal hunger in man. *Gut* **2016**, *65*, 214–224. [CrossRef] [PubMed]
16. Müller, T.D.; Finan, B.; Bloom, S.R.; D'Alessio, D.; Drucker, D.J.; Flatt, P.R.; Fritsche, A.; Gribble, F.; Grill, H.J.; Habener, J.F.; et al. Glucagon-like peptide 1 (GLP-1). *Mol. Metab.* **2019**, *30*, 72–130. [CrossRef] [PubMed]
17. Rehfeld, J.F. Cholecystokinin-from local gut hormone to ubiquitous messenger. *Front. Endocrinol.* **2017**, *8*, 47. [CrossRef] [PubMed]
18. Manning, S.; Batterham, R.L. The role of gut hormone peptide YY in energy and glucose homeostasis: Twelve years on. *Ann. Rev. Physiol.* **2014**, *76*, 585–608. [CrossRef] [PubMed]
19. Vahl, T.P.; Drazen, D.L.; Seeley, R.J.; D'Alessio, D.A.; Woods, S.C. Meal-anticipatory glucagon-like peptide-1 secretion in rats. *Endocrinology* **2010**, *151*, 569–575. [CrossRef]
20. Veedfald, S.; Plamboeck, A.; Deacon, C.F.; Hartmann, B.; Knop, F.K.; Vilsboll, T.; Holst, J.J. Cephalic phase secretion of insulin and other enteropancreatic hormones in humans. *Am. J. Physiol.* **2016**, *310*, G43–G51. [CrossRef] [PubMed]
21. Powley, T.L.; Phillips, R.J. Gastric satiation is volumetric, intestinal satiation is nutritive. *Physiol. Behav.* **2004**, *82*, 69–74. [CrossRef]
22. Page, A.J.; Kentish, S.J. Plasticity of gastrointestinal vagal afferent satiety signals. *Neurogastroenterol. Motil.* **2017**, *29*, e12973. [CrossRef]
23. Bai, L.; Mesgarzadeh, S.; Ramesh, K.S.; Huey, E.L.; Liu, Y.; Gray, L.A.; Aitken, T.J.; Chen, Y.; Beutler, L.; Ahn, J.S.; et al. Genetic identification of vagal sensory neurons that control feeding. *Cell* **2019**, *179*, 1129–1143.e23. [CrossRef] [PubMed]
24. Noah, T.K.; Donahue, B.; Shroyer, N.F. Intestinal development and differentiation. *Exp. Cell Res.* **2011**, *317*, 2702–2710. [CrossRef] [PubMed]
25. Egerod, K.L.; Engelstoft, M.S.; Grunddal, K.V.; Nøhr, M.K.; Secher, A.; Sakata, I.; Pedersen, J.; Windeløv, J.A.; Füchtbauer, E.-M.; Olsen, J.; et al. A major lineage of enteroendocrine cells coexpress CCK, secretin, GIP, GLP-1, PYY, and neurotensin but not somatostatin. *Endocrinology* **2012**, *153*, 5782–5795. [CrossRef]
26. Habib, A.M.; Richards, P.; Cairns, L.S.; Rogers, G.J.; Bannon, C.A.; Parker, H.E.; Morley, T.C.; Yeo, G.S.; Reimann, F.; Gribble, F.M. Overlap of endocrine hormone expression in the mouse intestine revealed by transcriptional profiling and flow cytometry. *Endocrinology* **2012**, *153*, 3054–3065. [CrossRef]
27. Gehart, H.; van Es, J.H.; Hamer, K.; Beumer, J.; Kretzschmar, K.; Dekkers, J.F.; Rios, A.; Clevers, H. Identification of enteroendocrine regulators by real-time single-cell differentiation mapping. *Cell* **2019**, *176*, 1158–1173.e16. [CrossRef]
28. Beumer, J.; Puschhof, J.; Martinez, J.B.; Martínez-Silgado, A.; Elmentaite, R.; James, K.R.; Ross, A.; Hendriks, D.; Artegiani, B.; Busslinger, G.A.; et al. High-resolution mRNA and secretome atlas of human enteroendocrine cells. *Cell* **2020**, *182*, 1062–1064. [CrossRef]

29. He, J.; Irwin, D.M.; Chen, R.; Zhang, Y.-P. Stepwise loss of motilin and its specific receptor genes in rodents. *J. Mol. Endocrinol.* **2010**, *44*, 37–44. [CrossRef] [PubMed]
30. Beumer, J.; Artegiani, B.; Post, Y.; Reimann, F.; Gribble, F.; Nguyen, T.N.; Zeng, H.; Van den Born, M.; Van Es, J.H.; Clevers, H. Enteroendocrine cells switch hormone expression along the crypt-to-villus BMP signalling gradient. *Nat. Cell Biol.* **2018**, *20*, 909–916. [CrossRef] [PubMed]
31. Farooqi, I.S.; O'Rahilly, S. 20 years of leptin: Human disorders of leptin action. *J. Endocrinol.* **2014**, *223*, T63–T70. [CrossRef]
32. Heymsfield, S.B.; Greenberg, A.S.; Fujioka, K.; Dixon, R.M.; Kushner, R.; Hunt, T.; Lubina, J.A.; Patane, J.; Self, B.; Hunt, P.; et al. Recombinant leptin for weight loss in obese and lean adults: A randomized, controlled, dose-escalation trial. *JAMA* **1999**, *282*, 1568–1575. [CrossRef] [PubMed]
33. Ye, Z.; Liu, G.; Guo, J.; Su, Z. Hypothalamic endoplasmic reticulum stress as a key mediator of obesity-induced leptin resistance. *Obes. Rev.* **2018**, *19*, 770–785. [CrossRef] [PubMed]
34. Chellappa, K.; Perron, I.J.; Naidoo, N.; Baur, J.A. The leptin sensitizer celastrol reduces age-associated obesity and modulates behavioral rhythms. *Aging Cell* **2019**, *18*, e12874. [CrossRef]
35. De Lartigue, G.; Diepenbroek, C. Novel developments in vagal afferent nutrient sensing and its role in energy homeostasis. *Curr. Opin. Pharmacol.* **2016**, *31*, 38–43. [CrossRef] [PubMed]
36. De Lartigue, G.; Ronveaux, C.C.; Raybould, H.E. Deletion of leptin signaling in vagal afferent neurons results in hyperphagia and obesity. *Mol. Metab.* **2014**, *3*, 595–607. [CrossRef] [PubMed]
37. Kentish, S.J.; O'Donnell, T.A.; Isaacs, N.J.; Young, R.L.; Li, H.; Harrington, A.; Brierley, S.M.; Wittert, G.; Blackshaw, L.A.; Page, A.J. Gastric vagal afferent modulation by leptin is influenced by food intake status. *J. Physiol.* **2013**, *591*, 1921–1934. [CrossRef] [PubMed]
38. Tschöp, M.; Weyer, C.; Tataranni, P.A.; Devanarayan, V.; Ravussin, E.; Heiman, M.L. Circulating ghrelin levels are decreased in human obesity. *Diabetes* **2001**, *50*, 707–709. [CrossRef] [PubMed]
39. English, P.J.; Ghatei, M.A.; Malik, I.A.; Wilding, J.P. Food fails to suppress ghrelin levels in obese humans. *J. Clin. Endocrinol. Metab.* **2002**, *87*, 2984. [CrossRef]
40. Dadan, J.; Hady, H.R.; Zbucki, R.L.; Iwacewicz, P.; Bossowski, A.; Kasacka, I. The activity of gastric ghrelin positive cells in obese patients treated surgically. *Folia Histochem. Cytobiol.* **2009**, *47*, 307–313. [CrossRef]
41. Cummings, D.E.; Weigle, D.S.; Frayo, R.S.; Breen, P.A.; Ma, M.K.; Dellinger, E.P.; Purnell, J.Q. Plasma ghrelin levels after diet-induced weight loss or gastric bypass surgery. *N. Engl. J. Med.* **2002**, *346*, 1623–1630. [CrossRef]
42. Shiiya, T.; Nakazato, M.; Mizuta, M.; Date, Y.; Mondal, M.S.; Tanaka, M.; Nozoe, S.; Hosoda, H.; Kangawa, K.; Matsukura, S. Plasma ghrelin levels in lean and obese humans and the effect of glucose on ghrelin secretion. *J. Clin. Endocrinol. Metab.* **2002**, *87*, 240–244. [CrossRef]
43. Zwirska-Korczala, K.; Konturek, S.J.; Sodowski, M.; Wylezol, M.; Kuka, D.; Sowa, P.; Adamczyk-Sowa, M.; Kukla, M.; Berdowska, A.; Rehfeld, J.F.; et al. Basal and postprandial plasma levels of PYY, ghrelin, cholecystokinin, gastrin and insulin in women with moderate and morbid obesity and metabolic syndrome. *J. Physiol. Pharmacol.* **2007**, *58* (Suppl. 1), 13–35.
44. Deloose, E.; Janssen, P.; Lannoo, M.; Van Der Schueren, B.; Depoortere, I.; Tack, J. Higher plasma motilin levels in obese patients decrease after Roux-en-Y gastric bypass surgery and regulate hunger. *Gut* **2016**, *65*, 1110–1118. [CrossRef] [PubMed]
45. Stewart, J.E.; Seimon, R.V.; Otto, B.; Keast, R.S.; Clifton, P.M.; Feinle-Bisset, C. Marked differences in gustatory and gastrointestinal sensitivity to oleic acid between lean and obese men. *Am. J. Clin. Nutr.* **2011**, *93*, 703–711. [CrossRef]
46. French, S.J.; Murray, B.; Rumsey, R.D.; Sepple, C.P.; Read, N.W. Preliminary studies on the gastrointestinal responses to fatty meals in obese people. *Int. J. Obes. Relat. Metab. Disord.* **1993**, *17*, 295–300. [PubMed]
47. Brennan, I.M.; Luscombe-Marsh, N.D.; Seimon, R.V.; Otto, B.; Horowitz, M.; Wishart, J.M.; Feinle-Bisset, C. Effects of fat, protein, and carbohydrate and protein load on appetite, plasma cholecystokinin, peptide YY, and ghrelin, and energy intake in lean and obese men. *Am. J. Physiol. Gastrointest. Liver Physiol.* **2012**, *303*, G129–G140. [CrossRef]
48. Faerch, K.; Torekov, S.; Vistisen, D.; Johansen, N.B.; Witte, D.R.; Jonsson, A.; Pedersen, O.; Hansen, T.; Lauritzen, T.; Sandbaek, A.; et al. GLP-1 response to oral glucose is reduced in prediabetes, screen-detected type 2 diabetes, and obesity and influenced by sex: The addition-pro study. *Diabetes* **2015**, *64*, 2513–2525. [CrossRef] [PubMed]
49. Ranganath, L.R.; Beety, J.M.; Morgan, L.M.; Wright, J.W.; Howland, R.; Marks, V. Attenuated GLP-1 secretion in obesity: Cause or consequence? *Gut* **1996**, *38*, 916–919. [CrossRef]
50. Vilsboll, T.; Krarup, T.; Deacon, C.F.; Madsbad, S.; Holst, J.J. Reduced postprandial concentrations of intact biologically active glucagon-like peptide 1 in type 2 diabetic patients. *Diabetes* **2001**, *50*, 609–613. [CrossRef] [PubMed]
51. Verdich, C.; Toubro, S.; Buemann, B.; Madsen, J.L.; Holst, J.J.; Astrup, A. The role of postprandial releases of insulin and incretin hormones in meal-induced satiety–effect of obesity and weight reduction. *Int. J. Obes. Relat. Metab. Disord.* **2001**, *25*, 1206–1214. [CrossRef]
52. Toft-Nielsen, M.B.; Damholt, M.B.; Madsbad, S.; Hilsted, L.M.; Hughes, T.E.; Michelsen, B.K.; Holst, J.J. Determinants of the impaired secretion of glucagon-like peptide-1 in type 2 diabetic patients. *J. Clin. Endocrinol. Metab.* **2001**, *86*, 3717–3723. [CrossRef]
53. Fukase, N.; Manaka, H.; Sugiyama, K.; Takahashi, H.; Igarashi, M.; Daimon, M.; Yamatani, K.; Tominaga, M.; Sasaki, H. Response of truncated glucagon-like peptide-1 and gastric inhibitory polypeptide to glucose ingestion in non-insulin dependent diabetes mellitus. Effect of sulfonylurea therapy. *Acta Diabetol.* **1995**, *32*, 165–169. [CrossRef]

54. Lee, S.; Yabe, D.; Nohtomi, K.; Takada, M.; Morita, R.; Seino, Y.; Hirano, T. Intact glucagon-like peptide-1 levels are not decreased in Japanese patients with type 2 diabetes. *Endocr. J.* **2010**, *57*, 119–126. [CrossRef] [PubMed]
55. Nauck, M.A.; Heimesaat, M.M.; Orskov, C.; Holst, J.J.; Ebert, R.; Creutzfeldt, W. Preserved incretin activity of glucagon-like peptide 1 [7–36 amide] but not of synthetic human gastric inhibitory polypeptide in patients with type-2 diabetes mellitus. *J. Clin. Investig.* **1993**, *91*, 301–307. [CrossRef] [PubMed]
56. Vollmer, K.; Holst, J.J.; Baller, B.; Ellrichmann, M.; Nauck, M.A.; Schmidt, W.E.; Meier, J.J. Predictors of incretin concentrations in subjects with normal, impaired, and diabetic glucose tolerance. *Diabetes* **2008**, *57*, 678–687. [CrossRef] [PubMed]
57. Batterham, R.L.; Heffron, H.; Kapoor, S.; Chivers, J.E.; Chandarana, K.; Herzog, H.; le Roux, C.W.; Thomas, E.L.; Bell, J.D.; Withers, D.J. Critical role for peptide YY in protein-mediated satiation and body-weight regulation. *Cell Metab.* **2006**, *4*, 223–233. [CrossRef]
58. Batterham, R.L.; Cohen, M.A.; Ellis, S.M.; Le Roux, C.W.; Withers, D.J.; Frost, G.S.; Ghatei, M.A.; Bloom, S.R. Inhibition of food intake in obese subjects by peptide YY3-36. *N. Engl. J. Med.* **2003**, *349*, 941–948. [CrossRef]
59. Gutierrez, J.A.; Solenberg, P.J.; Perkins, D.R.; Willency, J.A.; Knierman, M.D.; Jin, Z.; Witcher, D.R.; Luo, S.; Onyia, J.E.; Hale, J.E. Ghrelin octanoylation mediated by an orphan lipid transferase. *Proc. Natl. Acad. Sci. USA* **2008**, *105*, 6320–6325. [CrossRef]
60. Kojima, M.; Hosoda, H.; Date, Y.; Nakazato, M.; Matsuo, H.; Kangawa, K. Ghrelin is a growth-hormone-releasing acylated peptide from stomach. *Nature* **1999**, *402*, 656–660. [CrossRef]
61. Nakazato, M.; Murakami, N.; Date, Y.; Kojima, M.; Matsuo, H.; Kangawa, K.; Matsukura, S. A role for ghrelin in the central regulation of feeding. *Nature* **2001**, *409*, 194–198. [CrossRef]
62. Diano, S.; A Farr, S.; Benoit, S.C.; McNay, E.C.; Da Silva, I.; Horvath, B.; Gaskin, F.S.; Nonaka, N.; Jaeger, L.B.; A Banks, W.; et al. Ghrelin controls hippocampal spine synapse density and memory performance. *Nat. Neurosci.* **2006**, *9*, 381–388. [CrossRef] [PubMed]
63. Abizaid, A.; Liu, Z.-W.; Andrews, Z.B.; Shanabrough, M.; Borok, E.; Elsworth, J.D.; Roth, R.H.; Sleeman, M.W.; Picciotto, M.R.; Tschöp, M.H.; et al. Ghrelin modulates the activity and synaptic input organization of midbrain dopamine neurons while promoting appetite. *J. Clin. Investig.* **2006**, *116*, 3229–3239. [CrossRef]
64. Malik, S.; McGlone, F.; Bedrossian, D.; Dagher, A. Ghrelin modulates brain activity in areas that control appetitive behavior. *Cell Metab.* **2008**, *7*, 400–409. [CrossRef] [PubMed]
65. Zhao, T.-J.; Sakata, I.; Li, R.L.; Liang, G.; Richardson, J.A.; Brown, M.S.; Goldstein, J.L.; Zigman, J.M. Ghrelin secretion stimulated by {beta}1-adrenergic receptors in cultured ghrelinoma cells and in fasted mice. *Proc. Natl. Acad. Sci. USA* **2010**, *107*, 15868–15873. [CrossRef]
66. Mani, B.K.; Osborne-Lawrence, S.; Vijayaraghavan, P.; Hepler, C.; Zigman, J.M. β1-Adrenergic receptor deficiency in ghrelin-expressing cells causes hypoglycemia in susceptible individuals. *J. Clin. Investig.* **2016**, *126*, 3467–3478. [CrossRef] [PubMed]
67. Foster-Schubert, K.E.; Overduin, J.; Prudom, C.E.; Liu, J.; Callahan, H.S.; Gaylinn, B.D.; Thorner, M.O.; Cummings, D.E. Acyl and total ghrelin are suppressed strongly by ingested proteins, weakly by lipids, and biphasically by carbohydrates. *J. Clin. Endocrinol. Metab.* **2008**, *93*, 1971–1979. [CrossRef] [PubMed]
68. Callahan, H.S.; Cummings, D.E.; Pepe, M.S.; Breen, P.A.; Matthys, C.C.; Weigle, D.S. Postprandial suppression of plasma ghrelin level is proportional to ingested caloric load but does not predict intermeal interval in humans. *J. Clin. Endocrinol. Metab.* **2004**, *89*, 1319–1324. [CrossRef] [PubMed]
69. Kweh, F.A.; Miller, J.L.; Sulsona, C.R.; Wasserfall, C.; Atkinson, M.; Shuster, J.J.; Goldstone, A.P.; Driscoll, D.J. Hyperghrelinemia in Prader-Willi syndrome begins in early infancy long before the onset of hyperphagia. *Am. J. Med. Genet. A* **2015**, *167A*, 69–79. [CrossRef]
70. Cassidy, S.B.; Schwartz, S.; Miller, J.L.; Driscoll, D.J. Prader-Willi syndrome. *Genet. Med.* **2012**, *14*, 10–26. [CrossRef] [PubMed]
71. Widmayer, P.; Küper, M.; Kramer, M.; Königsrainer, A.; Breer, H. Altered expression of gustatory-signaling elements in gastric tissue of morbidly obese patients. *Int. J. Obes.* **2012**, *36*, 1353–1359. [CrossRef] [PubMed]
72. Ritze, Y.; Schollenberger, A.; Sinno, M.H.; Bühler, N.; Böhle, M.; Bárdos, G.; Sauer, H.; Mack, I.; Enck, P.; Zipfel, S.; et al. Gastric ghrelin, GOAT, leptin, and leptinR expression as well as peripheral serotonin are dysregulated in humans with obesity. *Neurogastroenterol. Motil.* **2016**, *28*, 806–815. [CrossRef] [PubMed]
73. Vancleef, L.; Thijs, T.; Baert, F.; Ceulemans, L.J.; Canovai, E.; Wang, Q.; Steensels, S.; Segers, A.; Farré, R.; Pirenne, J.; et al. Obesity impairs oligopeptide/amino acid-induced ghrelin release and smooth muscle contractions in the human proximal stomach. *Mol. Nutr. Food Res.* **2018**, *62*, 62. [CrossRef] [PubMed]
74. Wang, Q.; Liszt, K.I.; Deloose, E.; Canovai, E.; Thijs, T.; Farré, R.; Ceulemans, L.; Lannoo, M.; Tack, J.; Depoortere, I. Obesity alters adrenergic and chemosensory signaling pathways that regulate ghrelin secretion in the human gut. *FASEB J.* **2019**, *33*, 4907–4920. [CrossRef]
75. Uchida, A.; Zechner, J.F.; Mani, B.K.; Park, W.-M.; Aguirre, V.; Zigman, J.M. Altered ghrelin secretion in mice in response to diet-induced obesity and Roux-en-Y gastric bypass. *Mol. Metab.* **2014**, *3*, 717–730. [CrossRef] [PubMed]
76. Zigman, J.M.; Bouret, S.G.; Andrews, Z.B. Obesity impairs the action of the neuroendocrine ghrelin system. *Trends Endocrinol. Metab.* **2016**, *27*, 54–63. [CrossRef]
77. Mani, B.K.; Puzziferri, N.; He, Z.; Rodriguez, J.A.; Osborne-Lawrence, S.; Metzger, N.P.; Chhina, N.; Gaylinn, B.; Thorner, M.O.; Thomas, E.L.; et al. LEAP2 changes with body mass and food intake in humans and mice. *J. Clin. Investig.* **2019**, *129*, 3909–3923. [CrossRef]

78. Druce, M.R.; Wren, A.M.; Park, A.J.; Milton, J.E.; Patterson, M.; Frost, G.; Ghatei, M.A.; Small, C.; Bloom, S.R. Ghrelin increases food intake in obese as well as lean subjects. *Int. J. Obes.* **2005**, *29*, 1130–1136. [CrossRef] [PubMed]
79. Brown, J.C.; Cook, M.A.; Dryburgh, J.R. Motilin, a gastric motor activity-stimulating polypeptide: Final purification, amino acid composition, and C-terminal residues. *Gastroenterology* **1972**, *62*, 401–404. [CrossRef]
80. Tomasetto, C.; Wendling, C.; Rio, M.-C.; Poitras, P. Identification of cDNA encoding motilin related peptide/ghrelin precursor from dog fundus. *Peptides* **2001**, *22*, 2055–2059. [CrossRef]
81. Deloose, E.; Janssen, P.; Depoortere, I.; Tack, J. The migrating motor complex: Control mechanisms and its role in health and disease. *Nat. Rev. Gastroenterol. Hepatol.* **2012**, *9*, 271–285. [CrossRef] [PubMed]
82. Pieramico, O.; Malfertheiner, P.; Nelson, D.K.; Glasbrenner, B.; Ditschuneit, H. Interdigestive gastroduodenal motility and cycling of putative regulatory hormones in severe obesity. *Scand. J. Gastroenterol.* **1992**, *27*, 538–544. [CrossRef] [PubMed]
83. Koop, I.; Schindler, M.; Bosshammer, A.; Scheibner, J.; Stange, E.; Koop, H. Physiological control of cholecystokinin release and pancreatic enzyme secretion by intraduodenal bile acids. *Gut* **1996**, *39*, 661–667. [CrossRef] [PubMed]
84. Rogers, R.C.; Hermann, G.E. Mechanisms of action of CCK to activate central vagal afferent terminals. *Peptides* **2008**, *29*, 1716–1725. [CrossRef]
85. Fried, M.; Erlacher, U.; Schwizer, W.; Löchner, C.; Koerfer, J.; Beglinger, C.; Jansen, J.B.; Lamers, C.B.; Harder, F.; Bischof-Delaloye, A.; et al. Role of cholecystokinin in the regulation of gastric emptying and pancreatic enzyme secretion in humans. Studies with the cholecystokinin-receptor antagonist loxiglumide. *Gastroenterology* **1991**, *101*, 503–511. [CrossRef]
86. Ahrén, B.; Holst, J.J.; Efendic, S. Antidiabetogenic action of cholecystokinin-8 in type 2 diabetes. *J. Clin. Endocrinol. Metab.* **2000**, *85*, 1043–1048. [CrossRef] [PubMed]
87. De Krom, M.; van der Schouw, Y.T.; Hendriks, J.; Ophoff, R.A.; van Gils, C.H.; Stolk, R.P.; Grobbee, D.E.; Adan, R. Common genetic variations in CCK, leptin, and leptin receptor genes are associated with specific human eating patterns. *Diabetes* **2007**, *56*, 276–280. [CrossRef] [PubMed]
88. Marchal-Victorion, S.; Vionnet, N.; Escrieut, C.; Dematos, F.; Dina, C.; Dufresne, M.; Vaysse, N.; Pradayrol, L.; Froguel, P.; Fourmy, D. Genetic, pharmacological and functional analysis of cholecystokinin-1 and cholecystokinin-2 receptor polymorphism in type 2 diabetes and obese patients. *Pharmacogenetics* **2002**, *12*, 23–30. [CrossRef]
89. Lieverse, R.J.; Jansen, J.B.; A Masclee, A.; Lamers, C.B. Satiety effects of a physiological dose of cholecystokinin in humans. *Gut* **1995**, *36*, 176–179. [CrossRef]
90. Jordan, J.; Greenway, F.; Leiter, L.; Li, Z.; Jacobson, P.; Murphy, K.; Hill, J.; Kler, L.; Aftring, R. Stimulation of cholecystokinin—A receptors with GI181771X does not cause weight loss in overweight or obese patients. *Clin. Pharmacol. Ther.* **2008**, *83*, 281–287. [CrossRef]
91. Miller, L.J.; Desai, A.J. Metabolic actions of the type 1 cholecystokinin receptor: Its potential as a therapeutic target. *Trends Endocrinol. Metab.* **2016**, *27*, 609–619. [CrossRef]
92. Krieger, J.P. Intestinal glucagon-like peptide-1 effects on food intake: Physiological relevance and emerging mechanisms. *Peptides* **2020**, *131*, 170342. [CrossRef] [PubMed]
93. Seino, Y.; Fukushima, M.; Yabe, D. GIP and GLP-1, the two incretin hormones: Similarities and differences. *J. Diabetes Investig.* **2010**, *1*, 8–23. [CrossRef]
94. Migoya, E.M.; Bergeron, R.; Miller, J.L.; Snyder, R.N.K.; Tanen, M.; Hilliard, D.; Weiss, B.; Larson, P.; Gutiérrez, M.; Jiang, G.; et al. Dipeptidyl peptidase-4 inhibitors administered in combination with metformin result in an additive increase in the plasma concentration of active GLP-1. *Clin. Pharmacol. Ther.* **2010**, *88*, 801–808. [CrossRef]
95. Santos-Marcos, J.A.; Rangel-Zuñiga, O.A.; Jimenez-Lucena, R.; Quintana-Navarro, G.M.; Garcia-Carpintero, S.; Malagon, M.M.; Landa, B.B.; Tena-Sempere, M.; Perez-Martinez, P.; Lopez-Miranda, J.; et al. Influence of gender and menopausal status on gut microbiota. *Maturitas* **2018**, *116*, 43–53. [CrossRef]
96. Vaag, A.A.; Holst, J.J.; Vølund, A.; Beck-Nielsen, H. Gut incretin hormones in identical twins discordant for non-insulin-dependent diabetes mellitus (NIDDM)—evidence for decreased glucagon-like peptide 1 secretion during oral glucose ingestion in NIDDM twins. *Eur. J. Endocrinol.* **1996**, *135*, 425–432. [CrossRef]
97. Hira, T.; Pinyo, J.; Hara, H. What is GLP-1 really doing in obesity? *Trends Endocrinol. Metab.* **2020**, *31*, 71–80. [CrossRef] [PubMed]
98. Nauck, M.A.; Meier, J.J. Management of endocrine disease: Are all GLP-1 agonists equal in the treatment of type 2 diabetes? *Eur. J. Endocrinol.* **2019**, *181*, R211–R234. [CrossRef]
99. Ahrén, B. DPP-4 Inhibition and the path to clinical proof. *Front. Endocrinol.* **2019**, *10*, 376. [CrossRef] [PubMed]
100. Tatemoto, K. Isolation and characterization of peptide YY (PYY), a candidate gut hormone that inhibits pancreatic exocrine secretion. *Proc. Natl. Acad. Sci. USA* **1982**, *79*, 2514–2518. [CrossRef]
101. Gibbons, C.; Caudwell, P.; Finlayson, G.; Webb, D.-L.; Hellström, P.M.; Näslund, E.; Blundell, J.E. Comparison of postprandial profiles of ghrelin, active GLP-1, and total PYY to meals varying in fat and carbohydrate and their association with hunger and the phases of satiety. *J. Clin. Endocrinol. Metab.* **2013**, *98*, E847–E855. [CrossRef] [PubMed]
102. Batterham, R.L.; Cowley, M.A.; Small, C.J.; Herzog, H.; Cohen, M.A.; Dakin, C.L.; Wren, A.M.; Brynes, A.E.; Low, M.J.; Ghatei, M.A.; et al. Gut hormone PYY (3-36) physiologically inhibits food intake. *Nature* **2002**, *418*, 650–654. [CrossRef] [PubMed]
103. Tschöp, M.; Castaneda, T.R.; Joost, H.G.; Thöne-Reineke, C.; Ortmann, S.; Klaus, S.; Hagan, M.M.; Chandler, P.C.; Oswald, K.D.; Benoit, S.C.; et al. Physiology: Does gut hormone PYY3-36 decrease food intake in rodents? *Nature* **2004**, *430*, 165, p. 1 following 165, discussion p. 2, following 165. [CrossRef]

104. Gura, T. Obesity research. Labs fail to reproduce protein's appetite-suppressing effects. *Science* **2004**, *305*, 158–159. [CrossRef]
105. Lee, S.J.; Depoortere, I.; Hatt, H. Therapeutic potential of ectopic olfactory and taste receptors. *Nat. Rev. Drug. Discov.* **2019**, *18*, 116–138. [CrossRef] [PubMed]
106. Steensels, S.; Depoortere, I. Chemoreceptors in the Gut. *Ann. Rev. Physiol.* **2018**, *80*, 117–141. [CrossRef]
107. Vancleef, L.; Broeck, T.V.D.; Thijs, T.; Steensels, S.; Briand, L.; Tack, J.; Depoortere, I. Chemosensory signalling pathways involved in sensing of amino acids by the ghrelin cell. *Sci. Rep.* **2015**, *5*, 15725. [CrossRef]
108. Jang, H.-J.; Kokrashvili, Z.; Theodorakis, M.J.; Carlson, O.D.; Kim, B.-J.; Zhou, J.; Kim, H.H.; Xu, X.; Chan, S.L.; Juhaszova, M.; et al. Gut-expressed gustducin and taste receptors regulate secretion of glucagon-like peptide-1. *Proc. Natl. Acad. Sci. USA* **2007**, *104*, 15069–15074. [CrossRef]
109. Gorboulev, V.; Sch\ufcrmann, A.; Vallon, V.; Kipp, H.; Jaschke, A.; Klessen, D.; Friedrich, A.; Scherneck, S.; Rieg, T.; Cunard, R.; et al. Na(+)-D-glucose cotransporter SGLT1 is pivotal for intestinal glucose absorption and glucose-dependent incretin secretion. *Diabetes* **2012**, *61*, 187–196. [CrossRef] [PubMed]
110. Wang, Q.; Liszt, K.I.; Depoortere, I. Extra-oral bitter taste receptors: New targets against obesity? *Peptides* **2020**, *127*, 170284. [CrossRef] [PubMed]
111. Nunez-Salces, M.; Li, H.; Feinle-Bisset, C.; Young, R.L.; Page, A.J. The regulation of gastric ghrelin secretion. *Acta Physiol.* **2020**, *231*, e13588.
112. Nguyen, N.Q.; Debreceni, T.L.; Bambrick, J.E.; Chia, B.; Wishart, J.; Deane, A.M.; Rayner, C.K.; Horowitz, M.; Young, R.L. Accelerated intestinal glucose absorption in morbidly obese humans: Relationship to glucose transporters, incretin hormones, and glycemia. *J. Clin. Endocrinol. Metab.* **2015**, *100*, 968–976. [CrossRef]
113. Young, R.L.; Chia, B.; Isaacs, N.J.; Ma, J.; Khoo, J.; Wu, T.; Horowitz, M.; Rayner, C.K. Disordered control of intestinal sweet taste receptor expression and glucose absorption in type 2 diabetes. *Diabetes* **2013**, *62*, 3532–3541. [CrossRef]
114. Ichimura, A.; Hirasawa, A.; Poulain-Godefroy, O.; Bonnefond, A.; Hara, T.; Yengo, L.; Kimura, I.; Leloire, A.; Liu, N.; Iida, K.; et al. Dysfunction of lipid sensor GPR120 leads to obesity in both mouse and human. *Nature* **2012**, *483*, 350–354. [CrossRef] [PubMed]
115. Segers, A.; Depoortere, I. Circadian clocks in the digestive system. *Nat. Rev. Gastroenterol. Hepatol.* **2021**, *18*, 239–251.
116. Laermans, J.; Depoortere, I. Chronobesity: Role of the circadian system in the obesity epidemic. *Obes. Rev.* **2016**, *17*, 108–125. [CrossRef]
117. Yildiz, B.O.; Suchard, M.A.; Wong, M.-L.; McCann, S.M.; Licinio, J. Alterations in the dynamics of circulating ghrelin, adiponectin, and leptin in human obesity. *Proc. Natl. Acad. Sci. USA* **2004**, *101*, 10434–10439. [CrossRef] [PubMed]
118. Galindo Muñoz, J.S.; Jiménez Rodríguez, D.; Hernández Morante, J.J. Diurnal rhythms of plasma GLP-1 levels in normal and overweight/obese subjects: Lack of effect of weight loss. *J. Physiol. Biochem.* **2015**, *71*, 17–28. [CrossRef] [PubMed]
119. Chaix, A.; Manoogian, E.N.; Melkani, G.C.; Panda, S. Time-restricted eating to prevent and manage chronic metabolic diseases. *Ann. Rev. Nutr.* **2019**, *39*, 291–315. [CrossRef] [PubMed]
120. Cienfuegos, S.; Gabel, K.; Kalam, F.; Ezpeleta, M.; Wiseman, E.; Pavlou, V.; Lin, S.; Oliveira, M.L.; Varady, K.A. Effects of 4- and 6-h time-restricted feeding on weight and cardiometabolic health: A randomized controlled trial in adults with obesity. *Cell Metab.* **2020**, *32*, 366–378.e3. [CrossRef]
121. Sutton, E.F.; Beyl, R.; Early, K.S.; Cefalu, W.T.; Ravussin, E.; Peterson, C.M. Early time-restricted feeding improves insulin sensitivity, blood pressure, and oxidative stress even without weight loss in men with prediabetes. *Cell Metab.* **2018**, *27*, 1212–1221.e3. [CrossRef]
122. Briggs, D.I.; Lockie, S.H.; Wu, Q.; Lemus, M.B.; Stark, R.; Andrews, Z.B. Calorie-restricted weight loss reverses high-fat diet-induced ghrelin resistance, which contributes to rebound weight gain in a ghrelin-dependent manner. *Endocrinology* **2013**, *154*, 709–717. [CrossRef] [PubMed]
123. Sloth, B.; Due, A.; Larsen, T.M.; Holst, J.J.; Heding, A.; Astrup, A. The effect of a high-MUFA, low-glycaemic index diet and a low-fat diet on appetite and glucose metabolism during a 6-month weight maintenance period. *Br. J. Nutr.* **2009**, *101*, 1846–1858. [CrossRef]
124. Sumithran, P.; Prendergast, L.A.; Delbridge, E.; Purcell, K.; Shulkes, A.; Kriketos, A.; Proietto, J. Long-term persistence of hormonal adaptations to weight loss. *N. Engl. J. Med.* **2011**, *365*, 1597–1604. [CrossRef] [PubMed]
125. Chearskul, S.; Delbridge, E.; Shulkes, A.; Proietto, J.; Kriketos, A. Effect of weight loss and ketosis on postprandial cholecystokinin and free fatty acid concentrations. *Am. J. Clin. Nutr.* **2008**, *87*, 1238–1246. [CrossRef]
126. Rastelli, M.; Cani, P.D.; Knauf, C. The gut microbiome influences host endocrine functions. *Endocr. Rev.* **2019**, *40*, 1271–1284. [CrossRef]
127. Steensels, S.; Cools, L.; Avau, B.; Vancleef, L.; Farré, R.; Verbeke, K.; Depoortere, I. Supplementation of oligofructose, but not sucralose, decreases high-fat diet induced body weight gain in mice independent of gustducin-mediated gut hormone release. *Mol. Nutr. Food Res.* **2017**, *61*, 61. [CrossRef]
128. Parnell, J.A.; Reimer, R.A. Weight loss during oligofructose supplementation is associated with decreased ghrelin and increased peptide YY in overweight and obese adults. *Am. J. Clin. Nutr.* **2009**, *89*, 1751–1759. [CrossRef]
129. Chambers, E.S.; Viardot, A.; Psichas, A.; Morrison, D.J.; Murphy, K.G.; Zac-Varghese, S.E.K.; MacDougall, K.; Preston, T.; Tedford, C.; Finlayson, G.S.; et al. Effects of targeted delivery of propionate to the human colon on appetite regulation, body weight maintenance and adiposity in overweight adults. *Gut* **2015**, *64*, 1744–1754. [CrossRef]

130. Zhao, L.; Zhang, F.; Ding, X.; Wu, G.; Lam, Y.Y.; Wang, X.; Fu, H.; Xue, X.; Lu, C.; Ma, J.; et al. Gut bacteria selectively promoted by dietary fibers alleviate type 2 diabetes. *Science* **2018**, *359*, 1151–1156. [CrossRef]
131. Plovier, H.; Everard, A.; Druart, C.; Depommier, C.; Van Hul, M.; Geurts, L.; Chilloux, J.; Ottman, N.; Duparc, T.; Lichtenstein, L.; et al. A purified membrane protein from Akkermansia muciniphila or the pasteurized bacterium improves metabolism in obese and diabetic mice. *Nat. Med.* **2017**, *23*, 107–113. [CrossRef] [PubMed]
132. Ekberg, J.H.; Hauge, M.; Kristensen, L.V.; Madsen, A.N.; Engelstoft, M.S.; Husted, A.-S.; Sichlau, R.; Egerod, K.L.; Timshel, P.; Kowalski, T.J.; et al. GPR119, a Major enteroendocrine sensor of dietary triglyceride metabolites coacting in synergy with FFA1 (GPR40). *Endocrinology* **2016**, *157*, 4561–4569. [CrossRef]
133. Steensels, S.; Lannoo, M.; Avau, B.; Laermans, J.; Vancleef, L.; Farré, R.; Verbeke, K.; Depoortere, I. The role of nutrient sensing in the metabolic changes after gastric bypass surgery. *J. Endocrinol.* **2017**, *232*, 363–376. [CrossRef] [PubMed]
134. Seeley, R.J.; Berridge, K.C. The hunger games. *Cell* **2015**, *160*, 805–806. [CrossRef]
135. Peiris, M.; Aktar, R.; Raynel, S.; Hao, Z.; Mumphrey, M.B.; Berthoud, H.-R.; Blackshaw, L.A. Effects of obesity and gastric bypass surgery on nutrient sensors, endocrine cells, and mucosal innervation of the mouse colon. *Nutrients* **2018**, *10*, 1529. [CrossRef] [PubMed]
136. Moffett, R.C.; Docherty, N.G.; le Roux, C.W. The altered enteroendocrine reportoire following roux-en-Y-gastric bypass as an effector of weight loss and improved glycaemic control. *Appetite* **2021**, *156*, 104807. [CrossRef]
137. Peterli, R.; E Steinert, R.; Woelnerhanssen, B.; Peters, T.; Christoffel-Courtin, C.; Gass, M.; Kern, B.; Von Fluee, M.; Beglinger, C. Metabolic and hormonal changes after laparoscopic Roux-en-Y gastric bypass and sleeve gastrectomy: A randomized, prospective trial. *Obes. Surg.* **2012**, *22*, 740–748. [CrossRef] [PubMed]
138. Foschi, D.; Corsi, F.; Pisoni, L.; Vago, T.; Bevilacqua, M.; Asti, E.; Righi, I.; Trabucchi, E. Plasma cholecystokinin levels after vertical banded gastroplasty: Effects of an acidified meal. *Obes. Surg.* **2004**, *14*, 644–647. [CrossRef]
139. Goldstone, A.P.; Miras, A.; Scholtz, S.; Jackson, S.; Neff, K.J.; Pénicaud, L.; Geoghegan, J.; Chhina, N.; Durighel, G.; Bell, J.D.; et al. Link between increased satiety gut hormones and reduced food reward after gastric bypass surgery for obesity. *J. Clin. Endocrinol. Metab.* **2016**, *101*, 599–609. [CrossRef]
140. Orellana, E.R.; Covasa, M.; Hajnal, A. Neuro-hormonal mechanisms underlying changes in reward related behaviors following weight loss surgery: Potential pharmacological targets. *Biochem. Pharmacol.* **2019**, *164*, 106–114. [CrossRef]
141. Nauck, M.A.; Quast, D.R.; Wefers, J.; Meier, J.J. GLP-1 receptor agonists in the treatment of type 2 diabetes—State-of-the-art. *Mol. Metab.* **2021**, *46*, 101102. [CrossRef]
142. Wilding, J.P.; Batterham, R.L.; Calanna, S.; Davies, M.; Van Gaal, L.F.; Lingvay, I.; McGowan, B.M.; Rosenstock, J.; Tran, M.T.; Wadden, T.A.; et al. Once-weekly semaglutide in adults with overweight or obesity. *N. Engl. J. Med.* **2021**, *384*, 989. [CrossRef]
143. Brandt, S.J.; Müller, T.D.; DiMarchi, R.D.; Tschöp, M.H.; Stemmer, K. Peptide-based multi-agonists: A new paradigm in metabolic pharmacology. *J. Intern. Med.* **2018**, *284*, 581–602. [CrossRef]
144. Christensen, M.B.; Calanna, S.; Holst, J.J.; Vilsbøll, T.; Knop, F.K. Glucose-dependent insulinotropic polypeptide: Blood glucose stabilizing effects in patients with type 2 diabetes. *J. Clin. Endocrinol. Metab.* **2014**, *99*, E418–E426. [CrossRef] [PubMed]
145. Christensen, M.B. Glucose-dependent insulinotropic polypeptide: Effects on insulin and glucagon secretion in humans. *Dan. Med. J.* **2016**, *63*, 63.
146. Chia, C.W.; Carlson, O.D.; Kim, W.; Shin, Y.K.; Charles, C.P.; Kim, H.S.; Melvin, D.L.; Egan, J.M. Exogenous glucose-dependent insulinotropic polypeptide worsens post prandial hyperglycemia in type 2 diabetes. *Diabetes* **2009**, *58*, 1342–1349. [CrossRef]
147. Campbell, J.E. Targeting the GIPR for obesity: To agonize or antagonize? Potential mechanisms. *Mol. Metab.* **2021**, *46*, 101139. [CrossRef] [PubMed]
148. Calanna, S.; Christensen, M.; Holst, J.J.; Laferrère, B.; Gluud, L.L.; Vilsbøll, T.; Knop, F.K. Secretion of glucose-dependent insulinotropic polypeptide in patients with type 2 diabetes: Systematic review and meta-analysis of clinical studies. *Diabetes Care* **2013**, *36*, 3346–3352. [CrossRef] [PubMed]
149. Mroz, P.A.; Finan, B.; Gelfanov, V.; Yang, B.; Tschöp, M.H.; DiMarchi, R.D.; Perez-Tilve, D. Optimized GIP analogs promote body weight lowering in mice through GIPR agonism not antagonism. *Mol. Metab.* **2019**, *20*, 51–62. [CrossRef]
150. Nørregaard, P.K.; Deryabina, M.A.; Tofteng Shelton, P.; Fog, J.U.; Daugaard, J.R.; Eriksson, P.O.; Larsen, L.F.; Jessen, L. A novel GIP analogue, ZP4165, enhances glucagon-like peptide-1-induced body weight loss and improves glycaemic control in rodents. *Diabetes Obes. Metab.* **2018**, *20*, 60–68. [CrossRef]
151. Hartman, M.L.; Sanyal, A.J.; Loomba, R.; Wilson, J.M.; Nikooienejad, A.; Bray, R.; Karanikas, C.A.; Duffin, K.L.; Robins, D.A.; Haupt, A. Effects of novel dual GIP and GLP-1 receptor agonist tirzepatide on biomarkers of nonalcoholic steatohepatitis in patients with type 2 diabetes. *Diabetes Care* **2020**, *43*, 1352–1355. [CrossRef] [PubMed]
152. Kleinert, M.; Sachs, S.; Habegger, K.M.; Hofmann, S.M.; Müller, T.D. Glucagon regulation of energy expenditure. *Int. J. Mol. Sci.* **2019**, *20*, 5407. [CrossRef] [PubMed]
153. Kim, T.; Holleman, C.L.; Nason, S.; Arble, D.M.; Ottaway, N.; Chabenne, J.; Loyd, C.; Kim, J.-A.; Sandoval, D.; Drucker, D.J.; et al. Hepatic glucagon receptor signaling enhances insulin-stimulated glucose disposal in rodents. *Diabetes* **2018**, *67*, 2157–2166. [CrossRef]
154. Day, J.W.; Ottaway, N.; Patterson, J.; Gelfanov, V.; Smiley, D.; Gidda, J.; Findeisen, H.; Bruemmer, D.; Drucker, D.J.; Chaudhary, N.; et al. A new glucagon and GLP-1 co-agonist eliminates obesity in rodents. *Nat. Chem. Biol.* **2009**, *5*, 749–757. [CrossRef] [PubMed]

155. Henderson, S.J.; Konkar, A.; Hornigold, D.C.; Trevaskis, J.L.; Jackson, R.; Fredin, M.F.; Jansson-Löfmark, R.; Naylor, J.; Rossi, A.; Bednarek, M.A.; et al. Robust anti-obesity and metabolic effects of a dual GLP-1/glucagon receptor peptide agonist in rodents and non-human primates. *Diabetes Obes. Metab.* **2016**, *18*, 1176–1190. [CrossRef] [PubMed]
156. Laker, R.C. Cotadutide (MEDI0382): A dual receptor agonist with glucagon-like peptide-1 and glucagon activity, modulates hepatic glycogen and fat content. Presented at 80th Scientific Sessions of the American Diabetes Association, Relocated from Chicago to Cyberspace, Chicago, IL, USA, 12–16 June 2020. Available online: https://www.bjd-abcd.com/index.php/bjd/article/view/677/877 (accessed on 1 March 2021).
157. Holst, J.J.; Albrechtsen, N.J.; Gabe, M.B.N.; Rosenkilde, M.M. Oxyntomodulin: Actions and role in diabetes. *Peptides* **2018**, *100*, 48–53. [CrossRef]
158. Ma, T.; Huo, S.; Xu, B.; Li, F.; Wang, P.; Liu, Y.; Lei, H. A novel long-acting oxyntomodulin analogue eliminates diabetes and obesity in mice. *Eur. J. Med. Chem.* **2020**, *203*, 112496. [CrossRef]
159. Schmidt, J.B.; Gregersen, N.T.; Pedersen, S.D.; Arentoft, J.L.; Ritz, C.; Schwartz, T.W.; Holst, J.J.; Astrup, A.; Sjödin, A. Effects of PYY3-36 and GLP-1 on energy intake, energy expenditure, and appetite in overweight men. *Am. J. Physiol. Endocrinol. Metab.* **2014**, *306*, E1248–E1256. [CrossRef] [PubMed]
160. Field, B.C.; Wren, A.M.; Peters, V.; Baynes, K.C.; Martin, N.M.; Patterson, M.; Alsaraf, S.; Amber, V.; Wynne, K.; Ghatei, M.A.; et al. PYY3-36 and oxyntomodulin can be additive in their effect on food intake in overweight and obese humans. *Diabetes* **2010**, *59*, 1635–1639. [CrossRef]
161. Finan, B.; Yang, B.; Ottaway, N.; Smiley, D.L.; Ma, T.; Clemmensen, C.; Chabenne, J.; Zhang, L.; Habegger, K.M.; Fischer, K.; et al. A rationally designed monomeric peptide triagonist corrects obesity and diabetes in rodents. *Nat. Med.* **2015**, *21*, 27–36. [CrossRef] [PubMed]
162. Kim, J.K. Therapeutic efficacy of a novel long-acting GLP-1/GIP/Glucagon triple agonist (HM15211) in NASH and fibrosis animal models. In Proceedings of the EASD annual Meeting, Berlin, Germany, 3 October 2018.
163. Hanmi Pharmaceutical Company Ltd. Study to Evaluate Efficacy, Safety and Tolerability of HM15211 in Subjects. 2021. Available online: https://trialbulletin.com/lib/entry/ct-04505436 (accessed on 1 March 2021).

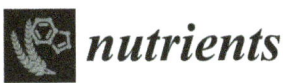

Review

Do Gut Hormones Contribute to Weight Loss and Glycaemic Outcomes after Bariatric Surgery?

Dimitris Papamargaritis [1] and Carel W. le Roux [2,3,*]

1. Diabetes Research Centre, Leicester General Hospital, University of Leicester, Leicester, LE5 4PW, UK; dp421@leicester.ac.uk
2. Diabetes Complications Research Centre, Conway Institute, University College of Dublin, Dublin 4, Ireland
3. Diabetes Research Group, School of Biomedical Sciences, Ulster University, Coleraine BT52 1SA, UK
* Correspondence: carel.leroux@ucd.ie

Abstract: Bariatric surgery is an effective intervention for management of obesity through treating dysregulated appetite and achieving long-term weight loss maintenance. Moreover, significant changes in glucose homeostasis are observed after bariatric surgery including, in some cases, type 2 diabetes remission from the early postoperative period and postprandial hypoglycaemia. Levels of a number of gut hormones are dramatically increased from the early period after Roux-en-Y gastric bypass and sleeve gastrectomy—the two most commonly performed bariatric procedures—and they have been suggested as important mediators of the observed changes in eating behaviour and glucose homeostasis postoperatively. In this review, we summarise the current evidence from human studies on the alterations of gut hormones after bariatric surgery and their impact on clinical outcomes postoperatively. Studies which assess the role of gut hormones after bariatric surgery on food intake, hunger, satiety and glucose homeostasis through octreotide use (a non-specific inhibitor of gut hormone secretion) as well as with exendin 9–39 (a specific glucagon-like peptide-1 receptor antagonist) are reviewed. The potential use of gut hormones as biomarkers of successful outcomes of bariatric surgery is also evaluated.

Keywords: gut hormones; bariatric surgery; GLP-1; PYY; ghrelin; Roux-en-Y gastric bypass; gastric band; sleeve gastrectomy

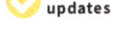

Citation: Papamargaritis, D.; le Roux, C.W. Do Gut Hormones Contribute to Weight Loss and Glycaemic Outcomes after Bariatric Surgery?. *Nutrients* **2021**, *13*, 762. https://doi.org/10.3390/nu13030762

Academic Editor: Christine Feinle-Bisset

Received: 29 December 2020
Accepted: 20 February 2021
Published: 26 February 2021

Publisher's Note: MDPI stays neutral with regard to jurisdictional claims in published maps and institutional affiliations.

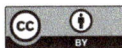

Copyright: © 2021 by the authors. Licensee MDPI, Basel, Switzerland. This article is an open access article distributed under the terms and conditions of the Creative Commons Attribution (CC BY) license (https://creativecommons.org/licenses/by/4.0/).

1. Introduction

Obesity is a complex, chronic, progressive and relapsing disease which affects currently approximately 650 million adults worldwide [1,2]. Complications of obesity include type 2 diabetes mellitus (T2D), cancer, sleep apnoea, cardiovascular, musculoskeletal, reproductive and psychological morbidities [3]. The cornerstone of prevention and treatment of obesity is behavioural changes together with diet and exercise (lifestyle changes) [4]. However, lifestyle approaches for treatment of severe obesity and its associated complications often do not achieve enough weight loss to reverse complications and weight loss maintenance remains a major challenge [5–7]. Current available pharmacotherapy in combination with the lifestyle changes can add a further weight loss of 2.6–8.8% [8] and help with weight maintenance [7,9], but newer medications promise more weight loss in the long term [10,11]. Even so, bariatric surgery remains a valuable tool for weight loss, leading to improvements in health, functionality and quality of life [12–15], especially for those that lifestyle- and medication-based approaches have proven ineffective to achieve and maintain clinically significant weight loss.

Currently, around 685,000 weight loss operations are performed every year worldwide [16] and the three most commonly performed procedures are the Roux-en-Y gastric bypass (RYGB), the sleeve gastrectomy (SG) and the adjustable gastric band (AGB) [16,17].

Bariatric surgery achieves successful weight loss and weight maintenance long-term as a result of reduced caloric intake postoperatively due to decreased hunger and increased satiety [18–22]. The changes in satiety are profound from the early postoperative period after RYGB and SG and, in some cases, there are also alterations in food preferences after these procedures [23,24]. These findings are different to what is observed after low-calorie diet, which can be very effective in the induction of weight loss, however, the vast majority of people fail to maintain the achieved weight loss in the long-term [6,7,25,26]. On a low-calorie diet, people usually report an increase in hunger, a decrease in satiety and an increased desire to eat [18,27,28] and this is likely due to robust compensatory processes that resist a drift of body fat stores below an established "set point" [29,30]. The alterations in gut hormone levels after diet-induced weight loss have been suggested as an important mediator of eating behaviours favouring weight regain in the long term [27,31]. More specifically, ghrelin, a hunger hormone, is increased after diet-induced weight loss when postprandial levels of satiety hormones are decreased [27,31].

In contrast, RYGB and SG lead to increased postprandial secretion of satiety hormones including glucagon-like peptide-1 (GLP-1), peptide YY (PYY), and oxyntomodulin (OXM) [23,32–34]. These changes in gut hormone secretion from the early period after RYGB and SG have been suggested as potential mediators of the increased satiety and reduced hunger postoperatively, indicating that bariatric surgery may address the dysfunctional appetite regulation in people with obesity. Moreover, significant improvements in glucose homeostasis and even remission of T2D occurs within days after bariatric surgery [35–37] due to well described changes in insulin secretion and sensitivity from the early postoperative period [38–40]. The known effect of GLP-1 on insulin secretion [41,42] combined with the elevated GLP-1 levels postoperatively further increases the interest about the gut hormones as potential mediators of these effects.

In this review, we will evaluate the currently available evidence from human studies on:

(a) The changes in gut hormones after bariatric surgery (Section 2);
(b) The role of gut hormones on weight loss outcomes after bariatric surgery (Section 3)—more specifically we will review their role as (i) biomarkers of successful weight loss postoperatively (Sections 3.1 and 3.2) and as (ii) mediators of the postoperative changes in food intake and appetite (Section 3.3);
(c) The role of GLP-1 after bariatric surgery on glycaemic outcomes (Section 4)—we will evaluate the role of GLP-1 as mediator (i) of type 2 diabetes improvement/remission (Section 4.1) and (ii) of postprandial hyperinsulinaemic hypoglycaemia (PHH) (Section 4.2).

Figure 1 demonstrates the three main sections of this review article for convenience of the readers. The focus for the sections exploring the role of gut hormones as mediators of weight loss and glycaemic outcomes after bariatric surgery will be on studies using either octreotide (a nonspecific inhibitor of gut hormones secretion) or exendin 9–39 (Ex-9, a specific GLP-1 antagonist).

2. Changes in Gut Hormones after Bariatric Surgery

Changes in gut hormone levels—especially those secreted from the L-cells with highest density in the ileum (such as GLP-1, PYY, OXM and glicentin)—have been consistently seen from the early postoperative period after RYGB and SG (Table 1). In contrast, gut hormone levels do not significantly change after AGB (Table 1).

2.1. Potential Explanations for the Increased Postprandial Gut Hormone Secretion from the Distal Gut after RYGB and SG

In people with severe obesity, gastric emptying and small intestinal transit time are slower compared to lean people and are associated with reduction in postprandial glucose absorption and glycaemic excursions as well as with reduced postprandial rise in GLP-1 and glucose-dependent insulinotropic polypeptide levels (GIP) [43].

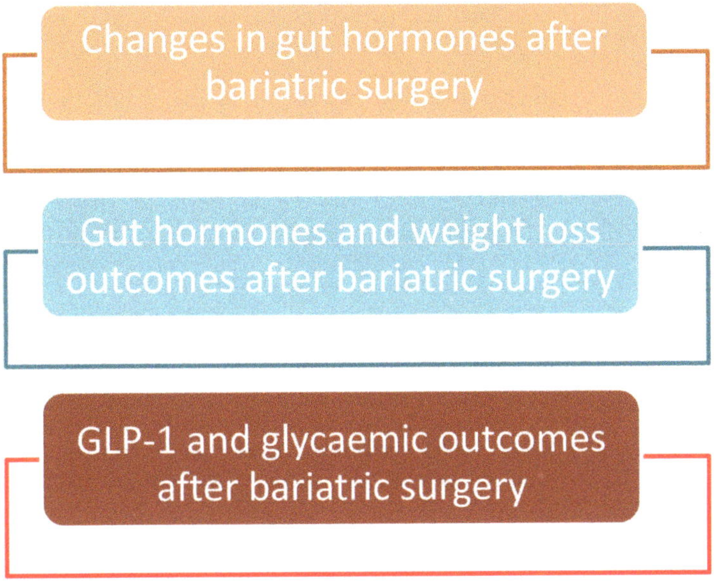

```
┌─────────────────────────────────────────┐
│   Changes in gut hormones after         │
│          bariatric surgery              │
└─────────────────────────────────────────┘

┌─────────────────────────────────────────┐
│   Gut hormones and weight loss          │
│   outcomes after bariatric surgery      │
└─────────────────────────────────────────┘

┌─────────────────────────────────────────┐
│   GLP-1 and glycaemic outcomes          │
│        after bariatric surgery          │
└─────────────────────────────────────────┘
```

Figure 1. Structure of the review article.

After RYGB, the rapid gastric emptying of both solids and liquids [44–47] and the bypass of the stomach and duodenum postoperatively result in accelerated nutrient delivery and absorption to the distal part of the gut [45] and subsequently to increased postprandial secretion of gut hormones [33,45,48,49]. After SG, there is increased gastric pressure [50,51], accelerated gastric emptying of nutrients [45,52,53] and accelerated small bowel transit [54] to induce an early and prolonged secretion of L-cell hormones from the intestine. In contrast, AGB does not alter the rate of gastric emptying for solids or liquids [55,56] and this is probably the reason that gut hormone secretion from the distal part of the gut is not significantly altered post-AGB [56].

There are differences between RYGB and SG on macronutrient absorption—glucose and protein absorption are accelerated after RYGB [57,58], when after SG glucose absorption is increased (but less compared to RYGB) and protein absorption is not modified [45]. These differences may account for the different hormonal profiles observed between the two procedures [34,45].

The nutrient absorption from the gut appears to be more important for the gut hormone secretion compared to the exposure of the gut to nutrients [59,60]. Further evidence on the importance of glucose absorption on GLP-1 secretion after RYGB comes from a study where sodium glucose co-transporters-1 (SGLT-1), a major mechanism of dietary glucose absorption from the gastrointestinal tract, were blocked in people who have undergone RYGB through canagliflozin, a dual SGLT-1/SGLT-2 inhibitor [61]. The study found that indeed dual SGLT-1/SGLT-2 inhibition could reduce glucose absorption and subsequently reduce peak GLP-1 levels and insulin secretion after RYGB [61].

High gastric emptying rates after RYGB for prolonged periods may also induce adaptive changes, such as an increase in enteroendocrine cell number and surface area [62,63]. Experiments with gastrostomy feeding and reversal of RYGB demonstrate acute reversal of excessive gut hormone secretion immediately after rerouting of nutrients to the stomach or after reversal of RYGB [64,65]. This supports the concept that the rapid delivery and absorption of the nutrients at the distal part of the gut constitutes a more potent stimulus for secretion of gut hormones after RYGB compared to the changes in the enteroendocrine cells.

Other mechanisms, such as changes in bile acid flow and bile acid plasma levels, may also play a role in gut hormone secretion after bariatric surgery, especially after RYGB [66–68]. However, further studies are required to define the role of bile acids on gut hormone secretion after bariatric surgery, particularly as evidence on changes of bile acid levels after SG is conflicting [69–73] and the time course of bile acid changes after RYGB is unclear [70,72–74].

2.2. Ghrelin

Ghrelin is mainly produced from the X/A like cells of the stomach and to a lesser degree from the small intestine. Ghrelin is considered to be most active in its acylated form, and is a known orexigenic hormone which stimulates appetite and food intake [75]. Furthermore, ghrelin inhibits insulin secretion in healthy people [75–77]. Plasma ghrelin levels are typically increased during prolonged fasting and suppressed immediately after food intake [75,78,79]. In states of increased adiposity, lower fasting plasma ghrelin levels are observed, coupled with blunted postprandial ghrelin suppression [80,81].

Changes in ghrelin levels after bariatric surgery are presented in Table 1 [33,34,82–94]. It is of note that during the first months after RYGB, fasting and postprandial ghrelin levels are decreased, but over the first postoperative year, ghrelin levels after RYGB gradually increase [34,86–90].

2.3. GIP

GIP is secreted from K cells found throughout the small intestine, but in highest proportion in the duodenum and jejunum. GIP increases insulin secretion following ingestion of oral glucose in healthy volunteers [41]. On the other hand, in people with T2D, the insulinotropic capacity of exogenous GIP is markedly attenuated, but it appears to be improved after near-normalisation of glycaemic control [41,95,96].

The changes in postprandial levels of GIP after RYGB and SG are inconsistent [33,48,83,97–101] (Table 1). On the other hand, GIP levels after AGB appear unchanged [33,56,102–104] (Table 1).

2.4. GLP-1

Glucagon-like peptide 1 (GLP-1) is secreted from L cells which predominate in the distal ileum and colon. GLP-1 stimulates insulin release in response to nutrient ingestion and reduces blood glucose levels in a glucose-dependent manner [41,105]. GLP-1 is rapidly inactivated by the enzyme dipeptidyl-peptidase-4 (DPP-4) [106]. Additionally, endogenous GLP-1 inhibits gastric emptying, inhibits glucagon secretion and has centrally mediated effects upon appetite [105,107].

Postprandial levels of GLP-1 are significantly elevated after RYGB and SG [32–34,45,83,85,90], but they remain stable after AGB [56,89,91,94] (Table 1). The increase in postprandial GLP-1 levels after RYGB is more profound compared to SG in some studies [34,45], but not in all [90,108].

2.5. PYY

PYY is a peptide secreted from intestinal endocrine L-cells of the distal gut following food ingestion along with GLP-1 [82,109]. Following cleavage in the circulation by the enzyme DPP-4, PYY 1–36 is converted to PYY 3–36 which is considered to promote satiety [81]. PYY is released postprandially in proportion to the calories ingested [110] and it increases satiety, reduces food intake, delays gastric emptying and reduces postprandial insulin secretion [111–113].

Alterations in PYY levels after bariatric surgery [21,32,34,45,83,85,89,91,94,108,114] are described in Table 1. Postprandial PYY levels are elevated after RYGB and SG, with more potent changes after RYGB [34,91,108,114].

2.6. Oxyntomodulin

Oxyntomodulin (OXM) is a peptide hormone which is structurally similar to glucagon and is produced by the L-cells of the gut [81,115]. OXM is a weak dual agonist of GLP-1 receptor and glucagon receptor [116]. A specific receptor for mediating the effect of OXM has not yet been identified in humans. Exogenous administration of OXM reduces food intake and increases energy expenditure in humans [117,118]. Few studies have assessed the changes in oxyntomodulin levels after bariatric surgery [23,33,97,119] and their results are presented in Table 1.

2.7. Glicentin

Glicentin contains the entire sequences of oxyntomodulin (and hence glucagon) and glicentin-related pancreatic peptide [120] and it is cleaved from the proglucagon prohormone in the L-cell. It is unclear whether glicentin is a metabolically inert by-product of proglucagon processing, which is co-secreted from the L-cell, or has a distinct function [120,121]. Currently, there is no known glicentin receptor in humans. Limited data is also available on the changes of glicentin levels after bariatric surgery [23,33,97], however postprandial glicentin levels appear to be elevated after RYGB (Table 1).

3. The Role of Gut Hormones on Weight Outcomes after Bariatric Surgery

3.1. Gut Hormone Levels as Predictors of Weight Loss before and after Bariatric Surgery

Werling et al. [122] reported that preoperative responses of GLP-1 and PYY to a mixed meal do not correlate with postoperative weight loss after RYGB surgery.

After RYGB and SG, the postprandial increase in oxyntomodulin and glicentin levels [% change of Area Under the Curve (AUC)]) during the first three to six months predict successful weight loss at twelve to eighteen months postoperatively [23,33] and it was also associated with favourable changes in eating behaviour [23]. The increase in glicentin levels was the strongest hormonal predictor of weight loss (was able to explain 22% of variation in weight loss at eighteen months [23]), but combining multiple gut hormones (including PYY, ghrelin, GLP-1, oxyntomodulin and glicentin) not surprisingly increased further the predictive power for postoperative weight loss, suggesting synergistic effects of gut hormones for weight loss after bariatric surgery [23]. These results may reflect that glicentin, because of its longer half-life, is probably the best marker for the secretion of proglucagon-derived hormones with already established effects on food intake and weight loss (such as GLP-1) rather than being indicative of a regulatory role for glicentin on food choice and weight loss [23]. Therefore, early postprandial responses of gut hormones, including glicentin, may be early markers of postoperative weight loss.

Table 1. Changes in gut hormones after the most commonly performed bariatric procedures.

H	RYGB	SG	AGB
Ghrelin	Fasting ↓ [85,87,88,90] or ↔ [33,34,48,88,89,91,92,94,108,114] or ↑ [86–88,91,108] Postprandial ↓ [48,85,90] or ↔ [33,34,48,89,94,108,114] or ↑ [89,91]	Fasting ↓↓ [23,33,34,83–85,90,93,108,114] Postprandial ↓ [23,33,85,90,114]	Fasting ↔ [33,84,89,91,94,104] or ↑ [84,91–93] Postprandial ↔ [9,91,94] or ↑ [91,94]
GIP	Fasting ↔ [33,97–99,101,103] Postprandial ↓ [33,103] or ↔ [48,97,101] or ↑ [98,101]	Fasting ↔ [33,83,104] Postprandial ↓ [33,104] or ↔ [105] or↑ [104]	Fasting ↔ [33,56,103,104] Postprandial ↔ [56,103]
GLP-1	Fasting ↔ [23,33,34,48,85,91,94,97–99,108] Postprandial ↑↑ [23,34,48,89,90,91,94,97–99,101,114]	Fasting ↔ [23,32–34,85,100,101,108,114] Postprandial ↑ [23,32–34,83,85,100,101]	Fasting ↔ [33,56,89,91,94,103,104] Postprandial ↔ [56,89,91,94,103]
PYY	Fasting ↔ [21,23,34,89,94,108,114] or ↑ [33,91,94,108] Postprandial ↑↑ [21,23,33,34,85,89–91,94,108,114]	Fasting ↔ [21,23,32–34,108,114] Postprandial ↑ [21,23,32–34,83,90,108,114]	Fasting ↔ [33,89,91,94] Postprandial ↔ [89,91,94] or ↑ [91,94]
OXM	Fasting ↔ [23,33,97,119] Postprandial ↑↑ [23,33,97,119]	Fasting ↔ [23,33] Postprandial ↔ [23] or ↑ [33]	Fasting ↔ [33] Postprandial NA
Glicentin	Fasting ↔ [33,97] or ↑ [23] Postprandial ↑↑ [23,33,97]	Fasting ↔ [23] or ↑ [33] Postprandial ↔ [23] or ↑ [33]	Fasting ↔ [33] Postprandial NA

RYGB: Roux-en-y gastric bypass, SG: Sleeve gastrectomy, AGB: Adjustable gastric band, GLP-1: Glucagon Like Peptide-1, PYY: Peptide YY, GIP: Glucose-dependent Insulinotropic Polypeptide, OXM: Oxyntomodulin, ↓ reduced compared to preoperatively, ↔ no change compared to preoperatively, ↑ increased compared to preoperatively, ↓↓ very reduced compared to preoperatively, ↑↑ very increased compared to preoperatively. NA: limited/no data available. Referenced studies are presented in brackets.

3.2. Gut Hormone Levels in Poor and Good Responders after Bariatric Surgery

As discussed, multiple satiety gut hormones are elevated after RYGB and SG, but is there a difference in gut hormone levels between "good" responders and "poor" responders to bariatric surgery? Almost all the studies which have addressed this question have been performed after RYGB. Despite the different definitions for "good" and "poor" responders between the studies, people with "poor" postoperative weight loss after RYGB have elevated ghrelin levels and reduced secretion of satiety gut hormones (mainly GLP-1 levels and in some cases PYY levels) compared to "good" responders to the operation [19,123–125]. Moreover, suppression of hunger was more pronounced in "good" responders to RYGB after a standardized meal compared to "poor" responders [19,125].

"Poor" responders to bariatric surgery can be further categorized as primary "poor" responders (people who have undergone bariatric surgery and achieved suboptimal maximum weight loss compared to the expected) and secondary "poor" responders (people who achieved good maximum weight loss, but then experienced significant weight regain). There is a lack of standardisation in definitions for primary and secondary "poor" responders and "good" responders [126,127]. The majority of people who are "poor" responders to bariatric surgery are secondary "poor" responders, with a 5% of bariatric surgery population being primary "poor" responders [126]. There may be a number of differences in physiology between primary and secondary "poor" responders compared to "good" responders to bariatric surgery.

De Hollanda et al. [124] evaluated whether there is a difference in gut hormones between people who are secondary "poor" responders to RYGB (n = 22) compared to "good" responders to RYGB (n = 32). They reported that secondary "poor" responders have lower GLP-1 and PYY levels and less suppression of ghrelin following a mixed meal test than "good" responders. Furthermore, ad libitum food intake (both absolute and body weight adjusted food intake) was increased in secondary "poor" responders compared to "good" responders to RYGB.

The main limitation in studies investigating differences between "good" and "poor" responders after bariatric surgery is the cross-sectional design. Thus, it is not possible to know whether the observed differences in gut hormones between "good" and "poor" responders were actually preceded the weight loss/weight gain postoperatively or are merely a consequence of the difference in body weight at the time of the study.

3.3. Gut Hormones and Their Role in Appetite and Food Intake after Bariatric Surgery

The increased levels of postprandial secretion of gut hormones (GLP-1, PYY) and their known role in food intake and appetite have predictably led to the hypothesis that changes in gut hormones are contributed to the observed changes in appetite and food intake after RYGB and SG. To demonstrate causality for the effect of gut hormones on satiety and food intake after bariatric surgery, a somatostatin analogue (octreotide) has been used to non-specifically attenuate the response of postprandial gut hormones (Table 2). The first evidence to strongly suggest a role for the exaggerated response of gut hormones was provided when increased food intake and reduced satiety was shown in patients after RYGB who received octreotide compared to saline (placebo) within a randomized controlled trial [19]. In contrast, patients who had undergone AGB (an operation with minimal effect on gut hormones), did not exhibit changes in appetite or food intake with octreotide administration [19].

De Hollanda et al. [124] also found that octreotide suppressed gut hormone secretion, increased food intake and suppressed satiety after RYGB. However, the observed changes in food intake and satiety were comparable in secondary "poor" responders and "good" responders to RYGB, suggesting that the role of gut hormones in the weight regain in secondary "poor" responders may be limited.

In a recently presented conference abstract, Bojsen-Moller et al. [128] reported that in primary "poor" responders to RYGB, octreotide attenuates gut hormone secretion but does not affect ad libitum food intake. In contrast, in "good" responders to the RYGB, there was an increase of 23% in ad libitum food intake with octreotide compared to placebo. Interestingly, in this study there was no significant difference in postprandial gut hormone levels (GLP-1, PYY or post-meal suppression of ghrelin) between primary "poor" responders and "good" responders. These observations suggest that impaired regulation of food intake by gut hormones may contribute to a primary "poor" response to RYGB.

As octreotide has non-specific effects to block gut hormone secretion, it is difficult to identify the main gut hormones contributing to food intake and appetite changes after RYGB. Moreover, octreotide has an inhibitory effect on gastrointestinal motility [129], which may improve postprandial symptoms and affect further the appetite postoperatively.

In an attempt to isolate the particular role of GLP-1 on inhibition of food intake after RYGB, Svane et al. [130] used the specific GLP-1 receptor antagonist Ex-9. Preoperatively, Ex-9 was associated with a 35% increased food intake in patients with obesity and T2D prior to RYGB compared to placebo. After RYGB, while food intake was less than preoperatively during Ex-9 and saline administration, there was no difference in food intake between Ex-9 and placebo. However, after administration of Ex-9, the already elevated postoperative GLP-1 and PYY levels were further increased. The increase in PYY levels was interpreted to indicate that while an inhibitory effect of GLP-1 on food intake may have been removed with the antagonist, at the same time an even greater PYY response occurs, which would favour inhibition of food intake so that the influence of Ex-9 on food intake after RYGB is neutral [130,131].

A subsequent study accordingly tried to block both GLP-1 and PYY actions [130]. Ex-9 was used to block GLP-1 actions, but as there is no available antagonist of PYY for use in humans, a DPP-4 inhibitor was used in order to inhibit the conversion of PYY 1–36 to PYY 3–36, which appears to be the actual satiety-promoting form of the hormone. In a crossover study patients after RYGB received placebo, Ex-9, sitagliptin (a DPP-4 inhibitor), and a combination of Ex-9 and sitagliptin. GLP-1 and PYY 3–36 levels were increased during placebo, and further increase following Ex-9 administration was observed as expected. The DPP-4 inhibitor caused further increases in active GLP-1 levels, but almost abolished the PYY 3–36 responses to food intake. The Ex-9 plus DPP-4 inhibitor in combination were associated with a significant increase of 20% in food intake [130,131]. These observations strongly support the concept that GLP-1 and PYY 3–36 are involved synergistically in the inhibition of appetite and food intake following RYGB.

Table 2. Studies using octreotide to assess food intake and satiety after bariatric surgery.

Author	Groups	No (% F)	Octreotide Dose/Saline	Meal	Age (years)	BMI Preop (kg/m²)	BMI at Assessment (kg/m²)	Time of Assessment (postoperative)	Food Intake with Octreotide vs. Placebo	Satiety/Fullness with Octreotide vs. Placebo
Le Roux 2007 [19]	RYGB	7 (NR)	100 mcg octreotide/ 1 mL saline	Ad libitum meal 60 min after octreotide/saline	43 ± 4.5	44.5 ± 2.9	33.2 ± 1.9	9.5 ± 1.5 months	↑NC RYGB ↔ AGB	↑NC RYGB (Fullness) ↔ AGB (Fullness)
	AGB	6 (NR)			41.1 ± 5.6	41.9 ± 7.5	29.6 ± 1.5	17.0 ± 1.4 months		
De Hollanda 2015 [124]	RYGB, secondary "poor" responders (EWL% <50%)	19 (68.4%)	100 mcg octreotide/ 1 mL saline	Ad libitum meal 60 min after octreotide/saline	43.9 ± 10.3	46.9 ± 5.0	39.9 ± 4.0	6.5 ± 1.1 years	+53.7% (↑ND) secondary "poor" responders	↓(satiety) in secondary "poor" responders
	RYGB, "good" responders (EWL >50%)	23 (78.3%)			42.1 ± 10	45.6 ± 5.6	28.7 ± 3.3	6.0 ± 2.1 years	+47.3% (↑) "good" responders	↓ (satiety) in "good" responders
Bojsen-Moller 2020 [128] (abstract)	RYGB, primary "poor" responders (EBLmax <50%)	20 (100%)	1 mcg/kg octreotide (max 100 mcg)/saline	Standardised MMTT 30 min after octreotide/saline and then ad libitum meal at 270 min	51 ± 9	43.1 ± 4.0	40 ± 4.1	4.8 ± 2.0 years	−0.5% (↔) primary "poor" responders	NR
	RYGB, "good" responders (EBLmax >60%)	20 (100%)			51 ± 9	43.0 ± 3.6	29.2 ± 3.3	4.8 ± 1.4 years	+23% (↑*) "good" responders	NR

Roux-en-Y gastric bypass, EWL%: Excess Weight Loss, EBLmax: Maximum Excess BMI Loss, F: Female, MMTT: Mixed Meal Tolerance Test, NR: Not Reported, ↑: increased with octreotide vs. placebo, ↔: no change with octreotide vs. placebo, ↓: reduced with octreotide vs. placebo,*: significant difference between study groups on the outcome change with octreotide vs. placebo, NC: no comparison performed between study groups on the outcome change with octreotide vs. placebo, ND: no difference between study groups on the outcome change with octreotide vs. placebo.

4. The Role of GLP-1 on Glycaemic Outcomes after Bariatric Surgery

4.1. GLP-1 as a Mediator of the Improvement in Glucose Homeostasis in People with Type 2 Diabetes after Bariatric Surgery

Yoshino et al. assessed the changes in glucose homeostasis before and after matched weight loss induced by RYGB (*n* = 22) or diet alone (*n* = 22) in people with obesity and T2D [132]. After 18% weight loss, they found similar improvements in insulin sensitivity and beta cell function with RYGB and diet, suggesting that weight loss is the main driver for the observed improvements in glycaemic parameters after RYGB [132]. However, after bariatric surgery, the improvement in glucose homeostasis for people with T2D is observed from the first postoperative days, supporting the existence of weight loss independent mechanisms [36,133].

During the first postoperative weeks, the improvement in hepatic insulin sensitivity and insulin clearance due to calorie restriction and reduction in liver fat are contributed to the improvement in glucose homeostasis [36,39,134]. Additionally, the existence of RYGB mechanisms relevant to improvement in postprandial glucose metabolism which are independent to weight loss and calorie restriction is supported by the example of a patient with insulin-treated T2D who had a gastrostomy tube inserted after RYGB [135]. Five weeks after RYGB, this patient was given identical meals orally or through the gastrostomy tube on 2 consecutive days. On the day of oral feeding (200 mL of liquid meal, 300 kcal, consumed over 10 min), he had normal glucose tolerance with large GLP-1 and insulin responses; on the day of gastrostomy feeding (same meal, given over 10 min), he had glucose levels consistent with T2D and low GLP-1 and insulin levels. This was later confirmed in a larger cohort of patients [65]. These observations suggest an effect of RYGB on insulin secretion and beta cell function which can be activated by diverting food via the duodenum and it is independent of weight loss and calorie restriction.

Indeed, immediately after RYGB, beta cell function in response to a meal improves in subjects with T2D accompanied by an increased postprandial GLP-1 secretion [133,136–138]. Studies with Ex-9, have demonstrated causality between the increased GLP-1 secretion and the increased postprandial insulin secretion after RYGB in people with T2D (Table 3). In every study where people with T2D preoperatively were given Ex-9 vs. placebo after RYGB, at any postoperative time point, postprandial insulin secretion (whether measured as insulin, c-peptide or insulin secretion rate) was significantly reduced following Ex-9 administration and compared to the non-operated control population [37,139–141] (Table 3). Similar findings have been reported in people with T2D remission two years after SG [142] and in people without T2D who have undergone RYBG or SG [142–146]. These findings confirm that postprandial GLP-1 action is key mediator of postprandial insulin secretion after RYGB and SG; however, whether this increased insulin secretion is fundamental to the improvement in postprandial glucose levels during the early postoperative period in people with T2D is more complex, as multiple other factors may contribute to glucose homeostasis. These factors include the improved hepatic insulin sensitivity and insulin clearance due to caloric restriction during the first weeks postoperatively and, subsequently, on the gradual improvement in peripheral insulin sensitivity due to weight loss [39,131].

4.1.1. Studies Using Exendin 9–39 during the Early Postoperative Period in People with Type 2 Diabetes after Bariatric Surgery

Jorgensen et al. [37] studied meal-induced responses in patients with obesity and T2D before, 1 week and 3 months after RYGB with or without simultaneous infusions of Ex-9. The Ex-9 administration impaired insulin secretion before, and particularly after, the operation; insulin secretion reverted to the preoperative values with the Ex-9 infusion at the first week and the third month postoperatively. As a result, with the administration of Ex-9 glucose tolerance worsened to preoperatively levels at the first week postoperative and was still impaired at 3 months. These findings strongly support a role of GLP-1 for improved beta cell function and improvement in glucose tolerance during the first postoperative weeks.

Another study by Shah et al. [141] assessed the role of GLP-1 action on insulin secretion and insulin clearance rate after an oral glucose tolerance test at 3 months post-RYGB, in people with T2D preoperatively ($n = 22$). Blockade of GLP-1 action with Ex-9 resulted as expected in 49% reduction in postprandial insulin levels and 51% reduction in insulin secretion rate compared to placebo as well as in 19% increase in postprandial insulin clearance rate [141]. However, this study did not have a non-surgical control group and did not report the changes in glucose levels.

On the other hand, a prospective case–control study compared the effects of Ex-9 on insulin secretion and postprandial glucose levels in 10 people with T2D after RYGB and 10 people with T2D who received an intensive lifestyle intervention after both groups have achieved 10% weight loss (12 kg) [140]. As expected, despite the comparable weight reduction between the two groups, RYGB was associated with a larger postprandial GLP-1 and insulin secretion compared to the intensive lifestyle intervention group. Ex-9 had a greater impact on insulin secretion reduction in people who have undergone RYGB than the intensive lifestyle group. Postprandial glucose levels and glucose tolerance deteriorated comparably in both RYGB and intensive lifestyle modification group during Ex-9 infusion. Therefore, this study confirms that in people with T2D preoperatively, GLP-1 action after RYGB has an important role on postoperative insulin secretion. However, the role of the excessive GLP-1 secretion after RYGB on the improvement of postprandial glucose levels and glucose tolerance after 10% weight loss may be limited compared to other factors such as the improved hepatic and peripheral insulin sensitivity, a finding in partial agreement with the study from Yoshino et al. [132]

An important factor that may contribute to the attenuated improvement in postprandial glucose levels after RYGB despite the substantial improvement in GLP-1 mediated insulin secretion is the paradoxical increase in postprandial glucagon levels after RYGB compared to the non-surgical groups, which increases further after administration of Ex-9 [37,140,147]. The underlying aetiology for the increased glucagon levels after gastrointestinal surgery is still under investigation. The glucagon concentrations after RYGB appear to follow closely the amino acid absorption and plasma amino acid concentrations [45], in agreement with recent evidence suggesting that glucagon and amino acids are linked in a mutual feedback cycle between the liver and the pancreatic a-cells [148]. Furthermore, there is evidence that part of the excessive postprandial glucagon concentration after RYGB might be gastrointestinally derived. More specifically, the expression of the glucagon gene in the small intestine appears to be increased after surgery and glucagon was identified in small intestine biopsy specimens obtained after, but not before RYGB [149]. These findings suggest that glucagon derived from small intestine enteroendocrine L cells may contribute to postprandial plasma concentrations of glucagon after RYGB [149]. Finally, accurate measurement of postprandial glucagon levels after RYGB can be challenging [150] and in some cases, the elevated plasma glucagon in people after gastrointestinal surgery may represent an assay artefact due to increased concentrations of cross-reacting proglucagon peptides [151].

Future research on the role of GLP-1 on T2D remission/improvement during the early postoperative period may also focus in people who have undergone SG. Currently there is limited number of studies with Ex-9 for people with T2D who have undergone SG (Table 3), despite that it is the most commonly performed procedure worldwide.

4.1.2. Studies Using Exendin 9–39 after the Early Postoperative Period in People with Type 2 Diabetes after Bariatric Surgery

Few studies have investigated the effect of endogenous GLP-1 action on postprandial glucose levels in subjects with T2D remission who had undergone RYGB or SG at least two years before assessment, with the use of Ex-9 (Table 3) [139,142]. Jimenez et al. [139], in a cross-sectional study, assessed eight people who had undergone RYGB and achieved T2D remission and 34% weight loss at the time of assessment. A control group of seven people without diabetes and normal BMI was also recruited. In the RYGB group, insulin and C-peptide secretion decrease with Ex-9 administration, by 52% and 24%, respectively, when there was no change in insulin and C-peptide levels with Ex-9 administration in the control group. Postprandial glucose levels in the RYGB group after administration of Ex-9 increased by approximately 2 mmol/l between 90' and 120' post-meal which was not observed in the control group [139]. This study accordingly confirmed a role of GLP-1 for increased insulin secretion in people with T2D remission even >2 years after RYGB. Moreover, it demonstrated that GLP-1 action is contributed to the improvements in postprandial glucose levels for people who achieve T2D remission after RYGB, even if the improvement in peripheral insulin sensitivity due to substantial weight loss appears to be the main mediator of the improvement in postprandial glucose levels and T2D remission at this time.

A subsequent study from the same group assessed eight people with obesity and T2D who underwent SG more than two years ago and had achieved T2D remission. There was a control group with six BMI-matched people without T2D preoperatively who have also undergone SG at least 2 years ago and a second control group of eight people without diabetes and normal BMI [142]. Ex-9 administration was associated with impaired insulin secretion in the SG groups (the T2D remission group and the control group without T2D) compared to the non-operated control group. The blockade of GLP-1 through Ex-9 resulted in a moderate deterioration of postprandial glucose levels in all the three groups. However, postprandial glucose levels after Ex-9 were comparable between the three groups suggesting a limited role for the excess GLP-1 secretion after SG on the improvement in postprandial glucose levels in people with T2D remission after significant weight loss through SG.

An important consideration to the above studies using Ex-9 to investigate the role of GLP-1 on insulin secretion and postprandial glucose levels in people with T2D after bariatric surgery is that almost all of them have been performed in people with short duration of T2D and presumably reasonable beta cell functional capacity [37,139,140,142]. People with impaired insulin secretion and beta cell function before and after surgery are those who do not achieve T2D remission [137,152], despite that postprandial GLP-1 levels are similar between people who achieve or do not achieve T2D remission [37,139,140,142,153]. Therefore, exaggerated GLP-1 responses after RYGB and SG are probably insufficient in individuals with poor functional capacity of beta cells to secrete enough insulin and to achieve important improvement in postprandial glucose levels postoperatively [153,154].

Another limitation of studies assessing the impact of Ex-9 on glucose homeostasis after bariatric surgery is the small number of participants (the majority of studies had less than 10 participants, Table 3) and therefore the results should be interpreted with caution. Other challenges regarding the interpretation of the results include the different amount of intravenous Ex-9 administered at different studies (Table 3), as well as the increased glucagon levels after Ex-9 administration in some cases [155], which as discussed before, may affect the postprandial glucose levels. Finally, the increased levels of PYY and GLP-1 after Ex-9 administration [130] may suggest that Ex-9 interfere with intestinal endocrine feedback loops [155] which may also affect the glucose levels.

Between the other gut hormones (except of GLP-1) which may contribute to changes in glucose homeostasis after bariatric surgery, GIP is of interest due to its known insulinotropic effect. Data on GIP action after bariatric surgery is limited and GIP levels are inconsistent after RYGB and SG. There are no studies with specific GIP antagonists to assess the role of GIP on glucose homeostasis after RYGB or SG. To determine whether GIP is important after RYGB, patients without diabetes who underwent RYGB were given the DPP-4 inhibitor sitagliptin to increase the bioavailability of both GLP-1 and GIP [146,156]. They then received Ex-9 (in combination with sitagliptin) in order to block GLP-1 action and consequently, isolate the impact of GIP signalling on glucose tolerance. Interestingly, sitagliptin did not improve glucose tolerance or *beta* cell function when GLP-1 receptor signalling was blocked [146]. In contrast, patients with T2D who have not undergone bariatric procedures fully responded to the DPP-4 inhibitor with improved glucose tolerance and insulin secretion, when DPP-4 inhibitor was combined with Ex-9 [156,157]. Together these data may suggest that RYGB shifts the balance of the incretin effect towards GLP-1 and away from GIP [156]. Nevertheless, a specific GIP antagonist for human use is currently available and its use in future studies may help us understand better the role of GIP as well as the role of the combined GIP/GLP-1 action on glucose homeostasis and diabetes remission after bariatric surgery [155].

4.2. GLP-1 and Postprandial Hypoglycaemia after Bariatric Surgery

Postprandial hyperinsulinaemic hypoglycaemia (PHH) is a well described condition after RYGB and SG, which is associated with reduced quality of life, high degree of functional disability (inability to work, drive and care for others) and weight regain [158–160]. The incidence of PHH ranges between 17–75% after RYGB and SG, depending on the definition of hypoglycaemia, the population studied and the diagnostic tool used to assess hypoglycaemia [161–168]. The vast majority (around 80%) of hypoglycaemic episodes after bariatric surgery detected with continuous glucose monitoring (CGM) are asymptomatic [162], however, data on self-reported hypoglycaemia symptoms in a general population after RYGB and SG suggests that the prevalence of severe symptomatic hypoglycaemia (defined as self-reported severe symptoms of hypoglycaemia in Edinburgh hypoglycaemia scale, hypoglycaemic episodes required assistance from others, episodes of syncope, seizure or medically confirmed hypoglycaemia) is 11.6% [164]. The incidence of hypoglycaemia seems to be comparable between RYGB and SG [163], but RYGB is associated with more severe hypoglycaemic episodes and symptoms [163,166]. RYGB is also associated with higher risk of hospitalisation due to symptomatic hypoglycaemia compared to a control population, but the actual proportion of RYGB patients presented to hospital with hypoglycaemia was low (0.2%) [169]. Currently, the treatment options for PHH after bariatric surgery are limited. Patients are commonly advised to follow dietary modifications of small and frequent meals with controlled portions of low glycaemic index carbohydrates [170].

The underlying pathophysiology of PHH after RYGB is poorly defined but several studies have shown that after RYGB people who experience PHH have higher postprandial peak glucose levels, higher peak insulin secretion and higher peak GLP-1 levels compared to those without PHH [171–173]. PHH is a condition which often affects people without T2D preoperatively and is likely to be the outcome of the altered nutrient delivery and altered glucose absorption after RYGB rather than inherent beta-cell hypertrophy or hyperfunction [64,164]. Per this theory, feeding through gastrostomy tube to the remnant stomach after RYGB or reversal of RYGB operation can lead to remission/improvement of PHH, as well as reduction in the peak glucose, GLP-1 and insulin levels [64].

Ex-9 has been used in order to demonstrate causality between the exaggerated GLP-1 secretion and the PHH [143,144,174]. Blockade of GLP-1 action through intravenous Ex-9 in individuals with PHH reduced postprandial insulin secretion by around 50–70% [143,144,175], increased the glucagon levels, increased the postprandial glucose levels (including the nadir glucose levels) and reduced the risk and symptoms of hypoglycaemia [143,144] (Table 3). Subjects with confirmed PHH after RYGB exhibited a greater glycaemic response to intravenous Ex-9 administration with a pronounced increase in postprandial glucose [144] (Table 3). In an early phase trial in people with PHH after RYGB, subcutaneous Ex-9 increased the postprandial glucose nadir by 66%, reduced peak insulin levels by 57%, and reduced neuroglycopenic symptoms by 80% [174] (Table 3). A phase 2 trial confirmed the safety, tolerability and efficacy of subcutaneous GLP-1 antagonist as a treatment for PHH [176]. More specifically, twice daily administration of subcutaneous exendin 9–39 for 3 days, effectively raised the nadir glucose levels by 39–47% and improved by 47% the symptoms suggestive of hypoglycaemia after an oral glucose tolerance test (see also Table 3) [176].

Table 3. Studies using the GLP-1 antagonist Exendin 9–39 to assess glycaemic outcomes in people with type 2 diabetes or postprandial hypoglycaemia after bariatric surgery.

Author	Groups	No (F%)	Meal	Ex-9 Dose/Placebo	Age (years)	BMI before Intervention (Kg/m²)	BMI at Assessment (Kg/m²)	Time of Assessment	T2D Duration (years)	Glucose Parameters with Ex-9 vs. Placebo	Insulin Parameters with Ex-9 vs. Placebo	C-Peptide Parameters with Ex-9 vs. Placebo
						Studies in Population with T2D Preoperatively.						
Jorgensen 2013 [37]	RYGB, T2D preoperatively	9 (33%)	MMTT, 300 kcal, 50% carbs, 35% fat, 15% protein	43,000 pmol/kg bolus and then 900 pmol/kg/min OR saline (IV)	50 ± 3		37.67 (mean)	1 week postop	5.7 ± 1.3	+64.6% (↑NC) AUC (0–240) +28.8% (↑NC) 2 h glucose	−22.9% (↓NC) AUC (0–240)	−28.4% (↓NC) AUC (0–240)
	RYGB, T2D preoperatively						34.03 (mean)	3 months postop		+39.2% (↔ NC) AUC (0–240) +29.2% (↑NC) 2 h glucose	−31.7% (↔ NC) AUC (0–240)	−25.5% (↓NC) AUC (0–240)
	Preoperative values used as control					39.2 ± 2.4		Preop		+49.7 (↑) AUC (0–240) +18% (↑) 2 h glucose	−2.9% (↔) AUC (0–240)	−2.1% (↔) AUC (0–240)
Vetter 2015 [140]	RYGB, T2D preoperatively	10 (90%)	MMTT, 240 Kcal, 55% carbs, 25% protein 20% fat	7500 pmol/kg bolus and then 750 pmol/kg/min OR saline (IV)	54 ± 6.6	43.2 ± 1.9	39.1 ± 1.4	58.9 ± 12.1 days postop	5.2 ± 3.3	+41.4% (↑ND) AUC (0–180)	−44.9% (↓ND) AUC (0–180)	−37.1% (↓*) AUC (0–180)
	Intensive lifestyle modification (ILM), T2D at baseline	10 (50%)			51.8 ± 11.6	41.8 ± 1.2	37.3 ± 1.4	85.5 ± 24.4 days post-ILM initiation	3.1 ± 2.7	+44.4% (↑) AUC (0–180)	−10% (↔) AUC (0–180)	−5.1% (↔) AUC (0–180)

Table 3. Cont.

	Groups	No (F%)	Meal	Ex-9 Dose/Placebo	Age (years)	BMI before Intervention (Kg/m²)	BMI at Assessment (Kg/m²)	Time of Assessment	T2D Duration (years)	Glucose Parameters with Ex-9 vs. Placebo	Insulin Parameters with Ex-9 vs. Placebo	C-Peptide Parameters with Ex-9 vs. Placebo
Shah 2019 [141]	RYGB, T2D preoperatively	22 (91%)	75 g of oral glucose	600 pmol/kg/min OR saline (IV)	44.1 ± 8.6	42.1 ± 5.1	34.9 ± 4.6	3 months	8.26 ± 7.6	NR	−48.8% (↓NA) in AUC (0–180)	−51.1% (↓NA) in ISR AUC (0–180)
	No control group											
Jimenez 2013 [139]	RYGB, T2D remission	8 (100%)	MMTT, 398 kcal, 50% carbs, 35% fat, 15% protein	7500 pmol/kg bolus and then 750 pmol/kg/min OR saline (IV)	54.1 ± 8.4	46.8 ± 6.6	30.8 ± 4.7	NR (>24 months postop)	2.1 ± 1.1	+10.07% (↑NC) AUC (0–120) +NR (↑NC) 2 h glucose	−53.8% (↓NC) AUC (0–120)	−24.9% (↓NC) in AUC (0–120)
	Healthy controls	7 (NR)		47.0 ± 10.8 pmol/kg/min OR saline (IV)		NA	21.1 ± 1.3	NA	NA	+9.3% (↑) AUC (0–120) +NR (↔) 2 h glucose	−4% (↔) in AUC (0–120)	−2.9% (↔) in AUC (0–120)

Author	Groups	No (F%)	Meal	Ex-9 Dose/Placebo	Age (years)	BMI before Intervention (Kg/m²)	BMI at Assessment (Kg/m²)	Time of Assessment	T2D Duration (years)	Glucose Parameters with Ex-9 vs. Placebo	Insulin Parameters with Ex-9 vs. Placebo	C-Peptide Parameters with Ex-9 vs. Placebo
Jimenez 2014 [142]	SG, T2D remission	8 (67%)	MMTT, 398 kcal, 50% carbs, 35% fat, 15% protein	7500 pmol/kg bolus and then 750 pmol/kg/min OR saline (IV)	49.8 ± 12.4	47.7 ± 5.5	32.7 ± 2.3	3.4 ± 0.9 year-spostop	2.8 ± 1.8	+12.4% (NR) in AUC (0–120) +23.7% (↑) in 2 h glucose	−18.4% (↓*) in total insulin output	−39.1% (↓) in b-cell glucose sensitivity
	SG, without T2D preop	6 (67%)			52.1 ± 13.1	44.9 ± 5.3	31.1 ± 4.2	2.9 ± 0.9 years postop	NA	+2.9% (NR) in AUC (0–120) +16.7% (↔) in 2 h glucose	−11.1% (↓*) in total insulin output	+3.3% (NR) in b-cell glucose sensitivity

Table 3. Cont.

	Healthy controls	8 (67%)		50 ± 13	NA	23.3 ± 2.0	NA	NA	+9.4% (NR) in AUC (0–120) +12.7% (↔) in 2 h glucose	+2.4% (↔) in total insulin output	−33.7% (NR) in b-cell glucose sensitivity

Studies in Populations with Postprandial Hyperinsulinaemic Hypoglycaemia

Salehi 2014 [144]	RYGB with established PHH	9 (100%)	MMTT, 350 kcal, 57% carbs, 28% fat, 15% protein	44.6 ± 4.5	48 ± 2.6	30.9 ± 2.5	3.9 ± 0.5 years postop	NA	+67.3% (NR) in nadir levels +250.4% (↑*,**) AUC (0–180)	−63.3% (↓*,**) AUC (0–180)	−46.8% (↓*,**) in ISR AUC (0–180)
	RYGB without symptoms of PHH	7 (43%)		47.6 ± 3.0	55 ± 2.6	33.8 ± 3.4	3.6 ± 0.7 years postop	NA	+14.3% (NR) in nadir levels +32.1% (↔ ND) AUC (0–180)	−19.2% (↔ ND) AUC (0–180)	−22.4% (↔ ND) in ISR AUC (0–180)
	BMI-matched controls	8 (88%)	7500 pmol/kg bolus and then 750 pmol/kg/min OR saline (IV)	33.1 ± 3.3	NA	32.8 ± 1.1	NA	NA	+9.8% (NR) in nadir levels +5.4% (↔) AUC (0–180)	−22.2% (↔) AUC (0–180)	−22.6% (↔) in ISR AUC (0–180)
Craig 2017 [143]	RYGB with established PHH	8 (100%)	75 g of oral glucose	46.4 ± 4	NR	31.2 ± 2	5 years postop	NA	+69.2% (↑) in nadir levels +21.1% (↑) AUC (0–180)	−56% (↓) in peak levels −57.1% (↓) AUC (0–180)	−51.4% (↓) AUC (0–180)
	BMI-matched controls	8 (100%)	7500 pmol/kg bolus and then 750 pmol/kg/min OR saline (IV)	47 ± 3	NA	31.0 ± 0	NA	NA	NA	NA	NA

Table 3. Cont.

Study	Group	N (%)	Meal	Drug dose	Col1	Col2	Col3	Time postop	Col4	Glucose/Insulin outcome	GLP-1/C-pep outcome	Additional outcome
Craig 2018 [174]	RYGB with established PHH	8 (100%)	75 g of oral glucose	0.13–0.38 mg/kg (subcut)	45 ± 3.8	49 ± 2.3	29 ± 1.3	6.9 years postop	NA	+66% (↑NA) in nadir levels +72% (↑NA) AUC (90–180)	−57% (↓) in peak levels −48% (↓) AUC (0–60)	−44% (↓) in peak levels −31% (↓) AUC (0–60)
	No control group											
Tan 2020 [176]	RYGB with established PHH (treated with Lyo Ex-9)	14 (100%)	75 g of oral glucose	0.05–0.46 mg/kg bd for 3 days (subcut)	45 ± 5	48 ± 3	28 ± 4	8.6 years postop	NA	+39% (↑NA) in nadir levels^ +79% (↑NA) AUC (90–180)^	−50% (↓) in peak levels^ −47% (↓) AUC (0–60)^	NA
	RYGB with established PHH (treated with Liq Ex-9)	5 (100%)		0.38 mg/kg bd for 3 days (subcut)	51 ± 3	50 ± 4	30 ± 4	10.2 years postop	NA	+47% (↑NA) in nadir levels +71% (↑) AUC (90–180)	−67% (↔) in peak levels −63% (↓) AUC (0–60)	NA
	No control group											
Salehi 2011 [175]	RYGB without symptoms of PHH	12 (75%)	MMTT with clamp MMTT, 57% carbs, 15% protein, 28% fat	7500 pmol/kg bolus and then 750 pmol/kg/min OR saline (IV)	47 ± 2	52 ± 2	33 ± 1	3.3 ± 0.3 years postop	NA	0% AUC (95–270) (clamp study)	−50% (↓*) AUC (95–270)	−28% (NR) AUC (95–270)
	RYGB with symptoms of PHH	12 (92%)			39 ± 2	52 ± 2	32 ± 2	3.7 ± 0.4 years postop	NA	0% AUC (95–270) (clamp study)	−54% (↓*) AUC (95–270)	−37% (NR) AUC (95–270)
	BMI matched controls	10 (80%)			43 ± 3		33 ± 2	NA	NA	0% AUC (95–270) (clamp study)	−16% (NR) AUC (95–270)	−12% (NR) AUC (95–270)

Roux-en-Y gastric bypass, T2D: Type 2 Diabetes Mellitus, F: Female, MMTT: Mixed Meal Tolerance Test, SG: Sleeve Gastrectomy, PHH: Postprandial Hyperinsulinaemic Hypoglycaemia, Ex-9: Exendin 9-39, AUC: Area Under the Curve, 2 h: 2 h, ISR: Insulin Secretion Rate, bd: twice daily, NA: Not Applicable, NR: Not Reported, ↑: increased with Ex-9 vs. placebo, ↔: no change with Ex-9 vs. placebo, ↓: reduced with Ex-9 vs. placebo, *: significant difference between surgical and non-surgical groups on the outcome change with Ex-9 vs. placebo, NC: no comparison performed between study groups on the outcome change with Ex-9 vs. placebo, ND: no difference between surgical and non-surgical group on the outcome change with Ex-9 vs. placebo, **: significant difference between surgical groups on the outcome change with Ex-9 vs. placebo, Lyo: Lyophilized Ex-9, Liq: Liquid form of Ex-9, IV: intravenous, subcut: subcutaneous. ^ the analysis is for a subgroup of 6 participants received ≥20 mg (≥0.35 mg/kg) of subcutaneous Lyophilized (Lyo) Ex-9.

5. Pharmaceutical Use of Gut Hormones after Bariatric Surgery

Multiple GLP-1 receptor analogues (GLP-1 RA) are currently available for the management of obesity and T2D. The GRAVITAS (GLP-1 Receptor Agonist interVentIon for poor responders after bariAtric Surgery) randomized controlled trial [177], demonstrated that in individuals with persistent or recurrent T2D after RYGB or SG, use of 1.8 mg liraglutide once daily in combination with lifestyle advice and support for 6 months reduced HbA1c by 1.2% and led to an additional weight loss of 4.2 kg compared to placebo [177]. Moreover, in a recent retrospective analysis of 2092 patients, the use of liraglutide 3.0 mg (licensed for treatment of obesity) was evaluated in patients who have had bariatric surgery (n = 188), as well as non-surgical patients [178]. Weight loss achieved was approximately 6% after $\geq$ 16 weeks, which was comparable between the surgical and non-surgical groups, confirming the potential effectiveness of liraglutide 3.0 mg after bariatric surgery [178]. Observational studies using liraglutide 3.0 mg after bariatric surgery have reported similar results regarding weight loss [179].

These findings suggest that despite the increased endogenous postprandial GLP-1 secretion after RYGB and SG, GLP-1 RA could still be effective after bariatric surgery on improving weight loss and glycaemic control in T2D. Currently, a number of clinical trials with liraglutide 3.0 mg are taking place for treatment of "poor" responders to bariatric surgery [180] or for treatment of weight regain after bariatric surgery [181].

6. Conclusions

Each bariatric procedure has a unique gut hormone profile. Changes in gut hormones after RYGB have an important and synergistic role to increase satiety and reduce food intake postoperatively. The best evidence currently exists for GLP-1 and PYY 3–36 to reduce food intake after surgery. Moreover, postprandial changes in glicentin and oxyntomodulin during the early postoperative period after RYGB and SG are associated with weight loss outcomes. These hormones have the potential to be used as early markers of inadequate postoperative weight loss to identify people who may require additional postoperative supportive care.

GLP-1 contributes also to increased insulin secretion after RYGB from the early postoperative period in people with and without T2D. GLP-1 may also be pivotal to PHH after RYGB and ongoing studies are assessing the safety and efficacy of a subcutaneous GLP-1 receptor antagonist (Ex-9) as a treatment option. Interpretation of the role of enhanced GLP-1 responses to improved postprandial glucose levels in people with preoperative T2D is confounded by the effects of caloric restriction on glucose homeostasis during the early postoperative setting and the effects of weight loss in the late postoperative setting.

Based on the described changes in gut hormones after RYGB and SG and the evidence of their synergistic action in reducing food intake and appetite, combinations of gut hormone receptor agonists aiming to replicate the hormonal changes after bariatric surgery are under development and may form the next generation of treatments for obesity and T2D [182].

Author Contributions: Conceptualization, D.P. and C.W.l.R.; Methodology, D.P. and C.W.l.R.; Investigation, D.P., C.W.l.R.; Writing—Original Draft Preparation, D.P.; Writing—Review and Editing, C.W.l.R.; Visualization, D.P. and C.W.l.R.; Supervision, C.W.l.R. All authors have read and agreed to the published version of the manuscript.

Funding: This research received no external funding.

Acknowledgments: D.P. is funded by a National Institute of Health Research Clinical Lectureship. C.W.l.R. is funded by the Health Research Board in Ireland and the Irish Research Council.

Conflicts of Interest: D.P. reports grants from the Novo Nordisk UK Research Foundation, the Academy of Medical Sciences and Health Education East Midlands. C.W.l.R. serves on advisory boards for Novo Nordisk, Boehringer Ingelheim, Herbalife, GI Dynamics, Keyron, and Johnson&Johnson.

References

1. Bray, G.A.; Kim, K.K.; Wilding, J.P.H. Obesity: A chronic relapsing progressive disease process. A position statement of the World Obesity Federation. *Obes. Rev.* **2017**, *18*, 715–723. [CrossRef] [PubMed]
2. W.H.O. Obesity and Overweight. Available online: https://www.who.int/news-room/fact-sheets/detail/obesity-and-overweight (accessed on 7 December 2020).
3. Haslam, D.W.; James, W.P. Obesity. *Lancet* **2005**, *366*, 1197–1209. [CrossRef]
4. Bray, G.A.; Frühbeck, G.; Ryan, D.H.; Wilding, J.P. Management of obesity. *Lancet* **2016**, *387*, 1947–1956. [CrossRef]
5. Purcell, K.; Sumithran, P.; Prendergast, L.A.; Bouniu, C.J.; Delbridge, E.; Proietto, J. The effect of rate of weight loss on long-term weight management: A randomised controlled trial. *Lancet Diabetes Endocrinol.* **2014**, *2*, 954–962. [CrossRef]
6. Wadden, T.A. Treatment of obesity by moderate and severe caloric restriction. Results of clinical research trials. *Ann. Intern. Med.* **1993**, *119*, 688–693. [CrossRef]
7. Johansson, K.; Neovius, M.; Hemmingsson, E. Effects of anti-obesity drugs, diet, and exercise on weight-loss maintenance after a very-low-calorie diet or low-calorie diet: A systematic review and meta-analysis of randomized controlled trials. *Am. J. Clin. Nutr* **2014**, *99*, 14–23. [CrossRef]
8. Khera, R.; Murad, M.H.; Chandar, A.K.; Dulai, P.S.; Wang, Z.; Prokop, L.J.; Loomba, R.; Camilleri, M.; Singh, S. Association of Pharmacological Treatments for Obesity With Weight Loss and Adverse Events: A Systematic Review and Meta-analysis. *JAMA* **2016**, *315*, 2424–2434. [CrossRef]
9. Wadden, T.A.; Hollander, P.; Klein, S.; Niswender, K.; Woo, V.; Hale, P.M.; Aronne, L. Weight maintenance and additional weight loss with liraglutide after low-calorie-diet-induced weight loss: The SCALE Maintenance randomized study. *Int. J. Obes.* **2013**, *37*, 1443–1451. [CrossRef]
10. Kushner, R.F.; Calanna, S.; Davies, M.; Dicker, D.; Garvey, W.T.; Goldman, B.; Lingvay, I.; Thomsen, M.; Wadden, T.A.; Wharton, S.; et al. Semaglutide 2.4 mg for the Treatment of Obesity: Key Elements of the STEP Trials 1 to 5. *Obesity* **2020**, *28*, 1050–1061. [CrossRef]
11. O'Neil, P.M.; Birkenfeld, A.L.; McGowan, B.; Mosenzon, O.; Pedersen, S.D.; Wharton, S.; Carson, C.G.; Jepsen, C.H.; Kabisch, M.; Wilding, J.P.H. Efficacy and safety of semaglutide compared with liraglutide and placebo for weight loss in patients with obesity: A randomised, double-blind, placebo and active controlled, dose-ranging, phase 2 trial. *Lancet* **2018**, *392*, 637–649. [CrossRef]
12. Miras, A.D.; Kamocka, A.; Patel, D.; Dexter, S.; Finlay, I.; Hopkins, J.C.; Khan, O.; Reddy, M.; Sedman, P.; Small, P.; et al. Obesity surgery makes patients healthier and more functional: Real world results from the United Kingdom National Bariatric Surgery Registry. *Surg. Obes. Relat. Dis.* **2018**, *14*, 1033–1040. [CrossRef] [PubMed]
13. Neff, K.J.; Chuah, L.L.; Aasheim, E.T.; Jackson, S.; Dubb, S.S.; Radhakrishnan, S.T.; Sood, A.S.; Olbers, T.; Godsland, I.F.; Miras, A.D.; et al. Beyond weight loss: Evaluating the multiple benefits of bariatric surgery after Roux-en-Y gastric bypass and adjustable gastric band. *Obes. Surg.* **2014**, *24*, 684–691. [CrossRef] [PubMed]
14. Miras, A.D.; Al-Najim, W.; Jackson, S.N.; McGirr, J.; Cotter, L.; Tharakan, G.; Vusirikala, A.; le Roux, C.W.; Prechtl, C.G.; Scholtz, S. Psychological characteristics, eating behaviour, and quality of life assessment of obese patients undergoing weight loss interventions. *Scand. J. Surg.* **2015**, *104*, 10–17. [CrossRef] [PubMed]
15. Andersen, J.R.; Aasprang, A.; Karlsen, T.I.; Natvig, G.K.; Våge, V.; Kolotkin, R.L. Health-related quality of life after bariatric surgery: A systematic review of prospective long-term studies. *Surg. Obes. Relat. Dis.* **2015**, *11*, 466–473. [CrossRef]
16. Angrisani, L.; Santonicola, A.; Iovino, P.; Vitiello, A.; Higa, K.; Himpens, J.; Buchwald, H.; Scopinaro, N. IFSO Worldwide Survey 2016: Primary, Endoluminal, and Revisional Procedures. *Obes. Surg.* **2018**, *28*, 3783–3794. [CrossRef]
17. Welbourn, R.; Hollyman, M.; Kinsman, R.; Dixon, J.; Liem, R.; Ottosson, J.; Ramos, A.; Våge, V.; Al-Sabah, S.; Brown, W.; et al. Bariatric Surgery Worldwide: Baseline Demographic Description and One-Year Outcomes from the Fourth IFSO Global Registry Report 2018. *Obes. Surg.* **2019**, *29*, 782–795. [CrossRef]
18. Al-Najim, W.; Docherty, N.G.; le Roux, C.W. Food Intake and Eating Behavior After Bariatric Surgery. *Physiol. Rev.* **2018**, *98*, 1113–1141. [CrossRef]
19. Le Roux, C.W.; Welbourn, R.; Werling, M.; Osborne, A.; Kokkinos, A.; Laurenius, A.; Lönroth, H.; Fändriks, L.; Ghatei, M.A.; Bloom, S.R.; et al. Gut hormones as mediators of appetite and weight loss after Roux-en-Y gastric bypass. *Ann. Surg.* **2007**, *246*, 780–785. [CrossRef]
20. le Roux, C.W.; Aylwin, S.J.; Batterham, R.L.; Borg, C.M.; Coyle, F.; Prasad, V.; Shurey, S.; Ghatei, M.A.; Patel, A.G.; Bloom, S.R. Gut hormone profiles following bariatric surgery favor an anorectic state, facilitate weight loss, and improve metabolic parameters. *Ann. Surg.* **2006**, *243*, 108–114. [CrossRef] [PubMed]
21. Valderas, J.P.; Irribarra, V.; Boza, C.; de la Cruz, R.; Liberona, Y.; Acosta, A.M.; Yolito, M.; Maiz, A. Medical and surgical treatments for obesity have opposite effects on peptide YY and appetite: A prospective study controlled for weight loss. *J. Clin. Endocrinol. Metab.* **2010**, *95*, 1069–1075. [CrossRef]
22. Mans, E.; Serra-Prat, M.; Palomera, E.; Suñol, X.; Clavé, P. Sleeve gastrectomy effects on hunger, satiation, and gastrointestinal hormone and motility responses after a liquid meal test. *Am. J. Clin. Nutr* **2015**, *102*, 540–547. [CrossRef]
23. Nielsen, M.S.; Ritz, C.; Wewer Albrechtsen, N.J.; Holst, J.J.; le Roux, C.W.; Sjödin, A. Oxyntomodulin and Glicentin May Predict the Effect of Bariatric Surgery on Food Preferences and Weight Loss. *J. Clin. Endocrinol. Metab.* **2020**, *105*. [CrossRef] [PubMed]

24. Makaronidis, J.M.; Neilson, S.; Cheung, W.H.; Tymoszuk, U.; Pucci, A.; Finer, N.; Doyle, J.; Hashemi, M.; Elkalaawy, M.; Adamo, M.; et al. Reported appetite, taste and smell changes following Roux-en-Y gastric bypass and sleeve gastrectomy: Effect of gender, type 2 diabetes and relationship to post-operative weight loss. *Appetite* **2016**, *107*, 93–105. [CrossRef] [PubMed]
25. Weiss, E.C.; Galuska, D.A.; Kettel Khan, L.; Gillespie, C.; Serdula, M.K. Weight regain in U.S. adults who experienced substantial weight loss, 1999–2002. *Am. J. Prev. Med.* **2007**, *33*, 34–40. [CrossRef]
26. Fildes, A.; Charlton, J.; Rudisill, C.; Littlejohns, P.; Prevost, A.T.; Gulliford, M.C. Probability of an Obese Person Attaining Normal Body Weight: Cohort Study Using Electronic Health Records. *Am. J. Public Health* **2015**, *105*, e54–e59. [CrossRef]
27. Sumithran, P.; Prendergast, L.A.; Delbridge, E.; Purcell, K.; Shulkes, A.; Kriketos, A.; Proietto, J. Long-term persistence of hormonal adaptations to weight loss. *N. Engl. J. Med.* **2011**, *365*, 1597–1604. [CrossRef] [PubMed]
28. Anton, S.D.; Han, H.; York, E.; Martin, C.K.; Ravussin, E.; Williamson, D.A. Effect of calorie restriction on subjective ratings of appetite. *J. Hum. Nutr. Diet.* **2009**, *22*, 141–147. [CrossRef]
29. Miras, A.D.; le Roux, C.W. Mechanisms underlying weight loss after bariatric surgery. *Nat. Rev. Gastroenterol. Hepatol.* **2013**, *10*, 575–584. [CrossRef] [PubMed]
30. Maclean, P.S.; Bergouignan, A.; Cornier, M.A.; Jackman, M.R. Biology's response to dieting: The impetus for weight regain. *Am. J. Physiol. Regul. Integr. Comp. Physiol.* **2011**, *301*, R581–R600. [CrossRef]
31. Zhao, X.; Han, Q.; Gang, X.; Lv, Y.; Liu, Y.; Sun, C.; Wang, G. The Role of Gut Hormones in Diet-Induced Weight Change: A Systematic Review. *Horm. Metab. Res.* **2017**, *49*, 816–825. [CrossRef]
32. Papamargaritis, D.; le Roux, C.W.; Sioka, E.; Koukoulis, G.; Tzovaras, G.; Zacharoulis, D. Changes in gut hormone profile and glucose homeostasis after laparoscopic sleeve gastrectomy. *Surg. Obes. Relat. Dis.* **2013**, *9*, 192–201. [CrossRef]
33. Perakakis, N.; Kokkinos, A.; Peradze, N.; Tentolouris, N.; Ghaly, W.; Pilitsi, E.; Upadhyay, J.; Alexandrou, A.; Mantzoros, C.S. Circulating levels of gastrointestinal hormones in response to the most common types of bariatric surgery and predictive value for weight loss over one year: Evidence from two independent trials. *Metabolism* **2019**, *101*, 153997. [CrossRef]
34. Yousseif, A.; Emmanuel, J.; Karra, E.; Millet, Q.; Elkalaawy, M.; Jenkinson, A.D.; Hashemi, M.; Adamo, M.; Finer, N.; Fiennes, A.G.; et al. Differential effects of laparoscopic sleeve gastrectomy and laparoscopic gastric bypass on appetite, circulating acyl-ghrelin, peptide YY3–36 and active GLP-1 levels in non-diabetic humans. *Obes. Surg.* **2014**, *24*, 241–252. [CrossRef]
35. Jackness, C.; Karmally, W.; Febres, G.; Conwell, I.M.; Ahmed, L.; Bessler, M.; McMahon, D.J.; Korner, J. Very low-calorie diet mimics the early beneficial effect of Roux-en-Y gastric bypass on insulin sensitivity and β-cell Function in type 2 diabetic patients. *Diabetes* **2013**, *62*, 3027–3032. [CrossRef]
36. Steven, S.; Hollingsworth, K.G.; Small, P.K.; Woodcock, S.A.; Pucci, A.; Aribasala, B.; Al-Mrabeh, A.; Batterham, R.L.; Taylor, R. Calorie restriction and not glucagon-like peptide-1 explains the acute improvement in glucose control after gastric bypass in Type 2 diabetes. *Diabet. Med.* **2016**, *33*, 1723–1731. [CrossRef]
37. Jørgensen, N.B.; Dirksen, C.; Bojsen-Møller, K.N.; Jacobsen, S.H.; Worm, D.; Hansen, D.L.; Kristiansen, V.B.; Naver, L.; Madsbad, S.; Holst, J.J. Exaggerated glucagon-like peptide 1 response is important for improved β-cell function and glucose tolerance after Roux-en-Y gastric bypass in patients with type 2 diabetes. *Diabetes* **2013**, *62*, 3044–3052. [CrossRef] [PubMed]
38. Pérez-Pevida, B.; Escalada, J.; Miras, A.D.; Frühbeck, G. Mechanisms Underlying Type 2 Diabetes Remission After Metabolic Surgery. *Front. Endocrinol.* **2019**, *10*, 641. [CrossRef] [PubMed]
39. Bojsen-Møller, K.N.; Dirksen, C.; Jørgensen, N.B.; Jacobsen, S.H.; Serup, A.K.; Albers, P.H.; Hansen, D.L.; Worm, D.; Naver, L.; Kristiansen, V.B.; et al. Early enhancements of hepatic and later of peripheral insulin sensitivity combined with increased postprandial insulin secretion contribute to improved glycemic control after Roux-en-Y gastric bypass. *Diabetes* **2014**, *63*, 1725–1737. [CrossRef] [PubMed]
40. Jacobsen, S.H.; Olesen, S.C.; Dirksen, C.; Jørgensen, N.B.; Bojsen-Møller, K.N.; Kielgast, U.; Worm, D.; Almdal, T.; Naver, L.S.; Hvolris, L.E.; et al. Changes in gastrointestinal hormone responses, insulin sensitivity, and beta-cell function within 2 weeks after gastric bypass in non-diabetic subjects. *Obes. Surg.* **2012**, *22*, 1084–1096. [CrossRef]
41. Drucker, D.J. The biology of incretin hormones. *Cell Metab.* **2006**, *3*, 153–165. [CrossRef]
42. Kreymann, B.; Williams, G.; Ghatei, M.A.; Bloom, S.R. Glucagon-like peptide-1 7–36: A physiological incretin in man. *Lancet* **1987**, *2*, 1300–1304. [CrossRef]
43. Nguyen, N.Q.; Debreceni, T.L.; Burgess, J.E.; Bellon, M.; Wishart, J.; Standfield, S.; Malbert, C.H.; Horowitz, M. Impact of gastric emptying and small intestinal transit on blood glucose, intestinal hormones, glucose absorption in the morbidly obese. *Int. J. Obes.* **2018**, *42*, 1556–1564. [CrossRef]
44. Stano, S.; Alam, F.; Wu, L.; Dutia, R.; Ng, S.N.; Sala, M.; McGinty, J.; Laferrère, B. Effect of meal size and texture on gastric pouch emptying and glucagon-like peptide 1 after gastric bypass surgery. *Surg. Obes. Relat. Dis.* **2017**, *13*, 1975–1983. [CrossRef] [PubMed]
45. Svane, M.S.; Bojsen-Møller, K.N.; Martinussen, C.; Dirksen, C.; Madsen, J.L.; Reitelseder, S.; Holm, L.; Rehfeld, J.F.; Kristiansen, V.B.; van Hall, G.; et al. Postprandial Nutrient Handling and Gastrointestinal Hormone Secretion After Roux-en-Y Gastric Bypass vs. Sleeve Gastrectomy. *Gastroenterology* **2019**, *156*, 1627–1641. [CrossRef] [PubMed]
46. Dirksen, C.; Damgaard, M.; Bojsen-Møller, K.N.; Jørgensen, N.B.; Kielgast, U.; Jacobsen, S.H.; Naver, L.S.; Worm, D.; Holst, J.J.; Madsbad, S.; et al. Fast pouch emptying, delayed small intestinal transit, and exaggerated gut hormone responses after Roux-en-Y gastric bypass. *Neurogastroenterol. Motil.* **2013**, *25*, 346–e255. [CrossRef]

47. Horowitz, M.; Cook, D.J.; Collins, P.J.; Harding, P.E.; Hooper, M.J.; Walsh, J.F.; Shearman, D.J. Measurement of gastric emptying after gastric bypass surgery using radionuclides. *Br. J. Surg.* **1982**, *69*, 655–657. [CrossRef]
48. Falkén, Y.; Hellström, P.M.; Holst, J.J.; Näslund, E. Changes in glucose homeostasis after Roux-en-Y gastric bypass surgery for obesity at day three, two months, and one year after surgery: Role of gut peptides. *J. Clin. Endocrinol. Metab.* **2011**, *96*, 2227–2235. [CrossRef]
49. Nguyen, N.Q.; Debreceni, T.L.; Bambrick, J.E.; Bellon, M.; Wishart, J.; Standfield, S.; Rayner, C.K.; Horowitz, M. Rapid gastric and intestinal transit is a major determinant of changes in blood glucose, intestinal hormones, glucose absorption and postprandial symptoms after gastric bypass. *Obesity* **2014**, *22*, 2003–2009. [CrossRef]
50. Yehoshua, R.T.; Eidelman, L.A.; Stein, M.; Fichman, S.; Mazor, A.; Chen, J.; Bernstine, H.; Singer, P.; Dickman, R.; Beglaibter, N.; et al. Laparoscopic sleeve gastrectomy—Volume and pressure assessment. *Obes. Surg.* **2008**, *18*, 1083–1088. [CrossRef]
51. Mion, F.; Tolone, S.; Garros, A.; Savarino, E.; Pelascini, E.; Robert, M.; Poncet, G.; Valette, P.J.; Marjoux, S.; Docimo, L.; et al. High-resolution Impedance Manometry after Sleeve Gastrectomy: Increased Intragastric Pressure and Reflux are Frequent Events. *Obes. Surg.* **2016**, *26*, 2449–2456. [CrossRef]
52. Melissas, J.; Daskalakis, M.; Koukouraki, S.; Askoxylakis, I.; Metaxari, M.; Dimitriadis, E.; Stathaki, M.; Papadakis, J.A. Sleeve gastrectomy-a "food limiting" operation. *Obes. Surg.* **2008**, *18*, 1251–1256. [CrossRef] [PubMed]
53. Melissas, J.; Koukouraki, S.; Askoxylakis, J.; Stathaki, M.; Daskalakis, M.; Perisinakis, K.; Karkavitsas, N. Sleeve gastrectomy: A restrictive procedure? *Obes. Surg.* **2007**, *17*, 57–62. [CrossRef]
54. Melissas, J.; Leventi, A.; Klinaki, I.; Perisinakis, K.; Koukouraki, S.; de Bree, E.; Karkavitsas, N. Alterations of global gastrointestinal motility after sleeve gastrectomy: A prospective study. *Ann. Surg.* **2013**, *258*, 976–982. [CrossRef] [PubMed]
55. De Jong, J.R.; van Ramshorst, B.; Gooszen, H.G.; Smout, A.J.; Tiel-Van Buul, M.M. Weight loss after laparoscopic adjustable gastric banding is not caused by altered gastric emptying. *Obes. Surg.* **2009**, *19*, 287–292. [CrossRef] [PubMed]
56. Usinger, L.; Hansen, K.B.; Kristiansen, V.B.; Larsen, S.; Holst, J.J.; Knop, F.K. Gastric emptying of orally administered glucose solutions and incretin hormone responses are unaffected by laparoscopic adjustable gastric banding. *Obes. Surg.* **2011**, *21*, 625–632. [CrossRef] [PubMed]
57. Bojsen-Møller, K.N.; Jacobsen, S.H.; Dirksen, C.; Jørgensen, N.B.; Reitelseder, S.; Jensen, J.E.; Kristiansen, V.B.; Holst, J.J.; van Hall, G.; Madsbad, S. Accelerated protein digestion and amino acid absorption after Roux-en-Y gastric bypass. *Am. J. Clin. Nutr.* **2015**, *102*, 600–607. [CrossRef]
58. Jacobsen, S.H.; Bojsen-Møller, K.N.; Dirksen, C.; Jørgensen, N.B.; Clausen, T.R.; Wulff, B.S.; Kristiansen, V.B.; Worm, D.; Hansen, D.L.; Holst, J.J.; et al. Effects of gastric bypass surgery on glucose absorption and metabolism during a mixed meal in glucose-tolerant individuals. *Diabetologia* **2013**, *56*, 2250–2254. [CrossRef]
59. Kuhre, R.E.; Frost, C.R.; Svendsen, B.; Holst, J.J. Molecular mechanisms of glucose-stimulated GLP-1 secretion from perfused rat small intestine. *Diabetes* **2015**, *64*, 370–382. [CrossRef]
60. Kuhre, R.E.; Christiansen, C.B.; Saltiel, M.Y.; Wewer Albrechtsen, N.J.; Holst, J.J. On the relationship between glucose absorption and glucose-stimulated secretion of GLP-1, neurotensin, and PYY from different intestinal segments in the rat. *Physiol. Rep.* **2017**, *5*. [CrossRef]
61. Martinussen, C.; Veedfald, S.; Dirksen, C.; Bojsen-Møller, K.N.; Svane, M.S.; Wewer Albrechtsen, N.J.; van Hall, G.; Kristiansen, V.B.; Fenger, M.; Holst, J.J.; et al. The effect of acute dual SGLT1/SGLT2 inhibition on incretin release and glucose metabolism after gastric bypass surgery. *Am. J. Physiol. Endocrinol. Metab.* **2020**, *318*, E956–E964. [CrossRef]
62. Rhee, N.A.; Wahlgren, C.D.; Pedersen, J.; Mortensen, B.; Langholz, E.; Wandall, E.P.; Friis, S.U.; Vilmann, P.; Paulsen, S.J.; Kristiansen, V.B.; et al. Effect of Roux-en-Y gastric bypass on the distribution and hormone expression of small-intestinal enteroendocrine cells in obese patients with type 2 diabetes. *Diabetologia* **2015**, *58*, 2254–2258. [CrossRef]
63. Gribble, F.M.; Reimann, F. Function and mechanisms of enteroendocrine cells and gut hormones in metabolism. *Nat. Rev. Endocrinol.* **2019**, *15*, 226–237. [CrossRef]
64. Davis, D.B.; Khoraki, J.; Ziemelis, M.; Sirinvaravong, S.; Han, J.Y.; Campos, G.M. Roux en Y gastric bypass hypoglycemia resolves with gastric feeding or reversal: Confirming a non-pancreatic etiology. *Mol. Metab.* **2018**, *9*, 15–27. [CrossRef] [PubMed]
65. Pournaras, D.J.; Aasheim, E.T.; Bueter, M.; Ahmed, A.R.; Welbourn, R.; Olbers, T.; le Roux, C.W. Effect of bypassing the proximal gut on gut hormones involved with glycemic control and weight loss. *Surg. Obes. Relat. Dis.* **2012**, *8*, 371–374. [CrossRef]
66. Patti, M.E.; Houten, S.M.; Bianco, A.C.; Bernier, R.; Larsen, P.R.; Holst, J.J.; Badman, M.K.; Maratos-Flier, E.; Mun, E.C.; Pihlajamaki, J.; et al. Serum bile acids are higher in humans with prior gastric bypass: Potential contribution to improved glucose and lipid metabolism. *Obesity* **2009**, *17*, 1671–1677. [CrossRef] [PubMed]
67. Nielsen, S.; Svane, M.S.; Kuhre, R.E.; Clausen, T.R.; Kristiansen, V.B.; Rehfeld, J.F.; Holst, J.J.; Madsbad, S.; Bojsen-Moller, K.N. Chenodeoxycholic acid stimulates glucagon-like peptide-1 secretion in patients after Roux-en-Y gastric bypass. *Physiol. Rep.* **2017**, *5*. [CrossRef] [PubMed]
68. Kuhre, R.E.; Wewer Albrechtsen, N.J.; Larsen, O.; Jepsen, S.L.; Balk-Møller, E.; Andersen, D.B.; Deacon, C.F.; Schoonjans, K.; Reimann, F.; Gribble, F.M.; et al. Bile acids are important direct and indirect regulators of the secretion of appetite- and metabolism-regulating hormones from the gut and pancreas. *Mol. Metab.* **2018**, *11*, 84–95. [CrossRef]
69. Belgaumkar, A.P.; Vincent, R.P.; Carswell, K.A.; Hughes, R.D.; Alaghband-Zadeh, J.; Mitry, R.R.; le Roux, C.W.; Patel, A.G. Changes in Bile Acid Profile After Laparoscopic Sleeve Gastrectomy are Associated with Improvements in Metabolic Profile and Fatty Liver Disease. *Obes. Surg.* **2016**, *26*, 1195–1202. [CrossRef]

70. Nemati, R.; Lu, J.; Dokpuang, D.; Booth, M.; Plank, L.D.; Murphy, R. Increased Bile Acids and FGF19 After Sleeve Gastrectomy and Roux-en-Y Gastric Bypass Correlate with Improvement in Type 2 Diabetes in a Randomized Trial. *Obes. Surg.* **2018**, *28*, 2672–2686. [CrossRef]
71. Chen, Y.; Lu, J.; Nemati, R.; Plank, L.D.; Murphy, R. Acute Changes of Bile Acids and FGF19 After Sleeve Gastrectomy and Roux-en-Y Gastric Bypass. *Obes. Surg.* **2019**, *29*, 3605–3621. [CrossRef] [PubMed]
72. Eiken, A.; Fuglsang, S.; Eiken, M.; Svane, M.S.; Kuhre, R.E.; Wewer Albrechtsen, N.J.; Hansen, S.H.; Trammell, S.A.J.; Svenningsen, J.S.; Rehfeld, J.F.; et al. Bilio-enteric flow and plasma concentrations of bile acids after gastric bypass and sleeve gastrectomy. *Int J. Obes.* **2020**, *44*, 1872–1883. [CrossRef] [PubMed]
73. Steinert, R.E.; Peterli, R.; Keller, S.; Meyer-Gerspach, A.C.; Drewe, J.; Peters, T.; Beglinger, C. Bile acids and gut peptide secretion after bariatric surgery: A 1-year prospective randomized pilot trial. *Obesity* **2013**, *21*, E660–E668. [CrossRef]
74. Dutia, R.; Embrey, M.; O'Brien, C.S.; Haeusler, R.A.; Agénor, K.K.; Homel, P.; McGinty, J.; Vincent, R.P.; Alaghband-Zadeh, J.; Staels, B.; et al. Temporal changes in bile acid levels and 12α-hydroxylation after Roux-en-Y gastric bypass surgery in type 2 diabetes. *Int J. Obe.s* **2015**, *39*, 806–813. [CrossRef] [PubMed]
75. Müller, T.D.; Nogueiras, R.; Andermann, M.L.; Andrews, Z.B.; Anker, S.D.; Argente, J.; Batterham, R.L.; Benoit, S.C.; Bowers, C.Y.; Broglio, F.; et al. Ghrelin. *Mol. Metab.* **2015**, *4*, 437–460. [CrossRef]
76. Tong, J.; Davis, H.W.; Gastaldelli, A.; D'Alessio, D. Ghrelin Impairs Prandial Glucose Tolerance and Insulin Secretion in Healthy Humans Despite Increasing GLP-1. *J. Clin. Endocrinol. Metab.* **2016**, *101*, 2405–2414. [CrossRef] [PubMed]
77. Tong, J.; Prigeon, R.L.; Davis, H.W.; Bidlingmaier, M.; Kahn, S.E.; Cummings, D.E.; Tschöp, M.H.; D'Alessio, D. Ghrelin suppresses glucose-stimulated insulin secretion and deteriorates glucose tolerance in healthy humans. *Diabetes* **2010**, *59*, 2145–2151. [CrossRef]
78. Cummings, D.E.; Frayo, R.S.; Marmonier, C.; Aubert, R.; Chapelot, D. Plasma ghrelin levels and hunger scores in humans initiating meals voluntarily without time- and food-related cues. *Am. J. Physiol. Endocrinol. Metab.* **2004**, *287*, E297–E304. [CrossRef]
79. Cummings, D.E.; Weigle, D.S.; Frayo, R.S.; Breen, P.A.; Ma, M.K.; Dellinger, E.P.; Purnell, J.Q. Plasma ghrelin levels after diet-induced weight loss or gastric bypass surgery. *N. Engl. J. Med.* **2002**, *346*, 1623–1630. [CrossRef]
80. Barazzoni, R.; Zanetti, M.; Nagliati, C.; Cattin, M.R.; Ferreira, C.; Giuricin, M.; Palmisano, S.; Edalucci, E.; Dore, F.; Guarnieri, G.; et al. Gastric bypass does not normalize obesity-related changes in ghrelin profile and leads to higher acylated ghrelin fraction. *Obesity* **2013**, *21*, 718–722. [CrossRef]
81. Meek, C.L.; Lewis, H.B.; Reimann, F.; Gribble, F.M.; Park, A.J. The effect of bariatric surgery on gastrointestinal and pancreatic peptide hormones. *Peptides* **2016**, *77*, 28–37. [CrossRef]
82. Papamargaritis, D.; Miras, A.D.; le Roux, C.W. Influence of diabetes surgery on gut hormones and incretins. *Nutr. Hosp.* **2013**, *28* (Suppl. S2), 95–103. [CrossRef]
83. McCarty, T.R.; Jirapinyo, P.; Thompson, C.C. Effect of Sleeve Gastrectomy on Ghrelin, GLP-1, PYY, and GIP Gut Hormones: A Systematic Review and Meta-analysis. *Ann. Surg.* **2020**, *272*, 72–80. [CrossRef] [PubMed]
84. Langer, F.B.; Reza Hoda, M.A.; Bohdjalian, A.; Felberbauer, F.X.; Zacherl, J.; Wenzl, E.; Schindler, K.; Luger, A.; Ludvik, B.; Prager, G. Sleeve gastrectomy and gastric banding: Effects on plasma ghrelin levels. *Obes. Surg.* **2005**, *15*, 1024–1029. [CrossRef]
85. Peterli, R.; Wölnerhanssen, B.; Peters, T.; Devaux, N.; Kern, B.; Christoffel-Courtin, C.; Drewe, J.; von Flüe, M.; Beglinger, C. Improvement in glucose metabolism after bariatric surgery: Comparison of laparoscopic Roux-en-Y gastric bypass and laparoscopic sleeve gastrectomy: A prospective randomized trial. *Ann. Surg.* **2009**, *250*, 234–241. [CrossRef] [PubMed]
86. Ybarra, J.; Bobbioni-Harsch, E.; Chassot, G.; Huber, O.; Morel, P.; Assimacopoulos-Jeannet, F.; Golay, A. Persistent correlation of ghrelin plasma levels with body mass index both in stable weight conditions and during gastric-bypass-induced weight loss. *Obes. Surg.* **2009**, *19*, 327–331. [CrossRef]
87. Sundbom, M.; Holdstock, C.; Engström, B.E.; Karlsson, F.A. Early changes in ghrelin following Roux-en-Y gastric bypass: Influence of vagal nerve functionality? *Obes. Surg.* **2007**, *17*, 304–310. [CrossRef]
88. Xu, H.C.; Pang, Y.C.; Chen, J.W.; Cao, J.Y.; Sheng, Z.; Yuan, J.H.; Wang, R.; Zhang, C.S.; Wang, L.X.; Dong, J. Systematic Review and Meta-analysis of the Change in Ghrelin Levels After Roux-en-Y Gastric Bypass. *Obes. Surg.* **2019**, *29*, 1343–1351. [CrossRef] [PubMed]
89. Bose, M.; Machineni, S.; Oliván, B.; Teixeira, J.; McGinty, J.J.; Bawa, B.; Koshy, N.; Colarusso, A.; Laferrère, B. Superior appetite hormone profile after equivalent weight loss by gastric bypass compared to gastric banding. *Obesity* **2010**, *18*, 1085–1091. [CrossRef]
90. Peterli, R.; Steinert, R.E.; Woelnerhanssen, B.; Peters, T.; Christoffel-Courtin, C.; Gass, M.; Kern, B.; von Fluee, M.; Beglinger, C. Metabolic and hormonal changes after laparoscopic Roux-en-Y gastric bypass and sleeve gastrectomy: A randomized, prospective trial. *Obes. Surg.* **2012**, *22*, 740–748. [CrossRef] [PubMed]
91. Tsouristakis, A.I.; Febres, G.; McMahon, D.J.; Tchang, B.; Conwell, I.M.; Tsang, A.J.; Ahmed, L.; Bessler, M.; Korner, J. Long-Term Modulation of Appetitive Hormones and Sweet Cravings After Adjustable Gastric Banding and Roux-en-Y Gastric Bypass. *Obes. Surg.* **2019**, *29*, 3698–3705. [CrossRef] [PubMed]
92. Stoeckli, R.; Chanda, R.; Langer, I.; Keller, U. Changes of body weight and plasma ghrelin levels after gastric banding and gastric bypass. *Obes. Res.* **2004**, *12*, 346–350. [CrossRef]
93. Wang, Y.; Liu, J. Plasma ghrelin modulation in gastric band operation and sleeve gastrectomy. *Obes. Surg.* **2009**, *19*, 357–362. [CrossRef]

94. Korner, J.; Inabnet, W.; Febres, G.; Conwell, I.M.; McMahon, D.J.; Salas, R.; Taveras, C.; Schrope, B.; Bessler, M. Prospective study of gut hormone and metabolic changes after adjustable gastric banding and Roux-en-Y gastric bypass. *Int. J. Obes.* **2009**, *33*, 786–795. [CrossRef]
95. Mentis, N.; Vardarli, I.; Köthe, L.D.; Holst, J.J.; Deacon, C.F.; Theodorakis, M.; Meier, J.J.; Nauck, M.A. GIP does not potentiate the antidiabetic effects of GLP-1 in hyperglycemic patients with type 2 diabetes. *Diabetes* **2011**, *60*, 1270–1276. [CrossRef]
96. Højberg, P.V.; Vilsbøll, T.; Rabøl, R.; Knop, F.K.; Bache, M.; Krarup, T.; Holst, J.J.; Madsbad, S. Four weeks of near-normalisation of blood glucose improves the insulin response to glucagon-like peptide-1 and glucose-dependent insulinotropic polypeptide in patients with type 2 diabetes. *Diabetologia* **2009**, *52*, 199–207. [CrossRef]
97. Alexiadou, K.; Cuenco, J.; Howard, J.; Wewer Albrechtsen, N.J.; Ilesanmi, I.; Kamocka, A.; Tharakan, G.; Behary, P.; Bech, P.R.; Ahmed, A.R.; et al. Proglucagon peptide secretion profiles in type 2 diabetes before and after bariatric surgery: 1-year prospective study. *BMJ Open Diabetes Res. Care* **2020**, *8*. [CrossRef]
98. Laferrère, B.; Heshka, S.; Wang, K.; Khan, Y.; McGinty, J.; Teixeira, J.; Hart, A.B.; Olivan, B. Incretin levels and effect are markedly enhanced 1 month after Roux-en-Y gastric bypass surgery in obese patients with type 2 diabetes. *Diabetes Care* **2007**, *30*, 1709–1716. [CrossRef]
99. Laferrère, B.; Teixeira, J.; McGinty, J.; Tran, H.; Egger, J.R.; Colarusso, A.; Kovack, B.; Bawa, B.; Koshy, N.; Lee, H.; et al. Effect of weight loss by gastric bypass surgery versus hypocaloric diet on glucose and incretin levels in patients with type 2 diabetes. *J. Clin. Endocrinol. Metab.* **2008**, *93*, 2479–2485. [CrossRef]
100. Prior, S.L.; Churm, R.; Min, T.; Dunseath, G.J.; Barry, J.D.; Stephens, J.W. Temporal Effects of Sleeve Gastrectomy on Glucose-Insulin Homeostasis and Incretin Hormone Response at 1 and 6 Months. *Obes. Surg.* **2020**, *30*, 2243–2250. [CrossRef] [PubMed]
101. Wallenius, V.; Dirinck, E.; Fändriks, L.; Maleckas, A.; le Roux, C.W.; Thorell, A. Glycemic Control after Sleeve Gastrectomy and Roux-En-Y Gastric Bypass in Obese Subjects with Type 2 Diabetes Mellitus. *Obes. Surg.* **2018**, *28*, 1461–1472. [CrossRef]
102. Rodieux, F.; Giusti, V.; D'Alessio, D.A.; Suter, M.; Tappy, L. Effects of gastric bypass and gastric banding on glucose kinetics and gut hormone release. *Obesity* **2008**, *16*, 298–305. [CrossRef] [PubMed]
103. Bunt, J.C.; Blackstone, R.; Thearle, M.S.; Vinales, K.L.; Votruba, S.; Krakoff, J. Changes in glycemia, insulin and gut hormone responses to a slowly ingested solid low-carbohydrate mixed meal after laparoscopic gastric bypass or band surgery. *Int. J. Obes.* **2017**, *41*, 706–713. [CrossRef]
104. Shak, J.R.; Roper, J.; Perez-Perez, G.I.; Tseng, C.H.; Francois, F.; Gamagaris, Z.; Patterson, C.; Weinshel, E.; Fielding, G.A.; Ren, C.; et al. The effect of laparoscopic gastric banding surgery on plasma levels of appetite-control, insulinotropic, and digestive hormones. *Obes. Surg.* **2008**, *18*, 1089–1096. [CrossRef] [PubMed]
105. Müller, T.D.; Finan, B.; Bloom, S.R.; D'Alessio, D.; Drucker, D.J.; Flatt, P.R.; Fritsche, A.; Gribble, F.; Grill, H.J.; Habener, J.F.; et al. Glucagon-like peptide 1 (GLP-1). *Mol. Metab.* **2019**, *30*, 72–130. [CrossRef]
106. Holst, J.J. The physiology of glucagon-like peptide 1. *Physiol. Rev.* **2007**, *87*, 1409–1439. [CrossRef] [PubMed]
107. Deane, A.M.; Nguyen, N.Q.; Stevens, J.E.; Fraser, R.J.; Holloway, R.H.; Besanko, L.K.; Burgstad, C.; Jones, K.L.; Chapman, M.J.; Rayner, C.K.; et al. Endogenous glucagon-like peptide-1 slows gastric emptying in healthy subjects, attenuating postprandial glycemia. *J. Clin. Endocrinol. Metab.* **2010**, *95*, 215–221. [CrossRef] [PubMed]
108. Gu, L.; Lin, K.; Du, N.; Ng, D.M.; Lou, D.; Chen, P. Differences in the effects of laparoscopic sleeve gastrectomy and laparoscopic Roux-en-Y gastric bypass on gut hormones: Systematic and meta-analysis. *Surg. Obes. Relat. Dis.* **2020**. [CrossRef] [PubMed]
109. Papamargaritis, D.; Panteliou, E.; Miras, A.D.; le Roux, C.W. Mechanisms of weight loss, diabetes control and changes in food choices after gastrointestinal surgery. *Curr. Atheroscler. Rep.* **2012**, *14*, 616–623. [CrossRef]
110. le Roux, C.W.; Batterham, R.L.; Aylwin, S.J.; Patterson, M.; Borg, C.M.; Wynne, K.J.; Kent, A.; Vincent, R.P.; Gardiner, J.; Ghatei, M.A.; et al. Attenuated peptide YY release in obese subjects is associated with reduced satiety. *Endocrinology* **2006**, *147*, 3–8. [CrossRef]
111. Chen, C.H.; Stephens, R.L., Jr.; Rogers, R.C. PYY and NPY: Control of gastric motility via action on Y1 and Y2 receptors in the DVC. *Neurogastroenterol. Motil.* **1997**, *9*, 109–116. [CrossRef]
112. Karra, E.; Chandarana, K.; Batterham, R.L. The role of peptide YY in appetite regulation and obesity. *J. Physiol.* **2009**, *587*, 19–25. [CrossRef]
113. Batterham, R.L.; Cohen, M.A.; Ellis, S.M.; Le Roux, C.W.; Withers, D.J.; Frost, G.S.; Ghatei, M.A.; Bloom, S.R. Inhibition of food intake in obese subjects by peptide YY3-36. *N. Engl. J. Med.* **2003**, *349*, 941–948. [CrossRef]
114. Arakawa, R.; Febres, G.; Cheng, B.; Krikhely, A.; Bessler, M.; Korner, J. Prospective study of gut hormone and metabolic changes after laparoscopic sleeve gastrectomy and Roux-en-Y gastric bypass. *PLoS ONE* **2020**, *15*, e0236133. [CrossRef]
115. Dimitriadis, G.K.; Randeva, M.S.; Miras, A.D. Potential Hormone Mechanisms of Bariatric Surgery. *Curr. Obes. Rep.* **2017**, *6*, 253–265. [CrossRef]
116. Pocai, A. Unraveling oxyntomodulin, GLP1's enigmatic brother. *J. Endocrinol.* **2012**, *215*, 335–346. [CrossRef]
117. Wynne, K.; Park, A.J.; Small, C.J.; Patterson, M.; Ellis, S.M.; Murphy, K.G.; Wren, A.M.; Frost, G.S.; Meeran, K.; Ghatei, M.A.; et al. Subcutaneous oxyntomodulin reduces body weight in overweight and obese subjects: A double-blind, randomized, controlled trial. *Diabetes* **2005**, *54*, 2390–2395. [CrossRef]
118. Wynne, K.; Park, A.J.; Small, C.J.; Meeran, K.; Ghatei, M.A.; Frost, G.S.; Bloom, S.R. Oxyntomodulin increases energy expenditure in addition to decreasing energy intake in overweight and obese humans: A randomised controlled trial. *Int. J. Obes.* **2006**, *30*, 1729–1736. [CrossRef] [PubMed]

119. Laferrère, B.; Swerdlow, N.; Bawa, B.; Arias, S.; Bose, M.; Oliván, B.; Teixeira, J.; McGinty, J.; Rother, K.I. Rise of oxyntomodulin in response to oral glucose after gastric bypass surgery in patients with type 2 diabetes. *J. Clin. Endocrinol. Metab.* **2010**, *95*, 4072–4076. [CrossRef] [PubMed]
120. Said, H. (Ed.) Chapter 2—Gastrointestinal hormones. In *Physiology of the Gastrointestinal Tract*, 6th ed.; Academic Press: Cambridge, MA, USA, 2018. [CrossRef]
121. Kokkinos, A.; Tsilingiris, D.; le Roux, C.W.; Rubino, F.; Mantzoros, C.S. Will medications that mimic gut hormones or target their receptors eventually replace bariatric surgery? *Metabolism* **2019**, *100*, 153960. [CrossRef]
122. Werling, M.; Fändriks, L.; Vincent, R.P.; Cross, G.F.; le Roux, C.W.; Olbers, T. Preoperative assessment of gut hormones does not correlate to weight loss after Roux-en-Y gastric bypass surgery. *Surg. Obes. Relat. Dis.* **2014**, *10*, 822–828. [CrossRef]
123. De Hollanda, A.; Jiménez, A.; Corcelles, R.; Lacy, A.M.; Patrascioiu, I.; Vidal, J. Gastrointestinal hormones and weight loss response after Roux-en-Y gastric bypass. *Surg. Obes. Relat. Dis.* **2014**, *10*, 814–819. [CrossRef] [PubMed]
124. de Hollanda, A.; Casals, G.; Delgado, S.; Jiménez, A.; Viaplana, J.; Lacy, A.M.; Vidal, J. Gastrointestinal Hormones and Weight Loss Maintenance Following Roux-en-Y Gastric Bypass. *J. Clin. Endocrinol. Metab.* **2015**, *100*, 4677–4684. [CrossRef]
125. Dirksen, C.; Jørgensen, N.B.; Bojsen-Møller, K.N.; Kielgast, U.; Jacobsen, S.H.; Clausen, T.R.; Worm, D.; Hartmann, B.; Rehfeld, J.F.; Damgaard, M.; et al. Gut hormones, early dumping and resting energy expenditure in patients with good and poor weight loss response after Roux-en-Y gastric bypass. *Int. J. Obes.* **2013**, *37*, 1452–1459. [CrossRef]
126. De Hollanda, A.; Ruiz, T.; Jiménez, A.; Flores, L.; Lacy, A.; Vidal, J. Patterns of Weight Loss Response Following Gastric Bypass and Sleeve Gastrectomy. *Obes. Surg.* **2015**, *25*, 1177–1183. [CrossRef] [PubMed]
127. Bonouvrie, D.S.; Uittenbogaart, M.; Luijten, A.; van Dielen, F.M.H.; Leclercq, W.K.G. Lack of Standard Definitions of Primary and Secondary (Non)responders After Primary Gastric Bypass and Gastric Sleeve: A Systematic Review. *Obes. Surg.* **2019**, *29*, 691–697. [CrossRef] [PubMed]
128. Abstract Discussion. *Obes. Rev.* **2020**, *21*, e13115. [CrossRef]
129. Farthing, M.J. Octreotide in dumping and short bowel syndromes. *Digestion* **1993**, *54* (Suppl. S1), 47–52. [CrossRef] [PubMed]
130. Svane, M.S.; Jørgensen, N.B.; Bojsen-Møller, K.N.; Dirksen, C.; Nielsen, S.; Kristiansen, V.B.; Toräng, S.; Wewer Albrechtsen, N.J.; Rehfeld, J.F.; Hartmann, B.; et al. Peptide YY and glucagon-like peptide-1 contribute to decreased food intake after Roux-en-Y gastric bypass surgery. *Int. J. Obes.* **2016**, *40*, 1699–1706. [CrossRef] [PubMed]
131. Holst, J.J.; Madsbad, S.; Bojsen-Møller, K.N.; Svane, M.S.; Jørgensen, N.B.; Dirksen, C.; Martinussen, C. Mechanisms in bariatric surgery: Gut hormones, diabetes resolution, and weight loss. *Surg. Obes. Relat. Dis.* **2018**, *14*, 708–714. [CrossRef] [PubMed]
132. Yoshino, M.; Kayser, B.D.; Yoshino, J.; Stein, R.I.; Reeds, D.; Eagon, J.C.; Eckhouse, S.R.; Watrous, J.D.; Jain, M.; Knight, R.; et al. Effects of Diet versus Gastric Bypass on Metabolic Function in Diabetes. *N. Engl. J. Med.* **2020**, *383*, 721–732. [CrossRef] [PubMed]
133. Jørgensen, N.B.; Jacobsen, S.H.; Dirksen, C.; Bojsen-Møller, K.N.; Naver, L.; Hvolris, L.; Clausen, T.R.; Wulff, B.S.; Worm, D.; Lindqvist Hansen, D.; et al. Acute and long-term effects of Roux-en-Y gastric bypass on glucose metabolism in subjects with Type 2 diabetes and normal glucose tolerance. *Am. J. Physiol. Endocrinol. Metab.* **2012**, *303*, E122–E131. [CrossRef]
134. Kotronen, A.; Vehkavaara, S.; Seppälä-Lindroos, A.; Bergholm, R.; Yki-Järvinen, H. Effect of liver fat on insulin clearance. *Am. J. Physiol. Endocrinol. Metab.* **2007**, *293*, E1709–E1715. [CrossRef]
135. Dirksen, C.; Hansen, D.L.; Madsbad, S.; Hvolris, L.E.; Naver, L.S.; Holst, J.J.; Worm, D. Postprandial diabetic glucose tolerance is normalized by gastric bypass feeding as opposed to gastric feeding and is associated with exaggerated GLP-1 secretion: A case report. *Diabetes Care* **2010**, *33*, 375–377. [CrossRef] [PubMed]
136. Kashyap, S.R.; Daud, S.; Kelly, K.R.; Gastaldelli, A.; Win, H.; Brethauer, S.; Kirwan, J.P.; Schauer, P.R. Acute effects of gastric bypass versus gastric restrictive surgery on beta-cell function and insulinotropic hormones in severely obese patients with type 2 diabetes. *Int. J. Obes.* **2010**, *34*, 462–471. [CrossRef]
137. Nannipieri, M.; Mari, A.; Anselmino, M.; Baldi, S.; Barsotti, E.; Guarino, D.; Camastra, S.; Bellini, R.; Berta, R.D.; Ferrannini, E. The role of beta-cell function and insulin sensitivity in the remission of type 2 diabetes after gastric bypass surgery. *J. Clin. Endocrinol. Metab.* **2011**, *96*, E1372–E1379. [CrossRef]
138. Martinussen, C.; Bojsen-Møller, K.N.; Dirksen, C.; Jacobsen, S.H.; Jørgensen, N.B.; Kristiansen, V.B.; Holst, J.J.; Madsbad, S. Immediate enhancement of first-phase insulin secretion and unchanged glucose effectiveness in patients with type 2 diabetes after Roux-en-Y gastric bypass. *Am. J. Physiol. Endocrinol. Metab.* **2015**, *308*, E535–E544. [CrossRef]
139. Jiménez, A.; Casamitjana, R.; Viaplana-Masclans, J.; Lacy, A.; Vidal, J. GLP-1 action and glucose tolerance in subjects with remission of type 2 diabetes after gastric bypass surgery. *Diabetes Care* **2013**, *36*, 2062–2069. [CrossRef] [PubMed]
140. Vetter, M.L.; Wadden, T.A.; Teff, K.L.; Khan, Z.F.; Carvajal, R.; Ritter, S.; Moore, R.H.; Chittams, J.L.; Iagnocco, A.; Murayama, K.; et al. GLP-1 plays a limited role in improved glycemia shortly after Roux-en-Y gastric bypass: A comparison with intensive lifestyle modification. *Diabetes* **2015**, *64*, 434–446. [CrossRef]
141. Shah, A.; Holter, M.M.; Rimawi, F.; Mark, V.; Dutia, R.; McGinty, J.; Levin, B.; Laferrère, B. Insulin Clearance After Oral and Intravenous Glucose Following Gastric Bypass and Gastric Banding Weight Loss. *Diabetes Care* **2019**, *42*, 311–317. [CrossRef]
142. Jiménez, A.; Mari, A.; Casamitjana, R.; Lacy, A.; Ferrannini, E.; Vidal, J. GLP-1 and glucose tolerance after sleeve gastrectomy in morbidly obese subjects with type 2 diabetes. *Diabetes* **2014**, *63*, 3372–3377. [CrossRef] [PubMed]
143. Craig, C.M.; Liu, L.F.; Deacon, C.F.; Holst, J.J.; McLaughlin, T.L. Critical role for GLP-1 in symptomatic post-bariatric hypoglycaemia. *Diabetologia* **2017**, *60*, 531–540. [CrossRef]

144. Salehi, M.; Gastaldelli, A.; D'Alessio, D.A. Blockade of glucagon-like peptide 1 receptor corrects postprandial hypoglycemia after gastric bypass. *Gastroenterology* **2014**, *146*, 669–680.e662. [CrossRef] [PubMed]
145. Shah, M.; Law, J.H.; Micheletto, F.; Sathananthan, M.; Dalla Man, C.; Cobelli, C.; Rizza, R.A.; Camilleri, M.; Zinsmeister, A.R.; Vella, A. Contribution of endogenous glucagon-like peptide 1 to glucose metabolism after Roux-en-Y gastric bypass. *Diabetes* **2014**, *63*, 483–493. [CrossRef] [PubMed]
146. Svane, M.S.; Bojsen-Møller, K.N.; Nielsen, S.; Jørgensen, N.B.; Dirksen, C.; Bendtsen, F.; Kristiansen, V.B.; Hartmann, B.; Holst, J.J.; Madsbad, S. Effects of endogenous GLP-1 and GIP on glucose tolerance after Roux-en-Y gastric bypass surgery. *Am. J. Physiol. Endocrinol. Metab.* **2016**, *310*, E505–E514. [CrossRef]
147. Douros, J.D.; Tong, J.; D'Alessio, D.A. The Effects of Bariatric Surgery on Islet Function, Insulin Secretion, and Glucose Control. *Endocr. Rev.* **2019**, *40*, 1394–1423. [CrossRef]
148. Holst, J.J.; Wewer Albrechtsen, N.J.; Pedersen, J.; Knop, F.K. Glucagon and Amino Acids Are Linked in a Mutual Feedback Cycle: The Liver-α-Cell Axis. *Diabetes* **2017**, *66*, 235–240. [CrossRef]
149. Jorsal, T.; Wewer Albrechtsen, N.J.; Christensen, M.M.; Mortensen, B.; Wandall, E.; Langholz, E.; Friis, S.; Worm, D.; Ørskov, C.; Støving, R.K.; et al. Investigating Intestinal Glucagon After Roux-en-Y Gastric Bypass Surgery. *J. Clin. Endocrinol. Metab.* **2019**, *104*, 6403–6416. [CrossRef] [PubMed]
150. Wewer Albrechtsen, N.J.; Hartmann, B.; Veedfald, S.; Windeløv, J.A.; Plamboeck, A.; Bojsen-Møller, K.N.; Idorn, T.; Feldt-Rasmussen, B.; Knop, F.K.; Vilsbøll, T.; et al. Hyperglucagonaemia analysed by glucagon sandwich ELISA: Nonspecific interference or truly elevated levels? *Diabetologia* **2014**, *57*, 1919–1926. [CrossRef]
151. Roberts, G.P.; Kay, R.G.; Howard, J.; Hardwick, R.H.; Reimann, F.; Gribble, F.M. Gastrectomy with Roux-en-Y reconstruction as a lean model of bariatric surgery. *Surg. Obes. Relat. Dis.* **2018**, *14*, 562–568. [CrossRef] [PubMed]
152. Nannipieri, M.; Baldi, S.; Mari, A.; Colligiani, D.; Guarino, D.; Camastra, S.; Barsotti, E.; Berta, R.; Moriconi, D.; Bellini, R.; et al. Roux-en-Y gastric bypass and sleeve gastrectomy: Mechanisms of diabetes remission and role of gut hormones. *J. Clin. Endocrinol. Metab.* **2013**, *98*, 4391–4399. [CrossRef] [PubMed]
153. Vidal, J.; de Hollanda, A.; Jiménez, A. GLP-1 is not the key mediator of the health benefits of metabolic surgery. *Surg. Obes. Relat. Dis.* **2016**, *12*, 1225–1229. [CrossRef]
154. Madsbad, S.; Holst, J.J. GLP-1 as a mediator in the remission of type 2 diabetes after gastric bypass and sleeve gastrectomy surgery. *Diabetes* **2014**, *63*, 3172–3174. [CrossRef]
155. Gasbjerg, L.S.; Bergmann, N.C.; Stensen, S.; Christensen, M.B.; Rosenkilde, M.M.; Holst, J.J.; Nauck, M.; Knop, F.K. Evaluation of the incretin effect in humans using GIP and GLP-1 receptor antagonists. *Peptides* **2020**, *125*, 170183. [CrossRef]
156. Hutch, C.R.; Sandoval, D. The Role of GLP-1 in the Metabolic Success of Bariatric Surgery. *Endocrinology* **2017**, *158*, 4139–4151. [CrossRef]
157. Nauck, M.A.; Kind, J.; Köthe, L.D.; Holst, J.J.; Deacon, C.F.; Broschag, M.; He, Y.L.; Kjems, L.; Foley, J. Quantification of the Contribution of GLP-1 to Mediating Insulinotropic Effects of DPP-4 Inhibition With Vildagliptin in Healthy Subjects and Patients With Type 2 Diabetes Using Exendin [9–39] as a GLP-1 Receptor Antagonist. *Diabetes* **2016**, *65*, 2440–2447. [CrossRef] [PubMed]
158. Emous, M.; Wolffenbuttel, B.H.R.; Totté, E.; van Beek, A.P. The short- to mid-term symptom prevalence of dumping syndrome after primary gastric-bypass surgery and its impact on health-related quality of life. *Surg. Obes. Relat. Dis.* **2017**, *13*, 1489–1500. [CrossRef]
159. Varma, S.; Clark, J.M.; Schweitzer, M.; Magnuson, T.; Brown, T.T.; Lee, C.J. Weight regain in patients with symptoms of post-bariatric surgery hypoglycemia. *Surg. Obes. Relat. Dis.* **2017**, *13*, 1728–1734. [CrossRef]
160. Øhrstrøm, C.C.; Worm, D.; Hansen, D.L. Postprandial hyperinsulinemic hypoglycemia after Roux-en-Y gastric bypass: An update. *Surg. Obes. Relat. Dis.* **2017**, *13*, 345–351. [CrossRef]
161. Papamargaritis, D.; Koukoulis, G.; Sioka, E.; Zachari, E.; Bargiota, A.; Zacharoulis, D.; Tzovaras, G. Dumping symptoms and incidence of hypoglycaemia after provocation test at 6 and 12 months after laparoscopic sleeve gastrectomy. *Obes. Surg.* **2012**, *22*, 1600–1606. [CrossRef]
162. Abrahamsson, N.; Edén Engström, B.; Sundbom, M.; Karlsson, F.A. Hypoglycemia in everyday life after gastric bypass and duodenal switch. *Eur. J. Endocrinol.* **2015**, *173*, 91–100. [CrossRef]
163. Capristo, E.; Panunzi, S.; De Gaetano, A.; Spuntarelli, V.; Bellantone, R.; Giustacchini, P.; Birkenfeld, A.L.; Amiel, S.; Bornstein, S.R.; Raffaelli, M.; et al. Incidence of Hypoglycemia After Gastric Bypass vs. Sleeve Gastrectomy: A Randomized Trial. *J. Clin. Endocrinol. Metab* **2018**, *103*, 2136–2146. [CrossRef]
164. Lee, C.J.; Clark, J.M.; Schweitzer, M.; Magnuson, T.; Steele, K.; Koerner, O.; Brown, T.T. Prevalence of and risk factors for hypoglycemic symptoms after gastric bypass and sleeve gastrectomy. *Obesity* **2015**, *23*, 1079–1084. [CrossRef]
165. Belligoli, A.; Sanna, M.; Serra, R.; Fabris, R.; Pra, C.D.; Conci, S.; Fioretto, P.; Prevedello, L.; Foletto, M.; Vettor, R.; et al. Incidence and Predictors of Hypoglycemia 1 Year After Laparoscopic Sleeve Gastrectomy. *Obes. Surg.* **2017**, *27*, 3179–3186. [CrossRef]
166. Lupoli, R.; Lembo, E.; Ciciola, P.; Schiavo, L.; Pilone, V.; Capaldo, B. Continuous glucose monitoring in subjects undergoing bariatric surgery: Diurnal and nocturnal glycemic patterns. *Nutr. Metab. Cardiovasc. Dis.* **2020**, *30*, 1954–1960. [CrossRef]
167. Emous, M.; Ubels, F.L.; van Beek, A.P. Diagnostic tools for post-gastric bypass hypoglycaemia. *Obes Rev.* **2015**, *16*, 843–856. [CrossRef] [PubMed]

168. Emous, M.; van den Broek, M.; Wijma, R.B.; de Heide, L.J.M.; van Dijk, G.; Laskewitz, A.; Totté, E.; Wolffenbuttel, B.H.R.; van Beek, A.P. Prevalence of hypoglycaemia in a random population after Roux-en-Y gastric bypass after a meal test. *Endocr Connect.* **2019**, *8*, 969–978. [CrossRef]
169. Marsk, R.; Jonas, E.; Rasmussen, F.; Näslund, E. Nationwide cohort study of post-gastric bypass hypoglycaemia including 5,040 patients undergoing surgery for obesity in 1986–2006 in Sweden. *Diabetologia* **2010**, *53*, 2307–2311. [CrossRef] [PubMed]
170. Suhl, E.; Anderson-Haynes, S.E.; Mulla, C.; Patti, M.E. Medical nutrition therapy for post-bariatric hypoglycemia: Practical insights. *Surg. Obes. Relat. Dis.* **2017**, *13*, 888–896. [CrossRef] [PubMed]
171. Tharakan, G.; Behary, P.; Wewer Albrechtsen, N.J.; Chahal, H.; Kenkre, J.; Miras, A.D.; Ahmed, A.R.; Holst, J.J.; Bloom, S.R.; Tan, T. Roles of increased glycaemic variability, GLP-1 and glucagon in hypoglycaemia after Roux-en-Y gastric bypass. *Eur. J. Endocrinol.* **2017**, *177*, 455–464. [CrossRef]
172. Goldfine, A.B.; Mun, E.C.; Devine, E.; Bernier, R.; Baz-Hecht, M.; Jones, D.B.; Schneider, B.E.; Holst, J.J.; Patti, M.E. Patients with neuroglycopenia after gastric bypass surgery have exaggerated incretin and insulin secretory responses to a mixed meal. *J. Clin. Endocrinol. Metab.* **2007**, *92*, 4678–4685. [CrossRef]
173. Vaurs, C.; Brun, J.F.; Bertrand, M.; Burcelin, R.; du Rieu, M.C.; Anduze, Y.; Hanaire, H.; Ritz, P. Post-prandial hypoglycemia results from a non-glucose-dependent inappropriate insulin secretion in Roux-en-Y gastric bypassed patients. *Metabolism* **2016**, *65*, 18–26. [CrossRef] [PubMed]
174. Craig, C.M.; Liu, L.F.; Nguyen, T.; Price, C.; Bingham, J.; McLaughlin, T.L. Efficacy and pharmacokinetics of subcutaneous exendin (9–39) in patients with post-bariatric hypoglycaemia. *Diabetes Obes. Metab.* **2018**, *20*, 352–361. [CrossRef] [PubMed]
175. Salehi, M.; Prigeon, R.L.; D'Alessio, D.A. Gastric bypass surgery enhances glucagon-like peptide 1-stimulated postprandial insulin secretion in humans. *Diabetes* **2011**, *60*, 2308–2314. [CrossRef]
176. Tan, M.; Lamendola, C.; Luong, R.; McLaughlin, T.; Craig, C. Safety, efficacy and pharmacokinetics of repeat subcutaneous dosing of avexitide (exendin 9–39) for treatment of post-bariatric hypoglycaemia. *Diabetes Obes. Metab.* **2020**, *22*, 1406–1416. [CrossRef]
177. Miras, A.D.; Pérez-Pevida, B.; Aldhwayan, M.; Kamocka, A.; McGlone, E.R.; Al-Najim, W.; Chahal, H.; Batterham, R.L.; McGowan, B.; Khan, O.; et al. Adjunctive liraglutide treatment in patients with persistent or recurrent type 2 diabetes after metabolic surgery (GRAVITAS): A randomised, double-blind, placebo-controlled trial. *Lancet Diabetes Endocrinol.* **2019**, *7*, 549–559. [CrossRef]
178. Suliman, M.; Buckley, A.; Al Tikriti, A.; Tan, T.; le Roux, C.W.; Lessan, N.; Barakat, M. Routine clinical use of liraglutide 3 mg for the treatment of obesity: Outcomes in non-surgical and bariatric surgery patients. *Diabetes Obes. Metab.* **2019**, *21*, 1498–1501. [CrossRef]
179. Wharton, S.; Kuk, J.L.; Luszczynski, M.; Kamran, E.; Christensen, R.A.G. Liraglutide 3.0 mg for the management of insufficient weight loss or excessive weight regain post-bariatric surgery. *Clin. Obes.* **2019**, *9*, e12323. [CrossRef]
180. Evaluation of Liraglutide 3.0mg in Patients With Poor Weight-loss and a Suboptimal Glucagon-like Peptide-1 Response (BARIOP-TIMISE). Available online: https://www.clinicaltrials.gov/ct2/show/NCT03341429 (accessed on 7 December 2020).
181. Clinical Efficacy and Safety of Using 3.0mg Liraglutide to Treat Weight Regain After Roux-en-Y Gastric Bypass Surgery. Available online: https://www.clinicaltrials.gov/ct2/show/NCT03048578 (accessed on 7 December 2020).
182. Alexiadou, K.; Anyiam, O.; Tan, T. Cracking the combination: Gut hormones for the treatment of obesity and diabetes. *J. Neuroendocrinol.* **2019**, *31*, e12664. [CrossRef]

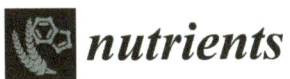

Review

Rational Use of Protein Supplements in the Elderly—Relevance of Gastrointestinal Mechanisms

Ian Chapman [1], Avneet Oberoi [1], Caroline Giezenaar [2] and Stijn Soenen [3,*]

1. Adelaide Medical School and Centre of Research Excellence (C.R.E.) in Translating Nutritional Science to Good Health, The University of Adelaide, Royal Adelaide Hospital, Adelaide, SA 5000, Australia; ian.chapman@adelaide.edu.au (I.C.); avneet.oberoi@adelaide.edu.au (A.O.)
2. Riddett Institute, Massey University, Palmerston North 9400, New Zealand; c.giezenaar@massey.ac.nz
3. Faculty of Health Sciences and Medicine, Bond University, Robina, QLD 4226, Australia
* Correspondence: stijn.soenen@adelaide.edu.au; Tel.: +61-07-55595-1390

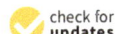

Citation: Chapman, I.; Oberoi, A.; Giezenaar, C.; Soenen, S. Rational Use of Protein Supplements in the Elderly—Relevance of Gastrointestinal Mechanisms. *Nutrients* 2021, 13, 1227. https://doi.org/10.3390/nu13041227

Academic Editor: Shanon L. Casperson

Received: 15 February 2021
Accepted: 1 April 2021
Published: 8 April 2021

Publisher's Note: MDPI stays neutral with regard to jurisdictional claims in published maps and institutional affiliations.

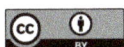

Copyright: © 2021 by the authors. Licensee MDPI, Basel, Switzerland. This article is an open access article distributed under the terms and conditions of the Creative Commons Attribution (CC BY) license (https://creativecommons.org/licenses/by/4.0/).

Abstract: Protein supplements are increasingly used by older people to maintain nutrition and prevent or treat loss of muscle function. Daily protein requirements in older people are in the range of 1.2 gm/kg/day or higher. Many older adults do not consume this much protein and are likely to benefit from higher consumption. Protein supplements are probably best taken twice daily, if possible soon after exercise, in doses that achieve protein intakes of 30 gm or more per episode. It is probably not important to give these supplements between meals, as we have shown no suppressive effects of 30 gm whey drinks, and little if any suppression of 70 gm given to older subjects at varying time intervals from meals. Many gastrointestinal mechanisms controlling food intake change with age, but their contributions to changes in responses to protein are not yet well understood. There may be benefits in giving the supplement with rather than between meals, to achieve protein intakes above the effective anabolic threshold with lower supplement doses, and have favourable effects on food-induced blood glucose increases in older people with, or at risk of developing, type 2 diabetes mellitus; combined protein and glucose drinks lower blood glucose compared with glucose alone in older people.

Keywords: aging; protein; whey; anorexia; appetite; supplements; sarcopenia

1. Introduction

This review will focus on appetite, feeding, and gastrointestinal responses to protein ingestion in older people. As a background, the high rates of under-nutrition, sarcopenia, and likely sub-optimal dietary protein intake in older people will be outlined, in support of the logical use of protein or protein-rich supplements by older people. The type, amount, and timing of such supplements, as well as possible side effects of these supplements, will be covered. The results of studies with whey protein by our group will be used to illustrate a number of gastrointestinal and cardiovascular responses to protein ingestion and to support some preliminary recommendations about beneficial use of protein supplements by older people. A number of issues remain unresolved.

1.1. Aging, Weight Loss, and Undernutrition

Healthy aging is associated with a physiological reduction in appetite and food intake, the so-called "anorexia of aging" [1]; people over 80 years consume about 30% less energy per day than those in their 20s [2]. Consequently, after about 65 years in developed countries, body weight tends to decrease [2]. This age-related weight loss, particularly when substantial and involuntary, has been associated with increased mortality [2]. Adverse factors prevalent in older people can be superimposed on the age-related changes to cause pathological under-nutrition, with even greater associated increases in morbidity and mortality [3]. Rates of under-nutrition increase with age and loss of independence; it is present in up to 45% of community dwelling elderly people, 50–80% in hospital, and 80–100% in residential facilities [3].

The major markers of existing or pending under-nutrition in older people are low body weight (particularly body mass index < 22 kg/m^2); loss of weight, particularly when involuntary and >5%; substantial loss of muscle mass, which can lead to sarcopenia (see below); reduced muscle strength and function; reduced appetite and food intake; and frailty [2,3].

1.2. Aging and Sarcopenia

The weight lost with increased aging is disproportionately made up of lean tissue, particularly skeletal muscle, but also bone mass. In contrast, fat mass increases with ageing, tending to mask the extent of lean tissue loss [2]. After approximately age 30 years, about 5% of lean muscle mass is lost per decade [2]. The loss of lean tissue, when large, can result in sarcopenia, an excessive and damaging loss of muscle. Sarcopenia is present in up to 15% of community-dwelling people over 85 years [4]. Sarcopenia has functional adverse consequences, with increased morbidity due to falls, fractures, infections and other conditions, as well as increased mortality [5].

2. Prevention and Management of Under-Nutrition and Sarcopenia in Older People

A greater appreciation of the high rates and significant adverse effects of undernutrition and sarcopenia, which often co-exist in older people, has led to attempts to prevent and treat these conditions. Both exercise and nutritional measures have been shown to have benefits, particularly when combined [6,7].

2.1. Nutritional Measures

Nutritional measures often start with encouragement and assistance to consume greater quantities of usual foods to maintain body weight, the so-called "Food First" approach [8]. These measures may include providing meals at home; supervising food intake and/or having the person eat with others in aged care settings (to counteract reduced appetite and reduced spontaneous food intake); increasing the nutrient and energy density of the food; adding flavour boosters; and fortifying the food with additional fats, protein, and carbohydrates [8].

2.2. Nutritional Supplements

While these "Food First" approaches may be sufficient, they may be difficult to implement because of the cost of foods or time/staffing/convenience constraints, and not always successful. Consequently, nutritional supplements are increasingly recommended for, and used by, older people, both as a means of increasing total energy intake (when harmful weight loss is a concern) and to increase protein intake. Mixed macronutrient supplements are used for the former, while supplements of pure protein or very high in protein are used more specifically for the latter.

The use of such supplements offers the opportunity to more closely tailor the timing and composition of added protein intake to what is likely to be most beneficial. It is often recommended that older people take nutritional supplement drinks between and well separated from regular meals so as not to reduce energy intake at those meals; maintenance of weight or even weight gain is a desirable outcome in the many older people with, or at risk of, under-nutrition.

Consequently, specific nutritional supplements, usually commercial preparations, are used widely by older people. When the aim is to maintain body weight and general nutrition, rather than specifically enhance skeletal muscle and function, these usually take the form of a mixture of macronutrients in a drink containing 1–1.5 kcal/mL of protein, fat, and carbohydrates. Frequently used preparations contain about 9–15 gm protein (15–17% of total energy) in a 200–240 mL serving.

2.3. Protein Nutritional Supplements

When the aim is to preferentially prevent and/or reverse aging-associated muscle loss and sarcopenia, the use of such mixed macronutrient nutrient supplements may not be sufficient and pure protein or high protein supplements may be used.

3. Dietary Protein Requirements in Older People

Recommended dietary protein intakes for adults of all ages, based on nitrogen balance studies, are 0.8 gm/kg body weight in most countries [9], with no adjustments for age or gender. There have been increasing calls, however, for the minimum recommended daily protein intake in older people to be higher than that [10,11]. One reason is concern that the traditional nitrogen balance study methods used to determine appropriate protein requirements in adults of any age underestimate true requirements, with requirements as determined by the newer indicator amino acid oxidation (IAAO) methods up to 25–75% higher [9]. The minimal protein intake for healthy younger adults determined by IAAO is approximately 1.0–1.2 gm/kg/day [9].

Secondly, older people are likely to need higher dietary protein intakes than younger adults for the maintenance of good health, for a number of reasons. These include an age-related reduction in muscle anabolic response to ingested protein; while digestion and absorption of dietary protein is not apparently affected by aging, there is evidence for an age-related reduction in the anabolic muscle response to ingested protein—anabolic resistance (see [10]). This is due to both a redistribution of ingested proteins away from the muscle to splanchnic tissues and a reduced anabolic effect on muscle of the amino acids that do reach the muscle. In addition, catabolic conditions associated with increased muscle breakdown and needs for dietary protein intake become more prevalent with increasing age. These include chronic diseases such as obstructive airways disease, heart failure, renal failure, malignancies, inflammatory forms of arthritis and polymyalgia rheumatica, and acute conditions such as infections and cardiovascular/cerebrovascular events.

Although not conclusive, there is some evidence from balance studies that older people do have higher dietary protein requirements than young adults. One meta-analysis was reported to show approximately 6% higher protein intakes needed to maintain nitrogen balance in people 60 year and older compared with those younger [12], and another approximately 26% higher intakes needed in those over 55 years compared with those younger [13], although neither difference achieved statistical significance due to small subject numbers. Using the indicator amino acid oxidation method mentioned above to study small numbers (12 or less per group) of subjects, protein requirements have been reported as 1.24 gm/kg/day in men over 65 years [14] and 1.15–1.29 gm/kg/day in women over 65 years [15].

3.1. Do Men and Women Have Different Dietary Protein Needs?

Women, on average, consume less protein than men, in absolute terms owing to lower body weight, and possibly also less compared with body weight. Women over 70 years in the 2003–4 U.S. NHANES study consumed about 10% less protein per kg body weight than men of the same age, with 50% of these older women reporting daily protein intakes ≤0.9 gm/kg ideal body weight/day, compared with only 25% of older men [16]. These reduced intakes in women are probably in line with reduced needs. The results of several meta-analyses of nitrogen balance studies indicate that adult women need approximately 10% less dietary protein per kg body weight than men to maintain nitrogen balance [12,13], probably because of lower muscle mass relative to body weight. Nevertheless, there were few older subjects in the studies examined in those meta-analyses, and not all studies show lower requirements in women [17]. While protein needs/kg body weight of older women may be lower than those of older men, the difference does not appear to be great. In the interests of simplicity and the absence of evidence that higher protein intakes, if achievable, do much harm (see below), it seems reasonable to maintain gender-neutral protein intake recommendations for older people at this time.

3.2. Summary Recommendations for Dietary Protein Intake in Older People

Total Daily Protein Intake

For reasons outlined above, recent recommendations for total daily protein intake in healthy older people are usually in the range of 1–1.5 gm/kg per day. The European PROT-AGE study group, for example, has recommended 1.0–1.2 gm/kg dietary protein for healthy older adults [11]. Others have suggested that even higher intakes (>1.2 gm/kg/day) are needed for maintenance of muscle mass and function [10]. Even higher intakes than these are likely to be needed at times of catabolic stress owing to acute or chronic illness, with the PROT-AGE group recommending 1.2–1.5 g/kg/day for those with acute or chronic illness, and up to 2.0 gm/kg/day for those with severe illness or injury or with marked malnutrition [11].

3.3. How Many Older People Need Supplements to Reach the Recommended Protein Intake?

It is unclear how many older adults consume less than the recommended protein intake (either current RDA Recommended Dietary Allowance or the newer recommendations), but probably a substantial proportion. The U.S. NHANES study of 2003–4 reported dietary protein intake substantially lower in healthy older than young adults; in people over 70 years, mean total protein intake was 64.7 gm with a mean intake of 1.0 gm/kg ideal body weight, 27% and 23% respectively, below reported intakes in adults 19–30 years [16]. Over 75% of people over 70 years reported intakes of less than 1.2 gm/kg ideal body weight [16]. Similarly, in the Quebec NuAge study, the mean protein intake of older subjects was very close to 1 gm/kg/day [17].

3.4. Possible Adverse Effects of Protein Supplements

Some concerns have been raised about increasing the dietary protein intakes of older people over current recommended levels. These include the following.

3.4.1. Renal Effects

Renal function declines with increasing age [18]. High protein intakes can increase renal filtration and accelerate the progression of established renal disease; restricted protein intakes of 0.3–0.8 gm/kg/day have been shown to delay the progression of established renal disease and are often prescribed for this indication. The adverse effects of high dietary protein intakes on impaired renal function appear to be increased in those with diabetes mellitus, hypertension, or obesity. It is possible, therefore, that increasing the dietary protein intake of older people, whose renal function has already undergone age-related declines, to levels of 1.2 gm/kg/day or higher may induce renal impairment or accelerate the progression of pre-existing renal disease. While this is possible, it is not established that older people with relatively good renal function and without significant risk factors are at such risk. Evidence does not support a relationship between increased dietary protein content and a decline in renal function [19], and high protein diets undertaken for up to 2 years have not been shown to impair renal function in otherwise healthy people [20]. Advanced age alone does not, therefore, appear to be a reason to avoid increased dietary protein intake when indicated, although caution should be exercised in those with pre-existing renal impairment or risk factors for renal function deterioration.

3.4.2. Bone Effects

Previous suggestions that increased dietary protein intake may have adverse effects on bone health by increasing bone mineral loss and increasing the risk of fractures have not been supported by more recent studies [9,21], which have, if anything, shown beneficial effects of dietary protein on bone health.

3.4.3. Post-Prandial Hypotension

Ingestion of nutrients leads to redirection of blood flow from other organs to the splanchnic circulation to aid digestion. As a result, blood pressure (BP) can drop. This is largely prevented in young, healthy adults by an increase in heart rate and other compensatory mechanisms, but in older people, these are less effective. As a result, older people have greater food-induced BP decreases than younger adults [22]. In some, this can be excessive and lead to symptoms of dizziness and, in some cases, falls and cardiovascular events [23]. The excessive drop in BP after food ingestion has been termed post-prandial hypotension and defined as a decrease in systolic BP of 20 mm Hg or more within 2 h of food ingestion [24]. Ingestion of all three macronutrients, alone or together, causes post-prandial BP falls in older people. Available evidence indicates that carbohydrate and protein have equivalent BP lowering effects, although the BP decreases occur sooner after carbohydrate than protein and fat [25]. We have recently reported substantial systolic BP decreases after ingestion of a 70 gm whey protein drink by healthy, older men, with 58% having a decrease of 20 mm of Hg systolic or more within three hours of protein ingestion, with maximum decreases occurring between two and three hours after the drink [26] In contrast, maximum decreases after carbohydrate alone, or mixed drinks, appear to occur earlier. Seventy grams of whey is a high dose, higher than is generally recommended or likely to be ingested by older people (see below), and the hypotensive effects of protein and other macronutrients do seem to be at least partly dose-responsive [27]. Nevertheless, high energy nutrient supplement drinks decrease BP in older people and the hypotensive effects of pure or high protein drinks may be quite prolonged and possibly greater in those already on antihypertensive medications. Appropriate advice and precautions are indicated after such drinks, particularly in at-risk individuals.

3.5. Evidence for Benefits of Nutritional Supplements in Older People

A detailed review of this matter is beyond the scope of this review (see [4]). Study methods and results are variable. Not all studies show benefits [17]. Nevertheless, in our view, a number of conclusions can be drawn; the use of such supplements is generally safe (see above) and relatively easy to implement. Few, if any, adverse effects of such supplements have been reported; the use of these supplements by older people improves nutritional intakes and is associated with weight gain and an increase in lean body mass in many cases and, in some cases, improvements in muscle function, hospitalisation rates, and even death rates [28]. The greatest benefits of taking nutritional supplements are obtained by the most undernourished older people [29].

For these reasons, and because many older people appear to have a suboptimal dietary protein intake, protein or protein-rich supplements are increasingly recommended to older people.

In summary, there is evidence of the following:

1. Older people have higher dietary protein needs than young adults, particularly if they have lost weight and/or are undernourished, are sarcopenic, or have acute or chronic medical conditions that contribute to muscle catabolism. These requirements are in the range of 1.2 gm/kg/day or higher.
2. Many (probably the majority of those >70 years) older people do not consume these minimum protein requirements. It can be difficult for older people to increase their dietary protein intake by increasing their intake of usual foods owing to anorexia and the cost of high protein foods.
3. Protein supplements increase muscle mass and strength, and may also reduce morbidity and mortality, particularly in undernourished and/or sarcopenic older people.

3.6. Does the Type of Protein or Amino Acid in the Supplement Matter?

Yes, it probably does. Not all ingested proteins are the same, particularly in terms of their anabolic effects on skeletal muscle (see [9] for review). The available evidence indicates that branched chain amino acids, particularly leucine, are the most effective amino acids in stimulating muscle protein synthesis (MPS). Consistent with this, in one longitudinal study, older people (>65 years) with dietary leucine intakes in the upper quartile had preservation of lean body mass over 6 years, whereas those with intakes in the lowest quartile had loss of lean body mass [30]. The extent of MPS is proportional to the peak leucine plasma concentration after protein ingestion [31].

Animal-derived dietary proteins appear to be stronger in stimulating MPS than plant-based proteins, and milk-based proteins in particular are a good source of leucine containing proteins [9]. Whey protein, obtained from milk in the cheese making process, is high in leucine, about 10–15%, and more rapidly absorbed than casein, factors that may contribute to its greater stimulatory effect than casein on MPS in older men [32]. The maximum stimulatory effects on MPS probably occur after ingestion of 2–2.5 gm leucine in young and middle aged adults, with little additional effect of higher intakes. Ingestion of 20 gm whey protein concentrate at one time is probably sufficient to optimise MPS in young and middle aged adults [33]. In contrast, because of anabolic resistance, older adults appear to need 30–35 gm or more of whey to achieve similar anabolic effects [34].

The effects of protein supplements to increase muscle mass and strength and to have functional benefits appear greatest in those most at risk; i.e., malnourished, sarcopenic, or at risk of sarcopenia. Several interventional studies have demonstrated that combined dietary supplements of whey protein and leucine increase muscle mass and strength and improve function in older sarcopenic adults; see [9]. A recent meta-analysis reported increased lean body mass without an increase in strength in sarcopenic older adults taking 2–7.8 gm of leucine supplements/day [35]. It is difficult to separate the effects of leucine supplements from those of other amino acids or proteins such as whey when they are given in combination. It may be, particularly in the case of already leucine-rich whey protein supplements, that they have benefits in addition to those of leucine, and that, when a sufficient amount is ingested, further leucine fortification has little further benefit.

3.7. How Much Protein Should There Be in the Supplement?

Owing to age-induced "anabolic resistance", older people probably require 30–45 gm protein per serving to stimulate muscle protein synthesis after that meal, whereas lower doses (≤20 gm) are sufficient in young adults (see above and [36]). The consumption of 1–2 daily meals with protein content of 30 to 45 g may be an important strategy for increasing and/or maintaining lean body mass and muscle strength with aging [36]. There is evidence that older men and women with more-evenly mealtime distributed protein intakes have higher muscle strength irrespective of their total protein intake [17]. It seems reasonable, therefore, that if protein supplements are being used for their effects on muscle, they be used in a way that provides at least 1.2 gm/kg/protein per day (food plus supplement) with at least two protein intake episodes/day (food plus supplement) containing at least 30 gm protein each. As the post protein BP drop, which could be potentially harmful, appears to be dose-responsive, it is also likely that smaller, twice daily or even more frequent, doses of protein supplement will have more beneficial effects on BP than once daily larger doses.

3.8. Timing of Protein Intake Relative to Exercise

Both protein ingestion and resistance exercise independently stimulate muscle protein synthesis in older people, although the response to both is blunted in the elderly [37,38]. These two stimuli have synergistic anabolic effects on MPS, particularly when the protein is ingested soon after the resistance exercise [39]. While ingestion of approximately 20 gm of a high quality protein is sufficient to maximize skeletal muscle protein synthesis rates during recovery from resistance-type exercise in younger adults, doses up to 40 gm or possibly even higher are needed in older adults [37,38].

4. Gastrointestinal Responses to Protein Ingestion: Effects of Aging

Appetite and food intake in free living humans are dependent on a complex interplay of environmental factors and central and peripheral physical mechanisms. The latter mechanisms include intra-gastric and small intestinal sensory and motor functions and their interactions [2]. Their study has been a focus of our group. We have used whey protein drinks and intra-duodenal infusions of whey protein to investigate peripheral responses to protein in young and older adults and have identified a number of age-related differences between these age groups in gastrointestinal responses to protein ingestion. These studies have involved older people predominantly of Anglo-Saxon background. The doses of oral whey used have mainly been 30 gm and/or 70 gm, which is of significance as 30 gm appears to approximate the amount required in older people to stimulate muscle protein synthesis (see above), while higher doses are used by some older people.

Older people have reduced appetite compared with young adults and consume less food. There is no change, however, with aging in the preference for particular macronutrients; i.e., the percentage of total energy ingested as protein does not seem to change with increasing age [40].

4.1. Effect of Aging on Appetite and Feeding Responses to Whey Protein

There is evidence that protein is the most satiating of the macronutrients in young adults [41], although this effect may be less in women than men [42]. Our studies have demonstrated that healthy aging is associated with a marked and significant reduction in the satiating effects of whey protein, administered by both intra-duodenal [43] and oral routes [44,45].

4.1.1. Intra-Duodenal Whey

Healthy aging is associated with a marked reduction in the suppressive effect of whey protein administered directly into the duodenum, on appetite and subsequent food intake. Sixty minute intra-duodenal infusions of 8 gm (0.5 kcal/min), 24 gm (1.5 kcal/min), and 48 gm (3 kcal/min) of whey had a dose-responsive suppressive effect on subsequent ad libitum food intake in young men, whereas older men experienced suppression of food intake only after the 48 gm infusion (~33% vs. 17% suppression by 48 gm whey in young vs. older, $p < 0.05$) [43]. Baseline hunger ratings were lower in the older than young men and were suppressed less by the protein infusions in the older than young men, consistent with the reduced effects of intra-duodenal fat and carbohydrate infusions on appetite in older people [46].

4.1.2. Oral Whey

We have reported that healthy, non-obese, young men, but not women, experience significant suppression of hunger ratings and ad libitum food intake three hours after 30 gm and 70 gm whey protein drinks [42,44,47]. In contrast, and consistent with their reduced responses to intra-duodenal whey, healthy, non-obese men and women over 65 years experience little reduction in hunger and no suppression of ad libitum food intake three hours after either 30 gm or 70 gm whey drinks [44,47–50].

This age-related reduction in the satiating effects of whey drinks is observed in our studies largely irrespective of the timing of the whey drink relative to later ad libitum food intake at test meals. Thirty gram whey protein drinks do not suppress appetite ratings or subsequent ad libitum food intake in healthy older people immediately after the drink, or 35 min, 1 h, 2 h, 3 h, 265 min, and 510 min after the drink [44,45,49–51]. In only one study have we detected any reduction in subsequent food intake by older people after a whey drink [45]. In that study, older men received a 30 gm or 70 gm whey drink and then ate adlibitum at breakfast (30 min later), lunch (265 min later), and dinner (510 min later). There was no reduction in food intake compared with the control day at any of the three meals on the 30 gm day. On the 70 gm day, there was no effect on breakfast intake, but a 15% reduction in lunch energy intake ($p < 0.05$ vs. control), followed by a compensatory 7% increase at dinner.

When intake from whey drinks plus subsequent food intake is calculated, absent (usually) or only minor suppression of subsequent food intake by whey drinks has resulted in consistent findings of increases in total energy intake and even greater proportional increases in protein intake after whey drinks in our short-term studies of older people. For example, in the study above, where whey drinks were taken before breakfast and men were studied for the rest of the day [45], there were non-significant 4% and 3% increases in total energy intake on the 30 gm and 70 gm days, respectively, compared with the control day. Total daily protein intake was increased significantly by the whey drinks in a dose-responsive manner, with increases almost equal to the protein content of the whey drinks (+31 gm on the 30 gm whey drink day, +62 gm on the 70 gm whey drink day, $p < 0.001$ vs. control [45]).

These findings suggest that it should be possible to give enough extra protein to older people to preserve or increase muscle mass and function without suppressing energy intake and promoting weight loss, particularly if they are encouraged to continue their usual non-supplement food (energy) intake.

4.2. What Is the Best Timing of the Protein Supplement Use by Older People?

Because older men can increase their protein intake in a single episode into the range of 30–40 gm, enough to maximize the protein's anabolic effects on muscle without the timing of that supplement's ingestion making much if any difference to subsequent appetite and food intake, these supplements can probably be ingested as a between-meal supplement, close to or even with meals. The effects in women are likely to be similar [50], but require further study. The effects of more frequent protein doses across the day also need to be determined.

Indeed, if the supplement is given with a protein-containing meal, instead of between meals, less supplementary protein is needed to reach the 30–40 gm anabolic threshold described above. Older men in the NuAge study, for example, had a mean daily protein intake of 1 gm/kg (mean of 18 gm at breakfast and 23 gm at lunch and dinner) [17]. Their protein intake could be increased to 1.33 gm/kg/day with a total protein intake of 35 gm per meal two meals a day by adding as little as 12 gm protein with each of lunch and dinner. A pragmatic measure, to allow for those with below average dietary protein intakes, would be to take 20 gm of a protein supplement with the two meals each day already containing the most protein. This dose is unlikely to have many, if any, side effects for most older people.

4.3. Effect of Aging on Gastric Function and Emptying

Healthy aging is associated with changes in gastric function. These include reduced perceptions of proximal gastric distension and delayed gastric accommodation [52], probable changes in the intra-gastric distribution of food after its ingestion, greater stimulation of phasic pyloric pressure waves by intra-duodenal lipid [46], and slowing of gastric emptying. It is unclear, however, how much, if at all, these changes contribute to the age-related reduction in the satiating effect of ingested protein and responses to protein supplements in older people. It is possible, however, that they may contribute to age-related reduced appetite and food intake.

4.3.1. Intra-Gastric Food Distribution and Antral Area

After food is ingested, it is distributed throughout the stomach, with varying amounts in the proximal versus distal stomach (antrum). Antral distension appears to be a greater determinant of satiety and satiation than proximal gastric distension; the more distal the intra-gastric distribution of food, the greater the antral distension, the greater the sensations of fullness, the less the hunger, and the lower the subsequent food intake [53]. Owing to impaired receptive relaxation of the gastric fundus [52] and other factors, food is distributed more distally in older people, as indicated by them having larger antral areas than young adults after ingestion of the same mixed macro-nutrient loads [53]. As a result, they probably experience greater fullness and lower hunger ratings. While the more distal movement of food after its ingestion thus probably contributes to reduced hunger and increased fullness in older people, it is unclear how these changes could contribute to the reduced suppression of appetite ratings and food intake after oral ingestion of protein, alone or combined with other nutrients.

4.3.2. Gastric Emptying

The oral ingestion of nutrients, irrespective of their type, slows gastric emptying. Gastric emptying of non-nutrient drinks is slightly slower in older than in young adults [44–54]. Whey protein drinks in doses of 30–70 gm slow gastric emptying in a dose-responsive manner [42,44,50], and probably slow it more in older than in young adults; the stomachs of healthy older men emptied whey into the duodenum at approximately 0.8 kcal/min compared with 1.0 kcal for young adult men ($p < 0.05$) in one study [44]. Gastric emptying of whey protein drinks is faster in young, non-obese men than women [42], but this sex difference is no longer present in healthy people over 65 years [50]. Gastric emptying of whey drinks occurs at a similar rate in obese young and older men [49], with neither age group having suppression of appetite or food intake 3 hours after ingestion of 30 gm whey—a suppressive dose in young, non-obese men [42,44]. The findings suggest that obesity may blunt the effects of whey on both food intake and the slowing of gastric emptying.

Delayed gastric emptying results in more food in the stomach at any given time after food ingestion than would otherwise be the case. This increases gastric distension and, depending on the distribution of the food within the stomach, might be expected to produce greater feelings of fullness and reduced subsequent food intake. Consistent with this, the intentional creation of gastric distension and fullness by implanting gastric balloons has had some success in the treatment of obesity [55]. Greater gastric distension after eating, due to slower gastric emptying, in older than in young adults, might thus be expected to cause greater post-eating suppression of appetite and food intake in older than in young adults. Existing evidence does not suggest, however, that this is so. Perceptions of gastric distension are less in older than young adults [52], and healthy older people have fullness ratings (unlike hunger ratings) 3 h after a whey drink, at the start of an ad libitum meal, that do not relate significantly to energy intake at that meal [44]. Furthermore, as outlined above, older people have less, not more, suppression of appetite and food intake by whey drinks than younger adults, despite slower gastric emptying and presumably greater gastric distension at any given time after the drinks. Our groups' studies have largely involved administering the ad libitum test meal 3 hours after the whey test drink, in order to allow the full effect of gastric mechanisms to be studied. The stomach is empty or almost empty by then after both 30 gm and 70 gm whey protein drinks [44]. While it is possible that, if the meal had been given earlier, greater suppressive effects on intake due to greater gastric distension would have been present, this is not supported by our finding of a lack of suppression by 30 gm whey of food intake immediately after the drink and hourly up to 3 hours after the drink [51].

4.3.3. Small Intestinal Satiety Mechanisms

As aging has similar qualitative effects on appetite and food intake after intra-duodenal protein (whey) to those of oral whey (see above), and the age-related changes in gastric mechanisms do not appear to explain the reduced suppression of appetite and food intake by protein in older people, it seems likely that the reduced age-related changes in response to protein are mediated mainly by reductions in the satiating effects of the protein after it enters the small intestine. Nevertheless, slower gastric emptying in older people may modify these post-gastric effects by delaying their onset and prolonging their duration. Sixty minute duodenal infusions of 0.5 kcal/min and 1.5 kcal whey/minute do not suppress subsequent food intake in healthy older men, but 3 kcal/min infusions do, albeit less in older than in younger men [43]. As healthy older men empty whey drinks from the stomach at a rate of approximately 0.8 kcal/min [44], it is likely that, even if a very high protein load is taken in drink form, for most older people, their age-related slowing of gastric emptying and markedly reduced effect of whey once it enters the duodenum combine to result in no suppression of appetite or subsequent energy intake. In contrast, duodenal infusions of whey in doses of 0.5, 1.5, and 3 kcal/in have dose-responsive suppressive effects on energy intake in young men, who empty whey drinks from the stomach faster than older men (~1 kcal/min) [44]. Together, these findings explain the suppressive effects of both 30 gm and 70 gm whey drinks on subsequent energy intake in young, but not older adults [44].

4.4. Selected Hormones

Ingestion of protein, either orally or by infusion directly into the duodenum, results in changes in circulating concentrations of a number of hormones with definite or possible effects on appetite and subsequent food intake. Among them, concentrations of cholecystokinin (CCK), insulin, glucagon, gastric inhibitory peptide (GIP), glucagon-like peptide-1 (GLP-1), peptide tyrosine-tyrosine (PYY), and amino acids increase, while glucose does not change and ghrelin concentrations decrease [42,47,48,50,56,57].

A number of these small intestinal responses to protein ingestion differ between healthy older and younger adults and these age-related changes in turn possibly affect the responses to protein or protein containing supplements in older people.

4.4.1. Cholecystokinin (CCK)

CCK is released by the small bowel after nutrient ingestion and acts to slow gastric emptying and reduce food intake. Circulating CCK concentrations increase less after oral protein ingestion in young women than in young men, which may be one reason for the lower satiating effect of whey protein in young women than men [42]. Circulating CCK concentrations are higher in healthy fasting older than young adults [58,59], and older adults retain their sensitivity to the satiating effects of exogenous CCK [60]. Increased CCK activity may thus be a cause of the anorexia of ageing and reduced hunger pre-meals observed in older adults. Increases in circulating CCK concentrations are at least as great [53], if not greater [58], after whey drinks in healthy older than young adult men and women. The cause of this possibly greater rise is not known; it may relate to slower transition of whey through the small bowel in older people and, therefore, more prolonged contact with the CCK releasing cells. Ageing-related increases in CCK secretion and action are unlikely, however, to contribute to the reduced suppression of appetite and food intake by whey protein observed in older people compared with young adults. The opposite might be expected. The exact role of CCK in mediating age-related responses to protein supplements remains to be determined.

4.4.2. Glucagon-Like Peptide 1 (GLP-1)

GLP-1 is released by the small bowel and colon in response to food ingestion. Like CCK, it slows gastric emptying and has satiating effects. Fasting GLP-1 concentrations are higher in healthy older than young ageing [58,59], which may thus contribute to lower basal (fasting) hunger in older people. Circulating GLP-1 concentrations appear to increase to a similar extent after whey drinks in young and older adults [54–56], which does not support a role for the lesser suppression of food intake by whey protein in older adults.

4.4.3. Gastric Inhibitory Peptide (GIP)

Along with GLP-1, GIP is an incretin that plays roles in the control of glucagon, insulin, and blood glucose concentrations. It is not clear what role GIP plays in the control of appetite and feeding, but it may have some effect to stimulate food intake [61]. Circulating fasting GIP concentrations are not affected by normal aging, but GIP concentrations increase more after oral whey ingestion in older than in young adults [45–54]. This greater increase might act to reduce the whey-induced suppression of food intake that would otherwise occur. It might also act to limit blood glucose concentration increases in older people after protein is co-ingested with other nutrients.

4.4.4. Insulin and Glucose

Insulin plays a key role in glucose homeostasis, while its role in appetite and feeding control is less clear. Oral ingestion of protein, including whey, stimulates insulin secretion in a dose-responsive manner [58]. While oral ingestion of protein on its own has little, if any, effect on blood glucose concentrations, its co-ingestion with glucose by non-elderly adults with type 2 diabetes results in significantly smaller increases in blood glucose concentrations than ingestion of the same amount of glucose on its own [62]. The stimulation of insulin secretion by whey drinks is not apparently affected by aging, and remains robust [58]. We have recently found that co-ingestion of 30 gm whey protein with 30 gm glucose in drink form significantly reduces the increase in blood glucose concentrations compared with ingestion of 30 gm glucose alone (peak glucose 7.4 vs. 9.0 mmol/L, $p < 0.01$) in men over 65 years [27], and are now extending these studies to older people with type 2 diabetes. These findings suggest that moderately high whey protein intake together with carbohydrate might improve postprandial glycaemia in older people, particularly those with diabetes, and provide an additional benefit of taking a protein supplement with, rather than between, meals.

4.4.5. Glucagon

Circulating concentrations of glucagon are not affected by aging [54–56]. Whey protein drinks act to increase glucagon concentrations, to a similar degree in older and young adults [58].

4.4.6. Ghrelin

Ghrelin is an orexigenic hormone secreted by the enteroendocrine cells of the gastrointestinal tract, particularly the stomach. Circulating concentrations are highest in the fasting state and decrease after food ingestion. Fasting circulating concentrations may be slightly lower in older than in young adults, and thus contribute to the anorexia of aging [63–65]. Ghrelin concentrations are suppressed to a similar degree after whey drinks in healthy older and young adults [58], so it is not clear what role, if any, ghrelin plays in mediating age-related reductions in feeding responses to protein supplements.

5. Future Directions

Future studies should focus on women as well as men to determine whether our findings in older men also apply to women. They should also determine whether the results of our short-term studies with protein supplements, such as post-supplement blood pressure drops and failure to suppress appetite and food intake, are replicated in studies of longer term protein supplement use. Further studies, both short- and longer-term, of the effect of protein when co-ingested with carbohydrates on glucose metabolism in older people with and without diabetes mellitus would also be of interest.

6. Conclusions

Nutritional supplements, including pure-protein or protein-enriched drinks, are increasingly used by older people to maintain body weight and nutrition, and specifically to prevent or treat loss of muscle function, sarcopenia, and frailty. Daily protein requirements in older people appear to be higher than those of young adults—in the range of 1.2 gm/kg/day or more. Many older adults do not consume this much protein in their usual diet and are likely to benefit from an increase. Protein supplements appear relatively safe, although care should be taken in those with or at risk of renal impairment, or prone to post-nutrient hypotension. Protein supplements (alone or in a mixed macronutrient supplement) in doses sufficient to reach the above daily intake are likely to be beneficial, perhaps best taken twice daily, if possible soon after resistance exercise, in doses that achieve protein intakes of 30 gm or more per episode. Our study results suggest that it is probably not important to give these supplements between meals, because they have little, if any, suppressive effect on appetite and later food intake in older people, owing to age-related changes in gastrointestinal and other mechanisms that are as yet poorly understood. Adding protein supplements to usual food intake is very unlikely to reduce energy intake and instead is likely to increase overall energy and protein intake, particularly if encouragement is given to continue usual food intake. There may even be benefits in giving the supplement with meals, to achieve protein intakes above the effective anabolic threshold with lower supplement doses, and have favorable effects on food-induced blood glucose increases in older people with, or at risk of, developing type 2 diabetes mellitus.

Further studies are indicated to determine the following:

1. The acute effects of whey and other proteins, when co-ingested with other macronutrients, with and between meals, on appetite and food intake in older people.
2. The longer term effects of protein ingestion, alone and combined with other macronutrients, on appetite, food intake, and glucose homoeostasis, in older people; i.e., whether effects observed in acute studies persist with longer-term administration.

A better understanding of the mechanisms underlying the reduced suppression of appetite and food intake by protein and other macronutrients in older compared with younger adults, whether gastro-intestinal, central, or both, can be used to develop ways of improving nutrition in at-risk older individuals. Although our studies with whey have identified a number of age-related changes in gastro-intestinal responses to protein ingestion, it is not yet clear exactly how they act to mediate age-related changes in appetite and feeding.

Author Contributions: Conceptualization, I.C.; Writing—original draft, I.C., A.O., C.G. and S.S.; Writing—review & editing, I.C., A.O., C.G. and S.S. All authors have read and agreed to the published version of the manuscript.

Funding: This research received no external funding.

Informed Consent Statement: Not applicable.

Conflicts of Interest: The authors declare no conflict of interest.

References

1. Morley, J.E.; Silver, A.J. Anorexia in the elderly. *Neurobiol. Aging* **1988**, *9*, 9–16. [CrossRef]
2. Soenen, S.; Chapman, I.M. Body weight, anorexia, and undernutrition in older people. *J. Am. Med. Dir. Assoc.* **2013**, *14*, 642–648. [CrossRef]
3. Visvanathan, R.; Chapman, I.M. Undernutrition and anorexia in the older person. *Gastroenterol. Clin. N. Am.* **2009**, *38*, 393–409. [CrossRef] [PubMed]
4. Castillo, E.M.; Gruen, D.G.; Silverstein, D.K.; Morton, D.J.; Wingard, D.L.; Connor, E.B. Sarcopenia in elderly men and women: The Rancho Bernardo study. *Am. J. Prev. Med.* **2003**, *25*, 226–231. [CrossRef]
5. Janssen, I. Evolution of sarcopenia research. *Appl. Physiol. Nutr. Meta.* **2010**, *35*, 707–712. [CrossRef] [PubMed]
6. Luo, D.; Lin, Z.; Li, S.; Liu, S.H. Effect of nutritional supplement combined with exercise intervention on sarcopenia in the elderly: A meta-analysis. *Int. J. Nurs. Sci.* **2017**, *4*, 389–401. [CrossRef]
7. Bell, K.E.; Snijders, T.; Zulyniak, M.; Kumbhare, D.; Parise, G.; Phillips, S.M. A whey protein-based multi-ingredient nutritional supplement stimulates gains in lean body mass and strength in healthy older men: A randomized controlled trial. *PLoS ONE* **2017**, *2*, e0181387. [CrossRef] [PubMed]
8. Roberts, H.C.; Lim, S.E.R.; Cox, N.J.; Ibrahim, K. The Challenge of Managing Undernutrition in Older People with Frailty. *Nutrients* **2019**, *11*, 808. [CrossRef] [PubMed]
9. Phillips, S.M. Current Concepts and Unresolved Questions in Dietary Protein Requirements and Supplements in Adults. *Front. Nutr.* **2017**, *4*, 13. [CrossRef] [PubMed]
10. Traylor, D.A.; Gorissen, S.H.M.; Phillips, S.M. Perspective: Protein Requirements and Optimal Intakes in Aging: Are We Ready to Recommend More Than the Recommended Daily Allowance? *Adv. Nutr.* **2018**, *9*, 171–182. [CrossRef] [PubMed]
11. Bauer, J.; Biolo, G.; Cederholm, T.; Cesari, M.; Jentoft, A.J.C.; Morley, J.E.; Phillips, S.; Sieber, C.; Stehle, P.; Teta, D.; et al. Evidence-based recommendations for optimal dietary protein intake in older people: A position paper from the PROT-AGE Study Group. *J. Am. Med. Dir. Assoc.* **2013**, *14*, 542–559. [CrossRef]
12. Li, M.; Sun, F.; Piao, J.H.; Yang, X.G. Protein requirements in healthy adults: A meta-analysis of nitrogen balance studies. *Biomed. Environ. Sci.* **2014**, *27*, 606–613. [PubMed]
13. Rand, W.M.; Pellett, P.L.; Young, V.R. Meta-analysis of nitrogen balance studies for estimating protein requirements in healthy adults. *Am. J. Clin. Nutr.* **2003**, *77*, 109–127. [CrossRef] [PubMed]

14. Rafii, M.; Chapman, K.; Elango, R.; Campbell, W.W.; Ball, R.O.; Pencharz, P.B.; Martin, G.C. Dietary Protein Requirement of Men >65 Years Old Determined by the Indicator Amino Acid Oxidation Technique Is Higher than the Current Estimated Average Requirement. *J. Nutr.* **2015**, *146*, 681–687. [CrossRef]
15. Rafii, M.; Chapman, K.; Elango, R.; Campbell, W.W.; Ball, R.O.; Pencharz, P.B.; Martin, G.C. Dietary protein requirement of female adults >65 years determined by the indicator amino acid oxidation technique is higher than current recommendations. *J. Nutr.* **2015**, *145*, 18–24. [CrossRef] [PubMed]
16. Fulgoni, V.L., 3rd. Current protein intake in America: Analysis of the National Health and Nutrition Examination Survey, 2003-2004. *Am. J. Clin. Nutr.* **2008**, *87*, 1554S–1557S. [CrossRef] [PubMed]
17. Farsijani, S.; Payette, H.; Morais, J.A.; Shatenstein, B.; Gaudreau, P.; Chevalier, S. Even mealtime distribution of protein intake is associated with greater muscle strength, but not with 3-y physical function decline, in free-living older adults: The Quebec longitudinal study on Nutrition as a Determinant of Successful Aging (NuAge study). *Am. J. Clin. Nutr.* **2017**, *106*, 113–124. [CrossRef] [PubMed]
18. Weinstein, J.R.; Anderson, S. The aging kidney: Physiological changes. *Adv. Chronic Kidney Dis.* **2010**, *17*, 302–307. [CrossRef] [PubMed]
19. Trumbo, P.; Schlicker, S.; Yates, A.A.; Poos, M. Dietary reference intakes for energy, carbohydrate, fiber, fat, fatty acids, cholesterol, protein and amino acids. *J. Am. Diet. Assoc.* **2002**, *102*, 1621–1630. [CrossRef]
20. Friedman, A.N.; Ogden, L.G.; Foster, G.D.; Klein, S.; Stein, R.; Miller, B.; Hill, J.O.; Brill, C.; Bailer, B.; Rosenbaum, D.R.; et al. Comparative effects of low-carbohydrate high-protein versus low-fat diets on the kidney. *Clin. J. Am. Soc. Nephrol.* **2012**, *7*, 1103–1111. [CrossRef]
21. Rizzoli, R.; Biver, B.; Bonjour, J.P.; Coxam, V.; Goltzman, D.; Kanis, J.A.; Lappe, J.; Rejnmark, L.; Sahni, S.; Weaver, C.; et al. Benefits and safety of dietary protein for bone health-an expert consensus paper endorsed by the European Society for Clinical and Economical Aspects of Osteopororosis, Osteoarthritis, and Musculoskeletal Diseases and by the International Osteoporosis Foundation. *Osteoporos. Int.* **2018**, *29*, 1933–1948. [PubMed]
22. Trahair, L.G.; Horowitz, M.; Jones, K.L. Postprandial hypotension: A systematic review. *J. Am. Med. Dir. Assoc.* **2014**, *15*, 394–409. [CrossRef] [PubMed]
23. Aronow, W.S.; Ahn, C. Association of postprandial hypotension with incidence of falls, syncope, coronary events, stroke, and total mortality at 29-month follow-up in 499 older nursing home residents. *J. Am. Geriatr. Soc.* **1997**, *45*, 1051–1053. [CrossRef] [PubMed]
24. Jansen, R.W.; Lipsitz, L.A. Postprandial hypotension: Epidemiology, pathophysiology, and clinical management. *Ann. Intern. Med.* **1995**, *122*, 286–295. [CrossRef] [PubMed]
25. Gentilcore, D.; Hausken, T.; Meyer, J.M.; Chapman, I.M.; Horowitz, M.; Jones, K.L. Effects of intraduodenal glucose, fat, and protein on blood pressure, heart rate, and splanchnic blood flow in healthy older subjects. *Am. J. Clin. Nutr.* **2008**, *87*, 156–161. [CrossRef]
26. Giezenaar, C.; Oberoi, A.; Jones, K.L.; Horowitz, M.; Chapman, I.; Soenen, S. Effects of age on blood pressure and heart rate responses to whey protein in younger and older men. *J. Am. Geriatr. Soc.* **2021**, in press. [CrossRef] [PubMed]
27. Oberoi, A.; Giezenaar, C.; Tippett, R.; Jones, K.L.; Chapman, I.; Soenen, S. Effects of whey protein and glucose intake on energy intake, gastric emptying and glycaemia in healthy older subjects. *EASD* **2020**.
28. Milne, A.C.; Potter, J.; Avenell, A. Protein and energy supplementation in elderly people at risk from malnutrition. *Cochrane Database Syst. Rev.* **2005**, CD003288. [CrossRef]
29. Milne, A.C.; Potter, J.; Vivanti, A.; Avenell, A. Protein and energy supplementation in elderly people at risk from malnutrition. *Cochrane Database Syst. Rev.* **2009**, CD003288. [CrossRef]
30. McDonald, C.K.; Ankarfeldt, M.Z.; Capra, S.; Bauer, J.; Raymond, K.; Heitmann, B.L. Lean body mass change over 6 years is associated with dietary leucine intake in an older Danish population. *Br. J. Nutr.* **2016**, *115*, 1556–1562. [CrossRef] [PubMed]
31. Norton, L.E.; Wilson, G.J.; Layman, D.K.; Bunpo, P.; Anthony, T.G.; Brana, D.V.; Garlick, P.J. The leucine content of a complete meal directs peak activation but not duration of skeletal muscle protein synthesis and mammalian target of rapamycin signaling in rats. *J. Nutr.* **2009**, *139*, 1103–1109. [CrossRef] [PubMed]
32. Pennings, B.; Boirie, Y.; Senden, J.M.G.; Gijsen, A.P.; Kuipers, H.; Loon, L.J.C.V. Whey protein stimulates postprandial muscle protein accretion more effectively than do casein and casein hydrolysate in older men. *Am. J. Clin. Nutr.* **2011**, *93*, 997–1005. [CrossRef] [PubMed]
33. Mitchell, C.J.; McGregor, R.A.; D'Souza, R.F.; Thorstensen, E.B.; Markworth, J.F.; Fanning, A.C.; Poppitt, S.D.; Smith, D.C. Consumption of Milk Protein or Whey Protein Results in a Similar Increase in Muscle Protein Synthesis in Middle Aged Men. *Nutrients* **2015**, *7*, 8685–8699. [CrossRef] [PubMed]
34. Pennings, B.; Groen, B.; Lange, A.D.; Gijsen, A.P.; Zorenc, A.H.; Senden, J.M.G.; Loon, L.J.C.V. Amino acid absorption and subsequent muscle protein accretion following graded intakes of whey protein in elderly men. *Am. J. Physiol. Endocrinol. Metab.* **2012**, *302*, E992–E999. [CrossRef] [PubMed]
35. Komar, B.; Schwingshackl, L.; Hoffmann, G. Effects of leucine-rich protein supplements on anthropometric parameter and muscle strength in the elderly: A systematic review and meta-analysis. *J. Nutr. Health Aging* **2015**, *19*, 437–446. [CrossRef] [PubMed]
36. Loenneke, J.P.; Loprinzi, P.D.; Murphy, C.H.; Phillips, S.M. Per meal dose and frequency of protein consumption is associated with lean mass and muscle performance. *Clin. Nutr.* **2016**, *35*, 1506–1511. [CrossRef] [PubMed]
37. Churchward-Venne, T.A.; Holwerda, A.M.; Phillips, S.M.; Loon, L.J.C.V. What is the Optimal Amount of Protein to Support Post-Exercise Skeletal Muscle Reconditioning in the Older Adult? *Sports Med.* **2016**, *46*, 1205–1212. [CrossRef]

38. Yang, Z.; Scott, C.A.; Mao, C.; Tang, J.; Farmer, A.J. Resistance exercise enhances myofibrillar protein synthesis with graded intakes of whey protein in older men. *Br. J. Nutr.* **2012**, *108*, 1780–1788. [CrossRef]
39. Esmarck, B.; Andersen, J.L.; Olsen, S.; Richter, E.A.; Mizuno, M.; Kjaer, M. Timing of postexercise protein intake is important for muscle hypertrophy with resistance training in elderly humans. *J. Physiol.* **2001**, *535*, 301–311. [CrossRef]
40. Grech, A.; Rangan, A.; Allman-Farinelli, M. Macronutrient Composition of the Australian Population's Diet; Trends from Three National Nutrition Surveys 1983, 1995 and 2012. *Nutrients* **2018**, *10*, 1045. [CrossRef] [PubMed]
41. Soenen, S.; Westerterp-Plantenga, M.S. Proteins and satiety: Implications for weight management. *Curr. Opin. Clin. Nutr. Metab. Care* **2008**, *11*, 747–751. [CrossRef] [PubMed]
42. Giezenaar, C.; Luscombe-Marsh, N.D.; Hutchison, A.T.; Lange, K.; Hausken, T.; Jones, K.L.; Horowitz, M.; Chapman, I.; Soenen, S. Effect of gender on the acute effects of whey protein ingestion on energy intake, appetite, gastric emptying and gut hormone responses in healthy young adults. *Nutr. Diabetes* **2018**, *8*, 40. [CrossRef]
43. Soenen, S.; Giezenaar, C.; Hutchison, A.T.; Horowitz, M.; Chapman, I.; Luscombe-Marsh, N. Effects of intraduodenal protein on appetite, energy intake, and antropyloroduodenal motility in healthy older compared with young men in a randomized trial. *Am. J. Clin. Nutr.* **2014**, *100*, 1108–1115. [CrossRef] [PubMed]
44. Giezenaar, C.; Trahair, L.G.; Rigda, R.; Hutchison, A.T.; Feinle-Bisset, C.; Luscombe-Marsh, N.D.; Hausken, T.; Jones, K.L.; Horowitz, M.; Chapman, I.; et al. Lesser suppression of energy intake by orally ingested whey protein in healthy older men compared with young controls. *Am. J. Physiol. Regul. Integr. Comp. Physiol.* **2015**, *309*, R845–R854. [CrossRef]
45. Oberoi, A.; Giezenaar, C.; Clames, A.; BØhler, K.; Lange, K.; Horowitz, M.; Jones, K.L.; Chapman, I.; Soenen, S. Whey Protein Drink Ingestion before Breakfast Suppressed Energy Intake at Breakfast and Lunch, but Not during Dinner, and Was Less Suppressed in Healthy Older than Younger Men. *Nutrients* **2020**, *12*, 3318. [CrossRef] [PubMed]
46. Cook, C.G.; Andrews, J.M.; Jones, K.L.; Wittert, G.A.; Chapman, I.M.; Morley, J.E.; Horowitz, M. Effects of small intestinal nutrient infusion on appetite and pyloric motility are modified by age. *Am. J. Physiol.* **1997**, *273*, R755–R761. [CrossRef]
47. Giezenaar, C.; Lange, K.; Hausken, T.; Jones, K.L.; Horowitz, M.; Chapman, I.; Soenen, S. Effects of Age on Acute Appetite-Related Responses to Whey-Protein Drinks, Including Energy Intake, Gastric Emptying, Blood Glucose, and Plasma Gut Hormone Concentrations-A Randomized Controlled Trial. *Nutrients* **2020**, *12*, 1008. [CrossRef]
48. Giezenaar, C.; Burgh, Y.V.D.; Lange, K.; Hatzinikolas, S.; Hausken, T.; Jones, K.L.; Horowitz, M.; Chapman, I.; Soenen, S. Effects of Substitution, and Adding of Carbohydrate and Fat to Whey-Protein on Energy Intake, Appetite, Gastric Emptying, Glucose, Insulin, Ghrelin, CCK and GLP-1 in Healthy Older Men-A Randomized Controlled Trial. *Nutrients* **2018**, *10*, 113. [CrossRef] [PubMed]
49. Oberoi, A.; Giezenaar, C.; Jensen, C.; Lange, K.; Hausken, T.; Jones, K.L.; Horowitz, M.; Chapman, I.; Soenen, S. Acute effects of whey protein on energy intake, appetite and gastric emptying in younger and older, obese men. *Nutr. Diabetes.* **2020**, *10*, 37. [CrossRef]
50. Giezenaar, C.; Trahair, L.G.; Luscombe-Marsh, N.D.; Hausken, T.; Standfield, S.; Jones, K.L.; Lange, K.; Horowitz, M.; Chapman, I.; Soenen, S. Effects of randomized whey-protein loads on energy intake, appetite, gastric emptying, and plasma gut-hormone concentrations in older men and women. *Am. J. Clin. Nutr.* **2017**, *106*, 865–877. [CrossRef] [PubMed]
51. Giezenaar, C.; Coudert, Z.; Baqeri, A.; Jensen, C.; Hausken, T.; Horowitz, M.; Chapman, I.; Soenen, S. Effects of Timing of Whey Protein Intake on Appetite and Energy Intake in Healthy Older Men. *J. Am. Med. Dir. Assoc.* **2017**, *18*, 898.e9–898.e13. [CrossRef]
52. Rayner, C.K.; MacIntosh, C.G.; Chapman, I.M.; Morley, J.E.; Horowitz, M. Effects of age on proximal gastric motor and sensory function. *Scand. J. Gastroenterol.* **2000**, *35*, 1041–1047. [PubMed]
53. Sturm, K.; Parker, B.; Wishart, J.; Feinle-Bisset, C.; Jones, K.L.; Chapman, I.; Horowitz, M. Energy intake and appetite are related to antral area in healthy young and older subjects. *Am. J. Clin. Nutr.* **2004**, *80*, 656–667. [CrossRef] [PubMed]
54. Clarkston, W.K.; Pantano, M.M.; Morley, J.E.; Horowitz, M.; Littlefield, J.M.; Burton, F.R. Evidence for the anorexia of aging: Gastrointestinal transit and hunger in healthy elderly vs. young adults. *Am. J. Physiol.* **1997**, *272*, R243–R248. [CrossRef] [PubMed]
55. Yasawy, M.I.; Al-Quorain, A.A.; Hussameddin, A.M.; Yasawy, Z.M.; Al-Sulaiman, R.M. Obesity and gastric balloon. *J. Family Community Med.* **2014**, *21*, 196–199. [CrossRef] [PubMed]
56. Giezenaar, C.; Luscombe-Marsh, N.D.; Hutchison, A.T.; Stanfield, S.; Feinle-Bisset, C.; Horowitz, M.; Chapman, I. Dose-Dependent Effects of Randomized Intraduodenal Whey-Protein Loads on Glucose, Gut Hormone, and Amino Acid Concentrations in Healthy Older and Younger Men. *Nutrients* **2018**, *10*, 78. [CrossRef] [PubMed]
57. Giezenaar, C.; Lange, K.; Hausken, T.; Jones, K.L.; Horowitz, M.; Chapman, I.; Soenen, S. Acute Effects of Substitution, and Addition, of Carbohydrates and Fat to Protein on Gastric Emptying, Blood Glucose, Gut Hormones, Appetite, and Energy Intake. *Nutrients* **2018**, *10*, 1451. [CrossRef]
58. Giezenaar, C.; Hutchison, A.T.; Luscombe-Marsh, N.D.; Chapman, I.; Horowitz, M.; Soenen, S. Effect of Age on Blood Glucose and Plasma Insulin, Glucagon, Ghrelin, CCK, GIP, and GLP-1 Responses to Whey Protein Ingestion. *Nutrients* **2017**, *10*, 2. [CrossRef]
59. MacIntosh, C.G.; Andrews, J.M.; Jones, K.L.; Wishart, J.M.; Morris, H.A.; Jansen, J.B.; Morley, J.E.; Horowitz, M.; Chapman, I.M. Effects of age on concentrations of plasma cholecystokinin, glucagon-like peptide 1, and peptide YY and their relation to appetite and pyloric motility. *Am. J. Clin. Nutr.* **1999**, *69*, 999–1006. [CrossRef]
60. MacIntosh, C.G.; Morley, J.E.; Wishart, J.; Morris, H.; Jansen, J.B.; Horowitz, M.; Chapman, I.M. Effect of exogenous cholecystokinin (CCK)-8 on food intake and plasma CCK, leptin, and insulin concentrations in older and young adults: Evidence for increased CCK activity as a cause of the anorexia of aging. *J. Clin. Endocrinol. Metab.* **2001**, *86*, 5830–5837. [CrossRef]

61. Miyawaki, K.; Yamada, Y.; Ban, N.; Ihara, Y.; Tsukiyama, K.; Zhou, H.; Fujimoto, S.; Oku, A.; Tsuda, K.; Toyokuni, S.; et al. Inhibition of gastric inhibitory polypeptide signaling prevents obesity. *Nat. Med.* **2002**, *8*, 738–742. [CrossRef] [PubMed]
62. Nuttall, F.Q.; Mooradian, A.D.; Gannon, M.C.; Billington, C.; Krezowski, P. Effect of protein ingestion on the glucose and insulin response to a standardized oral glucose load. *Diabetes Care.* **1984**, *7*, 465–470. [CrossRef]
63. Nass, R.; Farhy, L.S.; Liu, J.; Pezzoli, S.S.; Johnson, M.L.; Gaylinn, B.D.; Thorner, M.O. Age-dependent decline in acyl-ghrelin concentrations and reduced association of acyl-ghrelin and growth hormone in healthy older adults. *J. Clin. Endocrinol. Metab.* **2014**, *99*, 602–608. [CrossRef]
64. Sturm, K.; MacIntosh, C.G.; Parker, B.A.; Wishart, J.; Horowitz, M.; Chapman, I.M. Appetite, food intake, and plasma concentrations of cholecystokinin, ghrelin, and other gastrointestinal hormones in undernourished older women and well-nourished young and older women. *J. Clin. Endocrinol. Metab.* **2003**, *88*, 3747–3755. [CrossRef] [PubMed]
65. Rigamonti, A.E.; Pincelli, A.I.; Corra, B.; Viarengo, R.; Bonomo, S.M.; Galimberti, D.; Scacchi, M.; Scarpini, E.; Cavagnini, F.; Muller, E.E. Plasma ghrelin concentrations in elderly subjects: Comparison with anorexic and obese patients. *J. Endocrinol.* **2002**, *175*, R1–R5. [CrossRef] [PubMed]

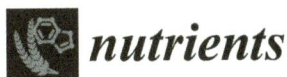

Article

The Effect of Isoleucine Supplementation on Body Weight Gain and Blood Glucose Response in Lean and Obese Mice

Rebecca O'Rielly [1], Hui Li [1,2], See Meng Lim [3,4], Roger Yazbeck [5], Stamatiki Kritas [6], Sina S. Ullrich [1,7], Christine Feinle-Bisset [1], Leonie Heilbronn [1,2] and Amanda J. Page [1,2,*]

[1] Adelaide Medical School, University of Adelaide, Adelaide, SA 5005, Australia; rebecca.orielly@adelaide.edu.au (R.O.); hui.li01@adelaide.edu.au (H.L.); sina.s.ullrich@gmail.com (S.S.U.); christine.feinle@adelaide.edu.au (C.F.-B.); leonie.heilbronn@adelaide.edu.au (L.H.)
[2] Nutrition, Diabetes and Gut Health, Lifelong Health Theme, South Australian Health and Medical Research Institute (SAHMRI), Adelaide, SA 5001, Australia
[3] School of Agriculture, Food and Wine, The University of Adelaide, Glen Osmond, SA 5064, Australia; seemeng.lim@adelaide.edu.au
[4] Centre for Community Health Studies, Faculty of Health Sciences, Universiti Kebangsaan Malaysia, Kuala Lumpur 50300, Malaysia
[5] College of Medicine and Public Health, Flinders Medical Centre, Flinders University, Bedford Park, SA 5042, Australia; roger.yazbek@flinders.edu.au
[6] Women's and Children's Hospital, North Adelaide, SA 5006, Australia; stamatiki.kritas@gmail.com
[7] Clinical Trial Unit, Department of Clinical Research, University of Basel and University Hospital Basel, 4031 Basel, Switzerland
* Correspondence: amanda.page@adelaide.edu.au; Tel.: +61-8-8128-4840

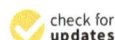

Received: 13 July 2020; Accepted: 12 August 2020; Published: 14 August 2020

Abstract: Chronic isoleucine supplementation prevents diet-induced weight gain in rodents. Acute-isoleucine administration improves glucose tolerance in rodents and reduces postprandial glucose levels in humans. However, the effect of chronic-isoleucine supplementation on body weight and glucose tolerance in obesity is unknown. This study aimed to investigate the impact of chronic isoleucine on body weight gain and glucose tolerance in lean and high-fat-diet (HFD) induced-obese mice. Male C57BL/6-mice, fed a standard-laboratory-diet (SLD) or HFD for 12 weeks, were randomly allocated to: (1) Control: Drinking water; (2) Acute: Drinking water with a gavage of isoleucine (300 mg/kg) prior to the oral-glucose-tolerance-test (OGTT) or gastric-emptying-breath-test (GEBT); (3) Chronic: Drinking water with 1.5% isoleucine, for a further six weeks. At 16 weeks, an OGTT and GEBT was performed and at 17 weeks metabolic monitoring. In SLD- and HFD-mice, there was no difference in body weight, fat mass, and plasma lipid profiles between isoleucine treatment groups. Acute-isoleucine did not improve glucose tolerance in SLD- or HFD-mice. Chronic-isoleucine impaired glucose tolerance in SLD-mice. There was no difference in gastric emptying between any groups. Chronic-isoleucine did not alter energy intake, energy expenditure, or respiratory quotient in SLD- or HFD-mice. In conclusion, chronic isoleucine supplementation may not be an effective treatment for obesity or glucose intolerance.

Keywords: obesity; amino acid; isoleucine; chronic supplementation; energy expenditure; oral glucose tolerance test; glycaemic control; gastric emptying breath test

1. Introduction

The branched-chain amino acids (BCAAs), isoleucine, leucine and valine, are essential amino acids accounting for ~35% of the essential amino acids comprising muscle proteins in humans and ~40% of the pre-formed amino acids required by all mammals [1]. In population studies, an elevated dietary intake of BCAAs was associated with a lower prevalence of overweight and obesity in adults [2,3]. Further, BCAA supplementation was demonstrated to preserve lean muscle mass during weight loss [4–6]. This evidence suggests a role for BCAA supplementation in the treatment of obesity. In particular, chronic isoleucine supplementation in rodents has been demonstrated to prevent high-fat diet (HFD)-induced obesity [7]. However, whether chronic isoleucine supplementation is an effective approach to ameliorate weight gain and promote weight loss in established obesity, is unknown.

Acute administration of isoleucine and leucine in rats improved glucose tolerance, with isoleucine showing greater effectiveness than leucine [8]. This was attributed to the synergistic action of isoleucine with endogenous insulin to enhance glucose uptake into tissues [9–11]. In addition, acute isoleucine supplementation improved glucose tolerance in leptin receptor-deficient (*db/db*) mice, a model of morbid obesity and hyperglycaemia [12]. This evidence suggests that isoleucine supplementation may be useful in the treatment of glucose intolerance. However, whether this glucose-lowering effect persists following a chronic supplementation regime is unknown.

It is known that postprandial blood glucose levels are influenced by the rate of gastric emptying [13]. In particpants with type 2 diabetes, consumption of whey protein before a meal slowed gastric emptying and was associated with lower postprandial blood glucose levels [14,15]. Further, in healthy lean participants, acute intragastric administration of isoleucine lowered the blood glucose response to a mixed nutrient drink, which was attributed to a slowing of gastric emptying [16]. Therefore, we hypothesised that chronic isoleucine supplementation will slow gastric emptying, improve glucose tolerance, and reduce body weight gain in mice.

The current study aimed to determine whether chronic dietary supplementation with the BCAA isoleucine, alters body weight gain, adiposity, glucose tolerance, and energy metabolism in mice with HFD-induced obesity.

2. Materials and Methods

2.1. Ethics Approval

This study was approved (Ethics approval: SAM237) by the South Australian Health and Medical Research Institute Animal Ethics Committee. All experimental protocols were performed in alignment with the Australian Code of Practice for the Care and Use of Animals for Scientific Purposes.

2.2. Study Design

Eight-week-old male C57BL/6 mice ($n = 54$) were group-housed in a 12:12 h light-dark cycle within a temperature (24 ± 1 °C) controlled facility. Mice were provided ad libitum access to either a standard laboratory diet (SLD; 12%, 23%, and 65% of energy from fat, protein, and carbohydrates, respectively; Specialty Feeds, Western Australia, Australia; $n = 30$) or HFD (60%, 20%, and 20% of energy from fat, protein, and carbohydrates, respectively; adapted from Research Diets Inc., New Brunswick, NJ, USA; $n = 24$). Consistent with the previous literature, the HFD-induced obese mouse model was chosen as both a model of obesity [17] and impaired glucose tolerance [18]. After 12 weeks on their respective diets, a sub-group of SLD ($n = 10$; SLD-Chronic (Ch)) and HFD-mice ($n = 8$; HFD-Ch) received ad libitum isoleucine (1.5% w/v; Purebulk Inc., Roseburg, OR, USA) supplemented in the drinking water. The remaining SLD ($n = 20$) and HFD-mice ($n = 16$) continued with ad libitum access to normal drinking water. At 16 weeks, all mice were singly housed and underwent an OGTT (at 1400 h) and gastric emptying breath test (at 0900 h) in random order with a three-day recovery between tests. In each diet group, the mice provided normal drinking water were subdivided into two groups, receiving either an oral gavage of water ($n = 10$, SLD-Control (C); $n = 8$, HFD-C) or isoleucine (300 mg/kg body weight; $n = 10$, SLD-Acute (A); $n = 8$, HFD-A) 30 min before the OGTT or GEBT. The SLD and HFD-Ch mice received an oral gavage of drinking water similar to the control groups. The doses for acute and chronic isoleucine treatments were chosen based on previous studies [8,12]. At 17 weeks, all mice were placed in metabolic monitoring cages. The body weight of all the mice was measured weekly, except the final two weeks due to the different interventions.

2.3. Oral Glucose Tolerance Test

Consistent with previous studies [19,20], mice were fasted for six hours (0800–1400 h) before receiving an oral gavage of either isoleucine (SLD/HFD-A groups) or water (SLD/HFD-C and SLD/HFD-Ch groups). After 30 min, all mice received an oral gavage of 20% D-glucose (1 g/kg BW), a dose chosen to ensure the HFD-mice did not experience a severe hyperglycemic response with blood glucose levels beyond the range of the glucose monitor. Blood was collected from a tail prick before isoleucine/water administration, considered as the baseline, and again at 15, 30, 45, 60, and 120 min post glucose administration. Blood glucose levels were determined with an ACCU CHEK Performa monitor (ACCU CHEK, New South Wales, Australia).

2.4. Gastric Emptying Breath Test

Gastric emptying of a solid meal was determined using a non-invasive breath test as previously described [21,22]. Mice were fasted overnight (1600–0900 h) prior to an oral gavage of either isoleucine (SLD/HFD-A) or water (SLD/HFD-C and SLD/HFD-Ch). After 30 min, all mice were provided 0.1 g of baked egg yolk containing ^{13}C-octanoic acid (1 µL/g; 99% enrichment, Cambridge Isotope Laboratories, Andover, MA, USA) to consume voluntarily within 1 min. Breath samples were collected before isoleucine administration (baseline; 0 min) and again at regular intervals (5 min intervals from 5–30 min and 15-min intervals from 30–150 min) after egg consumption. Breath samples were analysed for the $^{13}CO_2$ content using an isotope ratio mass spectrometer (Europa Scientific, Crewe, UK). The $^{13}CO_2$ excretion data were analysed by non-linear regression analysis for curve fitting and for calculation of gastric half emptying time (t $\frac{1}{2}$) [23]. Gastric half emptying time was not measured in the HFD-mice due to sampling difficulties; the egg yolk was not consumed within 1 min which invalidates results.

2.5. Metabolic Monitoring

Mice were individually housed in Promethium metabolic cages (Sable Systems International, North Las Vegas, NV, USA) for 72 h of continuous metabolic monitoring. Energy intake (kJ), energy expenditure (kJ/lean mass), respiratory quotient (RQ; VCO_2/VO_2), and total activity (meters, m) were measured and analysed using the ExpeData data analysis software (Sable Systems International, North Las Vegas, NV, USA).

2.6. Tissue Collection

Mice were fasted overnight (1600–0900 h) then anaesthetised with isoflurane (5% in medical oxygen). The nose-to-tail length and abdominal circumference of mice were measured. Blood was collected from the abdominal aorta and transferred to ethylenediaminetetraacetic acid (EDTA) tubes (Thermo Fisher Scientific, Victoria, Australia). Plasma was extracted by centrifugation at 1000 g and 4 °C for 15 min, and snap-frozen in liquid nitrogen prior to storage at −80 °C until further analysis. Liver, gonadal fat pads, and inter-scapula brown fat pads were collected and weighed. Lean mass was determined by the final body weight minus the weight of collected fat pads. A section of the liver was fixed in 4% paraformaldehyde for 4 h, cryoprotected overnight in 30% sucrose in a phosphate buffer, frozen in Tissue-Tek O.C.T. compound (Sakura Finetek USA Inc., Torrance, CA, USA) and stored at −80 °C before processing for histology.

2.7. Plasma Metabolites

Plasma total triglycerides, total cholesterol, and high-density lipoprotein (HDL)-cholesterol concentrations were measured using commercial enzymatic kits (OSR60118, OSR6116, and OSR6187, respectively (Beckman Coulter Inc., Georgia, USA)) on a Beckman AU480 clinical analyser (Beckman

Coulter Inc., Atlanta, GA, USA). Plasma low-density lipoprotein (LDL)-cholesterol concentrations were estimated using the Friedewald equation [24]:

LDL-cholesterol = Total cholesterol − (total triglyceride /2.2) − HDL-cholesterol

2.8. Liver Lipid Content

The histological lysochrome lipid stain Oil Red O was performed on liver sections using a standard protocol [25]. Slides were imaged using a NanoZoomer digital slide scanner (Hamamatsu Photonics, Hamamatsu City, Japan) and analysed for the average percentage of stained lipid per 1 mm^2 area using the ImageJ-win64 software.

2.9. Statistical Tests

Results are expressed as the mean ± SEM. A two-way ANOVA was performed to assess diet and isoleucine treatment effects with a Tukey's post hoc test for multiple comparisons, using the GraphPad Prism v8 software (GraphPad, California, USA). The OGTT$_{0-120\,min}$ blood glucose area under the curve (AUC) was generated using the IBM SPSS Statistics 26 software (IBM, New York, NY, USA). A correlation between gastric half emptying time (t $\frac{1}{2}$) and OGTT$_{0-120\,min}$ blood glucose AUC for SLD groups was performed in the GraphPad Prism v8 software. The coefficient of determination value (r^2) was considered significant at $p < 0.05$.

3. Results

3.1. Chronic Isoleucine Treatment Does Not Affect Weight Gain and Adiposity

At the beginning of week 12, prior to isoleucine supplementation, HFD-mice gained significantly more weight than SLD-mice ($p < 0.001$, unpaired *t*-test; Figure 1A). There was no difference in body weight between different treatment groups in mice fed a SLD or HFD prior to chronic isoleucine treatment ($p < 0.0001$, $F (1, 50) = 28.17$, diet effect; $p = 0.1262$, $F (1, 50) = 2.418$, isoleucine effect; SLD-C/A; 34.8 ± 0.7 g (*n* = 20), SLD-Ch; 37.2 ± 1.3 g (*n* = 10), HFD-C/A; 42.3 ± 1.6 g (*n* = 16), and HFD-Ch; 44.1 ± 1.7 g (*n* = 8)).

In weeks 12–15, HFD-mice continued to gain more weight compared to SLD-mice ($p < 0.0001$, $F (1, 50) = 19.21$, diet effect; Figure 1A), but there was no effect of chronic isoleucine treatment on weight gain (Figure 1A).

At week 18, abdominal circumference was greater in HFD-mice than SLD-mice, but was not affected by chronic isoleucine treatment ($p < 0.0001$, $F (1, 26) = 24.78$, diet effect; SLD-C, 9.3 ± 0.2 cm, SLD-Ch, 9.9 ± 0.5 cm, HFD-C, 11.4 ± 0.3 cm, and HFD-Ch, 11.2 ± 0.3 cm). In addition, HFD-mice had heavier gonadal fat pads and brown fat pads than SLD-mice (both $p < 0.01$, $F (1, 50) = 11.13$ and $F (1, 47) = 11.44$, respectively, diet effect; Figure 1(Bi,Bii)), but these parameters were not affected by the chronic isoleucine treatment.

3.2. Chronic Isoleucine Treatment Does Not Affect Liver Lipid Content

HFD-mice had heavier livers than SLD-mice ($p < 0.0001$, $F (1, 50) = 18.34$, diet effect; Figure 2A). The liver lipid content was greater in HFD-mice than SLD-mice ($p < 0.0001$, $F (1, 28) = 37.31$, diet effect; Figure 2B). There was no effect of the chronic isoleucine treatment on liver mass or lipid content (Figure 2A,B).

3.3. Chronic Isoleucine Treatment Does Not Alter Energy Intake, Energy Expenditure, Activity, and Respiratory Quotient

HFD-mice consumed more energy across 24 h ($p < 0.05$, $F (1, 50) = 4.157$, diet effect; Figure 3(Ai)) compared to SLD-mice, predominantly due to increased energy intake during the light phase ($p < 0.05$, $F (1, 50) = 5.715$, diet effect; Figure 3(Aii)). There was no effect of the chronic isoleucine treatment on total energy intake across 24 h, during the light phase or dark phase (Figure 3(Ai–Aiii)). HFD feeding and chronic isoleucine treatment had no effect on 24 h of total water intake (SLD-C; 3.5 ± 0.07 mL/day, SLD-Ch; 3.8 ± 0.17 mL/day, HFD-C; 3.5 ± 0.1 mL/day, and HFD-Ch; 3.6 ± 0.2 mL/day).

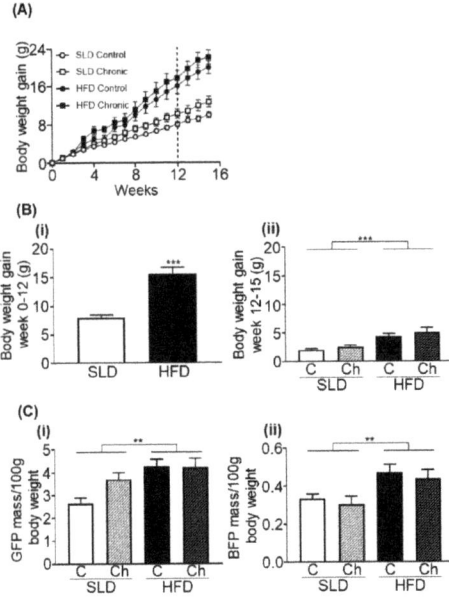

Figure 1. High fat diet (HFD) feeding but not the chronic isoleucine treatment increased weight gain and adiposity in mice. (**A**) Body weight gained during weeks 0–15 in mice fed a standard laboratory diet (SLD) or HFD (SLD/HFD-Control (C; control and acute groups pooled as no acute gavage of isoleucine had occurred at this point) n = 16–20; SLD/HFD-Chronic (Ch) n = 8–10). The dotted line indicates the onset of chronic isoleucine supplementation. (**B**) (**i**) Body weight gained during week 0–12 in SLD or HFD (n = 24–30/group; all HFD and SLD groups pooled as no chronic or acute isoleucine treatment had occurred at this point); *** $p < 0.001$ unpaired t-test. (**ii**) Body weight gained in week 12–15 (SLD/HFD-Control (C; control and acute groups pooled as no acute gavage of isoleucine had occurred at this point) n = 16–20; SLD/HFD-Chronic (Ch) n = 8–10). (**C**) (**i**) Gonadal fat pad (GFP) mass and (**ii**) brown fat pad (BFP) mass per 100 g of total body weight (n = 8–10/group). Values are mean ± SEM. ** $p < 0.01$, *** $p < 0.001$; diet effect, two-way ANOVA.

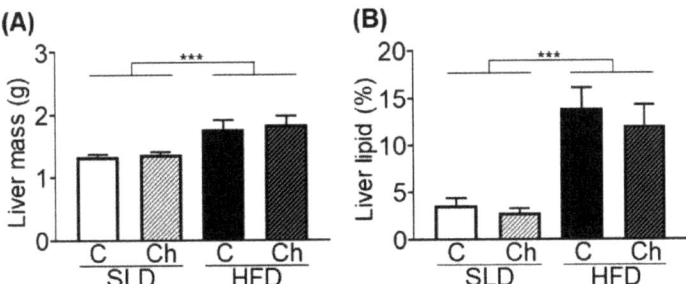

Figure 2. High fat diet (HFD) feeding but not chronic isoleucine treatment increased the liver mass and lipid content in mice. (**A**) Liver mass and (**B**) percentage lipid area per 1 mm^2 liver area of standard laboratory diet (SLD) and HFD-mice (SLD/HFD-Control (C) and SLD/HFD-Chronic (Ch), n = 8–10). Values are mean ± SEM. *** $p < 0.001$; diet effect, two-way ANOVA.

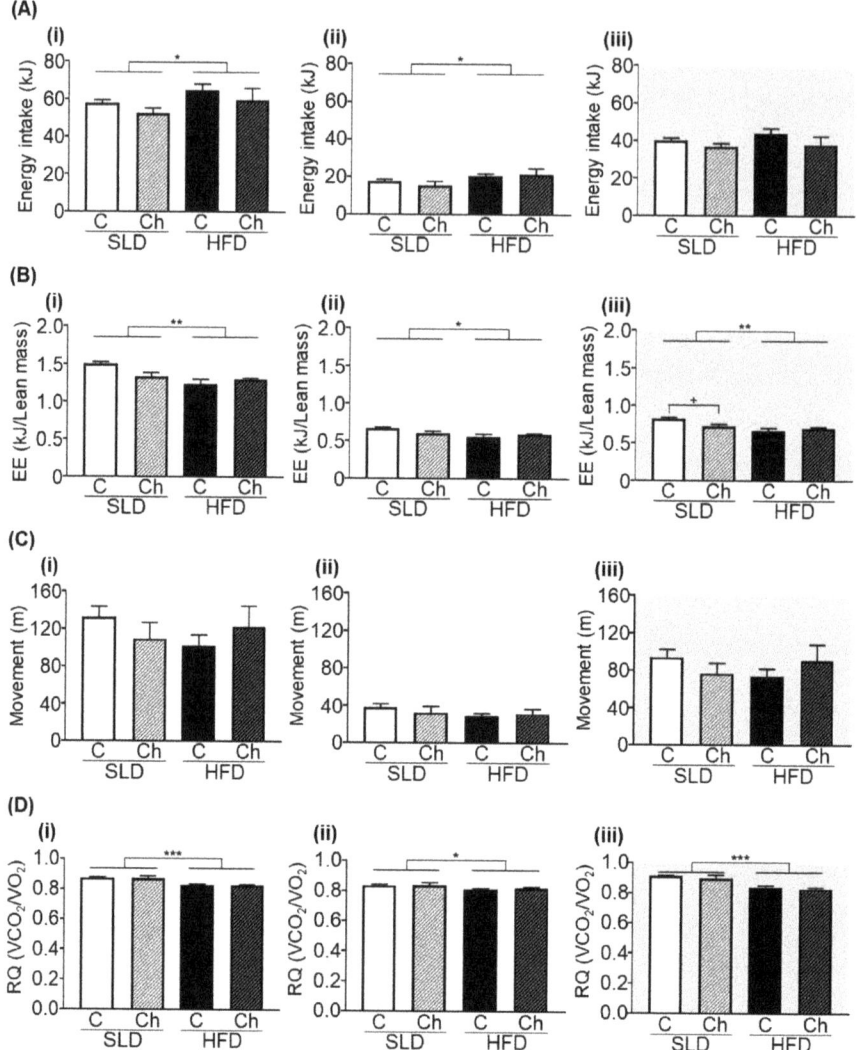

Figure 3. High fat diet (HFD) feeding but not the chronic isoleucine treatment affects energy balance in mice. (**A**) Energy intake, (**B**) energy expenditure (EE), (**C**) activity (distance of movement), and (**D**) respiratory quotients (RQ), across 24 h (**i**), 12 h of day (light phase) (**ii**), and 12 h of night (dark phase) (**iii**) in a standard laboratory diet (SLD) and HFD-mice (SLD/HFD-Control (C) n = 16–20, SLD/HFD-Chronic (Ch) n = 8–10). Values are mean ± SEM. * $p < 0.05$, ** $p < 0.01$, *** $p < 0.001$, diet effect; two-way ANOVA with Sidak's *post hoc* test, +$p < 0.05$.

HFD-mice had a significantly lower energy expenditure (normalised to lean body mass) compared to SLD-mice across 24 h, during the light phase or dark phase ($p < 0.01$, $F_{(1, 50)} = 9.151$, $p < 0.05$, $F_{(1, 50)} = 6.499$, $p < 0.01$, $F_{(1, 50)} = 11.25$, respectively, diet effect; Figure 3(Bi–Biii)). A significant diet by the chronic isoleucine treatment interaction was observed in energy expenditure across 24 h ($p < 0.05$, $F_{(1, 50)} = 5.416$, interaction; Figure 3(Bi)) and during the dark phase ($p < 0.05$, $F_{(1, 50)} = 6.468$, interaction; Figure 3(Biii)). During the dark phase, the chronic isoleucine treatment reduced energy expenditure in SLD-mice ($p < 0.05$, Sidak's post hoc test), but not in HFD-mice.

Total activity levels were not affected by HFD feeding or chronic isoleucine treatment across 24 h or during the light or dark phase (Figure 3(Ci–Ciii)).

HFD-mice had lower RQ values compared to SLD-mice across 24 h ($p < 0.001$, $F (1, 50) = 19.66$, diet effect; Figure 3(Ci)), during the light phase ($p < 0.05$, $F (1, 50) = 4.082$, diet effect; Figure 3(Cii)) and dark phase ($p < 0.001$, $F (1, 50) = 38.4$, diet effect; Figure 3(Ciii)). Average RQ values were not affected by the chronic isoleucine treatment across 24 h, during the light phase or dark phase (Figure 3(Ci–Ciii)).

3.4. Chronic Isoleucine Treatment Does Not Affect Plasma Lipid Metabolites

HFD-mice had elevated plasma total triglycerides ($p < 0.001$, $F (1, 30) = 31.28$, diet effect; Figure 4A), total cholesterol ($p < 0.001$, $F (1, 30) = 40.02$, diet effect; Figure 4B), HDL-cholesterol ($p < 0.001$, $F (1, 30) = 40.16$, diet effect; Figure 4C), and LDL-cholesterol ($p < 0.0001$, $F (1, 30) = 25.36$, diet effect; Figure 4D) compared to SLD-mice. There was no effect of chronic isoleucine treatment on these plasma lipid metabolites (Figure 4A–D).

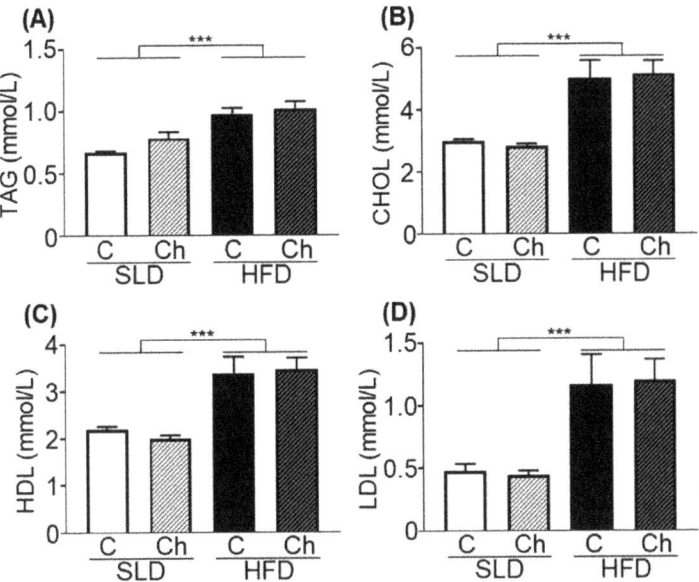

Figure 4. High fat diet (HFD) feeding but not the chronic isoleucine treatment elevated plasma lipid metabolites in mice. Plasma (**A**) total triglycerides (TAG), (**B**) total cholesterol (CHOL), (**C**) high density lipoprotein (HDL), and (**D**) low density lipoprotein (LDL) levels in a standard laboratory diet (SLD) and HFD-mice (SLD/HFD-Control (C) $n = 8$–10, SLD/HFD-Chronic (Ch) $n = 8$–10). Values are mean ± SEM *** $p < 0.001$, diet effect; two-way ANOVA.

3.5. Acute and Chronic Isoleucine Treatment Differentially Affect Glucose Tolerance in SLD- and HFD-Mice

HFD-mice had higher fasting blood glucose levels than SLD-mice ($p < 0.0001$, $F (1, 48) = 19.34$, diet effect; Figure 5(Ai,Bi)). There was no effect of the chronic isoleucine treatment on fasting blood glucose levels (Figure 5(Ai,Bi)).

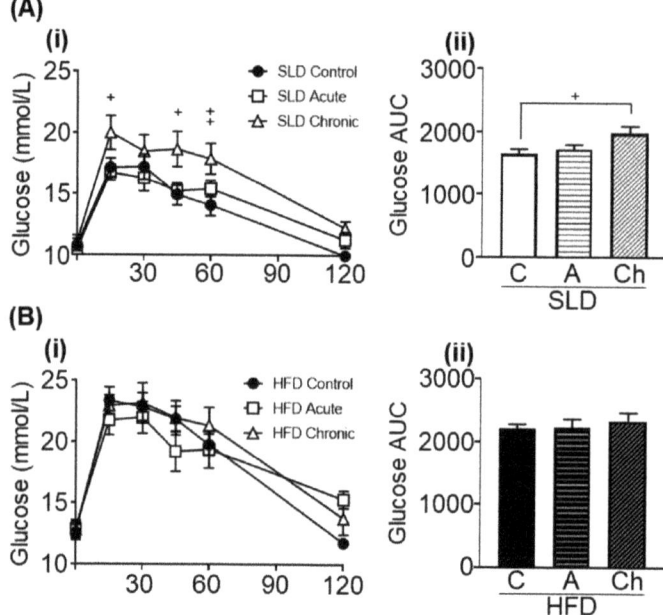

Figure 5. Acute (A) and chronic (Ch) isoleucine treatment differentially affects glucose tolerance. (i) Blood glucose levels in response to an oral glucose tolerance test and (ii) glucose area under curve (AUC) in (**A**) standard laboratory diet (SLD) and (**B**) high fat diet (HFD)-mice. (SLD/HFD-Control (C) n = 8–10, SLD/HFD-A n = 8–10 and SLD/HFD-Ch n = 8–10). Values are mean ± SEM. + $p < 0.05$, one-way ANOVA.

HFD-mice had a greater glucose AUC than SLD-mice ($p < 0.001$, $F (1, 48) = 34.44$, diet effect; Figure 5(Aii,Bii)). In SLD groups, an elevated glucose AUC was observed in chronic isoleucine treated mice compared to control mice ($p < 0.05$, one-way ANOVA; Figure 5(Aii)), but there was no difference between acute and chronic isoleucine treated mice. In HFD groups, there was no effect of acute or chronic isoleucine treatment on glucose AUC (Figure 5(Bii)).

3.6. Acute and Chronic Isoleucine Treatment Do Not Affect Gastric Emptying

There was no significant difference in the gastric half emptying time (t $\frac{1}{2}$) between different isoleucine groups in SLD-mice (SLD-C, 125.3 ± 13.2 min (n = 8); SLD-A, 144.4 ± 15.3 min (n = 8) and SLD-Ch, 126.7 ± 5.1 min (n = 7)).

There was no correlation between gastric half emptying time and blood glucose AUC in SLD-mice (correlation coefficient of determination value (r^2); SLD-C, $r^2 = 0.0197$, SLD-A, $r^2 = 0.2602$, and SLD-Ch, $r^2 = 0.004292$).

4. Discussion

Longitudinal population studies have demonstrated an inverse association between dietary BCAA consumption and the risk of obesity and diabetes [2,3], suggesting BCAA supplementation may be an effective dietary interevention to prevent obesity. In the current study, the acute isoleucine treatment had no beneficial effect on blood glucose levels in response to an OGTT. Further, chronic isoleucine supplementation was not an effective treatment for obesity and actually impaired glucose tolerance in SLD-mice.

In the current study, six weeks of chronic isoleucine treatment had no effect on body weight, gonadal fat pad mass, hepatic lipid content, and plasma lipid levels in SLD- and HFD-mice. Previously, four weeks of chronic isoleucine supplementation, protected mice from diet-induced weight gain and fat accumulation [7]. In that study, isoleucine supplementation was initiated after only two weeks of HFD feeding [7], which is arguably an insufficient time-course to establish obesity in mice [26]. Consistent with previous reports [27,28], 12 weeks of HFD feeding in the current study, led to significantly greater weight gain and adiposity compared to SLD-mice. Therefore, the findings suggest that isoleucine may be able to prevent diet-induced obesity, but may not be an effective treatment for reversing obesity.

Energy intake and energy expenditure are well-known effectors of body weight regulation [29]. In the current study, the chronic isoleucine treatment did not alter total energy expenditure, total energy intake, average RQ, or total activity in SLD- or HFD-mice. Previously, chronic isoleucine or leucine supplementation have been demonstrated to protect mice from diet-induced weight gain without reducing energy intake or increasing total activity levels [7,30]. Instead, leucine supplementation was observed to enhance total energy expenditure via an elevated 24 h oxygen consumption rate, normalised to body weight [30]. This elevated energy expenditure was attributed to an increased expression of uncoupling protein (UCP) 3 in thermogenic tissue [30]. In the isoleucine supplemented mice, energy expenditure was not directly measured [7]. However, expression of proteins involved in fatty acid uptake and oxidation were upregulated, namely FAT/CD36, PPARα and UCP2&3, in the liver and skeletal muscle [7]. This evidence suggests that chronic isoleucine or leucine supplementation in the previous reports may have protected from diet-induced fat gain through elevating fatty acid oxidation. However, in the current study, the chronic isoleucine treatment did not reduce 24 h RQ, suggesting no increase in lipid oxidation. Therefore, further investigation of lipid metabolism was not pursued. Indeed, the chronic supplementation of isoleucine in the current study, did not reverse the changes to energy expenditure observed in the HFD-induced obese mice.

In the current study, the chronic isoleucine treatment had no beneficial effect on fasting blood glucose levels in HFD-mice. This is consistent with a previous study where four weeks of isoleucine supplementation at a dose of 2.5%, did not affect fasting blood glucose levels in male mice fed a 45% HFD [7]. In contrast, six weeks of 2% chronic isoleucine supplementation significantly reduced fasting blood glucose levels compared to controls, in high-fat, high-sucrose fed female mice; a model of glucose intolerance [12]. These findings suggest that chronic isoleucine supplementation may be more effective in ameliorating fasting blood glucose elevated by high sucrose diets rather than high fat diets. In addition, there may be a difference in treatment effects between male and female mice. Future studies should, therefore, investigate the mechanisms of the effect of chronic isoleucine supplementation on glycaemic regulation, such as glucose uptake into tissues and hepatic glucose export. For example, acute administration of isoleucine to isolated myocytes stimulates the glucose uptake through enhanced recruitment of glucose transporters to the cell membrane [8]. Further, acute isoleucine administration in mice, suppressed key enzymes in hepatic gluconeogenesis, namely phosphoenolpyruvate carboxykinase and glucose 6-phosphatase [31,32], contributing to lower fasting blood glucose levels. Therefore, it is possible that the effect of isoleucine on these blood glucose regulatory mechanisms persists under a chronic supplementation regime. However, there was no difference in blood glucose levels in the OGTT after acute isoleucine treatment in either SLD- or HFD-mice and, therefore, this was not pursued in the current study but may warrant future investigation.

In the current study, acute isoleucine orally administered at a dose of 0.3 g/kg, had no effect on postprandial blood glucose levels in SLD- or HFD-mice. Previously, acute administration of 0.3 g/kg isoleucine in lean [8] and diet-induced obese mice (60% HFD for eight weeks) [12] induced a dose-dependent reduction in postprandial blood glucose levels. Further, acute isoleucine administration in obese leptin receptor-deficient (*db/db*) mice, significantly reduced blood glucose levels in response to an OGTT, albeit at a higher dose of 0.5 g/kg [12]. Considering this observed dose-dependent effect, a larger dose may have been necessary to reduce the blood glucose AUC in the current more chronic

(12 weeks) model of diet-induced obesity. However, this does not explain why no effect was observed in the SLD-mice.

Consistent with a previous report [12], the chronic isoleucine treatment had no beneficial effect on blood glucose levels in response to an OGTT in HFD-mice. In contrast, the chronic isoleucine supplementation impaired glucose tolerance in lean mice, suggesting an adverse effect of chronic isoleucine supplementation. It has been reported that a western diet low in BCAAs reduced the blood glucose AUC compared to mice fed a standard western diet [33]. Furthermore, consistent with the current study a western diet supplemented with BCAAs had no effect on blood glucose AUC compared to mice fed a standard western diet [33]. Further, there is some evidence that obesity-induced BCAA dysmetabolism may promote insulin resistance through mitochondria dysfunction and impaired fatty acid oxidation [34,35]. Whether chronic isoleucine supplementation induces BCAA dysmetabolism, and promotes insulin resistance in lean mice, requires further investigation.

Slowing gastric emptying allows for efficient digestion and absorption of nutrients, including glucose [13,36,37]. In the current study, the acute and chronic isoleucine treatment did not affect gastric emptying in SLD-mice. Further, there was no significant correlation between postprandial blood glucose levels and gastric emptying in any groups. Previously, the consumption of whey protein, rich in BCAAs, including isoleucine [38], before a meal has been demonstrated to slow gastric emptying and reduce postprandial hyperglycaemia in people with type 2 diabetes [14,15]. Similarly, intragastric adminsitartion of isoleucine slowed gastric emptying and reduced postprandial glucose levels in lean participants [16]. However, in rodent studies, the effect of isoleucine administration on gastric emptying is less clear. For example, in rats, oral administration of isoleucine reduced the $^{13}CO_2$ content in the breath following a gastric emptying breath test, but did not significantly affect the $^{13}CO_2$ AUC, Cmax, or Tmax values (peak concentration and the time at which it occurred) compared to controls [39].

5. Conclusions

The acute and chronic isoleucine supplementation had no beneficial effect to limit HFD-induced body weight gain, adiposity, fasting blood glucose levels, and glucose tolerance. In contrast, the chronic isoleucine treatment impaired glucose tolerance in SLD-mice. Therefore, the chronic isoleucine supplementation is unlikely to be an effective dietary intervention for the treatment of obesity and type 2 diabetes.

Author Contributions: R.O. performed the experiments, collected and analysed the data, and drafted the manuscript; H.L., S.M.L., R.Y., and S.K. contributed to data collection and analysis; S.S.U., C.F.-B., L.H., and A.J.P. supervised the project and provided input into the experimental design and analysis of data. All authors have read and agreed to the published version of the manuscript.

Funding: C.F-B. was supported by an NHMRC Senior Research Fellowship (grant 1103020, 2016-21).

Acknowledgments: We thank Cathryn Pape, research project officer at the Commonwealth Scientific and Industrial Research Organisation, for assistance in utilising their AU480 AU analyser to analyse mouse plasma and the Bioresources staff at SAHMRI for assistance in animal husbandary.

Conflicts of Interest: The authors declare no conflict of interest. The funders had no role in the design of the study; in the collection, analyses, or interpretation of data; in the writing of the manuscript, or in the decision to publish the results.

References

1. Holecek, M. Branched-Chain Amino Acids in Health and Disease: Metabolism, Alterations in Blood Plasma, and as Supplements. *Nutr. Metab.* **2018**, *15*, 33. [CrossRef] [PubMed]
2. Qin, L.; Xun, P.; Bujnowski, D.; Daviglus, M.L.; Van Horn, L.; Stamler, J.; He, K.; Intermap Cooperative Research Group. Higher Branched-Chain Amino Acid Intake Is Associated with a Lower Prevalence of Being Overweight or Obese in Middle-Aged East Asian and Western Adults. *J. Nutr.* **2011**, *141*, 249–254. [CrossRef] [PubMed]

3. Li, Y.; Li, Y.; Liu, L.; Chen, Y.; Zi, T.-Q.; Du, S.; Jiang, Y.-S.; Feng, R.-N.; Sun, C.H. The Ratio of Dietary Branched-Chain Amino Acids is Associated with a Lower Prevalence of Obesity in Young Northern Chinese Adults: An Internet-Based Cross-Sectional Study. *Nutrients* **2015**, *7*, 9573–9589. [CrossRef] [PubMed]
4. Lemon, P.W. Protein and Amino Acid Needs of the Strength Athlete. *Int. J. Sport Nutr.* **1991**, *1*, 127–145. [CrossRef] [PubMed]
5. Mero, A. Leucine supplementation and intensive training. *Sports Med.* **1999**, *27*, 347–358. [CrossRef] [PubMed]
6. Novin, Z.S.; Ghavamzadeh, S.; Mehdizadeh, A. The Weight Loss Effects of Branched Chain Amino Acids and Vitamin B6: A Randomized Controlled Trial on Obese and Overweight Women. *Int. J. Vitam. Nutr. Res.* **2018**, *88*, 80–89. [CrossRef]
7. Nishimura, J.; Masaki, T.; Arakawa, M.; Seike, M.; Yoshimatsu, H. Isoleucine Prevents the Accumulation of Tissue Triglycerides and Upregulates the Expression of Paralpha and Uncoupling Protein in Diet-Induced Obese Mice. *J. Nutr.* **2010**, *140*, 496–500. [CrossRef]
8. Doi, M.; Yamaoka, I.; Fukunaga, T.; Nakayama, M. Isoleucine, a potent plasma glucose-lowering amino acid, stimulates glucose uptake in C2C12 myotubes. *Biochem. Biophys. Res. Commun.* **2003**, *312*, 1111–1117. [CrossRef]
9. Nishitani, S.; Takehana, K.; Fujitani, S.; Sonaka, I. Branched-chain amino acids improve glucose metabolism in rats with liver cirrhosis. *Am. J. Physiol. Liver Physiol.* **2005**, *288*, G1292–G1300. [CrossRef]
10. Zhang, S.; Yang, Q.; Ren, M.; Qiao, S.; He, P.; Li, D.; Zeng, X. Effects of Isoleucine on Glucose Uptake through the Enhancement of Muscular Membrane Concentrations of Glut1 and Glut4 and Intestinal Membrane Concentrations of Na+/Glucose Co-Transporter 1 (Sglt-1) and Glut2. *Br. J. Nutr.* **2016**, *116*, 593–602. [CrossRef]
11. Watson, R.T.; Pessin, J.E. Bridging the GAP between Insulin Signaling and GLUT4 Translocation. *Trends Biochem. Sci.* **2006**, *31*, 215–222. [CrossRef] [PubMed]
12. Ikehara, O.; Kawasaki, N.; Maezono, K.; Komatsu, M.; Konishi, A. Acute and Chronic Treatment of L-isoleucine Ameliorates Glucose Metabolism in Glucose-Intolerant and Diabetic Mice. *Biol. Pharm. Bull.* **2008**, *31*, 469–472. [CrossRef] [PubMed]
13. Marathe, C.S.; Rayner, C.K.; Jones, K.L.; Horowitz, M. Relationships Between Gastric Emptying, Postprandial Glycemia, and Incretin Hormones. *Diabetes Care* **2013**, *36*, 1396–1405. [CrossRef] [PubMed]
14. Ma, J.; Jesudason, D.R.; Stevens, J.E.; Keogh, J.B.; Jones, K.L.; Clifton, P.M.; Horowitz, M.; Rayner, C.K. Sustained Effects of a Protein 'Preload' on Glycaemia and Gastric Emptying over 4 Weeks in Patients with Type 2 Diabetes: A Randomized Clinical Trial. *Diabetes Res. Clin. Pract.* **2015**, *108*, e31–e34. [CrossRef] [PubMed]
15. Ma, J.; Stevens, J.E.; Cukier, K.; Maddox, A.F.; Wishart, J.M.; Jones, K.L.; Clifton, P.M.; Horowitz, M.; Rayner, C.K. Effects of a Protein Preload on Gastric Emptying, Glycemia, and Gut Hormones After a Carbohydrate Meal in Diet-Controlled Type 2 Diabetes. *Diabetes Care* **2009**, *32*, 1600–1602. [CrossRef] [PubMed]
16. Ullrich, S.; Fitzgerald, P.C.; Schober, G.; Steinert, R.E.; Horowitz, M.C.; Feinle-Bisset, C. Intragastric Administration of Leucine or Isoleucine Lowers the Blood Glucose Response to a Mixed-Nutrient Drink by Different Mechanisms in Healthy, Lean Volunteers. *Am. J. Clin. Nutr.* **2016**, *104*, 1274–1284. [CrossRef]
17. Lang, P.; Hasselwander, S.; Li, H.; Xia, N. Effects of Different Diets Used in Diet-Induced Obesity Models on Insulin Resistance and Vascular Dysfunction in C57bl/6 Mice. *Sci. Rep.* **2019**, *9*, 19556. [CrossRef]
18. Winzell, M.S.; Ahrén, B. The High-Fat Diet–Fed Mouse: A Model for Studying Mechanisms and Treatment of Impaired Glucose Tolerance and Type 2. *Diabetes* **2004**, *53*, S215–S219. [CrossRef]
19. Andrikopoulos, S.; Blair, A.R.; DeLuca, N.; Fam, B.C.; Proietto, J. Evaluating the glucose tolerance test in mice. *Am. J. Physiol. Metab.* **2008**, *295*, E1323–E1332. [CrossRef]
20. Nagy, C.; Einwallner, E. Study of In Vivo Glucose Metabolism in High-fat Diet-fed Mice Using Oral Glucose Tolerance Test (OGTT) and Insulin Tolerance Test (ITT). *J. Vis. Exp.* **2018**, *131*, e56672. [CrossRef]
21. Symonds, E.L.; Butler, R.; Omari, T.I. Noninvasive breath tests can detect alterations in gastric emptying in the mouse. *Eur. J. Clin. Investig.* **2002**, *32*, 341–344. [CrossRef] [PubMed]
22. Symonds, E.L.; Butler, R.N.; Omari, T.I. Assessment of gastric emptying in the mouse using the [13C]-octanoic acid breath test. *Clin. Exp. Pharmacol. Physiol.* **2000**, *27*, 671–675. [CrossRef] [PubMed]

23. Ghoos, Y.F.; Maes, B.D.; Geypens, B.J.; Mys, G.; Hiele, M.I.; Rutgeerts, P.J.; Vantrappen, G. Measurement of gastric emptying rate of solids by means of a carbon-labeled octanoic acid breath test. *Gastroenterology* **1993**, *104*, 1640–1647. [CrossRef]
24. Friedewald, W.T.; Levy, R.I.; Fredrickson, D.S. Estimation of the Concentration of Low-Density Lipoprotein Cholesterol in Plasma, Without Use of the Preparative Ultracentrifuge. *Clin. Chem.* **1972**, *18*, 499–502. [CrossRef] [PubMed]
25. Mehlem, A.; Hagberg, C.; Muhl, L.; Eriksson, U.; Falkevall, A. Imaging of neutral lipids by oil red O for analyzing the metabolic status in health and disease. *Nat. Protoc.* **2013**, *8*, 1149–1154. [CrossRef]
26. Ciapaite, J.; van den Broek, N.M.; Brinke, H.T.; Nicolay, K.; Jeneson, J.A.; Houten, S.M.; Prompers, J.J. Differential Effects of Short- and Long-Term High-Fat Diet Feeding on Hepatic Fatty Acid Metabolism in Rats. *Biochim. Biophys. Acta* **2011**, *1811*, 441–451. [CrossRef]
27. Christie, S.; Vincent, A.D.; Li, H.; Frisby, C.L.; Kentish, S.J.; O'Rielly, R.; Wittert, G.A.; Page, A.J. A Rotating Light Cycle Promotes Weight Gain and Hepatic Lipid Storage in Mice. *Am. J. Physiol. Liver Physiol.* **2018**, *315*, G932–G942. [CrossRef]
28. Kentish, S.J.; Vincent, A.D.; Kennaway, D.J.; Wittert, G.A.; Page, A.J. High-Fat Diet-Induced Obesity Ablates Gastric Vagal Afferent Circadian Rhythms. *J. Neurosci. Off. J. Soc. Neurosci.* **2016**, *36*, 3199–3207. [CrossRef]
29. Dokken, B.B.; Tsao, T.S. The Physiology of Body Weight Regulation: Are We Too Efficient for Our Own Good? *Diabetes Spectr.* **2007**, *20*, 166–170. [CrossRef]
30. Zhang, Y.; Guo, K.; Leblanc, R.E.; Loh, D.; Schwartz, G.J.; Yu, Y.H. Increasing Dietary Leucine Intake Reduces Diet-Induced Obesity and Improves Glucose and Cholesterol Metabolism in Mice via Multimechanisms. *Diabetes* **2007**, *56*, 1647–1654. [CrossRef]
31. Doi, M.; Yamaoka, I.; Nakayama, M.; Sugahara, K.; Yoshizawa, F. Hypoglycemic Effect of Isoleucine Involves Increased Muscle Glucose Uptake and Whole Body Glucose Oxidation and Decreased Hepatic Gluconeogenesis. *Am. J. Physiol. Metab.* **2007**, *292*, E1683–E1693. [CrossRef] [PubMed]
32. Yoshizawa, F. New Therapeutic Strategy for Amino Acid Medicine: Notable Functions of Branched Chain Amino Acids as Biological Regulators. *J. Pharmacol. Sci.* **2012**, *118*, 149–155. [CrossRef] [PubMed]
33. Cummings, N.E.; Williams, E.M.; Kasza, I.; Konon, E.N.; Schaid, M.D.; Schmidt, B.A.; Poudel, C.; Sherman, D.S.; Yu, D.; Apelo, S.I.A.; et al. Restoration of metabolic health by decreased consumption of branched-chain amino acids. *J. Physiol.* **2017**, *596*, 623–645. [CrossRef] [PubMed]
34. Lynch, C.J.; Adams, S.H. Branched-chain amino acids in metabolic signalling and insulin resistance. *Nat. Rev. Endocrinol.* **2014**, *10*, 723–736. [CrossRef]
35. Nie, C.; He, T.; Zhang, W.-J.; Zhang, G.; Ma, X. Branched Chain Amino Acids: Beyond Nutrition Metabolism. *Int. J. Mol. Sci.* **2018**, *19*, 954. [CrossRef]
36. Cummings, D.E.; Overduin, J. Gastrointestinal regulation of food intake. *J. Clin. Investig.* **2007**, *117*, 13–23. [CrossRef]
37. Mihai, B.M.; Mihai, C.; Cijevschi-Prelipcean, C.; Grigorescu, E.D.; Dranga, M.; Drug, V.; Sporea, I.; Lăcătușu, C.M. Bidirectional Relationship between Gastric Emptying and Plasma Glucose Control in Normoglycemic Individuals and Diabetic Patients. *J. Diabetes Res.* **2018**, *2018*, 1–9. [CrossRef]
38. Gorissen, S.H.M.; Crombag, J.J.R.; Senden, J.M.G.; Waterval, W.A.H.; Bierau, J.; Verdijk, L.B.; van Loon, L.J.C. Protein content and amino acid composition of commercially available plant-based protein isolates. *Amino Acids* **2018**, *50*, 1685–1695. [CrossRef]
39. Uchida, M.; Kobayashi, O.; Iwasawa, K.; Shimizu, K. Effects of Straight Alkyl Chain, Extra Hydroxylated Alkyl Chain and Branched Chain Amino Acids on Gastric Emptying Evaluated Using a Non-Invasive Breath Test in Conscious Rats. *J. Smooth Muscle Res.* **2016**, *52*, 36–44. [CrossRef]

© 2020 by the authors. Licensee MDPI, Basel, Switzerland. This article is an open access article distributed under the terms and conditions of the Creative Commons Attribution (CC BY) license (http://creativecommons.org/licenses/by/4.0/).

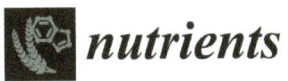

Article

Effect of Obesity on the Expression of Nutrient Receptors and Satiety Hormones in the Human Colon

Lucas Baumard [1], Zsa Zsa R. M. Weerts [2], Ad A. M. Masclee [2], Daniel Keszthelyi [2], Adina T. Michael-Titus [1] and Madusha Peiris [1,*]

1. Centre for Neuroscience, Surgery and Trauma, Blizard Institute, Barts and The London School of Medicine & Dentistry, Queen Mary University of London, London E1 2AT, UK; l.baumard@qmul.ac.uk (L.B.); a.t.michael-titus@qmul.ac.uk (A.T.M.-T.)
2. Division of Gastroenterology and Hepatology, Department of Internal Medicine, School for Nutrition and Translational Research in Metabolism, Maastricht University Medical Centre, 6229 Maastricht, The Netherlands; z.weerts@maastrichtuniversity.nl (Z.Z.R.M.W.); a.masclee@mumc.nl (A.A.M.M.); daniel.keszthelyi@maastrichtuniversity.nl (D.K.)
* Correspondence: m.peiris@qmul.ac.uk; Tel.: +44-207-882-2634

Citation: Baumard, L.; Weerts, Z.Z.R.M.; Masclee, A.A.M.; Keszthelyi, D.; Michael-Titus, A.T.; Peiris, M. Effect of Obesity on the Expression of Nutrient Receptors and Satiety Hormones in the Human Colon. *Nutrients* **2021**, *13*, 1271. https://doi.org/10.3390/nu13041271

Academic Editor: Christine Feinle-Bisset and Michael Horowitz

Received: 5 March 2021
Accepted: 9 April 2021
Published: 13 April 2021

Publisher's Note: MDPI stays neutral with regard to jurisdictional claims in published maps and institutional affiliations.

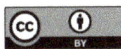

Copyright: © 2021 by the authors. Licensee MDPI, Basel, Switzerland. This article is an open access article distributed under the terms and conditions of the Creative Commons Attribution (CC BY) license (https://creativecommons.org/licenses/by/4.0/).

Abstract: Background: Receptors located on enteroendocrine cells (EECs) of the colon can detect nutrients in the lumen. These receptors regulate appetite through a variety of mechanisms, including hormonal and neuronal signals. We assessed the effect of obesity on the expression of these G-protein coupled receptors (GPCRs) and hormones at both mRNA and protein level. Methods: qPCR and immunohistochemistry were used to examine colonic tissue from cohorts of patients from the Netherlands (proximal and sigmoid tissue) and the United Kingdom (tissue from across the colon) and patients were grouped by body mass index (BMI) value (BMI < 25 and BMI ≥ 25). Results: The mRNA expression of the hormones/signaling molecules serotonin, glucagon, peptide YY (PYY), CCK and somatostatin were not significantly different between BMI groups. GPR40 mRNA expression was significantly increased in sigmoid colon samples in the BMI ≥ 25 group, but not proximal colon. GPR41, GPR109a, GPR43, GPR120, GPRC6A, and CaSR mRNA expression were unaltered between low and high BMI. At the protein level, serotonin and PYY containing cell numbers were similar in high and low BMI groups. Enterochromaffin cells (EC) showed high degree of co-expression with amino acid sensing receptor, CaSR while co-expression with PYY containing L-cells was limited, regardless of BMI. Conclusions: While expression of medium/long chain fatty acid receptor GPR40 was increased in the sigmoid colon of the high BMI group, expression of other nutrient sensing GPCRs and expression profiles of EECs involved in peripheral mechanisms of appetite regulation were unchanged. Collectively, these data suggest that in human colonic tissue, EEC and nutrient-sensing receptor expression profiles are not affected despite changes to BMI.

Keywords: nutrient sensing; enteroendocrine cells (EECs); appetite regulation; G-protein coupled receptors (GPCRs); obesity

1. Introduction

Obesity is a significant and growing health issue facing the Western world [1,2]. Obese adults are more susceptible to a wide range of comorbidities, including type 2 diabetes [3], metabolic disorders and abnormalities such as dyslipidaemia [4], cardiovascular disease [5]—including hypertension [6], stroke [7]—and a variety of cancers [8].

Appetite is regulated to balance energy intake and expenditure by the release of hunger and satiety signals [9]. Appetite regulation can begin before food enters the body; the cephalic phase is initiated by sights and smells of food and by environmental effects such as time of day [10]. Both mechanical and hormonal signals regulate food intake via central control from brain centres of appetite regulation, including the solitary tract nucleus in the brain stem [11,12]. Potent satiety hormones such as PYY and glucagon-like peptide 1 (GLP-1) are released from the small intestine to the colon, in response to dietary nutrients [13]. The colon is the main source of peripheral serotonin [14] and holds the highest number and diversity of microbiota, with bacterial by-products such as short chain fatty acids (SCFA) playing a role in nutrient sensing and obesity. Hormones such as PYY, CCK, and GLP-1 are released from the colon and can enter the circulation [15,16]. PYY can stimulate neurons within the hypothalamic arcuate nucleus: orexigenic neurons co-expresses agouti-related peptide (AgRP) and neuropeptide Y (NPY); anorexigenic neurons release pro-opiomelanocortin (POMC) and cocaine- and amphetamine-regulated transcript (CART) [9]. CCK can act on vagal fibres innervating the brain stem to alter gut motility, secretions from the pancreas and gall bladder activation [9].

Enteroendocrine cells (EECs) are a subset of epithelial cells expressed throughout gastrointestinal tissues and are classified according to their hormone/peptide content [17,18]. EECs express nutrient-sensing receptors and respond to luminal contents, leading to the release of anorectic hormones and mediators that act on the vagus nerve and hypothalamus, resulting in long-term satiation [18,19]. L cells, an EEC sub-type critical for appetite regulation, co-secrete the potent anorectic hormones PYY and GLP-1, and are highly expressed in the colon [20,21]. PYY acts on receptors within the hypothalamus to inhibit the release of the orexigenic peptide neuropeptide Y (NPY) [22]. These same receptors are also found on peripheral vagal afferents [10] and are likely to drive PYY's role in regulating gastric acid secretion and gastrointestinal motility [22]. GLP-1 receptors are also found within the hypothalamus and brain stem, where their activation reduces food intake [23]. In obesity, circulating levels of PYY and GLP-1 are decreased [24,25]. Enterochromaffin (EC) cells, a further population of EECs, secrete 95% of the body's serotonin in response to carbohydrate-rich foods and SCFAs [26]. Centrally released serotonin plays an important role in modulating food cravings and mood [27,28] whilst serotonin from the colon and periphery can activate small intestinal and colonic vagal afferent nerves to modulate gastrointestinal secretion and motility [14,28]. Drugs that can act as serotonin receptor agonists centrally have been shown to reduce weight gain in mice and caloric intake in lean and obese humans via the hypothalamic melanocortin system [29]. Serotonin is synthesised from tryptophan by the enzyme tryptophan hydroxylase 1 (TPH1), in a rate limiting process [30]. Cholecystokinin (CCK), released by I cells [31], strongly reduces food intake [32], and CCK administration reduces food intake in obese patients [33]. Finally, somatostatin is expressed in D cells [34] and inhibits the release of anorectic hormones like GLP-1 and PYY [35,36], demonstrating a critical cellular control mechanism. Collectively, various EECs are required for the normal processes of appetite regulation.

Importantly, to activate EECs and induce release of hormones/peptides, nutrients bind to and activate nutrient sensing G-protein coupled receptors (GPCRs) expressed on EECs [37]. SCFAs can bind to GPCRs via GPR41 [38], GPR43 [39], and GPR109a [40], medium/long chain fatty acids (M/LCFA) bind to GPR40 [41] and GPR120 [42] and amino acids bind to CaSR [43] and GPRC6a [44]. These receptors are expressed throughout the gastrointestinal tract, including the colon and rectum, in both mice and humans [45]. L-cells express the SCFA receptors GPR43, GPR41 [46], and CaSR [47] and colonic ECs have been shown to express GPR119, GPR120, GPR41, and GPR43 [48]. We have previously shown that agonist action at GPR41, GPR40, and GPR119 induces colonic EEC activation [49] and, importantly, that stimulation of GPR84 increases the release of GLP-1, PYY, and serotonin, demonstrating functional modulation of L and EC cells [45].

There is evidence to suggest that obesity alters peripheral pathways of appetite regulation. The mRNA expression and protein levels of GPR120 are decreased in the visceral adipose tissue of obese individuals [50], while GPR120 knockout mice demonstrate an obese phenotype [51]. mRNA expression of GPR41, GPR43, GPR40, and GPR120 increased in diet-induced obese mice compared to mice on a normal diet [49]. Additionally, postprandial release of hormones is altered, with lower circulating levels of PYY and GLP-1 reported in obesity [9,52], with levels remaining low after 10 weeks of sustained weight loss [53]. Collectively, these data suggest that obesity may alter peripheral mechanisms of appetite regulation.

The aim of this study was to assess expression profiles of EECs and nutrient-sensing GPCRs, to determine if weight gain alters the physiology of nutrient sensing at the cellular level, particularly in the colon.

2. Materials and Methods

2.1. Human Samples

Tissue specimens were collected in two centres: The Royal London Hospital, in London, UK, and the Maastricht University Medical Centre (MUMC), in Maastricht, the Netherlands.

In London, non-inflamed, non-cancerous (morphologically normal), full thickness, and mucosal samples were taken from the ascending, transverse, and descending colon of patients ($n = 30$) undergoing gastrointestinal cancer surgery.

In Maastricht, biopsies were taken from the right sided proximal and the sigmoid colon of patients with irritable bowel syndrome ($n = 30$) participating in the Maastricht IBS cohort study and undergoing routine colonoscopy. In addition, biopsies were taken from the sigmoid colon of healthy controls ($n = 7$) participating in an interventional study (placebo group). Inclusion and exclusion criteria of the Maastricht IBS cohort and the healthy control group are described elsewhere [54,55]. Biopsies were placed in Eppendorf tubes immediately and fresh frozen in liquid nitrogen to be stored at $-80\ °C$ until RNA isolation.

All participants gave written informed consent prior to inclusion. The studies were approved by the East London and The City HA Local Research Ethics Committee (NREC 09/H0704/2) and the University of Maastricht Medical Ethics Committee, respectively, and were performed in compliance with the revised Declaration of Helsinki (64th WMA General Assembly, Fortaleza, Brazil, 2013). All samples collected were from fasted subjects with tissue collection occurring in the morning. The study is registered in the US National Library of Medicine (http://www.clinicaltrials.gov, NCT00775060, 2008, accessed on 5 March 2021). Patient and healthy control characteristics are presented in Supplementary Tables S1 and S2, with the distribution of participant BMI from both research locations shown in Supplementary Graphs S1 and S2.

2.2. Immunohistochemistry

Patient samples used for immunohistochemistry were obtained from the Royal London Hospital as previously described. Full thickness samples were fixed in 4% paraformaldehyde/phosphate buffered saline (PBS) at $4\ °C$ overnight. Tissue was cryoprotected in 30% sucrose/PBS, then mounted in OCT embedding compound for cutting and subsequent storage at $-80\ °C$.

Cut tissue sections (10 μm) were washed with PBS, blocked with Trident Universal Protein Blocking Reagent (animal serum free) (Insight Biotechnology limited GTX 30963) and primary antibody was applied (Supplementary Table S3) for 18 h at $4\ °C$. Tissue was then washed in PBS and incubated for 1 h with species-specific Alexa Fluor conjugated secondary antibodies (Supplementary Table S4 (1:400)). Slides were cover-slipped with a mounting medium containing diamidino-2-phenylindole (DAPI) (VECTASHIELD, Vector laboratories H-1500). Negative controls were obtained by omitting the primary antibody. Sections were visualised and imaged on an epifluorescence microscope (Leica DM4000 Epi-Fluorescence Microscope) and images were acquired on a monochrome CCD digital camera system (Leica DFC365) using Metamorph imaging system software. Images were analysed using ImageJ (Rasband, W.S., ImageJ, U. S. National Institutes of Health, Bethesda, MD, USA, https://imagej.nih.gov/ij/, 1997–2018, accessed on 5 March 2021).

Cell counts were performed on stained sections from a colonic region and positively stained cells were manually counted. Counts were performed blinded to patient data, including BMI. A minimum of 10 field of views (FOV) were taken in each section, the number of cells and crypts were counted and the average value calculated for cells/crypt for each field of view and patient. Cells were counted based on the inclusion and exclusion criteria listed in Table 1.

Table 1. Inclusion and exclusion criteria for counting of stained cells.

Inclusion Criteria	Exclusion Criteria
Whole cells	Parts of cells visible within fields of view (FOV)
Cells clearly distinguishable with nucleus (shape, size)	Ambiguity in defining cell shape
Cells located within crypts	Cells located outside of crypts
Levels of background low	High background/noise across the FOV

2.3. Gene Expression Studies

Quantitative real-time reverse transcriptase PCR (RT-PCR) was used to assess the relative expression of nutrient GPCRs and hormone/peptides in human colonic tissue (Supplementary Table S6 for patient and tissue details).

Mucosal samples were stored in RNALater (Qiagen, Manchester, UK) at −80 °C prior to gene expression experiments. RNA was extracted from tissues using a RNeasy Mini kit (Qiagen). RNA quantity and quality were assessed using a NanoDrop machine. RNA was reverse transcribed into cDNA using the Quantitech RT kit (Qiagen) or the High-Capacity cDNA Reverse Transcription Kit with RNase inhibitor (Applied biosystems, Thermo Fisher Scientific) for the London and Maastricht samples, respectively.

cDNA samples from Maastricht were reverse transcribed using MultiScribe Reverse Transcriptase (ThermoFischer Scientific, Waltham, MA, USA). These samples were run on TaqMan PCR (Thermofisher TaqMan Array Micro Fluidic card Cat# 4342249) using a ViiA7 machine. For each patient, the relative gene expression of genes of interest and 2 positive controls (18s ribosomal RNA (18s) and glyceraldehyde-3-phosphate dehydrogenase (GAPDH)) were calculated for each plate. The relative expression of mRNA from the sigmoid and proximal colon was plotted separately against BMI. BMI values were used to divide patients into normal weight patients (BMI < 25) and obese/overweight patients (BMI ≥ 25). We also used regression analysis (Pearson r correlation and simple linear regression) with BMI as the co-variant, and similar results were obtained (data not shown). The patient group of BMI < 25 are all those patients below or equal to 24.9 BMI. Sigmoidal and proximal colon samples were analysed separately. Supplementary Table S1 shows the number of samples for each gene and colonic location and Supplementary Table S2 the BMI distribution of these patients.

For samples from the Royal London Hospital, SYBR green primers were purchased from Qiagen (Supplementary Table S5). Target gene expression was determined relative to the endogenous control, 18s ribosomal RNA, using the comparative cycle threshold method on an Applied Biosystems StepOnePLus real-time PCR system thermal cycling block.

2.4. Statistical Analysis

Data is expressed as mean ± SEM. Statistical analysis for mRNA expression and cell counting was performed using unpaired t tests (Mann-Whitney test) (GraphPad Prism, V.8, GraphPad Software Inc, San Diego, CA, USA), with $p < 0.05$ considered statistically significant.

3. Results

3.1. The mRNA Expression of Hormones and Peptides Involved in Appetite Regulation Is Unchanged between Healthy BMI (<25) and Overweight/Obese BMI (≥25)

In the proximal colon, there was no significant change in the expression of tryptophan hydroxylase 1 (TPH1), glucagon, PYY or somatostatin, between the healthy BMI (<25) or overweight/obese BMI group (≥25) (Figure 1A–E). We also assessed the expression of the leptin receptor and observed no change in expression in either tissues between BMI groups.

The sigmoid colon showed no change in the mRNA expression of the genes assessed, between the two BMI groups (Figure 1F–J).

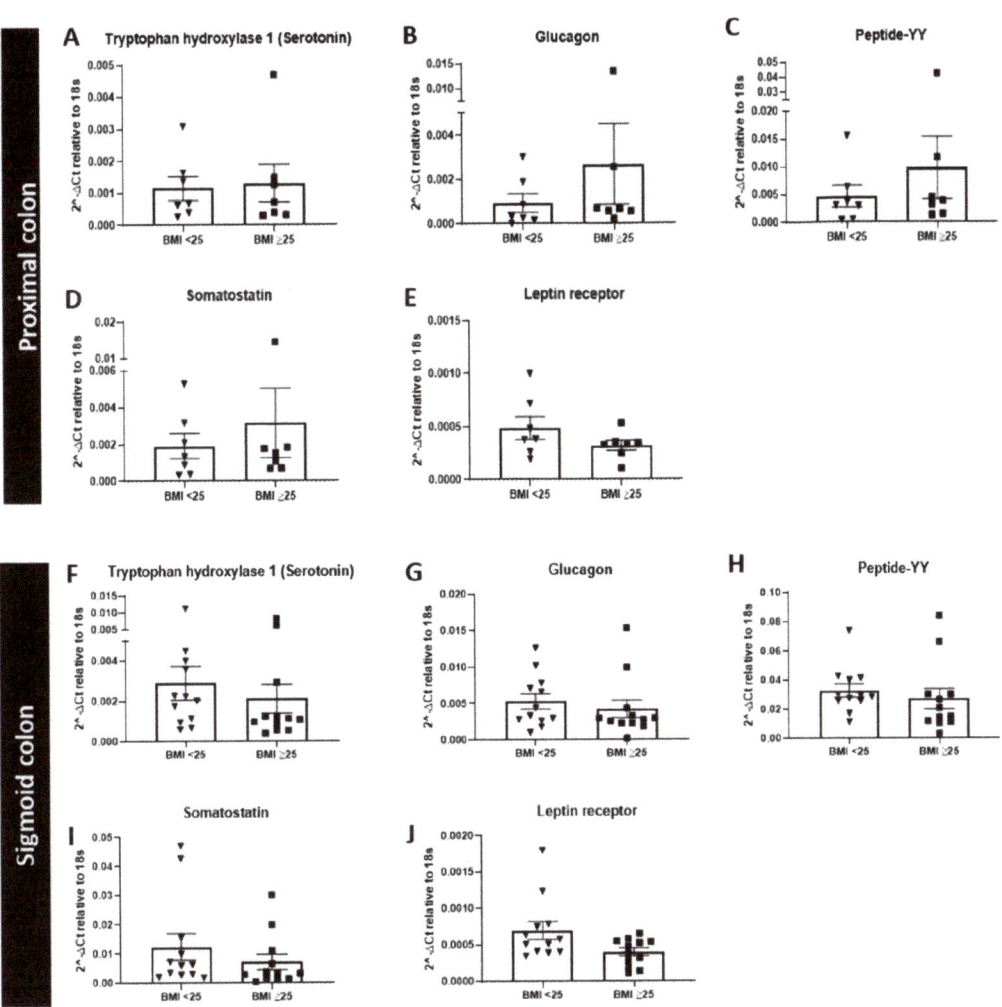

Figure 1. Relative mRNA expression of hormones and hormone receptors involved in satiety in the proximal and sigmoid colon. mRNA expression (relative to 18s) of hormone markers in the proximal (**A–E**), (body mass index (BMI) < 25 n = 7, BMI ≥ 25 n = 7), and sigmoid colon (**F–J**), (BMI < 25 n = 12, BMI ≥ 25 n = 12).

3.2. The Expression of PYY and Serotonin in Enterochromaffin and L-Cells Is Unchanged between Healthy BMI (<25) and Overweight/Obese BMI (≥25)

In colonic tissue samples (from the Royal London Hospital, London, UK) serotonin containing EC cells were present in colonic crypts in both the <25 and ≥25 BMI groups (Figure 2A,B, respectively). PYY positive L-cells were also present in colonic crypts in both BMI groups (Figure 2A,B). The quantification of EC and PYY cells showed no significant difference between BMI groups (Figure 2C).

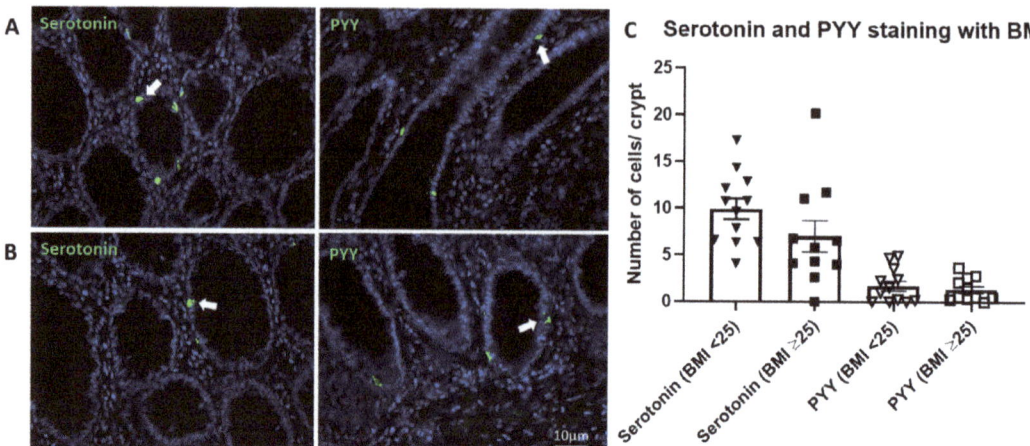

Figure 2. Serotonin and PYY immunohistochemistry expression in human colonic tissue of BMI < 25 and ≥25. (**A,B**): Representative images of serotonin and PYY expression in patients of BMI < 25 and BMI ≥ 25, respectively. Arrows denote serotonin and PYY positive cells. (**C**): Counts of cells per crypt stained positively for serotonin and PYY, grouped as BMI < 25 (n = 12) and BMI ≥ 25 (n = 11). Scale bars represent 10 µm.

3.3. mRNA Expression of GPR40 Is Significantly Increased in Sigmoid Colon of ≥25 BMI Group

In the proximal colon there was no significant difference in mRNA expression between BMI groups for the SCFA receptors GPR43, GPR41 and GPR109a (Figure 3A–C). There was no significant difference in mRNA expression of the LCFA receptor GPR120 (Figure 3E) and the M/LCFA receptor GPR40 (Figure 3D).

In the sigmoid colon, there was no significant difference in the mRNA expression of GPR43, GPR41, GPR109a, GPR120, or CaSR (Figure 3F–K). mRNA expression of GPR40 was significantly increased in the BMI ≥ 25 compared to BMI < 25 group (p = 0.0464) (Figure 3I).

Individual qPCR expression experiments were conducted on proximal colonic tissue obtained from patients attending the Royal London Hospital to assess mRNA levels that were at a low detection level in samples from Maastricht. There was no significant difference in the expression of the amino acid sensing GPCRs, CaSR or GPRC6A in the BMI groups assessed (Figure 4A,B). Expression of the anorectic hormone CCK was also not significantly changed between the two BMI groups assessed (Figure 4C).

3.4. CaSR Is Highly Expressed on Serotonin Positive ECs Irrespective of BMI

Serotonin containing EC cells co-stained with CaSR in both BMI groups (Figure 5A,B). Cell counting demonstrated no significant differences in individual CaSR or serotonin positive cells, or cells that were co-stained in the two BMI groups (Figure 5A,B). CaSR was expressed on 99% and 95% of serotonin containing EC cell in the normal BMI and obese/overweight groups, respectively (Figure 5C).

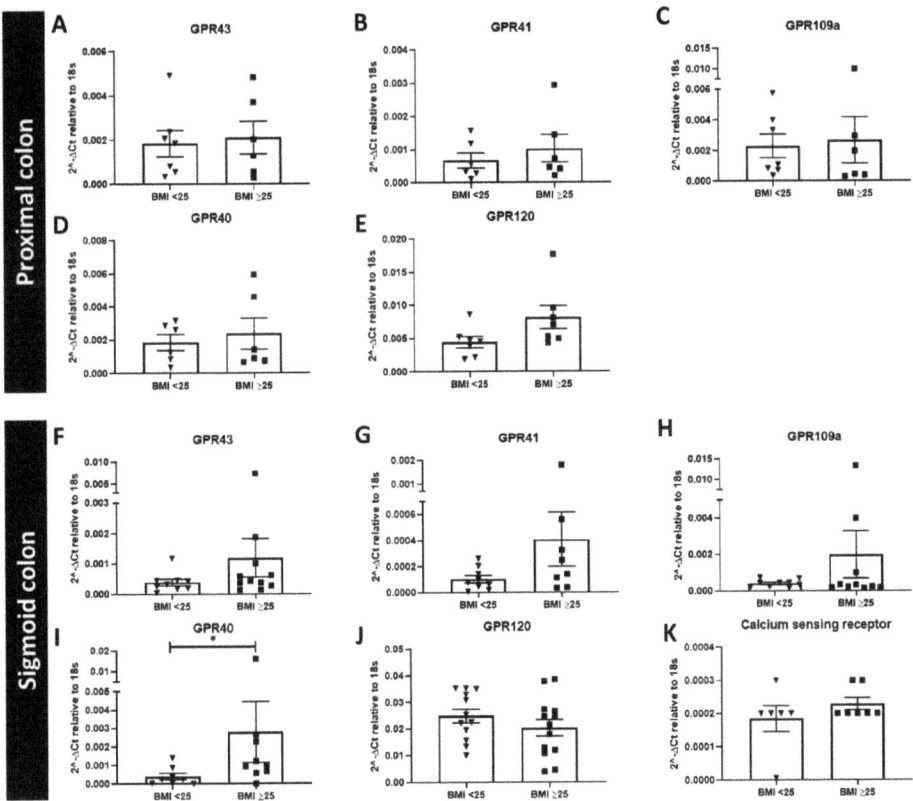

Figure 3. Relative mRNA expression of genes for nutrient receptors in the proximal and sigmoid colonic tissue from a Dutch cohort. Relative expression (against 18s) of nutrient receptors in the proximal (**A–E**, $n = 6$–7) and sigmoid colon (**F–K**, $n = 6$–13) with patients divided into those with a BMI < 25 and BMI ≥ 25, respectively, * significant increase.

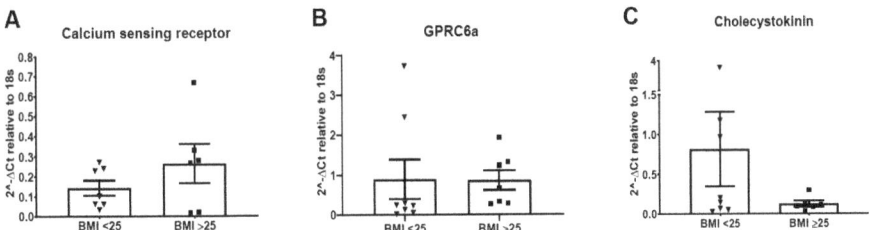

Figure 4. Relative mRNA expression of nutrient receptors in colonic tissue from a UK cohort. Relative expression (against 18s) of (**A**) CaSR ($n = 7$; $n = 6$), (**B**) GPRC6a ($n = 8$; $n = 7$) and (**C**) cholecystokinin ($n = 8$; $n = 6$) in a cohort of patients from the Royal London Hospital, divided into those with a BMI < 25 and BMI ≥ 25, respectively.

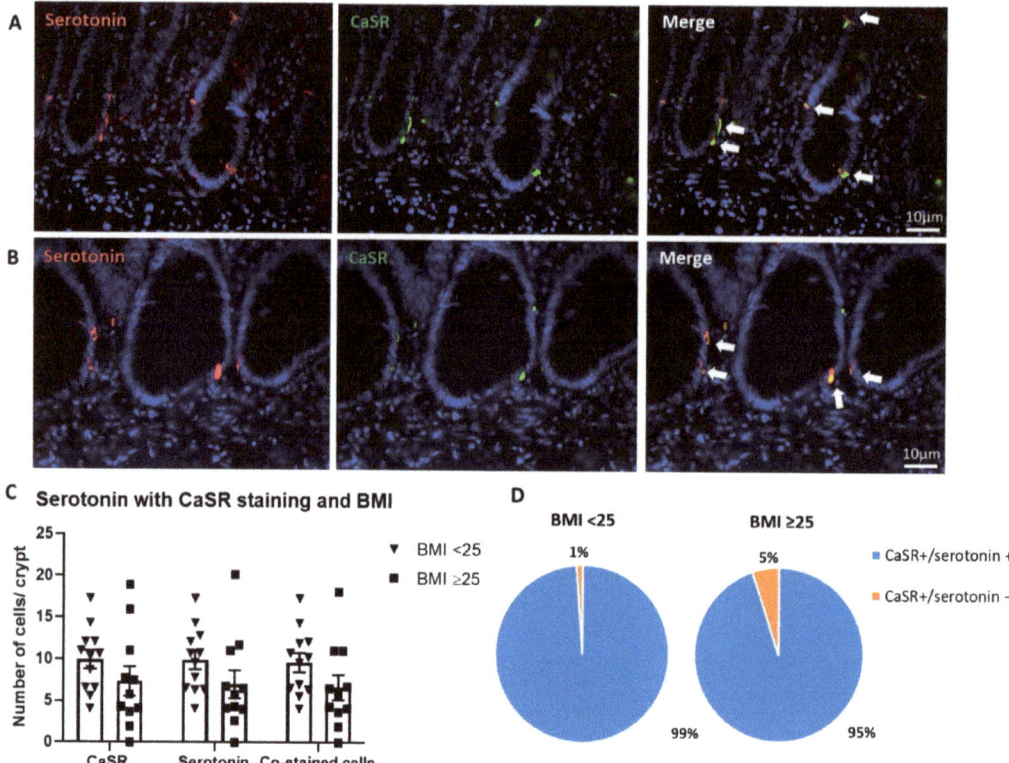

Figure 5. Serotonin and CaSR expression in human colonic samples according to BMI. (**A**): Representative image from BMI < 25 patient tissue staining for serotonin (red) and CaSR (green). (**B**): Representative image BMI ≥ 25 patient tissue staining for serotonin (red) and CaSR (green). Arrows denote serotonin and CaSR co-stained cells. (**C**): Quantification of positive cells per crypt for CaSR, serotonin and co-stained cells in BMI < 25 (n = 12) and BMI of ≥25 (n = 11). (**D**): Proportion of cells per crypt CaSR+/serotonin+ or CaSR+/serotonin- in patients with a BMI < 25 and BMI ≥ 25. Scale bars represent 10 μm.

3.5. Limited Expression of CaSR on PYY Expressing L-Cells

PYY and CaSR showed positive staining in our colonic tissue samples from both the healthy and overweight/obese groups (Figure 6A,B, respectively). Quantification of positively stained cells showed no significant changes in the expression of CaSR, PYY, or co-stained cells between healthy or overweight/obese BMI groups (Figure 6C). Co-staining of PYY with CaSR was infrequent—5% and 6% of cells in the healthy BMI and obese/overweight BMI groups, respectively (Figure 6D).

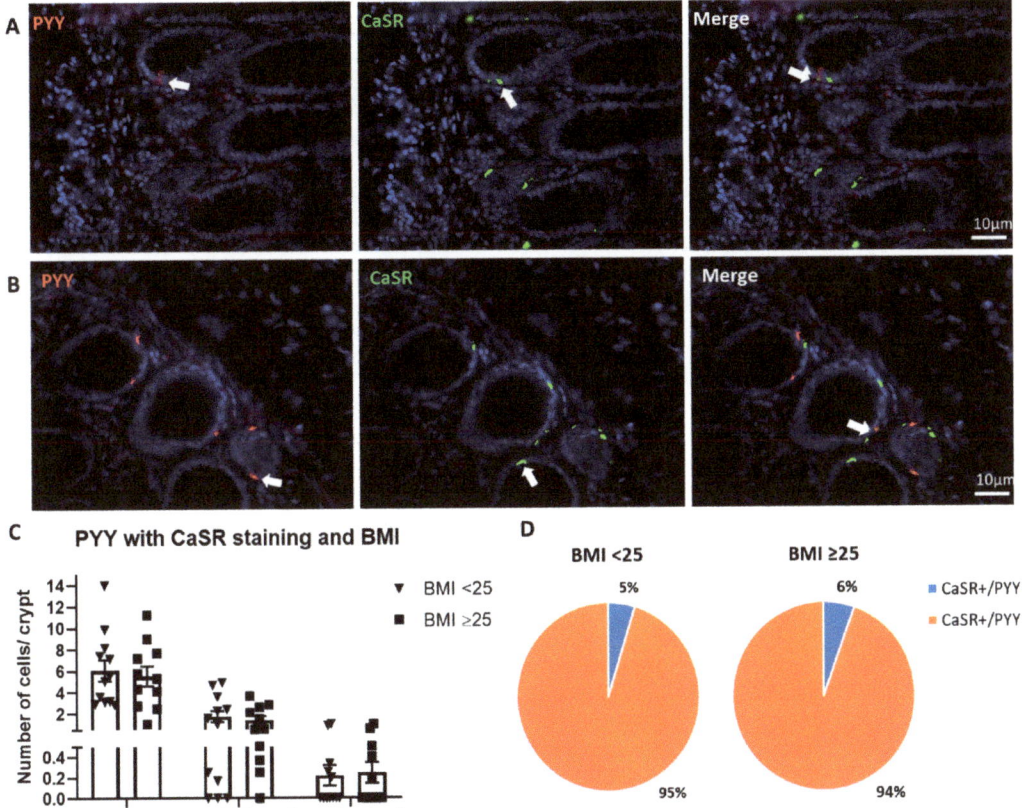

Figure 6. Serotonin and CaSR immunohistochemistry expression in human colon. (**A**): Representative image from BMI < 25 patient tissue staining for PYY (red) and CaSR (green). (**B**): Representative image BMI ≥ 25 patient tissue staining for serotonin (red) and CaSR (green). Arrows denote PYY and CaSR co-stained cells. (**C**): Number of cells per crypt for CaSR, PYY and cells co-stained with both PYY and CaSR, samples differentiated as BMI < 25 (n = 12) and BMI ≥ 25 (n = 11). (**D**): Proportion of cells per crypt that are CaSR+/serotonin+ or CaSR+/serotonin- in patients with a BMI < 25 and BMI ≥ 25. Scale bars represent 10 μm.

4. Discussion

We show that overall, overweight/obesity does not alter the gene expression of hormones/peptides, nutrient-sensing GPCRs for SCFAs, the LCFA GPR120, or amino acids. Similarly, at the protein level, the expression profile of EC and L cells is unchanged between healthy and overweight/obese BMI groups. However, we do show a modest increase in expression of the medium and long chain fatty acid receptor GPR40 in the sigmoid colon of patients in the BMI ≥ 25 group.

We report that both PYY mRNA expression and the number of PYY containing L cells are unchanged with increasing BMI. Our data suggests that the decreased circulating levels of PYY described previously [24,25] are not caused by reduced PYY mRNA expression or L-cell numbers, indicating that PYY release may be impaired. In addition, the mRNA expression of glucagon (a marker of GLP-1 production) is not significantly different between the two BMI groups, in either the sigmoid or proximal colon. GLP-1 and PYY have been shown to be co-expressed and co-released from secretory vesicles in L cells [23] therefore, it is expected that their release profile will be similar. Indeed, it has been demonstrated that obese individuals have decreased PYY and GLP-1 plasma levels that persisted for at least 12 months, despite weight loss [53]. Taken together with our data, this suggests that while the cells and receptors regulating cell function are unchanged in obesity, the cellular mechanisms leading to hormone release may be altered.

EC cells-mediated release of serotonin has been shown to be increased in obese vs. non-obese patients but the colonic mRNA expression of TPH1, an enzyme critical for serotonin production, is unchanged [56]. We similarly report no change in the expression of TPH1 and show that EC numbers in human colon do not change in response to BMI. These findings concur with a mouse study where EC numbers were unchanged in the jejunum between high and low fat diet animals [9]. However, our group has previously shown that expression of TPH-1 and the numbers of ECs were increased in the colons of an obese mouse group compared to a wild-type group (though this increase did not reach statistical significance) [49]. Collectively, these studies demonstrate that expression of TPH1 mRNA and serotonin containing EC cells are stable in humans despite weight changes. Furthermore, there may be changes at the genetic and protein levels in the murine colon, compared to the human colon.

Other hormones, such as the anorexigenic hormones leptin and CCK, were unchanged between the low and high BMI groups, as was the mRNA expression of somatostatin. Leptin, produced by adipose tissue, is increased in obesity (in serum and plasma) [57]. Our data shows that the colonic tissue has no impact on leptin changes. Unchanged levels of CCK may reflect the small population in the colon, as I cells expressing CCK are found primarily in the small intestine [31]. Somatostatin containing D cells are commonly found in the duodenum and stomach, while colonic populations constitute 3–5% of cells [34]; therefore, changes to somatostatin expression may occur primarily outside of the colon.

mRNA expression of nutrient-sensing GPCRs which activate and stimulate release of the cells described were similarly unchanged overall. However, there was a modest increase in GPR40 mRNA expression in the sigmoid colon of the overweight/obese BMI group. No change in GPR40 expression was observed in the proximal colon despite the previously reported equal distribution between the proximal and distal colon [45]. GPR40 binds to medium/long chain fatty acids and is expressed on human L cells, with agonist action increasing the release of GLP-1 [58]. The difference between the proximal and sigmoid colon expression of GPR40 may be attributed to its expression on L-cells, as density of these cells increases along the colon, with highest levels found in the rectum [18]. Therefore, it may be that greater numbers of cells expressing GPR40 are found in the sigmoid region, accounting for the small difference in expression observed. GPR120, another important MCFA sensing GPCR, was also unchanged in our study. This was a surprising result as absence of the gene encoding GPR120 induces an obese phenotype in humans [59] and mRNA expression is reportedly increased in the duodenum of obese and overweight humans [60]. However, in diet-induced obese mice, our group has previously shown a significant increase in mRNA expression of GPR120 and GPR40 between in obese mice [49]. Our data suggests that the colonic expression of GPR120 is stable and less likely to be influenced by increased caloric intake as most nutrients are absorbed in the small intestine.

Although reports suggest that the microbiome is altered in obesity [61] and that the luminal concentration of by-products of bacterial fermentation, i.e., SCFAs, may be altered [62], we report no change in the mRNA expression of the SCFA receptors GPR43, GPR41 or GPR109a. GRP43 and GPR41 knock-out mice have impaired L cell activity [63,64] suggesting that these receptors are involved in peripheral mechanisms of satiety and we have previously shown significant increase in expression of GPR41 or GPR43 in diet-induced obesity [49]. However, data from this study in human colonic tissue suggests that while the luminal environment may be altered in terms of bacterial populations and subsequent fermentation products, the expression of SCFA GPCRs remains stable.

To understand whether changes to GPCR and EEC expression patterns were affected by increasing BMI, we assessed co-expression via immunofluorescence. CaSR and EC cells were highly co-localised while a small population of PYY containing L-cells also expressed CaSR in human colonic tissue, regardless of BMI. We have previously reported a similar expression pattern of CaSR with PYY and serotonin in human colonic tissue [45]. Our data shows that obesity (BMI > 25) does not alter the expression of CaSR on EEC types. Activation of CaSR expressed on EECs has been shown to release gastrin, CCK, and GLP-1 [47,65] while L-cells from CaSR deficient mice show impaired release of CCK and Ca^{2+} in response to L-phenylalanine [47], suggesting that CaSR is crucial for their release. Our data suggests that agonists of CaSR may be an important target in obesity, as there is conservation of the cellular pathways which may be targeted for L-cell activation.

An important limitation of the current study is that the release of hormones from EECs cells or the ability of cells to become activated by nutrients binding to their corresponding nutrient receptors was not assessed. Clinical data has shown that circulating levels of these hormones is altered with obesity, therefore it is likely that hormone release is abrogated from these cells [24,25]. Importantly, maintenance of long-term satiety is critically dependent on PYY and GLP-1 [22,66]. Therefore, further studies are required to understand the capacity of EC and L cells from overweight/obese individuals to release their hormone content in response to nutrient stimulation. The focus of this study was the peripheral mechanisms regulating appetite in order to understand changes to molecular machinery in response to obesity. Lack of changes to expression of nutrient-sensing receptors and EECs does not exclude possible changes to downstream pathways in the periphery, including changes to hormone release profiles and afferent nerve activity, and warrants further investigation.

Overall, this study demonstrates that in human colonic tissue, the expression of nutrient sensing GPCRs, satiety hormones and EEC does not significantly change in the overweight/obese state. As previously discussed, obesity is characterised by an increased caloric load, changes to the microbial and luminal environment in obesity. However, our findings indicate that the expression pattern of the receptors and cells that sense luminal content is stable in the human colon.

Supplementary Materials: The following are available online at https://www.mdpi.com/article/10.3390/nu13041271/s1, Graphs S1: Distribution of BMI for patient samples from the Royal London Hospital, UK. BMI data from individuals (n = 32) from whom colonic tissue was collected is plotted alongside their assigned patient number., Graphs S2: Distribution of BMI for patient samples from the University of Maastricht. BMI data from individuals (n = 67) from whom colonic tissue was collected., Table S1: Patient demographics from the Royal London Hospital, U.K., Table S2: Details of patient samples recruited at the University of Maastricht, Netherlands., Table S3: Primary antibodies used for immunohistochemistry, Table S4: Secondary antibodies used for immunohistochemistry, Table S5: Primers for gene expression studies, Table S6: Distribution of patient samples by gene examined by Taqman qPCR.

Author Contributions: Conceptualization, M.P. and A.T.M.-T.; formal analysis, L.B.; investigation, L.B. and Z.Z.R.M.W.; writing—original draft preparation, L.B., A.T.M.-T., and M.P.; writing—review and editing, Z.Z.R.M.W., D.K., L.B., A.T.M.-T., and M.P.; supervision, A.A.M.M., A.T.M.-T., and M.P.; funding acquisition, M.P. All authors have read and agreed to the published version of the manuscript.

Funding: This research was funded by Bowel Research U.K. and BBSRC Institute Strategic Programme Gut Microbes and Health BB/R012490/1 and its constituent project (BBS/E/F/000PR10355).

Institutional Review Board Statement: The study was conducted according to the guidelines of the Declaration of Helsinki, and approved by the East London and The City HA Local Research Ethics Committee [NREC 09/H0704/2] and the University of Maastricht Medical Ethics Committee, respectively, and were performed in compliance with the revised Declaration of Helsinki (64th WMA General Assembly, Fortaleza, Brazil, 2013). The study is registered in the US National Library of Medicine (http://www.clinicaltrials.gov, NCT00775060, 2008, accessed on 5 March 2021).

Informed Consent Statement: Informed consent was obtained from all subjects involved in the study.

Data Availability Statement: All data relevant to this study is presented here or in the supplementary data associated with this publication.

Conflicts of Interest: The authors declare no conflict of interest.

References

1. Public Health England. *Health Matters: Getting Every Adult Active Every Day*; Public Health England: London, UK, 2016.
2. Public Health England. *Health Matters: Obesity and the Food Environment*; Public Health England: London, UK, 2019.
3. Nguyen, N.T.; Magno, C.P.; Lane, K.T.; Hinojosa, M.W.; Lane, J.S. Association of hypertension, diabetes, dyslipidemia, and metabolic syndrome with obesity: Findings from the National Health and Nutrition Examination Survey, 1999 to 2004. *J. Am. Coll. Surg.* **2008**, *207*, 928–934. [CrossRef]
4. Grundy, S.M.; Barnett, J.P. Metabolic and health complications of obesity. *Dis. Mon.* **1990**, *36*, 641–731.
5. Klein, S.; Burke, L.E.; Bray, G.A.; Blair, S.; Allison, D.B.; Pi-Sunyer, X.; Hong, Y.; Eckel, R.H.; American Heart Association Council on Nutrition; Physical Activity; et al. Clinical implications of obesity with specific focus on cardiovascular disease: A statement for professionals from the American Heart Association Council on Nutrition, Physical Activity, and Metabolism: Endorsed by the American College of Cardiology Foundation. *Circulation* **2004**, *110*, 2952–2967. [CrossRef]
6. Wilson, P.W.; D'Agostino, R.B.; Sullivan, L.; Parise, H.; Kannel, W.B. Overweight and obesity as determinants of cardiovascular risk: The Framingham experience. *Arch. Intern. Med.* **2002**, *162*, 1867–1872. [CrossRef]
7. Rexrode, K.M.; Hennekens, C.H.; Willett, W.C.; Colditz, G.A.; Stampfer, M.J.; Rich-Edwards, J.W.; Speizer, F.E.; Manson, J.E. A prospective study of body mass index, weight change, and risk of stroke in women. *JAMA* **1997**, *277*, 1539–1545. [CrossRef]
8. Calle, E.E.; Rodriguez, C.; Walker-Thurmond, K.; Thun, M.J. Overweight, obesity, and mortality from cancer in a prospectively studied cohort of U.S. adults. *N. Engl. J. Med.* **2003**, *348*, 1625–1638. [CrossRef]
9. Druce, M.; Bloom, S.R. The regulation of appetite. *Arch. Dis. Child.* **2006**, *91*, 183–187. [CrossRef]
10. Schloegl, H.; Percik, R.; Horstmann, A.; Villringer, A.; Stumvoll, M. Peptide hormones regulating appetite–focus on neuroimaging studies in humans. *Diabetes Metab. Res. Rev.* **2011**, *27*, 104–112. [CrossRef]
11. Wynne, K.; Stanley, S.; McGowan, B.; Bloom, S. Appetite control. *J. Endocrinol.* **2005**, *184*, 291. [CrossRef]
12. Oesch, S.; Rüegg, C.; Fischer, B.; Degen, L.; Beglinger, C. Effect of gastric distension prior to eating on food intake and feelings of satiety in humans. *Physiol. Behav.* **2006**, *87*, 903–910. [CrossRef]
13. Sun, E.W.L.; Martin, A.M.; Young, R.L.; Keating, D.J. The Regulation of Peripheral Metabolism by Gut-Derived Hormones. *Front. Endocrinol.* **2018**, *9*, 754. [CrossRef]
14. Gershon, M.D.; Tack, J. The serotonin signaling system: From basic understanding to drug development for functional GI disorders. *Gastroenterology* **2007**, *132*, 397–414. [CrossRef]
15. le Roux, C.W.; Bloom, S.R. Peptide YY, appetite and food intake. *Proc. Nutr. Soc.* **2005**, *64*, 213–216. [CrossRef]
16. Näslund, E.; Gutniak, M.; Skogar, S.; Rössner, S.; Hellström, P.M. Glucagon-like peptide 1 increases the period of postprandial satiety and slows gastric emptying in obese men. *Am. J. Clin. Nutr.* **1998**, *68*, 525–530. [CrossRef]
17. Sternini, C.; Anselmi, L.; Rozengurt, E. Enteroendocrine cells: A site of 'taste' in gastrointestinal chemosensing. *Curr. Opin. Endocrinol. Diabetes Obes.* **2008**, *15*, 73–78. [CrossRef]
18. Gunawardene, A.R.; Corfe, B.M.; Staton, C.A. Classification and functions of enteroendocrine cells of the lower gastrointestinal tract. *Int. J. Exp. Pathol.* **2011**, *92*, 219–231. [CrossRef] [PubMed]
19. Latorre, R.; Sternini, C.; De Giorgio, R.; Greenwood-Van Meerveld, B. Enteroendocrine cells: A review of their role in brain-gut communication. *Neurogastroenterol. Motil. Off. J. Eur. Gastrointest. Motil. Soc.* **2016**, *28*, 620–630. [CrossRef]
20. Sjolund, K.; Sanden, G.; Hakanson, R.; Sundler, F. Endocrine cells in human intestine: An immunocytochemical study. *Gastroenterology* **1983**, *85*, 1120–1130. [CrossRef]
21. Habib, A.M.; Richards, P.; Rogers, G.J.; Reimann, F.; Gribble, F.M. Co-localisation and secretion of glucagon-like peptide 1 and peptide YY from primary cultured human L cells. *Diabetologia* **2013**, *56*, 1413–1416. [CrossRef]
22. Batterham, R.L.; Bloom, S.R. The gut hormone peptide YY regulates appetite. *Ann. N. Y. Acad. Sci.* **2003**, *994*, 162–168. [CrossRef]
23. Holst, J.J. The physiology of glucagon-like peptide 1. *Physiol. Rev.* **2007**, *87*, 1409–1439. [CrossRef]
24. Alvarez Bartolome, M.; Borque, M.; Martinez-Sarmiento, J.; Aparicio, E.; Hernandez, C.; Cabrerizo, L.; Fernandez-Represa, J.A. Peptide YY secretion in morbidly obese patients before and after vertical banded gastroplasty. *Obes. Surg.* **2002**, *12*, 324–327. [CrossRef] [PubMed]
25. le Roux, C.W.; Batterham, R.L.; Aylwin, S.J.; Patterson, M.; Borg, C.M.; Wynne, K.J.; Kent, A.; Vincent, R.P.; Gardiner, J.; Ghatei, M.A.; et al. Attenuated peptide YY release in obese subjects is associated with reduced satiety. *Endocrinology* **2006**, *147*, 3–8. [CrossRef]
26. Spiller, R. Serotonin and GI clinical disorders. *Neuropharmacology* **2008**, *55*, 1072–1080. [CrossRef]
27. Morrison, S.F.; Madden, C.J.; Tupone, D. Central neural regulation of brown adipose tissue thermogenesis and energy expenditure. *Cell Metab.* **2014**, *19*, 741–756. [CrossRef]
28. Lund, M.L.; Egerod, K.L.; Engelstoft, M.S.; Dmytriyeva, O.; Theodorsson, E.; Patel, B.A.; Schwartz, T.W. Enterochromaffin 5-HT cells—A major target for GLP-1 and gut microbial metabolites. *Mol. Metab.* **2018**, *11*, 70–83. [CrossRef]
29. Halford, J.C.; Harrold, J.A.; Boyland, E.J.; Lawton, C.L.; Blundell, J.E. Serotonergic drugs: Effects on appetite expression and use for the treatment of obesity. *Drugs* **2007**, *67*, 27–55. [CrossRef]
30. France, M.; Skorich, E.; Kadrofske, M.; Swain, G.M.; Galligan, J.J. Sex-related differences in small intestinal transit and serotonin dynamics in high-fat-diet-induced obesity in mice. *Exp. Physiol.* **2016**, *101*, 81–99. [CrossRef]
31. Ritter, R.C. Gastrointestinal mechanisms of satiation for food. *Physiol. Behav.* **2004**, *81*, 249–273. [CrossRef]

32. Duca, F.A.; Lam, T.K. Gut microbiota, nutrient sensing and energy balance. *Diabetes Obes. Metab.* **2014**, *16* (Suppl. S1), 68–76. [CrossRef]
33. Crawley, J.N.; Corwin, R.L. Biological actions of cholecystokinin. *Peptides* **1994**, *15*, 731–755. [CrossRef]
34. Buffa, R.; Capella, C.; Fontana, P.; Usellini, L.; Solcia, E. Types of endocrine cells in the human colon and rectum. *Cell Tissue Res.* **1978**, *192*, 227–240. [CrossRef] [PubMed]
35. Reichlin, S. Secretion of somatostatin and its physiologic function. *J. Lab. Clin. Med.* **1987**, *109*, 320–326.
36. Patel, Y.C. Molecular pharmacology of somatostatin receptor subtypes. *J. Endocrinol. Investig.* **1997**, *20*, 348–367. [CrossRef] [PubMed]
37. Page, A.J.; Symonds, E.; Peiris, M.; Blackshaw, L.A.; Young, R.L. Peripheral neural targets in obesity. *Br. J. Pharmacol.* **2012**, *166*, 1537–1558. [CrossRef]
38. Tazoe, H.; Otomo, Y.; Karaki, S.; Kato, I.; Fukami, Y.; Terasaki, M.; Kuwahara, A. Expression of short-chain fatty acid receptor GPR41 in the human colon. *Biomed. Res.* **2009**, *30*, 149–156. [CrossRef]
39. McNabney, S.M.; Henagan, T.M. Short Chain Fatty Acids in the Colon and Peripheral Tissues: A Focus on Butyrate, Colon Cancer, Obesity and Insulin Resistance. *Nutrients* **2017**, *9*, 1348. [CrossRef]
40. Wong, T.P.; Chan, L.K.; Leung, P.S. Involvement of the Niacin Receptor GPR109a in the LocalControl of Glucose Uptake in Small Intestine of Type 2Diabetic Mice. *Nutrients* **2015**, *7*, 7543–7561. [CrossRef] [PubMed]
41. Lan, H.; Hoos, L.M.; Liu, L.; Tetzloff, G.; Hu, W.; Abbondanzo, S.J.; Vassileva, G.; Gustafson, E.L.; Hedrick, J.A.; Davis, H.R. Lack of FFAR1/GPR40 does not protect mice from high-fat diet-induced metabolic disease. *Diabetes* **2008**, *57*, 2999–3006. [CrossRef]
42. Paulsen, S.J.; Larsen, L.K.; Hansen, G.; Chelur, S.; Larsen, P.J.; Vrang, N. Expression of the fatty acid receptor GPR120 in the gut of diet-induced-obese rats and its role in GLP-1 secretion. *PLoS ONE* **2014**, *9*, e88227. [CrossRef] [PubMed]
43. Conigrave, A.D.; Brown, E.M. Taste receptors in the gastrointestinal tract. II. L-amino acid sensing by calcium-sensing receptors: Implications for GI physiology. *Am. J. Physiol. Gastrointest. Liver Physiol.* **2006**, *291*, G753–G761. [CrossRef] [PubMed]
44. Clemmensen, C.; Smajilovic, S.; Wellendorph, P.; Brauner-Osborne, H. The GPCR, class C, group 6, subtype A (GPRC6A) receptor: From cloning to physiological function. *Br. J. Pharmacol.* **2014**, *171*, 1129–1141. [CrossRef]
45. Symonds, E.L.; Peiris, M.; Page, A.J.; Chia, B.; Dogra, H.; Masding, A.; Galanakis, V.; Atiba, M.; Bulmer, D.; Young, R.L.; et al. Mechanisms of activation of mouse and human enteroendocrine cells by nutrients. *Gut* **2015**, *64*, 618–626. [CrossRef]
46. Chambers, E.S.; Viardot, A.; Psichas, A.; Morrison, D.J.; Murphy, K.G.; Zac-Varghese, S.E.; MacDougall, K.; Preston, T.; Tedford, C.; Finlayson, G.S.; et al. Effects of targeted delivery of propionate to the human colon on appetite regulation, body weight maintenance and adiposity in overweight adults. *Gut* **2015**, *64*, 1744–1754. [CrossRef]
47. Reimann, F.; Tolhurst, G.; Gribble, F.M. G-protein-coupled receptors in intestinal chemosensation. *Cell Metab.* **2012**, *15*, 421–431. [CrossRef]
48. Martin, A.M.; Lumsden, A.L.; Young, R.L.; Jessup, C.F.; Spencer, N.J.; Keating, D.J. The nutrient-sensing repertoires of mouse enterochromaffin cells differ between duodenum and colon. *Neurogastroenterol. Motil.* **2017**, *29*, e13046. [CrossRef] [PubMed]
49. Peiris, M.; Aktar, R.; Raynel, S.; Hao, Z.; Mumphrey, M.B.; Berthoud, H.R.; Blackshaw, L.A. Effects of Obesity and Gastric Bypass Surgery on Nutrient Sensors, Endocrine Cells, and Mucosal Innervation of the Mouse Colon. *Nutrients* **2018**, *10*, 1529. [CrossRef] [PubMed]
50. Rodriguez-Pacheco, F.; Garcia-Serrano, S.; Garcia-Escobar, E.; Gutierrez-Repiso, C.; Garcia-Arnes, J.; Valdes, S.; Gonzalo, M.; Soriguer, F.; Moreno-Ruiz, F.J.; Rodriguez-Canete, A.; et al. Effects of obesity/fatty acids on the expression of GPR120. *Mol. Nutr. Food Res.* **2014**, *58*, 1852–1860. [CrossRef] [PubMed]
51. Oh, D.Y.; Olefsky, J.M. Omega 3 fatty acids and GPR120. *Cell Metab.* **2012**, *15*, 564–565. [CrossRef]
52. le Roux, C.W.; Aylwin, S.J.; Batterham, R.L.; Borg, C.M.; Coyle, F.; Prasad, V.; Shurey, S.; Ghatei, M.A.; Patel, A.G.; Bloom, S.R. Gut hormone profiles following bariatric surgery favor an anorectic state, facilitate weight loss, and improve metabolic parameters. *Ann. Surg.* **2006**, *243*, 108–114. [CrossRef] [PubMed]
53. Sumithran, P.; Prendergast, L.A.; Delbridge, E.; Purcell, K.; Shulkes, A.; Kriketos, A.; Proietto, J. Long-term persistence of hormonal adaptations to weight loss. *N. Engl. J. Med.* **2011**, *365*, 1597–1604. [CrossRef] [PubMed]
54. Wilms, E.; Jonkers, D.M.A.E.; Savelkoul, H.F.J.; Elizalde, M.; Tischmann, L.; de Vos, P.; Masclee, A.A.M.; Troost, F.J. The Impact of Pectin Supplementation on Intestinal Barrier Function in Healthy Young Adults and Healthy Elderly. *Nutrients* **2019**, *11*, 1554. [CrossRef]
55. Vork, L.; Weerts, Z.; Mujagic, Z.; Kruimel, J.W.; Hesselink, M.A.M.; Muris, J.W.M.; Keszthelyi, D.; Jonkers, D.; Masclee, A.A.M. Rome III vs Rome IV criteria for irritable bowel syndrome: A comparison of clinical characteristics in a large cohort study. *Neurogastroenterol. Motil. Off. J. Eur. Gastrointest. Motil. Soc.* **2018**, *30*, e13189. [CrossRef] [PubMed]
56. Young, R.L.; Lumsden, A.L.; Martin, A.M.; Schober, G.; Pezos, N.; Thazhath, S.S.; Isaacs, N.J.; Cvijanovic, N.; Sun, E.W.L.; Wu, T.; et al. Augmented capacity for peripheral serotonin release in human obesity. *Int. J. Obes.* **2018**, *42*, 1880–1889. [CrossRef] [PubMed]
57. Schwartz, M.W.; Peskind, E.; Raskind, M.; Boyko, E.J.; Porte, D., Jr. Cerebrospinal fluid leptin levels: Relationship to plasma levels and to adiposity in humans. *Nat. Med.* **1996**, *2*, 589–593. [CrossRef]
58. Goldspink, D.A.; Lu, V.B.; Miedzybrodzka, E.L.; Smith, C.A.; Foreman, R.E.; Billing, L.J.; Kay, R.G.; Reimann, F.; Gribble, F.M. Labeling and Characterization of Human GLP-1-Secreting L-cells in Primary Ileal Organoid Culture. *Cell Rep.* **2020**, *31*, 107833. [CrossRef]

59. Ichimura, A.; Hirasawa, A.; Poulain-Godefroy, O.; Bonnefond, A.; Hara, T.; Yengo, L.; Kimura, I.; Leloire, A.; Liu, N.; Iida, K.; et al. Dysfunction of lipid sensor GPR120 leads to obesity in both mouse and human. *Nature* **2012**, *483*, 350–354. [CrossRef]
60. Little, T.J.; Isaacs, N.J.; Young, R.L.; Ott, R.; Nguyen, N.Q.; Rayner, C.K.; Horowitz, M.; Feinle-Bisset, C. Characterization of duodenal expression and localization of fatty acid-sensing receptors in humans: Relationships with body mass index. *Am. J. Physiol. Gastrointest. Liver Physiol.* **2014**, *307*, G958–G967. [CrossRef]
61. Liou, A.P.; Paziuk, M.; Luevano, J.M., Jr.; Machineni, S.; Turnbaugh, P.J.; Kaplan, L.M. Conserved shifts in the gut microbiota due to gastric bypass reduce host weight and adiposity. *Sci. Transl. Med.* **2013**, *5*, 178ra141. [CrossRef]
62. Tremaroli, V.; Backhed, F. Functional interactions between the gut microbiota and host metabolism. *Nature* **2012**, *489*, 242–249. [CrossRef]
63. Samuel, B.S.; Shaito, A.; Motoike, T.; Rey, F.E.; Backhed, F.; Manchester, J.K.; Hammer, R.E.; Williams, S.C.; Crowley, J.; Yanagisawa, M.; et al. Effects of the gut microbiota on host adiposity are modulated by the short-chain fatty-acid binding G protein-coupled receptor, Gpr41. *Proc. Natl. Acad. Sci. USA* **2008**, *105*, 16767–16772. [CrossRef]
64. Tolhurst, G.; Heffron, H.; Lam, Y.S.; Parker, H.E.; Habib, A.M.; Diakogiannaki, E.; Cameron, J.; Grosse, J.; Reimann, F.; Gribble, F.M. Short-Chain Fatty Acids Stimulate Glucagon-Like Peptide-1 Secretion via the G-Protein–Coupled Receptor FFAR2. *Diabetes* **2012**, *61*, 364–371. [CrossRef]
65. Tang, L.; Cheng, C.Y.; Sun, X.; Pedicone, A.J.; Mohamadzadeh, M.; Cheng, S.X. The Extracellular Calcium-Sensing Receptor in the Intestine: Evidence for Regulation of Colonic Absorption, Secretion, Motility, and Immunity. *Front. Physiol.* **2016**, *7*, 245. [CrossRef]
66. Guo, Y.; Ma, L.; Enriori, P.J.; Koska, J.; Franks, P.W.; Brookshire, T.; Cowley, M.A.; Salbe, A.D.; Delparigi, A.; Tataranni, P.A. Physiological evidence for the involvement of peptide YY in the regulation of energy homeostasis in humans. *Obesity* **2006**, *14*, 1562–1570. [CrossRef]

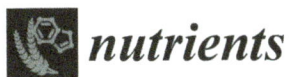

Article

Cannabinoid CB$_1$ Receptors in the Intestinal Epithelium Are Required for Acute Western-Diet Preferences in Mice

Bryant Avalos [1], Donovan A. Argueta [1,2], Pedro A. Perez [1], Mark Wiley [1], Courtney Wood [1] and Nicholas V. DiPatrizio [1,*]

1. Division of Biomedical Sciences, School of Medicine, University of California, Riverside, Riverside, CA 92521, USA; baval002@ucr.edu (B.A.); daarguet@hs.uci.edu (D.A.A.); Pedro.Perez@medsch.ucr.edu (P.A.P.); Mark.Wiley@medsch.ucr.edu (M.W.); cwood019@ucr.edu (C.W.)
2. Department of Medicine, School of Medicine, University of California, Irvine, Irvine, CA 92697, USA
* Correspondence: ndipatri@medsch.ucr.edu; Tel.: +1-951-827-7252

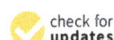

Received: 29 August 2020; Accepted: 17 September 2020; Published: 20 September 2020

Abstract: The endocannabinoid system plays an important role in the intake of palatable food. For example, endocannabinoid signaling in the upper small-intestinal epithelium is increased (i) in rats after tasting dietary fats, which promotes intake of fats, and (ii) in a mouse model of diet-induced obesity, which promotes overeating via impaired nutrient-induced gut–brain satiation signaling. We now utilized a combination of genetic, pharmacological, and behavioral approaches to identify roles for cannabinoid CB$_1$Rs in upper small-intestinal epithelium in preferences for a western-style diet (WD, high-fat/sucrose) versus a standard rodent diet (SD, low-fat/no sucrose). Mice were maintained on SD in automated feeding chambers. During testing, mice were given simultaneous access to SD and WD, and intakes were recorded. Mice displayed large preferences for the WD, which were inhibited by systemic pretreatment with the cannabinoid CB$_1$R antagonist/inverse agonist, AM251, for up to 3 h. We next used our novel intestinal epithelium-specific conditional cannabinoid CB$_1$R-deficient mice (IntCB$_1$−/−) to investigate if intestinal CB$_1$Rs are necessary for WD preferences. Similar to AM251 treatment, preferences for WD were largely absent in IntCB$_1$−/− mice when compared to control mice for up to 6 h. Together, these data suggest that CB$_1$Rs in the murine intestinal epithelium are required for acute WD preferences.

Keywords: endocannabinoid; cannabinoid CB$_1$ receptor; gut–brain; intestine; western diet; preference

1. Introduction

Humans and other mammals, when given a choice, generally prefer food that contains fats, sugars, or a combination of both [1]. Homeostatic and hedonic feeding are controlled by diverse, albeit overlapping, neural and molecular signaling pathways throughout the brain, including those regulated by the endocannabinoid (eCB) system [2–5]. Recent studies, however, suggest important roles for the peripheral eCB system in energy homeostasis and intake of palatable food [6–29]. For example, we reported that tasting dietary lipids was sufficient to increase levels of eCBs in the rat upper small-intestinal epithelium, which required an intact vagus nerve, and pharmacological inhibition of cannabinoid subtype-1 receptors (CB$_1$Rs) in the periphery blocked consumption of lipids [14,15]. Moreover, levels of eCBs in the upper small-intestinal epithelium were increased in mice maintained for eight weeks on a western-style diet high in fat and sugar (WD) when compared to mice fed a standard diet low in fat and sugar, and pharmacological inhibition of CB$_1$Rs in the periphery blocked overeating associated with WD-induced obesity [17].

Nutrients are sensed by gustatory cells in the oral cavity and enteroendocrine cells in the intestinal epithelium. In response, these cells release several satiation- and satiety-related molecules that communicate with the brain via a mechanism that includes the afferent vagus nerve [30–38]. We recently reported that eCB signaling in the gut controls nutrient-induced release of satiation peptides [16]. Gene transcripts for CB_1Rs were enriched in a subpopulation of enteroendocrine cells in the upper small-intestinal epithelium that secrete the satiation peptide, cholecystokinin [16,39]. Notably, the ability for nutrients to stimulate an increase in levels of circulating cholecystokinin was impaired in mice fed WD for eight weeks when compared to lean control mice, and pharmacological inhibition of overactive eCB signaling at peripheral CB_1Rs in mice fed WD restored the ability for nutrients to induce release of cholecystokinin [16]. Furthermore, the appetite-suppressing effects of peripheral CB_1R inhibition in mice maintained on WD were attenuated by co-treatment with an antagonist for cholecystokinin-A receptors [16], which are expressed by sensory vagal neurons and other organs [40]. Collectively, these studies suggest that eCB signaling in upper small-intestinal epithelium is dysregulated in WD-induced obese mice and promotes overeating by a mechanism that includes blocking nutrient-induced gut–brain satiation signaling.

In the current study, we used a novel conditional intestinal epithelium-specific CB_1R-deficient mouse model to investigate if CB_1Rs in the intestinal epithelium are required for WD preferences.

2. Materials and Methods

2.1. Animals

C57BL/6Tac male mice (Taconic, Oxnard, CA, USA) or transgenic mice (described below in Transgenic Mouse Generation) 8–10 weeks of age were group-housed with ad-libitum access to a standard rodent laboratory diet (SD; Teklad 2020x, Envigo, Huntingdon, UK; 16% kcal from fat, 24% kcal from protein, 60% kcal from carbohydrates) and water throughout all experiments. Mice were maintained on a 12-h dark/light cycle beginning at 1800 h. All procedures met the U.S. National Institute of Health guidelines for care and use of laboratory animals and were approved by the Institutional Animal Care and Use Committee (IACUC Protocol 20200023) of the University of California, Riverside.

2.2. Transgenic Mouse Generation

Conditional intestinal epithelium-specific CB_1R-deficient mice ($Cnr1^{tm1.1\,mrl}$/vil-cre ERT2) were generated by crossing Cnr1-floxed mice ($Cnr1^{tm1.1\,mrl}$; Taconic, Oxnard, CA, USA; Model # 7599) with Vil-CRE ERT2 mice donated by Dr. Randy Seeley (University of Michigan, Ann Arbor, MI, USA) with permission from Dr. Sylvie Robin (Curie Institute, Paris, France). Cre recombinase expression in the intestinal epithelium is driven by the villin promotor, which allows for conditional tamoxifen-dependent Cre recombinase action to remove the *Cnr1* gene from these cells, as described by el Marjou et al., [41]. When compared to other mouse lines that exhibit extra-intestinal expression of CRE recombinase, the Vil-CRE ERT2 mice used in our studies show selective expression in the intestinal epithelium with scattered expression in the testis [42]. $Cnr1^{tm1.1\,mrl}$/vil-cre ERT2 mice used in these experiments are referred to as $IntCB_1-/-$, and $Cnr1^{tm1.1\,mrl}$ control mice (lacking Cre recombinase) are referred to as $IntCB_1+/+$. Tail snips were collected from pups at weaning and DNA was extracted and analyzed by conventional PCR using the following primers (5′-3′): GCAGGGATTATGTCCCTAGC (CNR1-ALT), CTGTTACCAGGAGTCTTAGC (1415-35), GGCTCAAGGAATACACTTATACC (1415-37), GAACCTGATGGACATGTTCAGG (vilcre, AA), AGTGCGTTCGAACGCTAGAGCCTGT (vilcre, SS), TTACGTCCATCGTGG-ACAGC (vilcre, MYO F), TGGGCTGGGTGTTAGCCTTA (vilcre, MYO R).

2.3. Western Diet Preference Test

Mice were single-housed in two-hopper feeding chambers (TSE Systems, Chesterfield, MO, USA) for five days to acclimate, and received ad-libitum access to SD and water throughout behavioral testing. At the time of testing, mice were given access for the first time to the hopper containing

Western Diet (WD; Research Diets D12079B, New Brunswick, NJ, USA; 40% kcal from fat, 17% kcal from protein, 43% kcal from carbohydrates as mostly sucrose). Food weights were measured in real time and recorded every minute using Phenomaster software (TSE Systems). Preferences for WD versus SD (% total kcals from WD), total caloric intake of each diet (kcals), average meal size of each diet (kcals), and meal frequency were calculated from recorded data, beginning one hour before the dark cycle (1700 h). The criteria for a meal was consumption of a minimum of 0.1 g of food with an inter-meal interval less than 30 min.

2.4. Chemical Preparation and Administration

IntCB$_1$−/− and IntCB$_1$+/+ mice were administered tamoxifen (Intraperitoneal, 40 mg per kg) every 24 h for five consecutive days. Tamoxifen (Sigma-Aldrich, St. Louis, MO, USA) was dissolved in corn oil at a concentration of 10 mg per mL then stored at 37 °C protected from light until administration. Tamoxifen in corn oil was placed in a bath sonicator for 10 min prior to administration. Mice were group housed in disposable cages throughout the injection window and for a 3-day post-injection period. The CB$_1$R antagonist/inverse agonist, AM251 (Tocris, Minneapolis, MN, USA), was administered (Intraperitoneal, 3 mg per kg per 2 mL) 30 min prior to testing. The vehicle consisted of 7.5% dimethyl sulfoxide (DMSO, Sigma-Aldrich, St. Louis, MO, USA), 7.5% Tween 80 (Chem Implex Intl Inc., Wood Dale, IL, USA), and 85% sterile saline.

2.5. Immunohistochemistry

Proximal small intestinal tissue was collected from IntCB$_1$−/− and IntCB$_1$+/+ control mice 7 days after the completion of tamoxifen schedule. Tissue was flushed with ice-cold 4% paraformaldehyde/phosphate-buffered saline then fixed for 4 h at 4 °C. Cross sections of the upper small intestine were cut and frozen in embedding medium (Fisher Healthcare, Chino, CA, USA) on dry ice. Approximately 16 μm sections were obtained using a cryostat (Leica, Wetzlar, Germany) then mounted onto charged glass slides. Sections were permeabilized with 0.5% Tween20/PBS and then blocked with 0.1% Tween20 in casein solution (Thermo Fisher, Waltham, MA, USA). Primary antibodies for CB$_1$Rs (kindly provided by Dr. Ken Mackie, Indiana University, Bloomington, IL, USA) raised in rabbit were diluted 1:500 in blocking buffer, slides were incubated for 1 h at room temperature. Sections were washed three times with 0.1% Tween20/PBS solution then incubated for 1 h at room temperature with goat anti-rabbit secondary antibodies conjugated with alexafluor 647. Following repeated washes, coverslips were mounted with Prolong Gold Antifade reagent with DAPI (Thermo Fisher) for nuclear counterstaining. Images were obtained at room temperature using an Axio Observer Z1 Inverted Microscope (Zeiss, Oberkochen, Germany) as previously described [16].

2.6. Gene Expression

Total RNA from intestinal epithelium tissue was extracted using a RNeasy kit (Qiagen, Valencia, CA, USA) and first-strand cDNA was generated using M-MLV reverse transcriptase (Invitrogen, Carlsbad, CA, USA). Areas used for tissue collection and processing were sanitized with 70% ethanol solution then treated with an RNAse inhibitor (RNAse out, G-Biosciences, St. Louis, MO, USA). Reverse transcription of total RNA was performed as previously described [16]. Quantitative RT-PCR was performed using PrimePCR Assays (Biorad, Irvine, CA, USA) with primers for CB$_1$R (Cnr1), CB$_2$R (Cnr2), g-protein coupled receptor 55 (Gpr55), diacylglycerol lipase alpha (Dagla), diacylglycerol lipase beta (Daglb), monoacylglycerol lipase (Mgll), alpha beta hydrolase domain containing 6 (Abhd6), N-acyl-phosphatidylethanolamine-hydrolyzing phospholipase D (Napepld), and fatty acid amide hydrolase (Faah) gene transcripts under preconfigured SYBR Green assays (Biorad, Irvine, CA, USA). Relative quantification using the delta-delta ($2^{-\Delta\Delta Cq}$) method was used to compare changes in gene expression between IntCB$_1$−/− mice and control IntCB$_1$+/+ mice. Tissue specific housekeeping genes served as internal controls and were validated by verifying that expression was not affected between experimental conditions. Hprt was used as a housekeeping gene for stomach, duodenum intestinal epithelium, jejunum intestinal epithelium, ileum intestinal epithelium, small-intestinal submucosa/muscle/serosal layer, large intestinal epithelium, and liver; β-actin (Actb) as housekeeping gene for pancreas; and β2-microglobulin (B2m) as housekeeping gene for epididymal fat. Reactions were run in triplicate and values are expressed as relative mRNA expression.

2.7. Statistical Analysis

Data were analyzed by GraphPad Prism 8 software using unpaired Student's *t*-tests (two-tailed) or two-way ANOVA with Holm-Sidak's multiple comparisons post-hoc test when appropriate. Results are expressed as means ± S.E.M. and significance was determined at $p < 0.05$.

3. Results

3.1. Systemic Pharmacological Blockade of CB_1Rs Reduces Acute Preferences for Western Diet in Mice

We investigated roles for cannabinoid CB_1 receptors in preferences for Western Diet (WD). Naïve mice maintained on ad-libitum standard laboratory chow diet (SD) were administered the vehicle or the cannabinoid CB_1R antagonist/inverse agonist, AM251 (3mg per kg), and subjected to a 24 h preference test for WD versus SD. Vehicle-treated mice displayed robust preferences for WD when compared to SD, an effect inhibited by AM251 by 3 h (Figure 1a, from 84.7 ± 7.1% total kcals from WD in vehicle-treated mice compared to 58.7 ± 8.3% in AM251-treated mice; $p = 0.042$). These effects were absent during the 3–6 h interval (Figure 1b, from 92.4 ± 3.5% total kcals from WD in vehicle-treated mice compared to 81.9 ± 8.0% in AM251-treated mice; $p = 0.25$), and the 6–12 h interval (Figure 1c from 98.0 ± 1.9% total kcals from WD in vehicle-treated mice compared to 96.9 ± 2.1% in AM251-treated mice; $p = 0.69$) after initiation of the preference test. Vehicle-treated mice displayed significant reductions in preference for WD during the 12–24 h interval when compared to AM251-treated mice, (Figure 1d, from 70.9 ± 8.7% total kcals from WD in vehicle-treated mice compared to 93.85 ± 3.57% in AM251-treated mice; $p = 0.024$). Which was due to increases in SD intake in vehicle-treated mice during the 12–24 h interval (see Figure 1h) rather than an actual increase in preference for WD in AM251-treated mice.

Consistent with these data, vehicle-treated mice ate significantly more kcals from WD than from SD by 3 h (Figure 1e, $p = 0.046$), during the 6–12 h interval (Figure 1g, $p = 0.019$), and the 12–24 h interval (Figure 1h, $p = 0.009$), but not during the 3–6 h interval (Figure 1f, $p = 0.09$) after initiation of the preference test. These effects were absent in mice treated with AM251 by 3 h (Figure 1e, $p = 0.951$), during the 3–6 h interval (Figure 1f, $p = 0.588$), and the 12–24 h interval (Figure 1h, $p = 0.151$); however, mice consumed significantly more WD than SD during the 6–12 h interval (Figure 1g, $p = 0.028$). Moreover, vehicle-treated mice displayed larger meal sizes of WD versus SD by 3 h (Figure 1i, $p = 0.028$), an effect that failed to reach significance during the 3–6 h interval (Figure 1j, $p = 0.359$), the 6–12 h interval (Figure 1k, $p = 0.42$), and the 12–24 h interval after initiation of the preference test (Figure 1l, $p = 0.396$). Increases in meal size for WD by 3 h were absent in mice treated with AM251 (Figure 1i, $p = 0.816$). AM251 had no effect on meal frequency by 3h (Figure 1m, $p = 0.189$), during the 3–6 h interval (Figure 1n, $p = 0.629$), the 6–12 h interval (Figure 1o, $p = 0.071$) and the 12–24 h interval (Figure 1p, $p = 0.95$) after initiation of the preference test. In addition, there were no significant differences in total cumulative caloric intake (i.e., total kcals from WD + SD) between treatment groups by 3 h (Figure 1q, $p = 0.501$), during the 3–6 h interval (Figure 1r, $p = 0.569$), and the 6–12 h interval after initiation of the preference test (Figure 1s, $p = 0.619$). Despite large preferences for WD in AM251-treated mice during the 12–24 h interval (see Figure 1d), these mice consumed significantly less total calories during the 12–24 h interval after initiation of the preference test (Figure 1t, $p = 0.002$). Collectively, these results suggest that cannabinoid CB_1Rs control acute preferences for WD in mice.

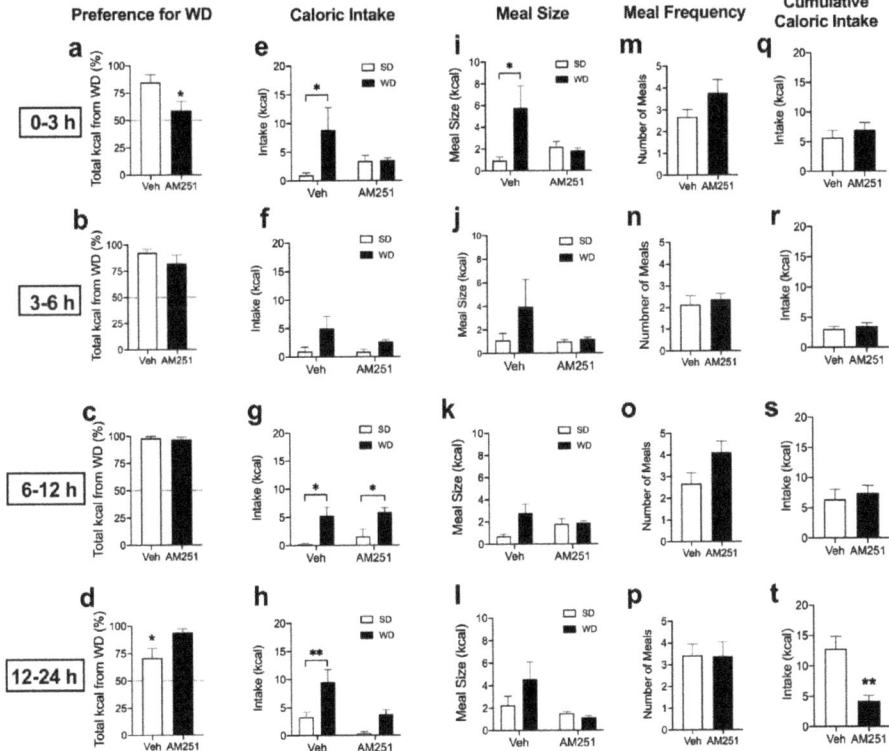

Figure 1. Cannabinoid CB_1Rs control acute preferences for Western Diet. Veh = vehicle treatment; AM251 = 3mg per kg; SD = standard rodent chow; WD = western diet. Unpaired Student's *t*-test, two-tailed (**a–d,m–t**); Two-way ANOVA with Holm-Sidak's multiple comparison tests (**e–l**); * = $p < 0.05$, ** = $p < 0.01$. Results are expressed as means ± S.E.M; $n = 7$–8 per condition.

3.2. Acute Preferences for Western Diet are Absent in Mice with CB_1R Deletion in the Intestinal Epithelium

Endocannabinoid signaling in the rodent upper small-intestinal epithelium is important for consumption of dietary fats based on their taste properties [14,15], re-feeding after a fast [10], and hyperphagia in a mouse model of WD-induced obesity via a mechanism that includes blocking nutrient-induced gut–brain satiation signaling [16,17]. We used our novel intestinal epithelium-specific conditional CB_1R-deficient mice (IntCB1−/−) to probe the necessity for CB_1Rs in the intestinal epithelium in preferences for WD. Moreover, AM251 is reported to have some off-target effects [43,44]; therefore, this mouse model allows for direct evaluation of roles for CB_1Rs in the intestinal epithelium in these processes. CB_1R deficiency in the intestinal epithelium of IntCB$_1$−/− mice was verified by immunohistochemistry (Figure 2a–d).

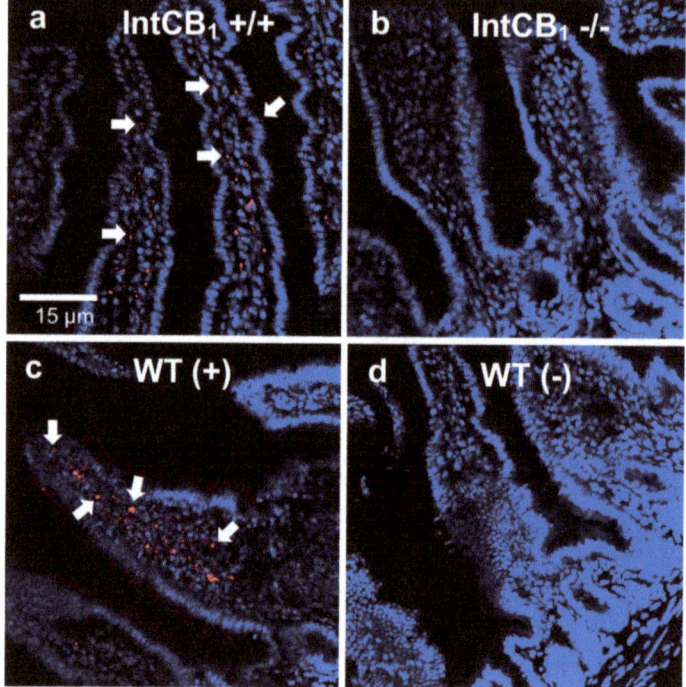

Figure 2. CB_1R immunoreactivity is absent in the upper small-intestinal epithelium of conditional intestinal epithelium-specific CB_1R-deficient mice. When compared to control mice (**a**, IntCB +/+), conditional intestinal epithelium-specific CB_1R-null mice (**b**, $IntCB_1-/-$) are deficient in immunoreactivity for CB_1Rs in the upper small-intestinal epithelium. Wild-type C57BL/6Tac mice display immunoreactivity for CB_1Rs in the upper small-intestinal epithelium (**c**, WT (+)), which is absent when the primary CB_1R antibody is not included (**d**, WT(-)). White arrows point to representative red immunoreactivity for CB_1Rs. Red = CB_1R immunoreactivity; blue = DAPI. WT = wild-type mice. (+) = with CB_1R primary antibody; (-) = without CB_1R primary antibody.

CB_1R deficiency in the intestinal epithelium of $IntCB_1-/-$ mice was further confirmed by qRT-PCR (Figure 3a,b). $IntCB_1-/-$ mice, when compared to $IntCB_1+/+$ controls, were deficient in expression of mRNA for CB_1Rs (*Cnr1*) in the jejunum epithelium (Figure 3a, $p = 0.031$). Expression of mRNA for other components of the endocannabinoid system in the jejunum epithelium was unaffected, including cannabinoid CB_2Rs (*Cnr2*; Figure 3a, $p = 0.892$), g-protein coupled receptor 55 (*Gpr55*; Figure 3a, $p = 0.736$), diacylglycerol lipase alpha (*Dagla*; Figure 3a, $p = 0.825$), diacylglycerol lipase beta (*Daglb*; Figure 3a, $p = 0.798$), monoacylglycerol lipase (*Mgll*; Figure 3a, $p = 0.872$), alpha beta hydrolase domain containing 6 (*Abhd6*; Figure 3a, $p = 0.314$), N-acyl-phosphatidylethanolamine-hydrolyzing phospholipase D (*Napepld*; Figure 3a, $p = 0.217$), and fatty acid amide hydrolase (*Faah*; Figure 3a, $p = 0.986$). In addition to the jejunum epithelium, $IntCB_1-/-$ mice were deficient in expression of mRNA for CB_1Rs (*Cnr1*) in the duodenum epithelium (Figure 3b, $p = 0.009$), ileum epithelium (Figure 3b, $p = 0.038$), large intestine epithelium (Figure 3b, $p = 0.039$), but not in the small-intestinal submucosa/muscle/serosal layers (Figure 3b, $p = 0.633$), stomach (Figure 3b, $p = 0.602$), liver (Figure 3b, $p = 0.593$), pancreas (Figure 3b, $p = 0.9$), and epididymal fat (Figure 3b, $p = 0.14$).

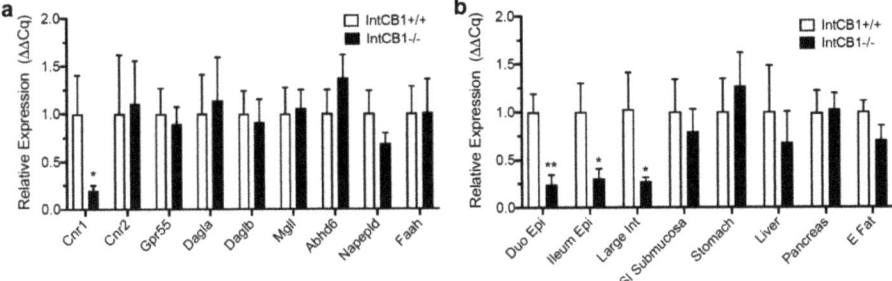

Figure 3. Expression of endocannabinoid system genes in conditional intestinal epithelium-specific CB_1R-deficient mice and controls. Expression of cannabinoid CB_1Rs (*Cnr1*) was reduced in the jejunum epithelium of conditional intestinal epithelium-specific CB_1R deficient mice ($IntCB_1-/-$) when compared to control mice ($IntCB_1+/+$) (**a**), and expression of mRNA for other components of the endocannabinoid system was unaffected, including cannabinoid CB_2Rs (*Cnr2*), g-protein coupled receptor 55 (*Gpr5*), diacylglycerol lipase alpha (*Dagla*), diacylglycerol lipase beta (*Daglb*), monoacylglycerol lipase (*Mgll*), alpha beta hydrolase domain containing 6 (*Abhd6*), N-acyl-phosphatidylethanolamine-hydrolyzing phospholipase D (*Napepld*), and fatty acid amide hydrolase (*Faah*) (**a**). $IntCB_1-/-$ mice, when compared to IntCB1+/+ controls, were deficient in expression of mRNA for CB_1Rs (*Cnr1*) in the duodenum epithelium (Duo Epi), ileum epithelium (Ileum Epi), large intestine (Large Int), but not in the small-intestinal submucosa/muscle/serosal layers (SI Submucosa), stomach, liver, pancreas, and epididymal fat (E Fat) (**b**). Unpaired Student's *t*-tests, two-tailed; * = $p < 0.05$, ** = $p < 0.01$. Results are expressed as means ± S.E.M; n = 5–8 per condition.

$IntCB_1-/-$ and $IntCB_1+/+$ control mice displayed similar body weights (Figure 4a, $p = 0.404$), and baseline 24-h caloric intake (Figure 4b, $p = 0.52$), 24-h water intake (Figure 4c, $p = 0.487$), average meal size (Figure 4d, $p = 0.653$), ambulation (Figure 4e, $p = 0.741$), and glucose clearance during an oral glucose tolerance test (Figure 4f,g; 15, 30, 60, 120 min; ns; total area under curve, $p = 0.847$).

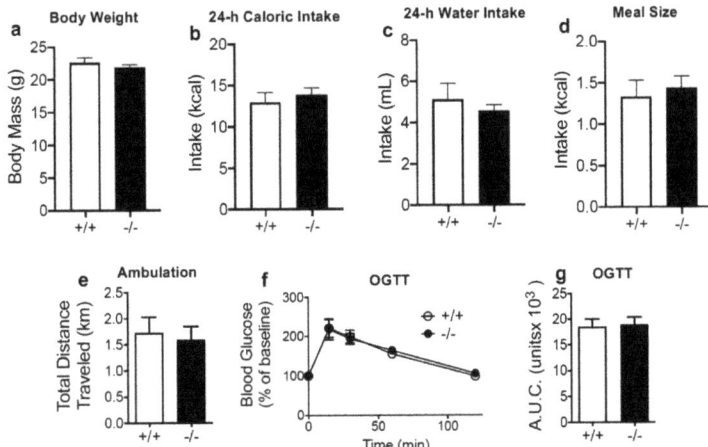

Figure 4. Conditional intestinal epithelium CB_1R-deficient mice display no changes in baseline feeding parameters, motor activity, or glucose clearance. Unpaired Student's *t*-test, two-tailed (**a–e,g**; $p > 0.05$); two-way Repeated Measures ANOVA with Holm-Sidak's multiple comparison tests (**f**; not significant). Results are expressed as means ± S.E.M; n = 7–8 per condition (**a–e**), n = 3–4 (**f,g**). +/+ = $IntCB_1+/+$ mice, −/− = $IntCB_1-/-$ mice; OGTT = oral glucose tolerance test; AUC = area under the curve.

Control IntCB$_1$+/+ mice displayed robust preferences for WD when compared to SD, an effect largely absent in IntCB$_1$−/− mice by 3 h (Figure 5a, from 92.8 ± 2.8% total kcals from WD in IntCB$_1$+/+ mice compared to 46.5 ± 12.5% in IntCB$_1$−/− mice; $p = 0.029$), and approaching significance during the 3–6 h interval (Figure 5b, from 96.2 ± 3.8% total kcals from WD in IntCB$_1$+/+ mice compared to 46.9 ± 16.5% in IntCB$_1$−/− mice; $p = 0.06$). Preferences for WD in IntCB$_1$−/− mice were not different from controls by the 6–12 h interval (Figure 5c, from 94.0 ± 3.8% total kcals from WD in IntCB$_1$+/+ mice compared to 87.6 ± 5.8% in IntCB$_1$−/− mice; $p = 0.49$) and the 12–24 h interval (Figure 5d, from 94.5 ± 5.5% total kcals from WD in IntCB$_1$+/+ mice compared to 89.5 ± 6.4% in IntCB$_1$−/− mice; $p = 0.633$) after initiation of the preference test.

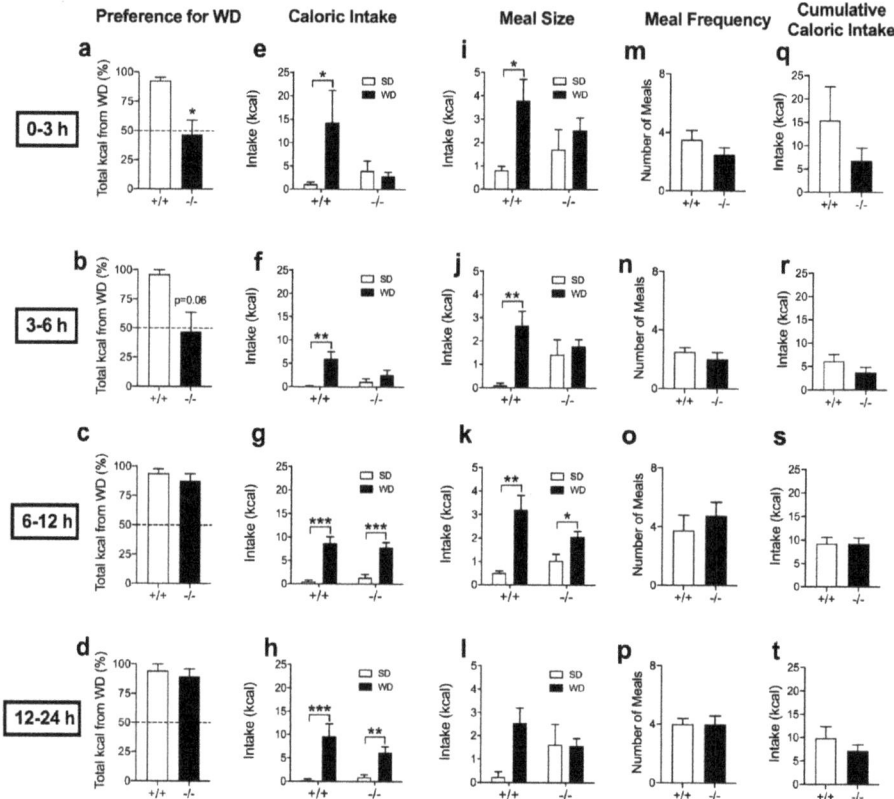

Figure 5. Acute preferences for western diet are absent in conditional intestinal epithelium-specific CB$_1$R-deficient mice. +/+ = IntCB$_1$+/+ control mice; −/− = IntCB$_1$−/− mice; SD = standard rodent chow; WD = western diet. Unpaired Student's t-test, two-tailed (**a–d,m–t**); Two-way ANOVA with Holm-Sidak's multiple comparison tests (**e–l**); * = $p < 0.05$, ** = $p < 0.01$, *** = $p < 0.001$. Results are expressed as means ± S.E.M; n = 4–8 per condition.

Congruent with these data, control IntCB$_1$+/+ mice ate significantly more kcals from WD when compared to SD by 3 h (Figure 5e, $p = 0.02$), during the 3–6 h interval (Figure 5f, $p = 0.004$), the 6–12 h interval (Figure 5g, $p < 0.001$), and the 12–24 h interval (Figure 5h, $p < 0.001$) after initiation of the preference test. These effects were absent in IntCB$_1$−/− mice by 3 h (Figure 5e, $p = 0.732$), and during the 3–6 h interval (Figure 5f, $p = 0.205$); however, intakes for WD rebounded in IntCB$_1$−/− mice by the 6–12 h interval (Figure 5g, $p < 0.001$) and during the 12–24 h interval (Figure 5h, $p = 0.002$). Moreover, IntCB$_1$+/+ mice displayed larger meal sizes of WD versus SD by 3 h (Figure 5i, $p = 0.031$), during the

3–6 h interval (Figure 5j, $p = 0.005$), and the 6–12 h interval (Figure 5k, $p = 0.002$), but not during the 12–24 h interval (Figure 5l, $p = 0.072$) after initiation of the preference test. These effects were absent in IntCB$_1$−/− mice by 3 h (Figure 5i, $p = 0.404$), during the 3–6 h interval (Figure 5j, $p = 0.589$), and the 12–24 h interval (Figure 5l, $p = 0.958$); however, meal size of WD versus SD was increased in IntCB$_1$−/− mice during the 6–12 h interval (Figure 5k, $p = 0.044$). No significant changes were found in meal frequency for IntCB$_1$−/− mice when compared to IntCB$_1$+/+ controls by 3 h (Figure 5m, $p = 0.239$), during the 3–6 h interval (Figure 5n, $p = 0.49$), the 6–12 h interval (Figure 5o, $p = 0.521$), and the 12–24 h interval (Figure 5p, $p = 0.99$) after initiation of the preference test. In addition, no significant changes were found in total cumulative caloric intake (i.e., total kcals from WD + SD) for IntCB$_1$−/− mice when compared to IntCB$_1$+/+ controls by 3 h (Figure 5q, $p = 0.196$), during the 3–6 h interval (Figure 5r, $p = 0.233$), the 6–12 h interval (Figure 5s, $p = 0.974$), and the 12–24 h interval (Figure 5t, $p = 0.305$) after initiation of the preference test.

4. Discussion

We report that acute preferences for WD (i) were inhibited by global pharmacological blockade of CB$_1$Rs, and (ii) were largely absent in mice conditionally deficient in CB$_1$Rs selectively in the intestinal epithelium. These results suggest that CB$_1$Rs in the intestinal epithelium are required for acute WD preferences in mice. Moreover, these studies expand our understanding of critical pathways for gut–brain communication in the control of preferences for palatable foods.

Dietary components are detected by receptors located throughout the oral cavity [36] and intestinal epithelium [45], which provide feedback associated with the nutritional content of food and contribute to determination of food preferences. For example, we reported that tasting dietary unsaturated lipids—but not sugar or protein—triggered production of endocannabinoids in the rat upper small-intestinal epithelium, and pharmacological inhibition of endocannabinoid signaling at CB$_1$Rs in the periphery blocked intake and preferences for fats in a sham-feeding model [14,15]. These studies suggest that endocannabinoid signaling in the gut contributes to the positive feedback control of fat intake based on its unique taste properties. Despite localized increases of endocannabinoids selectively in the upper small-intestinal epithelium and blockade of intake following pharmacological treatment with a peripherally-restricted neutral CB$_1$R antagonist, these studies were limited in their ability to identify necessity for CB$_1$Rs in the intestinal epithelium in food intake and dietary preferences. To overcome these challenges and examine whether CB$_1$Rs in the small-intestinal epithelium were required for WD preferences, we generated a novel conditional intestinal epithelium-specific CB$_1$R-deficient mouse. Notably, the WD used in these studies is composed of 40% kcals from fats and 43% from carbohydrates, which more closely matches the 35% fat and 47% carbohydrate composition of diets in humans [46] when compared to rodent studies that routinely use high-fat test diets containing 60% kcals from fat and relatively low levels of carbohydrates (e.g., Research Diets D12492). Robust preferences found for WD in control mice, when compared to a low-fat/no-sucrose chow, were largely absent in IntCB$_1$−/− mice during the first 12 h of preference testing. In addition, these effects were mimicked by systemic treatment with the globally acting CB$_1$R antagonist/inverse agonist, AM251, in wild-type mice. Collectively, these results provide evidence of a critical role for CB$_1$Rs in the rodent intestinal epithelium in acute preferences for food containing high levels of fats and sugars. Humans also display robust preferences for food that contains high levels of fats and sugar [1], and consumption of palatable food was associated with elevated levels of circulating endocannabinoids in humans [21]. It remains to be determined if consumption of palatable food in humans is controlled by gut–brain endocannabinoid signaling in a similar manner to rodents.

The specific mechanism(s) underlying intestinal epithelium CB$_1$R-mediated preferences for WD are unknown but may include CB$_1$R control of gut–brain signaling. We reported that hyperphagia and increased meal size associated with WD-induced obesity in mice are dependent on (i) elevated levels of endocannabinoids in the upper small-intestinal epithelium and (ii) CB$_1$R-mediated inhibition of nutrient-induced signaling of the satiation peptide, cholecystokinin [16]. Cholecystokinin is secreted from enteroendocrine cells in the upper small-intestinal epithelium when nutrients arrive in the lumen, and transmits satiation signals to the brain by interacting with cholecystokinin A receptors on the afferent vagus nerve [30,40,46–49] and possibly the brain [50,51]. Bohorquez and colleagues recently characterized enteroendocrine cells (i.e., neuropods) in the mouse intestinal epithelium that form functional synapses with afferent vagal fibers [33]. Neuropods sense nutrients in the lumen and in response, release glutamate and cholecystokinin, which activate afferent vagal neurons in a coordinated manner [52]. Moreover, afferent vagal neurons participate in reward-related behaviors—including flavor and place preferences—and control dopamine outflow in the mouse striatum [49]. Notably, however, studies suggest that the afferent vagus nerve is required for nutrient-induced negative feedback from the gut associated with satiation and satiety, but is dispensable for positive feedback (i.e., appetition [53]) associated with nutrient reinforcement and flavor-nutrient preference conditioning [54]. Nonetheless, it is possible that CB_1Rs in the intestinal epithelium participate in preferences for WD by a mechanism that includes control of nutrient-induced, neuropod-mediated, afferent vagal activity and recruitment of brain reward circuits. A direct test of this hypothesis and evaluation of distinct roles for intestinal CB_1Rs in satiation versus appetition remains for future studies.

We propose that CB_1Rs indirectly regulate afferent vagal activity by controlling nutrient sensing and release of satiation peptides from enteroendocrine cells in the small-intestinal epithelium that directly interact with the afferent vagus nerve [16,39]. Recent studies also suggest that CB_1Rs in the mouse stomach participate in alcohol intake by controlling formation of the appetite-stimulating hormone, ghrelin, which interacts with ghrelin receptors on afferent vagal fibers [55]. In addition to these indirect mechanisms, CB_1Rs may also directly control afferent vagal neurotransmission and food intake [56]. For example, Burdyga and colleagues reported that fasting was associated with increased expression of CB_1Rs in the rat vagal afferent neurons [57]. Refeeding or administration of cholecystokinin rapidly reversed fasting-induced expression of CB_1R [57], which was also blunted in rats maintained on a high-fat diet [58]. In addition, administration of ghrelin blocked the effects of refeeding on CB_1R expression [59]. Moreover, Christie and colleagues reported that low and high concentrations of methanandamide—a stable analog of anandamide—differentially modified mechanosensitivity of mouse gastric vagal afferents in vitro via a mechanism that included CB_1Rs, TRPV1, and ghrelin receptors [60], and these effects were dysregulated in mice fed a high-fat diet for 12 weeks [61]. These studies suggest that CB_1Rs on the afferent vagus nerve may participate in gut-brain signaling important for food intake and energy balance. Interestingly, mice with genetic deletion of CB_1Rs on afferent vagal neurons displayed no changes in body weight or food intake, irrespective of test diet (i.e., standard versus high-fat), which suggests that vagal CB_1Rs may not be necessary for long-term maintenance of body weight and feeding [62]. Further investigations are necessary to expand our understanding of physiological roles for the endocannabinoid system in vagal afferent neurons.

It is noteworthy that attenuation of preferences for WD were limited to the first 3 h in AM251-treated wild-type mice and the first 6 h in $IntCB_1-/-$ mice when compared to vehicle and $IntCB_1+/+$ mice, respectively. It is plausible that restricted temporal effects of AM251 in wild-type mice reflect the pharmacokinetic properties of this compound, which displays a half-life of 22 h in rats [63]. $IntCB_1-/-$ mice, however, displayed a similar restriction of preferences for WD, albeit to the first 6 h of the test when compared to control mice. The mechanism(s) in this restricted response to early time points remains unknown but may reflect a circadian pattern of activity or expression of the endocannabinoid system in the intestinal epithelium that controls gut–brain signaling important for food intake. A direct examination of roles for intestinal CB_1Rs in the circadian control of food intake remains for future studies. Moreover, post-prandial cues at later time-points may provide compensatory feedback and reinforcement and restore preferences for WD in the absence of CB_1Rs in the intestinal epithelium. One candidate in this proposed mechanism is the satiety factor oleoylethanolamide, which is synthesized in the intestinal epithelium from dietary fats and controls food intake and possibly reward through a mechanism that requires peroxisome proliferator-activated receptor α (PPARα) and the afferent vagus [64–66]. Studies examining interactions between orexigenic endocannabinoid and anorexic oleoylethanolamide signaling pathways in acute and long-term dietary preferences remain for future inquiry.

In summary, these studies extend our understanding beyond central roles for the endocannabinoid system in intake and reward value of palatable food [67–83], and provide evidence that CB_1Rs in the intestinal epithelium are an integral component of a gut–brain axis that controls dietary preferences. Future studies will be important to elucidate (i) specific mechanism(s) of intestinal CB_1R-mediated preferences for palatable food, (ii) roles for CB_1Rs in the intestinal epithelium in recruitment of brain reward circuits and the "wanting" or "liking" of palatable food [84], (iii) roles for intestinal CB_1Rs in satiation versus appetition, (iv) interactions between CB_1R and PPARa signaling pathways in preferences for palatable food, (v) roles CB_1Rs in the intestinal epithelium in development and maintenance of diet-induced obesity, (vi) physiological roles for CB_1Rs on vagal neurons, and (vii) possible circadian fluctuations in expression and function of the endocannabinoid system in the gut and its relationship with feeding behavior.

Author Contributions: B.A. and D.A.A. contributed equally. Conceptualization, B.A., D.A.A., N.V.D.; methodology, B.A., D.A.A., P.A.P., M.W., C.W., N.V.D.; formal analysis, B.A., D.A.A., P.A.P., N.V.D.; investigation, B.A., D.A.A., P.A.P., M.W., C.W.; resources, N.V.D.; data curation, B.A., D.A.A., P.A.P., M.W., C.W., N.V.D.; writing—original draft preparation, B.A. and N.V.D.; writing—review and editing, B.A., D.A.A., P.A.P., M.W., C.W., N.V.D.; supervision, N.V.D.; project administration, N.V.D.; funding acquisition, N.V.D. and D.A.A. All authors have read and agreed to the published version of the manuscript.

Funding: This study was funded by the National Institutes of Health, National Institute of Diabetes and Digestive and Kidney Diseases grants DK119498 and DK114978, and the Tobacco-Related Disease Research Program (TRDRP) from the University of California Office of the President grant T29KT0232 to N.V.D. In addition, we thank the Ford Foundation Dissertation Fellowship to D.A.

Conflicts of Interest: The authors declare no conflict of interest.

References

1. Levine, A.S.; Kotz, C.M.; Gosnell, B.A. Sugars and fats: The neurobiology of preference. *J. Nutr.* **2003**, *133*, 831S–834S. [CrossRef]
2. Lau, B.K.; Cota, D.; Cristino, L.; Borgland, S.L. Endocannabinoid modulation of homeostatic and non-homeostatic feeding circuits. *Neuropharmacology* **2017**, *124*, 38–51. [CrossRef]
3. Rossi, M.A.; Stuber, G.D. Overlapping Brain Circuits for Homeostatic and Hedonic Feeding. *Cell Metab.* **2018**, *27*, 42–56. [CrossRef] [PubMed]
4. DiPatrizio, N.V.; Piomelli, D. The thrifty lipids: Endocannabinoids and the neural control of energy conservation. *Trends Neurosci.* **2012**, *35*, 403–411. [CrossRef] [PubMed]
5. Di Marzo, V.; Ligresti, A.; Cristino, L. The endocannabinoid system as a link between homoeostatic and hedonic pathways involved in energy balance regulation. *Int. J. Obes. (Lond.)* **2009**, *33*, S18–S24. [CrossRef] [PubMed]
6. Gomez, R.; Navarro, M.; Ferrer, B.; Trigo, J.M.; Bilbao, A.; Del Arco, I.; Cippitelli, A.; Nava, F.; Piomelli, D.; Rodriguez de Fonseca, F. A peripheral mechanism for CB1 cannabinoid receptor-dependent modulation of feeding. *J. Neurosci.* **2002**, *22*, 9612–9617. [CrossRef] [PubMed]
7. Izzo, A.A.; Sharkey, K.A. Cannabinoids and the gut: New developments and emerging concepts. *Pharm. Ther.* **2010**, *126*, 21–38. [CrossRef]
8. Randall, P.A.; Vemuri, V.K.; Segovia, K.N.; Torres, E.F.; Hosmer, S.; Nunes, E.J.; Santerre, J.L.; Makriyannis, A.; Salamone, J.D. The novel cannabinoid CB1 antagonist AM6545 suppresses food intake and food-reinforced behavior. *Pharmacol. Biochem. Behav.* **2010**, *97*, 179–184. [CrossRef]
9. Cluny, N.L.; Vemuri, V.K.; Chambers, A.P.; Limebeer, C.L.; Bedard, H.; Wood, J.T.; Lutz, B.; Zimmer, A.; Parker, L.A.; Makriyannis, A.; et al. A novel peripherally restricted cannabinoid receptor antagonist, AM6545, reduces food intake and body weight, but does not cause malaise, in rodents. *Br. J. Pharmacol.* **2011**, *161*, 629–642. [CrossRef]

10. DiPatrizio, N.V.; Igarashi, M.; Narayanaswami, V.; Murray, C.; Gancayco, J.; Russell, A.; Jung, K.M.; Piomelli, D. Fasting stimulates 2-AG biosynthesis in the small intestine: Role of cholinergic pathways. *Am. J. Physiol. Regul. Integr. Comp. Physiol.* **2015**, *309*, R805–R813. [CrossRef]
11. Tam, J.; Vemuri, V.K.; Liu, J.; Batkai, S.; Mukhopadhyay, B.; Godlewski, G.; Osei-Hyiaman, D.; Ohnuma, S.; Ambudkar, S.V.; Pickel, J.; et al. Peripheral CB1 cannabinoid receptor blockade improves cardiometabolic risk in mouse models of obesity. *J. Clin. Investig.* **2010**, *120*, 2953–2966. [CrossRef] [PubMed]
12. Tam, J.; Szanda, G.; Drori, A.; Liu, Z.; Cinar, R.; Kashiwaya, Y.; Reitman, M.L.; Kunos, G. Peripheral cannabinoid-1 receptor blockade restores hypothalamic leptin signaling. *Mol. Metab.* **2017**, *6*, 1113–1125. [CrossRef] [PubMed]
13. Bellocchio, L.; Soria-Gomez, E.; Quarta, C.; Metna-Laurent, M.; Cardinal, P.; Binder, E.; Cannich, A.; Delamarre, A.; Haring, M.; Martin-Fontecha, M.; et al. Activation of the sympathetic nervous system mediates hypophagic and anxiety-like effects of CB1 receptor blockade. *Proc. Natl. Acad. Sci. USA* **2013**, *110*, 4786–4791. [CrossRef] [PubMed]
14. DiPatrizio, N.V.; Astarita, G.; Schwartz, G.; Li, X.; Piomelli, D. Endocannabinoid signal in the gut controls dietary fat intake. *Proc. Natl. Acad. Sci. USA* **2011**, *108*, 12904–12908. [CrossRef]
15. DiPatrizio, N.V.; Joslin, A.; Jung, K.M.; Piomelli, D. Endocannabinoid signaling in the gut mediates preference for dietary unsaturated fats. *FASEB J.* **2013**, *27*, 2513–2520. [CrossRef]
16. Argueta, D.A.; Perez, P.A.; Makriyannis, A.; DiPatrizio, N.V. Cannabinoid CB1 Receptors Inhibit Gut-Brain Satiation Signaling in Diet-Induced Obesity. *Front. Physiol.* **2019**, *10*, 704. [CrossRef] [PubMed]
17. Argueta, D.A.; DiPatrizio, N.V. Peripheral endocannabinoid signaling controls hyperphagia in western diet-induced obesity. *Physiol. Behav.* **2017**, *171*, 32–39. [CrossRef]
18. Niki, M.; Jyotaki, M.; Yoshida, R.; Yasumatsu, K.; Shigemura, N.; DiPatrizio, N.V.; Piomelli, D.; Ninomiya, Y. Modulation of sweet taste sensitivities by endogenous leptin and endocannabinoids in mice. *J. Physiol.* **2015**, *593*, 2527–2545. [CrossRef]
19. Ruiz de Azua, I.; Mancini, G.; Srivastava, R.K.; Rey, A.A.; Cardinal, P.; Tedesco, L.; Zingaretti, C.M.; Sassmann, A.; Quarta, C.; Schwitter, C.; et al. Adipocyte cannabinoid receptor CB1 regulates energy homeostasis and alternatively activated macrophages. *J. Clin. Investig.* **2017**, *127*, 4148–4162. [CrossRef]
20. Simon, V.; Cota, D. Mechanisms in Endocrinology: Endocannabinoids and metabolism: Past, present and future. *Eur. J. Endocrinol.* **2017**, *176*, R309–R324. [CrossRef]
21. Monteleone, P.; Piscitelli, F.; Scognamiglio, P.; Monteleone, A.M.; Canestrelli, B.; Di Marzo, V.; Maj, M. Hedonic eating is associated with increased peripheral levels of ghrelin and the endocannabinoid 2-arachidonoyl-glycerol in healthy humans: A pilot study. *J. Clin. Endocrinol. Metab.* **2012**, *97*, E917–E924. [CrossRef] [PubMed]
22. Price, C.A.; Argueta, D.A.; Medici, V.; Bremer, A.A.; Lee, V.; Nunez, M.V.; Chen, G.X.; Keim, N.L.; Havel, P.J.; Stanhope, K.L.; et al. Plasma fatty acid ethanolamides are associated with postprandial triglycerides, ApoCIII, and ApoE in humans consuming a high-fructose corn syrup-sweetened beverage. *Am. J. Physiol. Endocrinol. Metab.* **2018**, *315*, E141–E149. [CrossRef] [PubMed]
23. Little, T.J.; Cvijanovic, N.; DiPatrizio, N.V.; Argueta, D.A.; Rayner, C.K.; Feinle-Bisset, C.; Young, R.L. Plasma endocannabinoid levels in lean, overweight, and obese humans: Relationships to intestinal permeability markers, inflammation, and incretin secretion. *Am. J. Physiol. Endocrinol. Metab.* **2018**, *315*, E489–E495. [CrossRef] [PubMed]
24. Engeli, S.; Bohnke, J.; Feldpausch, M.; Gorzelniak, K.; Janke, J.; Batkai, S.; Pacher, P.; Harvey-White, J.; Luft, F.C.; Sharma, A.M.; et al. Activation of the peripheral endocannabinoid system in human obesity. *Diabetes* **2005**, *54*, 2838–2843. [CrossRef] [PubMed]
25. Bluher, M.; Engeli, S.; Kloting, N.; Berndt, J.; Fasshauer, M.; Batkai, S.; Pacher, P.; Schon, M.R.; Jordan, J.; Stumvoll, M. Dysregulation of the peripheral and adipose tissue endocannabinoid system in human abdominal obesity. *Diabetes* **2006**, *55*, 3053–3060. [CrossRef]
26. Cote, M.; Matias, I.; Lemieux, I.; Petrosino, S.; Almeras, N.; Despres, J.P.; Di Marzo, V. Circulating endocannabinoid levels, abdominal adiposity and related cardiometabolic risk factors in obese men. *Int. J. Obes. (Lond)* **2007**, *31*, 692–699. [CrossRef]

27. Di Marzo, V.; Cote, M.; Matias, I.; Lemieux, I.; Arsenault, B.J.; Cartier, A.; Piscitelli, F.; Petrosino, S.; Almeras, N.; Despres, J.P. Changes in plasma endocannabinoid levels in viscerally obese men following a 1 year lifestyle modification programme and waist circumference reduction: Associations with changes in metabolic risk factors. *Diabetologia* **2009**, *52*, 213–217. [CrossRef]
28. Matias, I.; Gatta-Cherifi, B.; Tabarin, A.; Clark, S.; Leste-Lasserre, T.; Marsicano, G.; Piazza, P.V.; Cota, D. Endocannabinoids measurement in human saliva as potential biomarker of obesity. *PLoS ONE* **2012**, *7*, e42399. [CrossRef]
29. Hillard, C.J. Circulating Endocannabinoids: From Whence Do They Come and Where are They Going? *Neuropsychopharmacology* **2017**, *43*, 155–172. [CrossRef]
30. Steinert, R.E.; Feinle-Bisset, C.; Asarian, L.; Horowitz, M.; Beglinger, C.; Geary, N. Ghrelin, CCK, GLP-1, and PYY(3-36): Secretory Controls and Physiological Roles in Eating and Glycemia in Health, Obesity, and After RYGB. *Physiol. Rev.* **2017**, *97*, 411–463. [CrossRef]
31. Schwartz, G.J. Roles for gut vagal sensory signals in determining energy availability and energy expenditure. *Brain Res.* **2018**, *1693*, 151–153. [CrossRef] [PubMed]
32. DiPatrizio, N.V.; Piomelli, D. Intestinal lipid-derived signals that sense dietary fat. *J. Clin. Investig.* **2015**, *125*, 891–898. [CrossRef] [PubMed]
33. Kaelberer, M.M.; Rupprecht, L.E.; Liu, W.W.; Weng, P.; Bohorquez, D.V. Neuropod Cells: The Emerging Biology of Gut-Brain Sensory Transduction. *Annu. Rev. Neurosci.* **2020**, *43*, 337–353. [CrossRef] [PubMed]
34. Berthoud, H.R. The vagus nerve, food intake and obesity. *Regul. Pept.* **2008**, *149*, 15–25. [CrossRef] [PubMed]
35. Dockray, G.J. Enteroendocrine cell signalling via the vagus nerve. *Curr. Opin. Pharmacol.* **2013**, *13*, 954–958. [CrossRef]
36. Roper, S.D. Taste buds as peripheral chemosensory processors. *Semin. Cell Dev. Biol.* **2013**, *24*, 71–79. [CrossRef]
37. Sclafani, A. From appetite setpoint to appetition: 50 years of ingestive behavior research. *Physiol. Behav.* **2018**, *192*, 210–217. [CrossRef]
38. Raybould, H.E. Gut chemosensing: Interactions between gut endocrine cells and visceral afferents. *Auton Neurosci.* **2010**, *153*, 41–46. [CrossRef]
39. Sykaras, A.G.; Demenis, C.; Case, R.M.; McLaughlin, J.T.; Smith, C.P. Duodenal enteroendocrine I-cells contain mRNA transcripts encoding key endocannabinoid and fatty acid receptors. *PLoS ONE* **2012**, *7*, e42373. [CrossRef]
40. Raybould, H.E. Mechanisms of CCK signaling from gut to brain. *Curr. Opin. Pharmacol.* **2007**, *7*, 570–574. [CrossRef]
41. El Marjou, F.; Janssen, K.P.; Chang, B.H.; Li, M.; Hindie, V.; Chan, L.; Louvard, D.; Chambon, P.; Metzger, D.; Robine, S. Tissue-specific and inducible Cre-mediated recombination in the gut epithelium. *Genesis* **2004**, *39*, 186–193. [CrossRef] [PubMed]
42. Rutlin, M.; Rastelli, D.; Kuo, W.T.; Estep, J.A.; Louis, A.; Riccomagno, M.M.; Turner, J.R.; Rao, M. The Villin1 Gene Promoter Drives Cre Recombinase Expression in Extraintestinal Tissues. *Cell Mol. Gastroenterol. Hepatol.* **2020**. online ahead of print. [CrossRef] [PubMed]
43. Henstridge, C.M. Off-target cannabinoid effects mediated by GPR55. *Pharmacology* **2012**, *89*, 179–187. [CrossRef] [PubMed]
44. Seely, K.A.; Brents, L.K.; Franks, L.N.; Rajasekaran, M.; Zimmerman, S.M.; Fantegrossi, W.E.; Prather, P.L. AM-251 and rimonabant act as direct antagonists at mu-opioid receptors: Implications for opioid/cannabinoid interaction studies. *Neuropharmacology* **2012**, *63*, 905–915. [CrossRef] [PubMed]
45. Gribble, F.M.; Reimann, F. Enteroendocrine Cells: Chemosensors in the Intestinal Epithelium. *Annu Rev. Physiol.* **2016**, *78*, 277–299. [CrossRef]
46. Schwartz, G.J.; Moran, T.H. CCK elicits and modulates vagal afferent activity arising from gastric and duodenal sites. *Ann. N. Y. Acad. Sci.* **1994**, *713*, 121–128. [CrossRef]
47. Smith, G.P.; Jerome, C.; Cushin, B.J.; Eterno, R.; Simansky, K.J. Abdominal vagotomy blocks the satiety effect of cholecystokinin in the rat. *Science* **1981**, *213*, 1036–1037. [CrossRef]
48. Smith, G.P.; Jerome, C.; Norgren, R. Afferent axons in abdominal vagus mediate satiety effect of cholecystokinin in rats. *Am. J. Physiol.* **1985**, *249*, R638–R641. [CrossRef]
49. Han, W.; Tellez, L.A.; Perkins, M.H.; Perez, I.O.; Qu, T.; Ferreira, J.; Ferreira, T.L.; Quinn, D.; Liu, Z.W.; Gao, X.B.; et al. A Neural Circuit for Gut-Induced Reward. *Cell* **2018**, *175*, 665–678. [CrossRef]

50. Reidelberger, R.D.; Hernandez, J.; Fritzsch, B.; Hulce, M. Abdominal vagal mediation of the satiety effects of CCK in rats. *Am. J. Physiol. Regul. Integr. Comp. Physiol.* **2004**, *286*, R1005–R1012. [CrossRef]

51. Ripken, D.; van der Wielen, N.; van der Meulen, J.; Schuurman, T.; Witkamp, R.F.; Hendriks, H.F.; Koopmans, S.J. Cholecystokinin regulates satiation independently of the abdominal vagal nerve in a pig model of total subdiaphragmatic vagotomy. *Physiol. Behav.* **2015**, *139*, 167–176. [CrossRef] [PubMed]

52. Kaelberer, M.M.; Buchanan, K.L.; Klein, M.E.; Barth, B.B.; Montoya, M.M.; Shen, X.; Bohorquez, D.V. A gut-brain neural circuit for nutrient sensory transduction. *Science* **2018**, *361*, eaat 5306. [CrossRef]

53. Sclafani, A. Gut-brain nutrient signaling. Appetition vs. satiation. *Appetite* **2013**, *71*, 454–458. [CrossRef] [PubMed]

54. Shechter, A.; Schwartz, G.J. Gut-brain nutrient sensing in food reward. *Appetite* **2018**, *122*, 32–35. [CrossRef] [PubMed]

55. Godlewski, G.; Cinar, R.; Coffey, N.J.; Liu, J.; Jourdan, T.; Mukhopadhyay, B.; Chedester, L.; Liu, Z.; Osei-Hyiaman, D.; Iyer, M.R.; et al. Targeting Peripheral CB1 Receptors Reduces Ethanol Intake via a Gut-Brain Axis. *Cell Metab.* **2019**, *29*, 1320–1333. [CrossRef] [PubMed]

56. Burdyga, G.; Varro, A.; Dimaline, R.; Thompson, D.G.; Dockray, G.J. Expression of cannabinoid CB1 receptors by vagal afferent neurons: Kinetics and role in influencing neurochemical phenotype. *Am. J. Physiol. Gastrointest. Liver Physiol.* **2010**, *299*, G63–G69. [CrossRef]

57. Burdyga, G.; Lal, S.; Varro, A.; Dimaline, R.; Thompson, D.G.; Dockray, G.J. Expression of cannabinoid CB1 receptors by vagal afferent neurons is inhibited by cholecystokinin. *J. Neurosci.* **2004**, *24*, 2708–2715. [CrossRef]

58. Cluny, N.L.; Baraboi, E.D.; Mackie, K.; Burdyga, G.; Richard, D.; Dockray, G.J.; Sharkey, K.A. High fat diet and body weight have different effects on cannabinoid CB(1) receptor expression in rat nodose ganglia. *Auton. Neurosci.* **2013**, *179*, 122–130. [CrossRef]

59. Burdyga, G.; Varro, A.; Dimaline, R.; Thompson, D.G.; Dockray, G.J. Ghrelin receptors in rat and human nodose ganglia: Putative role in regulating CB-1 and MCH receptor abundance. *Am. J. Physiol. Gastrointest. Liver Physiol.* **2006**, *290*, G1289–G1297. [CrossRef]

60. Christie, S.; O'Rielly, R.; Li, H.; Wittert, G.A.; Page, A.J. Biphasic effects of methanandamide on murine gastric vagal afferent mechanosensitivity. *J. Physiol.* **2020**, *598*, 139–150. [CrossRef]

61. Christie, S.; O'Rielly, R.; Li, H.; Nunez-Salces, M.; Wittert, G.A.; Page, A.J. Modulatory effect of methanandamide on gastric vagal afferent satiety signals depends on nutritional status. *J. Physiol.* **2020**, *598*, 2169–2182. [CrossRef] [PubMed]

62. Vianna, C.R.; Donato, J., Jr.; Rossi, J.; Scott, M.; Economides, K.; Gautron, L.; Pierpont, S.; Elias, C.F.; Elmquist, J.K. Cannabinoid receptor 1 in the vagus nerve is dispensable for body weight homeostasis but required for normal gastrointestinal motility. *J. Neurosci.* **2012**, *32*, 10331–10337. [CrossRef] [PubMed]

63. McLaughlin, P.J.; Winston, K.; Swezey, L.; Wisniecki, A.; Aberman, J.; Tardif, D.J.; Betz, A.J.; Ishiwari, K.; Makriyannis, A.; Salamone, J.D. The cannabinoid CB1 antagonists SR 141716A and AM 251 suppress food intake and food-reinforced behavior in a variety of tasks in rats. *Behav. Pharmacol.* **2003**, *14*, 583–588. [CrossRef] [PubMed]

64. Fu, J.; Gaetani, S.; Oveisi, F.; Lo Verme, J.; Serrano, A.; Rodriguez De Fonseca, F.; Rosengarth, A.; Luecke, H.; Di Giacomo, B.; Tarzia, G.; et al. Oleylethanolamide regulates feeding and body weight through activation of the nuclear receptor PPAR-alpha. *Nature* **2003**, *425*, 90–93. [CrossRef]

65. Schwartz, G.J.; Fu, J.; Astarita, G.; Li, X.; Gaetani, S.; Campolongo, P.; Cuomo, V.; Piomelli, D. The lipid messenger OEA links dietary fat intake to satiety. *Cell Metab.* **2008**, *8*, 281–288. [CrossRef]

66. Tellez, L.A.; Medina, S.; Han, W.; Ferreira, J.G.; Licona-Limon, P.; Ren, X.; Lam, T.T.; Schwartz, G.J.; de Araujo, I.E. A gut lipid messenger links excess dietary fat to dopamine deficiency. *Science* **2013**, *341*, 800–802. [CrossRef]

67. Higuchi, S.; Irie, K.; Yamaguchi, R.; Katsuki, M.; Araki, M.; Ohji, M.; Hayakawa, K.; Mishima, S.; Akitake, Y.; Matsuyama, K.; et al. Hypothalamic 2-arachidonoylglycerol regulates multistage process of high-fat diet preferences. *PLoS ONE* **2012**, *7*, e38609. [CrossRef]

68. Higuchi, S.; Ohji, M.; Araki, M.; Furuta, R.; Katsuki, M.; Yamaguchi, R.; Akitake, Y.; Matsuyama, K.; Irie, K.; Mishima, K.; et al. Increment of hypothalamic 2-arachidonoylglycerol induces the preference for a high-fat diet via activation of cannabinoid 1 receptors. *Behav. Brain Res.* **2011**, *216*, 477–480. [CrossRef]

69. Deshmukh, R.R.; Sharma, P.L. Stimulation of accumbens shell cannabinoid CB(1) receptors by noladin ether, a putative endocannabinoid, modulates food intake and dietary selection in rats. *Pharmacol. Res.* **2012**, *66*, 276–282. [CrossRef]
70. DiPatrizio, N.V.; Simansky, K.J. Activating parabrachial cannabinoid CB1 receptors selectively stimulates feeding of palatable foods in rats. *J. Neurosci.* **2008**, *28*, 9702–9709. [CrossRef]
71. DiPatrizio, N.V.; Simansky, K.J. Inhibiting parabrachial fatty acid amide hydrolase activity selectively increases the intake of palatable food via cannabinoid CB1 receptors. *Am. J. Physiol. Regul. Integr. Comp. Physiol.* **2008**, *295*, R1409–R1414. [CrossRef] [PubMed]
72. Mahler, S.V.; Smith, K.S.; Berridge, K.C. Endocannabinoid hedonic hotspot for sensory pleasure: Anandamide in nucleus accumbens shell enhances 'liking' of a sweet reward. *Neuropsychopharmacology* **2007**, *32*, 2267–2278. [CrossRef] [PubMed]
73. Wei, D.; Lee, D.; Li, D.; Daglian, J.; Jung, K.M.; Piomelli, D. A role for the endocannabinoid 2-arachidonoyl-sn-glycerol for social and high-fat food reward in male mice. *Psychopharmacology (Berl)* **2016**, *233*, 1911–1919. [CrossRef] [PubMed]
74. Mendez-Diaz, M.; Rueda-Orozco, P.E.; Ruiz-Contreras, A.E.; Prospero-Garcia, O. The endocannabinoid system modulates the valence of the emotion associated to food ingestion. *Addict. Biol.* **2012**, *17*, 725–735. [CrossRef] [PubMed]
75. De Luca, M.A.; Solinas, M.; Bimpisidis, Z.; Goldberg, S.R.; Di Chiara, G. Cannabinoid facilitation of behavioral and biochemical hedonic taste responses. *Neuropharmacology* **2012**, *63*, 161–168. [CrossRef] [PubMed]
76. Jarrett, M.M.; Scantlebury, J.; Parker, L.A. Effect of delta9-tetrahydrocannabinol on quinine palatability and AM251 on sucrose and quinine palatability using the taste reactivity test. *Physiol. Behav.* **2007**, *90*, 425–430. [CrossRef]
77. Melis, T.; Succu, S.; Sanna, F.; Boi, A.; Argiolas, A.; Melis, M.R. The cannabinoid antagonist SR 141716A (Rimonabant) reduces the increase of extra-cellular dopamine release in the rat nucleus accumbens induced by a novel high palatable food. *Neurosci. Lett.* **2007**, *419*, 231–235. [CrossRef]
78. Droste, S.M.; Saland, S.K.; Schlitter, E.K.; Rodefer, J.S. AM 251 differentially effects food-maintained responding depending on food palatability. *Pharmacol. Biochem. Behav.* **2010**, *95*, 443–448. [CrossRef]
79. South, T.; Deng, C.; Huang, X.F. AM 251 and beta-Funaltrexamine reduce fat intake in a fat-preferring strain of mouse. *Behav. Brain Res.* **2007**, *181*, 153–157. [CrossRef]
80. Thornton-Jones, Z.D.; Vickers, S.P.; Clifton, P.G. The cannabinoid CB1 receptor antagonist SR141716A reduces appetitive and consummatory responses for food. *Psychopharmacology (Berl)* **2005**, *179*, 452–460. [CrossRef]
81. Feja, M.; Leigh, M.P.K.; Baindur, A.N.; McGraw, J.J.; Wakabayashi, K.T.; Cravatt, B.F.; Bass, C.E. The novel MAGL inhibitor MJN110 enhances responding to reward-predictive incentive cues by activation of CB1 receptors. *Neuropharmacology* **2020**, *162*, 107814. [CrossRef] [PubMed]
82. Salamone, J.D.; McLaughlin, P.J.; Sink, K.; Makriyannis, A.; Parker, L.A. Cannabinoid CB1 receptor inverse agonists and neutral antagonists: Effects on food intake, food-reinforced behavior and food aversions. *Physiol. Behav.* **2007**, *91*, 383–388. [CrossRef] [PubMed]
83. Williams, C.M.; Kirkham, T.C. Anandamide induces overeating: Mediation by central cannabinoid (CB1) receptors. *Psychopharmacology (Berl)* **1999**, *143*, 315–317. [CrossRef]
84. Castro, D.C.; Berridge, K.C. Advances in the neurobiological bases for food 'liking' versus 'wanting'. *Physiol. Behav.* **2014**, *136*, 22–30. [CrossRef] [PubMed]

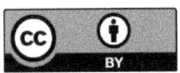

© 2020 by the authors. Licensee MDPI, Basel, Switzerland. This article is an open access article distributed under the terms and conditions of the Creative Commons Attribution (CC BY) license (http://creativecommons.org/licenses/by/4.0/).

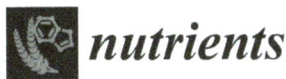

Article

Modulation of Food Intake by Differential TAS2R Stimulation in Rat

Carme Grau-Bové [1], Alba Miguéns-Gómez [1], Carlos González-Quilen [1], José-Antonio Fernández-López [2,3], Xavier Remesar [2,3], Cristina Torres-Fuentes [4], Javier Ávila-Román [4], Esther Rodríguez-Gallego [1], Raúl Beltrán-Debón [1], M Teresa Blay [1], Ximena Terra [1], Anna Ardévol [1,*] and Montserrat Pinent [1]

[1] MoBioFood Research Group, Department of Biochemistry and Biotechnology, Universitat Rovira i Virgili, 43007 Tarragona, Spain; carme.grau@urv.cat (C.G.-B.); alba.miguens@urv.cat (A.M.-G.); carlosalberto.gonzalez@urv.cat (C.G.-Q.); esther.rodriguez@urv.cat (E.R.-G.); raul.beltran@urv.cat (R.B.-D.); mteresa.blay@urv.cat (M.T.B.); ximena.terra@urv.cat (X.T.); montserrat.pinent@urv.cat (M.P.)
[2] Department of Biochemistry and Molecular Biomedicine, Faculty of Biology, University of Barcelona, Av. Diagonal 643, 08028 Barcelona, Spain; josfernandez@ub.edu (J.-A.F.-L.); xremesar@ub.edu (X.R.)
[3] CIBER Obesity and Nutrition, Institute of Health Carlos III, Av. Diagonal 643, 08028 Barcelona, Spain
[4] Nutrigenomics Research Group, Department of Biochemistry and Biotechnology, Universitat Rovira i Virgili, 43007 Tarragona, Spain; cristina.torres@urv.cat (C.T.-F.); franciscojavier.avila@urv.cat (J.Á.-R.)
* Correspondence: anna.ardevol@urv.cat; Tel.: +34-977-559-566

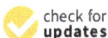

Received: 31 October 2020; Accepted: 4 December 2020; Published: 10 December 2020

Abstract: Metabolic surgery modulates the enterohormone profile, which leads, among other effects, to changes in food intake. Bitter taste receptors (TAS2Rs) have been identified in the gastrointestinal tract and specific stimulation of these has been linked to the control of ghrelin secretion. We hypothesize that optimal stimulation of TAS2Rs could help to modulate enteroendocrine secretions and thus regulate food intake. To determine this, we have assayed the response to specific agonists for hTAS2R5, hTAS2R14 and hTAS2R39 on enteroendocrine secretions from intestinal segments and food intake in rats. We found that hTAS2R5 agonists stimulate glucagon-like peptide 1 (GLP-1) and cholecystokinin (CCK), and reduce food intake. hTAS2R14 agonists induce GLP1, while hTASR39 agonists tend to increase peptide YY (PYY) but fail to reduce food intake. The effect of simultaneously activating several receptors is heterogeneous depending on the relative affinity of the agonists for each receptor. Although detailed mechanisms are not clear, bitter compounds can stimulate differentially enteroendocrine secretions that modulate food intake in rats.

Keywords: TAS2R5; TAS2R39; TAS2R14; agonist; food intake; GLP1; CCK; PYY

1. Introduction

Controlling food intake is a complex process that requires the combination of signals with very different origins. In animals, the nervous and hormonal systems play a role but in humans, feelings and sensations due to other environmental factors are also involved [1]. To study and monitor the regulation of food intake, numerous approaches involving diet, physical activity, medical devices, pharmacotherapy and metabolic (bariatric) surgery have been applied.

One of the most effective treatments against obesity and associated metabolic disorders is metabolic surgery [2], which leads to a huge change in metabolism and modifies the gastrointestinal secretome of patients. Enterohormones reach several targets in the body, including the brain and other peripheral tissues (e.g., adipose tissue, muscle and the gastrointestinal tract) [3]. The most consolidated effect of bariatric surgery in gastrointestinal secretome is an increase in glucagon-like peptide 1 (GLP-1) and peptide YY (PYY) [4]. Reproducing this enterohormone modulation without surgery could produce some of the beneficial effects of surgery without being so invasive. Several nutritional approaches cause enterohormone profile regulation [5]. However, they are not always effective at controlling food intake, probably because there is little control over the composition of the food components.

The bitter taste helps us to protect ourselves against unhealthy natural products [6]. Nevertheless, not all toxins are bitter and not all bitter compounds are toxic [7]. In fact, many bitter compounds have health benefits. It has even been suggested that healthier diets contain a higher proportion of bitter-tasting ingredients, such as bitter vegetables [8]. Recently, bitter taste receptors (TAS2Rs) have been identified in locations other than the mouth—where taste perception occurs—but a clear role for them there has not yet been defined [9,10]. Meyerhof et al. studied the association between bitter ligands and specific TAS2Rs using in vitro assays and calcium imaging [11]. Together with Di Pizio [12], they showed that humans and mice [13], which have a relatively large number of bitter taste receptors (25 in humans and 35 in mice), contain different types of receptors depending on their selectivity. Some selective receptors (such as hTAS2R3) only bind 1–3 ligands. In contrast, less selective receptors (such as hTAS2R39) and highly promiscuous receptors bind several ligands. A promiscuous TAS2R is one that can be activated by several ligands. In turn, ligands can be specific or unspecific for a certain receptor [12]. Species with a more limited number of bitter taste receptors contain only promiscuous receptors. Research is currently being conducted into the role of these bitter taste receptors that are located away from the lingual papillae where taste is perceived. They have been found in several locations, including the lungs [14] or stomach. Our group and others have shown that stimulating them induces ghrelin secretion in the murine ghrelinoma cell line [15] and in human fundic cells [16].

In this paper, we test whether a profile of enterohormones that limits food intake can be obtained by stimulating bitter taste receptors differentially. To do so, we used specific ligands for bitter taste receptors with different ranges of specificity, according to Meyerhof's definitions [11,17]. We also tested the effects of these ligands on enterohormone secretions in various segments of the rat intestine. Finally, we associated their effects on rat gastrointestinal secretome with their ability to modulate food intake in the whole animal.

2. Materials and Methods

2.1. Chemicals and Reagents

1,10-Phenantroline, (-)-epicatechin, Thiamine, Flufenamic acid, Vanillic acid and Protocatechuic acid were purchased from Sigma (Barcelona, Spain). Procyanidin B2 gallate, Epigallocatechin gallate (EGCG) and epicatechin gallate were purchased from Extrasynthese (Genay, France) and Procyanidin B2 was purchased from Adooq-Bioscience (Irvine, CA, USA).

We used Krebs–Ringer bicarbonate (KRB) buffer (Hepes 11.5 mM, $CaCl_2$ 2.6 mM, $MgCl_2$ 1.2 mM, KCl 5.5 mM, NaCl 138 mM, $NaHCO_3$ 4.2 mM, NaH_2PO_4 1.2 mM) pH 7.4, supplemented with either 10 mM D-Glucose (KRB-D-Glucose buffer) or 10 mM D-Mannitol (KRB-D-Mannitol buffer). For enterohormone secretion studies, KRB-D-Glucose was supplemented with protease inhibitors: 10 µM amastatin (Enzo Life Sciences, Madrid, Spain), 100 KIU aprotinin (Sigma, Barcelona, Spain) and 0.1% fatty acid free-bovine serum albumin.

2.2. Animals

We used 26 male Fischer-344 rats (Charles River Laboratories, Barcelona, Spain) and 20 female Wistar rats (Envigo, Barcelona, Spain). Most of these animals were housed at the animal housing facility of the Universitat Rovira i Virgili. Ten female Wistar rats were bred and housed at the Faculty of Biology of the Universitat de Barcelona. All rats were housed under standard conditions, i.e., they were caged in pairs at a room temperature of 23 °C with a standard 12-h light-dark cycle (lights on at 7 am), with ventilation, ad libitum access to tap water and a standard chow diet. The Fischer-344 rats were fed with a standard chow diet by SAFE (Cat No: A04, SAFE, Augy, France) while the Wistar rats were fed with a standard chow diet by Teklad (Cat No: Teklad 2014, Envigo, Barcelona, Spain). All procedures were approved by the Experimental Animal Ethics Committee of the autonomous government of Catalonia, Spain (Ministry of Territory and Sustainability, Directorate-General for Environmental Policy and the Natural Environment, project authorization code 10715) and the University of Barcelona (Ministry of Territory and Sustainability, Directorate-General for Environmental Policy and the Natural Environment, project authorization code 10769).

2.3. Ex Vivo Treatment of Intestinal Segments

We used 26 male Fischer-344 rats weighing 350–400 g. After a short fasting period (1–3 h), the rats were euthanized by decapitation and their intestines were excised. Samples were collected from the proximal duodenum and distal ileum. The tissue was rinsed with ice-cold KRB-D-Mannitol buffer and dissected into segments (0.5 cm diameter). After 15 min of washing, the tissue segments were placed in prewarmed (37 °C) KRB-D-Glucose buffer 0.1% Dimethyl Sulfoxide (DMSO) containing the compounds to be tested. Duodenal and ileal segments were treated with different compounds or a mix of compounds (Table S1) in a humidified incubator at 37 °C, 95% O_2 and 5% CO_2. After 30 min of treatment, the whole volume was frozen and stored at −80 °C for enterohormone quantification.

2.4. Studies of Food Intake

Ten female Wistar rats were housed in pairs for one week of adaptation. After this adaptation period, the animals were housed in single cages, introduced to daily 4 h food deprivation before light offset (3 p.m. to 7 p.m.) to habituate them to the experimental schedule, and trained for intragastric oral gavaging with tap water 1 h before dark onset (6 p.m.). One experiment per week was performed in a cross-over design for all food intake studies. For each experiment, the trained animals were treated with different compounds or a mix of compounds at defined concentrations (see Supplementary Table S1) intragastrically by oral gavage 1 h before dark onset (6 p.m.) using tap water as a vehicle. Parallel controls were performed by administering the vehicle intragastrically. Chow diet was administered at dark onset (7 p.m.) and chow intake was measured 3, 12 and 20 h later.

Determination of the effects of an acute dose of intragastric treatments in portal vein enterohormone secretion

Intragastric treatments were performed in two sets of animals. The first set comprised 10 female Wistar rats that received a specific intragastric dose of 1,10-Phenanthroline. The second set comprised 10 female Wistar rats that received an intragastric dose of (-)-Epicathechin. The same procedure (described earlier) was applied to both sets of rats. The animals were randomly divided into a control group and a treated group. The rats were fasted from 10 p.m. to 7 a.m. before treatment and anaesthetized 5 min later with either inhaled isoflurane (5% for induction, followed by 3% for maintenance) for the 1,10-Phenanthroline assay or pentobarbital (70 mg/kg) for the (-)-epicatechin assay. The abdominal cavity was incised through the midline and the portal vein was catheterized with a PE tube (Inner Diameter(I.D.) 0.28 mm, Outer Diameter (O.D.) 0.61 mm; Becton Dickinson, Sparks, MD, USA) following a standard procedure. The catheter was fixed with cyanoacrylate and the abdominal cavity was closed with surgical clamps. The body temperature was kept constant at 37 °C by a heated surgical table and overhead lamps. At time zero, 200 µL of blood were obtained and the catheter was refilled with saline. The specific treatment or tap water as the vehicle was punctured into the forestomach. Two portal blood samples (200 µL) were taken after treatment (described in the results) and each time the catheter was refilled with heparinized 0.9% NaCl. The blood was transferred to heparinized tubes containing a 1:100 volume of a 1:1 mix of commercial Dipeptidyl peptidase-4 inhibitor (DPPIV, Millipore, Madrid, Spain), to which a serine protease inhibitor (cOmplete™ ULTRA Tablets, Roche, Barcelona, Spain) was added. Plasma was collected by centrifugation at 1500× g over 15 min at 4 °C and frozen immediately at −80 °C for enterohormone quantification. The rats were sacrificed by bilateral thoracotomy.

2.5. Enterohormone Quantification

We measured enterohormone secretions from intestinal segments and plasma with commercial kits. Total and active GLP-1 were measured with ELISA kits from Millipore (Cat No: EZGLPT1-36k and EGLP-35K, respectively, Burlington, MA, USA). PYY was measured using a fluorescent immunoassay kit (Cat No: FEK-059-03, Phoenix Pharmaceuticals, Burlingame, CA, USA). Total CCK was measured with an ELISA kit (Cat No: EKE-069-04, Phoenix Pharmaceuticals, Burlingame, CA, USA).

2.6. Statistical Analysis

Our results are presented as mean ± SEM. Data were analyzed with XLSTAT 2020.1 (Addinsoft, Barcelona, Spain) statistical software. Statistical differences were assessed by Student t-tests, and $p < 0.05$ was considered statistically significant.

3. Results

3.1. Stimulation with Specific Agonists of hTA2R5 Increases GLP1 and CCK Secretions, While Stimulation with Specific Agonists of hTA2R39 Tends to Increase PYY and Decrease CCK

We tested the stimulation of different receptors with different degrees of selectivity. In humans, the most selective bitter taste receptors are hTAS2R3, hTAS2R5, hTAS2R13 and hTAS2R8. 1,10-Phenantroline is the only selective agonist for the hTAS2R5 receptor [12]. That is, this compound does not bind to other receptors in human TAS2Rs. We assayed the extent to which 1,10-Phenantroline, at around its minimum effective dose for hTAS2R5 (defined in Table 1), stimulated explants of various segments of rat intestine. Figure 1a shows that 1,10-Phenantroline increased total GLP1 (tGLP1) and CCK secretion with no statistical differences on PYY secretions.

Table 1. Comparison of the doses of the agonists and ligands assayed in the study and the individual binding parameters defined for each.

Compound (hTAS2R)	EC_{50} [1] (μM)	Effective Concentration [2] (μM)	Dose Administered to Rats	Dose for Treatment of Intestine Explants
1,10-Phenantroline (hTAS2R5) [18]	Not defined	100	290 μM	150 μM
Thiamine (hTAS2R39) [11]	Not defined	1000	7.5 mM	1 mM
ECg (hTAS2R39) [19]	88.2	Not defined	31 μM	-
Epicatechin (hTAS2R5) [19]	3210	1000	0.84/1 mM	1 mM
Epicatechin (hTAS2R39) [19]	3800	-	-	-
B2 gallate (hTAS2R5) [17]	6.3	Not defined	-	20 μM
B2 gallate (hTAS2R39) [17]	9.11	Not defined	-	-
Epigallocatechin Gallate (EGCG) (hTAS2R5) [17]	12.3	-	-	-
EGCG (hTAS2R39) [17]	8.5	Not defined	21/43 μM	300 μM
EGCG (hTAS2R39) [20]	181.6	10	-	-
Flufenamic acid (hTAS2R14) [11]	Not defined	10	50 μM	-
Protocatecuhic acid (hTAS2R14) [17]	156	Not defined	-	300 μM
Vanillic acid (hTAS2R14) [17]	151	Not defined	1.5 mM	300 μM
Procyanidin B2 [21]	Not defined	485 μM [3]	0.11 mM	67/300 μM

[1] EC_{50}: half-maximum effective concentrations. [2] Effective concentration: minimal concentration that elicited response. [3] Sensorial umbral, not effective concentration.

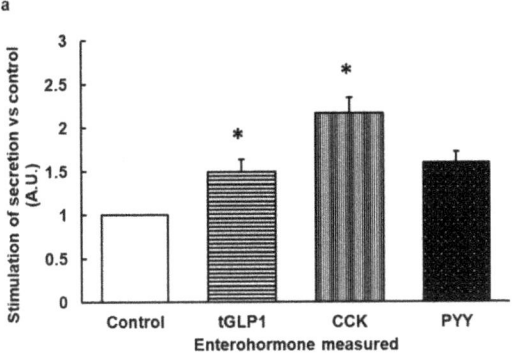

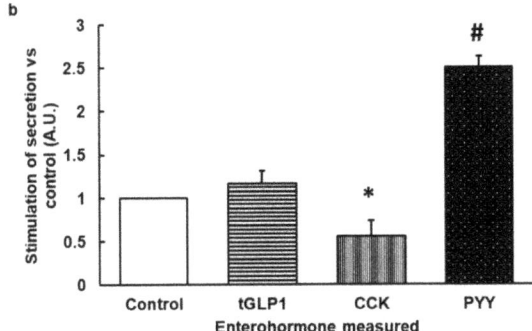

Figure 1. Ex vivo stimulation of enterohormone secretions induced by 1,10-Phenantroline (**a**) or Thiamine (**b**). Rat segments of duodenum (for cholecystokinin (CCK)) and ileum (for total glucagon-like peptide 1 (tGLP1) and peptide YY (PYY)) were treated with 1,10-Phenantroline 150 µM for 30 min (**a**) or Thiamine 1 mM for 30 min (**b**). Afterwards, medium was collected and respective enterohormones were quantified by ELISA (n = 6–10 segments). Results are calculated versus basal respective secretion in each hormone (Arbitrary Units, A.U.). Mean ± SEM. * denotes $p < 0.05$ vs. control; # indicate $p < 0.1$ vs. control.

According to Di Pizio et al. [12], hTAS2R39 is a less selective receptor. One of the selective agonists for it is Thiamine, though this compound also binds (h)TAS2R1 [11]. Treating rat intestine segments with the minimum effective dose of Thiamine for hTAS2R39 (Table 1) significantly reduced CCK secretion and tended to increase PYY secretion without affecting tGLP1 (Figure 1b).

3.2. When Bitter TAS2Rs Are Subjected to Simultaneous Stimulation, the Effect on Secretome Is Similar to the Effect on the Receptor with Lower EC50 Only

To understand responses closer to an in vivo situation, we assayed the simultaneous stimulation of hTAS2R5 and hTAS2R39 agonists with 1,10-Phenantroline plus Thiamine in rat intestinal segments at doses close to their minimally effective concentration (Table 1). Figure 2a shows that ileal tGLP1 secretion was clearly stimulated by simultaneous stimulation with 1,10-Phenantroline plus Thiamine. We then treated ileum segments with compounds that can bind both receptors but with a lower EC50 for hTAS2R5 than for hTAS2R39, i.e., B2gallate and (-)-epicatechin [19] (Table 1). B2 gallate tended to stimulate tGLP1 in ileum and CCK in the duodenum, while epicatechin significantly increased CCK secretion (Figure 2b).

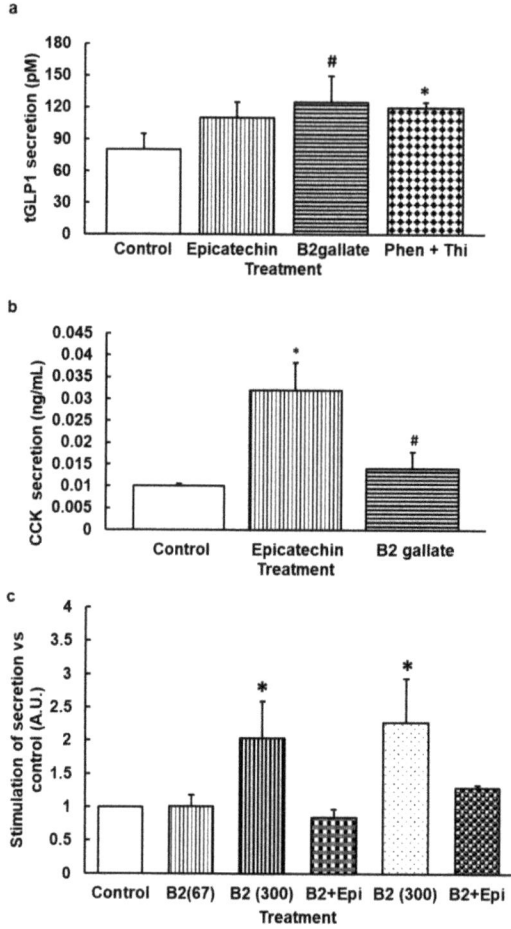

Figure 2. Ex vivo intestinal rat secretions induced by simultaneous stimulation by hTAS2R5 and hTAS2R39 agonist (**a**) and (**b**) or by Procyanidin B2 (**c**). (**a**) Segments of ileum were treated with epicatechin 1 mM, B2gallate 20 µM for 30 min or 1,10-Phenantroline 150 µM + Thiamine 1 mM for 45 min. (**b**) Segments of duodenum were treated with epicatechin 1 mM or B2gallate 20 µM for 30 min. (**c**) Segments of ileum (for tGLP1, vertical and squared lines) and duodenum (for CCK, dotted columns) were treated with B2 67 or 300 µM for 30 min, or B2 300 µM + epicatechin 1 mM for 45 min. Afterwards, medium was collected and respective enterohormones in the medium were quantified by ELISA (n = 6–10 segments). Mean ± SEM. (**c**) Results are calculated versus basal respective secretion in each hormone (Arbitrary Units, A.U.) * denotes $p < 0.05$ vs. control, # indicate $p < 0.1$ vs. control.

A different response was obtained with EGCG, which binds with lower EC50 to hTAS2R39 and also binds to TAS2R5 (Table 1) and hTAS2R43 [19]. EGCG 30 µM limits tGLP1 secretion in ileum segments (79.41 ±7.90 pM vs. control: 81.14 ± 13.41 pM, $p = 0.04$).

Finally, we tested Procyanidin B2, which has not yet been defined as a ligand for any TAS2R (though it has been identified as bitter with a threshold recognition of 0.485 mM [21]). Figure 2c shows that Procyanidin B2 increases tGLP1 and CCK at a dose of 300 µM. Its combination with epicatechin prevents these effects (Figure 2c).

3.3. Stimulation with Agonists of hTAS2R14 Increases GLP1 Secretion

One of the most promiscuous bitter taste receptors in humans is TAS2R14 [12]. Flufenamic acid is a selective agonist for this receptor, with a minimally effective concentration of 10 µM [11]. Rat intestine segments treated with Flufenamic (FFA) acid increased tGLP1 secretion (Figure 3), reduced CCK (0.60 ± 0.17 vs. control (1.00 ± 0.26); $p = 0.004$) and did not significantly modify PYY (1.15 ± 0.47 vs. control (1.00 ± 0.35); $p = 0.84$).

Vanillic acid (VAN), another selective ligand for TAS2R14 with an EC50 of 151.17 µM [17] also increased tGLP1 secretion in ileum segments, as did protocatechuic acid (PCA), another ligand of TAS2R14 (and TAS2R30) [17] (Figure 3).

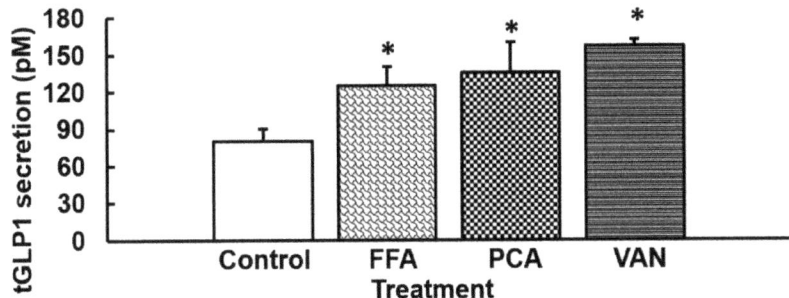

Figure 3. Ex vivo ileum rat total GLP1 secretion induced by hTAS2R14 agonists. Rat segments of ileum were treated with Flufenamic acid(FFA) 50 µM, protocatechuic acid(PCA) 300 µM or Vanillic acid(VAN) 300 µM for 30 min. Afterwards, the medium was collected and total GLP1 was quantified by ELISA ($n = 6$–10 segments). Mean ± SEM. * denotes $p < 0.05$ vs. control.

We also tested the effects of simultaneous activation with 1,10-Phenantroline (agonist for hTAS2R5) and Flufenamic acid (agonist for hTAS2R14), these being two stimulators of GLP1 secretion. Simultaneously treating ileum segments of rat intestine with the combination of Flufenamic acid (50 mM) and 1,10-Phenantroline (150 mM) did not induce tGLP1 secretion (control: 70.77 ± 7.47 vs. Phenantroline + Flufenamic acid: 104.01 ± 11.89 pM).

3.4. Agonists That Increase GLP1 and CCK Are More Effective in Limiting Food Intake

Acute administration of 1,10-Phenantroline to rats led to a reduction in food intake (Figure 4a). The same treatment tended to induce higher levels of active GLP1 in the portal vein thirty minutes after administration (t0 = 1.00 ± 0.15; t30 = 1.63 ± 0.4, p-value = 0.09, arbitrary units relative to secretion at t0). There were no clear effects on PYY or CCK at this time point (CCK ng/mL: t0 = 0.42 ± 0.04; t30 = 0.7 ± 0.07 control; t30 = 0.63 ± 0.10 1,10-Phenantroline; PYY pg/mL: t30 = 40.1 ± 3.15 control; t30 = 47.7 ± 8.9 1,10-Phenantroline). Neither was there a clear effect on glucose (results not shown).

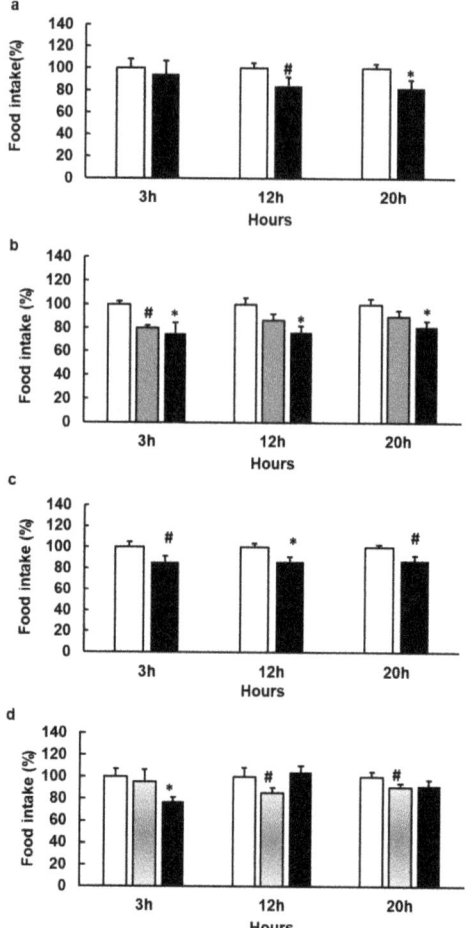

Figure 4. Food intake (FI) changes induced by acute doses of agonists of bitter taste receptors in female rats. Animals (n = 8–10/treatment) were treated one hour before dark period with an acute dose of 1,10-Phenantroline 200 mg/kg~ 290 µM (black columns) (**a**); 244 mg/kg~ 0.84 mM epicatechin (grey columns) or 300 mg/kg~ 1 mM epicatechin (black columns) (**b**); epicatechin + B2 + ECg (200 + 62 + 18 mg/kg) (black columns) (**c**); vanillic acid (252 mg/kg), grey columns) or Vanillic acid (252 mg/kg) + epicatechin (244 mg/kg) (black columns) (**d**); tap water as vehicle (white columns). Food intake was measured at the times indicated after the start of the dark period starts (Mean ± SEM). * denotes $p < 0.05$ vs. control; # indicate $p < 0.1$ vs. control.

An acute dose of around 0.84 mM of epicatechin tended to inhibit food intake, whereas an acute dose of around 1 mM clearly limited food intake (Figure 4b). This dose, increased levels of active GLP1 in the portal vein forty minutes after treatment (t0 = 1.00 ± 0.19; t20 = 1.56 ± 0.5; t40 = 4.69 ± 1.8, p-value = 0.03, arbitrary units relative to secretion at t0) and CCK secretion (CCK ng/mL: t0 = 0.68 ± 0.02; t40 = 0.78 ± 0.13 control; t40 = 0.96 ± 0.12 epicatechin). However, it did not change glycemia (results not shown).

Procyanidin B2 at a dose of 0.11 mM did not affect food intake (Figure S1). However, the same dose of B2 plus epicatechin (0.74 mM) and epicatechin gallate (ECg) at a total dose of 0.84 mM did reduce food intake (Figure 4c).

Vanillic acid tended to reduce food intake (Figure 4d). The combination of epicatechin with vanillic acid, both of them at doses that reduce food intake, was only effective three hours after treatment and was not effective thereafter (Figure 4d).

3.5. Stronger Agonism of hTAS2R39 Than hTAS2R5 Can Stimulate Food Intake

Rats treated with Thiamine (a selective hTAS2R39 ligand) at a dose of 7.5 mM, which is much higher than the effective concentration (Table 1), did not modify food intake (Figure S2). Neither did epicatechin gallate, which also binds hTAS2R39, with an EC50 of 88.2 µM [22] (Figure S3).

Stimulation with epicatechin 0.3 mM + 21.8 µM of EGCG (equivalent to simultaneous stimulation of hTAS2R39 and hTAS2R5) did not change food intake. We also found no effects when we doubled the epicatechin dose (0.78 mM) (Figure S4). Interestingly, when we added a selective hTAS2R39 agonist such as epicatechin gallate (at a dose that has no effect on food intake) to epicatechin to reach a total dose of 0.84 mM (at which epicatechin alone had no effect) we observed a stimulation of food intake (Figure 5a). This effect was also found with a simultaneous treatment of epicatechin plus procyanidin B2 (Figure 5b).

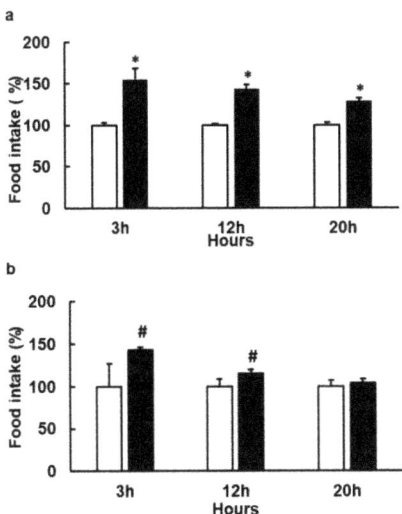

Figure 5. Changes in food intake (FI) induced by acute doses of agonists of bitter taste receptors in female rats. Animals (n = 8–10/treatment) were treated one hour before the dark period with an acute dose of epicatechin (234 mg/kg) + epicatechin gallate (14 mg/kg), a whole dose ~0.84 mM (black columns) (**a**); epicatechin (213 mg/kg) + B2 (62 mg/kg), a whole dose ~0.84 mM (**b**). White columns indicate the control group treated with tap water as vehicle. Food intake was measured at the times indicated after the start of the dark period starts (Mean ± SEM). * denotes $p < 0.05$ vs. control, # denotes $p < 0.1$ vs. control.

4. Discussion

We hypothesized that the specific stimulation of bitter taste receptors located in the gastrointestinal tract can produce a secretome that modulates food intake in rats. Knowledge of the role of these receptors in that location is scarce, though their ability to increase ghrelin secretion has been proven in two situations [15,16]. Here, we show that stimulation by some agonists for human TAS2R may be used as an on/off mechanism to elicit enterohormone secretions that modulate food intake in the organisms.

Our study is mainly based on the definitions by Meyerhof et al. [11] regarding the compounds that bind and activate human bitter taste receptors. To select the ligands, we worked with three receptors with different selectivities: a highly selective hTAS2R5, a moderately selective receptor such as hTAS2R39 and a highly promiscuous hTAS2R14. We stimulated intestinal segments with the agonists of the human TAS2Rs and measured their ability to induce gastrointestinal secretions that participate in the control of food intake. The most consolidated changes due to metabolic surgery (which modulates food intake) on the secretome in humans are increased GLP1 and PYY [4]. Here, we have found that in rats, the most effective changes in secretome for reducing food intake are increases in GLP1 and CCK, which do not affect PYY. The common denominator in these approaches is the increase in GLP1. In fact, the only approved drug for managing body weight via enterohormone mechanisms is based on GLP1 analogues such as liraglutide [23].

Increased GLP-1 is obtained with a specific agonist (1,10-Phenanthroline) or with agonists that preferentially bind to hTAS2R5 (epicatechin or B2 gallate). However, we also found an increase in GLP-1 via the stimulation of hTAS2R14—in this case together with a reduction in CCK, which, with vanillic acid, also tends to reduce food intake. There is no additive effect between epicatechin and vanillic acid and this cotreatment antagonizes their ability to stimulate tGLP1 secretion, which, as expected, limits their respective ability to inhibit food intake. Since we are working with theoretically defined receptors, we can postulate different interactions between these ligands to interfere with tGLP1 secretion. They could interfere intracellularly producing crosstalk between intracellular signaling [24], or there could be a desensitizing phenomenon, as has been defined for hTAS2R14 [25]. When the combination of epicatechin and vanillic acid was tested in vivo, at three hours we observed a reduction in food intake, probably due to epicatechin. Afterwards, when vanillic acids become effective (12 h onwards), the effects of the combination are lost, which could be due to heterologous desensitization. We obtained the same secretome profile (higher GLP1 and CCK) with procyanidin B2 at 300 μM. This procyanidin has not been shown to bind to any hTAS2R at the concentrations assayed (i.e., below 150 μM) [17]. When it was assayed at higher concentrations in intestinal segments, we found a similar secretome profile to that of epicatechin (a hTAS2R5 + hTAS2R39 agonist). Contrastingly, with the combination of procyanidin B2 with epicatechin assayed on intestinal segments, any differences on the secretion of neither GLP1 nor CCK were observed. This finding suggests that procyanidin B2 may act as a partial agonist of the effects of hTAS2R5. The effects of procyanidin B2 alone seem to correspond to those of agonists of hTAS2R5 and hTAS2R39 but in combination with another agonist, it cancels these effects [26]. When we used B2 alone with rats, we observed no effect. This was because we were working with a dose of 110 μM, which is closer to the dose of 67 μM (which was shown to be ineffective in the studies on secretome) than to the effective dose of 300 μM.

Stimulating only PYY secretion, as produced by specific hTAS2R39 stimulation, appears to be ineffective in reducing food intake in the rat. On the other hand, some combinations that preferentially target hTAS2R39 signaling (such as epicatechin plus epicatechin gallate) at a dose of over 0.84 mM do stimulate food intake. Previous studies with epicatechin showed a trend towards the stimulation of octanoyl ghrelin secretion in murine cells, while epicatechin gallate, a specific ligand for hTAS2R39, clearly stimulated octanoyl ghrelin—an effect that was abrogated by a specific antagonist for hTAS2R39 [15]. From these in vitro studies, it could be suggested that hTAS2R39 stimulates PYY and octanoyl ghrelin secretions. It was not possible to measure octanoyl ghrelin in our study because its presence in rat intestine is too low to be accurately measured. However, we cannot rule out the stimulation of ghrelin secretion in vivo that contributes to the orexigenic effect of this combination. We observed a similar stimulation of food intake when epicatechin plus procyanidin B2 was administered. We also treated ghrelin-producing cells with B2 or B2 gallate but octanoyl ghrelin secretion remained unchanged [15]. Therefore, if our hypothesis is that hTAS2R39 stimulation is related to the stimulation of food intake, we may suggest that B2 counteracts the effect of epicatechin in hTAS2R5 and allows only the stimulation of epicatechin in hTAS2R39.

Surprisingly, the combination of epicatechin plus procyanidin B2 and epicatechin gallate (all at non-effective doses for inhibiting food intake) leads to a reduction in food intake in the rat. To explain this finding, we postulate that all the ligands of hTAS2R39 in the mix compete amongst themselves at the level of the receptor or at other stages between the initial stimulation and the final effect on food intake, while the effects linked to hTAS2R5 remain unaltered. Nevertheless, we are unable to prove this with our data.

In addition to the different number of bitter taste receptors between species (25 in humans and 35 in rodents), there are different agonisms for the different sets of TAS2Rs possessed by each species [13]. 1,10-Phenantroline binds five bitter taste receptors in mice (mTas2r). Neither Thiamine nor Flufenamic acid has been tested in mice. Epicatechin binds two mTas2r while EGCG binds only one (mTas2144). In this study, we have been working on rats, about whom there is little information regarding TAS2R and their orthologues in humans, or their respective specificities against different ligands. Their proximity to mice can be used as a reference but extreme caution must be taken when extrapolating these results to humans. As an example, Avau et al. proved that intra-gastric stimulation induced a TAS2R-dependent delay in gastric emptying in mice that, when assayed in human volunteers, increased satiation [27]. Another aspect to address in the future should be gender effects since recently gender differences have been reported in humans [28,29]. Beyond these considerations, the importance of our study is the evidence that the stimulation with specific bitters produces enterohormone secretions linked to food intake modulation. However, specific attention must be paid to the possible differences between rat and human isoforms.

Finally, we used our hypothesis to explain the satiating effect of some doses of grape-seed derived procyanidins (GSPE), which we did not obtain when we used a very similar but slightly different (cocoa) extract [30]. Epicatechin, procyanidin B2, epicatechin gallate, vanillic acid and other ligands of hTAS2R5, hTAS2R14 and hTAS2R39 [17] are constituents of grape seeds. We showed that a grape-seed proanthocyanidin extract can increase GLP1 secretion, GIP and PYY [31,32] and limit food intake at doses above 350 mg/kg Bw [33]. Table S2 summarizes the abundance of ligands for hTAS2R5, hTAS2R14 and hTAS2R39 in GSPE, Cocoanox and the satiating combination (epicatechin + B2 + ECg). GSPE contains selective ligands for hTAS2R5 and very few amounts of ligands for hTAS2R14. The highest amounts of ligands are for hTAS2R5 and hTA2r39, together with selective ligands for hTAS2R39, which suggests competition by hTAS2R39 effects and enables the stimulation of enterohormones induced by hTAS2R5, which produces satiety. The case of Cocoanox resembles stimulation by epicatechin plus B2: either there is no effect or, depending on the ratio between both, food intake increases [30].

5. Conclusions

Food intake can be adjusted by gastrointestinal stimulation with compounds that bind to specific bitter taste receptors. This mechanism produces enterohormone secretions that can explain these effects on food intake. Specifically, the ligands of hTAS2R5 stimulation produce an anorexigenic effects in rats, whereas ligands of hTAS2R39 acts as an orexigenic. Further studies in humans are required to prove this strategy as means of controlling food intake.

6. Patents

There is a patent submitted on this manuscript P202030846.

Supplementary Materials: The following are available online at http://www.mdpi.com/2072-6643/12/12/3784/s1, Figure S1: Food intake after an acute dose of procyanidin B2 in female rats, Figure S2: Food intake after an acute dose of Thiamine in female rats, Figure S3: Food intake after an acute dose of epicatechin gallate in female rats, Figure S4: Food intake after an acute dose of epicatechin + EGCG in female rats. Table S1: Compounds tested for secretion in intestinal segments and food intake studies and their concentration, Table S2: Molarity of respective ligands of hTAS2R in GSPE and Cocoanox (mM).

Author Contributions: C.G.-B.: conceptualization, methodology, investigation, visualization, writing; A.M.-G. and C.G.-Q.: investigation and data acquisition; J.-A.F.-L. and X.R.: investigation, resources and review; C.T.-F. and J.Á.-R.: resources and critical review; E.R.-G. and R.B.-D.: methodology, critical review and funding; M.T.B.: conception of design and funding acquisition; X.T.: conception of design, formal analysis, funding acquisition; A.A. and M.P.: conceptualization, writing, funding acquisition and project administration. All authors have read and agreed to the published version of the manuscript.

Funding: This research was funded by Spanish Government grant number AGL2017-83477-R and R2B2018/03 co-funded by the FEDER program of the Generalitat de Catalunya and the URV. C. Grau-Bové received a doctoral research grant from the Martí Franques program of the Universitat Rovira i Virgili. C. González-Quilen received financial support through a FI-AGAUR grant, and C. Torres a Beatriu de Pinós grant, both from the autonomous government of Catalonia. M. Pinent and X. Terra are Serra Húnter fellows.

Acknowledgments: We would like to thank Niurka Llopiz for technical support. Thanks also to Eurecat, the Centre Tecnològic de Catalunya and the Unitat de Nutrició i Salut (Reus) for providing intestinal samples.

Conflicts of Interest: The authors declare no conflict of interest.

References

1. Blundell, J.E.; Finlayson, G.; Gibbons, C.; Caudwell, P.; Hopkins, M. The biology of appetite control: Do resting metabolic rate and fat-free mass drive energy intake? *Physiol. Behav.* **2015**, *152*, 473–478. [CrossRef]
2. Mulla, C.M.; Middelbeek, R.J.W.; Patti, M.E. Mechanisms of weight loss and improved metabolism following bariatric surgery. *Ann. N. Y. Acad. Sci.* **2018**, *1411*, 53–64. [CrossRef]
3. Gissey, L.C.; Mariolo, J.C.; Mingrone, G. Intestinal peptide changes after bariatric and minimally invasive surgery: Relation to diabetes remission. *Peptides* **2018**, *100*, 114–122. [CrossRef]
4. Sweeney, T.E.; Resident, S.; Morton, J.M.; Bariatric, C. Metabolic surgery: Action via hormonal milieu changes, changes in bile acids or gut microbiota? A summary of the literature. *Best Pract. Res. Clin. Gastroenterol.* **2014**, *28*, 727–740. [CrossRef]
5. Serrano, J.; Casanova-Martí, À.; Blay, M.T.; Terra, X.; Pinent, M.; Ardévol, A. Strategy for limiting food intake using food components aimed at multiple targets in the gastrointestinal tract. *Trends Food Sci. Technol.* **2017**, *68*, 113–129. [CrossRef]
6. Glendinning, J.I. Is the bitter rejection response always adaptive? *Physiol. Behav.* **1994**, *56*, 1217–1227. [CrossRef]
7. Nissim, I.; Dagan-Wiener, A.; Niv, M.Y. The taste of toxicity: A quantitative analysis of bitter and toxic molecules. *IUBMB Life* **2017**, *69*, 938–946. [CrossRef]
8. Duffy, V.B.; Hayes, J.E.; Davidson, A.C.; Kidd, J.R.; Kidd, K.K.; Bartoshuk, L.M. Vegetable Intake in College-Aged Adults Is Explained by Oral Sensory Phenotypes and TAS2R38 Genotype. *Chemosens. Percept.* **2010**, *3*, 137–148. [CrossRef]
9. Jeruzal-Świątecka, J.; Fendler, W.; Pietruszewska, W. Clinical role of extraoral bitter taste receptors. *Int. J. Mol. Sci.* **2020**, *21*, 5156. [CrossRef]
10. Foster, S.R.S.R.; Roura, E.; Thomas, W.G.W.G. Extrasensory perception: Odorant and taste receptors beyond the nose and mouth. *Pharmacol. Ther.* **2014**, *142*, 41–61. [CrossRef]
11. Meyerhof, W.; Batram, C.; Kuhn, C.; Brockhoff, A.; Chudoba, E.; Bufe, B.; Appendino, G.; Behrens, M. The Molecular Receptive Ranges of Human TAS2R Bitter Taste Receptors. *Chem. Senses* **2010**, *35*, 157–170. [CrossRef]
12. Di Pizio, A.; Niv, M.Y. Bioorganic & Medicinal Chemistry Promiscuity and selectivity of bitter molecules and their receptors. *Bioorg. Med. Chem.* **2015**, *23*, 4082–4091. [CrossRef]
13. Lossow, K.; Hübner, S.; Roudnitzky, N.; Slack, J.P.; Pollastro, F.; Behrens, M.; Meyerhof, W. Comprehensive analysis of mouse bitter taste receptors reveals different molecular receptive ranges for orthologous receptors in mice and humans. *J. Biol. Chem.* **2016**, *291*, 15358–15377. [CrossRef]
14. Grassin-Delyle, S.; Salvator, H.; Mantov, N.; Abrial, C.; Brollo, M.; Faisy, C.; Naline, E.; Couderc, L.J.L.-J.; Devillier, P. Bitter Taste Receptors (TAS2Rs) in Human Lung Macrophages: Receptor Expression and Inhibitory Effects of TAS2R Agonists. *Front. Physiol.* **2019**, *10*, 1–13. [CrossRef]
15. Serrano, J.; Casanova-Martí, À.; Depoortere, I.; Blay, M.T.M.T.; Terra, X.; Pinent, M.; Ardévol, A. Subchronic treatment with grape-seed phenolics inhibits ghrelin production despite a short-term stimulation of ghrelin secretion produced by bitter-sensing flavanols. *Mol. Nutr. Food Res.* **2016**, *60*, 2554–2564. [CrossRef]
16. Wang, Q.; Liszt, K.I.K.I.K.I.; Deloose, E.; Canovai, E.; Thijs, T.; Farré, R.; Ceulemans, L.J.L.J.; Lannoo, M.; Tack, J.; Depoortere, I. Obesity alters adrenergic and chemosensory signaling pathways that regulate ghrelin secretion in the human gut. *FASEB J.* **2019**, *33*, 4907–4920. [CrossRef] [PubMed]
17. Soares, S.; Silva, M.S.M.S.; García-Estevez, I.; Großmann, P.; Brás, N.; Brandão, E.; Mateus, N.; De Freitas, V.; Behrens, M.; Meyerhof, W. Human Bitter Taste Receptors Are Activated by Different Classes of Polyphenols. *J. Agric. Food Chem.* **2018**, *66*, 8814–8823. [CrossRef] [PubMed]

18. Wiener, A.; Shudler, M.; Levit, A.; Niv, M.Y. BitterDB: A database of bitter compounds. *Nucleic Acids Res.* **2012**, *40*, 413–419. [CrossRef]
19. Soares, S.; Kohl, S.; Thalmann, S.; Mateus, N.; Meyerhof, W.; De Freitas, V. Different Phenolic Compounds Activate Distinct Human Bitter Taste Receptors. *J. Agric. Food Chem.* **2013**, *61*, 1525–1533. [CrossRef]
20. Narukawa, M.; Noga, C.; Ueno, Y.; Sato, T.; Misaka, T.; Watanabe, T. Evaluation of the bitterness of green tea catechins by a cell-based assay with the human bitter taste receptor hTAS2R39. *Biochem. Biophys. Res. Commun.* **2011**, *405*, 620–625. [CrossRef] [PubMed]
21. Hufnagel, J.C.; Hofmann, T. Orosensory-Directed Identification of Astringent Mouthfeel and Bitter-Tasting Compounds in Red Wine. *J. Agric. Food Chem.* **2008**, *56*, 1376–1386. [CrossRef]
22. Drewnowski, A.; Gomez-Carneros, C. Bitter taste, phytonutrients, and the consumer: A review. *Am. J. Clin. Nutr.* **2000**, *72*, 1424–1435. [CrossRef]
23. Srivastava, G.; Apovian, C.M. Current pharmacotherapy for obesity. *Nat. Rev. Endocrinol.* **2018**, *14*, 12–24. [CrossRef]
24. Oswald, C.; Rappas, M.; Kean, J.; Doré, A.S.; Errey, J.C.; Bennett, K.; Deflorian, F.; Christopher, J.A.; Jazayeri, A.; Mason, J.S.; et al. Intracellular Allosteric Antagonism of the CCR9 Receptor. *Nat. Publ. Gr.* **2016**, *540*, 462–465. [CrossRef]
25. Woo, J.A.; Castaño, M.; Goss, A.; Kim, D.; Lewandowski, E.M.; Chen, Y.; Liggett, S.B. Differential long-term regulation of TAS2R14 by structurally distinct agonists. *FASEB J.* **2019**, *33*, 12213–12225. [CrossRef]
26. Kenakin, T.P. Chapter 4—Drug Antagonism: Orthosteric Drug Effects. In *Pharmacology in Drug Discovery and Development*, 2nd ed.; Academic Press: New York, NY, USA, 2017; pp. 65–100, ISBN 978-0-12-803752-2.
27. Avau, B.; Rotondo, A.; Thijs, T.; Andrews, C.N.; Janssen, P.; Tack, J.; Depoortere, I. Targeting extra-oral bitter taste receptors modulates gastrointestinal motility with effects on satiation. *Sci. Rep.* **2015**, *5*, 15985. [CrossRef]
28. Hayes, J.E.J.E.; Wallace, M.R.; Knopik, V.S.V.S.; Herbstman, D.M.D.M.; Bartoshuk, L.M.L.M.; Duffy, V.B.V.B. Allelic variation in TAS2R bitter receptor genes associates with variation in sensations from and ingestive behaviors toward common bitter beverages in adults. *Chem. Senses* **2011**, *36*, 311–319. [CrossRef]
29. Coltell, O.; Sorlí, J.V.; Asensio, E.M.; Fernández-Carrión, R.; Barragán, R.; Ortega-Azorín, C.; Estruch, R.; González, J.I.; Salas-Salvadó, J.; Lamon-Fava, S.; et al. Association between taste perception and adiposity in overweight or obese older subjects with metabolic syndrome and identification of novel taste-related genes. *Am. J. Clin. Nutr.* **2019**, *109*, 1709–1723. [CrossRef]
30. Serrano, J.; Casanova-Martí, À.; Gil-Cardoso, K.; Blay, M.T.; Terra, X.; Pinent, M.; Ardévol, A. Acutely administered grape-seed proanthocyanidin extract acts as a satiating agent. *Food Funct.* **2016**, *7*, 483–490. [CrossRef]
31. Casanova-martí, À.; Serrano, J.; Portune, K.J.; Sanz, Y. Function microbiota and enteroendocrine secretions in. *Food Funct.* **2019**, *10*, 4062–4070. [CrossRef]
32. González-Abuín, N.; Martínez-Micaelo, N.; Blay, M.; Ardévol, A.; Pinent, M. Grape-Seed Procyanidins Prevent the Cafeteria-Diet-Induced Decrease of Glucagon-Like Peptide-1 Production. *J. Agric. Food Chem.* **2014**, *62*, 1066–1072. [CrossRef]
33. Serrano, J.; Casanova-Martí, À.; Blay, M.; Terra, X.; Ardévol, A.; Pinent, M. Defining conditions for optimal inhibition of food intake in rats by a grape-seed derived proanthocyanidin extract. *Nutrients* **2016**, *8*, 652. [CrossRef]

Publisher's Note: MDPI stays neutral with regard to jurisdictional claims in published maps and institutional affiliations.

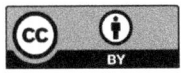

© 2020 by the authors. Licensee MDPI, Basel, Switzerland. This article is an open access article distributed under the terms and conditions of the Creative Commons Attribution (CC BY) license (http://creativecommons.org/licenses/by/4.0/).

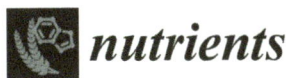

Article

Acute Effects of Lixisenatide on Energy Intake in Healthy Subjects and Patients with Type 2 Diabetes: Relationship to Gastric Emptying and Intragastric Distribution

Ryan Jalleh [1], Hung Pham [2], Chinmay S. Marathe [1,2], Tongzhi Wu [1,2], Madeline D. Buttfield [3], Seva Hatzinikolas [2], Charles H. Malbert [4], Rachael S. Rigda [2], Kylie Lange [2], Laurence G. Trahair [2], Christine Feinle-Bisset [2], Christopher K. Rayner [2,5], Michael Horowitz [1,2] and Karen L. Jones [1,2,*]

1. Endocrine and Metabolic Unit, Royal Adelaide Hospital, Adelaide SA 5000, Australia; ryan.jalleh@sa.gov.au (R.J.); chinmay.marathe@adelaide.edu.au (C.S.M.); tongzhi.wu@adelaide.edu.au (T.W.); michael.horowitz@adelaide.edu.au (M.H.)
2. Adelaide Medical School, Centre of Research Excellence in Translating Nutritional Science to Good Health, The University of Adelaide, Adelaide SA 5000, Australia; hung.pham@adelaide.edu.au (H.P.); seva.hatzinikolas@adelaide.edu.au (S.H.); rachael.tippett@adelaide.edu.au (R.S.R.); kylie.lange@adelaide.edu.au (K.L.); laurence.trahair@adelaide.edu.au (L.G.T.); christine.feinle@adelaide.edu.au (C.F.-B.); chris.rayner@adelaide.edu.au (C.K.R.)
3. School of Health Sciences, University of South Australia, Adelaide SA 5001, Australia; madeline.buttfield@bensonradiology.com.au
4. Aniscan, Institut National de la Rechercher Agronomique, 35590 Saint-Gilles, France; charles-henri.malbert@inra.fr
5. Department of Gastroenterology and Hepatology, Royal Adelaide Hospital, Adelaide SA 5000, Australia
* Correspondence: karen.jones@adelaide.edu.au; Tel.: +61-8-83137821

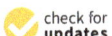

Received: 30 May 2020; Accepted: 29 June 2020; Published: 1 July 2020

Abstract: Glucagon-like peptide-1 receptor agonists induce weight loss, which has been suggested to relate to the slowing of gastric emptying (GE). In health, energy intake (EI) is more strongly related to the content of the distal, than the total, stomach. We evaluated the effects of lixisenatide on GE, intragastric distribution, and subsequent EI in 15 healthy participants and 15 patients with type 2 diabetes (T2D). Participants ingested a 75-g glucose drink on two separate occasions, 30 min after lixisenatide (10 mcg) or placebo subcutaneously, in a randomised, double-blind, crossover design. GE and intragastric distribution were measured for 180 min followed by a buffet-style meal, where EI was quantified. Relationships of EI with total, proximal, and distal stomach content were assessed. In both groups, lixisenatide slowed GE markedly, with increased retention in both the proximal ($p < 0.001$) and distal ($p < 0.001$) stomach and decreased EI ($p < 0.001$). EI was not related to the content of the total or proximal stomach but inversely related to the distal stomach at 180 min in health on placebo ($r = -0.58$, $p = 0.03$) but not in T2D nor after lixisenatide in either group. In healthy and T2D participants, the reduction in EI by lixisenatide is unrelated to changes in GE/intragastric distribution, consistent with a centrally mediated effect.

Keywords: lixisenatide; intragastric meal retention; energy intake; type 2 diabetes

1. Introduction

Glucagon-like peptide-1 (GLP-1) receptor agonists (RAs)—both 'short' and 'long' acting—induce moderate weight loss in obese subjects with or without type 2 diabetes (T2D) [1–5]. The mechanisms underlying this weight loss are poorly defined. 'Short-acting' GLP-1RAs slow gastric emptying markedly [6,7], which appears to be primarily responsible for their effect to diminish postprandial glycaemia substantially [8]. 'Long-acting' GLP-1RAs, which are used widely in the management of obesity, probably have a lesser effect on gastric emptying, so that both preprandial and postprandial glucose lowering may be attributable primarily to their insulinotropic and glucagonostatic properties [9]; however, it is now clear that long-acting GLP-1RAs do slow gastric emptying [10]. GLP-1, secreted from L-cells in the epithelium of the small intestine, binds to GLP-1 receptors that are expressed in multiple organs, including the pancreatic islets, kidneys, lungs, heart, and central and peripheral nervous systems [11]. Circulating GLP-1 is able to access central GLP-1 receptors in areas not fully blocked by the blood–brain barrier, such as the subfornical organ and area postrema [12,13]. Most GLP-1RAs are able to activate central GLP-1 receptors expressing neurons. Larger molecule GLP-1RAs that are unable to cross the blood–brain barrier appear to act via secondary signals from the vagus nerve [14], while smaller molecule GLP-1RAs, including lixisenatide, pass through the blood–brain barrier directly [15]. Possible mechanisms underlying weight loss by GLP-1RAs include satiation induced by the slowing of gastric emptying and a consequent prolongation of gastric distension, centrally-mediated anorexia, and the induction of nausea as an adverse effect [16]. The stomach comprises distinct anatomical regions—the fundus, body (corpus), antrum and pylorus, with the proximal stomach incorporating the fundus and proximal corpus and the distal stomach incorporating the distal corpus and antrum. The proximal stomach is primarily responsible for the storage of food and relaxes in response to eating to accommodate a meal with only a modest change in intragastric pressure, whereas the antrum grinds solid food into small particles, usually <1 mm in size, that are delivered into the small intestine at a rate that optimises digestion and absorption. Accordingly, each region plays a coordinated role in the regulation of gastric emptying. In health, antral—rather than proximal or total—intragastric content is most closely related to energy-intake suppression in young and older subjects, probably indicative of an effect of antral distension [17]. The effects of GLP-1RAs on intragastric meal distribution and the relationship of changes in energy intake with gastric emptying/intragastric distribution have not been evaluated.

The aims of this study were to evaluate the acute effects of lixisenatide on intragastric distribution and subsequent energy intake in health and T2D. This was a prespecified secondary analysis from a study evaluating the effects of lixisenatide on gastric emptying and blood pressure in these groups [8].

2. Materials and Methods

Twenty-four 'healthy' participants and 74 participants with T2D, managed by diet or a stable dose of metformin alone, were 'prescreened' by phone or email interview. Participants were required to be 40–80 years of age, with BMI 19–35 kg/m^2 and, for T2D patients, have an HbA1c < 8.5% (<69 mmol/mol). Three healthy participants and 47 T2D participants were excluded. Full exclusion criteria have been published [8]. The remaining participants attended the Royal Adelaide Hospital (RAH) for a screening visit and had a venous blood sample taken for measurement of HbA1c, liver function, creatinine, glucose, and biochemistry and, for females, a urine test for pregnancy. Of the 21 'healthy' participants, 18 were enrolled and 3 were excluded; of the 27 participants with T2D, 16 were enrolled. Of the healthy participants, 2 withdrew due to adverse events (nausea soon after administration of lixisenatide) and 1 was withdrawn on the first study day because of a low baseline blood pressure. Of the T2D participants, 1 was withdrawn due to inability to attend the RAH on the two study days.

Hence, a total of 15 healthy participants (9 male, 6 female; age: 67.2 ± 2.3 years; body mass index: 25.4 ± 0.8 kg/m^2) and 15 participants with T2D managed by diet or metformin alone (9 male, 6 female; age: 61.9 ± 2.3 years; BMI: 30.3 ± 0.7 kg/m^2; duration of known diabetes: 5.3 ± 1.2 years; HbA$_1$c: 6.9 ± 0.2% (51.8 ± 2.3 mmol/mol) were studied. Ten of the 15 participants in the T2D group were taking metformin (plasma half-life: 4–9 h [18]) that was withheld for 48 h prior to the study because of its potential effect on gastric emptying [19]. The other 5 participants were managed by diet alone. Antihypertensive medication (used by 3 age-matched, non-diabetic controls and 4 participants with T2D) was also held for 48 h. All participants were nonsmokers, and none had a history of gastrointestinal disease or surgery, significant respiratory, cardiac, hepatic and/or renal disease, alcohol consumption >20 g per day or epilepsy, and none were unable to withhold any medication likely to influence blood pressure or gastrointestinal function. The sample size was based on a primary outcome presented in a previous published study [8] and this is a secondary analysis, as stated previously.

2.1. Protocol

The study followed a randomised, double-blind, placebo-controlled, crossover design. Using a stratified (healthy/T2D), randomised permuted-blocks (block size of 2) method, participants were allocated to their respective groups by Sanofi. Participants attended the Department of Nuclear Medicine, Positron Emission Tomography and Bone Densitometry at the RAH at 8.30 am after an overnight fast (14 h for solids, 12 h for liquids) on two separate occasions.

Participants received either lixisenatide (10 mcg) or placebo subcutaneously (sc), and 27 min later ingested a drink comprising 75 g glucose (280.5 kcal) radiolabelled with 20 MBq ^{99m}Tc-Calcium Phytate (Radpharm Scientific, Belconnen, ACT, Australia), made up to 300 mL water, within 3 min ($t = 0$ min was defined as the end of drink ingestion).

2.2. Measurements

Gastric emptying was measured by scintigraphy for 180 min. Data was acquired every minute for the first hour, then every 3 min for the subsequent 2 h. A region-of-interest was drawn around the total stomach, which was then divided into proximal and distal stomach regions to determine intragastric distribution, i.e., retention of the drink in the proximal and distal stomach regions, whereby the proximal region corresponded to the fundus and proximal corpus and the distal stomach region corresponded to the antrum and distal corpus [20]. Data were analysed, using purpose-built software (CH Malbert, LabView, National Instruments (NI), Dallas TX, USA, 2013), by two experienced nuclear medicine technologists (MDB, KLJ), blinded to the study conditions.

Energy intake was assessed from $t = 180$ min when each participant was offered a cold, buffet-style meal on a tray and allowed to eat for 30 min until they felt comfortably full [21]. The buffet meal comprised four slices (125 g) of wholemeal bread, four slices (125 g) of white bread, 100 g sliced ham, 100 g sliced chicken, 85 g sliced cheddar cheese, 100 g lettuce, 100 g sliced tomato, 100 g sliced cucumber, 20 g mayonnaise, 20 g margarine, 170 g apple, 190 g banana, 200 g strawberry yogurt, 150 g chocolate custard, 140 g fruit salad, 600 mL iced coffee, 500 mL orange juice and 600 mL water with a total energy content of 11 808 kJ. Food was weighed prior to consumption and the amount (kcal) of energy consumed was derived using commercial software (Foodworks 3.01, Xyris Software, Highgate Hill, QLD, Australia), based on the weight of the remaining food on the tray at the end of the 30-min period [21].

Nausea was assessed using a validated 100 mm visual analog questionnaire [22], prior to study-drug administration, before consumption of the glucose drink and at 15-min intervals during the gastric emptying measurement. These data, together with plasma glucose, insulin, C-peptide, and glucagon concentrations, have previously been reported [8].

The protocol was approved by the Human Research Ethics Committee of the Royal Adelaide Hospital, and each participant provided written, informed consent. All studies were carried out in accordance with the Declaration of Helsinki. The study was registered on clinicaltrials.gov (NCT: 02308254).

2.3. Statistics

Effects of treatment and group were assessed with two-way repeated measures analysis of variance (ANOVA), with treatment as a within-subject factor and group as a between-subject factor, including treatment and group main effects and the treatment by group interaction. Relationships between energy intake and the content of the total, proximal and distal stomach after placebo and lixisenatide were assessed using linear regression analysis. Data were analysed using SPSS Statistics (SPSS, Chicago, IL, USA) and are presented as means ± SEMs. A value of $p < 0.05$ was considered significant.

3. Results

The studies were well tolerated. As reported, scores for nausea were uniformly very low with no difference between placebo and lixisenatide, and lixisenatide slowed gastric emptying markedly in both groups ($p < 0.001$). The proximal stomach retention at 180 min in the healthy group was 6.6 ± 3.5% with placebo vs. 40.9 ± 4.6% with lixisenatide ($p < 0.001$) and in the T2D group was 6.3 ± 4.1% with placebo vs. 34.8 ± 24.5% with lixisenatide ($p < 0.001$). The distal stomach retention at 180 min in health was 9.4 ± 9.1% with placebo vs. 18.6 ± 11.1% with lixisenatide ($p < 0.001$) and in T2D was 8.2 ± 4.2% with placebo vs. 19.6 ± 10.4% with lixisenatide ($p < 0.001$) (Figure 1). There was no difference in the effect of lixisenatide on intragastric distribution between the two groups.

Lixisenatide decreased energy intake ($p < 0.001$) in both healthy participants and T2D (Figure 2) by −29.2 ± 4.0% and −27.1 ± 8.2%, respectively. On the placebo day, there was no relationship between energy intake and the content of the proximal ($r = 0.005$, $p = 0.99$ in healthy participants; $r = 0.11$, $p = 0.70$ in T2D) or total stomach ($r = −0.47$, $p = 0.09$ in healthy participants; $r = −0.11$, $p = 0.70$ in T2D) at $t = 180$ min after placebo. However, energy intake was inversely related to the distal stomach content at $t = 180$ min in health ($r = −0.58$, $p = 0.03$) but not in T2D ($r = −0.31$, $p = 0.27$). On the lixisenatide day, there was no relationship between energy intake and the distal stomach content in healthy participants ($r = −0.16$, $p = 0.58$) or T2D ($r = −0.004$, $p = 0.99$) (Figure 3). Similarly, there was no relationship between energy intake and the proximal stomach content ($r = −0.16$, $p = 0.58$ in healthy participants; $r = 0.10$, $p = 0.71$ in T2D) or total stomach content ($r = −0.23$, $p = 0.42$ in healthy participants; $r = 0.09$, $p = 0.75$ in T2D).

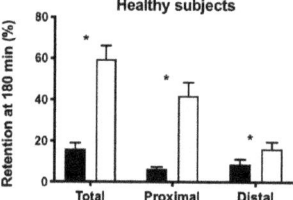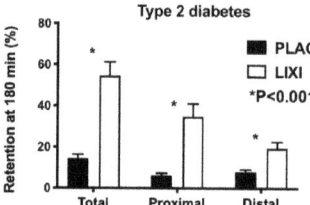

Figure 1. Intragastric distribution of gastric content (retention in the total, proximal, and distal stomach regions) at $t = 180$ min following a 75-g glucose drink radiolabelled with 20 MBq ^{99m}Tc-Calcium Phytate in health and type 2 diabetes (T2D) following lixisenatide (10 mcg sc) or placebo (sc). $p < 0.001$ treatment difference in two-way repeated measures ANOVA. Treatment-by-group interactions all nonsignificant ($p > 0.05$).

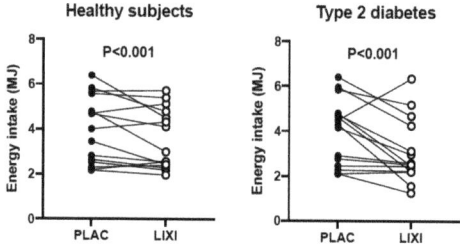

Figure 2. Effect of lixisenatide (10 mcg sc) (open circles) vs. placebo (sc) (black circles) on energy intake (MJ) at a buffet-style meal in healthy participants and patients with T2D $p < 0.001$ for both (placebo vs. lixisenatide). $p < 0.001$ treatment difference in two-way repeated measures analysis of variance (ANOVA). Treatment-by-group interaction nonsignificant ($p > 0.05$).

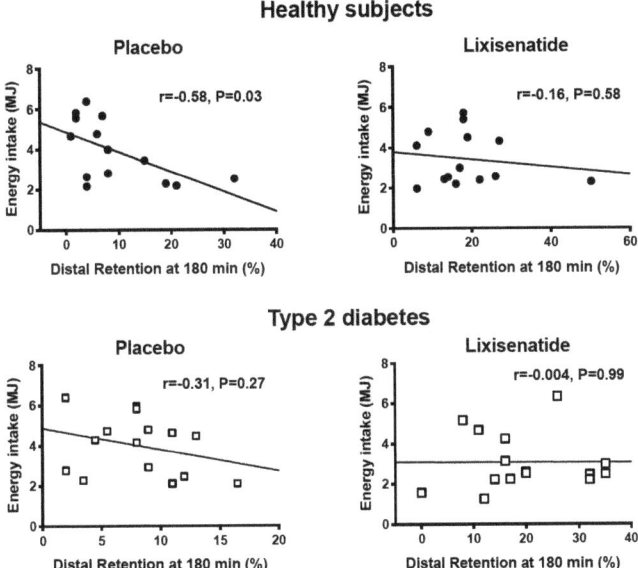

Figure 3. Relationships between energy intake (MJ) consumed at the buffet-style meal and retention in the distal stomach at 180 min after a drink containing 75 g glucose in healthy participants (black circles) following placebo ($r = -0.58$, $p = 0.03$) and lixisenatide ($r = -0.16$, $p = 0.58$) and patients with T2D (open squares) following placebo ($r = -0.31$, $p = 0.27$) and lixisenatide ($r = 0.004$, $p = 0.99$).

4. Discussion

Our study evaluated the acute effects of the 'short-acting' GLP-1RA lixisenatide on energy intake at a buffet meal, intragastric distribution of a glucose drink, and the relationship between them. We used a lower dose of lixisenatide (10 mcg) compared to the dose used clinically as monotherapy (titrated gradually to 20 mcg) to maximise tolerability. Doses of lixisenatide less than 20 mcg are, however, frequently used in practice, particularly in combination with insulin glargine, which has been shown to be well tolerated and associated with weight loss [23,24].

We have reported that lixisenatide at a dose of 10 mcg slows gastric emptying markedly in both health and well-controlled T2D, associated with a reduction in glycaemia [8]. The current study establishes that lixisenatide also affects intragastric distribution by increasing retention in both the proximal and distal stomach and reduces energy intake at a subsequent buffet meal. However, the effect of lixisenatide on energy intake was unrelated to its profound effects on intragastric distribution or total stomach emptying, strongly supporting the concept that the observed reduction of energy intake is primarily centrally mediated. We confirmed that, in health, the suppression of energy intake following a nutrient preload is closely related to the content of the distal—but not the total or proximal—stomach, presumably indicative of antral distension being a key determinant [17].

Intracerebroventricular injection of GLP-1 inhibits feeding in fasted rats [25], and radioligand binding studies in rats have shown high densities of GLP-1 receptors in the brain, including areas thought to be responsible for satiation [26]. In humans, cells positive for GLP-1 mRNA are expressed widely in the brain, including the hypothalamus, which is pivotal to the regulation of appetite [27]. One study, using functional MRI, has reported diminished responses in appetite- and reward-related brain areas after administration of intravenous exenatide in normoglycemic obese and T2D subjects, correlating with a reduction in food intake [28]. It has also been hypothesised that GLP-1 has peripherally mediated effects on appetite [16], particularly via slowing of gastric emptying, with consequent activation of gastric mechano-receptors which relay action potentials via the vagal nerves to the nucleus of the solitary tract to suppress appetite [29]. Our study does not support this hypothesis, given the absence of a relationship between energy intake and the increased retention of gastric content after lixisenatide. It has been suggested that weight loss resulting from GLP-1RAs represents an adverse effect due to the induction of nausea [30,31]. This was clearly not the case in our study, where there was minimal nausea after treatment with either lixisenatide or placebo.

Our study has several strengths, including the randomised, double-blind, placebo controlled, cross-over design in both health and T2D and use of the 'gold standard' technique of scintigraphy to measure gastric emptying and intragastric distribution.

Limitations relate to the 'proof-of-concept' design, the use of a glucose drink rather than a more physiologic mixed solid/liquid meal and that only the effects of a single, low dose of lixisenatide—instead of sustained administration—were assessed. Evidence to suggest that the suppression of energy intake by lixisenatide is centrally mediated is also indirect, and other mechanisms that could contribute to a reduction in energy intake by lixisenatide, including stimulation of brown adipose tissue activity, were not evaluated [32,33]. It should also be appreciated that the failure to observe a significant relationship between energy intake and the distal stomach content in the T2D group on the placebo days may reflect the modest number of participants, particularly given the relative heterogeneity of this group.

5. Conclusions

In conclusion, acute administration of 10 mcg lixisenatide reduces energy intake in the absence of nausea, slows gastric emptying of a glucose drink, and increases retention in the distal and proximal stomach. The reduction in energy intake by lixisenatide was unrelated to changes in gastric emptying/intragastric distribution, consistent with a centrally mediated effect.

Author Contributions: R.J. was involved in the data interpretation, statistical analysis and writing of the manuscript. H.P., C.H.M., L.G.T. and, C.F.-B. assisted with data analysis and interpretation. C.S.M. was involved in data analysis and interpretation. R.S.R. and S.H. were involved in participant recruitment, data collection, and data interpretation. M.D.B. and S.H. were involved in scintigraphic data analysis. K.L. performed the statistical analysis and was involved in data interpretation. K.L.J., M.H., C.K.R. and T.W. were involved in the conception and design of the study, data interpretation, and writing of the manuscript. K.L.J. and M.H. are the guarantors of this work and, as such, had full access to all the data in the study and take responsibility for the integrity of the data and the accuracy of the data analysis. Sanofi-Aventis provided study medicine (lixisenatide) and matching placebo. All authors critically reviewed the manuscript and have approved the publication of this final version of the manuscript.

Funding: This study was supported by investigator-initiated funds provided by Sanofi-Aventis (LIXISL06486). Study medication (lixisenatide and matching placebo) was also provided by Sanofi-Aventis. K.L.J is supported by a William T. Southcott Research Fellowship. C.S.M. is supported by an NHMRC Early Career Fellowship. T.W. is supported by a Royal Adelaide Hospital Research Committee Florey Fellowship. C.F.-B. is supported by an NHMRC Senior Research Fellowship. The Centre of Research Excellence in Translating Nutritional Science to Good Health is supported by funding from The Hospital Research Foundation.

Acknowledgments: We thank the staff of the Department of Nuclear Medicine, PET, and Bone Densitometry at the Royal Adelaide Hospital for the use of their gamma camera and the Royal Adelaide Hospital Pharmacy for dispensing the medication.

Conflicts of Interest: K.L.J. has received research funding from Sanofi and AstraZeneca and drug supplies from Merck Sharp & Dohme. T.W. has received travel support from Novartis and research funding from AstraZeneca. C.K.R. has received research funding from AstraZeneca, Merck Sharp & Dohme, Eli Lilly and Company, Novartis, and Sanofi. M.H. has participated in advisory boards and/or symposia for Novo Nordisk, Sanofi, Novartis, Eli Lilly and Company, Merck Sharp & Dohme, Boehringer Ingelheim, and AstraZeneca and has received honoraria for this activity. No other potential conflicts of interest relevant to this article are reported.

References

1. Meier, J.J.; Rosenstock, J.; Hincelin-Méry, A.; Roy-Duval, C.; Delfolie, A.; Coester, H.-V.; Menge, B.A.; Forst, T.; Kapitza, C. Contrasting effects of lixisenatide and liraglutide on postprandial glycemic control, gastric emptying, and safety parameters in patients with type 2 diabetes on optimized insulin glargine with or without metformin: A randomized, open-label trial. *Diabetes Care* **2015**, *38*, 1263–1273. [CrossRef]
2. Halawi, H.; Khemani, D.; Eckert, D.; O'Neill, J.; Kadouh, H.; Grothe, K.; Clark, M.M.; Burton, D.D.; Vella, A.; Acosta, A.; et al. Effects of liraglutide on weight, satiation, and gastric functions in obesity: A randomised, placebo-controlled pilot trial. *Lancet Gastroenterol. Hepatol.* **2017**, *2*, 890–899. [CrossRef]
3. Hjerpsted, J.B.; Flint, A.; Brooks, A.; Axelsen, M.B.; Kvist, T.; Blundell, J. Semaglutide improves postprandial glucose and lipid metabolism, and delays first-hour gastric emptying in subjects with obesity. *Diabetes Obes. Metab.* **2018**, *20*, 610–619. [CrossRef]
4. Acosta, A.; Camilleri, M.; Burton, D.; O'Neill, J.; Eckert, D.; Carlson, P.; Zinsmeister, A.R. Exenatide in obesity with accelerated gastric emptying: A randomized, pharmacodynamics study. *Physiol. Rep.* **2015**, *3*, 12610. [CrossRef]
5. Astrup, A.; Rossner, S.; Van Gaal, L.; Rissanen, A.; Niskanen, L.; Al Hakim, M.; Madsen, J.; Rasmussen, M.F.; Lean, M.E. Effects of liraglutide in the treatment of obesity: A randomised, double-blind, placebo-controlled study. *Lancet* **2009**, *374*, 1606–1616. [CrossRef]
6. Lorenz, M.; Pfeiffer, C.; Steinsträsser, A.; Becker, R.H.; Rütten, H.; Ruus, P.; Horowitz, M. Effects of lixisenatide once daily on gastric emptying in type 2 diabetes—Relationship to postprandial glycemia. *Regul. Pept.* **2013**, *185*, 1–8. [CrossRef]
7. Linnebjerg, H.; Park, S.; Kothare, P.A.; Trautmann, M.E.; Mace, K.; Fineman, M.; Wilding, I.; Nauck, M.; Horowitz, M. Effect of exenatide on gastric emptying and relationship to postprandial glycemia in type 2 diabetes. *Regul. Pept.* **2008**, *151*, 123–129. [CrossRef]
8. Jones, K.L.; Rigda, R.S.; Buttfield, M.D.M.; Hatzinikolas, S.; Pham, H.T.; Marathe, C.S.; Wu, T.; Lange, K.; Trahair, L.G.; Rayner, C.K.; et al. Effects of lixisenatide on postprandial blood pressure, gastric emptying and glycaemia in healthy people and people with type 2 diabetes. *Diabetes Obes. Metab.* **2019**, *21*, 1158–1167. [CrossRef]
9. Gentilella, R.; Pechtner, V.; Corcos, A.; Consoli, A. Glucagon-like peptide-1 receptor agonists in type 2 diabetes treatment: Are they all the same? *Diabetes Metab. Res. Rev.* **2019**, *35*, 3070. [CrossRef]
10. Jones, K.L.; Huynh, L.Q.; Hatzinikolas, S.; Rigda, R.S.; Phillips, L.K.; Pham, H.T.; Marathe, C.S.; Wu, T.; Malbert, C.H.; Stevens, J.E.; et al. Exenatide once weekly slows gastric emptying of solids and liquids in healthy, overweight people at steady-state concentrations. *Diabetes Obes. Metab.* **2020**, *22*, 788–797. [CrossRef]
11. Drucker, D.J. The biology of incretin hormones. *Cell Metab.* **2006**, *3*, 153–165. [CrossRef] [PubMed]
12. Kastin, A.J.; Akerstrom, V.; Pan, W. Interactions of glucagon-like peptide-1 (GLP-1) with the blood-brain barrier. *J. Mol. Neurosci.* **2002**, *18*, 7–14. [CrossRef]
13. Chaudhri, O.; Small, C.; Bloom, S. Gastrointestinal hormones regulating appetite. *Philos. Trans. R. Soc. B Boil. Sci.* **2006**, *361*, 1187–1209. [CrossRef] [PubMed]
14. Paternoster, S.; Falasca, M. Dissecting the physiology and pathophysiology of glucagon-like peptide-1. *Front. Endocrinol.* **2018**, *9*, 584. [CrossRef]
15. Hunter, K.; Hölscher, C. Drugs developed to treat diabetes, liraglutide and lixisenatide, cross the blood brain barrier and enhance neurogenesis. *BMC Neurosci.* **2012**, *13*, 33. [CrossRef]
16. Holst, J.J. Incretin hormones and the satiation signal. *Int. J. Obes.* **2013**, *37*, 1161–1168. [CrossRef] [PubMed]
17. Sturm, K.; Parker, B.; Wishart, J.; Feinle-Bisset, C.; Jones, K.L.; Chapman, I.; Horowitz, M. Energy intake and appetite are related to antral area in healthy young and older subjects. *Am. J. Clin. Nutr.* **2004**, *80*, 656–667. [CrossRef] [PubMed]
18. Scheen, A.J. Clinical pharmacokinetics of metformin. *Clin. Pharmacokinet.* **1996**, *30*, 359–371. [CrossRef] [PubMed]
19. Borg, M.J.; Bound, M.; Grivell, J.; Sun, Z.; Jones, K.L.; Horowitz, M.; Rayner, C.K.; Wu, T. Comparative effects of proximal and distal small intestinal administration of metformin on plasma glucose and glucagon-like peptide-1, and gastric emptying after oral glucose, in type 2 diabetes. *Diabetes, Obes. Metab.* **2019**, *21*, 640–647. [CrossRef]

20. Jones, K.L.; Horowitz, M.; Wishart, M.J.; Maddox, A.F.; Harding, P.E.; Chatterton, B.E. Relationships between gastric emptying, intragastric meal distribution and blood glucose concentrations in diabetes mellitus. *J. Nucl. Med.* **1995**, *36*, 2220–2228.
21. Nair, N.S.; Brennan, I.M.; Little, T.J.; Gentilcore, D.; Hausken, T.; Jones, K.L.; Wishart, J.M.; Horowitz, M.; Feinle-Bisset, C. Reproducibility of energy intake, gastric emptying, blood glucose, plasma insulin and cholecystokinin responses in healthy young males. *Br. J. Nutr.* **2009**, *101*, 1094–1102. [CrossRef] [PubMed]
22. Parker, B.A.; Sturm, K.; MacIntosh, C.G.; Feinle, C.; Horowitz, M.; Chapman, I.M. Relation between food intake and visual analogue scale ratings of appetite and other sensations in healthy older and young subjects. *Eur. J. Clin. Nutr.* **2004**, *58*, 212–218. [CrossRef]
23. Aroda, V.R.; Rosenstock, J.; Wysham, C.; Unger, J.; Bellido, D.; González-Gálvez, G.; Takami, A.; Guo, H.; Niemoeller, E.; Souhami, E.; et al. Efficacy and safety of LixiLan, a titratable fixed-ratio combination of insulin glargine plus lixisenatide in type 2 diabetes inadequately controlled on basal insulin and metformin: The LixiLan-L randomized trial. *Diabetes Care* **2016**, *39*, 1972–1980. [CrossRef] [PubMed]
24. Rosenstock, J.; Aronson, R.; Grunberger, G.; Hanefeld, M.; Piatti, P.; Serusclat, P.; Cheng, X.; Zhou, T.; Niemoeller, E.; Souhami, E.; et al. Benefits of LixiLan, a titratable fixed-ratio combination of insulin glargine plus lixisenatide, versus insulin glargine and lixisenatide monocomponents in type 2 diabetes inadequately controlled on oral agents: The LixiLan-O randomized trial. *Diabetes Care* **2016**, *39*, 2026–2035. [CrossRef] [PubMed]
25. Turton, M.D.; O'Shea, D.; Gunn, I.; Beak, S.A.; Edwards, C.M.; Meeran, K.; Choi, S.J.; Taylor, G.M.; Heath, M.M.; Lambert, P.D.; et al. A role for glucagon-like peptide-1 in the central regulation of feeding. *Nature* **1996**, *379*, 69–72. [CrossRef] [PubMed]
26. Göke, R.; Larsen, P.J.; Mikkelsen, J.D.; Sheikh, S.P. Distribution of GLP-1 binding sites in the rat brain: Evidence that exendin-4 is a ligand of brain GLP-1 binding sites. *Eur. J. Neurosci.* **1995**, *7*, 2294–2300. [CrossRef] [PubMed]
27. Alvarez, E.; Martínez, M.D.; Roncero, I.; Chowen, J.A.; Garcia-Cuartero, B.; Gispert, J.D.; Sanz, C.; Vazquez, P.; Maldonado, A.; De Cáceres, J.; et al. The expression of GLP-1 receptor mRNA and protein allows the effect of GLP-1 on glucose metabolism in the human hypothalamus and brainstem. *J. Neurochem.* **2005**, *92*, 798–806. [CrossRef]
28. Van Bloemendaal, L.; Ijzerman, R.G.; Ten Kulve, J.S.; Barkhof, F.; Konrad, R.J.; Drent, M.L.; Veltman, D.J.; Diamant, M. GLP-1 receptor activation modulates appetite- and reward-related brain areas in humans. *Diabetes* **2014**, *63*, 4186–4196. [CrossRef]
29. Shah, M.; Vella, A. Effects of GLP-1 on appetite and weight. *Rev. Endocr. Metab. Disord.* **2014**, *15*, 181–187. [CrossRef]
30. Lean, M.E.J.; Carraro, R.; Finer, N.; Hartvig, H.; Lindegaard, M.L.; Rössner, S.; Van Gaal, L.; Astrup, A. Tolerability of nausea and vomiting and associations with weight loss in a randomized trial of liraglutide in obese, non-diabetic adults. *Int. J. Obes.* **2014**, *38*, 689–697. [CrossRef]
31. Horowitz, M.; Aroda, V.R.; Han, J.; Hardy, E.; Rayner, C.K. Upper and/or lower gastrointestinal adverse events with glucagon-like peptide-1 receptor agonists: Incidence and consequences. *Diabetes Obes. Metab.* **2017**, *19*, 672–681. [CrossRef] [PubMed]
32. Baggio, L.L.; Drucker, D.J. Glucagon-like peptide-1 receptors in the brain: Controlling food intake and body weight. *J. Clin. Investig.* **2014**, *124*, 4223–4226. [CrossRef] [PubMed]
33. Geloneze, B.; De Lima-Júnior, J.C.; Velloso, L.A. Glucagon-like peptide-1 receptor agonists (GLP-1RAs) in the brain-adipocyte axis. *Drugs* **2017**, *77*, 493–503. [CrossRef] [PubMed]

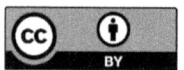

© 2020 by the authors. Licensee MDPI, Basel, Switzerland. This article is an open access article distributed under the terms and conditions of the Creative Commons Attribution (CC BY) license (http://creativecommons.org/licenses/by/4.0/).

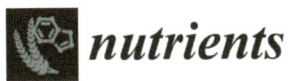

Article

Abdominothoracic Postural Tone Influences the Sensations Induced by Meal Ingestion

Dan M. Livovsky [1,2], Claudia Barber [1], Elizabeth Barba [3], Anna Accarino [1] and Fernando Azpiroz [1,*]

1. Digestive System Research Unit, University Hospital Vall d'Hebron, Centro de Investigación Biomédica en Red de Enfermedades Hepáticas y Digestivas (Ciberehd), Departament de Medicina, Universitat Autònoma de Barcelona, 08193 Bellaterra (Cerdanyola del Vallès), Spain; danlivo@yahoo.com (D.M.L.); claudiabarbercaselles@gmail.com (C.B.); aaccarino@telefonica.net (A.A.)
2. Faculty of Medicine, Hebrew University of Jerusalem, Digestive Diseases Institute, Shaare Zedek Medical Center, Jerusalem 9103401, Israel
3. Neurogastroenterology Motility Unit, Hospital Clínic, University of Barcelona, 08007 Barcelona, Spain; ebarbaorozco@gmail.com
* Correspondence: azpiroz.fernando@gmail.com; Tel.: +34-93-274-6259

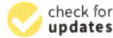

Citation: Livovsky, D.M.; Barber, C.; Barba, E.; Accarino, A.; Azpiroz, F. Abdominothoracic Postural Tone Influences the Sensations Induced by Meal Ingestion. Nutrients 2021, 13, 658. https://doi.org/10.3390/nu13020658

Received: 22 January 2021
Accepted: 15 February 2021
Published: 18 February 2021

Publisher's Note: MDPI stays neutral with regard to jurisdictional claims in published maps and institutional affiliations.

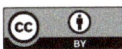

Copyright: © 2021 by the authors. Licensee MDPI, Basel, Switzerland. This article is an open access article distributed under the terms and conditions of the Creative Commons Attribution (CC BY) license (https://creativecommons.org/licenses/by/4.0/).

Abstract: Postprandial objective abdominal distention is frequently associated with a subjective sensation of abdominal bloating, but the relation between both complaints is unknown. While the bloating sensation has a visceral origin, abdominal distention is a behavioral somatic response, involving contraction and descent of the diaphragm with protrusion of the anterior abdominal wall. Our aim was to determine whether abdominal distention influences digestive sensations. In 16 healthy women we investigated the effect of intentional abdominal distention on experimentally induced bloating sensation (by a meal overload). Participants were first taught to produce diaphragmatic contraction and visible abdominal distention. After a meal overload, sensations of bloating (0 to 10) and digestive well-being (-5 to $+5$) were measured during 30-s. maneuvers alternating diaphragmatic contraction and diaphragmatic relaxation. Compared to diaphragmatic relaxation, diaphragmatic contraction was associated with diaphragmatic descent (by $21 + 3$ mm; $p < 0.001$), objective abdominal distention ($32 + 5$ mm girth increase; $p = 0.001$), more intense sensation of bloating ($7.3 + 0.4$ vs. $8.0 + 0.4$ score; $p = 0.010$) and lower digestive well-being ($-0.9 + 0.5$ vs. $-1.9 + 0.5$ score; $p = 0.028$). These results indicate that somatic postural tone underlying abdominal distention worsens the perception of visceral sensations (ClinicalTrials.gov ID: NCT04691882).

Keywords: meal ingestion; postprandial responses; hedonic sensations; homeostatic sensations; abdominal wall activity; abdominal distension

1. Introduction

Abdominal bloating and distention are the major and most bothersome complaints in patients with functional gut disorders, such as functional dyspepsia and irritable bowel syndrome [1]. In the past 20 years several studies have investigated the relation between these tandem complaints [2].

Abdominal bloating, i.e., the sensation of abdominal pressure/fullness, is a subjective sensation of visceral origin. Abdominal bloating in healthy subjects can be induced by experimental increments of gut contents, for instance by inflation of a gastric balloon [3], intestinal gas infusion [4] or a meal overload [5]. Patients with functional gut disorders complaining of bloating have increased visceral sensitivity, so that physiological volumes, well tolerated by healthy subjects, reproduce their customary symptoms [6,7]. Hence, bloating sensation may be induced by large intraluminal loads and/or increased sensitivity of the gut.

It has been consistently shown that patients complaining of abdominal distention exhibit an objective increase in girth [2]. Abdominal distention is a behavioural somatic response featuring diaphragmatic contraction and descent coupled with relaxation and protrusion of the anterior abdominal wall [8–10].

The relation between bloating and distention is not clear. In the past both terms were used indistinctively, and this unprecise terminology contributed to the confusion [1]. However, patients clearly distinguish between the subjective sensation of increased abdominal pressure/fullness (i.e., bloating) and visible abdominal distension [11–13]. Since patients frequently relate distension to bloating sensation, it could be speculated that the somatic response is a conditioned protective attempt to mitigate the visceral sensation, somewhat analogous to the abdominal contraction covering peritoneal irritation, but the attempt turns out ineffective and the distension becomes then a major complaint. The potential interactions between abdominal bloating and distension are highly relevant for the management of patients in clinical practice, and our specific aim was to determine the effect of abdominal distension on visceral sensation. To this aim, we measured the effect of intentional abdominal distension on experimentally induced bloating sensation in healthy subjects.

2. Material and Methods

2.1. Participants

Sixteen healthy, non-obese, non-dieting and weight-stable women without history of gastrointestinal symptoms were recruited by public advertising to participate in the study. Exclusion criteria were chronic health conditions, prior obesity, previous abdominal surgery, use of medications (except occasional use of NSAIDs and antihistamines), history of anosmia and ageusia, current dieting or any pattern of selective eating such as vegetarianism, alcohol abuse and use of recreational drugs. Absence of current digestive symptoms was verified using a standard abdominal symptom questionnaire (no symptom > 2 on a 0–10 scale). Psychological and eating disorders were excluded using the following tests: Hospital Anxiety and Depression scale (HAD), Dutch Eating Behavior Questionnaire (DEBQ—Emotional eating, External eating, Restrained eating), and Physical Anhedonia Scale (PAS). Candidates were asked whether they liked the test meal to be tested (see below) and those who did not were not included.

The research was conducted according to the Declaration of Helsinki. The protocol for the study had been previously approved by the Institutional Review Board of the University Hospital Vall d'Hebron, (Comitè d'Ètica d'Investigació Clinica, Vall d'Hebron Insitiut de Recerca; protocol number PR(AG)338/2016 approved 28 October 2016, revised 11 December 2020) and all participants provided written informed consent.

2.2. Experimental Design

Single-center study performed at the Vall d'Hebron University Hospital, comparing postprandial digestive sensations (abdominal bloating and digestive well-being) during consecutive maneuvers of diaphragmatic contraction (i.e., descent) versus diaphragmatic relaxation (i.e., ascent) in a cross-over randomized design. Outcomes were the effect of somatic maneuvers on abdominal bloating sensation (primary outcome) and on digestive well-being (secondary outcome). The study protocol was registered at ClinicalTrials.gov (ID: NCT04691882). All co-authors had access to the study data and reviewed and approved the final manuscript.

2.3. General Procedure

Participants were instructed to refrain from strenuous physical activity the day prior to the study, to consume only a light breakfast at home after an overnight fast and to report to the laboratory, where the probe meal was administered 4 h after breakfast (only water was allowed until 2 h before the study). Studies were conducted in a quiet, isolated room. First, participants were taught to control the postural tone of the abdominal wall and maintain two different positions for 30-s episodes: (a) diaphragmatic contraction and anterior abdominal wall relaxation (visible abdominal protrusion) and (b) diaphragmatic relaxation and anterior wall contraction (flat abdomen); after a 30-min training period all participants effectively learned the abdominothoracic maneuvers. Second, a probe meal was administered up to maximal satiation in order to induce abdominal bloating sensation. Immediately after ingestion participants were asked to stand up and lean on a high bench in a comfortable position and were instructed to sequentially perform 30-s maneuvers alternating diaphragmatic contraction and diaphragmatic relaxation. Two sequences of 4 alternating maneuvers starting with a different order were performed separated by a 1-min rest interval; in random allocation; half of the participants started with one maneuver and the other half in with the other. Digestive sensations were scored immediately before meal ingestion, every 4 min during meal ingestion, and at the end of each abdominal maneuver in the postprandial period.

2.4. Probe Meal

The probe meal consisted of a mixture of nutrients (Fresubin®Protein Energy—Fresenius Kabi, Germamy; 1.5 kcal/mL) and non-absorbable polyethylenglycol 4000 (27 g/L) to prevent water absorption. The nutrient drink is presented in 3 flavors (chocolate, vanilla and cappuccino) and participants were asked to select their choice. Participants were then instructed to drink the probe meal at a standard rate (75 mL/min) until maximal satiety.

2.5. Perception Measurements

Two 10 cm scales graded from −5 to + 5 were used to measure hunger/satiety (extremely hungry/completely satiated) and digestive well-being (extremely unpleasant sensation/extremely pleasant sensation); abdominal bloating-fullness sensation was measured using a 10 cm scale graded from 0 (not at all) to 10 (very much). Subjects received standard instructions on how to fill-out the scales [14].

2.6. Ancillary Validation Study

A subset of the participants (n = 6) underwent a second study on a separate day measuring the physiological effects of the somatic maneuvers. Following the same experimental procedure, the following outcomes were measured.

2.6.1. Abdominal Girth

The method has been previously described in detail [15]. Briefly, a non-stretch belt (48 mm wide) was placed over the umbilicus and fixed to the skin on the back to prevent slipping. The overlapping ends of the belt were adjusted carefully by two elastic bands to maintain the belt constantly adapted to the abdominal wall. Girth measurements during the study were taken directly with a metric tape measure fixed to the belt. Measurements were obtained before meal ingestion, immediately after ingestion, and during the somatic maneuvers without manipulation of the belt-tape assembly. Previous studies validated the reproducibility of the measurements and sensitivity of this method to consistently detect the small variations in girth induced by various experimental conditions [15–23].

2.6.2. Position of the Diaphragm

In previous studies, we showed that displacement of the diaphragm can be equally evaluated by monitoring the position of either the right liver dome by CT scan or the right lower margin imaged by ultrasonography [4]. As previously described, the position of the lower margin of the right liver lobe at the right anterior axillary line was identified by ultrasonography (Eco 1, Chison Medical Technologies, Jiangsu, China) using a 3.5 MHz curved array transducer held over the edge of the costal wall in a coronal plane with the shaft held in a horizontal position and the head in an axial direction. At each determination (before ingestion, after ingestion and during somatic maneuvers) participants were instructed to breathe normally and the mid-point between the end-inspiratory and end-expiratory position of the liver margin, assessed over a period of six respiratory cycles, was marked on the overlying skin, then the differences between determinations were measured.

2.6.3. Intragastric Pressure and Respiratory Rate

A manometric catheter (Latitude®Esophageal Motility Catheter, Unisensor AG, Attikon, Switzerland, model GIM600E) (2.7 mm outside diameter) with 4 micro-balloons at 5 cm intervals was introduced through the nose and placed with 2 recording sites above and 2 below the gastroesophageal junction at the beginning of the experiments; the balloons were filled with air and intraluminal pressures were continuously recorded. Intrathoracic (esophageal) and intraabdominal (intragastric) pressures and respiratory rate were measured before and after meal ingestion and during each somatic maneuver.

2.6.4. Heart Rate and Heart Rate Variability (Vagal Tone)

Continuous heart rate monitoring with high quality inter-beat data was recorded during the entire experiment using a Bluetooth heart rate strap (H10, Polar Electro, Kempele, Finland). R-R intervals and cardiac interbit intervals were obtained. Heart rate variability (HRV) was assessed at the beginning of the experiments before and during intubation, before and after meal ingestion, and during each somatic maneuver. Measurements before intubation and before meal ingestion were performed over a period of 5 min; measurements after meal ingestion and during the somatic maneuvers were performed over 30-s periods; the validity of this ultrashort period of HRV analysis has been shown in several setting [24–29]. HRV analysis of the exported data was performed on a computer using a dedicated HRV software (Kubios Premium ver. 3.4.2). Prior to HRV computation all IBI data were visually inspected for correctness and then underwent automatic artifact correction to calculate mean values of root mean square of the successive differences between normal heartbeats (RMSSD) as a marker of vagal tone (higher RMSSD reflects higher vagal tone). The RMSSD is obtained by calculating each successive time difference between heartbeats in ms. Each of the values is squared and the result is averaged, then the square root of the total is obtained [30–32].

2.6.5. Galvanic Skin Responses (Sympathetic Activity)

Two 11 mm Ag/AgCl dry electrodes were secured on the index and middle fingers of the right hand, with Velcro straps and electrodermal activity (EDA) was continuously recorded (MySignals, Libelium Comunicaciones Distribuidas, Zaragoza, Spain). Galvanic skin responses (GSR) were measured as in EDA phasic changes within 1–5 s following different conditions: intubation, meal ingestion and somatic maneuvers [30]. EDA depends on the activity of sweat glands, and hence, the conductance of electrical signals through the skin; GSR reflect sympathetic activity.

2.7. Statistical Analysis

Statistical analysis was performed using IBM statistics SPSS v25; a significance level of 5% (two tails) was used in all analyses. Descriptive statistics were used to define baseline demographic characteristics of participants. Data are presented as mean values ± standard error. The Shapiro-Wilk Test was used to determine normality of data distribution. Parametric normally distributed data were compared by paired or unpaired Student's t-test, as corresponded; otherwise, the Wilcoxon signed rank test was used for paired data, and the Mann-Whitney U test was used for unpaired data. The association of parameters was analyzed using Pearson's R test.

3. Results

3.1. Demographics and Study Conduction

Participants had a mean age of 30 ± 2 years, 62 ± 3 Kg body weight, 164 ± 2 cm height and 22.5 ± 0.7 Kg/m^2 body mass index. All participants had a normal bowel habit and scored HAD, PAS, and DEBQ within the normal range. Each study day, participants confirmed compliance with the dietary instructions. All participants completed the studies and were included for analysis.

3.2. Responses to Meal Ingestion

Before ingestion, participants were hungry with sensation of digestive well-being. During the ingestion period, baseline hunger declined and the hunger/satiation axis progressively shifted towards maximal satiation by the end of the meal. The amount of food tolerated was 839 ± 29 mL. No significant correlations were found between food tolerance and body mass index (BMI) (r = −0.228; p = 0.396) or weight (Pearson r = −0.212; p = 0.430). By the end of the meal, participants experienced abdominal bloating and negative sensation of digestive well-being. (Figure 1).

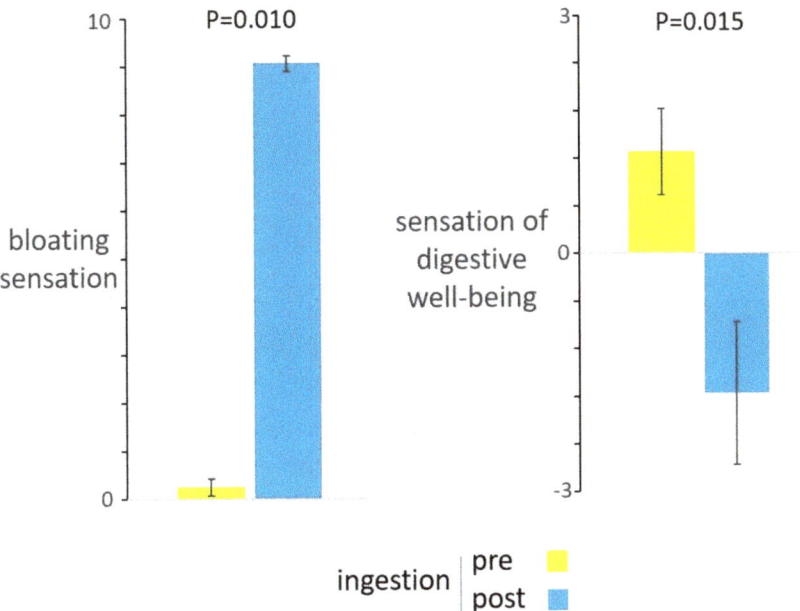

Figure 1. Responses to meal ingestion. The challenge meal induced bloating sensation and impaired sensation of digestive well-being.

During the ingestion period in the validation studies, intragastric pressure initially decreased, and then gradually increased, but the changes were not statistically significant. Meal ingestion was associated with a significant increase in girth (by 13 + 3 mm; p = 0.009), accent of the diaphragm (by 9 + 4 mm; p = 0.057), decrease in vagal tone (by 7.4 ± 1.2 ms RMSSD; p = 0.013), increase in heart rate (by 9.6 ± 2.6 beats per min; p = 0.014) and respiratory rate (by 3.5 ± 1.3 breaths per min; p = 0.047), without significant changes in intrathoracic pressure (0.3 + 0.7 mmHg difference; p = 0.767) and sympathetic activity (0.1 + 0.4 µS difference; p = 0.817).

3.3. Effect of Thoracoabdominal Postural Tone on Postprandial Sensations

Compared to diaphragmatic relaxation, diaphragmatic contraction was associated with more intense sensation of bloating (by 0.7 ± 0.2 score; p = 0.010) and lower digestive well-being (by 1 ± 0.4 score; p = 0.028). (Figure 2). The order of the maneuvers did not influence the results (no differences were detected between the subjects allocated to either sequence, i.e., initiating with diaphragmatic contraction or relaxation).

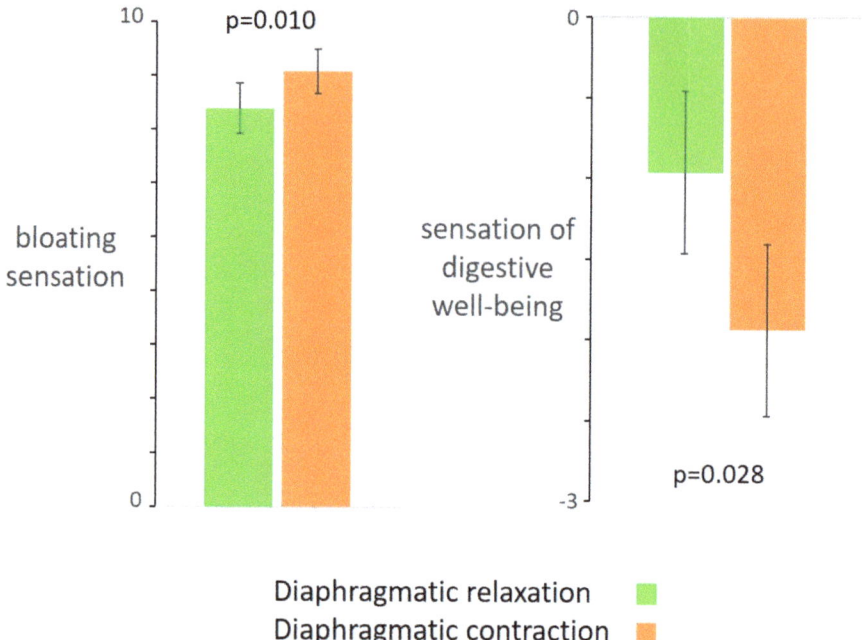

Figure 2. Effect of somatic maneuvers on digestive sensations. Diaphragmatic contraction (i.e., intentional abdominal distension) was associated with increased postprandial bloating and impaired digestive well-being.

3.4. Effect of Thoracoabdominal Postural Tone on Physiological Parameters (Validation Study)

As compared to diaphragmatic relaxation, maneuvers of diaphragmatic contraction produced anterior protrusion of the abdominal wall with significant girth increment (by 32 ± 5 mm; $p = 0.001$), diaphragmatic descent (by 21 + 3 mm; $p < 0.001$), increase in intragastric pressure (by 8 ± 2 mmHg; $p = 0.016$) and a mild decrease in heart rate (by 3 ± 1 beats per minute; $p = 0.033$) without significant changes in intrathoracic pressures 0.4 ± 0.8 mmHg; $p = 0.628$), respiratory frequency (-0.6 ± 0.4; breaths per minute; $p = 0.422$) and vagal tone (2.5 ± 1.6 ms RMSSD; $p = 0.195$). In contrast to the significant sympathetic arousal produced by nasopharyngeal stimulation during intubation with the manometry catheter (3.6 ± 0.8 μS increment; $p = 0.004$), the somatic maneuvers did not elicit a galvanic response (0.04 ± 0.08 μS difference; $p = 0.207$)

4. Discussion

Our data demonstrate that the activity of the abdominal wall influences perception of visceral stimuli, specifically, intentional abdominal distention heightens bloating sensation induced by a meal overload.

In normal conditions meal ingestion induces physiological responses that accomplish the digestion, as well as homeostatic (satiety, fullness) and hedonic sensations (digestive well-being and improved mood) [33]. Postprandial sensations depend on the characteristics of the meal and the appropriate digestive response, as well as on constitutive and inducible factors of the host, the latter influenced by a variety of conditioning mechanisms [34].

The meal load is determinant in the sensations induced by ingestion; the meal load bears a direct relation with homeostatic sensations and a bimodal relation with hedonic sensations: small comfort meals up to a certain level induce satisfactory homeostatic sensations (satiation, mild fullness, digestive well-being and consummatory reward), whereas larger meals induce aversive fullness sensation [34,35]. In this study we used a challenge meal to induce bloating sensation and dissatisfaction, mimicking postprandial symptoms in patients with functional gut disorders. This experimental model has been previously validated in our laboratory [6], and it has been shown that the homogeneous liquid meal induces stronger homeostatic sensations and less satisfaction than normal mixed meals with similar caloric and volume loads [36].

The intercostal muscles, diaphragm and the anterior abdominal muscles exert phasic rhythmic activity related to respiration (lung ventilation). These phasic contractions are superimposed on a tonic, i.e., sustained, muscular activity (postural tone). Muscular tone in this chain of muscles (intercostals, diaphragm and anterior abdominal wall) is finely coordinated, allowing a physiological redistribution of thoracoabdominal contents [4,37] without affecting respiratory function (tidal volume and the physiological dead space of the lungs): an upwards shift of contents is orchestrated by elevation of the costal wall (increase in intercostal tone), diaphragmatic ascent (decrease in tone) and flat abdomen (tight anterior abdominal wall), so that the abdominal cavity is elongated in cranial direction and the lungs accommodate into the upper chest. Conversely, a caudal shift involves descent of the costal wall (intercostal relaxation), diaphragmatic descent (increase in tone) and anterior wall protrusion (reduced tone).

As described before (see Introduction), abdominal distension with objective anterior wall protrusion in patients is due to an uncontrolled increase in diaphragmatic tone and blockade of the diaphragm in caudad position with downwards displacement of abdominal contents (abdominophrenic dyssynergia) [6,8,38,39]. Patients can be trained to control abdomino-phrenic postural tone, release the diaphragmatic blockade and correct abdominal distension, but the learning process, based on visual biofeedback signalling of abdominal thoracic muscular activity, is rather complex [8,38]. In contrast to patients, healthy subjects readily learned to master abdomino-phrenic tone and shift the balance back and forth from diaphragmatic relaxation/flat abdomen to diaphragmatic contraction/abdominal distension. In this experimental model we showed that during diaphragmatic contraction perception of gut stimuli is higher than during diaphragmatic relaxation, and intragastric content produced more severe postprandial bloating sensation with impaired digestive well-being.

Several mechanisms may be involved in this effect. We previously showed that sympathetic arousal released by lower body negative pressure (blood sequestration in the lower extremities) increases intestinal sensitivity and heightens perception of intestinal distension [40]. The lack of galvanic response to the somatic manoeuvres in the present study makes this mechanism unlikely; furthermore, no changes in vagal tone and minor changes in cardiorespiratory function were detected. Diaphragmatic contraction produced a relatively small but consistent increase in intragastric pressure. Conceivably, the external compression of the diaphragm over the full stomach heightened perception of intragastric content, in a similar way as abdominal palpation might do. Hence, the exploratory mechanistic outcomes of our study suggest that the somato-visceral interaction is mediated by mechanical factors.

We wish to acknowledge some limitations of our study. First, we cannot ascertain whether our results are extensible to men, because this proof-of-concept study was performed in women. Women were selected because previous studies showed that they are more susceptible to conditioning of postprandial sensations and probably this may explain the female preponderance of functional digestive disorders [35,41,42]. Second, this study was performed in healthy subjects mimicking the situation in patients with meal-related symptoms and abdominal distension, yet we cannot ascertain to what extent the experimental procedures in healthy subjects reproduced real-life clinical conditions. Third, abdominal symptoms were induced by a meal overload, and it is not clear whether somatic activity may also influence symptoms of a different origin, e.g., colonic distension.

The clinical relevance and importance of the somato-visceral interaction evidenced by our study helps to explain the relation between abdominal bloating and distension in patients with functional gut disorders. It could be speculated that bloating sensation elicits the somatic behavioural response leading to abdominal distension, as a protective mechanism attempting to reduce the visceral sensation; however, our data show that abdominal distention (increased diaphragmatic tone) worsens bloating sensation. Conversely, we have previously shown that correction of abdomino-phrenic dyssynergia by biofeedback effectively prevented abdominal distention [8,38]. That study showed that correction of distension was associated with improvement of digestive symptoms, and our current data explain this unexpected effect.

5. Conclusions

Our proof-of-concept study indicates that the somatic postural tone underlying abdominal distention worsens the perception of visceral sensations; these data in healthy subjects help to understand the somato-visceral interactions and the pathophysiological relation of abdominal bloating to distension, two major complaints in patients with functional gut disorders.

Author Contributions: D.M.L. Study design, study management, conduction of experiments, data analysis and manuscript preparation. C.B. Conduction of experiments. E.B. Data interpretation. A.A. Supervision of studies. F.A. Study design, data interpretation and manuscript revision. All authors have read and agreed to the published version of the manuscript.

Funding: This work was supported in part by the Spanish Ministry of Economy and Competitiveness (Dirección General de Investigación Científica y Técnica, SAF 2016-76648-R). Ciberehd is funded by the Instituto de Salud Carlos III. Dan M. Livovsky received support from the Israeli Medical Association and from Israel Gastroenterological Association 2020 fellowship grants.

Informed Consent Statement: Not applicable.

Data Availability Statement: Not applicable.

Acknowledgments: The authors thank Gloria Santaliestra for secretarial assistance.

Conflicts of Interest: The authors declare no conflict of interest.

References

1. Azpiroz, F.; Malagelada, J. Abdominal Bloating. *Gastroenterology* **2005**, *129*, 1060–1078. [CrossRef]
2. Azpiroz, F. Intestinal gas. In *Sleisenger and Fordtran's Gastrointestinal and Liver Disease: Pathophysiology, Diagnosis, Management*; Feldman, M.F.L., Brand, L.J., Eds.; Elsevier: Philadelphi, PA, USA, 2020.
3. Caldarella, M.P.; Azpiroz, F.; Malagelada, J.-R. Selective effects of nutrients on gut sensitivity and reflexes. *Gut* **2007**, *56*, 37–42. [CrossRef] [PubMed]
4. Burri, E.; Cisternas, D.; Villoria, A.; Accarino, A.; Soldevilla, A.; Malagelada, J.-R.; Azpiroz, F. Accommodation of the abdomen to its content: Integrated abdomino-thoracic response. *Neurogastroenterol. Motil.* **2012**, *24*, 312-e162. [CrossRef] [PubMed]
5. Burri, E.; Cisternas, D.; Villoria, A.; Accarino, A.; Soldevilla, A.; Malagelada, J.-R.; Azpiroz, F. Abdominal accommodation induced by meal ingestion: Differential responses to gastric and colonic volume loads. *Neurogastroenterol. Motil.* **2013**, *25*, 339–e253. [CrossRef] [PubMed]
6. Burri, E.; Barba, E.; Huaman, J.W.; Cisternas, D.; Accarino, A.; De, G.F.; Malagelada, J.-R.; Azpiroz, F. Mechanisms of postprandial abdominal bloating and distension in functional dyspepsia. *Gut* **2014**, *63*, 395–400. [CrossRef] [PubMed]
7. Enck, P.; Azpiroz, F.; Boeckxstaens, G.; Elsenbruch, S.; Feinle-Bisset, C.; Holtmann, G.; Lackner, J.M.; Ronkainen, J.; Schemann, M.; Stengel, A.; et al. Functional dyspepsia. *Nat. Rev. Dis. Primers* **2017**, *3*, 17081. [CrossRef]
8. Barba, E.; Burri, E.; Accarino, A.; Cisternas, D.; Quiroga, S.; Monclus, E.; Navazo, I.; Malagelada, J.R.; Azpiroz, F. Abdomino-thoracic mechanisms of functional abdominal distension and correction by biofeedback. *Gastroenterology* **2015**, *148*, 732–738. [CrossRef] [PubMed]
9. Barba, E.; Accarino, A.; Azpiroz, F. Correction of Abdominal Distension by Biofeedback-Guided Control of Abdominothoracic Muscular Activity in a Randomized, Placebo-Controlled Trial. *Clin. Gastroenterol. Hepatol.* **2017**, *15*, 1922–1929. [CrossRef]
10. Barba, E.; Sánchez, B.; Burri, E.; Accarino, A.; Monclus, E.; Navazo, I.; Guarner, F.; Margolles, A.; Azpiroz, F. Abdominal distension after eating lettuce: The role of intestinal gas evaluated in vitro and by abdominal CT imaging. *Neurogastroenterol. Motil.* **2019**, *31*, e13703. [CrossRef]
11. Chassany, O.; Tugaut, B.; Marrel, A.; Guyonnet, D.; Arbuckle, R.; Duracinsky, M.; Whorwell, P.J.; Azpiroz, F. The Intestinal Gas Questionnaire: Development of a new instrument for measuring gas-related symptoms and their impact on daily life. *Neurogastroenterol. Motil.* **2015**, *27*, 885–898. [CrossRef]

12. Huaman, J.-W.; Mego, M.; Manichanh, C.; Cañellas, N.; Cañueto, D.; Segurola, H.; Jansana, M.; Malagelada, C.; Accarino, A.; Vulevic, J.; et al. Effects of Prebiotics vs. a Diet Low in FODMAPs in Patients with Functional Gut Disorders. *Gastroenterology* **2018**, *155*, 1004–1007. [CrossRef] [PubMed]
13. Le Nevé, B.; De La Torre, A.M.; Tap, J.; Derrien, M.; Cotillard, A.; Barba, E.; Mego, M.; Ruiz, A.N.; Hernandez-Palet, L.; Dornic, Q.; et al. A Fermented Milk Product with B. lactis CNCM I-2494 and Lactic Acid Bacteria Improves Gastrointestinal Comfort in Response to a Challenge Diet Rich in Fermentable Residues in Healthy Subjects. *Nutrients* **2020**, *12*, 320. [CrossRef]
14. Malagelada, C.; Accarino, A.; Molne, L.; Méndez, S.; Campos, E.; Gonzalez, A.; Malagelada, J.R.; Azpiroz, F. Digestive, cognitive and hedonic responses to a meal. *Neurogastroenterol. Motil.* **2015**, *27*, 389–396. [CrossRef] [PubMed]
15. Tremolaterra, F.; Villoria, A.; Azpiroz, F.; Serra, J.; Aguadé, S.; Malagelada, J. Impaired Viscerosomatic Reflexes and Abdominal-Wall Dystony Associated With Bloating. *Gastroenterology* **2006**, *130*, 1062–1068. [CrossRef]
16. Passos, M.C.; Serra, J.; Azpiroz, F.; Tremolaterra, F.; Malagelada, J.-R. Impaired reflex control of intestinal gas transit in patients with abdominal bloating. *Gut* **2005**, *54*, 344–348. [CrossRef]
17. Hernando-Harder, A.C.; Serra, J.; Azpiroz, F.; Malagelada, J.-R. Sites of symptomatic gas retention during intestinal lipid perfusion in healthy subjects. *Gut* **2004**, *53*, 661–665. [CrossRef]
18. Salvioli, B.; Serra, J.; Azpiroz, F.; Malagelada, J.-R. Impaired Small Bowel Gas Propulsion in Patients with Bloating During Intestinal Lipid Infusion. *Am. J. Gastroenterol.* **2006**, *101*, 1853–1857. [CrossRef]
19. Merletti, R.; Hermens, H.J. Detection and conditioning of the surface EMG signal. In *Electromyography—Physiology, Engineering, and Noninvasive Applications*, 1st ed.; Merletti, R., Parker, P., Eds.; John Wiley & Sons, Inc.: Hoboken, NJ, USA, 2004; pp. 107–131.
20. Ng, J.K.; Kippers, V.; Richardson, C.A. Muscle fibre orientation of abdominal muscles and suggested surface EMG electrode positions. *Electromyogr. Clin. Neurophysiol.* **1998**, *38*, 51–58. [PubMed]
21. Caldarella, M.P.; Serra, J.; Azpiroz, F.; Malagelada, J.-R. Prokinetic effects in patients with intestinal gas retention. *Gastroenterology* **2002**, *122*, 1748–1755. [CrossRef]
22. Salvioli, B.; Serra, J.; Azpiroz, F.; Lorenzo, C.; Aguade, S.; Castell, J.; Malagelada, J.-R. Origin of gas retention and symptoms in patients with bloating. *Gastroenterology* **2005**, *128*, 574–579. [CrossRef] [PubMed]
23. Harder, H.; Serra, J.; Azpiroz, F.; Passos, M.C.; Aguadé, S.; Malagelada, J.-R. Intestinal gas distribution determines abdominal symptoms. *Gut* **2003**, *52*, 1708–1713. [CrossRef] [PubMed]
24. Oliveira, V.; Von Rosenberg, W.; Montaldo, P.; Adjei, T.; Mendoza, J.; Shivamurthappa, V.; Mandic, D.; Thayyil, S. Early Postnatal Heart Rate Variability in Healthy Newborn Infants. *Front. Physiol.* **2019**, *10*, 922. [CrossRef]
25. Laborde, S.; Mosley, E.; Thayer, J.F. Heart Rate Variability and Cardiac Vagal Tone in Psychophysiological Research—Recommendations for Experiment Planning, Data Analysis, and Data Reporting. *Front. Psychol.* **2017**, *8*, 213. [CrossRef]
26. Salahuddin, L.; Cho, J.; Jeong, M.G.; Kim, D. Ultra Short Term Analysis of Heart Rate Variability for Monitoring Mental Stress in Mobile Settings. In Proceedings of the 2007 29th Annual International Conference of the IEEE Engineering in Medicine and Biology Society, Lyon, France, 22–26 August 2007; pp. 4656–4659.
27. Castaldo, R.; Montesinos, L.; Melillo, P.; James, C.; Pecchia, L. Ultra-short term HRV features as surrogates of short term HRV: A case study on mental stress detection in real life. *BMC Med. Inform. Decis. Mak.* **2019**, *19*, 1–13. [CrossRef]
28. Esco, M.R.; Flatt, A.A. Ultra-Short-Term Heart Rate Variability Indexes at Rest and Post-Exercise in Athletes: Evaluating the Agreement with Accepted Recommendations. *J. Sports Sci. Med.* **2014**, *13*, 535–541.
29. Munoz, M.L.; Van Roon, A.; Riese, H.; Thio, C.; Oostenbroek, E.; Westrik, I.; De Geus, E.J.C.; Gansevoort, R.; Lefrandt, J.; Nolte, I.M.; et al. Validity of (Ultra-)Short Recordings for Heart Rate Variability Measurements. *PLoS ONE* **2015**, *10*, e0138921. [CrossRef]
30. Hoshikawa, Y.; Fitzke, H.; Sweis, R.; Fikree, A.; Saverymuttu, S.; Kadirkamanathan, S.; Iwakiri, K.; Yazaki, E.; Aziz, Q.; Sifrim, D. Rumination syndrome: Assessment of vagal tone during and after meals and during diaphragmatic breathing. *Neurogastroenterol. Motil.* **2020**, *32*, e13873. [CrossRef] [PubMed]
31. Shaffer, F.; Ginsberg, J.P. An Overview of Heart Rate Variability Metrics and Norms. *Front. Public Health* **2017**, *5*, 258. [CrossRef]
32. Task Force of the European Society of Cardiology the North American Society of Pacing Electrophysiology. Heart rate variability: Standards of measurement, physiological interpretation and clinical use. *Circulation* **1996**, *93*, 1043–1065. [CrossRef]
33. Critchley, H.D. Review: Electrodermal Responses: What Happens in the Brain. *Neuroscientist* **2002**, *8*, 132–142. [CrossRef] [PubMed]
34. Livovsky, D.M.; Pribic, T.; Azpiroz, F. Food, Eating, and the Gastrointestinal Tract. *Nutrients* **2020**, *12*, 986. [CrossRef]
35. Monrroy, H.; Pribic, T.; Galan, C.; Nieto, A.; Amigo, N.; Accarino, A.; Correig, X.; Azpiroz, F. Meal Enjoyment and Tolerance in Women and Men. *Nutrients* **2019**, *11*, 119. [CrossRef]
36. Ciccantelli, B.; Pribic, T.; Malagelada, C.; Accarino, A.; Azpiroz, F. Relation between cognitive and hedonic responses to a meal. *Neurogastroenterol. Motil.* **2017**, *29*. [CrossRef] [PubMed]
37. Villoria, A.; Azpiroz, F.; Soldevilla, A.; Perez, F.; Malagelada, J.-R. Abdominal Accommodation: A Coordinated Adaptation of the Abdominal Wall to Its Content. *Am. J. Gastroenterol.* **2008**, *103*, 2807–2815. [CrossRef]
38. Barba, E.; Quiroga, S.; Accarino, A.; Lahoya, E.M.; Malagelada, C.; Burri, E.; Navazo, I.; Malagelada, J.-R.; Azpiroz, F. Mechanisms of abdominal distension in severe intestinal dysmotility: Abdomino-thoracic response to gut retention. *Neurogastroenterol. Motil.* **2013**, *25*. [CrossRef]
39. Villoria, A.; Azpiroz, F.; Burri, E.; Cisternas, D.; Soldevilla, A.; Malagelada, J.R. Abdomino-phrenic dyssynergia in patients with abdominal bloating and distension. *Am. J. Gastroenterol.* **2011**, *106*, 815–819. [CrossRef]

40. Iovino, P.; Azpiroz, F.; Domingo, E.; Malagelada, J.R. The sympathetic nervous system modulates perception and reflex responses to gut distension in humans. *Gastroenterology* **1995**, *108*, 680–686. [CrossRef]
41. Monrroy, H.; Borghi, G.; Pribic, T.; Galan, C.; Nieto, A.; Amigo, N.; Accarino, A.; Correig, X.; Azpiroz, F. Biological Response to Meal Ingestion: Gender Differences. *Nutrients* **2019**, *11*, 702. [CrossRef] [PubMed]
42. Masihy, M.; Monrroy, H.; Borghi, G.; Pribic, T.; Galan, C.; Nieto, A.; Accarino, A.; Azpiroz, F. Influence of Eating Schedule on the Postprandial Response: Gender Differences. *Nutrients* **2019**, *11*, 401. [CrossRef] [PubMed]

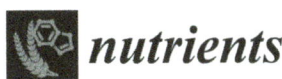

Article

Appetite Control across the Lifecourse: The Acute Impact of Breakfast Drink Quantity and Protein Content. The Full4Health Project

Daniel R. Crabtree [1,*,†], William Buosi [2,†], Claire L. Fyfe [2], Graham W. Horgan [3], Yannis Manios [4], Odysseas Androutsos [5], Angeliki Giannopoulou [4], Graham Finlayson [6], Kristine Beaulieu [6], Claire L. Meek [7], Jens J. Holst [8], Klaske Van Norren [9], Julian G. Mercer [2], Alexandra M. Johnstone [2] and on behalf of the Full4Health-Study Group

1. Centre for Health Science, Division of Biomedical Sciences, University of the Highlands and Islands, Old Perth Road, Inverness IV2 3JH, UK
2. The Rowett Institute, University of Aberdeen, Foresterhill Road, Aberdeen AB25 2ZD, UK; williambuosi@hotmail.fr (W.B.); c.fyfe@abdn.ac.uk (C.L.F.); j.mercer@abdn.ac.uk (J.G.M.); alex.johnstone@abdn.ac.uk (A.M.J.)
3. Biomathematics and Statistics Scotland, Foresterhill Road, Aberdeen AB25 2ZD, UK; g.horgan@abdn.ac.uk
4. Department of Nutrition-Dietetics, School of Health Science & Education, Harokopio University Athens, 70 El. Venizelou Avenue, 17671 Kallithea, Greece; manios@hua.gr (Y.M.); agiann@hua.gr (A.G.)
5. Department of Nutrition and Dietetics, School of Physical Education, Sport Science and Dietetics, University of Thessaly, 42100 Trikala, Greece; oandroutsos@uth.gr
6. School of Psychology, University of Leeds, Leeds LS2 9JT, UK; g.s.finlayson@leeds.ac.uk (G.F.); k.beaulieu@leeds.ac.uk (K.B.)
7. Institute of Metabolic Science, Metabolic Research Laboratories, University of Cambridge, Addenbrooke's Hospital, Box 289, Hills Road, Cambridge CB2 0QQ, UK; clm70@cam.ac.uk
8. Department of Biomedical Sciences and Novo Nordisk Foundation Center for Basic Metabolic Research, University of Copenhagen, DK-2200 Copenhagen, Denmark; jjholst@sund.ku.dk
9. Nutritional Biology, Human Nutrition and Health, Wageningen University, 6708 WE Wageningen, The Netherlands; klaske.vannorren@wur.nl
* Correspondence: daniel.crabtree@uhi.ac.uk; Tel.: +44-(0)1-4632-79405
† These authors contributed equally to this work.

Received: 16 October 2020; Accepted: 27 November 2020; Published: 30 November 2020

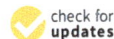

Abstract: Understanding the mechanisms of hunger, satiety and how nutrients affect appetite control is important for successful weight management across the lifecourse. The primary aim of this study was to describe acute appetite control across the lifecourse, comparing age groups (children, adolescents, adults, elderly), weight categories, genders and European sites (Scotland and Greece). Participants ($n = 391$) consumed four test drinks, varying in composition (15% (normal protein, NP) and 30% (high protein, HP) of energy from protein) and quantity (based on 100% basal metabolic rate (BMR) and 140% BMR), on four separate days in a double-blind randomized controlled study. Ad libitum energy intake (EI), subjective appetite and biomarkers of appetite and metabolism (adults and elderly only) were measured. The adults' appetite was significantly greater than that of the elderly across all drink types ($p < 0.004$) and in response to drink quantities ($p < 0.001$). There were no significant differences in EI between age groups, weight categories, genders or sites. Concentrations of glucagon-like peptide 1 (GLP-1) and peptide YY (PYY) were significantly greater in the elderly than the adults ($p < 0.001$). Ghrelin and fasting leptin concentrations differed significantly between weight categories, genders and sites ($p < 0.05$), while GLP-1 and PYY concentrations differed significantly between genders only ($p < 0.05$). Compared to NP drinks, HP drinks significantly increased postprandial GLP-1 and PYY ($p < 0.001$). Advanced age was concomitant with reduced appetite and elevated anorectic hormone release, which may contribute to the development of malnutrition. In addition, appetite hormone concentrations differed between weight categories, genders and geographical locations.

Keywords: appetite; lifecourse; gut hormones; hunger; protein

1. Introduction

Nutrition-related noncommunicable diseases are associated with increased morbidity and mortality at all stages of life [1,2]. Physiological and psychological responses to food change as we age, with impact on food choices and preferences, but little is known about how appetite control varies across the lifecourse [3]. This is a critical issue in combatting food intake-related chronic disease, commonly driven by over-consumption, but also in consideration of relative under-nutrition in the elderly and the clinically compromised.

Food intake and appetite are governed across the lifecourse by complex interactions between peripherally synthesized gut hormones and their central receptors [4]. These interactions are subject to external influences, including hedonic cues and the environment [5]. Short-acting gastrointestinal signals include the anorexigenic peptides glucagon-like peptide 1 (GLP-1) and peptide YY (PYY) and the orexigenic hormone ghrelin, while leptin maintains long-term energy homeostasis [6]. Homeostatic systems can, however, be overridden by hedonic signals, resulting in appetite control dysfunction, excess energy consumption and obesity [7]. There may be key periods in the lifecourse when appetite can be modulated for optimal health. For example, the onset of overweight and obesity starts as early as childhood and can track into adulthood [8]. Environmental factors contribute towards weight gain, if rewarding energy-dense foods are freely available and integrated into local culture, creating an obesogenic environment [9]. With advancing age, food reward signals are altered [10,11], food craving behavior declines, particularly in females [12] and food intake is suppressed [13,14], all contributing to a condition termed the "anorexia of ageing" [15]. Cross-sectional research reports a peak in calorie intake during late adolescence, followed by a decline, with calorie intake reducing by 1300 kcal/day on average between 20 and 80 years of age for males and 600 kcal/day for females [16]. Understanding how dietary interventions influence physiological and behavioral mediators of appetite at different stages of life is vital for effective long-term weight control [17]. High-protein diets are often recommended for weight management, as they are highly satiating [18–20], and in the prevention and treatment of malnutrition, particularly in elderly populations [21]. Protein-induced satiety has been observed acutely, within single meals that contained 25% to 81% of energy from protein, associated with reductions in subsequent energy intake (EI) compared to lower protein alternatives [22]. In children and adolescents, studies have reported either an appetite suppressant effect of increased protein content [23] or no effect [24]. In addition, breakfasts high in protein have been shown to induce greater hunger suppression compared to breakfasts with a lower protein content in adults [25]. It is not well understood how interactions between protein and appetite control differ between children, adolescents, adults and the elderly since studies are rarely conducted across the lifecourse.

The primary aim of this study was to describe the acute regulation of appetite across the lifecourse, thus being able to detect differences between four different age groups (children, adolescents, adults and elderly), two different weight categories (normal weight and overweight), the two genders (male and female) and two European sites (Aberdeen, Scotland and Athens, Greece). The secondary aim was to examine the short-term effects of breakfast test drinks varying in protein composition and quantity on appetite control. Our study is unique in that it applies an individualized appetite challenge across the lifecourse in lean and overweight males and females in northern and southern Europe.

2. Materials and Methods

2.1. Participants

Normal weight and overweight/obese and male and female child, adolescent, adult and elderly participants (age range 7–77 years) were recruited in Scotland and Greece as part of an identical, dual-site within-day dietary intervention study, thereby creating four groups: age (children, adolescents, adults and elderly), weight category (normal weight and overweight), gender (male and female) and site (Scotland and Greece). Recruitment of volunteers was by public advertisement using radio, newspapers and social media, and was conducted from May 2012 to August 2015. When requested, study information sessions were conducted at schools, health care centers and day care centers for the elderly. Participants were individuals who were motivated to actively respond to the volunteer request. Exclusion criteria included: smokers; morbid obesity (BMI $\geq$ 40 kg/m^2); pregnancy; obesity of known endocrine origin; neurological disorders; medication known to influence appetite (including orlistat, oral antidiabetics, insulin, digoxin, anti-arrhythmics, sibutramine, antidepressants); self-reported fever/systemic infection; participation in medical or surgical weight loss program within 1 month of selection; history of cerebrovascular disease; current major depressive disorder; history of cardiovascular disease; chronic obstructive pulmonary disease; an allergy to any of the test drink components and partaking in >6 h of vigorous physical activity per week. This study was conducted according to the guidelines laid down in the Declaration of Helsinki [26]. Ethical approval in Aberdeen was granted by the National Health Service North of Scotland Research Ethics Service. Ethical approval in Athens was granted by the Bioethics Committee of Harokopio University and the Greek Ministry of Education for the implementation of the study in schools. The study received ethical approval from NHS Grampian, Aberdeen, Scotland, UK and the Research Ethics Committee (reference number: 12/NS/0007). All participants provided written informed consent before entering the study and, in addition, the parents/guardians of the children consented for their child to participate.

2.2. Experimental Procedures and Protocol

Data on children and adolescents were collected at schools and adults and elderly attended the Rowett Institute, University of Aberdeen, Scotland (ABDN) and the Department of Nutrition-Dietetics, Harokopio University Athens, Greece (HUA). Prior to the main experimental trials, preliminary anthropometric measures were carried out under standardized conditions. During the main experimental trials, participants consumed four test drinks for breakfast on four separate occasions using a double-blind randomized controlled crossover design, with at least a 4 day period between trials. On the morning of each trial, participants arrived following an overnight fast (10 h) and having refrained from alcohol consumption and strenuous exercise for 12 h. Test drinks were consumed immediately following baseline measures (0 min), then at 120 min post-baseline, ad libitum EI was measured by means of a 30 min buffet-style test meal, after which participants were free to leave. Subjective appetite sensations were assessed using visual analog scales (VASs) at 0, 30, 60, 90 and 120 min (pre-meal), pleasantness and satisfaction VASs were also completed immediately post-test drink. Blood samples were taken at 0, 30, 60 and 120 min to determine biomarker concentrations. The true aims of the study were concealed from the participants; however, all participants were fully debriefed following their completion of the study. See Figure 1 for an overview of the experimental protocol. This trial was registered at clinicaltrials.gov as NCT01597024.

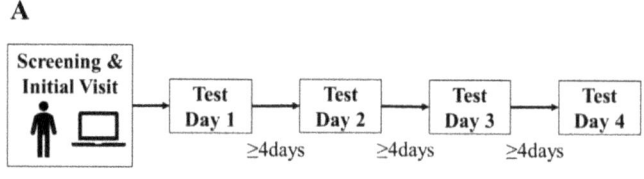

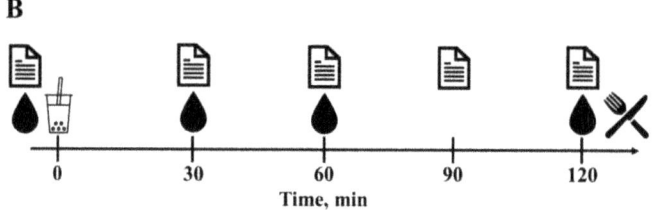

Figure 1. Experimental design (**A**) and test day protocol (**B**). 🚶 anthropometric measurements, 💻 LFPQ, 📄 appetite ratings (Likert scale, children and adolescents; VAS, adult and elderly), 💧 blood sampling (adult and elderly cohorts only), 🥤 randomized test drink intake (NPMT, NPWL, HPMT or HPWL), ✗ ad libitum food intake from buffet-style test meal; (HPMT) high-protein maintenance, HPWL: high-protein weight loss, LFPQ: Leeds Food Preference Questionnaire, NPMT: normal-protein maintenance, NPWL: normal-protein weight loss, VAS: visual analog scale.

2.3. Anthropometric Measures

Height, body mass, waist circumference and body composition were measured in the fasted state and after voiding as described previously [27]. Height was measured to the nearest 0.1 cm using a portable stadiometer (Model 213, SECA, Hamburg, Germany). Body mass, measured to the nearest 0.1 kg, and body composition were assessed using a multi frequency segmental body composition analyzer (Model BC-418-MA, Tanita Corporation, Tokyo, Japan). Body mass index was calculated for each participant and compared against the age- and gender-matched thresholds for normal weight and overweight, as defined by the World Health Organization [28]. In addition, waist circumference and visceral fat percentage measures were performed using abdominal bioelectrical impedance analysis (AB 140 Viscan, Tanita Corporation, Tokyo, Japan), with participants in the supine position.

2.4. Test Drinks

The test drinks provided for the study were designed by Nutricia (Danone, Utrecht, The Netherlands) to taste, look and smell identical. One test drink was created with a normal-protein (NP) composition (15% energy from protein) and the other was created with a high-protein (HP) composition (30% energy from protein). The test drink compositions are presented in Table 1 and compared with whole milk. The test drink quantity either corresponded to 100% of the participant's estimated basal metabolic rate (BMR, kcal/day; weight loss requirements, WL) or 140% of the participant's estimated BMR (weight maintenance requirements, MT). Basal metabolic rate was estimated for all age groups according to equations derived by Schofield [29], suitable for children and adults (see Table S1 for the equations used to estimate BMR). When calculating participant energy requirements for the MT drinks, BMR was multiplied by a correction factor of 1.4, whereas when calculating energy requirements for the WL drinks, BMR was multiplied by a correction factor of 1. In addition, for the purposes of this study, breakfast was defined as the first meal of the day consisting of 25% of the participant's daily energy requirements, which is similar to previous studies [30,31]. Therefore, when calculating participant energy requirements for both drinks, daily BMR was multiplied by 0.25. The following formulas give the energy requirements (ER) for the MT and WL test drinks, respectively:

$$ER_{MT} = BMR \times 1.4 \times 0.25 \qquad (1)$$

$$ER_{WL} = BMR \times 1 \times 0.25 \qquad (2)$$

Table 1. Composition of the high-protein and normal-protein test drinks per 100 mL compared to whole milk.

Product (per 100 mL)		HP Drink	NP Drink	Whole Milk
Total Energy	(kcal)	130	130	63
Protein	(g)	10.0	5.0	3.4
	Energy (%)	30.7	15.3	21.9
	Casein (g)	8.0	4.0	2.7
	Whey (g)	2.0	1.0	0.7
Fat	(g)	3.5	3.5	3.6
	Energy (%)	24.2	24.2	50.6
Carbohydrate	(g)	14.7	19.7	4.6
	Energy (%)	45.1	60.5	27.9
	Lactose (g)	<0.06	<0.06	4.6

HP: high-protein test drink, NP: normal-protein test drink.

The quantity of each drink to be served was calculated considering the energy density of the drinks. The energy density of the drinks in kcal/100 mL ($ED_{kcal/100\ mL}$) was:

$$ED_{kcal/100\ mL} = 130\ kcal/100\ mL \qquad (3)$$

The physical density (d) of the drinks was 1.088 kg/L. Therefore, the energy density of the drinks in kcal/100 g ($ED_{kcal/100\ g}$) was:

$$ED_{kcal/100\ g} = (ED_{kcal/100\ mL} \div d \times 100) \times 100 \qquad (4)$$

$$ED_{kcal/100\ g} = 130 \div 1.09 = 119\ kcal/100\ g \qquad (5)$$

Finally, the quantity of drink to be served was as follows:

$$Quantity\ (g) = (ER \div ED_{kcal/100\ g}) \times 100 = (ER \div 119) \times 100 \qquad (6)$$

Each participant consumed the four different types of test drink: normal-protein weight loss (NPWL), normal-protein weight maintenance (NPMT), high-protein weight loss (HPWL) and high-protein weight maintenance (HPMT) in a randomized order and at a standardized time. The composition of the test drinks was double-blinded and the drinks were labeled A, B, C and D. Nutricia labeled the drinks and generated the random allocation sequence. The drinks were weighed to the nearest gram and placed into neutral sealed cups with a straw. Participants were required to consume at least 80% of each drink and failure to do so would result in their withdrawal from the study. The composition of the drinks was unblinded to the researchers after the final participant completed the study.

2.5. Ad Libitum EI

The ad libitum buffet-style test meal consisted of a counter-balanced selection of 25 sweet and savory, high- and low-calorie food and drink items, all of which were provided in excess (Table S2). All food and drink items were chosen to be commercially available in the UK and Greece. Buffet items were offered either in transparent plastic containers or in their original packaging. The buffet was provided 120 min after test drink consumption, participants were given access to the buffet for 30 min and instructed to consume as much or as little of each buffet item as they wanted until they were satisfied. All foods and drinks were presented identically on each occasion and covertly weighed before and after the buffet. Ad libitum energy and macronutrient intakes were calculated using nutritional values provided by the manufacturer, or by using an electronic version of McCance and Widdowson's The Composition of Foods [32]; NETWISP™ software (version 3.0 for Windows, Tinuviel Software, Anglesey, UK).

2.6. Subjective Appetite Assessment

Appetite perceptions (hunger, fullness and prospective food consumption (PFC)) were measured in adult and elderly participants using previously validated 100mm visual analog scales (VASs, [33]). Participants indicated their subjective feelings of appetite by marking a vertical line on the VAS. A composite appetite score was calculated at each time of measurement using the following formula:

$$[Hunger + (100 - fullness) + prospective\ consumption]/3 \qquad (7)$$

Higher composite appetite scores relate to elevated feelings of appetite. The composite appetite score is increasingly used in the literature for ease of data analysis and presentation [25,34].

Children and adolescents used a 9-point Likert scale to rate fullness (How full do you feel?) and PFC (How much do you think you could eat now?), with 1 representing "Not at all full"/"Nothing at all" and 9 representing "As full as I've ever felt"/"A large amount" for fullness and PFC, respectively. Participants were not permitted to view their previous ratings when completing the scales.

2.7. Test Drink Pleasantness and Satisfaction

After consuming the test drinks, participants rated the drinks for pleasantness and satisfaction. The adult and elderly participants used a 100 mm VAS to rate the drinks, with "Not at all pleasant"/"Not at all satisfying" on the left side and "Extremely pleasant"/"Very satisfying" on the right side of the pleasantness and satisfaction scales. Children and adolescents used a 9-point Likert scale adapted from Jansen et al. [35] to rate the drinks for pleasantness and satisfaction. The scale consisted of 5 cartoon faces (smileys). The first cartoon face on the left (unhappy) reflecting low perceived pleasantness/satisfaction was scored 1 and the last face (very happy) on the right of the scale, reflecting high perceived pleasantness/satisfaction, was scored 9. Participants could rate in between two faces, creating a 9-point scale.

2.8. Food Reward: Leeds Food Preference Questionnaire (LFPQ)

The Leeds Food Preference Questionnaire [36] provided a baseline measure of liking and wanting along dimensions of fat and taste. Participants were presented with an array of pictures of individual food items common in the diet. Foods were chosen by the local research team from a validated database to be either predominantly high (>50% energy) or low (<20% energy) in fat, sweet or savory in taste, but similar in familiarity, protein content and cultural suitability for the study population [37]. The LFPQ has been validated in previous studies investigating dietary protein [38–40]. Explicit liking was measured by participants rating the extent to which they liked each food using a 100 mm VAS ("How pleasant would it be to taste this food now?"). Implicit wanting was assessed using a forced choice methodology so that every image from each of the four food types was compared to every other type over 96 trials (food pairs). Reaction times for all responses were covertly recorded for each food type after adjusting for frequency of selection [37]. Fat bias scores for liking and wanting were calculated as the difference between the high-fat scores and the low-fat scores. Sweet bias scores were calculated as the difference between the sweet and savory scores. Positive values indicated greater liking/wanting for high fat > low fat or sweet > savory and negative values indicated the reverse.

2.9. Blood Sampling and Processing

At all test visits, glucose, insulin, total ghrelin, PYY and GLP-1 were measured fasted and postprandially (at 30, 60 and 120 min after eating), while leptin was measured at the first test visit only. An intravenous cannula (BD Venflon, BD, UK) was inserted into an antecubital vein for the collection of venous blood samples. During the trials, the cannula was kept patent with 2mL flushes of 0.9% NaCl(aq) isotonic saline solution (Baxter Healthcare, UK) after each bloodletting. At each time point, a venous blood sample was collected into a 4.9mL EDTA-coated monovette (S-Monovette, Sarstedt, Nümbrecht, Germany) for the measurement of plasma total ghrelin, PYY and GLP-1 concentrations. A second venous blood sample was collected into a 2.7 mL lithium heparin-coated monovette (S-Monovette, Sarstedt, Nümbrecht, Germany) for the measurement in plasma of leptin, glucose and insulin. Immediately after blood collection, collection tubes were placed in ice and 160μL of a preservative containing 4-(2-aminoethyl) benzenesulfonylfluoride hydrochloride (Roche, Basel, Switzerland), dipeptidyl peptidase-4 inhibitor (Merck Millipore, Darmstadt, Germany) and protease inhibitor cocktail (Sigma-Aldrich, St. Louis, MO, USA) were added to EDTA-coated monovettes. After gentle inversion, both monovettes were spun at 1000g for 15 min in a centrifuge at 4 °C and plasma was stored at −80 °C for batch analysis at the conclusion of the study. Identical blood sampling and processing procedures were followed at ABDN and HUA. Blood samples were collected from adult and elderly participants only. No samples were collected from children, as gaining ethical approval for blood samples in this vulnerable group was challenging.

2.10. Biomarker Analysis

2.10.1. Appetite Hormones

Total ghrelin concentrations were measured using a human-specific radioimmunoassay kit (Linco Research, St. Charles, MO, USA) at the laboratory of JJ Holst. The lowest concentration of ghrelin detectable using this assay was 93 pg/mL. The limit of linearity for this assay was 6000 pg/mL. All samples were read using a gamma counter. The between- and within-volunteer CVs were 39% and 14%, respectively. Total PYY and GLP-1 were measured in duplicate using an electrochemical luminescence immunoassay kit (Meso Scale Discovery, Rockville, Maryland, USA) on the Meso Scale Discovery® multiarray assay platform (Meso Scale Discovery, Rockville, Maryland, USA) at the Core Biomedical Assay Laboratory (CBAL), Cambridge. The PYY immunoassay measured both PYY_{1-36} and PYY_{3-36} with a range of 30–3000 pg/mL. Inter-assay CVs of 7.8–16.4% were obtained. The GLP-1 immunoassay measures all endogenous forms of GLP-1 (including GLP-11-36, GLP-11-37, GLP-17-36, GLP-17-37, GLP-19-36 and GLP-19-37) and has a range of 1.4–1000 pg/mL and CVs of 5.2–8.2% for most of the analytical range. Leptin analysis was performed at CBAL using an in-house two-site DELFIA® assay, which used a monoclonal capture antibody and a polyclonal detection antibody with fluorescent detection using europium-labeled streptavidin [41,42]. The antibodies and standards were sourced from R&D Systems (R&D Systems Europe, Abingdon, UK). This assay had a lower limit of detection of 0.1 ng/mL and intra-assay CVs of 3.9–7.1%.

2.10.2. Glucose Homeostasis

Glucose and insulin plasma analysis was conducted at the University of Aberdeen, Rowett Institute, Technical Services department. Glucose concentrations were measured using a hexokinase method on a Dimension® clinical chemistry analyzer (Siemens Healthcare GmbH, Erlangen, Germany) with CVs of <2% within the reference range. Insulin was detected using a Liaison® XL automated immunoassay analyzer (DiaSorin, Italy) with a chemiluminescence immunoassay, which had a range of 20–3470 pmol/L and intra-assay CVs of 5.0–6.0% across the analytical range. The homeostatic model assessment [43] was used to estimate hepatic insulin resistance (HOMA-IR):

$$IR_{insulin}: \text{fasting glucose (mmol/L)} \times \text{fasting insulin (mU/L)}/22.5 \tag{8}$$

β-cell function was measured using an early insulin secretion function index (insulinogenic index (IGI)):

$$\text{IGI: (Insulin\_0 min} - \text{Insulin\_30 min)/(Glucose\_0 min} - \text{Glucose\_30 min)} \quad (9)$$

Insulin to glucose ratio (IGR) was also calculated.

2.11. Statistical Analysis

It was calculated that 16 participants in each group (defined by age, BMI, gender and study site) would give approximately 80% power to detect group and treatment differences in any variable comparable to the unpredictable variation between groups or within individuals, i.e., to detect a standard effect size of approximately 1.0. Main factor effect comparisons are based on combinations of groups and so larger volunteer numbers had the power to detect smaller effect sizes.

Variables were analyzed by linear mixed models using residual maximum likelihood with random effect terms for volunteer and fixed effect terms for test drink type, age group, BMI group, gender, site and all two-way and three-way interactions. An additional analysis was carried out in each case in which the drink effect was decomposed into its factorial components of composition (HP vs. NP) and quantity (WL vs. MT). Where data were collected at several timepoints in a day (appetite scores and gut hormones), an additional random effect term for day, and fixed effect term for time, were included in the models. Significance of fixed effect terms was assessed by F statistics calculated from Wald statistics, with estimated denominator degrees of freedom. Drinks were compared with post hoc tests based on least significant differences. A *p* value < 0.05 was considered to indicate statistical significance. Analyses were carried out using Genstat v17 (VSN International, Hemel Hempstead, UK). Data are presented as mean ± the standard error of the differences of the mean (SED) unless stated otherwise.

3. Results

3.1. Participants

In total, 424 members of the public were enrolled in the study (See the Consolidated Standards of Reporting Trials (CONSORT) flow diagram (Figure S1) summarizing the participant flow). Thirty-three participants discontinued the study after randomization, of which five were excluded as they consumed <80% of at least one of the test drinks. Therefore, 391 participants across ABDN and HUA completed the study, as 103 children, 109 adolescents, 97 adults and 82 elderly. The characteristics of the participants from ABDN and HUA who completed the study are presented in Table 2. In addition, Supplementary Materials Table S3 presents the number of participants allocated to each group at both sites.

Table 2. Participant characteristics by age group and site [1].

	Children			Adolescents			Adults			Elderly		
	ABDN (n = 39)	HUA (n = 64)	All (n = 103)	ABDN (n = 45)	HUA (n = 64)	All (n = 109)	ABDN (n = 46)	HUA (n = 51)	All (n = 97)	ABDN (n = 36)	HUA (n = 46)	All (n = 82)
Age (years)	8.72 ± 0.69	9.20 ± 0.65	9.02 ± 0.70	15.4 ± 1.28	14.5 ± 1.33	14.9 ± 1.37	29.9 ± 7.34	32.8 ± 6.71	31.4 ± 7.13	68.0 ± 3.82	68.5 ± 3.88	68.3 ± 3.84
Height (m)	1.37 ± 0.08	1.40 ± 0.06	1.39 ± 0.07	1.65 ± 0.09	1.67 ± 0.09	1.66 ± 0.09	1.71 ± 0.09	1.71 ± 0.10	1.71 ± 0.09	1.64 ± 0.08	1.62 ± 0.08	1.62 ± 0.08
Weight (kg)	31.6 ± 6.94	38.3 ± 8.39	35.7 ± 8.49	60.3 ± 12.3	65.7 ± 10.4	63.4 ± 11.5	71.0 ± 14.2	76.1 ± 14.4	73.7 ± 14.5	68.6 ± 11.9	75.7 ± 14.4	72.6 ± 13.7
BMI (kg/m^2)	16.7 ± 2.41	19.5 ± 3.33	18.4 ± 3.31	22.2 ± 4.23	23.5 ± 2.82	23.0 ± 3.51	24.3 ± 4.07	25.9 ± 4.33	25.1 ± 4.27	25.5 ± 3.58	28.9 ± 4.71	27.4 ± 4.55
BMR [2] (MJ)	4.93 ± 0.62	5.52 ± 0.82	5.30 ± 0.8	6.70 ± 1.02	7.14 ± 1.04	6.96 ± 1.05	6.67 ± 1.04	7.18 ± 1.17	6.94 ± 1.13	5.73 ± 0.74	6.54 ± 1.00	6.19 ± 0.98
Body fat [3] (%)	22.8 ± 5.70	25.4 ± 5.93	24.4 ± 5.95	24.8 ± 8.47	24.8 ± 7.54	24.8 ± 7.90	23.6 ± 10.1	26.2 ± 9.95	24.9 ± 10.1	32.4 ± 6.78	35.4 ± 6.78	34.2 ± 6.90
Waist Circumference [4] (cm)	64.5 ± 8.56	71.8 ± 12.4	69.6 ± 11.8	81.6 ± 10.9	84.9 ± 9.75	83.7 ± 10.3	91.4 ± 13.0	96.9 ± 12.4	94.4 ± 12.9	100 ± 14.0	109 ± 12.8	106 ± 14.0
Visceral Fat [4] (%)	3.67 ± 2.23	4.95 ± 3.25	4.58 ± 3.03	5.43 ± 3.67	6.05 ± 3.28	5.81 ± 3.43	7.72 ± 4.92	9.64 ± 4.64	8.76 ± 4.84	10.4 ± 4.25	15.1 ± 6.76	13.2 ± 6.29

[1] Values are means ± SD; [2] calculated by Schofield equation; [3] measured by whole body BIA; [4] measured by abdominal VISCAN bio-impedance; ABDN: Scotland, BIA: bioelectrical impedance analysis, BMR: basal metabolic rate, HUA: Greece.

3.2. Test Drinks

The average test drink energy (kcal) and protein (g) consumption, corrected for mass consumed, varied significantly between age groups ($p < 0.001$; Table 3).

Table 3. Test drink energy and protein consumption [1].

		NPWL	NPMT	HPWL	HPMT	SED$_{type}$	p_{type} [2]
Energy (kcal)	Children ($n = 102$)	306	425	304	425	10	<0.001
	Adolescents ($n = 108$)	406	565	402	557		
	Adults ($n = 97$)	399	553	395	548		
	Elderly ($n = 82$)	348	483	343	478		
Protein (g)	Children ($n = 102$)	11.4	15.9	23.3	32.6	0.6	<0.001
	Adolescents ($n = 108$)	15.2	21.1	30.8	42.7		
	Adults ($n = 97$)	14.9	20.6	30.3	42.0		
	Elderly ($n = 82$)	13.0	18.0	26.3	36.6		

[1] Corrected for mass consumed. Mean data are presented for drink type (NPWL, NPMT, HPWL, HPMT); [2] determined by ANOVA, differences are statistically significant when $p < 0.05$; HPMT: high-protein maintenance, HPWL: high-protein weight loss, NPMT: normal-protein maintenance, NPWL: normal-protein weight loss.

3.3. Ad Libitum EI

Differences in mean ad libitum EI after the test drinks between age groups, weight categories, genders and sites are presented in Table 4. Differences between age groups in response to the quantity of drink provided (WL vs. MT) approached significance ($p = 0.074$).

Table 4. Ad libitum EI (kcal) [1].

	Group	NPWL	NPMT	HPWL	HPMT	SED$_{type}$	p_{type} [2]	NP	HP	SED$_{composition}$	$p_{composition}$ [2]	WL	MT	SED$_{quantity}$	$p_{quantity}$ [2]
Age	Children ($n = 103$)	718	641	679	646	29	0.483	679	663	21	0.941	699	644	21	0.074
	Adolescents ($n = 109$)	950	876	940	852			914	895			945	864		
	Adults ($n = 97$)	672	603	641	627			639	634			658	615		
	Elderly ($n = 82$)	526	522	478	500			524	490			502	510		
BMI	Normal Weight ($n = 221$)	701	644	656	636	21	0.928	672	646	15	0.700	677	639	15	0.858
	Overweight ($n = 170$)	732	677	715	675			706	696			725	677		
Gender	Males ($n = 171$)	825	751	773	744	21	0.166	789	758	15	0.220	799	749	15	0.123
	Females ($n = 220$)	608	569	598	567			589	581			603	567		
Site	HUA ($n = 225$)	806	766	797	756	21	0.245	787	778	15	0.272	801	761	15	0.897
	ABDN ($n = 166$)	627	555	572	555			591	565			600	555		

[1] $n = 391$. Mean data are presented for drink type (NPWL, NPMT, HPWL, HPMT), drink composition (NP, HP) and drink quantity (WL, MT); [2] determined by ANOVA (with age, BMI, gender and site as fixed factors), differences are statistically significant when $p < 0.05$; ABDN: Scotland, EI: energy intake, HP: high protein, HPMT: high-protein maintenance, HPWL: high-protein weight loss, HUA: Greece, MT: weight maintenance, NP: normal protein, NPMT: normal-protein maintenance, NPWL: normal-protein weight loss, WL: weight loss.

There were no significant differences between weight categories, genders or sites. Furthermore, there were no significant differences in total caloric intake (test drink EI + ad libitum EI) between age groups, weight categories, genders or sites in response to drink type, composition or quantity (Table 5).

Table 5. Total caloric intake (kcal) [1].

	Group	NPWL	NPMT	HPWL	HPMT	SED$_{type}$	p_{type} [2]	NP	HP	SED$_{composition}$	$p_{composition}$ [2]	WL	MT	SED$_{quantity}$	$p_{quantity}$ [2]
Age	Children (n = 103)	1022	1075	991	1077			1049	1034			1007	1076		
	Adolescents (n = 109)	1372	1461	1352	1416	50	0.562	1416	1384	46	0.793	1362	1438	46	0.143
	Adults (n = 97)	1078	1168	1048	1186			1123	1117			1063	1177		
	Elderly (n = 82)	885	1022	835	993			953	914			860	1008		
BMI	Normal Weight (n = 221)	1235	1325	1,85	1314	31	0.625	1280	1249	29	0.499	1210	1319	29	0.940
	Overweight (n = 170)	943	1038	928	1023			991	975			936	1030		
Gender	Males (n = 171)	1044	1126	996	1112	31	0.775	1085	1054	29	0.751	1020	1119	29	0.455
	Females (n = 220)	1134	1237	1117	1225			1185	1171			1125	1231		
Site	HUA (n = 225)	995	1075	942	1063	30	0.287	1035	1002	28	0.239	968	1069	28	0.862
	ABDN (n = 166)	1183	1288	1171	1274			1236	1222			1177	1281		

[1] n = 391. Mean data are presented for drink type (NPWL, NPMT, HPWL, HPMT), drink composition (NP, HP) and drink quantity (WL, MT); [2] determined by ANOVA (with age, BMI, gender and site as fixed factors), differences are statistically significant when $p < 0.05$; ABDN: Scotland, EI: energy intake, HP: high protein, HPMT: high-protein maintenance, HPWL: high-protein weight loss, HUA: Greece, MT: weight maintenance, NP: normal protein, NPMT: normal-protein maintenance, NPWL: normal-protein weight loss, WL: weight loss.

The data for mean ad libitum energy and macronutrient intake with all participants combined are reported in Table S4, to explore drink effects. Ad libitum EI was significantly greater after consuming the NPWL drink, in comparison to the other drink types ($p < 0.001$). There were small but statistically significant differences in energy and macronutrient intakes between drinks fed at WL or MT quantities, reflected by higher intakes after WL (all $p < 0.001$). There were no differences in ad libitum energy or nutrient intakes between the NP and HP drinks.

Visit number had a significant effect on ad libitum EI, with EI significantly greater for visits 2, 3 and 4 compared to visit 1 for all participants combined (Supplementary Materials Table S5; $p = 0.001$). In addition, the effect of visit number on ad libitum EI differed significantly between age groups ($p < 0.001$).

3.4. Subjective Appetite Assessment

Table 6 presents the fullness and PFC ratings for drink type, composition and quantity × time interactions for children and adolescents. Fullness did not differ between children and adolescents in response to drink type ($p = 0.252$), composition ($p = 0.220$) or quantity ($p = 0.554$). There were no significant differences in ratings of PFC in response to drink type ($p = 0.332$), composition ($p = 0.209$) or quantity ($p = 0.653$) when comparing children and adolescents. There were no significant differences in fullness or PFC ratings between weight categories, genders or sites (data not shown).

Table 7 presents the composite appetite score for drink type, composition and quantity × time interactions for adults and elderly. The adults' appetite score was significantly greater than that of the elderly across all drink types ($p < 0.004$) and in response to both drink quantities ($p < 0.001$). There were no significant differences between adult and elderly appetite scores in response to drink composition ($p = 0.624$). There were no significant differences in composite appetite scores between weight categories, genders or sites (data not shown).

Table 6. Children [1] and adolescent [2] motivation to eat at baseline and in response to test drink type, composition and quantity.

		Time (mins)	NPWL	NPMT	HPWL	HPMT	SED$_{type}$	Type.Time Interaction p [3]	NP	HP	SED$_{composition}$	Composition.Time Interaction p [3]	WL	MT	SED$_{quantity}$	Quantity.Time Interaction p [3]
Fullness	Children	0	2.25	2.02	1.77	2.19			2.13	1.98			2.01	2.10		
		30	3.73	3.86	3.37	3.71			3.79	3.54			3.55	3.78		
		60	3.06	3.14	3.02	2.83	0.21	0.252	3.10	2.92	0.16	0.220	3.04	2.98	0.16	0.554
		90	2.60	2.75	2.52	2.51			2.68	2.51			2.56	2.63		
		120	2.13	2.28	2.33	2.19			2.21	2.26			2.23	2.23		
	Adolescents	0	2.69	2.90	2.95	2.95			2.80	2.95			2.82	2.92		
		30	4.49	4.85	5.06	5.13			4.67	5.10			4.78	4.99		
		60	4.15	4.44	4.52	4.59	0.18		4.29	4.56	0.14		4.33	4.52	0.14	
		90	3.65	3.94	3.91	4.06			3.80	3.98			3.78	4.00		
		120	3.28	3.53	3.59	3.59			3.40	3.59			3.43	3.56		
PFC	Children	0	6.61	6.89	7.05	7.16			6.75	7.10			6.83	7.02		
		30	6.00	6.00	6.22	5.90			6.00	6.06			6.11	5.95		
		60	6.70	6.55	6.54	6.96	0.19	0.332	6.62	6.75	0.16	0.209	6.62	6.76	0.16	0.653
		90	7.14	7.14	7.05	7.26			7.14	7.16			7.10	7.20		
		120	7.62	7.65	7.55	7.60			7.64	7.57			7.58	7.63		
	Adolescents	0	6.19	6.06	6.05	5.90			6.13	5.98			6.12	5.98		
		30	5.08	4.63	4.58	4.31			4.85	4.44			4.83	4.47		
		60	5.47	5.05	5.08	4.96	0.21		5.26	5.02	0.14		5.27	5.01	0.14	
		90	5.85	5.66	5.61	5.61			5.76	5.61			5.73	5.64		
		120	6.42	6.08	6.07	6.10			6.25	6.09			6.25	6.09		

[1] $n = 103$ for children; [2] $n = 109$ for adolescents; [3] determined by ANOVA between age groups, differences are statistically significant when $p < 0.05$. Mean data are presented for drink type (NPWL, NPMT, HPWL, HPMT), drink composition (NP, HP) and drink quantity (WL, MT); HP: high protein, HPMT: high-protein maintenance, HPWL: high-protein weight loss, MT: weight maintenance, NP: normal protein, NPMT: normal-protein maintenance, NPWL: normal-protein weight loss, PFC: prospective food consumption, WL: weight loss.

Table 7. Adult[1] and elderly[2] composite appetite scores at baseline and in response to test drink type, composition and quantity.

		Time (mins)	NPWL	NPMT	HPWL	HPMT	SED$_{type}$	Type.Time Interaction p[3]	NP	HP	SED$_{composition}$	Composition.Time Interaction p[3]	WL	MT	SED$_{quantity}$	Quantity.Time Interaction p[3]
Appetite Score (mm)	Adults	0	63.2	65.6	61.5	62.8			64.4	62.1			62.3	64.2		
		30	42.6	35.5	41.2	34.8	2.1	0.004	39.0	38.0	1.6	0.624	41.9	35.1	1.6	<0.001
		60	46.7	40.3	44.6	37.9			43.5	41.3			45.7	39.1		
		90	52.0	44.8	49.6	42.4			48.4	46.0			50.8	43.6		
		120	55.9	50.9	54.6	48.1			53.4	51.4			55.3	49.5		
	Elderly	0	44.5	43.7	45.4	43.9			44.1	44.6			44.9	43.8		
		30	31.4	28.6	29.7	31.3	2.7		30.0	30.5	2.1		30.5	30.0	2.1	
		60	35.2	33.7	34.7	33.0			34.4	33.9			35.0	33.3		
		90	40.9	37.5	39.1	36.5			39.2	37.8			40.0	37.0		
		120	44.3	41.9	43.2	38.3			43.1	40.8			43.7	40.1		

[1] $n = 97$ for adults; [2] $n = 82$ for elderly; [3] determined by ANOVA between age groups, differences are statistically significant when $p < 0.05$. Mean data are presented for drink type (NPWL, NPMT, HPWL, HPMT), drink composition (NP, HP) and drink quantity (WL, MT); HP: high protein, HPMT: high-protein maintenance, HPWL: high-protein weight loss, MT: weight maintenance, NP: normal protein, NPMT: normal-protein maintenance, NPWL: normal-protein weight loss, VAS: visual analog scale, WL: weight loss.

3.5. Test Drink Pleasantness and Satisfaction

There was a significant difference in pleasantness ratings between drinks for the children and adolescents and the adults and elderly, with a significantly higher rating for the NPWL drink, in comparison to the NPMT, HPWL and HPMT drinks (children and adolescents (n = 212): 5.14, 4.80, 4.97, 4.60, respectively; $p < 0.001$; SED: 0.12; adults and elderly (n = 179): 68.4, 64.6, 64.7, 62.5 mm, respectively; p = 0.002; SED: 1.9). Participants also preferred the NP over HP composition (children and adolescents: 4.97, 4.78, respectively; p = 0.032; SED: 0.09; adults and elderly: 66.5, 63.6 mm, respectively; p = 0.012; SED: 1.3) and the WL over the MT quantity (children and adolescents: 5.05, 4.70, respectively; $p < 0.001$; SED: 0.09; adults and elderly: 66.5, 63.6 mm, respectively; p = 0.04; SED: 1.3). Average pleasantness ratings were significantly higher in the ABDN children and adolescent cohort (n = 84) compared to the HUA cohort (n = 128; 5.86, 3.89, respectively; $p < 0.001$; SED: 0.22).

Average satisfaction ratings were significantly higher in the children (n = 103) compared to the adolescents (n = 109; 5.17, 4.27, respectively; p = 0.009; SED: 0.20). Children and adolescent females (n = 107) reported significantly higher average satisfaction ratings compared to males (n = 105; 4.95, 4.49, respectively; p = 0.037; SED: 0.20), and average satisfaction ratings were higher in the ABDN children and adolescent cohort (n = 84) compared to the HUA cohort (n = 128; 5.45, 3.99, respectively; $p < 0.001$; SED: 0.20). There were no differences between age groups, weight categories, genders or sites and no effect of drink on satisfaction ratings in the adults and elderly (n = 179; data not shown).

3.6. Food Reward: LFPQ

Fat bias scores (liking and wanting scores for high-fat relative to low-fat foods) and sweet bias scores (scores for sweet relative to savory foods) were compared according to age, BMI, gender and site (Table S6). There was a main effect of age group on liking (p = 0.001) and wanting ($p < 0.001$) for high-fat food. Post hoc analyses showed that the elderly had the lowest fat preference, followed by adults, and that both groups showed a clear preference (liking and wanting) for low-fat relative to high-fat foods. Adolescents showed a greater liking and wanting for high-fat relative to low-fat food. There was also an effect of age group on wanting for sweet foods ($p < 0.001$), with a greater wanting for sweet in children, adolescents and elderly compared to adults ($p < 0.05$). For BMI, while there were no group differences for liking and wanting fat bias, liking (p = 0.047) and wanting (p = 0.059) sweet bias tended to be greater in normal weight than overweight participants. There was no main effect of gender. There was a main effect of site on liking and wanting for sweet (both p = 0.019) and high-fat (both $p < 0.001$) foods, with the ABDN population showing a greater sweet and fat preference compared to HUA.

3.7. Biomarkers

Note that, of the 179 adult and elderly participants, four normal weight adults and three normal weight elderly from ABDN were unable to provide blood samples, therefore, 172 participants were included in the biomarker analyses.

3.7.1. Appetite Hormones

Differences in GLP-1, PYY and ghrelin concentrations between age groups, weight categories, genders and sites in response to all test drinks combined are presented in Figure 2 (GLP-1), Figure 3 (PYY) and Figure 4 (ghrelin). GLP-1 and PYY baseline concentrations did not differ significantly between groups for age, BMI, gender or site comparisons. Ghrelin baseline concentrations did not differ significantly between age groups, but baseline differences are reported for gender, BMI and site comparisons (all $p < 0.001$). Plasma concentrations of GLP-1 (Figure 2A) and PYY (Figure 3A) were significantly greater in the elderly than the adults (both $p < 0.001$), however, there were no significant differences in ghrelin release between age groups (Figure 4A; p = 0.119). There were no significant differences in GLP-1 (Figure 2B; p = 0.996) or PYY (Figure 3B; p = 0.826) responses between normal weight and overweight participants, however, normal weight participants exhibited significantly greater ghrelin concentrations when compared to overweight participants (Figure 4B; $p < 0.001$). Concentrations of all three hormones were greater in females in comparison to males ($p = 0.039$, $p = 0.028$ and $p < 0.001$ for GLP-1 (Figure 2C), PYY (Figure 3C) and ghrelin (Figure 4C), respectively). There were no differences in GLP-1 (Figure 2D) or PYY (Figure 3D) concentrations between ABDN and HUA participants, though ghrelin concentrations were greater in the ABDN cohort compared to the HUA cohort (Figure 4D; $p < 0.001$). Interestingly, ghrelin differences between sites could not be explained by differences in body composition or gender.

Table 8 presents the gut hormones (GLP-1, PYY and ghrelin) drink type, composition and quantity x time interactions for all participants combined. There was a significant effect of drink type on concentrations of GLP-1 and PYY (both $p < 0.001$) and ghrelin ($p < 0.005$). The HP test drinks elicited a significantly greater increase in GLP-1 and PYY (both $p < 0.001$) in comparison to the NP drinks, however, protein content did not significantly affect ghrelin ($p = 0.710$). The MT test drinks elicited a significantly greater increase in GLP-1 and PYY (both $p < 0.001$) in comparison to the WL drinks (both $p < 0.001$), while ghrelin was suppressed to a significantly greater extent in response to the MT drinks compared to the WL drinks ($p < 0.001$).

Pooled data from adults and elderly demonstrated that GLP-1 and PYY concentrations were negatively associated with ad libitum EI (both $p < 0.001$), while there was no significant association between ghrelin and ad libitum EI ($p = 0.770$). PYY concentrations were negatively associated with composite appetite score ($p = 0.028$), while the association between GLP-1 concentrations and composite appetite score approached significance ($p = 0.052$). There was no significant association between ghrelin concentrations and composite appetite score ($p = 0.605$).

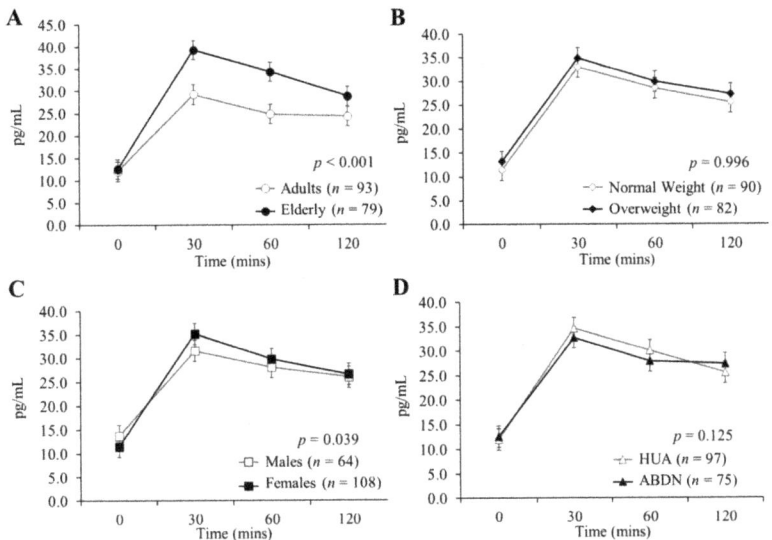

Figure 2. Plasma concentrations of GLP-1 in the adult and elderly cohorts in response to all test drinks combined. Data are presented as mean ± SED, $n = 172$; seven ABDN participants (four normal weight adults, three normal weight elderly) did not complete this measurement. Determined using an electrochemical luminescence immunoassay kit, values were analyzed as repeated measurements using ANOVA, differences are statistically significant when $p < 0.05$. (**A**) Comparison of age group, (**B**) comparison of BMI group, (**C**) comparison of gender, (**D**) comparison of site. ABDN: Scotland, GLP-1: glucagon-like peptide 1, HUA: Greece.

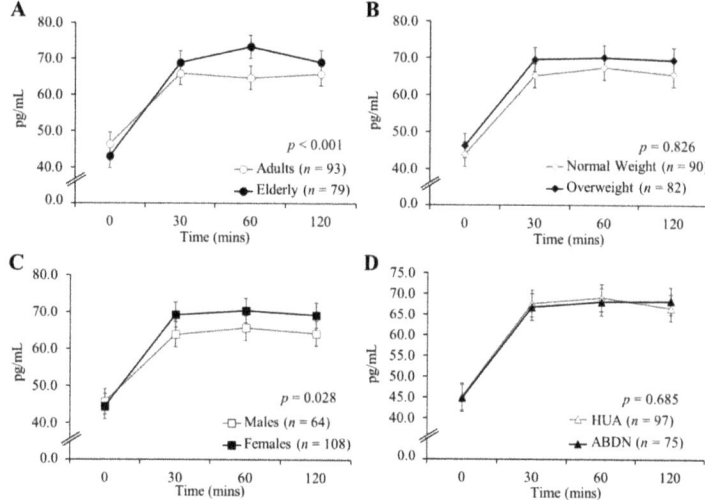

Figure 3. Plasma concentrations of PYY in the adult and elderly cohorts in response to all test drinks combined. Data are presented as mean ± SED, $n = 172$; seven ABDN participants (four normal weight adults, three normal weight elderly) did not complete this measurement. Determined using an electrochemical luminescence immunoassay kit, values were analyzed as repeated measurements using ANOVA, differences are statistically significant when $p < 0.05$. (**A**) Comparison of age group, (**B**) comparison of BMI group, (**C**) comparison of gender, (**D**) comparison of site. ABDN: Scotland, HUA: Greece, PYY: peptide YY.

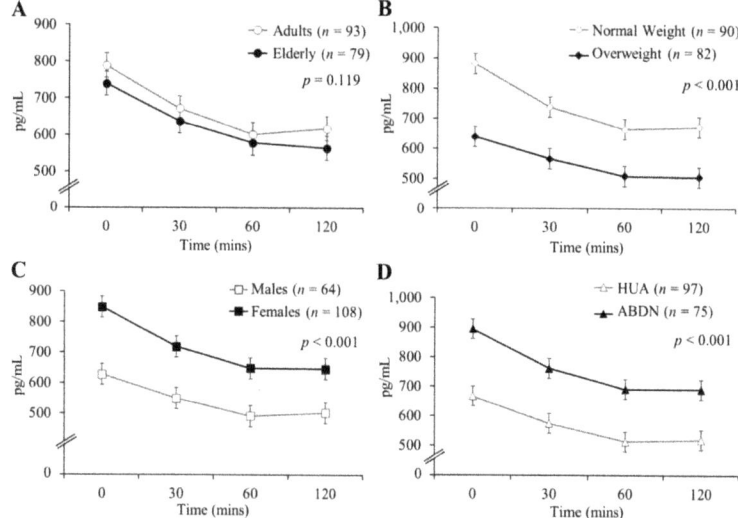

Figure 4. Plasma concentrations of ghrelin in the adult and elderly cohorts in response to all test drinks combined. Data are presented as mean ± SED, $n = 172$; seven ABDN participants (four normal weight adults, three normal weight elderly) did not complete this measurement. Determined using a human-specific radioimmunoassay kit, values were analyzed as repeated measurements using ANOVA, differences are statistically significant when $p < 0.05$. (**A**) Comparison of age group, (**B**) comparison of BMI group, (**C**) comparison of gender, (**D**) comparison of site. ABDN: Scotland, HUA: Greece.

Table 8. Combined adult and elderly[1] appetite hormone concentrations at baseline and in response to test drink type, composition and quantity.

Drink	Time (min)	GLP-1 (pg/mL)	SED	Drink.Time Interaction, p[2]	PYY (pg/mL)	SED	Drink.Time Interaction, p[2]	Ghrelin (pg/mL)	SED	Drink.Time Interaction, p[2]
NPWL	0	12.7			46.1			773		
	30	33.1			68.3			651		
	60	26.6			69.6			596		
	120	21.8			65.2			604		
NPMT	0	11.9			43.5			762		
	30	37.1			71.3			659		
	60	31.3			74.3			584		
	120	28.7	1.3	<0.001	73.4	1.9	<0.001	574	12	<0.005
HPWL	0	12.1			44.9			767		
	30	31.3			63.2			661		
	60	27.6			63.4			603		
	120	26.3			64.2			622		
HPMT	0	12.5			45.2			763		
	30	33.9			66.4			653		
	60	31.1			67.3			578		
	120	28.7			66.5			572		
NP	0	12.3			44.8			767		
	30	35.1			69.8			655		
	60	29.0			72.0			590		
	120	25.2	1.1	<0.001	69.3	1.5	<0.001	589	9	0.710
HP	0	12.3			45.1			765		
	30	32.6			64.8			657		
	60	29.4			65.4			591		
	120	27.5			65.3			597		
WL	0	12.4			45.5			770		
	30	32.2			65.7			656		
	60	27.1			66.5			599		
	120	24.1	1.1	<0.001	64.7	1.5	<0.001	613	9	<0.001
MT	0	12.2			44.4			763		
	30	35.5			68.8			656		
	60	31.2			70.8			581		
	120	28.7			69.9			573		

[1] n = 172; seven ABDN participants (four normal weight adults, four normal weight elderly) did not complete this measurement; [2] determined by ANOVA, differences are statistically significant when p < 0.05. Mean data are presented for drink type (NPWL, NPMT, HPWL, HPMT), drink composition (NP, HP) and drink quantity (WL, MT); GLP-1: glucagon-like peptide 1, HP: high protein, HPMT: high-protein maintenance, HPWL: high-protein weight loss, MT: weight maintenance, NP: normal protein, NPMT: normal-protein maintenance, NPWL: normal-protein weight loss, PYY: pancreatic peptide YY, WL: weight loss.

There were no significant differences in fasting leptin concentrations between adult and elderly participants (adults: 18.21 ng/mL; elderly: 20.86 ng/mL; $p = 0.408$; SED: 2.08). It is well established that obesity enhances the synthesis and release of leptin and, as anticipated, leptin concentrations were significantly higher in overweight participants compared to normal weight participants (overweight: 29.49 ng/mL; normal weight: 10.26 ng/mL; $p < 0.001$; SED: 2.04). Females exhibited significantly greater concentrations of leptin than males (females: 26.55 ng/mL; males: 7.40 ng/mL; $p < 0.001$; SED: 2.12). Leptin concentrations were also significantly greater in HUA participants compared to the ABDN cohort (HUA: 21.36 ng/mL; ABDN: 16.93 ng/mL; $p = 0.016$; SED: 1.98). The gender and site differences can be explained by differences in body composition.

3.7.2. Glucose Homeostasis

Table S7 presents the group × time interactions for glucose and insulin concentrations, and includes HOMA-IR, IGI and IGR. Elderly participants exhibited significantly greater concentrations of glucose ($p < 0.001$), insulin ($p < 0.001$) and HOMA-IR ($p < 0.001$) compared to adults. As expected, glucose homeostasis was significantly influenced by BMI, with glucose ($p < 0.001$), insulin ($p < 0.001$), HOMA-IR ($p < 0.001$) and IGR ($p = 0.006$) greater in overweight compared to normal weight participants. Glucose ($p = 0.036$) and IGR ($p = 0.005$) were significantly greater in females compared to males. Glucose ($p = 0.008$), insulin ($p = 0.005$), HOMA-IR ($p = 0.017$) and IGR ($p = 0.005$) were significantly greater in the HUA cohort compared to the ABDN cohort. These significant group × time interactions were due to delayed insulin responses in elderly, overweight and HUA participants. Furthermore, differences in insulin concentrations between sites can be explained by differences in body composition.

There were significant drink type ($p < 0.001$), composition ($p < 0.05$) and quantity ($p < 0.001$) × time interaction effects for glucose, insulin, HOMA-IR, IGI and IGR (Table S8).

4. Discussion

In relation to the primary aim of this study, the current novel findings demonstrate that ad libitum EI did not differ significantly between age groups, BMIs, genders or geographical locations, though composite appetite score was lower in the elderly subjects compared to the younger adults in response to drink type and quantity. The elderly group exhibited greater postprandial levels of GLP-1 and PYY than the adult group, but ghrelin release was not affected by age. Concentrations of all appetite hormones were greater in females compared to males, while ghrelin levels were lower and fasting leptin levels were higher in overweight compared to normal weight participants. Furthermore, elevated ghrelin release and suppressed fasting leptin levels were observed in the ABDN cohort in comparison to the HUA cohort. As regards the secondary aim, ad libitum EI was not affected by drink composition, though concentrations of GLP-1 and PYY were higher in response to the HP compared to the NP test drinks. In addition, as might be expected, in response to the WL drink quantity, ad libitum EI was elevated, GLP-1 and PYY levels were lower and ghrelin concentrations were higher in comparison to the MT drink quantity.

4.1. Ad Libitum EI and Subjective Appetite

In the present study, there were no significant effects of the test meal on ad libitum EI between weight categories, gender, site or age; albeit we noted a trend towards differences between age groups in response to the quantity of drink provided below or at maintenance requirements. This approached significance, in part explained by the lower intakes in the elderly participants, which was also detected in their significantly lower subjective appetite score. Other authors have highlighted differences in appetite suppression between young and older healthy participants in response to protein and energy load [44], and this warrants further investigation to explore the influence of ageing on mechanisms of protein-induced satiety. Although we assessed subsequent ad libitum EI 2 h after the breakfast drink, we did not measure 24 h EI, so it may be that energy compensation occurred later in the day. Belza et al. [25] also examined the effects of consuming an NP vs. HP test drink in adults. The HP drink led to reduced hunger and increased satiety compared to the NP drink. This might be because the HP drink that Belza et al. [25] used provided 50% energy from protein or 88.4g protein per dose; there may be a threshold absolute concentration of protein required to stimulate protein-induced satiety, and the amount of protein supplied in our HP drink (10 g) may have fallen below this threshold. Furthermore, food form could be important for appetite control across the lifecourse. Indeed, Leidy et al. [23] demonstrated that a solid meal reduced lunch intake by approximately 480 kJ compared to a liquid meal in adolescents. By the nature of our current study design, we did not investigate the form of protein delivery and it is unclear as to whether a solid version would elicit greater changes.

To the authors' knowledge, this is one of the few studies to report the effects of study visit number on ad libitum EI. Interestingly, we observed that the children's ad libitum EI was lower on the final visit compared to the first visit, in agreement with previous research [45], while the adult and elderly ad libitum EI was higher. Possible explanations for these findings may include children habituating to the buffet items following their initial, novel exposure to the buffet during visit 1, and the older age groups initially experiencing heightened feelings of anxiety before acclimatizing to the environment, as demonstrated previously [46]. Future studies may consider incorporating a familiarization/acclimatization session when assessing ad libitum EI, to reduce the effects of study visit order.

4.2. Food Reward: LFPQ

A greater liking and wanting for low-fat relative to high-fat foods and non-sweet relative to sweet foods was shown in the Greek participants. This difference may reflect in part the cultural norms for consuming sweet foods in the morning in Scotland but may also be due to the greater availability of fresh fruit and vegetables and the more traditional rather than "'westernized" diet in Greece [47,48]. Indeed, a north–south European differentiation in food habits consistent with these findings has previously been proposed [49]. We also found an age effect, with adults and the elderly having a greater liking and wanting for low-fat food compared to children and adolescents, and adults having a lower wanting of sweet foods compared to similarly high sweet wanting scores in children, adolescents and the elderly. Very few studies have examined food preferences across the lifecourse and, to our knowledge, no studies have examined both dimensions of fat and sweet taste in food. The findings on sweet taste preference are consistent with one psychophysical study showing that optimally preferred sucrose concentrations were higher for the elderly than for other age groups, except for the children [50]. As regards fat preferences, it is noted that the ability to accurately assess the fat content of foods is limited in humans, but adults may be more responsive to visual cues indicating the healthiness of food, which could influence food choice [51].

4.3. Biomarkers

GLP-1 is co-secreted with PYY by L cells in the lower intestine, with concentrations of both hormones increasing in response to a meal and inducing acute satiety [52–54]. Deficiencies in GLP-1 and PYY have been reported in obese individuals [55–58], although not consistently [59–61] and not in the present study. We do, however, report higher postprandial concentrations of GLP-1 and PYY in the elderly and in females, which in the long term could partially facilitate weight reduction. Ageing modifies the gastrointestinal tract, causing alterations in gut hormone secretion and feedback mechanisms, which slow gastric emptying [62]. Furthermore, authors have observed slower gastric emptying rates in females compared to males [63,64]. Elevated concentrations of GLP-1 and PYY contribute to delayed gastric emptying and prolonged satiety [56,65]. Therefore, we speculate that slower gastric emptying in the elderly and female groups may have partially accounted for elevated postprandial levels of GLP-1 and PYY. In addition, gastric emptying and satiety hormones have been shown to fluctuate depending on the phase of the menstrual cycle [66–68], highlighting the important role of sex hormones in appetite control.

Ghrelin is the only known gastrointestinal hormone to increase food intake [69]. Its concentrations peak prior to meal initiation and are suppressed by nutrient intake [69]. We report elevated fasting ghrelin concentrations in the normal weight compared to overweight participants and in females vs. males, as shown previously [70], however, postprandial patterns of response were similar. Ghrelin concentrations did not differ between adults and elderly, which agrees with previous data [71–75], though findings to the contrary have also been reported [76–79]. Ghrelin exists as two isoforms: acyl ghrelin, which stimulates energy intake [80,81] and des-acyl ghrelin, which may act independently from acyl ghrelin [82]. Most studies, including the present study, reporting no differences in ghrelin concentrations between younger and older adults [71–73,75], have measured total ghrelin (acyl and des-acyl ghrelin) only. However, studies measuring acyl ghrelin observe lower concentrations and an impaired postprandial response in the elderly [77–79]. Therefore, the form of ghrelin measured may contribute to discrepancies in the literature and merits further investigation.

Although insulin is predominantly considered a principal regulator of glucose metabolism, it also acts on the arcuate nucleus of the hypothalamus to signal satiety [83]. Studies demonstrating increased satiety with age also report greater postprandial insulin concentrations in older compared to younger adults [73,78,84], in agreement with our findings. Insulin modulates changes in the circulation of leptin [85] and ghrelin [86] and may induce satiety indirectly by amplifying the anorectic actions of leptin and/or suppressing ghrelin secretion [86,87]. In the present study, we did not observe differences in leptin or ghrelin concentrations between adults and the elderly, suggesting that greater insulin secretion in the elderly was not sufficient to cause age-related differences in leptin and ghrelin release.

This is one of the few studies to compare appetite control in different geographical locations. We observed lower ghrelin concentrations in HUA participants compared to those in ABDN. However, differences at baseline were accountable for postprandial differences between each "site". Interestingly, we also observed elevated fasting leptin concentrations and postprandial insulin concentrations in the HUA cohort compared to the ABDN cohort, which may have partially modulated ghrelin expression. These are novel findings and not likely due to technical issues since processing, storage and analysis were identical, instead, differences in leptin and insulin levels appear to be associated with differences in body composition between the two locations, though body composition did not account for differences in ghrelin concentrations and neither did gender. Future studies may consider the influence of geographical location on variations in appetite control, as other authors have suggested that differences are not related to habitual diet [88].

In the current study, we observed a significant decrease in ghrelin concentrations in response to the caloric load, but not the protein amount. This lack of protein-induced dose-dependent effect is reported by other authors [25,89]. It has been suggest that the postprandial decrease in ghrelin may be mediated through stimulation of gastric inhibitory polypeptide (GIP) and glucagon [25,90,91], possibly linked to gastric emptying, but also the carbohydrate content of the meal [25,91]. We also suggest that interactions between the protein and carbohydrate content is likely to influence ghrelin release, and that dietary carbohydrate may be a more potent stimulator than protein. Interestingly, in the current study, the HP drinks increased GLP-1 and PYY in comparison to the NP drinks. Belza et al. [25] provide a concise commentary on this aspect and suggest that these two hormones, in combination, do affect appetite after a protein-rich meal.

4.4. Strengths and Limitations

The present study has several strengths, which include having a controlled diet intervention study conducted as a randomized crossover design in a large cohort taking account of age, body size, gender and geographical location. For some factors (such as drink), this study has the strengths of a crossover design, whereas for others (such as age), there are the unavoidable limitations of studying observable factors. As with any lab-based dietary intervention study, there are limitations, such as limited ecological validity, the amount and type of protein and many phenotypic effects which have not been investigated. The iso-energetic load for the meals was achieved by reducing carbohydrate content, so we cannot rule out the effect of this lower carbohydrate nutrient profile of the high-protein meal to contribute to the study results. We presented unadjusted p-values for comparing treatment groups in tests of several variables, to preserve the power of the study, so although there are clear patterns of significant differences, there is a risk that a small proportion of these are type I errors. Therefore, significant p-values presented within the present study come with this caveat, which should be considered when interpreting our findings. We recruited people motivated to respond to a diet trial and, consequently, this is not a truly random sample. Furthermore, had we recruited a much larger sample size, this may have allowed the statistical results to be generalized to a larger population or phenotype. Finally, long-term intervention and monitoring across the lifecourse to assess the mechanisms underlying changes in appetite control were out with the scope of this study.

5. Conclusions

The primary aim of this study was to describe the acute regulation of appetite across the lifecourse, thus being able to detect differences between four different age groups (children, adolescents, adult and elderly), two different weight categories (normal weight and overweight), the two genders (male and female) and two European sites (Aberdeen, Scotland and Athens, Greece). The present study shows that the elderly reported lower subjective appetite ratings in response to the different drink types and quantities in comparison to the adults. Furthermore, in agreement with Di Francesco et al. [73], postprandial anorexigenic signals prevailed over orexigenic signals in the elderly, which over time could induce an energy deficit and accentuate the anorexia of ageing. In addition to age, differences in appetite hormone concentrations between BMIs, genders and geographical locations were also observed, the latter of which being of particular interest, as location is rarely considered in the context of acute appetite control. Future research may consider expanding upon our findings and examining the role of appetitive neuronal circuits in food–gut–brain interactions across the lifecourse.

Supplementary Materials: The following are available online at http://www.mdpi.com/2072-6643/12/12/3710/s1, Table S1: Schofield equations for estimating BMR, Table S2: Nutritional values of the foods and drinks served at the ad libitum buffet-style test meal, Table S3: Number of participants completed within each group at both sites, Table S4: Buffet-style test meal ad libitum energy and macronutrient intake (n = 391), Table S5: Effect of visit number on ad libitum EI, Table S6: Mean food reward (liking and wanting) results, Table S7: Combined adult and elderly glucose homeostasis, by group, at baseline and post-test drink consumption, Table S8: Combined adult and elderly glucose homeostasis at baseline and in response to test drink type, composition and quantity, Figure S1: CONSORT diagram summarizing participant flow. The number of participants from both study sites who were recruited, enrolled, allocated to intervention, discontinued, included in the analyses and completed are presented. ABDN: Scotland, HUA: Greece.

Author Contributions: Y.M., J.G.M. and A.M.J. conceptualization; D.R.C., W.B., C.L.F, O.A. and A.G. data curation; G.W.H., G.F. and K.B. formal analysis; Y.M., J.G.M. and A.M.J. funding acquisition; D.R.C., W.B., C.L.F, O.A., A.G., C.L.M., J.J.H. and A.M.J. investigation; D.R.C., W.B., O.A., G.F., C.L.M., J.J.H., K.V.N. and A.M.J. methodology; G.W.H. project administration; G.F., C.L.M., J.J.H. and K.V.N. resources; Y.M. and J.G.M. supervision; D.R.C., W.B., C.L.F., G.F. and A.M.J. writing—original draft; G.W.H., Y.M., O.A., A.G., K.B., C.L.M., J.J.H., K.V.N. and J.G.M. writing—review & editing. All authors have read and agreed to the published version of the manuscript.

Funding: This research was funded by the European Union's Seventh Framework Programme FP7-KBBE-2010-4 under grant agreement No: 266408. Authors from the University of Aberdeen, Rowett Institute gratefully acknowledge financial support from the Scottish Government as part of the RESAS Strategic Research Programme at the Rowett Institute.

Acknowledgments: We thank Sylvia Stephen, Karen Taylor, Ruth Melican, Rachel Malone, Tara Lyons Argyri Tsipra, Charlotte Zeller, Miroslaw Kasprzak, Niamh Maloney, Evie Nikokavoura, Laura Bardon, Zahra Mansy and the staff at the Human Nutrition Unit for their assistance with the dietary preparation and participant data collection. The authors would also like to thank all the participants for their time and effort.

Conflicts of Interest: Dr Klaske van Norren worked as a Wageningen University consultant for Nutricia Research in Utrecht, a medical Nutrition company. No other author has a conflict of interest to declare. The founding sponsors had no role in the design of the study; in the collection, analyses, or interpretation of data; in the writing of the manuscript, and in the decision to publish the results.

References

1. World Health Organization. *Diet, Nutrition and the Prevention of Chronic Diseases. Report of a Joint WHO/FAO Expert Consultation*; WHO Technical Report Series No. 916; World Health Organization: Geneva, Switzerland, 2003.
2. Darnton-Hill, I.; Nishida, C.; James, W.P.T. A life course approach to diet, nutrition and the prevention of chronic diseases. *Public Health Nutr.* **2004**, *7*, 101–121. [CrossRef] [PubMed]
3. Donaldson, A.I.C.; Johnstone, A.M.; de Roos, B.; Myint, P.K. Role of protein in healthy ageing. *Eur. J. Integr. Med.* **2018**, *23*, 32–36. [CrossRef]
4. Zac-Varghese, S.; Tan, T.; Bloom, S.R. Hormonal interactions between gut and brain. *Discov. Med.* **2010**, *10*, 543–552. [PubMed]
5. Bilman, E.; van Kleef, E.; van Trijp, H. External cues challenging the internal appetite control system—Overview and practical implications. *Crit. Rev. Food Sci. Nutr.* **2017**, *57*, 2825–2834. [CrossRef] [PubMed]
6. Murphy, K.G.; Bloom, S.R. Gut hormones in the control of appetite. *Exp. Physiol.* **2004**, *89*, 507–516. [CrossRef]
7. Simpson, K.A.; Bloom, S.R. Appetite and Hedonism: Gut Hormones and the Brain. *Endocrinol. Metab. Clin.* **2010**, *39*, 729–743. [CrossRef] [PubMed]
8. Juonala, M.; Magnussen, C.G.; Berenson, G.S.; Venn, A.; Burns, T.L.; Sabin, M.A.; Srinivasan, S.R.; Daniels, S.R.; Davis, P.H.; Chen, W.; et al. Childhood Adiposity, Adult Adiposity, and Cardiovascular Risk Factors. *N. Engl. J. Med.* **2011**, *365*, 1876–1885. [CrossRef]
9. Rendina, D.; Campanozzi, A.; De Filippo, G. Methodological approach to the assessment of the obesogenic environment in children and adolescents: A review of the literature. *Nutr. Metab. Cardiovasc. Dis.* **2019**, *29*, 561–571. [CrossRef]
10. Marschner, A.; Mell, T.; Wartenburger, I.; Villringer, A.; Reischies, F.M.; Heekeren, H.R. Reward-based decision-making and aging. *Brain Res. Bull.* **2005**, *67*, 382–390. [CrossRef]
11. Dreher, J.-C.; Meyer-Lindenberg, A.; Kohn, P.; Berman, K.F. Age-related changes in midbrain dopaminergic regulation of the human reward system. *Proc. Natl. Acad. Sci. USA* **2008**, *105*, 15106–15111. [CrossRef]
12. Pelchat, M.L. Food Cravings in Young and Elderly Adults. *Appetite* **1997**, *28*, 103–113. [CrossRef] [PubMed]
13. Koehler, K.M. The New Mexico Aging Process Study. *Nutr. Rev.* **1994**, *52*, S34–S37. [CrossRef] [PubMed]
14. Zhu, K.; Devine, A.; Suleska, A.; Tan, C.Y.; Toh, C.Z.J.; Kerr, D.; Prince, R.L. Adequacy and change in nutrient and food intakes with aging in a seven-year cohort study in elderly women. *J. Nutr. Health Aging* **2010**, *14*, 723–729. [CrossRef]
15. Morley, J.E. Anorexia of aging: Physiologic and pathologic. *Am. J. Clin. Nutr.* **1997**, *66*, 760–773. [CrossRef] [PubMed]
16. Briefel, R.R.; McDowell, M.A.; Alaimo, K.; Caughman, C.R.; Bischof, A.L.; Carroll, M.D.; Johnson, C.L. Total energy intake of the US population: The third National Health and Nutrition Examination Survey, 1988-1991. *Am. J. Clin. Nutr.* **1995**, *62*, 1072S–1080S. [CrossRef] [PubMed]
17. Mercer, J.G.; Johnstone, A.M.; Halford, J.C.G. Approaches to influencing food choice across the age groups: From children to the elderly. *Proc. Nutr. Soc.* **2015**, *74*, 149–157. [CrossRef]
18. Nickols-Richardson, S.M.; Coleman, M.D.; Volpe, J.J.; Hosig, K.W. Perceived Hunger Is Lower and Weight Loss Is Greater in Overweight Premenopausal Women Consuming a Low-Carbohydrate/High-Protein vs High-Carbohydrate/Low-Fat Diet. *J. Am. Diet. Assoc.* **2005**, *105*, 1433–1437. [CrossRef]
19. Lejeune, M.P.; Westerterp, K.R.; Adam, T.C.; Luscombe-Marsh, N.D.; Westerterp-Plantenga, M.S. Ghrelin and glucagon-like peptide 1 concentrations, 24-h satiety, and energy and substrate metabolism during a high-protein diet and measured in a respiration chamber. *Am. J. Clin. Nutr.* **2006**, *83*, 89–94. [CrossRef]
20. Johnstone, A.M.; Horgan, G.W.; Murison, S.D.; Bremner, D.M.; Lobley, G.E. Effects of a high-protein ketogenic diet on hunger, appetite, and weight loss in obese men feeding ad libitum. *Am. J. Clin. Nutr.* **2008**, *87*, 44–55. [CrossRef]
21. Wolfe, R.R. The role of dietary protein in optimizing muscle mass, function and health outcomes in older individuals. *Br. J. Nutr.* **2012**, *108* (Suppl. 2), S88–S93. [CrossRef]
22. Veldhorst, M.; Smeets, A.; Soenen, S.; Hochstenbach-Waelen, A.; Hursel, R.; Diepvens, K.; Lejeune, M.; Luscombe-Marsh, N.; Westerterp-Plantenga, M. Protein-induced satiety: Effects and mechanisms of different proteins. *Physiol. Behav.* **2008**, *94*, 300–307. [CrossRef] [PubMed]

23. Leidy, H.J.; Bales-Voelker, L.I.; Harris, C.T. A protein-rich beverage consumed as a breakfast meal leads to weaker appetitive and dietary responses v. a protein-rich solid breakfast meal in adolescents. *Br. J. Nutr.* **2011**, *106*, 37–41. [CrossRef] [PubMed]
24. Nguo, K.; Bonham, M.; Truby, H.; Barber, E.; Brown, J.; Huggins, C. Effect of Macronutrient Composition on Appetite Hormone Responses in Adolescents with Obesity. *Nutrients* **2019**, *11*, 340. [CrossRef] [PubMed]
25. Belza, A.; Ritz, C.; Sørensen, M.Q.; Holst, J.J.; Rehfeld, J.F.; Astrup, A. Contribution of gastroenteropancreatic appetite hormones to protein-induced satiety. *Am. J. Clin. Nutr.* **2013**, *97*, 980–989. [CrossRef] [PubMed]
26. Association, W.M. World Medical Association Declaration of Helsinki: Ethical Principles for Medical Research Involving Human Subjects. *JAMA* **2013**, *310*, 2191–2194. [CrossRef]
27. Johnstone, A.M.; Murison, S.D.; Duncan, J.S.; Rance, K.A.; Speakman, J.R. Factors influencing variation in basal metabolic rate include fat-free mass, fat mass, age, and circulating thyroxine but not sex, circulating leptin, or triiodothyronine. *Am. J. Clin. Nutr.* **2005**, *82*, 941–948. [CrossRef]
28. World Health Organization. *Physical Status: The Use and Interpretation of Anthropometry. Report of a WHO Expert Committee*; Technical Report Series no. 854; World Health Organization: Geneva, Switzerland, 1995.
29. Schofield, W.N. Predicting basal metabolic rate, new standards and review of previous work. *Hum. Nutr. Clin. Nutr.* **1985**, *39* (Suppl. 1), 5–41.
30. Chowdhury, E.A.; Richardson, J.D.; Tsintzas, K.; Thompson, D.; Betts, J.A. Carbohydrate-rich breakfast attenuates glycaemic, insulinaemic and ghrelin response to ad libitum lunch relative to morning fasting in lean adults. *Br. J. Nutr.* **2015**, *114*, 98–107. [CrossRef]
31. Leidy, H.J.; Racki, E.M. The addition of a protein-rich breakfast and its effects on acute appetite control and food intake in 'breakfast-skipping' adolescents. *Int. J. Obes.* **2010**, *34*, 1125–1133. [CrossRef]
32. McCance, R.A.; Widdowson, E.M. *McCance and Widdowson's the Composition of Foods*, 7th ed.; Royal Society of Chemistry: London, UK, 2015.
33. Flint, A.; Raben, A.; Blundell, J.E.; Astrup, A. Reproducibility, power and validity of visual analogue scales in assessment of appetite sensations in single test meal studies. *Int. J. Obes.* **2000**, *24*, 38–48. [CrossRef]
34. Anderson, G.H.; Catherine, N.L.A.; Woodend, D.M.; Wolever, T.M.S. Inverse association between the effect of carbohydrates on blood glucose and subsequent short-term food intake in young men. *Am. J. Clin. Nutr.* **2002**, *76*, 1023–1030. [CrossRef]
35. Jansen, A.; Theunissen, N.; Slechten, K.; Nederkoorn, C.; Boon, B.; Mulkens, S.; Roefs, A. Overweight children overeat after exposure to food cues. *Eat. Behav.* **2003**, *4*, 197–209. [CrossRef]
36. Finlayson, G.; King, N.; Blundell, J. The role of implicit wanting in relation to explicit liking and wanting for food: Implications for appetite control. *Appetite* **2008**, *50*, 120–127. [CrossRef] [PubMed]
37. Oustric, P.; Thivel, D.; Dalton, M.; Beaulieu, K.; Gibbons, C.; Hopkins, M.; Blundell, J.; Finlayson, G. Measuring food preference and reward: Application and cross-cultural adaptation of the Leeds Food Preference Questionnaire in human experimental research. *Food Qual. Prefer.* **2020**, *80*, 103824. [CrossRef]
38. Griffioen-Roose, S.; Mars, M.; Siebelink, E.; Finlayson, G.; Tomé, D.; de Graaf, C. Protein status elicits compensatory changes in food intake and food preferences. *Am. J. Clin. Nutr.* **2011**, *95*, 32–38. [CrossRef] [PubMed]
39. Griffioen-Roose, S.; Mars, M.; Finlayson, G.; Blundell, J.E.; de Graaf, C. The effect of within-meal protein content and taste on subsequent food choice and satiety. *Br. J. Nutr.* **2011**, *106*, 779–788. [CrossRef] [PubMed]
40. Karl, J.P.; Cole, R.E.; Berryman, C.E.; Finlayson, G.; Radcliffe, P.N.; Kominsky, M.T.; Murphy, N.E.; Carbone, J.W.; Rood, J.C.; Young, A.J.; et al. Appetite Suppression and Altered Food Preferences Coincide with Changes in Appetite-Mediating Hormones During Energy Deficit at High Altitude, But Are Not Affected by Protein Intake. *High Alt. Med. Biol.* **2018**, *19*, 156–169. [CrossRef] [PubMed]
41. Patel, S.; Alvarez-Guaita, A.; Melvin, A.; Rimmington, D.; Dattilo, A.; Miedzybrodzka, E.L.; Cimino, I.; Maurin, A.-C.; Roberts, G.P.; Meek, C.L.; et al. GDF15 Provides an Endocrine Signal of Nutritional Stress in Mice and Humans. *Cell Metab.* **2019**, *29*, 707–718.e8. [CrossRef]
42. Cheke, L.G.; Bonnici, H.M.; Clayton, N.S.; Simons, J.S. Obesity and insulin resistance are associated with reduced activity in core memory regions of the brain. *Neuropsychologia* **2017**, *96*, 137–149. [CrossRef]
43. Matthews, D.R.; Hosker, J.P.; Rudenski, A.S.; Naylor, B.A.; Treacher, D.F.; Turner, R.C. Homeostasis model assessment: Insulin resistance and β-cell function from fasting plasma glucose and insulin concentrations in man. *Diabetologia* **1985**, *28*, 412–419. [CrossRef]

44. Giezenaar, C.; Trahair, L.G.; Rigda, R.; Hutchison, A.T.; Feinle-Bisset, C.; Luscombe-Marsh, N.D.; Hausken, T.; Jones, K.L.; Horowitz, M.; Chapman, I.; et al. Lesser suppression of energy intake by orally ingested whey protein in healthy older men compared with young controls. *Am. J. Physiol. Integr. Comp. Physiol.* **2015**, *309*, R845–R854. [CrossRef]
45. Brindal, E.; Baird, D.; Danthiir, V.; Wilson, C.; Bowen, J.; Slater, A.; Noakes, M. Ingesting breakfast meals of different glycaemic load does not alter cognition and satiety in children. *Eur. J. Clin. Nutr.* **2012**, *66*, 1166–1171. [CrossRef] [PubMed]
46. Chandarana, K.; Drew, M.E.; Emmanuel, J.; Karra, E.; Gelegen, C.; Chan, P.; Cron, N.J.; Batterham, R.L. Subject Standardization, Acclimatization, and Sample Processing Affect Gut Hormone Levels and Appetite in Humans. *Gastroenterology* **2009**, *136*, 2115–2126. [CrossRef] [PubMed]
47. Trichopoulou, A.; Naska, A.; Costacou, T. DAFNE III Group Disparities in food habits across Europe. *Proc. Nutr. Soc.* **2002**, *61*, 553–558. [CrossRef] [PubMed]
48. Yannakoulia, M.; Karayiannis, D.; Terzidou, M.; Kokkevi, A.; Sidossis, L.S. Nutrition-related habits of Greek adolescents. *Eur. J. Clin. Nutr.* **2004**, *58*, 580–586. [CrossRef] [PubMed]
49. Rumm-Kreuter, D. Comparison of the eating and cooking habits of northern Europe and the Mediterranean countries in the past, present and future. *Int. J. Vitam. Nutr. Res.* **2001**, *71*, 141–148. [CrossRef]
50. Zandstra, E.H.; de Graaf, C. Sensory perception and pleasantness of orange beverages from childhood to old age. *Food Qual. Prefer.* **1998**, *9*, 5–12. [CrossRef]
51. Wadhera, D.; Capaldi-Phillips, E.D. A review of visual cues associated with food on food acceptance and consumption. *Eat. Behav.* **2014**, *15*, 132–143. [CrossRef]
52. Flint, A.; Raben, A.; Astrup, A.; Holst, J.J. Glucagon-like peptide 1 promotes satiety and suppresses energy intake in humans. *J. Clin. Investig.* **1998**, *101*, 515–520. [CrossRef]
53. Adrian, T.E.; Ferri, G.-L.; Bacarese-Hamilton, A.J.; Fuessl, H.S.; Polak, J.M.; Bloom, S.R. Human distribution and release of a putative new gut hormone, peptide YY. *Gastroenterology* **1985**, *89*, 1070–1077. [CrossRef]
54. De Silva, A.; Salem, V.; Long, C.J.; Makwana, A.; Newbould, R.D.; Rabiner, E.A.; Ghatei, M.A.; Bloom, S.R.; Matthews, P.M.; Beaver, J.D.; et al. The Gut Hormones PYY3-36 and GLP-17-36 amide Reduce Food Intake and Modulate Brain Activity in Appetite Centers in Humans. *Cell Metab.* **2011**, *14*, 700–706. [CrossRef] [PubMed]
55. Holst, J.J.; Schwartz, T.W.; Lovgreen, N.A.; Pedersen, O.; Beck-Nielsen, H. Diurnal profile of pancreatic polypeptide, pancreatic glucagon, gut glucagon and insulin in human morbid obesity. *Int. J. Obes.* **1983**, *7*, 529–538. [PubMed]
56. Näslund, E.; Barkeling, B.; King, N.; Gutniak, M.; Blundell, J.E.; Holst, J.J.; Rössner, S.; Hellström, P.M. Energy intake and appetite are suppressed by glucagon-like peptide-1 (GLP-1) in obese men. *Int. J. Obes.* **1999**, *23*, 304–311. [CrossRef] [PubMed]
57. Bartolomé, M.A.; Borque, M.; Martinez-Sarmiento, J.; Aparicio, E.; Hernández, C.; Cabrerizo, L.; Fernández-Represa, J.A. Peptide YY Secretion in Morbidly Obese Patients Before and After Vertical Banded Gastroplasty. *Obes. Surg.* **2002**, *12*, 324–327. [CrossRef] [PubMed]
58. Batterham, R.L.; Cohen, M.A.; Ellis, S.M.; Le Roux, C.W.; Withers, D.J.; Frost, G.S.; Ghatei, M.A.; Bloom, S.R. Inhibition of food intake in obese subjects by peptide YY3-36. *N. Engl. J. Med.* **2003**, *349*, 941–948. [CrossRef] [PubMed]
59. Vilsbøll, T.; Krarup, T.; Sonne, J.; Madsbad, S.; Vølund, A.; Juul, A.G.; Holst, J.J. Incretin Secretion in Relation to Meal Size and Body Weight in Healthy Subjects and People with Type 1 and Type 2 Diabetes Mellitus. *J. Clin. Endocrinol. Metab.* **2003**, *88*, 2706–2713. [CrossRef]
60. Kim, B.J.; Carlson, O.D.; Jang, H.J.; Elahi, D.; Berry, C.; Egan, J.M. Peptide YY is secreted after oral glucose administration in a gender-specific manner. *J. Clin. Endocrinol. Metab.* **2005**, *90*, 6665–6671. [CrossRef]
61. Vazquez Roque, M.I.; Camilleri, M.; Stephens, D.A.; Jensen, M.D.; Burton, D.D.; Baxter, K.L.; Zinsmeister, A.R. Gastric Sensorimotor Functions and Hormone Profile in Normal Weight, Overweight, and Obese People. *Gastroenterology* **2006**, *131*, 1717–1724. [CrossRef]
62. Morley, J.E.; Silver, A.J. Anorexia in the elderly. *Neurobiol. Aging* **1988**, *9*, 9–16. [CrossRef]
63. Datz, F.L.; Christian, P.E.; Moore, J. Gender-related differences in gastric emptying. *J. Nucl. Med.* **1987**, *28*, 1204–1207.

64. Giezenaar, C.; Trahair, L.G.; Luscombe-Marsh, N.D.; Hausken, T.; Standfield, S.; Jones, K.L.; Lange, K.; Horowitz, M.; Chapman, I.; Soenen, S. Effects of randomized whey-protein loads on energy intake, appetite, gastric emptying, and plasma gut-hormone concentrations in older men and women. *Am. J. Clin. Nutr.* **2017**, *106*, 865–877. [CrossRef] [PubMed]
65. Savage, A.P.; Adrian, T.E.; Carolan, G.; Chatterjee, V.K.; Bloom, S.R. Effects of peptide YY (PYY) on mouth to caecum intestinal transit time and on the rate of gastric emptying in healthy volunteers. *Gut* **1987**, *28*, 166–170. [CrossRef]
66. Brennan, I.M.; Feltrin, K.L.; Nair, N.S.; Hausken, T.; Little, T.J.; Gentilcore, D.; Wishart, J.M.; Jones, K.L.; Horowitz, M.; Feinle-Bisset, C. Effects of the phases of the menstrual cycle on gastric emptying, glycemia, plasma GLP-1 and insulin, and energy intake in healthy lean women. *Am. J. Physiol. Gastrointest. Liver Physiol.* **2009**, *297*, 602–610. [CrossRef]
67. Hirschberg, A.L. Sex hormones, appetite and eating behaviour in women. *Maturitas* **2012**, *71*, 248–256. [CrossRef] [PubMed]
68. Campolier, M.; Thondre, S.P.; Clegg, M.; Shafat, A.; Mcintosh, A.; Lightowler, H. Changes in PYY and gastric emptying across the phases of the menstrual cycle and the influence of the ovarian hormones. *Appetite* **2016**, *107*, 106–115. [CrossRef] [PubMed]
69. Cummings, D.E.; Purnell, J.Q.; Frayo, R.S.; Schmidova, K.; Wisse, B.E.; Weigle, D.S. A preprandial rise in plasma ghrelin levels suggests a role in meal initiation in humans. *Diabetes* **2001**, *50*, 1714–1719. [CrossRef] [PubMed]
70. Beasley, J.M.; Ange, B.A.; Anderson, C.A.M.; Miller, E.R., III; Holbrook, J.T.; Appel, L.J. Characteristics Associated With Fasting Appetite Hormones (Obestatin, Ghrelin, and Leptin). *Obesity* **2009**, *17*, 349–354. [CrossRef]
71. Sturm, K.; MacIntosh, C.G.; Parker, B.A.; Wishart, J.; Horowitz, M.; Chapman, I.M. Appetite, food intake, and plasma concentrations of cholecystokinin, ghrelin, and other gastrointestinal hormones in undernourished older women and well-nourished young and older women. *J. Clin. Endocrinol. Metab.* **2003**, *88*, 3747–3755. [CrossRef]
72. Bertoli, S.; Magni, P.; Krogh, V.; Ruscica, M.; Dozio, E.; Testolin, G.; Battezzati, A. Is ghrelin a signal of decreased fat-free mass in elderly subjects? *Eur. J. Endocrinol.* **2006**, *155*, 321–330. [CrossRef]
73. Di Francesco, V.; Zamboni, M.; Zoico, E.; Mazzali, G.; Dioli, A.; Omizzolo, F.; Bissoli, L.; Fantin, F.; Rizzotti, P.; Solerte, S.B.; et al. Unbalanced serum leptin and ghrelin dynamics prolong postprandial satiety and inhibit hunger in healthy elderly: Another reason for the "anorexia of aging". *Am. J. Clin. Nutr.* **2006**, *83*, 1149–1152. [CrossRef]
74. Schneider, S.M.; Al-Jaouni, R.; Caruba, C.; Giudicelli, J.; Arab, K.; Suavet, F.; Ferrari, P.; Mothe-Satney, I.; Van Obberghen, E.; Hébuterne, X. Effects of age, malnutrition and refeeding on the expression and secretion of ghrelin. *Clin. Nutr.* **2008**, *27*, 724–731. [CrossRef] [PubMed]
75. Giezenaar, C.; Luscombe-Marsh, N.D.; Hutchison, A.T.; Standfield, S.; Feinle-Bisset, C.; Horowitz, M.; Chapman, I.; Soenen, S. Dose-dependent effects of randomized intraduodenal whey-protein loads on glucose, gut hormone, and amino acid concentrations in healthy older and younger men. *Nutrients* **2018**, *10*, 78. [CrossRef]
76. Rigamonti, A.E.; Pincelli, A.I.; Corrá, B.; Viarengo, R.; Bonomo, S.M.; Galimberti, D.; Scacchi, M.; Scarpini, E.; Cavagnini, F.; Müller, E.E. Plasma ghrelin concentrations in elderly subjects: Comparison with anorexic and obese patients. *J. Endocrinol.* **2002**, *175*, R1–R5. [CrossRef]
77. Di Francesco, V.; Fantin, F.; Residori, L.; Bissoli, L.; Micciolo, R.; Zivelonghi, A.; Zoico, E.; Omizzolo, F.; Bosello, O.; Zamboni, M. Effect of age on the dynamics of acylated ghrelin in fasting conditions and in response to a meal. *J. Am. Geriatr. Soc.* **2008**, *56*, 1369–1370. [CrossRef] [PubMed]
78. Bauer, J.M.; Haack, A.; Winning, K.; Wirth, R.; Fischer, B.; Uter, W.; Erdmann, J.; Schusdziarra, V.; Sieber, C.C. Impaired postprandial response of active ghrelin and prolonged suppression of hunger sensation in the elderly. *J. Gerontol. Ser. A Biol. Sci. Med. Sci.* **2010**, *65*, 307–311. [CrossRef] [PubMed]
79. Nass, R.; Farhy, L.S.; Liu, J.; Pezzoli, S.S.; Johnson, M.L.; Gaylinn, B.D.; Thorner, M.O. Age-dependent decline in acyl-ghrelin concentrations and reduced association of acyl-ghrelin and growth hormone in healthy older adults. *J. Clin. Endocrinol. Metab.* **2014**, *99*, 602–608. [CrossRef]
80. Kojima, M.; Hosoda, H.; Date, Y.; Nakazato, M.; Matsuo, H.; Kangawa, K. Ghrelin is a growth-hormone-releasing acylated peptide from stomach. *Nature* **1999**, *402*, 656–660. [CrossRef] [PubMed]

81. Wren, A.M.; Small, C.J.; Ward, H.L.; Murphy, K.G.; Dakin, C.L.; Taheri, S.; Kennedy, A.R.; Roberts, G.H.; Morgan, D.G.A.; Ghatei, M.A.; et al. The Novel Hypothalamic Peptide Ghrelin Stimulates Food Intake and Growth Hormone Secretion. *Endocrinology* **2000**, *141*, 4325–4328. [CrossRef] [PubMed]
82. Fernandez, G.; Cabral, A.; Cornejo, M.P.; De Francesco, P.N.; Garcia-Romero, G.; Reynaldo, M.; Perello, M. Des-Acyl Ghrelin Directly Targets the Arcuate Nucleus in a Ghrelin-Receptor Independent Manner and Impairs the Orexigenic Effect of Ghrelin. *J. Neuroendocrinol.* **2016**, *28*. [CrossRef]
83. Könner, A.C.; Klöckener, T.; Brüning, J.C. Control of energy homeostasis by insulin and leptin: Targeting the arcuate nucleus and beyond. *Physiol. Behav.* **2009**, *97*, 632–638. [CrossRef]
84. Serra-Prat, M.; Palomera, E.; Clave, P.; Puig-Domingo, M. Effect of age and frailty on ghrelin and cholecystokinin responses to a meal test. *Am. J. Clin. Nutr.* **2009**, *89*, 1410–1417. [CrossRef]
85. Doucet, E.; St-Pierre, S.; Alméras, N.; Mauriège, P.; Després, J.-P.; Richard, D.; Bouchard, C.; Tremblay, A. Fasting Insulin Levels Influence Plasma Leptin Levels Independently from the Contribution of Adiposity: Evidence from Both a Cross-Sectional and an Intervention Study1. *J. Clin. Endocrinol. Metab.* **2000**, *85*, 4231–4237. [CrossRef] [PubMed]
86. Saad, M.F.; Bernaba, B.; Hwu, C.-M.; Jinagouda, S.; Fahmi, S.; Kogosov, E.; Boyadjian, R. Insulin Regulates Plasma Ghrelin Concentration. *J. Clin. Endocrinol. Metab.* **2002**, *87*, 3997–4000. [CrossRef] [PubMed]
87. Saad, M.F.; Khan, A.; Sharma, A.; Michael, R.; Riad-Gabriel, M.G.; Boyadjian, R.; Jinagouda, S.D.; Steil, G.M.; Kamdar, V. Physiological insulinemia acutely modulates plasma leptin. *Diabetes* **1998**, *47*, 544–549. [CrossRef]
88. Ellis, A.C.; Chandler-Laney, P.; Casazza, K.; Goree, L.L.; McGwin, G.; Gower, B.A. Circulating ghrelin and GLP-1 are not affected by habitual diet. *Regul. Pept.* **2012**, *176*, 1–5. [CrossRef] [PubMed]
89. Erdmann, J.; Lippl, F.; Schusdziarra, V. Differential effect of protein and fat on plasma ghrelin levels in man. *Regul. Pept.* **2003**, *116*, 101–107. [CrossRef]
90. Veedfald, S.; Wu, T.; Bound, M.; Grivell, J.; Hartmann, B.; Rehfeld, J.F.; Deacon, C.F.; Horowitz, M.; Holst, J.J.; Rayner, C.K. Hyperosmolar Duodenal Saline Infusion Lowers Circulating Ghrelin and Stimulates Intestinal Hormone Release in Young Men. *J. Clin. Endocrinol. Metab.* **2018**, *103*, 4409–4418. [CrossRef] [PubMed]
91. Blom, W.A.M.; Lluch, A.; Stafleu, A.; Vinoy, S.; Holst, J.J.; Schaafsma, G.; Hendriks, H.F.J. Effect of a high-protein breakfast on the postprandial ghrelin response. *Am. J. Clin. Nutr.* **2006**, *83*, 211–220. [CrossRef]

Publisher's Note: MDPI stays neutral with regard to jurisdictional claims in published maps and institutional affiliations.

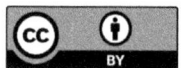

© 2020 by the authors. Licensee MDPI, Basel, Switzerland. This article is an open access article distributed under the terms and conditions of the Creative Commons Attribution (CC BY) license (http://creativecommons.org/licenses/by/4.0/).

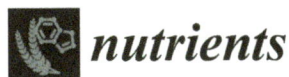

Article

Whey Protein Drink Ingestion before Breakfast Suppressed Energy Intake at Breakfast and Lunch, but Not during Dinner, and Was Less Suppressed in Healthy Older than Younger Men

Avneet Oberoi [1], Caroline Giezenaar [2], Alina Clames [1], Kristine Bøhler [1], Kylie Lange [1], Michael Horowitz [1], Karen L. Jones [1], Ian Chapman [1] and Stijn Soenen [1,3,*]

1. Adelaide Medical School and Centre of Research Excellence in Translating Nutritional Science to Good Health, The University of Adelaide, Adelaide, Royal Adelaide Hospital, Adelaide, SA 5000, South-Australia, Australia; avneet.oberoi@adelaide.edu.au (A.O.); alina.clames@adelaide.edu.au (A.C.); kristine.bohler@adelaide.edu.au (K.B.); kylie.lange@adelaide.edu.au (K.L.); michael.horowitz@adelaide.edu.au (M.H.); karen.jones@adelaide.edu.au (K.L.J.); ian.chapman@adelaide.edu.au (I.C.)
2. Riddet Institute, Massey University, Palmerston North 9430, New Zealand; c.giezenaar@massey.ac.nz
3. Faculty of Health Sciences & Medicine, Bond University, Gold Coast 4229, Queensland, Australia
* Correspondence: stijn.soenen@adelaide.edu.au; Tel.: +61-487-333-418

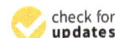

Received: 24 September 2020; Accepted: 27 October 2020; Published: 29 October 2020

Abstract: Ageing is associated with changes in feeding behavior. We have reported that there is suppression of energy intake three hours after whey protein drink ingestion in young, but not older, men. This study aimed to determine these effects over a time period of 9 h. Fifteen younger (27 ± 1 years, 25.8 ± 0.7 kg/m^2) and 15 older (75 ± 2 years, 26.6 ± 0.8 kg/m^2) healthy men were studied on three occasions on which they received, in a randomized order, a 30 g/120 kcal, 70 g/280 kcal whey-protein, or control (~2 kcal) drink. Ad-libitum energy intake (sum of breakfast, lunch, and dinner) was suppressed in a protein load responsive fashion ($P = 0.001$). Suppression was minimal at breakfast, substantial at lunch (~−16%, $P = 0.001$), no longer present by dinner, and was less in older than younger men (−3 ± 4% vs. −8 ± 4%, $P = 0.027$). Cumulative protein intake was increased in the younger and older men (+20% and +42%, $P < 0.001$). Visual analogue scale ratings of fullness were higher and desire to eat and prospective food consumption were lower after protein vs. control, and these effects were smaller in older vs. younger men (interaction effect $P < 0.05$). These findings support the use of whey-protein drink supplements in older people who aim to increase their protein intake without decreasing their overall energy intake.

Keywords: whey protein; energy intake; gastric emptying; appetite

1. Introduction

The number of older people with malnutrition, both under- and over-nutrition, is rising [1]. Healthy ageing is associated with a reduction in appetite and food intake, including protein intake, which predisposes older people to loss of body weight and in particular, skeletal muscle mass [2,3]. The latter is associated with a decrease in function and quality of life [4]. The causes of the reduction in food intake during healthy ageing are likely to be heterogeneous, including changes in gastrointestinal mechanisms induced by nutrient intake, such as slowing of gastric emptying [5,6].

A common strategy to increase energy intake and body weight in undernourished older people is the use of >25–30 g whey protein-enriched supplements [7], which may result in preserved or even increased muscle mass and strength [7,8]. We reported that in healthy older adults, when compared to younger adults, the acute suppression (up to 3 h following ingestion) of energy intake by protein administered orally or infused directly into the duodenum is less, resulting in an increase of overall energy and protein intake in the older adults [9–11]. In healthy, younger adults, protein is considered to be the most satiating macronutrient and protein-rich supplements and diets are often recommended as a weight loss strategy in obese, younger individuals. There is a lack of definitive evidence on their efficacy [12,13], especially in older adults.

In this study, we aimed to characterize the effect of ageing on the suppression of food intake at breakfast, lunch, and dinner over a time period of 9 h by a pre-breakfast whey protein load (30 g and 70 g) compared to a control drink in healthy younger and older men. We hypothesized that suppression of energy intake by whey protein when compared to control would be less in healthy older than younger adults, resulting in an increase in cumulative energy and protein intake in the older men.

2. Materials and Methods

2.1. Subjects

The study included 15 healthy younger men (mean ± standard error of the mean (SEM) age: 27 ± 1 years; body weight: 76.1 ± 2.0 kg; height: 1.73 ± 0.02 m; body mass index (BMI): 25.8 ± 0.7 kg/m^2) and 15 healthy older men (75 ± 2 years; 80.7 ± 2.9 kg; 1.75 ± 0.01 m; 26.6 ± 0.8 kg/m^2). Body weight and BMI of the younger and older men did not differ significantly ($P > 0.05$). Subjects were recruited by online advertisement and by flyers placed on notice boards at the University of Adelaide, Adelaide, Australia.

Exclusion criteria included smoking; alcohol intake of >2 standard drinks on >5 days per week; being vegetarian; intake of any illicit substance; use of prescribed or non-prescribed medications that may affect appetite, body weight, gastrointestinal function, or energy metabolism; food allergy(s); diabetes mellitus (fasting glucose concentration >6.9 mmol/L); epilepsy; gallbladder, pancreatic, cardiovascular, or respiratory diseases; significant gastrointestinal symptoms, disease, or surgery; any other illness deemed significant by the investigator; and an inability to comprehend the study protocol. Inclusion criteria included being weight stable (<5% fluctuation in their body weight) at study entry, as assessed by their self-reported weight in the preceding 3 months, and maintenance of usual physical activity level.

All subjects gave written informed consent for inclusion before they participated in the study. The study was conducted in accordance with the Declaration of Helsinki and the protocol was approved by the Ethics Committee of The Royal Adelaide Hospital (HREC/18/CALHN/132) and registered under trial registration number ACTRN12618000881235.

2.2. Protocol

Each participant was studied on three occasions, separated by ~3–10 days. On each occasion, they received, in a randomized order (using the method of randomly permuted blocks; www.randomization.com), a single drink of either flavoured water (control; ~2 kcal), 30 g whey protein (120 kcal), or 70 g whey protein (280 kcal). The drinks were equivolaemic (~450 mL) and contained different quantities of food-grade unflavoured whey protein isolate (Bulk Nutrients, Tasmania, Australia) dissolved in varying amounts of distilled water, sodium chloride, and low-calorie lime cordial (Bickford's "diet lime" cordial) [11].

Volunteers arrived at the laboratory at ~8.00 a.m. after fasting for ~12 h overnight and refraining from strenuous exercise and alcohol for 24 h. The subjects were provided with a standard meal the night before each study day (beef lasagne, McCain Foods Pty Ltd., Wendouree, VIC, Australia ~591 kcal). Subjects were told that we were assessing perceptions of appetite around the 3 meals, but not that we measured their food/energy intake.

At baseline (t = −5 min), perceptions of appetite were assessed by visual analogue scales (VAS) and the antral area of the stomach (cm^2) was measured with a LogiqTM e-ultrasound machine

(GE Healthcare Technologies, Sydney, NSW, Australia). Subsequently, the drink was administered at t = −2 min (~8.30 a.m.) and was served in an opaque cup to ensure that the volunteers were blinded. Participants were asked to ingest the drink within 2 min. Following consumption of the drink (t = 0 min), palatability of the drink and perceptions of appetite were assessed by VAS. The antral area of the stomach was measured at several time points between the drink and breakfast (t = 0, 5, 20, 35 min) and not thereafter. Energy intake was measured at breakfast (t = 35–65 min; ~9 a.m.), lunch (t = 275–305 min; ~1 p.m.), and dinner (t = 515–545 min; ~5 p.m.). Breakfast and lunch consisted of a cold buffet-style meal (Table 1) and dinner consisted of a warm meal and a small variation of buffet items (Table 2). Subjects were instructed to consume food until they were comfortably full. Before and after consumption of the meals, perceptions of appetite, in terms of hunger, fullness, desire to eat, and prospective food consumption, were assessed (t = 0, 5, 20, 35, 65, 80, 95, 275, 305, 320, 335, 515, 545, 560, 575 min). Subjects were not permitted to consume any food or drink between ingesting the study drink and the end of the study day, except at the breakfast, lunch, and dinner meals provided during the study day. Water intake in between meals was allowed, but not within 30 min before their next meal.

Table 1. Composition of the cold buffet-style breakfast and lunch meal.

Food Items	Amount Served (g)	Energy Content (kcal)	Protein (g)	Carbohydrate (g)	Fat (g)
Whole meal bread, 4 slices *	125	308	13.8	54.8	4.9
White bread, 4 slices *	125	304	11.1	61.4	2.7
Cheese, sliced [†]	85	346	22.6	0.9	29.2
Ham, sliced [‡]	100	95	17.1	3.5	1.8
Chicken, sliced [§]	100	104	19.4	3.7	1.7
Margarine [∥]	20	108	0.0	0.0	12.4
Mayonnaise [¶]	20	137	0.4	0.7	15.2
Tomato, sliced	100	13	1.0	2.0	0.1
Cucumber, sliced	100	11	0.5	2.0	0.1
Lettuce	100	5	0.9	0.4	0.0
Apple	170	89	0.5	2.0	0.1
Banana	190	166	3.3	39.0	0.2
Fruit salad **	140	81	0.4	17.7	1.3
Strawberry yogurt [††]	175	162	9.1	25.0	3.4
Chocolate custard [‡‡]	100	105	3.3	16.9	3.1
Milky Way [§§]	12	52	0.3	9.0	1.9
Orange juice, unsweetened [∥∥]	300	117	1.9	22.6	2.7
Iced coffee [¶¶]	375	254	12.4	38.3	6.6
Water	600	0	0.0	0.0	0.0
Total		2457	19%	49%	32%

* Sunblest, Tiptop, George Weston Foods Ltd., Enfield, NSW, Australia. [†] Coon Tasty Cheese slices, Australian Cooperative Foods Ltd., Sydney Olympic Park, NSW, Australia. [‡] KR Castlemaine boneless leg ham, George Weston Foods Ltd., Enfield, NSW, Australia. [§] Inghams chicken breast, Inghams Enterprises Pty Ltd., Burton, SA, Australia. [∥] Vita-Lite canola, Peerless Holdings Pty Ltd., Braybook, VIC, Australia. [¶] MasterFoods, Mars Food Australia, Berkeley Vale, NSW, Australia. ** Goulburn Valley, SPC, Ardmona Operations Ltd., Shepparton, VIC, Australia. [††] Yoplait, LD&D Foods Pty Ltd., Docklands, VIC, Australia. [‡‡] Yogo, LD&D Foods Pty Ltd., Docklands, VIC, Australia. [§§] Mars Chocolate Australia, Wendouree, VIC, Australia. [∥∥] Golden Circle Orange juice, Golden Circle Limited, QLD, Australia. [¶¶] Farmers Union, LD&D Foods Pty Ltd., Docklands, VIC, Australia.

Table 2. Composition of the dinner meal.

Food Items	Amount Served (g)	Energy Content (kcal)	Protein (g)	Carbohydrate (g)	Fat (g)
Pasta with Meatballs [o]	500	720	27.7	78.4	35.0
Whole meal bread, 4 slices *	125	308	14.0	55.5	4.9
Margarine [ǁ]	20	108	0.0	0.0	12.5
Philadelphia cream cheese [°]	68	175	3.8	2.1	17.3
Apple	170	89	0.5	2.0	0.1
Banana	190	166	3.3	39.5	0.2
Fruit salad **	140	81	0.4	17.9	1.4
Strawberry yogurt [††]	175	162	9.2	25.3	3.4
Chocolate custard [‡‡]	100	105	3.3	17.1	3.1
Muesli bar [ᵌ]	35	185	5.6	12.5	13.1
Orange juice, unsweetened [ǁǁ]	300	117	1.9	22.9	2.7
Water	600	0	0.0	0.0	0.0
Total		2216	13%	49%	38%

[o] Man Size Spaghetti and Meatballs, McCain Foods Pty Ltd., Wendouree, VIC, Australia. * Sunblest, Tiptop, George Weston Foods Ltd., Enfield, NSW, Australia. [ǁ] Vita-Lite canola, Peerless Holdings Pty Ltd., Braybook, VIC, Australia. [°] Philadelphia Spreadable Cream Cheese snack tubs, Consumer Advisory Service, Melbourne, VIC, Australia. ** Goulburn Valley, SPC, Ardmona Operations Ltd., Shepparton, VIC, Australia. [††] Yoplait, LD&D Foods Pty Ltd., Docklands, VIC, Australia. [‡‡] Yogo, LD&D Foods Pty Ltd., Docklands, VIC, Australia. [ᵌ] Coles Nut bars, choc coated, Coles Supermarkets Australia Pty Ltd., Hawthorn East, VIC, Australia. [ǁǁ] Golden Circle Orange juice, Golden Circle Limited, QLD, Australia.

2.3. Measurements

The primary outcome of the study was ad libitum energy intake at the buffet-style meal and secondary outcomes include antral area and appetite.

2.3.1. Energy Intake

To quantify the amount eaten, the weights of the food items were recorded before and after they was offered to the subjects [11]. Energy intake and macronutrient composition was calculated using commercially available software (Foodworks 3.01, Xyris Software, Highgate Hill, QLD, Australia). Absolute (kcal) and percentage suppression of energy intake (expressed as % of energy intake of the control day) by protein were calculated.

2.3.2. Antral Area

Gastric emptying (gastric retention) was determined by measuring the antral area of the stomach. The circumference of the antral area was measured with a LogiqTM e-ultrasound machine (GE Healthcare Technologies, Sydney, NSW, Australia) by using a 3.5 C broad spectrum 2.5–4 MHz convex linear array transducer. Antral area (cm^2) was determined with the use of a caliper and calculation program built into the ultrasound machine. Volunteers were seated on a chair and were asked to be still during the measurement. The transducer was positioned vertically to obtain a parasagittal image of the antrum, with the superior mesenteric vein and the abdominal aorta in a longitudinal section. If gastric contractions were observed, the acquisition was paused until the contraction wave had passed. To calculate meal retention in the whole stomach, the fasting antral area (measured at baseline) was subtracted from subsequent measurements performed after ingestion of the drinks [14]. Gastric retention was then calculated at a given time point as:

$$\text{Retention (\%)} = [AA(t) - AA(f)]/[AA(max) - AA(f)] \times 100,$$

where $AA(t)$ = antral area measured at a given time point, $AA(f)$ = fasting antral area, and $AA(max)$ = maximum antral area recorded after drink ingestion [11].

2.3.3. Perceptions of Appetite and Palatability

Perceptions of appetite in terms of hunger, fullness, desire to eat, and prospective consumption were assessed by use of a VAS questionnaire [15]. The questionnaire consisted of 100 mm horizontal lines, where 0 represented that the sensation was "not felt at all" and 100 represented that the sensation was "felt the greatest." Volunteers placed a vertical mark on each horizontal line to signify the strength of each sensation at the specified time points. Baseline fasting ratings were calculated as the mean of the three study days. Total AUC was calculated over 0–180 min [11].

Palatability of the drink was assessed by ratings of pleasantness, intenseness, full of taste, sweetness, saltiness, sour, bitterness, umami, and creaminess immediately after drink intake; palatability of the meal was assessed by like of taste, like of aftertaste, and enjoyability of the meal by use of a VAS questionnaire.

2.4. Data and Statistical Analysis

Statistical analyses were performed using SPSS software (version 24; IBM, Armonk, NY, USA). Power calculations were performed for the primary outcome of energy intake using measures of variance obtained from previous data (SD of 181 kcal) [11] to detect a minimum difference in suppression of energy intake by the treatment condition compared with the control of 251 kcal between younger and older subjects. Age and protein load main effects and the age by protein load interaction on outcomes were determined by using two-way repeated-measures analysis of variance (ANOVA). Residuals from all models were checked for normality and constant variance and all assumptions were found to be met. When significant treatment and/or interaction effects were present, Bonferroni corrected post hoc tests were performed to determine which specific drink conditions were different between age groups. Statistical significance was accepted at $P < 0.05$. All data are presented as means ± SEMs.

3. Results

The study protocol was well tolerated by all subjects.

3.1. Energy Intake

Energy intake after the drink (sum of breakfast, lunch, and dinner; Figure 1) was suppressed by whey protein compared to control (protein load main effect on energy intake $P = 0.012$), driven by the suppression of the 70 g whey protein drink (young: −251 ± 117 kcal, −8 ± 4%; older: −184 ± 96 kcal, −5 ± 4%; post-hoc test $P = 0.023$), which was greater ($P = 0.027$) when compared with the 30 g protein drink (young: −88 ± 108 kcal, −3 ± 4%; older: −5 ± 99 kcal, 0 ± 4%; Table 3). Suppression of energy intake by the 70 g whey protein compared to control (protein load main effect, $P = 0.007$) was greatest at lunch (young: −181 ± 83 kcal, −17 ± 8%; older: −154 ± 49 kcal, −15 ± 5%; $P = 0.001$; Figure 2). Protein intake of the drink, before breakfast, did not affect ad libitum energy intake at dinner in either age group. Suppression of energy intake (sum of breakfast, lunch, and dinner) by whey protein was less in healthy older men: −94 ± 82 kcal when compared to younger men −169 ± 100 kcal (there was a main effect of age on suppression of energy intake by protein compared to control $P = 0.027$).

Cumulative energy intake (sum of energy in test drink, breakfast, lunch, and dinner) was not significantly different between study days and age groups (young: control: 2929 ± 131 kcal, 30 g whey protein: 2961 ± 161 kcal and 70 g whey protein: 2958 ± 163 kcal; older: 2878 ± 165 kcal, 2993 ± 122 kcal and 2974 ± 148 kcal, all $P > 0.05$).

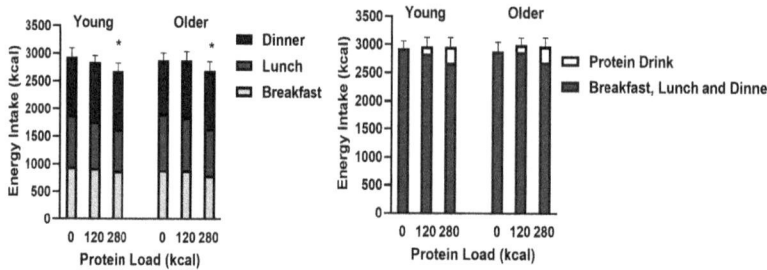

Figure 1. Energy intake at breakfast, lunch, and dinner following whey protein ingestion in healthy young and older men. Mean (± SEM) ad libitum energy intake (kcal; left) at breakfast (light grey bars), lunch (dark grey bars), and dinner (black bars) following drink ingestion containing flavored water (control, ~2 kcal) or whey protein (30 g/120 kcal or 70 g/280 kcal) and cumulative energy intake (kcal; right; sum total energy intake at breakfast, lunch, and dinner combined (dark grey bars) and protein drink (white bars)) in young (left; n = 15) and older (right; n = 15) men. Age and protein load main effects and interaction effects were determined by repeated measures ANOVA. * The 70 g protein drink suppressed energy intake (sum of breakfast, lunch, and dinner) compared with the control (protein load effect P = 0.012, post-hoc P = 0.023).

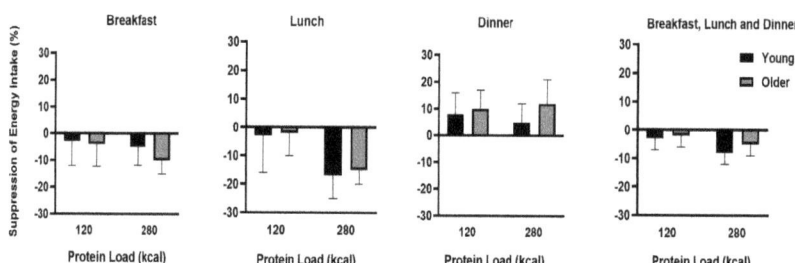

Figure 2. Suppression of energy intake by whey protein at breakfast, lunch, and dinner and total suppression of energy intake in healthy young and older men. Mean (± SEM) suppression of energy intake (kcal) at breakfast, lunch, and dinner following whey protein (30 g/120 kcal or 70 g/280 kcal) ingestion compared to control (~2 kcal) in young (black shading; n = 15) and older (grey shading; n = 15) men. Age and protein load main effects and interaction effects were determined by using repeated-measures ANOVA. Energy intake was suppressed by protein (protein load main effect P = 0.012). Suppression of energy intake by 70 g protein (P = 0.007) was evident, particularly at lunch (P = 0.001). Suppression of energy intake (sum of breakfast, lunch, and dinner) by protein was less in healthy older than younger men (main effect of age P = 0.027).

Table 3. Energy intake at and macronutrient composition of breakfast, lunch, and dinner following whey protein drink ingestion in healthy young and older men.

	Young (n = 15)				Older (n = 15)			
	Breakfast	Lunch	Dinner	Total	Breakfast	Lunch	Dinner	Total
Control drink								
Energy intake (kcal)	947 ± 64	933 ± 74	1049 ± 68	2929 ± 131	896 ± 74	1007 ± 62	975 ± 79	2878 ± 165
Fat (energy %)	34 ± 1	34 ± 2	36 ± 2		29 ± 2	33 ± 6	39 ± 2	
Carbohydrate (energy %)	43 ± 2	43 ± 2	50 ± 2		51 ± 2	46 ± 2	47 ± 2	
Protein (energy %)	23 ± 1	23 ± 1	14 ± 1		20 ± 1	21 ± 1	14 ± 1	
30 g (120 kcal) protein drink								
Energy intake (kcal)	925 ± 67	848 ± 89	1068 ± 48	2841 ± 161	888 ± 60	962 ± 84	1023 ± 66	2873 ± 122
Fat (energy %)	34 ± 2	30 ± 3	38 ± 2		30 ± 1	34 ± 1	38 ± 2	
Carbohydrate (energy %)	43 ± 2	48 ± 4	47 ± 1		51 ± 3	46 ± 2	48 ± 1	
Protein (energy %)	23 ± 1	22 ± 2	15 ± 0		19 ± 1	20 ± 1	14 ± 1	
70 g (280 kcal) protein drink								
Energy intake (kcal)	874 ± 70	752 ± 85 *	1052 ± 56	2678 ± 163	794 ± 72	853 ± 69 *	1047 ± 82	2694 ± 148
Fat (energy %)	34 ± 1	27 ± 2	48 ± 2		30 ± 2	32 ± 1	38 ± 2	
Carbohydrate (energy %)	43 ± 2	54 ± 3	47 ± 1		51 ± 4	46 ± 2	48 ± 1	
Protein (energy %)	23 ± 1	19 ± 2	15 ± 0		19 ± 1	22 ± 1	14 ± 0	

Mean (±SEM) ad libitum energy intake (kcal) at and macronutrient composition (energy percentage) of breakfast, lunch, and dinner, following drink ingestion containing flavoured water (control, ~2 kcal) or whey protein (30 g/120 kcal or 70 g/280 kcal) in young (left; n = 15) and older (right; n = 15) men. Age and protein load main effects and interaction effects were determined by using repeated-measures ANOVA. * Energy intake was suppressed by protein compared to control (protein load main effect $P = 0.012$). Suppression of energy intake by 70 g protein compared to control ($P = 0.007$) occurred particularly during lunch ($P = 0.001$).

3.2. Protein Intake

1. The sum of breakfast, lunch, and dinner protein intake after the test drinks decreased after the 70 g (P = 0.023), but not 30 g, whey protein drink when compared to the control day (protein load main effect P = 0.009, main effect of age P = 0.71, interaction effect P = 0.54).
2. Cumulative protein intake (sum of protein in the drink plus protein intake at the meals) was increased in a protein load responsive fashion (young: control: 143 ± 10 g, 30 g whey protein: +17%, 167 ± 9 g and 70 g whey protein: +36%, 195 ± 9 g; older: control: 133 ± 10 g, 30 g whey protein: +23%, 164 ± 10 g and 70 g whey protein: +47%, 195 ± 9 g; P < 0.001) comparably in the healthy younger and older men (main effect of age P = 0.71, interaction effect of age x protein load P = 0.54; Figure 3).

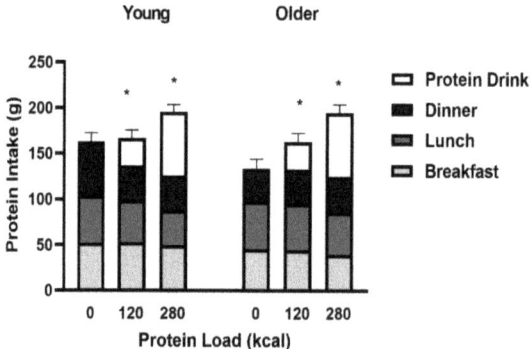

Figure 3. Mean (± SEM) protein intake (g) at breakfast (light grey bars), lunch (dark grey bars), and dinner (black bars) following drink ingestion containing flavored water (control, ~2 kcal) or whey protein (30 g/120 kcal or 70 g/280 kcal; white bars) in young (left; n = 15) and older (right; n = 15) men. Age and protein load main effects and interaction effects were determined by using repeated-measures ANOVA. * Cumulative protein intake (sum of protein drink plus protein intake at meals) was increased in a protein load responsive fashion comparably in the healthy young and older men (main effect of age P = 0.71, protein load main effect P < 0.001, interaction effect P = 0.54).

3.3. Gastric Emptying

Antral areas following overnight fasting (control: 3.4 ± 0.8 cm^2; 30 g whey protein: 2.8 ± 0.7 cm^2; 70 g whey protein: 2.9 ± 0.8 cm^2; protein load main effect P = 0.21) and immediately after drink consumption (control: 15.6 ± 0.8 cm^2; 30 g whey protein: 16.2 ± 0.8 cm^2; 70 g whey protein: 16.4 ± 0.8 cm^2; protein load main effect P = 0.76) were comparable between the study days for both the age groups. Gastric retention was greater after both protein drinks compared to control (main effect of age P = 0.27, protein load main effect P < 0.001, interaction effect P = 0.091; Figure 4).

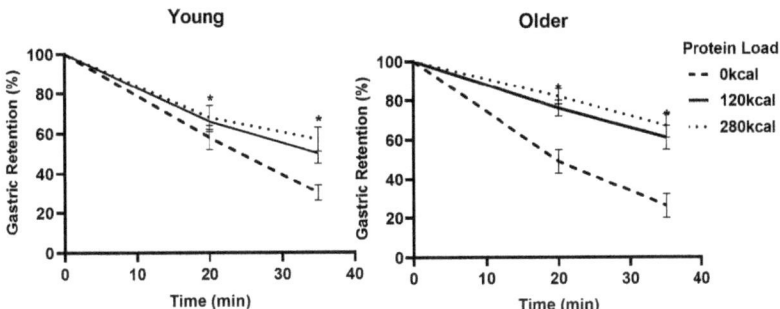

Figure 4. Mean (± SEM) Gastric Retention (%) of drinks containing flavored water (control, ~2 kcal) or whey protein (30 g/120 kcal or 70 g/280 kcal; open bars) in young (left; $n = 15$) and older (right; $n = 15$) men. Age and protein load main effects and interaction effects were determined by using repeated-measures ANOVA. * Gastric Retention, calculated based on the antral areas, were larger after both protein drinks compared to control (main effect of age $P = 0.27$, protein main effect $P < 0.001$, interaction effect $P = 0.091$).

3.4. Appetite

Baseline perceptions of appetite in terms of hunger (young: 61 ± 8 mm; older: 59 ± 9 mm), fullness (13 ± 4 mm; 5 ± 2 mm), desire to eat (61 ± 7 mm; 52 ± 8 mm), and prospective food consumption (67 ± 5 mm; 55 ± 6 mm) were not significantly different between study days and age groups after overnight fasting (all $P > 0.05$). Protein drink ingestion affected fullness (protein main effect $P < 0.001$), desire to eat ($P < 0.001$), and prospective food consumption ($P = 0.002$; Figure 5) in a protein load related fashion; fullness was higher (AUC, both $P < 0.001$) and desire to eat (AUC, $P = 0.035$ and $P = 0.009$) and prospective food consumption (immediately before lunch, $P = 0.025$, $P = 0.006$) were lower after the 70 g whey protein drink compared to control and the 30 g protein drink. Older compared to younger men had a lesser desire to eat (main effect of age $P = 0.028$) but also less fullness (main effect of age $P = 0.003$, interaction effect of age x protein load $P < 0.001$) throughout the day (Figure 5).

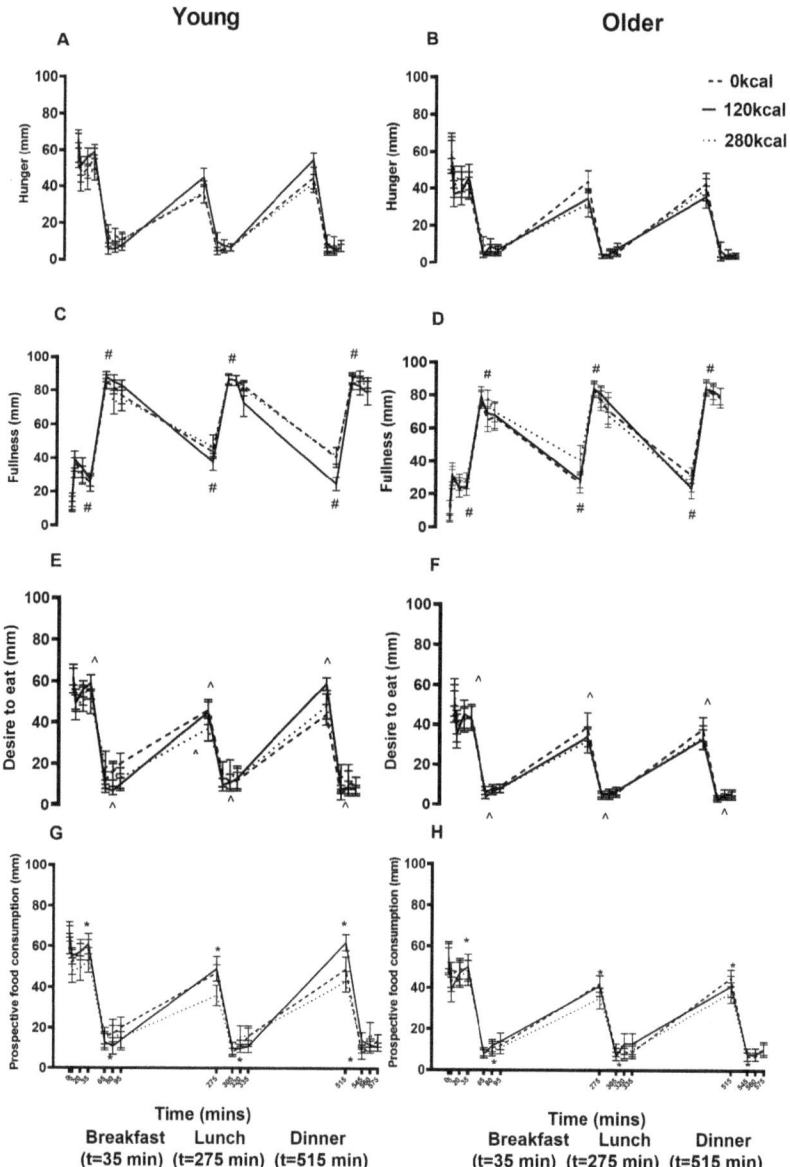

Figure 5. Mean (± SEM) visual analogue scores (VAS; 0–545 min) of hunger (**A**,**B**), fullness (**C**,**D**), desire to eat (**E**,**F**), and prospective food consumption (**G**,**H**) following overnight fasting (t = −5) and after drink ingestion (t = 0, 5, 20, 35, 65, 80, 95, 275, 305, 320, 335, 515, 545, 560, 575 min) containing flavored water (control, ~2 kcal) or whey protein (30 g/120 kcal or 70 g/280 kcal; open bars) and immediately before and after breakfast (B), lunch (L), and dinner (D) in young (left; n = 15) and older (right; n = 15) men. Age and protein load main effects and interaction effects were determined using repeated-measures ANOVA. Protein affected # fullness (protein load main effect $P < 0.001$), ^ desire to eat ($P < 0.001$), and * prospective food consumption ($P = 0.002$) in a protein load related fashion. Older compared to younger men had lower desire to eat (main effect of age $P = 0.028$) and fullness ($P = 0.003$, interaction effect $P < 0.001$).

3.5. Palatability of Drinks and Meals

The 70 g whey protein drink was perceived to be creamier when compared to the flavored control drink ($P = 0.016$). Ratings of pleasantness, intenseness, full of taste, sweetness, saltiness, sour, bitterness, umami, and creaminess of the drinks were not significantly different (main effect of protein $P > 0.05$). The healthy younger men rated the drinks as more bitter than the older men (young: 19±4 mm; older: 26 ± 3 mm, main effect of age $P = 0.037$). All other palatability ratings of the drinks were comparable between the age groups: pleasant (young: 47 ± 5 mm; older: 44 ± 4 mm), intense (51 ± 4 mm; 55 ± 3 mm), fullness (59 ± 4 mm; 59 ± 3 mm), sweet (53 ± 3 mm; 48 ± 3 mm), salty (31 ± 6 mm; 37 ± 4 mm), sour (34 ± 6 mm; 39 ± 4 mm), umami (34 ± 5 mm; 35 ± 3 mm), refreshing (40 ± 6 mm; 41 ± 4 mm), creaminess (27 ± 5 mm; 31 ± 3 mm, main effect of age all $P > 0.05$). Palatability of the meals, assessed as ratings of taste, aftertaste, and enjoyability, were comparable between study days and age groups (control, 30 g, 70 g protein: young: taste: 73 ± 5 mm, 75 ± 5 mm, 72 ± 6 mm, after taste: 73 ± 5 mm, 72 ± 5 mm, 73 ± 5 mm, enjoyable: 73 ± 5 mm, 75 ± 5 mm, 74 ± 5 mm; older: taste: 72 ± 4 mm, 74 ± 3 mm, 72 ± 4 mm, after taste: 71 ± 3 mm, 71 ± 3 mm, 72 ± 4 mm, enjoyable: 73 ± 4 mm, 76 ± 3 mm, 73 ± 4 mm; main effects of age, protein load main effects and interaction effects all $P > 0.05$).

4. Discussion

This study compared the acute effects of ingestion of whey protein drinks containing 30 g and 70 g to those of a flavored control drink consumed 35 min before breakfast on ad libitum energy intake at breakfast, lunch, and dinner, perceptions of appetite throughout the day, and gastric emptying (antral area) in healthy younger and older men. Energy intake (sum of breakfast, lunch, and dinner) was suppressed in a protein load-responsive fashion at breakfast and in particular, at lunch, but not at dinner. Suppression of combined energy intake at breakfast, lunch, and dinner by the protein drink was less in healthy older (−3%) when compared to younger (−7%) men. Cumulative protein intake (sum of protein drink plus protein intake at the meals) was increased in a protein load responsive fashion (+20% and +42%) in the healthy younger and older men. Gastric emptying of the protein drinks in the 35 min before breakfast was slower than that of the control. Fullness was higher and desire to eat and prospective food consumption lower after protein intake when compared with the control in a protein load related fashion. Older compared to younger men had a lower desire to eat but also lower fullness throughout the day, suggesting that older people experience lower sensitivity of the appetite-suppressing effects of a protein drink and may have a decreased perception of gastric distension as seen in our previous study [16,17].

Overall, suppression of energy intake by protein was less in healthy older than younger men in this study, confirming the results of our previous studies [11,18–21], e.g., in a study with a comparable design, suppression of energy intake by oral whey protein ingestion was ~−15% in healthy young compared to ~−1% in older men. In the present study, energy intake (sum of breakfast, lunch, and dinner) was suppressed most by the 70 g whey protein load compared to control (~7%) and at lunch, 4 h 35 min after the drink (~−20% in young and ~−15% in older men). In contrast, there was no suppression of energy intake by pre-breakfast protein at dinner time, 8 h 35 min after the drink, in either age group (~+7% compared to control dinner). We reported previously that in healthy older people, the timing of a 30 g whey protein drink (3 h, 2 h, 1 h, and immediately before the buffet-style meal) does not affect subsequent energy intake in older people. The effect of the whey protein ingestion on energy intake throughout the day may be associated with the slightly slower gastric emptying, reported by us and others in previous studies measuring gastric emptying for a period of 3 h in healthy older, when compared with younger, people [11,18–20]. Gastric emptying may be associated with postprandial satiety by affecting plasma gut hormone concentrations [22] in healthy younger adults [14,16,23,24].

The cumulative energy intake (sum of drink, breakfast, lunch, and dinner) was comparable between study days while cumulative protein intake was elevated during the protein conditions in both age groups. Cumulative energy intake on the protein days compared to control was slightly higher in older (+4%) than younger men (−1%), as was reported in our previous studies determining *ad libitum* energy intake 3 h after oral whey protein ingestion [11] and following 1 h whey protein infusions directly into the small intestine [9]. The insignificant effect of the whey drink on cumulative daily energy intake in this study may indicate that the ingestion of a single daily dose of whey protein, in doses up to 70 g, is unlikely to be a successful weight loss strategy to achieve a negative energy balance, without taking the effects on energy expenditure and muscle anabolism into account. Even if whey protein was given more than once a day, we have no evidence that this would have resulted in a greater cumulative energy deficit, particularly in older adults. The energy content of the protein drink would have equalled or outweighed suppression of energy intake produced by the protein drink. Given our finding with one protein drink before breakfast, it is likely that suppression of cumulative energy intake with multiple drinks would have been even less [25]. The subjects in this study were not aware, however, that we were interested in or measuring their ad libitum meal energy intake throughout the day in response to the different drinks. Young adults using protein supplements to lose weight may have different responses to those in this study. Cumulative protein intake was significantly increased by the 30 g and 70 g whey protein loads, particularly in the older men (young: +17% and +36% and older: +23% and +47%), reaching meaningful amounts sufficient to result in postprandial muscle anabolism in older adults [8,26]—the 70 g whey protein drink increased protein intake by 62 g, or ~0.8 g/kg body weight, in the older men.

A limitation of the study was that we only studied men. This was to enable comparisons with the results of our previous studies conducted in men which clearly showed the effect of protein load. As men generally show greater variations in appetite and food intake in response to energy manipulation than women [27,28], the effects of the protein drinks may be different in women and it would be appropriate to perform further studies including women. The healthy older participants were well nourished, unrestrained eaters, had an active lifestyle, and comparable energy intake on the control day to the younger men. It has been reported numerous times that healthy ageing is associated with reduced food intake [21,29] and hunger [21,30,31] and a blunting of the regulation of food intake [27,32] as suggested by the findings of this study, i.e., less suppression of energy intake by protein. The suppressive effect of whey protein in younger adults may be affected by having dietary restraints or actively trying to lose body weight [33,34]. Furthermore, the overall suppressive effect of protein supplements may be influenced by protein supplement intake before each meal of the day. The significant increase in cumulative protein intake and slight increase in cumulative energy intake in the older men suggests that whey protein can be given at breakfast, and possibly also at other meals, without decreasing overall daily energy intake, which would benefit malnourished, frail, older people—further studies are warranted. Another possible limitation was that the study was limited to 9 h after drink ingestion. As the effect of the pre breakfast drink on energy and protein intake had worn off by dinner, however, it seems unlikely that it would have had any effect after that.

5. Conclusions

Energy intake was suppressed by whey protein drinks in a protein load-responsive fashion at breakfast and particularly, at lunch, but not at dinner, and suppression of energy intake by protein was less in healthy older than younger men. Cumulative protein intake was increased in a protein load responsive fashion. These findings support the use of whey-protein drink supplements in healthy older patients who aim to increase their protein intake without decreasing their overall energy intake.

Author Contributions: C.G., A.C., and K.B. performed the study days; A.O., C.G., A.C., and K.L. analyzed the data; A.O., C.G., A.C., K.L.J., M.H., I.C., and S.S. interpreted the results; A.O., A.C., and K.B. drafted the manuscript; C.G., K.L., M.H., K.L.J., I.C., and S.S. edited and revised the manuscript; A.O., C.G., A.C., K.B., K.L., M.H., K.L.J., I.C., and S.S. approved the final version of the manuscript; K.L., M.H., I.C., and S.S. conception and design of the research. All authors have read and agreed to the published version of the manuscript.

Funding: This research was funded by Royal Adelaide Hospital Endocrine Unit Gum Bequest Grant. Royal Adelaide Hospital Research Foundation did not have any input in the design, implementation, analysis, or interpretation of the data.

Acknowledgments: We thank Bulk Nutrients, Tasmania, Australia for providing whey protein and the members of the Centre of Clinical Research Excellence in Translating Nutritional Research to Good Health, Adelaide Medical School, The University of Adelaide, Royal Adelaide Hospital for all provided support during this study.

Conflicts of Interest: The authors declare no conflict of interest.

References

1. Leslie, W.; Hankey, C. Aging, nutritional status and health. *Healthcare* **2015**, *3*, 648–658. [CrossRef] [PubMed]
2. Soenen, S.; Chapman, I.M. Body weight, anorexia, and undernutrition in older people. *J. Am. Med. Dir. Assoc.* **2013**, *14*, 642–648. [CrossRef]
3. Giezenaar, C.; Chapman, I.; Luscombe-Marsh, N.; Feinle-Bisset, C.; Horowitz, M.; Soenen, S. Ageing is associated with decreases in appetite and energy intake—A meta-analysis in healthy adults. *Nutrients* **2016**, *8*, 28. [CrossRef] [PubMed]
4. Siparsky, P.N.; Kirkendall, D.T.; Garrett, W.E., Jr. Muscle changes in aging: Understanding sarcopenia. *Sports Health* **2014**, *6*, 36–40. [CrossRef] [PubMed]
5. Soenen, S.; Rayner, C.K.; Horowitz, M.; Jones, K.L. Gastric emptying in the elderly. *Clin. Geriatr. Med.* **2015**, *31*, 339–353. [CrossRef] [PubMed]
6. Soenen, S.; Rayner, C.K.; Jones, K.L.; Horowitz, M. The ageing gastrointestinal tract. *Curr. Opin. Clin. Nutr. Metab. Care.* **2016**, *19*, 12–18. [CrossRef] [PubMed]
7. Cawood, A.; Elia, M.; Stratton, R. Systematic review and meta-analysis of the effects of high protein oral nutritional supplements. *Ageing Res. Rev.* **2012**, *11*, 278–296. [CrossRef] [PubMed]
8. Malafarina, V.; Uriz-Otano, F.; Iniesta, R.; Gil-Guerrero, L. Effectiveness of nutritional supplementation on muscle mass in treatment of sarcopenia in old age: A systematic review. *J. Am. Med. Dir. Assoc.* **2013**, *14*, 10–17. [CrossRef]
9. Soenen, S.; Giezenaar, C.; Hutchison, A.T.; Horowitz, M.; Chapman, I.; Luscombe-Marsh, N.D. Effects of intraduodenal protein on appetite, energy intake, and antropyloroduodenal motility in healthy older compared with young men in a randomized trial. *Am. J. Clin. Nutr.* **2014**, *100*, 1108–1115. [CrossRef]
10. Giezenaar, C.; Coudert, Z.; Baqeri, A.; Jensen, C.; Hausken, T.; Horowitz, M.; Chapman, I.; Soenen, S. Effects of timing of whey protein intake on appetite and energy intake in healthy older men. *J. Am. Med. Dir. Assoc.* **2017**, *18*, 898.e9–898.e13. [CrossRef]
11. Giezenaar, C.; Trahair, L.G.; Rigda, R.; Hutchison, A.T.; Feinle-Bisset, C.; Luscombe-Marsh, N.D.; Hausken, T.; Jones, K.L.; Horowitz, M.; Chapman, I.; et al. Lesser suppression of energy intake by orally ingested whey protein in healthy older men compared with young controls. *Am. J. Physiol. Regul. Integr. Comp. Physiol.* **2015**, *309*, R845–R854. [CrossRef] [PubMed]
12. Keri, M.N. Therapeutic applications of whey protein. *Altern. Med. Rev.* **2004**, *9*, 136–156.
13. Smithers, G.W. Whey and whey proteins—From 'gutter-to-gold'. *Int. Dairy J.* **2008**, *18*, 695–704. [CrossRef]
14. Hveem, K.; Jones, K.; Chatterton, B.; Horowitz, M. Scintigraphic measurement of gastric emptying and ultrasonographic assessment of antral area: Relation to appetite. *Gut* **1996**, *38*, 816–821. [CrossRef] [PubMed]
15. Parker, B.A.; Sturm, K.; MacIntosh, C.G.; Feinle, C.; Horowitz, M.; Chapman, I.M. Relation between food intake and visual analogue scale ratings of appetite and other sensations in healthy older and young subjects. *Eur. J. Clin. Nutr.* **2004**, *58*, 212–218. [CrossRef]
16. Rayner, C.K.; MacIntosh, C.G.; Chapman, I.M.; Morley, J.E.; Horowitz, M. Effects of age on proximal gastric motor and sensory function. *Scand. J. Gastroenterol.* **2000**, *35*, 1041–1047.
17. Giezenaar, C.; Lange, K.; Hausken, T.; Jones, K.L.; Horowitz, M.; Chapman, I.; Soenen, S. Effects of Age on Acute Appetite-Related Responses to Whey-Protein Drinks, Including Energy Intake, Gastric Emptying, Blood Glucose, and Plasma Gut Hormone Concentrations—A Randomized Controlled Trial. *Nutrients* **2020**, *12*, 1008. [CrossRef]

18. Giezenaar, C.; Trahair, L.G.; Luscombe-Marsh, N.D.; Hausken, T.; Standfield, S.; Jones, K.L.; Lange, K.; Horowitz, M.; Chapman, I.; Soenen, S. Effects of randomized whey-protein loads on energy intake, appetite, gastric emptying, and plasma gut-hormone concentrations in older men and women. *Am. J. Clin. Nutr.* **2017**, *106*, 865–877. [CrossRef]
19. Giezenaar, C.; Van Der Burgh, Y.; Lange, K.; Hatzinikolas, S.; Hausken, T.; Jones, K.L.; Horowitz, M.; Chapman, I.; Soenen, S. Effects of Substitution, and Adding of Carbohydrate and Fat to Whey-Protein on Energy Intake, Appetite, Gastric Emptying, Glucose, Insulin, Ghrelin, CCK and GLP-1 in Healthy Older Men—A Randomized Controlled Trial. *Nutrients* **2018**, *10*, 113. [CrossRef]
20. Hutchison, A.T.; Piscitelli, D.; Horowitz, M.; Jones, K.L.; Clifton, P.M.; Standfield, S.; Hausken, T.; Feinle-Bisset, C.; Luscombe-Marsh, N.D. Acute load-dependent effects of oral whey protein on gastric emptying, gut hormone release, glycemia, appetite, and energy intake in healthy men. *Am. J. Clin. Nutr.* **2015**, *102*, 1574–1584. [CrossRef]
21. Sturm, K.; Parker, B.; Wishart, J.; Feinle-Bisset, C.; Jones, K.L.; Chapman, I.; Horowitz, M. Energy intake and appetite are related to antral area in healthy young and older subjects. *Am. J. Clin. Nutr.* **2004**, *80*, 656–667. [CrossRef] [PubMed]
22. Giezenaar, C.; Hutchison, A.T.; Luscombe-Marsh, N.D.; Chapman, I.; Horowitz, M.; Soenen, S. Effect of age on blood glucose and plasma insulin, glucagon, ghrelin, CCK, GIP, and GLP-1 responses to whey protein ingestion. *Nutrients* **2017**, *10*, 2. [CrossRef]
23. Janssen, P.; Vanden, B.P.; Verschueren, S.; Lehmann, A.; Depoortere, I.; Tack, J. The role of gastric motility in the control of food intake. *Aliment. Pharmacol. Ther.* **2011**, *33*, 880–894. [CrossRef] [PubMed]
24. Jones, K.L.; Doran, S.M.; Hveem, K.; Bartholomeusz, F.D.; E Morley, J.; Sun, W.M.; E Chatterton, B.; Horowitz, M. Relation between postprandial satiation and antral area in normal subjects. *Am. J. Clin. Nutr.* **1997**, *66*, 127–132. [CrossRef]
25. E Rigamonti, A.; Leoncini, R.; Casnici, C.; Marelli, O.; De Col, A.; Tamini, S.; Lucchetti, E.; Cicolini, S.; Abbruzzese, L.; Cella, S.; et al. Whey Proteins Reduce Appetite, Stimulate Anorexigenic Gastrointestinal Peptides and Improve Glucometabolic Homeostasis in Young Obese Women. *Nutrients* **2019**, *11*, 247. [CrossRef] [PubMed]
26. Paddon, J.D.; Leidy, H. Dietary protein and muscle in older persons. *Curr. Opin. Clin. Nutr. Metab. Care* **2014**, *17*, 5. [CrossRef]
27. Rolls, B.J.; Dimeo, K.A.; Shide, D.J. Age-related impairments in the regulation of food intake. *Am. J. Clin. Nutr.* **1995**, *62*, 923–931. [CrossRef]
28. Giezenaar, C.; Luscombe-Marsh, N.D.; Hutchison, A.T.; Lange, K.; Hausken, T.; Jones, K.L.; Horowitz, M.; Chapman, I.; Soenen, S. Effect of gender on the acute effects of whey protein ingestion on energy intake, appetite, gastric emptying and gut hormone responses in healthy young adults. *Nutr. Diabetes* **2018**, *8*, 40. [CrossRef]
29. Wurtman, J.J.; Lieberman, H.; Tsay, R.; Nader, T.; Chew, B. Calorie and nutrient intakes of elderly and young subjects measured under identical conditions. *J. Gerontol.* **1988**, *43*, B174–B180. [CrossRef]
30. Clarkston, W.; Pantano, M.; Morley, J.; Horowitz, M.; Littlefield, J.; Burton, F. Evidence for the anorexia of aging: Gastrointestinal transit and hunger in healthy elderly vs. young adults. *Am. J. Physiol. Regul. Integr. Comp. Physiol.* **1997**, *272*, R243–R248. [CrossRef]
31. Sturm, K.; MacIntosh, C.G.; Parker, B.A.; Wishart, J.; Horowitz, M.; Chapman, I.M. Appetite, food intake, and plasma concentrations of cholecystokinin, ghrelin, and other gastrointestinal hormones in undernourished older women and well-nourished young and older women. *J. Clin. Endocrinol. Metab.* **2003**, *88*, 3747–3755. [CrossRef] [PubMed]
32. Roberts, S.B.; Fuss, P.; Heyman, M.B.; Evans, W.J.; Tsay, R.; Rasmussen, H.; Fiatarone, M.; Cortiella, J.; Dallal, G.E.; Young, V.R. Control of food intake in older men. *JAMA* **1994**, *272*, 1601–1606. [CrossRef] [PubMed]

33. Griffin, H.; Cheng, H.; O'connor, H.; Rooney, K.; Petocz, P.; Steinbeck, K. Higher protein diet for weight management in young overweight women: A 12-month randomized controlled trial. *Diabetes. Obes. Metab.* **2013**, *15*, 572–575. [CrossRef] [PubMed]
34. Leidy, H.J.; Carnell, N.S.; Mattes, R.D.; Campbell, W.W. Higher protein intake preserves lean mass and satiety with weight loss in pre-obese and obese women. *Obesity* **2007**, *15*, 421–429. [CrossRef]

Publisher's Note: MDPI stays neutral with regard to jurisdictional claims in published maps and institutional affiliations.

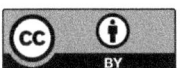

© 2020 by the authors. Licensee MDPI, Basel, Switzerland. This article is an open access article distributed under the terms and conditions of the Creative Commons Attribution (CC BY) license (http://creativecommons.org/licenses/by/4.0/).

MDPI
St. Alban-Anlage 66
4052 Basel
Switzerland
Tel. +41 61 683 77 34
Fax +41 61 302 89 18
www.mdpi.com

Nutrients Editorial Office
E-mail: nutrients@mdpi.com
www.mdpi.com/journal/nutrients

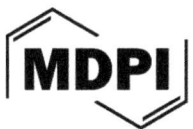

www.ingramcontent.com/pod-product-compliance
Lightning Source LLC
LaVergne TN
LVHW070127100526
838202LV00016B/2242